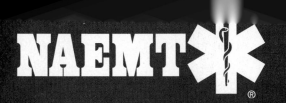

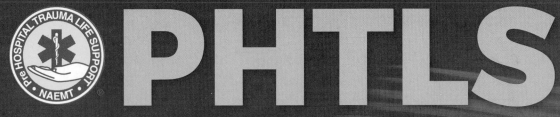

PHTLS
Prehospital Trauma Life Support
MILITARY NINTH EDITION

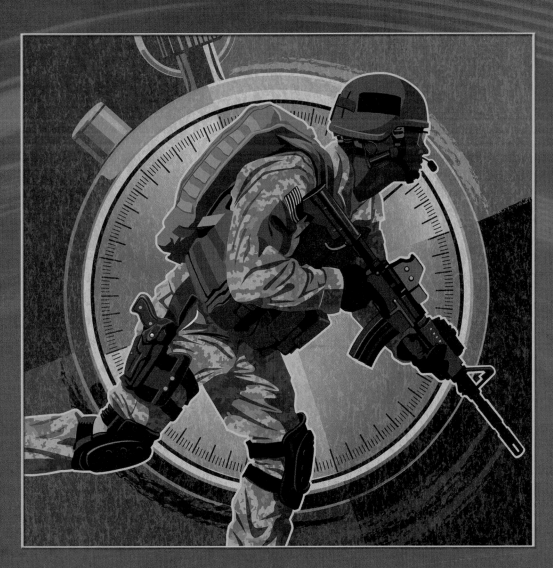

"The fate of the wounded rests in the hands of the one who applies the first dressing."

—Nicholas Senn, MD (1844–1908)
American Surgeon (Chicago, Illinois)
Founder, Association of Military Surgeons of the United States

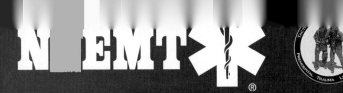

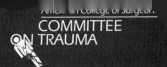

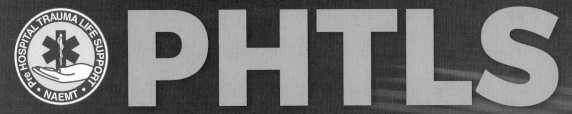

PHTLS

Prehospital Trauma Life Support

MILITARY NINTH EDITION

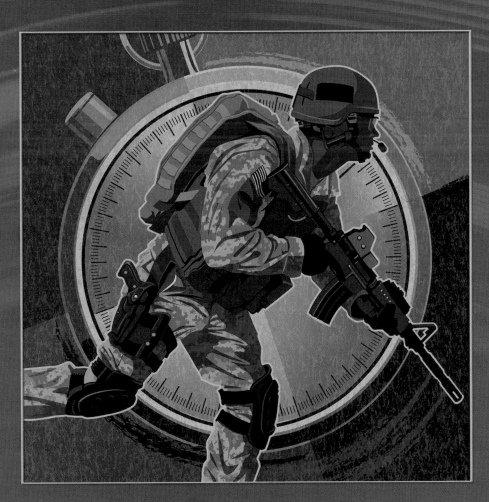

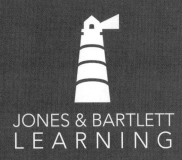

JONES & BARTLETT
LEARNING

World Headquarters
Jones & Bartlett Learning
5 Wall Street
Burlington, MA 01803
978-443-5000
info@jblearning.com
www.jblearning.com

Jones & Bartlett Learning books and products are available through most bookstores and online booksellers. To contact Jones & Bartlett Learning directly, call 800-832-0034, fax 978-443-8000, or visit our website, www.jblearning.com.

Substantial discounts on bulk quantities of Jones & Bartlett Learning publications are available to corporations, professional associations, and other qualified organizations. For details and specific discount information, contact the special sales department at Jones & Bartlett Learning via the above contact information or send an email to specialsales@jblearning.com.

21411-6

Production Credits

General Manager and Executive Publisher: Kimberly Brophy
VP, Product Development: Christine Emerton
Senior Managing Editor: Donna Gridley
Product Manager: Tiffany Sliter
Content Development Editor: Ashley Procum
Senior Project Specialist: Dan Stone
Digital Project Specialist: Angela Dooley
Director of Marketing Operations: Brian Rooney
VP, Manufacturing and Inventory Control: Therese Connell

Composition: S4Carlisle Publishing Services
Cover Design: Kristin E. Parker
Text Design: Kristin E. Parker
Media Development Editor: Troy Liston
Rights & Media Specialist: Maria Leon Maimone
Cover Image (Title Page, Chapter Opener):
 © Ralf Hiemisch/Getty Images
Printing and Binding: LSC Communications
Cover Printing: LSC Communications

Library of Congress Cataloging-in-Publication Data
Library of Congress Cataloging-in-Publication Data unavailable at time of printing.

Library of Congress Control Number: 2019910047

6048

Printed in the United States of America
23 22 21 20 19   10 9 8 7 6 5 4 3 2 1

Brief Contents

Table of Contents

Chapter 6 Patient Assessment and Management 167

Chapter 7 Airway and Ventilation . . . 199

Division 3 Specific Injuries   255

Chapter 8 Head Trauma 257

Division 4 Prevention   493

Chapter 16 Injury Prevention 495

Division 5 Mass Casualties and Terrorism   517

Chapter 17 Disaster Management . . 519

Division 7 Military Medicine   727

Chapter 24 Care Under Fire 749

Chapter 25 Tactical Field Care 763

Chapter 26 Tactical Evacuation Care 857

Specific Skills Table of Contents

Acknowledgments

Contributors

Medical Editor–Ninth Edition

Andrew N. Pollak, MD
The James Lawrence Kernan Professor and Chairman
Department of Orthopaedics
University of Maryland School of Medicine
Chief of Orthopaedics
University of Maryland Medical System
Baltimore, Maryland

Editors–Military Edition

Frank K. Butler, Jr., MD
Capt., MC, USN (Retired)
Chairperson
Committee on Tactical Combat Casualty Care
Joint Trauma System

Stephen D. Giebner, MD, MPH
Capt., MC, USN (Retired)
Past Chairperson
Developmental Editor
Committee on Tactical Combat Casualty Care
Joint Trauma System

Chapter Editors–Ninth Edition

Heidi Abraham, MD, EMT-B, EMT-T, FAEMS
Medical Director
New Braunfels Fire Department
San Antonio AirLIFE
New Braunfels, Texas

Faizan H. Arshad, MD
EMS Medical Director Health Quest Systems
Lead Author, All Hazards Disaster Response
NAEMT PHT Committee, EMS Physician Representative
Host and Producer of EMS Nation podcast
Evaluations Subcommittee Chair, Hudson Valley REMAC
Hudson Valley, New York

Luke Brown, MD
Orthopaedic Spine Research Fellow
University of Maryland Medical Center
Baltimore, Maryland

Ian Bussey, BS
R Adams Cowley Shock Trauma Center
Department of Orthopaedics
University of Maryland School of Medicine
Baltimore, Maryland

Thomas Colvin, NREMT-P
Firefighter/Paramedic
Houston Fire Department
Houston, Texas

Ann Dietrich, MD, FAAP, FACEP
Pediatric Medical Advisor, Medflight of Ohio
Education Director, Ohio ACEP
Clinical Skills Liaison Year 1, Co-IOR Acute Care, Ohio University Heritage College of Medicine
Medical Director, NAEMT Emergency Pediatric Care Committee
NAEMT Representative, American Academy of Pediatrics PEPP Steering Committee
Athens, Ohio

Alexander L. Eastman, MD, MPH, FACS, FAEMS
PHTLS Medical Director
Medical Director and Chief, The Rees-Jones Trauma Center at Parkland Memorial Hospital
Division of Burns, Trauma, and Critical Care at UT Southwestern Medical Center
Lieutenant and Chief Medical Officer, Dallas Police Department
Dallas, Texas

Richard Ellis, MSEDM, NRP
Program Chair, Paramedic Technology, Central Georgia Technical College
Tactical Medic, Bibb County Sheriff's Office
Macon, Georgia

Blaine Enderson, MD, MBA, FACS, FCCM
Professor of Surgery
University of Tennessee Graduate School of Medicine
Knoxville, Tennessee

Mark Gestring, MD, FACS
Medical Director, Kessler Trauma Center
Professor of Surgery, Emergency Medicine and Pediatrics
University of Rochester School of Medicine
Rochester, New York

Bruno Goulesque, MD
Medical Director, PHTLS France
Medical Director, Centre Hospitalier de Mulhouse
Wittenheim, France

Seth Hawkins, MD
Assistant Professor of Emergency Medicine, Wake Forest University
Medical Director, Burke County EMS & Burke County Communications
Medical Director, Western Piedmont Community College Emergency Services Programs
Medical Director, North Carolina State Parks
Chief, Appalachian Mountain Rescue Team
Winston-Salem, North Carolina

Michael Holtz, MD
EMS Physician
University of Pittsburgh Medical Center
Pittsburgh, Pennsylvania

Spogmai Komak, MD
Assistant Professor, Department of Surgery
UT Houston Health Science Center
McGovern School of Medicine
Houston, Texas

Michael Lohmeier, MD
Associate Professor, Department of Emergency Medicine
University of Wisconsin-Madison
Madison, Wisconsin

Steven C. Ludwig, MD
Professor of Orthopaedics
Chief of the Division of Spine Surgery
Fellowship Director
Department of Orthopaedics
University of Maryland Medical Center
Baltimore, Maryland

Lauren MacCormick, MD
Department of Orthopaedic Surgery
University of Minnesota
Minneapolis, Minnesota

Michael Mancera, MD, FAEMS
Associate EMS Medical Director
Assistant Professor, Department of
    Emergency Medicine
University of Wisconsin School of
    Medicine & Public Health
Madison, Wisconsin

Craig Manifold, DO, FACEP, FAAEM
Assistant Professor, Department of
    Emergency Health Sciences
School of Health Professions at the
    University of Texas Health Science
    Center in San Antonio
Joint Surgeon, Texas Air National Guard
Medical Director, NAEMT
San Antonio, Texas

Catherine L. McKnight, MD
Assistant Professor, Trauma and Critical
    Care
Department of Surgery
University of Tennessee Medical Center
    at Knoxville
Knoxville, Tennessee

Faroukh Mehkri, DO, AEMT
Resident-Physician, Department of
    Emergency Medicine
University of Connecticut Integrated
    Program in Emergency Medicine
Hartford, Connecticut

Vince Mosesso, MD, FACEP, FAEMS
Medical Director, NAEMT AMLS
    Committee
Professor of Emergency Medicine
Associate Chief, Division of EMS
Medical Director, UPMC Prehospital
    Care
University of Pittsburgh Medical Center
Pittsburgh, Pennsylvania

Jessica Naiditch, MD
Trauma Medical Director
Dell Children's Medical Center of
    Central Texas
Assistant Professor of Surgery &
    Perioperative Care
University of Texas–Austin
Austin, Texas

Alyssa Nash, BS
UMOA Spine Clinical Research
    Coordinator
University of Maryland Medical Center
Baltimore, Maryland

Daniel P. Nogee, MD
PGY-2 Emergency Medicine
Yale-New Haven Hospital
New Haven, Connecticut

Robert O'Toole, MD
Professor and Head
Division of Orthopaedic Traumatology
University of Maryland School of
    Medicine
Chief of Orthopaedics
R Adams Cowley Shock Trauma Center
Baltimore, Maryland

Jean-Cyrille Pitteloud, MD
At-Large Member, PHT Committee
Head of Anesthesiology, HJBE Hospital
    Bern County, Switzerland
Chair of the Board for Acute Care
    Anesthesia, the Swiss Society of
    Anesthesiology (SGAR)
Sion, Switzerland

David Potter, MD
Orthopedic Trauma Surgeon
Sanford University of South Dakota
    Medical Center
Sioux Falls, South Dakota

Christine Ramirez, MD
Trauma/Surgical Critical Care Fellow
University of Maryland Medical Center
Baltimore, Maryland

**Katherine Remick, MD, FAAP,
    FACEP, FAEMS**
Medical Director, San Marcos Hays
    County EMS System
Executive Lead, National EMS
    for Children Innovation and
    Improvement Center
Associate Medical Director, Austin-Travis
County EMS System
Assistant Professor of Pediatrics, Dell
    Medical School at the University of
    Texas at Austin
EMS Director, Pediatric Emergency
    Medicine Fellowship, Dell Medical
    School
Medical Director, NAEMT Emergency
    Pediatric Care Committee
Austin, Texas

Thomas Scalea, MD
Physician in Chief, R Adams Cowley
    Shock Trauma Center
Distinguished Francis X. Kelly Professor
    of Trauma
University of Maryland School of
    Medicine
Baltimore, Maryland

Andrew Schmidt, MD
Chairman of the Department of
    Orthopaedic Surgery
Hennepin County Medical Center
Co-editor of Surgical Treatment of
    Orthopaedic Trauma
Minneapolis, Minnesota

Manish Shah, MD, MPH
Associate Professor of Emergency
    Medicine, Public Health Sciences, and
    Medicine (Geriatrics and Gerontology)
University of Wisconsin–Madison
Vice-Chair for Research, Department of
    Emergency Medicine
Madison, Wisconsin

**R. Bryan Simon, RN, MSc, DiMM,
    FAWM**
Co-owner of Vertical Medicine
    Resources
Adjunct Professor, Salem University
Senior Editor, American Alpine Club
Director, Appalachian Mountain Rescue
    Team
Director, New River Alliance of Climbers
Climbing Columnist, Wilderness
    Medicine Magazine
Salem, West Virginia

Will Smith, MD, Paramedic
Medical Director, Teton County Search
    and Rescue Team
Medical Director, Grand Teton National
    Park
Medical Director, Teton County Search
    and Rescue, Jackson Hole Fire/EMS,
    NPS-SE AZ Group, USFS-BTNF
Clinical Faculty, University of
    Washington School of Medicine
Emergency Medicine, St. John's Medical
    Center, Jackson, Wyoming
Lt. Colonel, MC, U.S. Army
    Reserve–62A (Emergency Medicine)
Jackson, Wyoming

Deborah Stein, MD
The R Adams Cowley Professor in Shock
    and Trauma
University of Maryland Medical Center
Chief of Trauma and Director of
    Neurotrauma Critical Care
R Adams Cowley Shock Trauma Center
Baltimore, Maryland

Steven Stolle, EMT-P, NR-P, FP-C
Critical Care Flight Paramedic
AirLIFE
San Antonio, Texas

Ronald Tesoriero, MD, FACS
Assistant Professor of Surgery
University of Maryland School of
    Medicine
Chief of Critical Care
Associate Program Director, Surgical
    Critical Care & Acute Care Surgery
    Fellowship
R Adams Cowley Shock Trauma Center
University of Maryland Medical Center
Baltimore, Maryland

John Trentini, MD, PhD, FAWM
Major, USAF, MC
United States Air Force
Las Vegas, Nevada

David Tuggle, MD
Associate Trauma Medical Director
Dell Children's Medical Center in Texas
Former Vice-Chair of Surgery and Chief
    of Pediatric Surgery, OU Medical
    Center
Austin, Texas

Jason Weinberger, DO
Trauma/Surgical Critical Care Fellow
Department of Surgical Critical Care
R Adams Cowley Shock Trauma Center
University of Maryland Medical Center
Baltimore, Maryland

Patrick Wick
National Coordinator, NAEMT France:
    PHTLS, EPC, TCCC, TECC
President
Life Support France
Dietwiller, France

Brian H. Williams, MD, FACS
Medical Director, Parkland Community
    Health Institute
Parkland Health & Hospital System
Dallas, Texas

**Chapter Editors–Military
Edition**

Frank Anders, MD
Colonel, U.S. Army (Retired) (Hon.)

Col. Kimberlie Biever, ANC
Commander
Fort Leonard Wood Army Community
    Hospital
Fort Leonard Wood, Missouri

Frank K. Butler, Jr., MD
Captain, U.S. Navy (Retired) (Hon.)
Chairperson
Committee on Tactical Combat Casualty
    Care
Joint Trauma System

Leopoldo Cancio, MD
Colonel, U.S. Army (Retired)
U.S. Army Institute of Surgical Research
    Burn Center
San Antonio, Texas

Howard Champion, MD, FRCS, FACS
Senior Advisor in Trauma
Professor of Surgery
Uniformed Services University of
    Health Sciences
Bethesda, Maryland

Col. Kevin Chung, MD
U.S. Army Institute of Surgical Research
    Burn Center
San Antonio, Texas

Col. Peter J. Cuenca, MD
Brook Army Medical Center
San Antonio, Texas

Robert A. De Lorenzo, MD, MSM, MSCI
Colonel, U.S. Army (Retired)
U.S. Army Institute of Surgical Research
San Antonio, Texas

Brian J. Eastridge, MD, FACS
Colonel, U.S. Army (Retired)
Director, Joint Theater Trauma System
U.S. Army Institute of Surgical Research
San Antonio, Texas

Maj. Andy Fisher
U.S. Army Second Year Medical Student
Texas A+M College of Medicine
1st Battalion, 141st Infantry Regiment,
    Texas ANG
Former Regimental PA
75th Ranger Regiment
BSM V Recipient
Purple Heart Recipient
Army PA of the Year 2010

John Gandy, MD
Lt. Colonel, U.S. Air Force (Retired)
Uniformed Services University of the
    Health Sciences
Bethesda, MD

Keith S. Gates, MD, FACEP
Director, EMS Fellowship
Assistant Professor
Department of Emergency Medicine
The University of Texas
Health Science Center at Houston
Houston, Texas

Robert T. Gerhardt, MD, MPH
Colonel, U.S. Army (Retired)
Brook Army Medical Center
San Antonio, Texas

Maj. John Graybill, MD
U.S. Army Institute of Surgical Research
    Burn Center
San Antonio, Texas

Col. Jennifer Gurney
U.S. Army Institute of Surgical Research
Chairperson
Defense Committee on Trauma
Joint Trauma System
Defense Health Agency
Fort Sam Houston, Texas

John Holcomb, MD, FACS
Colonel, U.S. Army (Retired)
Vice Chair and Professor of Surgery
Chief, Division of Acute Care Surgery
Director, Center for Translational Injury
    Research
The University of Texas
Health Science Center at Houston
Houston, Texas

Col. Jay Johannigman, MD, FACS
Professor of Surgery
Chief, Division of Trauma and Surgical
    Critical Care
University Hospital
Cincinnati, Ohio

Col. Booker King
Director, U.S. Army Institute of Surgical
    Research Burn Center
San Antonio, Texas

Russ Kotwal, MD, MPH, FAAFP
Colonel, U.S. Army (Retired)
Regimental Surgeon, 75th Ranger
 Regiment
Adjunct Assistant Professor, Department
 of Military and Emergency Medicine
Uniformed Services University of the
 Health Sciences
Bethesda, Maryland
Adjunct Assistant Professor, Department
 of Family and Community Medicine
Texas A&M Health Center
College Station, Texas

Lt. Col. Jonathan Lundy, MD
U.S. Army Institute of Surgical Research
 Burn Center
San Antonio, Texas

Col. Robert Mabry, MD, FACEP
Commander
Joint Medical Augmentation Unit
Joint Special Operations Command
Fort Bragg, North Carolina

Harold Montgomery, NREMT, ATP
Master Sgt., U.S. Army (Retired)
Regimental Senior Medic, 75th Ranger
 Regiment
U.S. Army Special Operations
 Committee
Fort Bragg, North Carolina

Lt. Col. Wylan Peterson, MD
U.S. Army Institute of Surgical Research
 Burn Center
San Antonio

Evan Renz, MD
Colonel, U.S. Army (Retired)
Commander, San Antonio Military
 Medical Center
San Antonio, Texas

Col. Stacy Shackleford, MD
USAF Trauma Surgeon
Joint Trauma System—PI Director
Former Deputy CDR for Clinical Services
Craig Theater Hospital—BAF
Former Staff—C-STARS Program
Baltimore Shock Trauma Attending
Former Deployed Director, JTTS

SMSgt. Travis Shaw
USAF Pararescueman
ACC Pararescue Medical Programs
 Manager
USAF PJ Team Leader
Multiple Combat Deployments as a PJ

D. Eric Sine, NREMT, ATP
Command Master Chief Petty Officer,
 U.S. Marines (Retired)
3d Marine Division
Okinawa, Japan

National Association of Emergency Medical Technicians 2019 Board of Directors

Officers
President: Matt Zavadsky
President-Elect: Bruce Evans
Secretary: Troy Tuke
Treasurer: Terry L. David
Immediate Past President: Dennis Rowe

Directors
Region 1:
Sean J. Britton
Robert Luckritz
Region II:
Susan Bailey
Cory Richter
Region III:
Jason Scheiderer
Chris Way
Region IV:
William Justice
Karen Larsen
At Large:
Charlene Cobb
Jonathan Washko
Medical Director:
Craig A. Manifold, DO, FACEP, FAAEM,
 FAEMS

PHTLS/PHT Committee—Chairs

2018–Present: John Phelps, MA, NRP,
 LP, ACHE,
2017–2018: Dennis Rowe, EMT-P
2016–2017: Julie Chase, MSEd, FAWM,
 FP-C
2015–2016: Greg Chapman, BS, RRT,
 REMT-P
1996–2014: Will Chapleau, EMT-P, RN,
 TNS
1992–1996: Elizabeth M. Wertz, RN,
 BSN, MPM
1991–1992: James L. Paturas, EMT-P
1990–1991: John Sinclari, EMT-P
1988–1990: David Wuertz, EMT-P
1985–1988: James L. Paturas, EMT-P
1983–1985: Richard Vomacka,
 NREMT-P[†]
[†]Deceased

PHTLS—Medical Director

Alexander L. Eastman, MD, MPH, FACS, FAEMS
Senior Medical Officer, U.S. Department
 of Homeland Security
Countering Weapons of Mass
 Destruction Office
Lieutenant and Chief Medical Officer,
 Dallas Police Department
Dallas, Texas

PHT Committee

Faizan H. Arshad, MD
At-Large Member, PHT Committee
EMS Medical Director Health Quest
 Systems
Lead Author, All Hazards Disaster
 Response
NAEMT PHT Committee, EMS Physician
 Representative
Host and Producer of EMS Nation
 podcast
Evaluations Subcommittee Chair,
 Hudson Valley REMAC
Hudson Valley, New York

Frank Butler, MD
Military Medical Advisor, PHT
 Committee
Capt., MC, USN (Retired)
Chairperson, Committee on Tactical
 Combat Casualty Care
Joint Trauma System

Warren Dorlac, MD, FACS
Tactical Medical Director, PHT
 Committee
Col. (Retired), USAF, MC, FS
Medical Director, Trauma and Acute
 Care Surgery
Medical Center of the Rockies
University of Colorado Health
Loveland, Colorado

Amie Fuller, NRP
PHTLS Affiliate Faculty
Lieutenant, Frederick County Fire and
 Rescue
Winchester, Virginia

Anthony Harbour, BSN, MEd, RN, NRP
Virginia PHTLS State Coordinator
 (1989–2016)
PHTLS Affiliate Faculty
Acute Care/EMS Educator, Center for
Trauma and Critical Care Education
Virginia Commonwealth University,
 School of Medicine
Director, Southern Virginia EMS
Roanoke, Virginia

Jim McKendry, BSc, MEM
PHTLS Affiliate Faculty
Director, Paramedic Association of
  Manitoba
Instructor, Paramedicine, Red River
  College
Winnipeg, Manitoba, Canada

John C. Phelps II, MA, NRP, ACHE
PHTLS Course Editor; Chair, PHT
  Committee
NAEMT State Education Coordinator,
  Texas
Assistant Professor, Department of
  Emergency Health Sciences
UT Health San Antonio
San Antonio, Texas

Jean-Cyrille Pitteloud, MD
At-Large Member, PHT Committee
Head of Anesthesiology in HJBE Hospital
  Bern County, Switzerland
Chair of the Board for Acute Care
  Anesthesia of the Swiss Society of
  Anesthesiology (SGAR)
Sion, Switzerland

Andrew N. Pollak, MD
The James Lawrence Kernan Professor
  and Chairman
Department of Orthopaedics
University of Maryland School of
  Medicine
Chief of Orthopaedics
University of Maryland Medical System
Baltimore, Maryland

**The Committee on Tactical
Combat Casualty Care (CoTCCC)**
CoTCCC Staff
Chairperson: Frank K. Butler, Jr., MD
Developmental Editor: Stephen Giebner,
  MD, MPH
Operational Liaison: MSG (Retired)
  Harold Montgomery, ATP
TCCC Course Appraisal Specialist: SFC
  (Retired) Dominque Greydanus
Senior Administrative Assistant:
  Ms. Danielle Davis

Voting Members
SMSgt. Shawn Anderson
Dr. Jim Bagian
Col. Jeff Bailey
Capt. Sean Barbabella
HMCM Mark Boyle
Dr. Frank Butler
Master Sgt. Curt Conklin

Lt. Col. Cord Cunningham
Col. Jim Czarnik
Lt. Col. Steve DeLellis
Col. John Dorsch
Capt. Brendon Drew
Col. Joe Dubose
Col. Brian Eastridge
Dr. Erin Edgar
Maj. Andy Fisher
Col. Kirby Gross
Dr. Jay Johannigman
Mr. Win Kerr
Capt. Lanny Littlejohn
Lt. Col. Bob Mabry
Lt. Col. Dave Marcozzi
SOCS Matt McClain
Lt. Col. Ethan Miles
Master Sgt. Danny Morissette
Col. Shawn Nessen
Maj. D. Marc Northern
Cmdr. Dana Onifer
Dr. Mel Otten
Mr. Don Parsons
Mr. Gary Pesquera
Col. Todd Rasmussen
Master Sgt. Mike Remley
Lt. Col. Jamie Riesberg
HSCM Glenn Royes
Col. Stacy Shackelford
SMSgt. Travis Shaw
CSM Tim Sprunger
Mr. Rick Strayer
Cmdr. Matt Tadlock
Capt. Jeff Timby
HMCS Jeremy Torrisi

**Designated Tactical Combat
Casualty Care Subject
Matter Experts**
Dr. Frank Anders
Dr. Brad Bennett
Dr. Jeff Cain
Dr. Dave Callaway
Dr. Howard Champion
Dr. Paul Cordts
Dr. Warren Dorlac
Mr. Bill Donovan
Dr. Jim Dunne
Dr. Rocky Farr
Dr. Steve Flaherty
Dr. John Gandy
Dr. John Holcomb
Dr. Don Jenkins
Dr. Jim Kirkpatrick
Dr. Russ Kotwal
Dr. Norman McSwain
Dr. Peter Rhee

Special Thanks

Special thanks and gratitude are
extended to the medics, corpsmen, and
pararescuers who may be called upon to
risk their lives on the battlefield in order
to use these Tactical Combat Casualty
Care (TCCC) guidelines to save their
wounded teammates.

Reviewers

Alberto Adduci, MD, ED
Molinette Hospital
Turin, Italy

J. Adam Alford, BS, NRP
Old Dominion EMS Alliance
Bon Air, Virginia

Justin Arnone, BS, NRP, NCEE, TP-C
East Baton Rouge Parish EMS
Baton Rouge, Louisiana

Hector Arroyo
New York City Fire Department Bureau
  of Training
Bayside, New York

Ryan Batenhorst, MEd, NRP
Southeast Community College
Lincoln, Nebraska

Nick Bourdeau, RN, Paramedic I/C
Huron Valley Ambulance
Ypsilanti, Michigan

**Dr. Susan Smith Braithwaite, EdD,
NRP**
Western Carolina University
Cullowhee, North Carolina

Lawrence Brewer, MPH, NRP, FP-C
Rogers State University/Tulsa LifeFlight
Claremore, Oklahoma

Aaron R. Byington, MA, NRP
Davis Technical College
Kaysville, Utah

Bernadette Cekuta
Dutchess Community College
Wappingers Falls, New York

Ted Chialtas
Fire Captain/Paramedic, Paramedic
  Program Coordinator
San Diego Fire-Rescue Department
  Paramedic Program
San Diego, California

Hiram Colon
New York City Fire Department Bureau
of EMS
New York, New York

Kevin Curry, AS, NRP, CCEMT-P
United Training Center
Lewiston, Maine

Charlie Dixon, NRP, NCEE
Nucor Steel Berkeley
Huger, South Carolina

John A. Flora, FF/Paramedic, EMS-I
Urbana Fire Division
Urbana, Ohio

Fidel O. Garcia, EMT-P
Professional EMS Education
Grand Junction, Colorado

Jeff Gilliard, NRP/CCEMT-P/FPC, BS
President/CEO, Central Florida Office
Emergency Medical Education &
Technology Systems Inc.
Rockledge, Florida

David Glendenning, EMT-P
Education & Outreach Officer
New Hanover Regional EMS
Wilmington, North Carolina

Conrad M. Gonzales, Jr., NREMT-P
San Antonio Fire Department (Retired)
San Antonio, Texas

David M. Gray, BS, EMTP-IC
Knoxville Fire Department
Knoxville, Tennessee

**Jamie Gray, BS, AAS, FF, NRP
(NAEMT/NAEMSE/ATOA)**
State of Alabama Office of EMS
Montgomery, Alabama

Kevin M. Gurney, MS, CCEMT-P, I/C
Delta Ambulance
Waterville, Maine

**Jason D. Haag, CCEMT-P, CIC,
Tactical Medic**
Finger Lakes Ambulance
Clifton Springs, New York
Wayne County Advanced Life Support
Services
Marion, New York
Finger Lakes Regional Emergency
Medical Services Council
Geneva, New York

Poul Anders Hansen, MD
Medical Director
EMS North Denmark Region
Chairman PHTLS Denmark

**Anthony S. Harbour, BSN, MEd, RN,
NRP**
Executive Director
Southern Virginia Emergency Medical
Services
Roanoke, Virginia

Brad Haywood, NRP, FP-C, CCP-C
Fairfax County Fire and Rescue
Academy
Fairfax, Virginia

Greg Henington
Terlingua Fire & EMS
Terlingua, Texas

Paul Hitchcock, NRP
Front Royal, Virginia

Sandra Hultz, NREMT-P
Holmes Community College
Ridgeland, Mississippi

**Joseph Hurlburt, BS, NREMT-P,
EMT-P I/C**
Instructor Coordinator/Training Officer
Rapid Response EMS
Romulus, Michigan

Melanie Jorgenson
Regions Hospital EMS
Oakdale, Minnesota

Travis L. Karicofe, NREMT-P
EMS Officer
City of Harrisonburg Fire Department
Harrisonburg, Virginia

Brian Katcher NRP, FP-C
Warrenton, Virginia

Alan F. Kicks, EMT
PHTLS Instructor
Bergen County EMS Training Center
Paramus, New Jersey

Jared Kimball, NRP
Tulane Trauma Education
New Orleans, Louisiana

Timothy M. Kimble, AAS, NRP
Education Coordinator
Carilion Clinic Life Support Training
Center
Craig County Emergency Services
New Castle, Virginia

Don Kimlicka, NRP, CCEMT-P
Executive Director
Clintonville Area Ambulance Service
Clintonville, Wisconsin

Jim Ladle, BS, FP-C, CCP-C
South Jordan City Fire Department
South Jordan, Utah

Frankie S. Lobner
Mountain Lakes Regional EMS Council
Queensbury, New York

Robert Loiselle, MA, NRP, EMSIC
Bay City, Michigan

Joshua Lopez, BS-EMS, NRP
University of New Mexico EMS Academy
Albuquerque, New Mexico

Kevin M. Lynch, NREMT, NYS CIC
Greenburgh Police Department: EMS
White Plains, New York

Christopher Maeder, BA, EMT-P
Chief
Fairview Fire District
Fairview, New York

Jeanette S. Mann, BSN, RN, NRP
Director of EMS Programs
Dabney S. Lancaster Community College
Clifton Forge, Virginia

Michael McDonald, RN, NRP
Loudoun County Fire Rescue
Leesburg, Virginia

Jeff McPhearson, NRP
Southside Regional Medical Center
Petersburg, Virginia

David R. Murack, NREMT-P, CCP
EMS Educator
Lakeshore Technical College
Assistant Chief of Emergency Operations
City of Two Rivers Fire/Rescue
Cleveland, Wisconsin

**Stephen Nacy, FP-C, TP-C, CCEMT-P,
NRP, DMT**
Leesburg, Virginia

**Gregory S. Neiman, MS, NRP, NCEE,
CEMA(VA)**
VCU Health System
Richmond, Virginia

**Norma Pancake, BS, MEP,
NREMT-P**
Pierce County EMS
Tacoma, Washington

Deb Petty
St. Charles County Ambulance District
St. Peter's, Missouri

Mark Podgwaite, NECEMS I/C
Waterbury Ambulance Service
Waterbury, Vermont

Jonathan R. Powell, BS, NRP
University of South Alabama
Mobile, Alabama

Kevin Ramdayal
New York City Fire Department Bureau
   of EMS
New York, New York

Christoph Redelsteiner, PhD, MSW, MS, EMT-P
Academic Director Social Work (MA)
Danube University, Krems Austria
Scientific Director
Emergency Health Services Management
   Program
University of Applied Sciences St. Pölten

Les Remington, EMT-P, I/C, FI1
EMS Educator, Trauma Course
   Coordinator Genesys EMS and
   Employee Education
Grand Blanc, Michigan

Ian T.T. Santee, MPA, MICT
City and County of Honolulu
Honolulu, Hawaii

Edward Schauster, NREMT-P
Air Idaho Rescue
Idaho Falls, Idaho

Justin Schindler, BS, NRP
Monroe Ambulance
Rochester, New York

Kimberly Singleton, APRN, MSN, FNP-C
Gwinnett Medical Center
Lawrenceville, Georgia

Jennifer TeWinkel Smith, BA, AEMT
Regions Hospital Emergency Medical
   Services
Oakdale, Minnesota

Josh Steele, MBAHA, BS, AAS, NRP, FP-C, I/C
Hospital Wing (Memphis Medical Center
   Air Ambulance, Inc.)
Memphis, Tennessee

Richard Stump, NRP
Central Carolina Community College
Erwin, North Carolina

William Torres, Jr., NRP
Marcus Daly Memorial Hospital
Hamilton, Montana

Brian Turner, CCEMT-P, RN
Genesis Medical Center
Davenport, Iowa

Scott Vanderkooi, BS, NRP
Department of EMS Education
University of South Alabama
Mobile, Alabama

Gary S. Walter, NRP, BA, MS
Union College
International Rescue & Relief
Lincoln, Nebraska

Mitchell R. Warren, NRP
Children's Hospital and Medical Center
Omaha, Nebraska

David Watson, NRP, CCEMT-P, FP-C
Pickens County EMS
Pickens, South Carolina

Jackilyn E. Williams, RN, MSN, NRP
Portland Community College Paramedic
   Program
Portland, Oregon

Earl M. Wilson, III, BIS, NREMT-P
Nunez Community College
Chalmette, Louisiana

Rich Wisniewski, BS, NRP
Columbia, South Carolina

Karen "Keri" Wydner Krause, RN, CCRN, EMT-P
Lakeshore Technical College
Cleveland, Wisconsin

Dawn Young
Bossier Parish School for Technology
   and Innovative Learning
Bossier City, Louisiana

Photoshoot Acknowledgments
We would like to thank the following
people and institutions for their
collaboration on the photoshoot for
this project. Their assistance was
appreciated greatly.

Technical Consultants and Institutions
UMass Memorial Paramedics, Worcester
   EMS
Worcester, Massachusetts
Richard A. Nydam, AS, NREMT-P
Training and Education Specialist, EMS
UMass Memorial Paramedics, Worcester
   EMS
Worcester, Massachusetts

Southbridge Fire Department
Southbridge, Massachusetts

Jerry Flanagan
Account Manager
BoundTree Medical
Dublin, Ohio

Foreword

PHTLS

As we embark on this ninth edition of the *Prehospital Trauma Life Support (PHTLS)* textbook, we reflect on 37 years of incremental progress and improvements in prehospital care. PHTLS rolled out in 1981, around the time of the inception of Advanced Trauma Life Support (ATLS), and it complemented ATLS very well.

As with cardiopulmonary resuscitation (CPR), for many years in the 1970s and 1980s, research on trauma care was directed at advanced life support endeavors. Progress was made, but an apparent gap in prehospital survivability remained. It was not until the window of prehospital cardiac care was dissected that we finally realized that the scope of prehospital activity needed to be far greater than just calling 9-1-1 and transporting. For CPR, it was the recognition that prehospital or bystander CPR, initiated early, was a determinative factor in overall survival. The data from early studies clearly supported training all people in basic life support, and the resulting improvement in survival for out-of-hospital cardiac arrest was astounding.

As we studied and learned more about the prehospital incremental variables that decrease morbidity and mortality of the injured patient, it was also apparent that a well-vetted and memorialized body of prehospital knowledge—from extrication, to rapid identification and treatment of life-threatening injuries like loss of airway and exsanguination, to safe transport procedures—could be coupled as a best practices continuum of care that would result in improved patient outcomes. Hence, PHTLS has become the world standard of prehospital care.

Although the basic PHTLS concepts have remained the same over the years, the "all hazard" challenges that our prehospital care providers are facing today have become more complex, and they often appear as military-like combat injuries, sometimes including the need for rapid triage. This ninth edition of PHTLS includes this broader coverage. The PHTLS program continues to grow and become stronger due to the leadership, commitment, and partnership of the American College of Surgeons (ACS) and the National Association of Emergency Medical Technicians (NAEMT). In addition, numerous new and evolving emergency-related courses and training programs support and have incorporated PHTLS concepts into their curriculums. These include, but are not limited to, Tactical Emergency Medical Support (TEMS), Counter Narcotics and Terrorism Operational Medical Support (CONTOMS), Tactical Combat Casualty Care (TCCC), PHTLS for First Responders, Tactical Emergency Casualty Care (TECC), Bleeding Control (B-CON), and the military system of "buddy care."

As with the understanding of all-hazard preparedness and evolving practices to meet our current threats, it is clear that PHTLS must continue to renew itself for decades to come due to an apparently more complex and unstable world unfolding before us. As a former military and civilian first responder in peacetime and in war, I recognize firsthand the immense contribution that PHTLS has made to significantly reducing morbidity and mortality from all-hazard threats.

For many years, PHTLS was guided by a dear friend and colleague whose iconic presence lives on in prehospital and trauma care. For many decades, Dr. Norm McSwain led and served selflessly; he will be sorely missed by all of us. As we move forward, we are fortunate to gain the leadership of one of the next generation of PHTLS medical directors, Dr. Alex Eastman, a gifted young trauma surgeon and former firefighter/EMT whom I have known for decades.

The doctor is in, and we are in very good, capable hands as we chart our course into the collective PHTLS future.

Richard Carmona, MD, MPH, FACS
VADM Public Health Service Commissioned Corps (Retired)
17th Surgeon General of the United States
Distinguished Professor, University of Arizona

PHTLS Military

If you are a combatant wounded on the battlefield, the most critical phase of your care is the period from the time of injury until the time that you arrive at a surgically capable medical treatment facility (MTF). Almost 90% of American service men and women who die from combat wounds do so before they arrive at an MTF, thus highlighting the importance of the battlefield trauma care that is provided by our combat medics, corpsmen, and pararescuemen (PJs), as well as by the casualties themselves and their fellow combatants.

Most of the U.S. military went to war in Afghanistan and Iraq with battlefield trauma care strategies that were not based on Tactical Combat Casualty Care (TCCC)—medics in 2001 had no tourniquets, no hemostatic dressings, no intraosseous devices, and Civil War–vintage analgesia (IM morphine) and treated hemorrhagic shock with large-volume crystalloid fluid replacement.

Only a select few Special Operations and conventional units went to war with a robust TCCC capability. The 75th Ranger Regiment, for example, taught the concepts of TCCC to everyone in the Regiment as part of their TCCC-based Casualty Response Plan. As a result, the Regiment documented a preventable prehospital death rate of 0%, an unprecedented success in optimizing casualty survival on the battlefield. In contrast, the overall incidence of preventable prehospital deaths among U.S. combat fatalities was 24%, as documented by Col. Brian Eastridge in his landmark 2012 paper.

Once the U.S. Special Operations Command mandated that TCCC would be used in all of its units, the rest of the U.S. military began to take notice and to follow that example. As a result, prehospital trauma care in the military has undergone an unprecedented transformation since the beginning of the conflicts in Afghanistan and Iraq. A 2018 U.S. Department of Defense Instruction has officially established TCCC as the standard for battlefield trauma care in the U.S. military and requires that all service members receive TCCC training as appropriate for their role in helping to provide this care.

Combat medical personnel in the U.S. military (and those of most of our coalition partners) are now trained to manage combat trauma on the battlefield using the TCCC Guidelines. TCCC started as a biomedical research project in the U.S. Special Operations Command (USSO-COM). The largely tradition-based trauma care practices that were in place in 1993 were systematically re-evaluated. Many aspects of prehospital care were found to not be well supported by the available evidence and in need of revision. TCCC was introduced as a new framework on which to build trauma care guidelines customized for the battlefield. The original TCCC paper came out in Military Medicine in 1996 and provided a foundation, but TCCC has evolved steadily over the past 18 years and will always be a work in progress. These trauma care guidelines customized for use on the battlefield are now reviewed and updated by the Committee on TCCC (CoTCCC) on an ongoing basis. The CoTCCC is composed of trauma surgeons, emergency medicine physicians, combatant unit physicians, and combat medics, corpsmen, and PJs. There are also physician assistants and military medical educators among the members. At present the CoTCCC has representation from all of the U.S. armed services, and 100% of the voting membership has experience deploying in support of combat operations.

The CoTCCC was first located at the Naval Operational Medicine Institute (NOMI) through the leadership of Capt. Doug Freer, the Commander, and Capt. Steve Giebner, the first Chairman of the group. It remained at NOMI for 7 years before being relocated to become Defense Health Board in 2008. In 2013, the CoTCCC was moved again to function as part of the Joint Trauma System, which is in turn part of the Combat Support Directorate at the Defense Health Agency.

Changes in the TCCC Guidelines are based on direct input from combat medical personnel, an ongoing review of published prehospital trauma care literature, new research coming from military medical research organizations, lessons learned from U.S. and allied service medical departments, and trauma conferences conducted by the Joint Trauma System and the Armed Forces Medical Examiners System.

The CoTCCC publishes its recommendations in both the *Journal of Special Operations Medicine* and the *Prehospital Trauma Life Support Textbook*. The TCCC Guidelines are the only set of battlefield trauma care best-practice guidelines to have received the triple endorsement of the American College of Surgeons Committee on Trauma (ACS-COT), the National Associations of Emergency Medical Technicians (NAEMT), and the Department of Defense (DoD).

As the CoTCCC has continued to work to improve battlefield trauma care, it has formed strategic partnerships with other organizations that seek to improve prehospital trauma care in non-combat settings. TCCC began its partnership with the Prehospital Trauma Life Support (PHTLS) Committee in 1998 and continues to work with this internationally recognized group of leaders in prehospital trauma care. The PHTLS organization teaches TCCC courses around the world and has recently established a program to provide TCCC training to law enforcement agencies and the militaries of allied countries when these groups request it.

TCCC established a strategic partnership with the U.S. Army Institute of Surgical Research (USAISR) in 2004. At the request of USSOCOM, USAISR undertook the first preventable death review on all Special Operations fatalities from Afghanistan and Iraq that had occurred from the start of the conflict in Afghanistan until November 2004, which helped to highlight the critical need for all combatants to be trained in basic TCCC interventions. The USAISR subsequently developed a research effort with a strong focus on battlefield first responder care and published breakthrough reports on items such as tourniquets, hemostatic agents, junctional tourniquets, chest seals, and prehospital fluid resuscitation. This ongoing work has since firmly established USAISR as the Department of Defense leader in developing and evaluating battlefield trauma care technology and management strategies. The USAISR also led the very successful USSOCOM-sponsored TCCC Transition Initiative that was undertaken to ensure that deploying Special Operations units had the latest TCCC equipment and were trained to use it before deploying. The TCCC Transition Initiative also gathered feedback about the training, the equipment provided, and the outcomes from TCCC-recommended interventions when the units returned from their combat deployments. It was the success of that project that provided the impetus for the eventual adoption of TCCC by conventional forces in the U.S. military in addition to Special Operations units.

Meetings of the CoTCCC are now attended by representatives from combat units, the service Surgeons General offices, liaisons from allied nations, stakeholders from non-DoD government agencies, and representatives from federal law enforcement agencies. The Defense Health Agency—Medical Logistics Office is also represented to ensure that TCCC equipment issues, both in procurement and performance, are tracked by and discussed with the group. All of the above participants have played key roles in proposing, refining, and gaining approval for recent changes in the TCCC Guidelines. This robust interaction has helped to ensure that TCCC continues to reflect the state of the art in battlefield trauma care and reaches non-military organizations that may have to treat individuals with traumatic injuries.

The TCCC Guidelines are best-practice trauma care guidelines customized for use on the battlefield and are updated in real time as additional combat experience is gained. BUT they are guidelines only—there are no rigid protocols in combat, including TCCC. If the recommended TCCC combat trauma management plan doesn't work for the specific tactical setting that a combat medic, corpsman, or PJ encounters, then the plan must be modified to best fit the tactical situation.

TCCC is a combination of good medicine and good tactics, and both scenario-based training and planning are critically important to optimizing outcomes for combat casualties.

Frank K. Butler, Jr., MD
Captain, U.S. Army (Retired)
Chairman
Committee on Tactical Combat Casualty Care
Joint Trauma System
Defense Health Agency

Preface

Prehospital care providers must accept the responsibility to provide patient care that is as close to perfect as possible. This can only be achieved by possessing a thorough knowledge of the basic principles of evaluation and treatment of injured patients. We must remember that patients do not choose to be injured. On the other hand, prehospital care providers choose to take care of trauma patients. Prehospital care providers are therefore obligated to give 100% effort during contact with every patient. The patient has had a bad day; the prehospital care provider must be both compassionate and competent.

The patient is the focus of the efforts at the scene of an emergency. There is no time to think about the order in which the patient assessment is performed or what treatments should take priority over others. There is no time to practice a skill before using it on a patient. There is no time to think about where equipment or supplies are housed within the medic unit. There is no time to think about where to transport the injured patient. All this information and more must be preprogrammed in the prehospital care provider's mind, and all supplies and equipment must be present in the jump kit or on the rig when the provider arrives on the scene. Without the proper knowledge and equipment, the prehospital care provider may not be able to do what is necessary to save the patient's life. The stakes are simply too high not to be thoroughly prepared in advance.

Those who deliver care in the prehospital setting are integral members of the trauma patient care team, as are the nurses and physicians in the emergency department, operating room, intensive care unit, ward, and rehabilitation unit. Prehospital care providers must be practiced in their skills so that they can move the patient quickly and efficiently out of the environment of the emergency and transport the patient quickly to the closest appropriate facility.

Why PHTLS?

Course Education Philosophy

Prehospital Trauma Life Support (PHTLS) focuses on principles, not preferences. By focusing on the principles of good trauma care, PHTLS promotes critical thinking. The PHT Committee of the National Association of Emergency Medical Technicians (NAEMT) believes that emergency medical services (EMS) practitioners make the best decisions on behalf of their patients when prepared with a sound foundation of key principles and evidence-based knowledge. Rote memorization of mnemonics is discouraged. Furthermore, there is no one "PHTLS way" of performing a specific skill. The principle of the skill is taught, and then one acceptable method of performing the skill that meets the principle is presented. The authors realize that no one method can apply to the myriad unique situations encountered in the prehospital setting.

Up-to-Date Information

Development of the PHTLS program began in 1981, on the heels of the inception of the Advanced Trauma Life Support (ATLS) program for physicians. As the ATLS course is revised every 4 to 5 years, pertinent changes are incorporated into the next edition of PHTLS. This ninth edition of the PHTLS program has been revised based on the 2017 ATLS course and the tenth edition of the ATLS textbook, as well as subsequent publications in the medical literature. Although following the ATLS principles, PHTLS is specifically designed to prepare learners to address the unique challenges encountered when caring for trauma outside of the hospital. All chapters have been extensively revised and the table of contents streamlined. Video clips of critical skills and an eBook are available online.

Scientific Base

The authors and editors have adopted an evidence-based approach that includes references from medical literature supporting the key principles, and additional position papers published by national organizations are cited when applicable. Many references have been added, allowing those prehospital care providers with inquisitive minds to read the original scientific papers that form the evidentiary basis for our recommendations.

PHTLS—Commitment and Mission

As we continue to pursue the potential of the PHTLS course and the worldwide community of prehospital care providers, we must remember the goals and objectives of the PHTLS program:

- To provide a description of the physiology and kinematics of injury
- To provide an understanding of the need for and techniques of rapid assessment of the trauma patient
- To advance the participant's level of knowledge with regard to examination and diagnostic skills
- To enhance the participant's performance in the assessment and treatment of the trauma patient
- To advance the participant's level of competence in regard to specific prehospital trauma intervention skills
- To provide an overview and establish a management method for the prehospital care of the multisystem trauma patient
- To promote a common approach for the initiation and transition of care beginning with civilian first responders continuing up and through the levels of care until the patient is delivered to the definitive treatment facility

It is also fitting to reprise our mission statement, which was written during a marathon session at the NAEMT conference in 1997:

> *The Prehospital Trauma Life Support (PHTLS) program of the National Association of Emergency Medical Technicians (NAEMT) serves trauma victims through the global education of prehospital care providers of all levels. With medical oversight from the American College of Surgeons Committee on Trauma (ACS-COT), the PHTLS programs develop and disseminate educational materials and scientific information and promote excellence in trauma patient management by all providers involved in the delivery of prehospital care.*

The PHTLS mission also enhances the achievement of the NAEMT mission. The PHTLS program is committed to quality and performance improvement. As such, PHTLS is always attentive to changes in technology and methods of delivering prehospital trauma care that may be used to enhance the value of this program.

Support for NAEMT

NAEMT provides the administrative structure for the PHTLS program. All profits from the PHTLS program are reinvested into NAEMT to support programs that are of prime importance to EMS professionals, such as educational conferences and advocacy efforts on behalf of prehospital care providers and their patients.

PHTLS Is a World Leader

Because of the unprecedented success of the prior editions of *PHTLS*, the program has continued to grow rapidly. PHTLS courses continue to proliferate across civilian and military sectors the United States. It has also been taught worldwide in more than 68 nations, and many others are now expressing interest in bringing PHTLS to their countries in efforts to improve prehospital trauma care.

Prehospital care providers have the responsibility to assimilate this knowledge and these skills in order to use them for the benefit of their patients. The editors and authors of this material and the PHT Committee of NAEMT hope that you will incorporate this information into your practice and that you will rededicate yourself to the care of trauma patients.

National Association of Emergency Medical Technicians

Founded in 1975, the National Association of Emergency Medical Technicians (NAEMT) is the only national organization in the United States that represents and serves the professional interests of EMS practitioners, including paramedics, emergency medical technicians, emergency medical responders, and other professionals providing prehospital and out-of-hospital emergent, urgent, or preventive medical care. NAEMT members work in all sectors of EMS, including government service agencies, fire departments, hospital-based ambulance services, private companies, industrial and special operations settings, and the military.

NAEMT serves its members by advocating on issues that impact their ability to provide quality patient care, providing high-quality education that improves the knowledge and skills of practitioners, and supporting EMS research and innovation.

One of NAEMT's principal activities is EMS education. The mission of NAEMT education programs is to improve patient care through high-quality, cost-effective, evidence-based education that strengthens and enhances the knowledge and skills of EMS practitioners.

NAEMT strives to provide the highest quality education programs. All NAEMT education programs are developed by highly experienced EMS educators, clinicians, and medical directors. Course content incorporates the latest research, newest techniques, and innovative approaches in EMS learning. All NAEMT education programs promote critical thinking as the foundation for providing quality care. This is based on the belief that EMS practitioners make the best decisions on behalf of their patients when given a sound foundation of evidence-based knowledge and key principles.

Once developed, education programs are tested and refined to ensure that course materials are clear, accurate, and relevant to the needs of EMS practitioners. Finally, all education programs are reviewed and updated every 4 years to ensure that the content reflects the most up-to-date research and practices.

NAEMT provides ongoing support to its instructors and the EMS training sites that hold its courses. Over 2,000 training centers, including colleges, EMS agencies, hospitals, and other medical training facilities located in the United States and more than 70 other countries, offer NAEMT education programs. NAEMT headquarters staff work with the network of education program faculty engaged as committee members; authors; national, regional, and state coordinators; and affiliate faculty to provide administrative and educational support.

Andrew N. Pollak, MD, FAAOS
Medical Editor

Dedication

I am honored to write this memoriam in honor of Dr. Norman McSwain, the founder of PHTLS and a godfather of prehospital trauma care. Dr. McSwain passed away at his home in New Orleans on July 28, 2015. No physician has been a bigger advocate for the medic or had a larger impact on international prehospital trauma care than Dr. McSwain. I am lucky to have known him in several capacities, from my time years ago as a paramedic in New Orleans, to learning from him as a trauma fellow, and finally in working with him as his surgical partner in the trauma center that he helped build. He expected a lot but gave a lot in return, both in knowledge and in friendship.

In addition to being the founder of PHTLS, Dr. McSwain was the trauma director for the Spirit of Charity Trauma Center in New Orleans and professor of surgery at Tulane School of Medicine. He was a fellow of the American College of Surgeons and an active member of the Committee on Trauma. He served as the surgeon for the New Orleans Police Department and was always available for an officer in need. Dr. McSwain was especially proud of his work with the U.S. military to promulgate the TCCC course and developed a pathway for Naval Special Warfare medics to train in our civilian trauma center. He served as a founding member of the Hartford Consensus Group, leading to the development of the Stop the Bleed campaign that continues to grow around the world.

Today I operated on a gunshot wound to the aorta—Norman's favorite surgical case. It brought back a lot of great memories of my mentor and friend. A gunshot aorta is among the most challenging cases a trauma surgeon can encounter—the blood wells up from deep in the abdomen, flowing at the rate of a garden hose, and it is almost impossible to control. Patients lose blood so quickly they stop clotting as they slowly lose the fight to survive. Norman loved it because it required the best of a surgeon's abilities. Cut fast, be decisive, be technically skillful, stop the bleeding, and do whatever it takes to keep the patient alive. These are all lessons he has taught to generations of young surgeons. He believed the medic should have the same mindset as a trauma surgeon—know everything about the disease process you are treating, be aggressive, treat your patient as you would a family member, and never stop learning. These are the very principles upon which Norman based PHTLS when he developed the course in the early 1980s.

Norman will be remembered for many things—his cowboy boots, turtleneck shirts, and bear claw necklace. He loved all things New Orleans, including Mardi Gras, Jazz Fest, and his home on Bourbon Street. He will be remembered for the way he treated everyone—it didn't matter to him if you were a chairman of surgery, a tired medical student, or a medic on the street—all received a kind word and were shown the same respect. He was always willing to give of himself, his time, and his energy. Norman's accolades are numerous and may never be surpassed, but those who knew him best will remember him for the great person he was and the special way he treated them.

Dr. McSwain will never be forgotten. His memory lives on in the trauma center we recently named after him, in the PHTLS courses held around the world, and in the countless soldiers' lives saved on distant battlefields thanks to his teachings. He was the consummate surgeon, patient advocate, teacher, mentor, and friend. Keep a little of Norman alive in your heart by always asking yourself, "What have you done for the good of mankind today?"

Lance E. Stuke, MD, MPH, FACS
Norman E. McSwain, Jr., MD
Spirit of Charity Trauma Center
Louisiana State University Department of Surgery
New Orleans, Louisiana

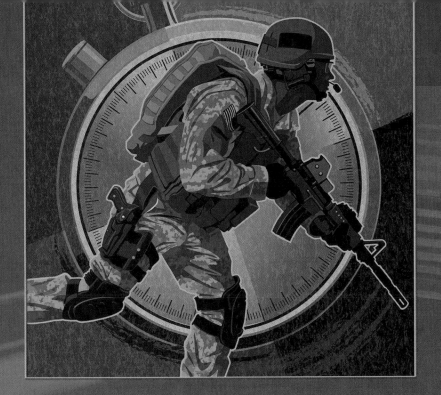

Introduction

CHAPTER 1

PHTLS: Past, Present, and Future

Lead Editors:
Richard Ellis, MSEDM, NRP
Patrick Wick

CHAPTER OBJECTIVES   At the completion of this chapter, you will be able to do the following:

- Understand the history and evolution of prehospital trauma care.
- Recognize the magnitude of the problem both in human and financial terms caused by traumatic injury.
- Understand the three phases of trauma care.

INTRODUCTION

Our patients did not choose us. We chose them. We could have chosen another profession, but we did not. We have accepted the responsibility for patient care in some of the worst situations—when we are tired or cold, when it is rainy and dark, when we cannot predict what conditions we will encounter. We must either accept this responsibility or surrender it. We must give to our patients the very best care that we can—not while we are daydreaming, not with unchecked equipment, not with incomplete supplies, and not with yesterday's knowledge. We cannot know what medical information is current, we cannot purport to be ready to care for our patients if we do not read and learn each day. The Prehospital Trauma Life Support (PHTLS) course provides a part of that knowledge to the working prehospital care provider, but, more importantly, it ultimately benefits the person who needs our all—the patient. At the end of each run, we should feel that the patient received nothing short of our very best.

History of Trauma Care in Emergency Medical Services (EMS)

The stages and development of the management of the trauma patient can be divided into roughly four time periods, as described by Norman McSwain, MD, in the Scudder Oration of the American College of Surgeons in 1999.[1] These time periods are (1) the ancient period, (2) the Larrey period, (3) the Farrington era, and (4) the modern era. This text, the entire PHTLS course, and care of the trauma patient are based on the principles developed and taught by the early pioneers of prehospital care. The list of these innovators is long; however, a few deserve special recognition.

Ancient Period

All of the medical care that was accomplished in Egypt, Greece, and Rome, by the Israelites, and up to the time of

Napoleon is classified as premodern EMS. Most of the medical care was accomplished within some type of rudimentary medical facility; little was performed by prehospital care providers in the field. The most significant contribution to our knowledge of this period is the Edwin Smith papyrus from approximately 4,500 years ago, which describes the medical care in a series of case reports.

Larrey Period (Late 1700s to Approximately 1950)

In the late 1700s, Baron Dominique Jean Larrey, Napoleon's chief military physician, recognized the need for prompt prehospital care. In 1797, he noted that "the remoteness of our ambulances deprive the wounded of the requisite attention. I was authorized to construct a carriage which I call flying ambulances."[2] He developed these horse-drawn "flying ambulances" for timely retrieval of warriors injured on the battlefield and introduced the premise that individuals working in these "flying ambulances" should be trained in medical care to provide on-scene and en route care for patients.

By the early 1800s, he had established the following elements of the basic theory of prehospital care that we continue to use to this day:

- The "flying" ambulance
- Proper training of medical personnel
- Movement into the field during battle for patient care and retrieval
- Field control of hemorrhage
- Transport to a nearby hospital
- Provision of care en route
- Development of frontline hospitals

He developed hospitals that were close to the front lines (much like the military of today) and stressed the rapid movement of patients from the field to medical care. Baron Larrey is now recognized by many as the father of EMS in the modern era.

Unfortunately, the type of care developed by Larrey was not used by the Union Army in the United States 60 years later at the beginning of the American Civil War. At the First Battle of Bull Run in August 1861, the wounded lay in the field—3,000 for 3 days, 600 for up to a week.[1] Jonathan Letterman was appointed Surgeon General and created a separate medical corps with better organized medical care (**Figure 1-1**). At the Second Battle of Bull Run a year later, there were 300 ambulances, and attendants collected 10,000 wounded in 24 hours.[3]

In August 1864, the International Red Cross was created at the First Geneva Convention. The convention recognized the neutrality of hospitals, of the sick and wounded, of all involved personnel, and of ambulances, and it guaranteed safe passage for ambulances and medical

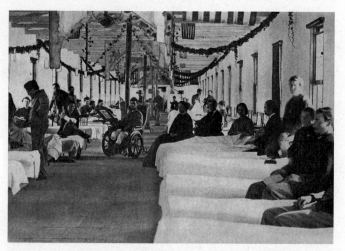

Figure 1-1 During the American Civil War, patient care practices for soldiers developed by Larrey, such as building temporary hospitals near the front lines, were put in place.
Unknown/Alamy Stock Photo.

personnel to move the wounded. It also stressed the equality of medical care provided, regardless of which side of the conflict the victim was on. This convention marked the first step toward the Code of Conduct used by the U.S. military today. This Code of Conduct is an important component of the Tactical Combat Casualty Care (TCCC) Course, which is now an integral part of the PHTLS program.

Hospitals, Military, and Mortuaries

In 1865, the first private ambulance service in the United States was created in Cincinnati, Ohio, at Cincinnati General Hospital.[3] Soon thereafter, several EMS systems were developed in the United States: Bellevue Hospital Ambulance[3] in New York in 1867; Grady Hospital Ambulance Service (the oldest continuously operating hospital-based ambulance) in Atlanta in the 1880s; Charity Hospital Ambulance Services in New Orleans, created in 1885 by a surgeon, Dr. A. B. Miles; and numerous other facilities in the United States. These ambulance services were run primarily by hospitals, the military, or mortuaries up until 1950.[1]

In 1891, Nicholas Senn, MD, the founder of the Association of Military Surgeons, said, "The fate of the wounded rests in the hands of one who applies the first dressing." Although prehospital care was rudimentary when Dr. Senn made his statement, the words still hold true, as prehospital care providers address the specific needs of trauma patients in the field.

Some changes in medical care occurred during the various wars up until the end of World War II, but generally the system and the type of care rendered prior to arrival at the Battalion Aid Station (Echelon II) in the military or at the back door of the civilian hospital remained unchanged until the mid-1950s.

During this period, many ambulances in the major cities that had teaching hospitals were staffed by interns who were beginning their first year of training. The last ambulance service to require physicians on ambulance runs was Charity Hospital in New Orleans in the 1960s. Despite the fact that physicians were present, most of the trauma care was primitive. The equipment and supplies had not changed from those used during the American Civil War.[1]

Farrington Era (Approximately 1950 to 1970)

The era of J. D. "Deke" Farrington, MD (1909 to 1982), began in 1950. Dr. Farrington, the father of EMS in the United States, stimulated the development of improved prehospital care with his landmark article, "Death in a Ditch."[4] In the late 1960s, Dr. Farrington and other early leaders, such as Oscar Hampton, MD, and Curtis Artz, MD, brought the United States into the modern era of EMS and prehospital care.[1] Dr. Farrington was actively involved in all aspects of ambulance care. His work as chairman of the committees that produced three of the initial documents establishing the basis of EMS—the essential equipment list for ambulances of the American College of Surgeons,[4] the design specifications of the Department of Transportation (DOT),[5] and the first emergency medical technician (EMT) basic training program—also propelled the idea and development of prehospital care. In addition to the efforts of Dr. Farrington, others actively helped to promote the importance of prehospital care for the trauma victim. Robert Kennedy, MD, was the author of *Early Care of the Sick and Injured Patient.*[6] Sam Banks, MD, along with Dr. Farrington, taught the first prehospital training course to the Chicago Fire Department in 1957, which initiated proper care of the trauma patient.

A 1965 text edited and compiled by George J. Curry, MD, a leader of the American College of Surgeons and its Committee on Trauma, stated:

> Injuries sustained in accidents affect every part of the human body. They range from simple abrasions and contusions to multiple complex injuries involving many body tissues. This demands efficient and intelligent primary appraisal and care, on an individual basis, before transport. It is obvious that the services of trained ambulance attendants are essential. If we are to expect maximum efficiency from ambulance attendants, a special training program must be arranged.[7]

The landmark white paper, *Accidental Death and Disability: The Neglected Disease of Modern Society,* further accelerated the process in 1967.[8] The National Academy of Sciences/National Research Council (NAS/NRC) issued this paper just 1 year after Dr. Curry's call to action.

Modern Era of Prehospital Care (Approximately 1970 to Today)

1970s

The modern era of prehospital care began with the Dunlap and Associates report to the DOT in 1968 defining the curriculum for EMT-Ambulance Training. This training first became known as EMT-Basic; it is known as EMT today.

The National Registry of EMTs (NREMT) was established in 1970, and it developed the standards for testing and registration of trained EMS personnel as advocated in the NAS/NRC white paper. Rocco Morando was the leader of the NREMT for many years and was associated with Drs. Farrington, Hampton, and Artz.

Dr. Curry's call for specialized training of ambulance attendants *for trauma* was initially answered by using the educational program developed by Drs. Farrington and Banks, by the publication of *Emergency Care and Transportation of the Sick and Injured* (the "Orange Book") by the American Academy of Orthopaedic Surgeons (AAOS), by the EMT training programs from the National Highway Traffic Safety Administration (NHTSA), and by the PHTLS training program during the past 25 years. The first training efforts were primitive; however, they have progressed significantly in a relatively brief time.

The first textbook of this era was *Emergency Care and Transportation of the Sick and Injured.* It was the brainchild of Walter A. Hoyt, Jr., MD, and was published in 1971 by the AAOS.[1] The text is now in its 11th edition.

During this same period, the Glasgow Coma Scale was developed in Glasgow, Scotland, by Dr. Graham Teasdale and Dr. Bryan Jennett for research purposes. Dr. Howard Champion brought it into the United States and incorporated it into the care of the trauma patient for assessment of the continued neurologic status of the patient.[2] The Glasgow Coma Scale is a sensitive indicator of improvement or deterioration of such patients.

In 1973, federal EMS legislation was created to promote the development of comprehensive EMS systems. The legislation identified 15 individual components that were needed to have an integrated EMS system. Dr. David Boyd, under the Department of Health and Human Services (DHHS), was placed in charge of implementing this legislation. One of these components was education. This became the basis for the development of training curricula for EMT-Basic, EMT-Intermediate, and EMT-Paramedic care throughout the United States. Today, these levels of training are called Emergency Medical Technician (EMT), Advanced Emergency Medical Technician (AEMT), and Paramedic. The curriculum was initially defined by the DOT in the NHTSA and became known as the National Standard Curriculum or the DOT curriculum.

Dr. Nancy Caroline defined the standards and the curriculum for the first paramedic program, and she wrote the initial textbook, *Emergency Care in the Streets*, used in the training of paramedics. This text is now in its eighth edition.

The Blue Star of Life was designed by the American Medical Association (AMA) as the symbol for a "Medic Alert"—an indication that a patient had an important medical condition that should be noted by EMS. Later, the AMA gave this symbol to the NREMT to use as their logo. Because the American Red Cross would not allow the "Red Cross" logo to be used on ambulances as an emergency symbol, Lew Schwartz, the chief of NHTSA's EMS branch, asked Dr. Farrington, the chairman of the NREMT board, to allow NHTSA to use the symbol for ambulances. Permission was granted by Dr. Farrington and Rocco Morando, the executive director of NREMT. The Blue Star of Life has since become an international symbol of EMS systems.[1]

The National Association of Emergency Medical Technicians (NAEMT) was established in 1975 with the financial support of NREMT (**Figure 1-2**). NAEMT is the nation's only organization dedicated solely to representing the professional interests of all EMS practitioners, including paramedics, AEMTs, EMTs, emergency medical responders, and other professionals working in prehospital emergency medicine.

1980s

In the mid-1980s it became apparent that trauma patients were different from cardiac patients. Trauma surgeons such as Frank Lewis, MD, and Donald Trunkey, MD, recognized the key distinction between these two groups: For cardiac

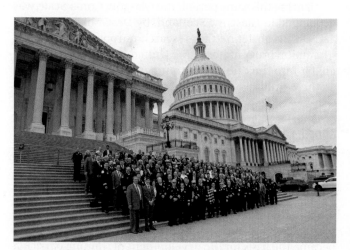

Figure 1-2 Formed in 1975, NAEMT is the only national association representing the professional interests of all emergency and mobile healthcare practitioners, including EMTs, AEMTs, emergency medical responders, paramedics, advanced practice paramedics, critical care paramedics, flight paramedics, community paramedics, and mobile integrated healthcare practitioners.
Courtesy of National Association of Emergency Medical Technicians (NAEMT).

patients, all or most of the tools needed for reestablishment of cardiac output (cardiopulmonary resuscitation [CPR], external defibrillation, and supportive medications) were available to properly trained paramedics in the field. For trauma patients, however, the most important tools (surgical control of internal hemorrhage and replacement of blood) were not available in the field. The importance of moving patients rapidly to the correct hospital became apparent to both prehospital care providers and EMS medical directors. A well-prepared facility incorporated a well-trained trauma team comprising emergency physicians, surgeons, trained nurses, and operating room (OR) staff; a blood bank; registration and quality assurance processes; and all of the components necessary for the management of trauma patients. All of these resources needed to be ready and waiting for the arrival of the patient, with the surgical team standing by to take the patient directly into the OR. Over time, these standards were modified to include such concepts as permissive hypotension (Dr. Ken Mattox) and a transfusion ratio close to one part red blood cells for one part plasma (1:1).[9-12] However, the bottom line of rapid availability of a well-equipped OR has not changed.

Rapid treatment of trauma patients depends on a prehospital care system that offers easy access to the system. This access is aided by a single emergency phone number (e.g., 9-1-1 in the United States), a good communication system to dispatch emergency medical units, and well-prepared and well-trained prehospital care providers. Many people have been taught that early access and early CPR save the lives of those experiencing cardiac arrest. Trauma can be approached in the same way. The principles just listed are the basis for good patient care; to these basic principles has been added the importance of internal hemorrhage control, which cannot be accomplished outside of the trauma center and OR. Thus, rapid assessment, proper packaging, and rapid delivery of the patient to a facility with OR resources immediately available has become the additional principle that was not understood until the mid-1980s. These basic principles remain the bedrock of EMS care today.

The accomplishments of these great physicians, prehospital care providers, and organizations stand out; however, there are many others, too numerous to mention, who contributed to the development of EMS. To all of them, we owe a great debt of gratitude.

Advances in the New Millennium

Every period of armed conflict gives rise to major advances in trauma care, and the past 20 years have been no exception. The military engagements of the past two decades have seen some of the most substantial changes in battlefield management of wounded military personnel in recent history. Some of the key organizations driving these advancements include the Department of Defense Joint Trauma System and the Committee on Tactical Combat

Casualty Care. The Department of Defense established the Joint Trauma System with aim of providing the optimal chance for survival and maximal chance for functional recovery to every service person wounded in battle. To this end, the Department of Defense established a Trauma Registry (previously known as the Joint Theater Trauma Registry) to collect data and statistics regarding wounded military personnel and the care they receive. The Committee on Tactical Combat Casualty Care uses these data and additional resources as a basis for research that can then be implemented into clinical practice guidelines. These clinical practice guidelines are deployed to medical personnel in the field for use in the treatment and stabilization of wounded military personnel. Implementing best practices for the care of those wounded in battle has become an agile process that adapts to changing circumstances on the front lines.

The result of this ongoing process has been lives saved. Mortality rates for those wounded in battle have decreased by over half when compared to previous conflicts. The survival rate for those wounded in combat has increased to over 90%.[13,14] In patients where massive transfusion is necessary, typically the most gravely wounded, the implementation of damage control resuscitation (discussed later in this chapter) has reduced mortality from 40% down to 20%.[15]

The benefit of these advancements in trauma care is not limited to military healthcare. The civilian world is rapidly adopting these changes for use in hospitals far away from the front lines. The use of damage control resuscitation in large trauma centers is becoming a standard of care. Tourniquet use, once considered a last resort, is rapidly becoming the primary intervention for severe bleeding in the field and during stabilization in the emergency department. The lessons learned from treating wounded military personnel over the past twenty years will have a significant impact on the quality and delivery of civilian trauma care for decades to come.

Philosophy of PHTLS

PHTLS provides an understanding of anatomy and physiology, zthe pathophysiology of trauma, the assessment and care of the trauma patient using the XABCDE approach, and the skills needed to provide that care—no more and no less. Patients who are bleeding or breathing inadequately have a limited amount of time before their condition results in severe disability or becomes fatal (**Box 1-1**). Prehospital care providers must possess and apply critical thinking skills to make and carry out decisions that will enhance the survival of the trauma patient. PHTLS does not train prehospital care providers to memorize a "one-size-fits-all" approach. Rather, PHTLS teaches an understanding of trauma care and critical thinking. Each prehospital care

---

> **Box 1-1** XABCDE
>
> ABCDE is a traditional mnemonic used to remember the steps in the primary survey (Airway, Breathing, Circulation, Disability, Expose/Environment). This textbook introduces a new approach to the primary survey that recognizes the immediate and potentially irreversible threat posed by exsanguinating extremity or junctional hemorrhage. The "X" placed before the traditional "ABCDE" describes the need to address exsanguinating hemorrhage immediately after establishing scene safety and before addressing airway. Severe exsanguinating hemorrhage, particularly arterial bleeding, has the potential to lead to complete loss of total or near total blood volume in a relatively short period of time. Depending on the pace of the bleeding, that time can be just a few minutes. Furthermore, in the prehospital environment, absent the ability to respond with blood transfusion, it will be impossible to correct the problem after the blood volume has been lost because crystalloid resuscitation will not restore the capacity to transport oxygen to the cells. Thus even prior to airway stabilization, controlling severe bleeding from a limb or other compressible external site takes precedence. Managing airway threats, ensuring adequate breathing, assessing circulatory status, disability, and exposing the body to allow a thorough evaluation follow.

---

provider–patient contact involves a unique set of circumstances. If the prehospital care provider understands the basis of medical care and the specific needs of the individual patient given the circumstances at hand, then precise patient care decisions can be made that ensure the greatest chance of survival for that patient.

The overarching tenets of PHTLS are that prehospital care providers must have a good foundation of knowledge, must be critical thinkers, and must have appropriate technical skills to deliver excellent patient care, even in less-than-optimal circumstances. PHTLS neither proscribes nor prescribes specific actions for the prehospital care provider; instead, it supplies the appropriate knowledge and skills to enable the prehospital care provider to use critical thinking to arrive at the best care for each patient.

The opportunity for a prehospital care provider to help a patient can be profound. Because trauma impacts people who are often in the most productive years of their lives, the societal impact of survival of a trauma patient who receives excellent trauma care, in both the prehospital and the hospital setting, is so compelling. The prehospital care provider can lengthen the life span and productive years of the trauma patient and benefit society by virtue of the care provided. By delivering effective care to trauma victims, prehospital care providers can have a significant positive impact on society.

Epidemiology and Financial Burden

Worldwide, injury has a profound effect on society. Each day some 14,000 people will die as a result of injury. Unintentional injury is the leading cause of death in people between 1 and 45 years of age.[16] Over 5 million people die annually as a result of injury, accounting for 9% of deaths.[16] The combined total of deaths caused by diseases such as tuberculosis, malaria, and HIV/AIDS amounts to only around half the number of deaths resulting from injury.[1] While it is not difficult to see that trauma is a problem of epidemic proportions, understanding the cause of traumatic injury remains complicated, despite the abundance of data available on the subject.

In the United States, the Centers for Disease Control and Prevention (CDC) reports fatalities as the result of trauma under the umbrella term "unintentional injury."[17] When attempting to research trauma as a cause of death, these data are confounded by the fact that not all unintentional injury is traumatic. Unintentional injury encompasses a number of proximate causes, including drowning, poisoning, firearms, falls, and motor vehicle crashes. Consider the fact that poisoning is a cited cause of unintentional injury, and deaths as a result of opioid overdose are frequently listed in this category.[17] This example demonstrates how careful analysis of the available data is necessary to fully understand the problem at hand.

To provide important context, it is helpful to evaluate the trends regarding some of the most common unintentional injury causes of death across the spectrum of age. When this approach is taken, areas of emphasis for prevention, training, and public education efforts can be identified. A few of these areas can be seen in **Figure 1-3** and **Figure 1-4**, which clearly illustrate that drowning and motor vehicle crashes are significant causes of death early in life. As age increases, the number of deaths secondary to drowning begins to fall, and motor vehicle crashes surge to become the leading cause of death until around 25 years of age, when poisoning emerges as the leading cause of unintentional injury leading to death.[18] Both poisoning and motor vehicle crashes remain the leading causes of death due to unintentional injury until approximately 65 to 70 years of age, when the leading cause becomes falls.[18]

When the data are broken down in this manner, it becomes clear that across the spectrum of age, motor vehicle crashes persist as a major cause of death, while the most likely cause of death early in life is drowning. While not traumatic, poisoning is growing as a leading cause of death secondary to unintentional injury, a trend that is likely to continue into the future if the opioid epidemic persists.

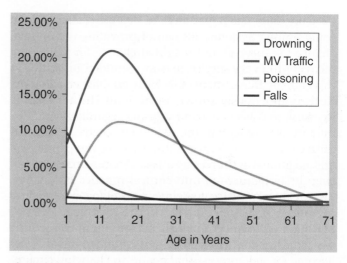

Figure 1-3 Percentage of all deaths by selected cause—ages 1 to 85 years.

Data from the National Center for Injury Prevention and Control: WISQARS. Leading Causes of Death Reports 1981-2015. Centers for Disease Control and Prevention. https://webappa.cdc.gov/sasweb/ncipc/leadcause.html.

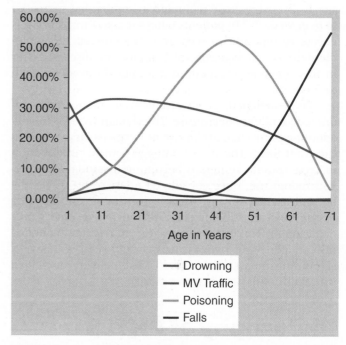

Figure 1-4 Percentage of unintentional injury deaths by selected cause—ages 1 to 85 years.

Data from the National Center for Injury Prevention and Control: WISQARS. Leading Causes of Death Reports 1981-2015. Centers for Disease Control and Prevention. https://webappa.cdc.gov/sasweb/ncipc/leadcause.html.

These statistics demonstrate alarming trends with regard to the causes of unintentional injury, and while the trends may not be new, the regions in the world that are most affected by these trends are changing. Efforts to reduce fatalities caused by motor vehicle crashes have led to an overall decrease from previous decades in developed countries, yet the overall number of deaths globally due to motor vehicle crashes is expected to increase by the year 2030.[16] This trend is largely a result of the rapidly rising use of motorized vehicles in developing countries, outpacing the ability of local infrastructure and resources (including EMS) to respond to the demands presented by the increased traffic. A similar pattern is expected in the coming decades with regard to deaths resulting from fall-related injuries. In 2015, falls caused a total of 34,488 deaths in the United States, of which 80% occurred in people 65 years of age and older.[19] In response to the increasing mortality from falls each year, developed countries have initiated fall risk screening, education, and prevention programs. Meanwhile, the average life span in developing regions of the world continues to rise, in part due to improved access to basic health care interventions such as immunizations and HIV/AIDS prevention and treatment.[20] The increasing number of older patients presents a different type of burden on the health care infrastructures of developing countries, where there has not previously been a pressing need to treat a geriatric population.

Analyzing the deaths that result from falls and motor vehicle crashes illuminates some of the complexities of trying to address unintentional injury and trauma on a global scale. Among the leading causes of death, falls and motor vehicle crashes are the only traumatic causes of death that are predicted to increase worldwide by the year 2030.[16]

While the loss of life due to trauma is staggering, so too is the financial burden incurred while caring for those victims who survive. Billions of dollars are spent on the management of trauma patients, not including the dollars lost in wages, insurance administration costs, property damage, and employer costs. The National Safety Council estimated that the economic impact in 2015 from both fatal and nonfatal trauma was approximately $886.4 billion in the United States.[21] Lost productivity and wages due to trauma totaled approximately $458 billion annually. The prehospital care provider has an opportunity to reduce the societal costs of trauma. For example, proper protection of the fractured cervical spine by a prehospital care provider may make the difference between lifelong quadriplegia and a productive, healthy life of unrestricted activity.

The following data come from the World Health Organization (WHO):

- *Road traffic injuries are a huge public health problem.* Road traffic crashes kill 1.25 million people per year worldwide, with an average of 3,400 people every day. They are the number one cause of death among persons 15 to 29 years of age. Road traffic crashes rank as the ninth leading cause of death overall and the number one cause of trauma deaths, accounting for nearly 4% of all deaths globally. WHO predicts that without improvements in prevention, road traffic accidents will rise to become the seventh leading cause of death worldwide by the year 2030.[22]
- *The majority of road traffic injuries affect people in low-income and middle-income countries, with three out of four road deaths occurring among men.* While individuals in low- and

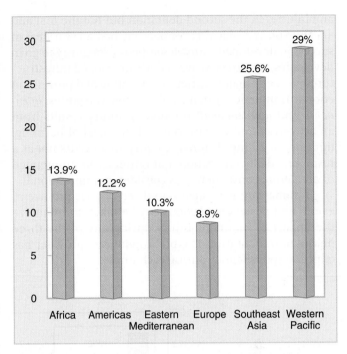

Figure 1-5 Worldwide distribution of road traffic deaths.
Data from World Health Organization (WHO) Road Traffic Injuries Fact Sheet No. 358.

middle-income countries own only 50% of the world's vehicles, these countries are responsible for 90% of all road traffic deaths (**Figure 1-5**).[22]

- *Worldwide, over 5 million people die annually from injury, both unintentional and intentional.* While road traffic incidents are the most common cause of death (24%), suicide (16%) and falls (14%) are the number two and three causes, respectively.[16]

As these statistics clearly show, trauma is a worldwide problem. Although the specific events that lead to injuries and deaths differ from country to country, the consequences do not. The impact of preventable injuries is global.

We who work in the trauma community have an obligation to our patients to prevent injuries, not just to treat them after the injuries occur. An often-told story about EMS best illustrates this point. On a long, winding mountain road, there was a curve where cars would often slide off the road and plummet 100 feet (30.5 meters) to the ground below. The community decided to station an ambulance at the bottom of the cliff to care for the patients involved in these crashes. The better alternative would have been to place guardrails along the curve to prevent the incident from occurring in the first place.

The Phases of Trauma Care

Trauma is no accident, even though it is often referred to as such. An accident is often defined as either a chance event or an event caused by carelessness. Most trauma deaths and injuries fit the second definition but not the first and are thus preventable. Prevention has had a great deal of success in developed countries but has a long way to go in developing countries, where poorly developed infrastructures present a major barrier for education and prevention efforts. Traumatic incidents fall into two categories: *intentional* and *unintentional*. Intentional injury results from an act carried out on purpose with the goal of harming, injuring, or killing. Traumatic injury that occurs not as a result of a deliberate action, but rather as an unintended or accidental consequence, is considered unintentional.

Trauma care is divided into three phases: pre-event, event, and postevent. Actions can be taken to minimize the impact of traumatic injury during any of the three phases of trauma care. The prehospital care provider has critical responsibilities during each phase.

Pre-event Phase

The **pre-event phase** involves the circumstances leading up to an injury. Efforts in this phase are primarily focused on injury prevention. To achieve maximum effect, strategies to address traumatic death and injury in the pre-event phase should focus on the most significant contributors to mortality and morbidity. According to the most recent data available, unintentional injury is the fourth overall leading cause of death among all ages annually in the United States. Almost half of the deaths caused by injury in the United States are a result of either a motor vehicle crash, a fall, or a firearm. (**Figure 1-6**).[17]

Over 95% of Americans currently own a mobile phone of some type, with the number of people who own a smartphone more than doubling since 2011.[23] With an

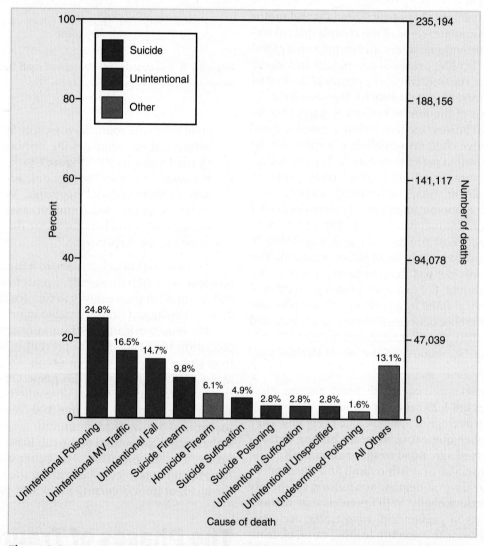

Figure 1-6 Motor vehicle trauma, falls, and firearms account for almost half of the deaths that result from injury.

Data from the National Center for Injury Prevention and Control: WISQARS. Leading Causes of Death Reports 2016. Centers for Disease Control and Prevention. https://webappa.cdc.gov/sasweb/ncipc/leadcause.html.

estimated 660,000 drivers using a cell phone while operating their vehicle during any given day, it is not surprising that distracted driving led to nearly 3,500 deaths in the United States in 2015.[24] The number of deaths pales in comparison to the nearly 400,000 injuries that were caused as a result of distracted driving, including texting while driving, that year.[24] Prevention efforts involving public awareness campaigns such as "It Can Wait" have been developed in recent years with the goal of curbing this rising trend.[25] In some states, these programs have been combined with laws targeting the use of cell phones and mobile devices while operating a motor vehicle. Currently, 15 states and the District of Columbia have primary enforcement laws in place banning the use of handheld phones by all individuals while driving, although hands-free use is acceptable in groups of drivers in those states.[26] The use of cell phones by novice drivers (drivers younger than 18 years) has been banned entirely in 38 states. This type of graded legal enforcement by age and experience is aimed specifically at preventing traffic accidents in these vulnerable groups.[26]

Another preventable cause of motor vehicle crashes is driving while intoxicated with alcohol.[27] There has been significant effort aimed at targeting this issue during the pre-event phase. As a result of increased public awareness, education, and pressure to change state laws regarding the minimum blood alcohol content at which individuals are considered legally intoxicated, the number of drunk drivers involved in fatal crashes has been consistently decreasing since 1989.

Promoting programs that raise awareness among populations at risk for falling is also an area of significant effort. The CDC has developed the STEADI (Stopping Elderly Accidents, Deaths, and Injuries) initiative for health care providers to identify individuals at risk for falling, recognize any risk factors that are modifiable for those individuals, and offer effective methods to prevent falls before they occur. Prehospital care providers are in a unique position to play a role in fall prevention. With one of the leading risk factors for a fall resulting in injury or death among older adults being a previous fall incident,[28] it is entirely possible that local EMS personnel are encountering at-risk individuals during calls for lift assistance or minor injury. These calls present an important opportunity for local public safety departments to collaborate with other health care providers and organizations to develop an evidence-based fall prevention program in the community.[29]

Increasing water safety education, especially in underserved and lower socioeconomic populations, must remain a priority.[30] It is estimated that three children die each day as a result of drowning.[31] Local code enforcement guidelines that require fencing around swimming pools have been implemented in cities across the United States. Additionally, programs that offer guidance to parents and swimmers

---

Box 1-2 Preparation

Preparation includes proper and complete education with updated information to provide the most current medical care. Just as you must update your home computer or handheld device with the latest software, you must update your knowledge with current medical practices and insights. In addition, you must review the equipment on the response unit at the beginning of every shift and review with your partner the individual responsibilities and expectations of who will carry out what duties. It is just as important to review the conduct of the care when you arrive on the scene as it is to decide who will drive and who will be in the back with the patient.

While unintentional injury may never be eliminated completely, it is possible that through programs such as those mentioned, the magnitude of unintentional injury as a significant cause of death may be minimized. EMS personnel will continue to play a crucial role in prevention efforts during the pivotal pre-event phase.

---

regarding safe practices around the water are widely available.[32-35] Given the level of trust and the unique position in local communities that is held by public safety agencies, their participation in these outreach programs is crucial to addressing the problem of drowning.

Another critical component of the pre-event phase is preparation by prehospital care providers for the events that are not prevented by public safety awareness programs (**Box 1-2**).

Event Phase

The **event phase** is the moment of the actual trauma. Actions taken during the event phase are aimed at minimizing injury as the result of the trauma. The use of safety equipment has significant influence on the severity of injury caused by the traumatic event. Motor vehicle safety restraint systems, airbags, and motorcycle helmets commonly play a role in injury reduction and avoidance during the event phase.

The history surrounding motorcycle helmet laws offers a good illustration of the impact that laws mandating the use of certain safety equipment can have on the incidence and severity of traumatic injury. In 1966, the U.S. Congress gave the DOT the authority to penalize states that failed to pass legislation mandating the use of motorcycle helmets.[36] Over the next 10 years, 47 states enacted universal helmet laws. Congress rescinded this authority from the DOT in 1975, and, incrementally, states began repealing their universal helmet laws. While motorcycle deaths had been steadily declining since the early 1980s, by 1998, just over two decades after the threat of penalty for states with no motorcycle helmet law had been lifted, those rates began to rise. As of October 2017, only 19 states and the District of Columbia have laws in place requiring all riders to wear helmets, 28 states have partial laws in place requiring some riders (generally persons 17 years of age and younger) to wear helmets, and 3 states (Illinois, Iowa, and New Hampshire) have no laws regulating helmet use for any riders, regardless of age or license status.[37] This is the lowest number of states having helmet laws since Congress originally granted authority to the DOT to influence states to pass helmet law legislation. The number of deaths related to motorcycle accidents has more than doubled from where it was in 1997 (2,056 deaths in 1997 vs. 4,693 deaths in 2015).[38] The complex history regarding helmet law legislation over the past 50 years is just one example of how legal statute and enforcement regarding the use of certain safety equipment can dramatically alter patient outcomes during the event phase of trauma care.

Another way to minimize the potential for traumatic injury is through the use of child safety seats. Many trauma centers, law enforcement organizations, and EMS and fire systems conduct programs to educate parents in the correct installation and use of child safety seats. When correctly installed and properly used, child safety seats offer infants and children the best protection during the event phase of trauma care.

Certain steps taken by EMS personnel play a large role in the outcome of the event phase. "Do no further harm" is the admonition for good patient care. Whether driving a personal vehicle or an emergency vehicle, prehospital care providers need to protect themselves and teach by example. You are responsible for yourself, your partner, and the patients under your care while in your ambulance vehicle; therefore, prevent injury by safe and attentive driving. The same level of attention you give to your patient care must be given to your driving. Always use the personal protective devices available, such as vehicle restraints, in the driving compartment and in the passenger or patient care compartment.

Postevent Phase

The **postevent phase** deals with the outcome of the traumatic event. Obviously, the worst possible outcome of a traumatic event is death of the patient. Trauma surgeon Donald Trunkey, MD, has described a trimodal distribution of trauma deaths.[39] The *first phase* of deaths occurs within the first few minutes and up to an hour after an incident. Many of these deaths occur immediately or within seconds

after the traumatic injury. Some, however, occur due to massive hemorrhage during the short period of time that elapses while waiting for medical care to arrive. The best way to combat these deaths is through injury prevention strategies and public education programs. Recent public awareness campaigns include education on the use of tourniquets by lay responders and the increased presence of hemorrhage control kits available in public areas and in police cruisers.[40] The *second phase* of deaths occurs within the first few hours of an incident. These deaths can often be prevented by good prehospital care and hospital care. The *third phase* of deaths occurs several days to several weeks after the incident. These deaths are generally caused by multiple organ failure. Recent studies suggest that this phase is being eliminated by modern trauma and critical care.[41] Damage control resuscitation is an evolving trend in trauma care that addresses third-phase deaths by combining staged surgical intervention with intensive care unit (ICU) stabilization in patients with massive trauma.[42-44] The evidence indicates that patient outcomes are improved when the initial surgical intervention is brief and only addresses major sources of bleeding, allowing the patient to be transferred to the trauma ICU where the patient can be physiologically stabilized to an appropriate metabolic state.[45-47] Once this ICU stabilization is complete, additional surgical interventions can be performed in a staged fashion with intermittent ICU stabilization as needed by the patient. Early and aggressive management of shock in the prehospital setting also plays a major role in preventing some of these deaths (**Figure 1-7**).

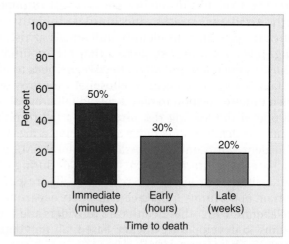

Figure 1-7 Immediate deaths can be prevented by injury-prevention public emergency response education. Early deaths can be prevented through timely, appropriate prehospital care to reduce mortality and morbidity. Late deaths can be prevented only through prompt transport to a hospital appropriately staffed for trauma care.

In regions of the world where access to combined ICU and trauma care is available, early intervention by EMS with aggressive control of hemorrhage along with damage control resuscitation in the hospital setting may improve outcomes in trauma patients.

R Adams Cowley, MD, founder of the Maryland Institute of Emergency Medical Services Systems (MIEMSS), one of the first trauma centers in the United States, defined what he called the Golden Hour.[48] Based on his research, Dr. Cowley believed that patients who received definitive care soon after an injury had a much higher survival rate than those whose care was delayed. One reason for this improvement in survival is prompt treatment of hemorrhage and preservation of the body's ability to produce energy to maintain organ function. For the prehospital care provider, this translates into maintaining oxygenation and perfusion and providing rapid transport to a facility that is prepared to continue the process of resuscitation using blood and plasma (damage control resuscitation) and to provide access to the immediate surgical intervention necessary to achieve prompt hemorrhage control.

Because this critical period of time is not literally 1 hour, the Golden Hour is often referred to as the "Golden Period." Some patients have less than an hour in which to receive care, whereas others have more time. In many urban prehospital systems in the United States, the average time between activation of EMS and arrival to the scene is 8 to 9 minutes, not including the time between injury and call to the public safety answering point. A typical transport time to the receiving facility is another 8 to 9 minutes. If the prehospital care providers spend only 10 minutes on the scene, over 30 minutes of time will have already passed by the time a patient arrives at the receiving facility. Every additional minute spent on the scene is additional time that the patient is bleeding, and valuable time is ticking away from the Golden Period.

Research data support the concept of rapid transport to definitive care.[49,50] One of these studies showed that critically injured patients had a significantly lower mortality rate (17.9% vs. 28.2%) when transported to the hospital by a private vehicle rather than an ambulance.[49] This unexpected finding was most likely the result of prehospital care providers spending too much time on the scene.

In the 1980s and 1990s, a trauma center documented that EMS scene times averaged 20 to 30 minutes for patients injured in motor vehicle crashes and for victims of penetrating trauma. This finding brings to light the questions that all prehospital care providers need to ask when caring for trauma victims: "Is what I am doing going to benefit the patient? Does that benefit outweigh the risk of delaying transport?"

One of the most important responsibilities of a prehospital care provider is to spend as little time on the scene as possible and instead expedite the field care and transport of the patient. In the first precious minutes after arrival at a scene, a prehospital care provider rapidly assesses the patient, performs lifesaving maneuvers, and prepares the patient for transport. In the 2000s, following the tenets of PHTLS, prehospital scene times have decreased by allowing all providers (fire, police, and EMS) to perform as a cohesive unit in a uniform style by having a standard methodology across emergency services. As a result, patient survival has increased. A second responsibility is transporting the patient to an appropriate facility. A factor that is extremely critical to a compromised patient's survival is the length of time that elapses between the incident and the provision of definitive care. For a cardiac arrest patient, definitive care is the return of spontaneous circulation that can occur in the field. For a patient whose airway is compromised, definitive care is the restoration of the airway and restoration of adequate ventilation.[50-54]

With the management of trauma patients, however, time from injury to arrival at the appropriate trauma center is critical to survival. Definitive care for trauma patients usually involves control of hemorrhage and restoration of adequate perfusion by replacement of fluids as near to whole blood as possible. Administration of reconstituted whole blood (packed red blood cells and plasma, in a ratio of 1:1) to replace lost blood has produced impressive results by the military in Iraq and Afghanistan and now in the civilian community. These fluids replace the lost oxygen-carrying capacity, the clotting components, and the oncotic pressure to prevent fluid loss from the vascular system. They are not currently available for use in the field and are an important reason for rapid transport to the hospital. En route to the hospital, balanced resuscitation (see the Shock: Pathophysiology of Life and Death chapter) has proven to be important. Hemostasis (hemorrhage control) cannot always be achieved in the field or in the emergency department (ED); often, it can be achieved only in the OR. Therefore, when determining an appropriate facility to which a patient should be transported, it is important that the prehospital care provider use the critical thinking process and consider the transport time to a given facility and the capabilities of that facility.

A trauma center that has a surgeon available either before or shortly after the arrival of the patient, a well-trained and trauma-experienced emergency medicine team, and an OR team immediately available can have a trauma patient with life-threatening hemorrhage in the OR within 10 to 15 minutes of the patient's arrival (and often faster), and this can make the difference between life and death (**Box 1-3**).

On the other hand, a hospital without in-house surgical capabilities must await the arrival of the surgeon

The American College of Surgeons (ACS) establishes the requirements for trauma centers in a document entitled *Resources for Optimal Care of the Injured Patient.* State and local jurisdictions utilize these requirements, and the ACS Committee on Trauma (COT) Verification Review Committee's reports from trauma site surveys designate trauma centers at varying levels. According to the ACS, there should be no difference in clinical requirements for level I and level II trauma centers. The primary difference between the two levels is that medical education, research, specialty services, and patient volume are higher at level I trauma centers. Level I trauma centers serve as a hub for organizing trauma care in a given region. Level III trauma centers generally have fewer resources and are typically located in suburban or rural areas. Their primary role is immediate treatment and stabilization, combined with rapid and efficient transport to the higher level of care provided at a level I or II trauma center. Level IV trauma centers have few resources other than a 24-hour staffed emergency room, and their major role is to serve as a guide for immediate basic care and stabilization with rapid transfer to a higher level trauma center.[55]

It is important to note that the ACS *does not* designate which institutions are considered trauma centers; they simply verify that hospitals meet the recommended criteria for a specific level of trauma service. The decision to designate a particular hospital as a trauma center, and what level trauma center that hospital will be designated as, lies with state and local government, usually after verification from the ACS that certain criteria have been met.

and the surgical team before transporting the patient from the ED to the OR. Additional time may then elapse before the hemorrhage can be controlled, resulting in an associated increase in mortality rate (**Figure 1-8**). There is a significant increase in survival if nontrauma centers are bypassed and all severely injured patients are taken to the trauma center.[56-64]

Experience, in addition to the initial training in surgery and trauma, is important. Studies have demonstrated that the more experienced surgeons in a busy trauma center have a better outcome than trauma surgeons with less experience.[64,65]

PHTLS—Past, Present, Future

Advanced Trauma Life Support

As happens so often in life, a personal experience brought about the changes in emergency care that resulted in the birth of the Advanced Trauma Life Support (ATLS) course, and eventually, the PHTLS program. ATLS started in 1978, 2 years after a private plane crash in a rural area of Nebraska. The ATLS course was born out of that mangled mass of metal, the injured, and the dead. An orthopaedic surgeon, his wife, and his four children were flying in their twin-engine airplane when it crashed. His wife was killed instantly. The children were critically injured. They waited for help to arrive, but it never did. After approximately 8 hours, the orthopaedic surgeon walked more than half a mile along a dirt road to a highway. After two trucks passed him by, he flagged down a car. Together, they drove to the accident site, loaded the injured children into the car, and drove to the closest hospital, a few miles south of the crash site.

When they arrived at the emergency room door of the local rural hospital, they found it was locked. The on-duty nurse called the two general practitioners in the small farming community who were on call. After examining the children, one of the doctors carried one of the injured children by the shoulders and the knees to the x-ray room. Later, he returned and announced that the x-rays showed no skull fracture. An injury to the child's cervical spine had not been considered. The doctor then began suturing a laceration the child had sustained. The orthopedic surgeon called his physician partner in Lincoln, Nebraska, and told him what had happened. His partner said that he would arrange to get the surviving family members to Lincoln as soon as possible.

The doctors and staff in this little rural hospital had little or no preparation for assessing and managing multiple patients with traumatic injuries. Unfortunately, there was a lack of training and experience on triage and on assessment and management of traumatic injuries. In the years that followed, the Nebraska orthopaedic surgeon and his colleagues recognized that something needed to be done about the general lack of a trauma care delivery system to treat acutely injured patients in a rural setting. They decided that rural physicians needed to be trained in a systematic manner on treating trauma patients. They chose to use a format similar to Advanced Cardiovascular Life Support (ACLS) and call it Advanced Trauma Life Support (ATLS).

A syllabus was created and organized into a logical approach to manage trauma. The "treat as you go" methodology was developed as well as the ABCs of trauma (airway, breathing, and circulation) to prioritize the order

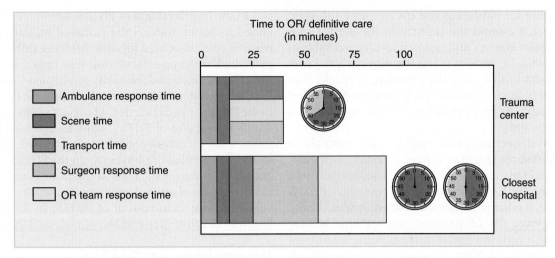

Figure 1-8 In locations in which trauma centers are available, bypassing hospitals not committed to the care of trauma patients can significantly improve patient care. In severely injured trauma patients, definitive patient care generally occurs in the OR. An extra 10 to 20 minutes spent en route to a hospital with an in-house surgeon and in-house OR staff will significantly reduce the time to definitive care in the OR. (Blue, EMS response time. Purple, on-scene time. Red, EMS transport time. Orange, surgical response time from out of hospital. Yellow, OR team response time from out of hospital.)

© National Association of Emergency Medical Technicians (NAEMT).

of assessment and treatment. In 1978, the ATLS prototype was field tested in Auburn, Nebraska, with the help of many surgeons. Next, the course was presented to the University of Nebraska and eventually to the American College of Surgeons Committee on Trauma.

Since that first ATLS course in Auburn, Nebraska, over three decades have passed and ATLS keeps spreading and growing. What was originally intended as a course for rural Nebraska has become a course for the whole world and for all types of trauma settings. It is this course that is the basis of PHTLS.

PHTLS

As Dr. Richard H. Carmona, former U.S. Surgeon General, stated in his foreword to the sixth edition of PHTLS:

> It has been said that we stand on the shoulders of giants in many apparent successes, and PHTLS is no different. With great vision and passion, as well as challenges, a small group of leaders persevered and developed PHTLS over a quarter of a century ago.

In 1958, Dr. Farrington convinced the Chicago Fire Department that fire fighters should be trained to manage emergency patients. Working with Dr. Sam Banks, Dr. Farrington started the Trauma Training Program in Chicago. Millions have been trained following the guidelines developed in this landmark program. Dr. Farrington continued to work at every level of EMS, from the field, to education, to legislation, to help expand and improve EMS as a profession. The principles of trauma care set

forth by Dr. Farrington's work form an important part of the nucleus of PHTLS.

The first chairman of the ATLS ad hoc committee for the American College of Surgeons and Chairman of the Prehospital Care Subcommittee on Trauma for the American College of Surgeons, Dr. Norman E. McSwain, Jr., FACS, knew that ATLS would have a profound effect on the outcomes of trauma patients. Moreover, he had a strong sense that an even greater effect could come from bringing this type of critical training to prehospital care providers.

Dr. McSwain, a founding member of the board of directors of NAEMT, gained the support of the association's president, Gary LaBeau, and began to lay plans for a prehospital version of ATLS.[66] President LaBeau directed Dr. McSwain and Robert Nelson, NREMT-P, to determine the feasibility of an ATLS-type program for prehospital care providers.

As a professor of surgery at Tulane University School of Medicine in New Orleans, Louisiana, Dr. McSwain gained the university's support in putting together the draft curriculum of what was to become PHTLS. With this draft in place, a PHTLS committee was established in 1983. This committee continued to refine the curriculum, and later that same year, pilot courses were conducted in Lafayette and New Orleans, Louisiana; the Marian Health Center in Sioux City, Iowa; the Yale University School of Medicine in New Haven, Connecticut; and the Norwalk Hospital in Norwalk, Connecticut.

Richard W. Vomacka (1946 to 2001) was a part of the task force that developed the initial PHTLS course.

PHTLS became his passion as the course came together, and he traveled around the country in the early 1980s conducting pilot courses and regional faculty workshops. He worked with Dr. McSwain and the other original task force members to fine-tune the program. Vomacka was instrumental in forging a relationship between PHTLS and the U.S. military. He also worked on the first international PHTLS course sites.

National dissemination of PHTLS began with three intensive workshops taught in Denver, Colorado; Bethesda, Maryland; and Orlando, Florida, between September 1984 and February 1985. The graduates of these early PHTLS courses formed what would be the "barnstormers." These individuals were PHTLS national and regional faculty members who traveled the country training additional faculty members, spreading the word on the core PHTLS principles. Alex Butman, NREMT-P, along with Vomacka worked diligently, frequently using money out of their own pockets, to bring the first two editions of the PHTLS program to fruition.

Throughout the growth process, medical oversight has been provided through the American College of Surgeons Committee on Trauma. For over 30 years, the partnership between the American College of Surgeons and NAEMT has ensured that PHTLS course participants receive the opportunity to help give trauma patients their best chance at survival.

Between 1994 and 2001, Dr. Scott B. Frame, FACS, FCCM (1952 to 2001), was the associate medical director for the PHTLS program. His major emphasis was in the development of the audiovisuals for PHTLS and its promulgation internationally. At the time of his death, he had assumed responsibility for the fifth edition of the PHTLS course. This included the revision of not only the textbook but also of the instructor's manual and all of the associated teaching materials. He was appointed as medical director of the PHTLS course when the fifth edition was published. The PHTLS program grew tremendously under Dr. Frame's leadership, and its continuation into the future owes much to his efforts and the part of his life that he lent to PHTLS and to his patients.

It is on the shoulders of these individuals and other individuals too numerous to mention, that PHTLS stands and continues to grow.

PHTLS in the Military

Beginning in 1988, the U.S. military aggressively set out to train its combat medics in PHTLS. Coordinated by the Defense Medical Readiness Training Institute (DMRTI) at Fort Sam Houston in Texas, PHTLS was taught to combat medics in the United States and stationed overseas. In 2001, the Army's 91WB program standardized the training of over 58,000 combat medics to include PHTLS.

In the fourth edition of PHTLS, a military chapter was added to better address the needs of military providers treating combat-related injuries. After the fifth edition was published, a strong relationship was forged between the PHTLS committee and the newly established Committee on Tactical Combat Casualty Care of the Defense Health Board in the Department of Defense. As a result of this relationship, a military version of PHTLS, with an extensively revised military chapter, was published as a revised fifth edition in 2005. This collaboration between the PHTLS committee and the Committee on Tactical Combat Casualty Care led to the creation of multiple military chapters for the military version of the sixth edition of PHTLS. In 2010, NAEMT began to offer the Department of Defense's TCCC course.

International PHTLS

The sound principles of prehospital trauma management emphasized in the PHTLS course have led prehospital care providers and physicians outside the United States to request the importation of the program to their various countries. Beginning in the early 1990s, PHTLS was launched internationally, first in the United Kingdom and Mexico, and then in other countries.

In 2016, over 12,800 international prehospital providers received PHTLS education. As of the publication of this edition, PHTLS has been taught in more than 60 countries across the globe.

Translations

Our growing international family has spawned translations of the PHTLS text, which is currently available in languages including Arabic, Dutch, English, French, German, Greek, Italian, Korean, Norwegian, Portuguese, Simplified Chinese, Spanish, and Turkish.

Vision for the Future

The PHTLS program will continue its mission to provide the highest quality prehospital trauma education to all who need and desire this opportunity. PHTLS is always driven by the latest evidence in prehospital trauma, and we are committed to seeking out this evidence from all reputable sources.

As prehospital trauma care evolves and improves, so too must the PHTLS program. We are dedicated to ongoing evaluation of the program to identify and implement improvements wherever needed. We will pursue new methods and technology for delivering PHTLS to enhance the clinical and service quality of the program.

We will strive to ensure that our program meets the needs of prehospital patients in all countries. Since 2010, PHTLS faculty in Europe have met to discuss methods for measuring program quality and to identify areas for improvement. Since 2012, the World Trauma Symposium has been held to present the latest evidence, trends, and controversies in prehospital trauma care. In 2017, NAEMT participated in the first EMSWORLD Américas congress, where several NAEMT courses were offered and faculty from throughout Latin America discussed trends in EMS education. These programs bring the work of practitioners and researchers from around the globe together to examine the continuing evolution of trauma care. Their contributions, as well as the contributions of the PHTLS family of instructors, medical directors, coordinators, authors, and reviewers worldwide, all volunteering countless hours of their lives, will ensure that the PHTLS program continues to thrive and grow.

PHTLS will maintain its unwavering commitment to our patients by ensuring that PHTLS providers are able to do the following:

- Assess their patients rapidly and accurately.
- Identify shock and hypoxemia.
- Initiate the right interventions at the right time.
- Transport their patients to the right place for the right care.

SUMMARY

- Prehospital care as we know it today can be traced back to the late 1700s, when Baron Dominique Jean Larrey, Napoleon's chief military physician, recognized the need for prompt prehospital care. Progress in prehospital care was relatively slow until about 1950, when J. D. "Deke" Farrington, MD, stimulated the development of improved prehospital care. Ever since, improving prehospital trauma care has been a steady and ongoing effort.
- The overarching tenets of Prehospital Trauma Life Support (PHTLS) are that prehospital care providers must have a good foundation of knowledge, must be critical thinkers, and must have appropriate technical skills to deliver excellent patient care, even in less-than-optimal circumstances.
- Worldwide, injury is a leading cause of death and disability, impacting not only the people directly involved, but, due to its financial ramifications, society as a whole.
- Trauma care is divided into three phases: pre-event, event, and postevent. Actions can be taken to minimize the impact of traumatic injury during any of the three phases of trauma care. The prehospital care provider has critical responsibilities during each phase.
- The concept of a Golden Period guides prehospital care. Research has shown that prompt transport to definitive care is a key to improving patient outcomes.
- The PHTLS course is modeled after the Advanced Trauma Life Support (ATLS) course created in 1978, which emphasized rapid patient transport and treatment en route. As PHTLS has grown, medical oversight has been provided through the American College of Surgeons Committee on Trauma. For over 30 years, the partnership between the American College of Surgeons and the National Association of Emergency Medical Technicians has ensured that PHTLS course participants receive the opportunity to help give trauma patients their best chance at survival.

References

1. McSwain NE. Prehospital care from Napoleon to Mars: the surgeon's role. *J Am Coll Surg.* 2005;200(44):487-504.
2. Larrey DJ. *Mémoires de Chirurgie Militaire, et Campagnes* [*Memoirs of Military Surgery and Campaigns of the French Armies*]. Paris, France: J. Smith and F. Buisson; 1812-1817. English translation with notes by R. W. Hall of volumes 1-3 in 2 volumes, Baltimore, MD, 1814. English translation of volume 4 by J. C. Mercer, Philadelphia, PA, 1832.
3. Rockwood CA, Mann CM, Farrington JD, et al. History of emergency medical services in the United States. *J Trauma.* 1976;16(4):299-308.
4. Farrington JD. Death in a ditch. *Bull Am Coll Surg.* 1967;52(3):121-132.
5. Federal Specifications for Ambulance, KKK-A-1822D. United States General Services Administration, Specifications Section, November 1994.
6. Kennedy R. *Early Care of the Sick and Injured Patient.* Chicago, IL: American College of Surgeons; 1964.
7. Curry G. *Immediate Care and Transport of the Injured.* Springfield, IL: Charles C. Thomas Publisher; 1965.
8. Committee on Trauma and Committee on Shock, Division of Medical Sciences. *Accidental Death and Disability: The*

Neglected Disease of Modern Society. Washington, DC: National Academy of Sciences/National Research Council; 1966.

9. Holcomb JB, Jenkins D, Rhee P, et al. Damage control resuscitation: directly addressing the early coagulopathy of trauma. *J Trauma*. 2007;62(2):307-310.

10. Holcomb JB, Tilley BC, Baraniuk S, et al. Transfusion of plasma, platelets, and red blood cells in a 1:1:1 vs a 1:1:2 ratio and mortality in patients with severe trauma: the PROPPR randomized clinical trial. *JAMA*. 2015;313(5):471-482.

11. Borgman MA, Spinella PC, Perkins JG, et al. The ratio of blood products transfused affects mortality in patients receiving massive transfusions at a combat support hospital. *J Trauma*. 2007;63(4):805-813.

12. Holcomb JB, Wade CE, Michalek JE, et al. Increased plasma and platelet to red blood cell ratios improves outcome in 466 massively transfused civilian trauma patients. *Ann Surg*. 2008;248(3):447-458.

13. Eastridge BJ, Jenkins D, Flaherty S, et al. Trauma system development in a theater of war: experiences from Operation Iraqi Freedom and Operation Enduring Freedom. *J Trauma*. 2006;61(6):1366-1372.

14. Ling GS, Rhee P, Ecklund JM. Surgical innovations arising from the Iraq and Afghanistan wars. *Annu Rev Med*. 2010;61:457-468.

15. Borden Institute. *Emergency War Surgery 2014*. 4th ed. Fort Sam Houston, TX: Office of the Surgeon General; 2014.

16. World Health Organization. Injuries and violence: the facts, 2014. http://apps.who.int/iris/bitstream/10665 /149798/1/9789241508018_eng.pdf. Published 2014. Accessed November 1, 2017.

17. Centers for Disease Control and Prevention. Key injury and violence data. https://www.cdc.gov/injury/wisqars/overview /key_data.html. Updated September 19, 2016. Accessed November 1, 2017.

18. Centers for Disease Control and Prevention, National Center for Injury Prevention and Control. Leading causes of death reports, 1981-2015. WISQARS. https://webappa.cdc.gov /sasweb/ncipc/leadcause.html. Accessed October 24, 2017.

19. Centers for Disease Control and Prevention, National Center for Injury Prevention and Control. WISQARS. Fatal injury reports: national, regional, and state, 1981–2015. https:// webappa.cdc.gov/sasweb/ncipc/mortrate.html. Accessed October 24, 2017.

20. World Health Organization. Global Health Observatory (GHO) data: life expectancy. http://www.who.int/gho /mortality_burden_disease/life_tables/situation_trends _text/en/. Accessed October 24, 2017.

21. National Safety Council. *Injury Facts*. 2017 ed. Itasca, IL: National Safety Council; 2017.

22. World Health Organization. World traffic injuries: the facts. http://www.who.int/violence_injury_prevention /road_safety_status/2015/magnitude_A4_web.pdf?ua=1. Accessed October 24, 2017.

23. Pew Research Center. Mobile fact sheet. http://www.pew internet.org/fact-sheet/mobile/. Accessed October 24, 2017.

24. U.S. Department of Transportation, National Highway Traffic Safety Administration. Distracted driving. https:// www.nhtsa.gov/risky-driving/distracted-driving. Accessed October 24, 2017.

25. It Can Wait. Distracted driving is never OK. https://www .itcanwait.com. Accessed October 24, 2017.

26. Governors Highway Safety Association. Distracted driving. http://www.ghsa.org/state-laws/issues/Distracted-Driving. Accessed October 24, 2017.

27. Mothers Against Drunk Driving. http://www.madd.org/. Accessed October 24, 2017.

28. Centers for Disease Control and Prevention, National Center for Injury Prevention and Control. Fact sheet: risk factors for falls. https://www.cdc.gov/steadi/pdf/risk_factors_for_falls -a.pdf. Published 2017. Accessed October 24, 2017.

29. Centers for Disease Control and Prevention, National Center for Injury Prevention and Control. Preventing falls: a guide to implementing effective community-based fall prevention programs. https://www.cdc.gov/homeandrecreationalsafety /pdf/falls/fallpreventionguide-2015-a.pdf. Published 2015. Accessed October 24, 2017.

30. American Red Cross. Red Cross launches anti-drowning campaign. http://www.redcross.org/news/article/co/denver /Red-Cross-Launches-Anti-Drowning-Campaign. Published May 23, 2014. Accessed October 24, 2017.

31. Centers for Disease Control and Prevention, National Center for Injury Prevention and Control, Division of Unintentional Injury Prevention. Protect the ones you love: child injuries are preventable; drowning prevention. https://www.cdc .gov/safechild/drowning/index.html. Updated April 30, 2016. Accessed October 24, 2017.

32. Ramos W, Beale A, Chambers P, Dalke S, Fielding R. Primary and secondary drowning interventions: The American Red Cross Circle of Drowning Prevention and Chain of Drowning Survival. *Int J Aquatic Res Educ*. 2015;9(1):89-101.

33. American Red Cross. Water safety. http://www.redcross .org/get-help/how-to-prepare-for-emergencies/types-of -emergencies/water-safety. Accessed October 24, 2017.

34. Association of Aquatic Professionals. Drowning prevention education. https://aquaticpros.org/drowning-prevention -education. Accessed October 24, 2017.

35. YMCA. Safety around water. http://www.ymca.net/water safety. Accessed October 24, 2017.

36. Goodwin A, Kirley B, Sandt L, et al., eds. *Countermeasures That Work: A Highway Safety Countermeasure Guide for State Highway Safety Offices*. 7th ed. Washington, DC: National Highway Traffic Safety Administration; 2013:5-7.

37. Insurance Institute of Highway Safety. Motorcycles: motorcycle helmet use. http://www.iihs.org/iihs/topics/laws /helmetuse/helmethistory?topicName=Motorcycles#table Data. Published 2017. Accessed November 1, 2017.

38. Insurance Institute of Highway Safety. Motorcycles: motorcycles and ATVs. http://www.iihs.org/iihs/topics/t/motor cycles/fatalityfacts/motorcycles. Published 2016. Accessed November 1, 2017.

39. Trunkey DD. Trauma. *Sci Am*. 1983;249(2):28-35.

40. U.S. Department of Homeland Security. Stop the bleed. https://www.dhs.gov/stopthebleed. Published June 16, 2017. Accessed November 1, 2017.

41. Cuschieri J, Johnson JL, Sperry J, et al. Benchmarking outcomes in the critically injured trauma patient and the effect of implementing standard operating procedures. *Ann Surg*. 2012;255(5):993-999.

42. Rotondo MF, Zonies DH. The damage control sequence and underlying logic. *Surg Clin North Am*. 1997;77(4):761-777.

43. Sugrue M, D'Amours SK, Joshipura M. Damage control surgery and the abdomen. *Injury*. 2004;35(7):642-648.

44. Beldowicz BC. The evolution of damage control in concept and practice. *Clin Colon Rectal Surg*. 2018;31(1):30-35.

45. Rotondo MF, Schwab CW, McGonigal MD, et al. "Damage control": an approach for improved survival in exsanguinating penetrating abdominal injury. *J Trauma*. 1993;35(3): 375-382.

46. Schreiber MA. Damage control surgery. *Crit Care Clin*. 2004; 20(1):101-118.

47. Parr MJ, Alabdi T. Damage control surgery and intensive care. *Injury*. 2004;35(7):713-722.

48. R Adams Cowley Shock Trauma Center: tribute to R Adams Cowley, MD. http://umm.edu/programs/shock-trauma/about /history. Accessed November 1, 2017.

49. Demetriades D, Chan L, Cornwell EE, et al. Paramedic vs. private transportation of trauma patients: effect on outcome. *Arch Surg*. 1996;131(2):133-138.

50. Cornwell EE, Belzberg H, Hennigan K, et al. Emergency medical services (EMS) vs. non-EMS transport of critically injured patients: a prospective evaluation. *Arch Surg*. 2000;135(3):315-319.

51. Smith S, Hildebrandt D. Effect of workday vs. after-hours on door to balloon time with paramedic out-of-hospital catheterization laboratory activation for STEMI. *Acad Emerg Med*. 2007;14(5)(suppl 1):S126-S127.

52. Tantisiriwat W, Jiar W, Ngamkasem H, et al. Clinical outcomes of fast track managed care system for acute ST elevation myocardial infarction (STEMI) patients: Chonburi Hospital experience. *J Med Assoc Thai*. 2008;91(6):822-827.

53. So DY, Ha AC, Turek MA, et al. Comparison of mortality patterns in patients with ST-elevation myocardial infarction arriving by emergency medical services vs. self-transport (from the Prospective Ottawa Hospital STEMI Registry). *Am J Cardiol*. 2006;97(4):458-461.

54. Bjorklund E, Stenestrand U, Lindback J, et al. Prehospital diagnosis and start of treatment reduces time delay and mortality in real-life patients with STEMI. *J Electrocardiol*. 2005;38(4)(suppl):186.

55. American Academy of Surgeons. *Resources for Optimal Care of the Injured Patient*. 6th ed. Chicago, IL: American

College of Surgeons; 2014. https://www.facs.org/~/media /files/quality%20programs/trauma/vrc%20resources /resources%20for%20optimal%20care.ashx. Accessed March 12, 2018.

56. Bio-Medicine.org. Trauma victims' survival may depend on which trauma center treats them. http://news.bio-medicine .org/medicine-news-3/Trauma-victims-survival-may-depend -on-which-trauma-center-treats-them-8343-1/. Published October 2005. Accessed December 11, 2017.

57. Peleg K, Aharonson-Daniel L, Stein M, et al. Increased survival among severe trauma patients: the impact of a national trauma system. *Arch Surg*. 2004;139(11):1231-1236.

58. Edwards W. Emergency medical systems significantly increase patient survival rates, Part 2. *Can Doct*. 1982;48(12): 20-24.

59. Haas B, Jurkovich GJ, Wang J, et al. Survival advantage in trauma centers: expeditious intervention or experience? *J Am Coll*. 2009;208(1):28-36.

60. Scheetz LJ. Differences in survival, length of stay, and discharge disposition of older trauma patients admitted to trauma centers and nontrauma center hospitals. *J Nurs Scholarsh*. 2005;37(4):361-366.

61. Norwood S, Fernandez L, England J. The early effects of implementing American College of Surgeons level II criteria on transfer and survival rates at a rurally based community hospital. *J Trauma*. 1995;39(2):240-244; discussion 244-245.

62. Kane G, Wheeler NC, Cook S, et al. Impact of the Los Angeles county trauma system on the survival of seriously injured patients. *J Trauma*. 1992;32(5):576-583.

63. Hedges JR, Adams AL, Gunnels MD. ATLS practices and survival at rural level III trauma hospitals, 1995-1999. *Prehosp Emerg Care*. 2002;6(3):299-305.

64. Konvolinka CW, Copes WS, Sacco WJ. Institution and per-surgeon volume vs. survival outcome in Pennsylvania's trauma centers. *Am J Surg*. 1995;170(4):333-340.

65. Margulies DR, Cryer HG, McArthur DL, et al. Patient volume per surgeon does not predict survival in adult level I trauma centers. *J Trauma*. 2001;50(4):597-601; discussion 601-603.

66. McSwain NE. Judgment based on knowledge: a history of Prehospital Trauma Life Support, 1970-2013. *J Trauma Acute Care Surg*. 2013;75:1-7.

Suggested Reading

Callaham M. Quantifying the scanty science of prehospital emergency care. *Ann Emerg Med*. 1997;30:785.

Cone DC, Lewis RJ. Should this study change my practice? *Acad Emerg Med*. 2003;10:417.

Haynes RB, McKibbon KA, Fitzgerald D, et al. How to keep up with the medical literature: II. Deciding which journals to read regularly. *Ann Intern Med*. 1986;105:309.

Keim SM, Spaite DW, Maio RF, et al. Establishing the scope and methodological approach to out-of-hospital outcomes and effectiveness research. *Acad Emerg Med*. 2004;11:1067.

Lewis RJ, Bessen HA. Statistical concepts and methods for the reader of clinical studies in emergency medicine. *J Emerg Med*. 1991;9:221.

MacAvley D. Critical appraisal of medical literature: an aid to rational decision making. *Fam Pract*. 1995;12:98.

Reed JF III, Salen P, Bagher P. Methodological and statistical techniques: what do residents really need to know about statistics? *J Med Syst*. 2003;27:233.

Sackett DL. How to read clinical journals: V. To distinguish useful from useless or even harmful therapy. *Can Med Assoc J*. 1981;124:1156.

CHAPTER 2

© Ralf Hiemisch/Getty Images.

Golden Principles, Preferences, and Critical Thinking

Lead Editor:
Blaine Enderson, MD, MBA, FACS, FCCM

CHAPTER OBJECTIVES

At the completion of this chapter, you will be able to do the following:

- Describe the difference between principles and preferences in relation to decision making in the field.
- Given a trauma scenario, discuss the principles of trauma care for the specific situation.
- Given a trauma scenario, use critical-thinking skills to determine the preferred method for accomplishing the principles of emergency trauma care.
- Relate the four principles of ethical decision making to prehospital trauma care.

- Given a trauma scenario, discuss the ethical issues involved and how to address them.
- Relate the importance of the "Golden Hour" or "Golden Period."
- Discuss the 14 "Golden Principles" of prehospital trauma care.
- Identify the components and importance of prehospital research and literature.

SCENARIO

You and your partner (a paramedic and an EMT) arrive at the scene of a two-vehicle T-bone collision. You are currently the only available unit. In a pickup truck, there is a young, unrestrained male driver who smells strongly of alcohol and has an obvious forearm deformity. The truck struck the passenger's side front door of a small sedan, with significant intrusion into vehicle. There is an older adult female in the front passenger seat who does not appear to be breathing; the windshield is starred directly in front of her. The female driver of the sedan is also injured but conscious and extremely anxious. In the rear seats, there are two children restrained in car seats. The child on the passenger side appears to be approximately 3 years old and is unconscious and slumped over in the car seat. On the driver's side, a restrained 5-year-old boy is crying hysterically in a booster seat and appears to be uninjured.

(continued)

INTRODUCTION

Medicine has changed a great deal since the painting by Sir Luke Fildes that shows a concerned and frustrated physician sitting at the bedside of a sick child (**Figure 2-1**). At that time, there were no antibiotics, only a superficial understanding of most diseases and illness, and rudimentary surgery. Medication consisted primarily of herbal remedies. For many years, medicine was not an exact science but more of an art form. Now, considerable advancements have been made in our understanding of disease, development of pharmaceuticals, and application of technology. Research has allowed us to provide better patient care through evidence-based medicine. However, even though the practice of medicine has become more science-based and less of an art form, the art remains.

It was not until the 1950s that consideration went into training individuals who encounter patients prior to arrival to the emergency room. The training of prehospital care providers has significantly advanced over the years. Along with this growth comes the responsibility that each provider must remain up-to-date with a continually developing medical knowledge and skill set. Proficiency is maintained by reading and attending continuing medical education (CME) classes. Skills improve with experience and critique, like those of a surgeon or an airplane pilot. Just as a pilot does not fly solo after one flight, the emergency medical technician (EMT) does not mature from using a skill only once or in only one type of situation.

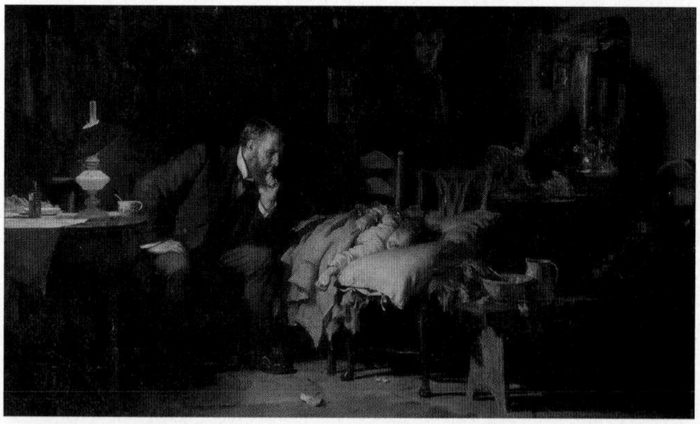

As discussed throughout this text, the science of prehospital care involves a working knowledge of the following:

1. Anatomy—the organs, bones, muscles, arteries, nerves, and veins of the human body
2. Physiology, including how the body produces and maintains heat, Frank-Starling law of the heart (increasing end diastolic volume increases stroke volume), and the Fick principle (which describes cardiac output and oxygen delivery and extraction to organs)
3. Pharmacology and the physiologic actions produced by various drugs and their interaction with each other inside the body
4. The relationship among these components and how they affect one another

By applying one's understanding of these elements, providers can make evidence-based decisions when treating their patients.

Major improvements in the science of medicine include technological advancements and the evolution of diagnostic tools. The ability to assess, diagnose, and treat a patient has dramatically improved with the imaging techniques of computed tomography (CT) scans, ultrasound, and magnetic resonance imaging (MRI); clinical laboratories can measure almost any electrolyte, hormone, or substance found in the human body. The pharmaceutical industry is continuously developing new medications. Treatments are becoming less invasive and less morbid through endovascular and interventional radiologic techniques. The emergency medical services (EMS) communications system has dramatically improved, and the global positioning system (GPS) helps find patients even in more remote areas. Rural outreach and response times have decreased, and overall

Figure 2-1 "The Doctor" by Sir Luke Fildes shows a concerned physician sitting by the bedside of an ill child. The relatively primitive state of health care offered few options for intervention beyond hopeful waiting and watching.

© Tate, London 2014.

patient care has improved secondary to advancements in the science of medicine.

Despite all of the scientific medical advances, the emergency first responder provides the art of medicine by linking the science with the delivery of the best care to the patient. Prehospital care providers need to be able to determine which patients are seriously injured and need rapid transport to which level of care; they need to be able to balance the amount of care to deliver at the scene versus during transport. Being able to choose which adjuncts and techniques to use to accomplish the end goal, which is end-organ perfusion, is critical. These functions are all examples of the art of medicine.

Medicine, like all other artistic endeavors, has guiding principles. This chapter concludes with an exploration of the Golden Principles of Trauma Care. The foundation of the PHTLS program is that patient care should be *judgment* driven and not *protocol* driven—hence the Golden Principles that assist prehospital care providers in improving patient outcomes by making rapid assessments, applying key field interventions, and rapidly transporting trauma patients to the closest appropriate facilities.

Principles and Preferences

The science of medicine provides the **principles** of medical care. Simply stated, principles define the duties required of the prehospital care provider in optimizing patient survival and outcome. How these principles are implemented by the individual provider to most efficiently manage the patient depends on the **preferences**, which describe how a system and its individual providers choose to apply scientific principles to the care of patients. This is how the *science* and *art* of medicine come together for the good of patient care.

An example such as airway management can illustrate the difference between principle and preference. The *principle* is that air, containing oxygen, must be moved through an open airway into the alveoli of the lungs to facilitate oxygen–carbon dioxide exchange with red blood cells (RBCs) so they may deliver oxygen to other tissues. This principle is true for all patients. The *preference* is how airway management is carried out in a particular patient. In some cases, patients will manage their own airway; in other patients, the prehospital care provider will have to decide which adjunct is best to facilitate airway management. In other words, the provider will determine the best method to ensure that the air passages are open to get oxygen into the lungs and, secondarily, to get carbon dioxide out. The art, or preference, is how the provider makes this determination and carries it out to achieve the principle. Much of this art is based on experience and anecdote, although there are standards of care that all must follow in applying scientific principles to the care of individual patients.

Box 2-1 Principles Versus Preferences

Principle—a fundamental scientific or evidence-based tenet for patient improvement or survival

Preference—how the specific prehospital care provider achieves the principle

The preference used to accomplish the principle depends on several factors:

- Situation that exists
- Condition of the patient
- Fund of knowledge, skills, and experience of the prehospital care provider
- Local protocols
- Equipment available

The preferences of how to accomplish the principles depend on several factors: the situation; the patient's condition; the provider's knowledge base, skills, and experience; local protocols; and the equipment available (**Box 2-1**).

The foundation of Prehospital Trauma Life Support (PHTLS) is to teach the prehospital care provider to make appropriate decisions for patient care based on knowledge and not on protocol. The goal of patient care is to achieve the principle. How this is achieved (i.e., the decision made by the provider to manage the patient) is the preference based on the situation, patient condition, fund of knowledge and skill, local protocols, and equipment available at the time—the several components outlined in Box 2-1.

The philosophy of the PHTLS program is that each situation and patient is different. PHTLS teaches the importance of having a strong understanding of the subject matter and the skills necessary to accomplish necessary interventions. The judgments and decisions made on scene should be individualized to the needs of the specific patient being managed at *that* specific time and in *that* specific situation. Protocols are helpful for guidance and direction, but they must be sufficiently flexible when there is variability in an event. Appropriate decisions can be made by understanding the principles involved and using critical-thinking skills to achieve the end goal.

Given that the preference is the way an individual prehospital care provider achieves the end goal, the principle will not be accomplished the same way every time. Not all providers have skill mastery in every technique. The equipment to carry out these techniques is not available at every emergency. Just because one instructor, lecturer, or physician director prefers one technique does not mean it is the best technique for *every* provider in *every* situation. The important point is to achieve the principle. How this is done and how the care is provided to the patient depend on the factors listed in Box 2-1. These factors are described in more detail in the following sections.

Situation

The situation involves all of the factors at a scene that can affect what care is provided to a patient. These factors include, but are not limited to, the following:

- Hazards on the scene
- Number of patients involved
- Location of the patient
- Position of the vehicle
- Contamination or hazardous materials concerns
- Fire or potential for fire
- Weather
- Scene control and security by law enforcement
- Time/distance to medical care, including the capabilities of the closest hospital versus the nearest trauma center
- Number of prehospital care providers and other possible helpers on the scene
- Bystanders
- Transportation available on the scene
- Other transportation available at a distance (i.e., helicopters, additional ambulances)

All of these conditions and circumstances, as well as many others, may be constantly changing and will affect the way a prehospital care provider can respond to the needs of the patient.

Take, for example, the following situation: a single-vehicle crash into a tree on a rural road in a wooded area. The weather is clear and dark (time 0200 hours). The transport time by ground to the trauma center is 35 minutes. A medical helicopter can be requested by prehospital care providers on the scene with approval of medical control. Startup time for the helicopter is 5 minutes, and travel time is 15 minutes; a nontrauma center hospital is 15 minutes away and has a helistop. Do you transport by ground, stop at the helistop, or stay on scene and wait for the helicopter?

Some examples of how the situation affects a procedure such as spinal immobilization include the following:

Situation 1:

- Automobile crash
- Bull's-eye fracture of the windshield
- Warm, sunny day
- No traffic on the road

Management:

- Patient examined in the car—significant back pain and lower extremity weakness noted
- Cervical collar applied
- Patient secured to the short backboard
- Rotated onto the long backboard
- Removed from the car
- Placed on the stretcher
- Physical assessment completed
- Patient transported to the hospital

Situation 2:

- Same as Situation 1, except gasoline is dripping from the gas tank
- Concern for fire

Management:

- Rapid extraction techniques used
- Patient moved significant distance from the vehicle
- Patient examined and need for implementation of spinal motion restriction determined
- Physical assessment completed
- Patient transported to the hospital

Situation 3:

- House fully involved in flames
- Patient unable to move

Management:

- No assessment
- Patient dragged from the fire
- Placed on backboard
- Moved quickly to a safe distance away from the fire
- Patient assessment completed
- Patient transported quickly to the hospital, depending on the patient's condition

Situation 4:

- Combat situation with nearby perpetrator or enemy combatants actively shooting
- Officer (or soldier) with gunshot wound to the knee and significant bleeding

Management:

- Assessment from a distance (binoculars)
- Presence of other wounds
- Patient still able to fire his weapon
- Tell patient to apply tourniquet on upper leg
- Tell patient to crawl to a protected position
- Rescue the patient when conditions permit

Condition of the Patient

The next component of the decision-making process concerns the medical condition of the patient. The major question that will affect decision making is "How sick is the patient?" Some information points that will facilitate this determination include the age of the patient, physiologic factors that affect end-organ perfusion (blood pressure, pulse, ventilatory rate, skin temperature, etc.), the cause of the trauma, the patient's medical condition prior to the event, medication that the patient is using, illicit drug use, and alcohol use. These factors and more require critical thinking to determine what needs to be done before and during transport and what method of transportation should be used.

Let us return to the scenario of the single-vehicle crash with a tree: The patient is breathing with difficulty at a rate of 30 breaths/minute, his heart rate is 110 beats/minute, his blood pressure is 90 millimeters of mercury (mm Hg) by palpation, and his Glasgow Coma Scale (GCS) score is 11 (E3V3M5); he is in his mid-20s, he was not wearing a seat belt, and his position is against the dash away from the driver-side air bag; he has a deformed right leg at mid-thigh and an open left ankle fracture with significant hemorrhage. There is approximately 1 liter of blood on the floorboard near the ankle.

Fund of Knowledge of the Prehospital Care Provider

The fund of knowledge of the prehospital care provider comes from several sources, including initial training, CME courses, local protocols, overall experience, and skill set.

Let us use airway management as an example again. The level of knowledge and experience a prehospital care provider possesses makes a significant impact on the choice of preference. The comfort level of performing a skill depends on the frequency with which it has been performed in the past. As the provider, you might consider: Can the patient maintain his or her own airway? If not, what devices are available, and of those, which ones do you feel comfortable using? When was the last time you performed an intubation? How comfortable are you with the laryngoscope? How comfortable are you with the anatomy of the oropharynx? How many times have you done a cricothyroidotomy on a live patient or even an animal training model? Without the appropriate skills and experience, the patient would likely be better off and the provider would be more comfortable choosing a nasopharyngeal or oropharyngeal airway plus bag-mask device rather than a more advanced intervention such as endotracheal intubation or a surgical airway as the preference for management.

Returning to the example of the patient in the single-vehicle crash, the responding prehospital care providers have been working together for 2 years. Both are nationally registered paramedics (NRPs). Their last update training for endotracheal (ET) intubation was 1 year ago. One paramedic last placed an ET tube 2 months ago; his partner placed one a month ago. They are not authorized to use paralytic drugs for ET insertion, but they can use sedation if necessary. They were just trained on hemorrhage control using tourniquets and hemostatic agents. How will their training impact what will be done to manage the patient in the field?

Local Protocols

Local protocols define what a PHTLS provider is credentialed to do in the field and under what circumstances. While these protocols should not and cannot describe in cookbook fashion how to care for every patient, they are intended to guide the approach to patients in a way that is systematic and consistent with best practices, local resources, and training. In the scenario of the single-vehicle crash, rapid-sequence induction with intubation may be valuable and indicated in some situations, but if the skill set is not included in the local protocols, the paramedics will not have it at their disposal. Local protocols often dictate which procedures and transport destinations the provider should select. They may, for example, indicate spinal immobilization or transport to a specific trauma center.

Equipment Available

The experience of a prehospital care provider does not matter if he or she does not have the appropriate equipment available. The provider must use the equipment or supplies that are available. As an example, blood may be the best resuscitation fluid for trauma victims. However, blood is not always available in the field; therefore, crystalloid may be the best resuscitative fluid of choice due to its availability. Another consideration is whether permissive hypotension would be a better choice given the nature of the patient's injuries. This particular issue is discussed in more detail in the Shock: Pathophysiology of Life and Death chapter.

Once again let us return to the patient in the single-vehicle crash: There is complete paramedic equipment that was checked at the beginning of the shift. It includes ET tubes, laryngoscopes, tourniquets, and other equipment and supplies as included in the American College of Surgeons/American College of Emergency Physicians (ACS/ACEP) equipment list. The paramedics have all the appropriate medications, including hemostatic agents. They apply manual pressure to the bleeding ankle and are able to control the hemorrhage. They splint the patient's femur and transport him to the nearby trauma center.

Another example is when a nonbreathing patient is encountered, the *principle* is that the airway must be opened and oxygen delivered to the lungs. The *preference* chosen depends on the preference factors (situation, patient condition, fund of knowledge, protocols and experience/skill, equipment available). A bystander on the street with only cardiopulmonary resuscitation (CPR) training may perform mouth-to-mask ventilation; the EMT may choose an oral airway and bag-mask ventilation; the paramedic may choose to place an ET tube or may decide that it is more advantageous to use the bag-mask device with rapid transport; the corpsman in combat may choose a cricothyroidotomy or nothing at all if the enemy fire is too intense; and the physician in the emergency department (ED) may choose paralytic drugs or fiber-optic–guided ET tube placement. None of the choices is wrong at a specific point in time for a given patient; applying the same logic in reverse, none is correct all of the time.

This concept of principle and preference for the care of the trauma patient has its most dramatic application in the combat situation in the military. For this reason, the Tactical Combat Casualty Care Committee (TCCC) wrote the military component of the PHTLS program. For the military provider, the scene situation will include whether or not there is active combat, the location of the enemy, the tactical situation, the weapons currently being used, and protection available for sheltering the wounded. Although obvious alterations are made in preference for patient care in combat situations, similar considerations exist in the civilian setting for tactical emergency medical support providers and those prehospital care providers who work in hazardous environments such as fire scenes. For example, in the middle of a house that is fully involved in fire, a fire fighter–paramedic discovers a patient who is down. He or she cannot stop to check the basic principles of patient assessment, such as airway or hemodynamics. The first step is to get the patient outside and away from the immediate danger of the fire and only then check the patient's airway and pulse.

For the military medic who is potentially involved in combat, the three-step process for casualty management developed by the TCCC is:

1. *Care under fire*—management in the middle of a fire fight
2. *Tactical field care*—management after the shooting is over but danger still exists
3. *Tactical evacuation care*—treatment of the casualty once the situation has been controlled and is considered safe

While the principles of patient care are not changed, the preferences of patient care may be dramatically different due to one or more of these factors. For further discussion, details, and clarification, refer to the Tactical Emergency Medical Support (TEMS) chapter or the military version of PHTLS. (These situational differences are described in more detail in the Scene Management chapter.)

Critical Thinking

To successfully accomplish the principle needed for a particular patient and to choose the best preference to implement the principle, critical-thinking skills are crucial. Critical thinking in medicine is a process in which the health care provider assesses the situation, the patient, and all of the resources

---

> **Box 2-2** Components of Critical Thinking in Emergency Medical Care
>
> 1. Assess the situation.
> 2. Assess the patient.
> 3. Assess the available resources.
> 4. Analyze the possible solutions.
> 5. Select the best answer to manage the situation and patient.
> 6. Develop the plan of action.
> 7. Initiate the plan of action.
> 8. Reassess the response of the patient to the plan of action.
> 9. Make any needed adjustments or changes to the plan of action.
> 10. Continue with steps 8 and 9 until this phase of care is completed.

---

that are available (**Box 2-2**). This information is then rapidly analyzed and combined to provide the best care possible to the patient. The critical-thinking process requires that the health care provider develop a plan of action, initiate this plan, reassess the plan as the process of caring for the patient moves forward, and make adjustments in the plan as the patient's condition changes until that phase of care is completed (**Box 2-3**). Critical thinking is a learned skill that improves with use and experience.[1] If prehospital care providers are to function successfully, they must be equipped with the lifelong learning and critical-thinking skills necessary to acquire and process information in a rapidly and ever-changing world.[2]

For the prehospital care provider, this process begins with the initial information provided at the time of dispatch and continues until the patient is handed off at the hospital. Critical thinking is also involved in the selection of receiving facility level, resources available, and the transport time. All of these critical decisions are based on the situation, the patient condition, the fund of knowledge of the provider, and the equipment available.

The critical-thinking process cannot be dogmatic or gullible; it must be open-minded with skepticism.[3] The prehospital care provider must question the scientific accuracy of all approaches. This is the reason why the provider must have a strong, well-grounded fund of knowledge that can be used to make appropriate decisions. However, the questioning cannot be taken too far as to delay care. Aristotle suggested that one should not require more certainty than the subject allows.[4] When a provider is assessing and caring for a patient, withholding action in hopes of securing absolute certainty in the patient's diagnosis would be foolish; such certainty is impossible, and seeking it would only delay needed interventions. A provider must make

---

Box 2-3 Steps in Critical Thinking Assessment

What is going on? What needs to be done? What are the resources to achieve the goal? Analysis will involve:

- Scene assessment
- Identification of any hazards to either the patient or the prehospital care provider
- Condition of the patient
- Rapidity required for resolution
- Location of the care (in the field, during transport, and after arrival to the hospital)
- Number of patients on the scene
- Number of transport vehicles required
- Need for more rapid transport
- Destination of the patient for the appropriate care

Analysis

Each of these conditions must be individually and rapidly analyzed, and they must be cross-referenced with the prehospital care provider's fund of knowledge and the resources available. Steps must be defined to provide the best care.

Construction of a Plan

The plan to achieve the best outcome for the patient is developed and critically reviewed. Is any step false? Are the planned steps all achievable? Are the resources available that will allow the plan to move forward? Will they, more likely than not, lead to a successful outcome?

Action

The plan is initiated and put into motion. This is done decisively and with assertiveness so that there is no confusion regarding what needs to be accomplished or who is in command and making the decisions. If the decisions are not effective for the outcome of the patient, the prehospital care provider in command must make appropriate changes. Suggestions for change can come from the commander or from other participants.

Reassessment

Is the patient progressing correctly? Has the situation on scene changed? Does anything in the action plan need to be changed? What is the patient's condition and has it changed? Has the treatment plan improved the patient's condition or has it worsened?

Changes Along the Way

Any changes that are identified by the prehospital care provider are assessed and analyzed as described here, and alterations are made accordingly to continue the best possible care for the patient. Alterations in decision making and reassessment of the patient should not be perceived as weakness as the patient and situation are ever-changing and may call for a change in plan. Having the ability to think critically and remain dynamic based on the situation is a sign of strength in a leader.

---

the most informed assessment and decision possible given the information available at the time.

The basis of appropriate medical care advocated by PHTLS relies on critical thinking: "judgment based on knowledge." Robert Carroll described critical thinking as concepts and principles, not hard-and-fast rules or step-by-step procedures.[3] The emphasis throughout PHTLS education is that protocols promoting recall but discouraging critical thinking are not beneficial for patient management. The guidelines for patient care must be flexible. Critical thinking requires that flexibility. Protocols should simply serve as guidelines to assist prehospital care providers in aligning their thought process.

Using Critical Thinking to Control Biases

All health care providers have biases that can affect the critical-thinking process and decision making about the patients. These biases must be recognized and not allowed to influence the patient care process. Biases usually arise

from several sources. A previous experience that resulted in either a significant positive or negative impact could be a source. Two thought processes help protect patients: (1) Assume the worst-case scenario until proven otherwise, and (2) uphold the Hippocratic Oath—"primum non nocere," or "first do no harm." The patient's treatment plan is designed regardless of the opinion of the prehospital care provider regarding the "apparent" conditions that might have led to the current circumstances. For example, the initial impression that a driver is intoxicated may be correct, but other conditions may exist as well. Because a patient is found to be intoxicated does not mean he or she is not injured as well. Because the patient is impaired from intoxication does not mean that some of the alteration in mental status might not be due to brain injury or decreased cerebral perfusion because of shock.

Frequently, the complete picture cannot be seen at initial presentation; therefore, the critical thinking and response of the prehospital care provider must be based on worst-case scenario. Judgments must be made on the best information available. The critical thinker is constantly looking for "other information" as it becomes available and acting on it. The critical-thinking process must continue throughout the assessment of the patient, the situation, and the conditions. The provider should always be anticipating and thinking several steps ahead.

Using Critical Thinking in Rapid Decision Making

EMS is a field of quick action and reliance on the innate ability of the prehospital care provider to respond decisively to varying presentations and varying diseases in a timely manner. Efficiency and accuracy are important. Combining protocol and preference efficiently is optimal.

Critical thinking at the site of an emergency must be swift, thorough, flexible, and objective. The prehospital care provider at the site of an emergency may have only seconds to assess the situation, the condition of the patient(s), and the resources available to make decisions and commence patient care. Sometimes the provider may have optimal time to think through a situation and should take advantage of the luxury of time, but this is often not the case.

Using Critical Thinking in Data Analysis

Information is gathered using four of the five senses: vision, smell, touch, and hearing. (This will be taught in the Patient Assessment and Management chapter.) The prehospital care provider then analyzes this information or data obtained based on the primary survey and determines the overall plan of care for the patient until handed off to a hospital provider.

Typically, the evaluation of a trauma patient begins with the primary survey of XABCDE (exsanguinating hemorrhage, airway, breathing, circulation, disability, expose/environment), but critical thinking guides the prehospital care provider to the most critical condition first. If the patient is in shock because of external hemorrhage, then applying direct pressure over the source of hemorrhage is the appropriate initial step after assessment. Critical thinking is the recognition that following the standard XABCDE priority for medical patients may lead to a trauma patient who has an airway but who has now exsanguinated; so, instead of attention to the airway, control of the bleeding was the appropriate first step. Critical thinking is the process of recognizing that if direct pressure is not working, then something else needs to be done. Critical thinking is based on the data collection of the situation, the condition of the patient, the fund of knowledge of the provider, the skills of the provider, and the equipment available.

> Critical thinking is a pervasive skill that involves scrutinizing, differentiating, and appraising information and reflecting on the information gained in order to make judgments and inform clinical decisions.[5]

Using Critical Thinking Throughout the Phases of Patient Care

The art and science of medicine, the knowledge of principles, and the appropriate application of preferences will lead to the anticipated outcome of the best care possible for the patient in the circumstances in which the care is provided. There are essentially four phases in the process of caring for patients with acute injuries:

- The prehospital phase
- The initial (resuscitative) phase in the hospital
- The stabilization and definitive care phase
- The long-term resolution and rehabilitation to return the patient to a functional status

All of these phases use the same principles of patient care in each step. All of the health care providers throughout the phases of the patient's care must use critical thinking. Critical thinking continues from the time of the injury until the time that the patient goes home. EMS personnel are directly involved in the initial prehospital phase of care but must use critical thinking and be aware of the entire process in order to produce seamless patient care as the patient moves through the system. The prehospital care provider must think beyond the current situation to the definitive care needs and the patient's ultimate outcome. The goal is to manage the patient's injuries so that they heal and the patient can return to his or her highest level of function possible—ideally just as before he or she was injured, or even better. For example, critical thinking involves recognizing that while splinting the fractured forearm of a multisystem trauma patient is not one of the initial priorities of care, when considering the definitive outcome of the patient and his or her ability to lead a productive life, the preservation of limb function (and thus splinting of the limb) is an important concern in the patient's prehospital treatment.

Ethics

Prehospital professionals face many ethically challenging scenarios that are both emergent and time sensitive. However, the lack of prehospital-specific ethics education can leave prehospital care providers feeling both unprepared and unsupported when confronted with ethical challenges.[6] Critical-thinking skills can provide a sound basis for making many of the difficult ethical decisions required of providers.

The goal of this section is to use bioethical principles and concepts to begin to develop ethical awareness and ethical reasoning skills and to provide common frameworks and vocabulary to think through and discuss even the most ethically challenging cases. This section will rely on the traditional elements of basic bioethics education, which are familiar to most health care providers, but will use prehospital examples and cases to provide content that is authentic, practical, and applicable to the field setting. Additionally, by exposing prehospital care providers to common bioethics principles and concepts, ethics conversations across health care disciplines and settings will be encouraged and promoted.

Ethical Principles

Everyone uses some set of values, beliefs, or social rules to make decisions. These rules are generally accepted beliefs about moral behavior and are often referred to as principles. Ethics is using a set of moral principles to assist in determining what is the right thing to do. In medicine, the set of principles that is often relied on to ensure ethically appropriate behavior, to guide clinical practice, and to assist in ethical decision making includes elements of **autonomy**, **nonmaleficence**, **beneficence**, and **justice**. The use of these four principles, often referred to as **principlism (Box 2-4)**, provides a framework within which one can weigh and balance benefits and burdens, generally within the context of treating a specific patient, in order to do what is in the patient's best interest.[4]

Autonomy

The word *autonomy* is from the Greek words *auto* and *nomos*, meaning "self-rule." In medicine, it refers to the patient's right to direct his or her own health care free from interference or undue influence.[4] In other words, competent adults get to make their own health care decisions. Respect for autonomy is the source from which informed consent and confidentiality developed. However, the unknown and emergent nature of the prehospital care provider's encounter with a patient can compromise a patient's autonomy. The provider should make the best decision possible for the patient with the information that is available. Not every piece of information will be available at the initial presentation.

Informed consent is a process through which a medical practitioner provides a patient who has decision-making capacity, or a surrogate decision maker (a person who is chosen to make health care decisions on the patient's behalf if the patient is not able to make decisions for himself or herself),[4] with the information necessary to provide

informed consent for, or refusal of, the medical treatment being offered. While many think of informed consent as a legal form, in reality, it is only a record of the consent conversation. There is an ethical obligation on the part of a health care provider to give patients the appropriate medical information to allow them to make health decisions based on their own values, beliefs, and wishes.

In order for an informed consent to be valid, the following must be true for patients:

1. Must have decision-making capacity
2. Must have the ability to communicate their understanding of their diagnosis, prognosis, and treatment options
3. Must be able to give consent or refusal voluntarily
4. Must actively refuse or consent to treatment[4,7,8]

Assessing any one of these elements can be hard enough to accomplish in a controlled clinical setting, but in an emergency situation, it is especially difficult. Although many people use the terms *competence* and *decision-making capacity* interchangeably, **competence** is a legal term referring to a person's general ability to make good decisions for himself or herself, and decision-making capacity refers to a patient's ability to make decisions regarding a specific set of medical treatment options or therapies.

Assessing the capacity of a patient is particularly difficult in an emergency situation. There is rarely knowledge of the patient's baseline on initial presentation, and the assessment is often made when the patient is sick, scared, or in pain. When assessing the decision-making capacity of an adult patient, it is necessary to attempt to determine his or her level of understanding. Can the patient understand the medical options and weigh the risks and benefits associated with those options? Patients should also have the capacity to appreciate the anticipated outcomes of their choices as well as be able to express their wishes to the health care provider. While the informed consent process respects the rights of patients to make their own decisions, the informed consent requirement may be overridden in emergency situations under certain conditions:

1. The patient lacks decision-making capacity due to unconsciousness or significant cognitive impairment and there is no surrogate available.
2. The condition is life or health threatening and the patient may suffer irreversible damage in the absence of treatment.
3. A reasonable person would consent to the treatment, in which case a health care provider may proceed with treatment in the absence of an autonomous consent from the patient or a surrogate.[7]

Privacy and Confidentiality

In the health care context, **privacy** refers to the right of patients to control who has access to their personal health

---

Box 2-4 Principlism: Guide to Ethical Decision Making

- Autonomy
- Nonmaleficence
- Beneficence
- Justice

information. **Confidentiality** refers to the obligation of health care providers not to share patient information that is disclosed to them within the patient–provider relationship to any individuals other than those the patient has authorized, other medical professionals involved in the patient's care, and agencies responsible for processing state and/or federally mandated reporting, such as in cases of child or elder abuse.

Depending on the circumstances, prehospital care providers may need to rely on and interact with people other than an incapacitated patient (family, friends, or neighbors) in order to gain the information necessary to care for the patient. However, great effort should be made to protect patient information from those who are not health care providers, such as observers or news media who may be at the scene of an event involving traumatic injury or loss of life, and to limit information given to others until an appropriate surrogate decision maker is identified.

Truth Telling

Truth telling can also present ethical challenges.[8] Truthfulness is both an expectation and a necessary part of building a trusting patient–provider relationship. Communicating honestly shows respect for the patient and enables decision making based on truthful information. However, especially in the prehospital setting, there are situations in which telling a patient the truth has the potential to cause great harm, such as in cases of multivictim trauma in which survivors are inquiring about the condition of nonsurviving or critically injured loved ones. At such times, the immediate obligation to tell the truth may sometimes be outweighed by the obligation to do no harm, depending on the level of injury and the condition of the patient who is asking.[6]

Advance Directives

The right of patients to make their own health decisions does not necessarily cease to exist when they become incapacitated or can no longer make competent decisions for themselves. Similarly, children and adults who have never been competent have the right to have their best interests protected by a competent decision maker. Protecting these rights is the role of advance directives (living will and medical power of attorney), out-of-hospital medical orders such as the physician's order for life-sustaining treatment (POLST), and surrogate decision makers. In order to protect and respect the rights of incompetent patients, it is important to have a working knowledge of these resources.

Advance directives allow patients to make decisions regarding their medical care in the event that they become incapacitated. They can be established informally through statements to family or friends or formally through written documents. The two types of written advance directives

most often encountered in a medical situation are a living will and a medical power of attorney. A **living will** is a document that expresses end-of-life treatment wishes, such as whether a person would want mechanical ventilation, CPR, dialysis, or other types of life-prolonging or life-sustaining treatments. While advance directive law varies from state to state, living wills do not generally go into effect unless the patient lacks decision-making capacity and has been certified by a health care professional, usually a doctor, to be either terminally ill or permanently unconscious. Because prehospital care providers often lack an extensive knowledge of a patient's medical history and are reacting to an emergent medical situation, it is difficult to determine if a living will is operative, and therefore the provider may be unable to rely on it to provide medical direction.

A **medical power of attorney (MPOA)** is an advance directive document used by competent adults to appoint someone to make medical decisions for them in the event that they are unable to make such decisions for themselves. Unlike living wills, MPOAs go into effect immediately any time a patient is incapable of making his or her own decisions, regardless of preexisting conditions, and become inactive again when and if the patient regains decision-making capacity. The person designated by the MPOA is authorized to make only medical decisions on the patient's behalf. These two advance directives, a living will and an MPOA, attempt to protect and respect the rights and wishes of formerly competent patients when they are no longer able to speak for themselves.

An **out-of-hospital medical order**, or **do-not-resuscitate (DNR) order**, is an order given by a physician to ensure that paramedics or other emergency personnel do not perform CPR on a terminally ill patient at home, or in some other community or nonclinical setting, against the patient's previously expressed wishes. The DNR order must be completed on the form specified by the state where the emergency occurs. Each state has its own DNR forms, and most states do not recognize DNR orders from other states. Unlike advance directives, DNR orders go into effect immediately upon being signed by a doctor or authorized health care professional and remain valid regardless of setting.

While the DNR form addresses only the withholding of CPR, a **physician's order for life-sustaining treatment (POLST)** is broader in scope and is meant "to improve the quality of care people receive at the end of life. It is based on effective communication of patient wishes, documentation of medical orders on a brightly colored form and a promise by health care professionals to honor these wishes."[9] The POLST allows for the acceptance or refusal of a wide variety of life-sustaining treatments, such as CPR, medical nutrition and hydration, and ventilator support, and allows prehospital care providers to access an active physician order regarding the end-of-life wishes of the terminally ill and frail elderly. Note that different states may use different names and abbreviations for this form, such as medical orders on scope of treatment (MOST) and physician's orders on scope of treatment (POST).

Nonmaleficence

Just as health care providers are legally and ethically obligated to respect a patient's autonomy, there is also an obligation to avoid putting patients at risk. The principle of nonmaleficence obligates the medical practitioner not to take actions that are likely to harm the patient. The maxim "do no harm," often attributed to the Greek physician Hippocrates and reflected in the Hippocratic Oath, is the essence of the principle of nonmaleficence.[4] If a patient tells a prehospital care provider that she is allergic to a particular medication and the provider disregards the patient's warning and gives the medication anyway and the patient has an allergic reaction, the provider has physically harmed the patient.

Additionally, prehospital care providers have an obligation not only to "do no harm" but also to avoid putting patients in harm's way. When transporting a trauma patient with minor injuries from the scene of an accident to the hospital, the principle of nonmaleficence would dictate that the driver proceed cautiously and without the use of emergency lights and siren while driving.

Beneficence

Beneficence involves taking an action to benefit another. Beneficence means "to do good" and requires prehospital care providers to act in a manner that maximizes the benefits and minimizes the risks to the patient. For example, a provider may have to start an intravenous line to administer medications or fluids. The needlestick inflicts pain but is necessary to benefit the patient. Additionally, when done carefully, providers can reduce the risk of additional harms such as bruising, swelling, or multiple needlesticks.

Beneficence can also include going above and beyond what is required by professional practice standards to benefit the patient. For example, making sure the patient is transported at a comfortable temperature and providing extra blankets to keep the patient comfortable may not be included in a prehospital protocol, but such actions are done to care for and benefit the patient.[4]

Justice

Justice, commonly thought of as that which is fair or just, usually refers to how we distribute medical resources when it is discussed with regard to health care. Distributive justice is the fair distribution of goods or services based on a socially agreed-upon set of moral guidelines or rules.[4] While many assume justice, or treating others fairly, means to treat all people equally regardless of age, race, gender, or ability to pay, treating everyone equally is not always ethically justifiable. For example, when triaging an emergency multiple casualty incident, those with the greatest medical needs are prioritized over those with less critical needs. Thus, the most vulnerable are often given a greater portion of health care goods and services based on a shared community value of caring for the sick and marginalized.

In a mass-casualty incident, triage is based partially on probability of survival, and some of the sickest or most vulnerable are moved to an expectant category to allow for resources to be focused on those with survivable injuries. Therefore, what is most just in a particular situation may depend on the availability of resources and the fairest way of using and distributing those resources in that specific case.[10]

The Golden Hour or Period

In the late 1960s, R Adams Cowley, MD, conceived the idea of a crucial time period during which it is important to begin definitive patient care for a critically injured trauma patient. In an interview he said:

> There is a "golden hour" between life and death. If you are critically injured, you have less than 60 minutes to survive. You might not die right then—it may be three days or two weeks later—but something has happened in your body that is irreparable.[11]

Dr. Cowley definitely had the correct concept; however, it is important to realize that a patient does not always have the luxury of a "Golden Hour." The "hour" was intended to be figurative and not a literal description of a period of time. A patient with a penetrating wound to the heart may have only a few minutes to reach definitive care before the shock caused by the injury becomes irreversible, but a patient with slow, ongoing internal hemorrhage from an isolated femur fracture may have several hours or longer to reach definitive care and resuscitation.

Because the Golden *Hour* is not a strict 60-minute time frame and varies from patient to patient based on the injuries, another commonly employed term is *Golden Period*. If a critically injured patient is able to obtain definitive care—that is, hemorrhage control and resuscitation—within that particular patient's Golden Period, the chance of survival is improved greatly.[12] The American College of Surgeons Committee on Trauma has used this concept to emphasize the importance of transporting trauma patients to facilities where expert trauma care is available in a timely manner.

The management of prehospital trauma must reflect these contingencies. The goals, however, do not change:

1. Gain access to the patient.
2. Identify and treat life-threatening injuries.
3. Package and transport the patient to the closest appropriate facility in the least amount of time.

The majority of the techniques and principles discussed are not new, and most are taught in initial training programs. PHTLS is different in the following ways:

1. It provides current, evidence-based management practices for the trauma patient.
2. It provides a systematic approach for establishing priorities of patient care for trauma patients who have sustained injury to multiple body systems.
3. It provides an organizational scheme for interventions.

Why Trauma Patients Die

Studies that analyze the causes of death in trauma patients reveal several common themes. A study from Russia of more than 700 trauma deaths found that most patients who rapidly succumbed to their injuries fall into one of three categories: massive acute blood loss (36%), severe injury to vital organs such as the brain (30%), and airway obstruction and acute ventilatory failure (25%).[13] A study published in 2010 documented that 76% of patients who died rapidly did so from nonsurvivable injuries to the head, aorta, or heart.[14] A study published in 2013 found a reduction in deaths from multiple organ failure, or the third phase of death (see the PHTLS: Past, Present, and Future chapter).[15] This reduction in deaths may be attributed to improvements in modern trauma care both in the field and in the hospital.

But what is happening to these patients on a cellular level? The metabolic processes of the human body are driven by energy, similar to any other machine. This is discussed further in the Shock: Pathophysiology of Life and Death chapter. Shock is viewed as a failure of energy production in the body. As with machines, the human body generates its own energy but must have fuel to do so. Fuel for the body is oxygen and glucose. The body can store glucose as complex carbohydrates (glycogen) and fat to use at a later time. However, oxygen cannot be stored. It must be constantly supplied to the cells of the body. Atmospheric air, containing oxygen, is drawn into the lungs by the action of the diaphragm and intercostal muscles. Oxygen diffuses across the alveolar and capillary walls, where it binds to the hemoglobin in the RBCs and is then transported to the body's tissues by the circulatory system. In the presence of oxygen, the cells of the tissues then "burn" glucose through a complex series of metabolic processes (glycolysis, Krebs cycle, and electron transport) to produce the energy needed for all body functions. This energy is stored as adenosine triphosphate (ATP). Without sufficient energy in the form of ATP, essential metabolic activities cannot occur normally, and cells begin to die and organ failure occurs.

The sensitivity of the cells to oxygen deprivation varies from organ to organ (**Box 2-5**). The cells within an organ

---

Box 2-5 Shock

When the heart is deprived of oxygen, the myocardial cells cannot produce enough energy to pump blood to the other tissues. For example, a patient has lost a significant number of RBCs and blood volume following a gunshot wound to the aorta. The heart continues to beat for several minutes before failing. Refilling the vascular system after the heart has been without oxygen for too long will not restore the function of the injured cells.

Although ischemia, as seen in severe shock, may result in damage to any tissues, the damage to the organs does not become apparent initially. In the lungs, acute respiratory distress syndrome often develops up to 48 hours after an ischemic insult, whereas acute renal failure and hepatic failure typically occur several days later. Although all body tissues are affected by insufficient oxygen, some tissues are more sensitive to ischemia. For example, a patient who has sustained a brain injury due to shock and anoxia may develop permanent brain damage. Although brain cells cease to function and die, the rest of the body can survive for years.

---

can be fatally damaged but can continue to function for a period of time (see the Shock: Pathophysiology of Life and Death chapter for complications of prolonged shock). This delayed death of cells, leading to organ failure, is what Dr. Cowley was referring to in his earlier quote. Shock results in death if a patient is not treated promptly, which is why Dr. Cowley advocated the rapid transport of the patient to the operating room for control of internal hemorrhage.

The Golden Hour or Period represents a crucial interval during which the cascade of events can worsen the long-term survival and overall outcomes of the patient; if proper care is received rapidly during this period, much of the damage is reversible. Failure to initiate appropriate interventions aimed at improving oxygenation and controlling hemorrhage allows shock to progress, eventually leading to death. For trauma patients to have the best chance of survival, interventions should start with an easily accessible and functional emergency communications system. Trained dispatchers can begin the process of providing care in the field by offering prearrival instructions such as hemorrhage control. Care in the field continues with the arrival of prehospital care providers and proceeds to the ED, the operating room, and the intensive care unit. Trauma is a "team sport." The patient "wins" when all members of the trauma team—from those in the field to those in the trauma center—work together to care for the individual patient.

The Golden Principles of Prehospital Trauma Care

This text discusses the assessment and management of patients who have sustained injury to specific body systems. Although the body systems are presented individually, most severely injured patients have injury to more than one body system—hence the term *multisystem trauma* patient (also known as *polytrauma*). A prehospital care provider needs to recognize and prioritize the treatment of patients with multiple injuries, following the Golden Principles of prehospital trauma care. Note, that these principles may not necessarily be performed in the exact order listed, but they must all be accomplished for optimal care of the injured patient. The Golden Principles are reviewed briefly in the following discussion. References are given to specific chapters in which each principle is more directly applied to prehospital trauma care. **Table 2-1** offers a quick reference to these principles.

1. Ensure the Safety of the Prehospital Care Providers and the Patient

Scene safety remains the highest priority on arrival to all calls for medical assistance. Prehospital care providers must develop and practice situational awareness of all scene types (**Figure 2-2**). This awareness includes not only the safety

Table 2-1 Reference Guide for the 14 Golden Principles	
Golden Principle	**Related Chapter(s)**
1. Ensure the safety of the prehospital care providers and the patient.	Chapter 5, Scene Management Chapter 16, Injury Prevention
2. Assess the scene situation to determine the need for additional resources.	Chapter 5, Scene Management Chapter 17, Disaster Management Chapter 18, Explosions and Weapons of Mass Destruction
3. Recognize the physics of trauma that produced the injuries.	Chapter 4, The Physics of Trauma
4. Use the primary survey approach to identify life-threatening conditions.	Chapter 6, Patient Assessment and Management
5. Provide appropriate airway management while maintaining cervical spine stabilization as indicated.	Chapter 7, Airway and Ventilation Chapter 8, Head Trauma Chapter 9, Spinal Trauma
6. Support ventilation and deliver oxygen to maintain an Spo_2 greater than or equal to 94%.	Chapter 7, Airway and Ventilation Chapter 8, Head Trauma
7. Control any significant external hemorrhage.	Chapter 3, Shock: Pathophysiology of Life and Death Chapter 11, Abdominal Trauma Chapter 12, Musculoskeletal Trauma Chapter 21, Wilderness Trauma Care Chapter 22, Civilian Tactical Emergency Medical Support (TEMS)
8. Provide basic shock therapy, including appropriately splinting musculoskeletal injuries and restoring and maintaining normal body temperature.	Chapter 3, Shock: Pathophysiology of Life and Death Chapter 12, Musculoskeletal Trauma Chapter 19, Environmental Trauma I: Heat and Cold Chapter 21, Wilderness Trauma Care

(continued)

Golden Principle	Related Chapter(s)
Table 2-1 Reference Guide for the 14 Golden Principles (*continued*)	
9. Maintain manual spinal stabilization until the patient is immobilized or it is clear that spinal immobilization is not necessary.	Chapter 9, Spinal Trauma
10. For critically injured trauma patients, initiate transport to the closest appropriate facility as soon as possible after EMS arrival on scene.	Chapter 6, Patient Assessment and Management Chapter 8, Head Trauma Chapter 13, Burn Injuries
11. Initiate warmed intravenous fluid replacement en route to the receiving facility.	Chapter 3, Shock: Pathophysiology of Life and Death Chapter 13, Burn Injuries
12. Ascertain the patient's medical history, and perform a secondary survey when life-threatening problems have been satisfactorily managed or have been ruled out.	Chapter 6, Patient Assessment and Management
13. Provide adequate pain relief.	Chapter 6, Patient Assessment and Management Chapter 10, Thoracic Trauma Chapter 11, Abdominal Trauma Chapter 12, Musculoskeletal Trauma Chapter 13, Burn Injuries Chapter 14, Pediatric Trauma Chapter 15, Geriatric Trauma
14. Provide thorough and accurate communication regarding the patient and the circumstances of the injury to the receiving facility.	Chapter 6, Patient Assessment and Management

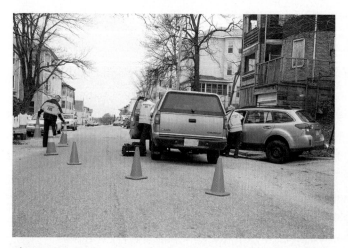

Figure 2-2 Ensure the safety of the prehospital care providers and the patient.

© Jones & Bartlett Learning. Photographed by Darren Stahlman.

of the patient but also the safety of all emergency responders. Based on information provided by dispatch, potential threats can often be anticipated before arrival at the scene. Chapters that discuss this principle include the Injury Prevention chapter and the Scene Management chapter.

2. Assess the Scene Situation to Determine the Need for Additional Resources

During the response to the scene and immediately upon arrival, prehospital care providers should perform a quick assessment to determine the need for additional or specialized resources. Examples include additional EMS units to accommodate the number of patients, fire suppression equipment, special rescue teams, power company personnel, medical helicopters, and physicians to aid in the triage of a large number of patients. The need for these resources should be anticipated and requested as soon as possible, and a designated communications channel should be secured. The Scene Management chapter discusses this principle in detail.

3. Recognize the Physics of Trauma That Produced the Injuries

The Physics of Trauma chapter provides the reader with a foundation of how kinetic energy can translate into injury to the trauma patient. As the prehospital care provider approaches the scene and the patient, he or she should be noting the physics of trauma of the situation (**Figure 2-3**). Knowledge of specific injury patterns aids in predicting injuries and knowing where to examine. Consideration of the physics of trauma should not delay the initiation of patient assessment and care but can be included in the global scene assessment and in the questions directed to the patient and bystanders. The physics of trauma may also play a key role in determining the destination facility for a given trauma patient (**Box 2-6**).

4. Use the Primary Survey to Identify Life-Threatening Conditions

This brief survey allows vital functions to be rapidly assessed and life-threatening conditions to be identified through systematic evaluation of the XABCDEs (**Box 2-7**). The primary survey involves a "treat as you go" philosophy. As life-threatening problems are identified, care is initiated at the earliest possible time, with many aspects of the primary

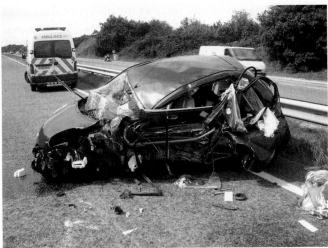

Figure 2-3 Recognize the physics of trauma that produced the injuries.
Courtesy of Dr. Mark Woolcock.

Box 2-6 Mechanism of Injury Criteria for Triage to Trauma Centers

- Falls
  - Adults: Greater than 20 feet (6.1 meters [m]) (one story is equal to 10 feet)
  - Children: Greater than 10 feet (3 m), or two or three times the child's height
- High-risk auto crash
  - Intrusion, including roof: Greater than 12 inches (0.3 m) occupant site; greater than 18 inches (0.5 m) any site
  - Ejection (partial or complete) from automobile
  - Death in same passenger compartment
  - Vehicle telemetry data consistent with a high risk of injury
  - Vehicle versus pedestrian or bicyclist who is thrown, run over, or significantly impacted (at greater than 20 miles per hour [mph])
- Motorcycle crash at greater than 20 mph

Source: Adapted from the Field Triage Decision Scheme: The National Trauma Triage Protocol, U.S. Department of Health and Human Services, Centers for Disease Control and Prevention.

Box 2-7 Critical or Potentially Critical Trauma Patient: Scene Time of 10 Minutes or Less

Presence of any of the following life-threatening conditions:

1. Inadequate or threatened airway
2. Impaired ventilation as demonstrated by any of the following:
   - Abnormally fast or slow ventilatory rate
   - Hypoxia (oxygen saturation [SpO_2] $\geq$ 94% even with supplemental oxygen)
   - Dyspnea
   - Open pneumothorax or flail chest
   - Suspected pneumothorax
   - Suspected tension pneumothorax
3. Significant external hemorrhage or suspected internal hemorrhage
4. Shock, even if compensated
5. Abnormal neurologic status
   - GCS score of 13 or less
   - Seizure activity
   - Sensory or motor deficit
6. Penetrating trauma to the head, neck, or torso, or proximal to the elbow and knee in the extremities

(continued)

Box 2-7 Critical or Potentially Critical Trauma Patient: Scene Time of 10 Minutes or Less (*continued*)

7. Amputation or near-amputation proximal to the fingers or toes
8. Any trauma in the presence of the following:
   · History of serious medical conditions (e.g., coronary artery disease, chronic obstructive pulmonary disease, bleeding disorder)
   · Age greater than 55 years
   · Children
   · Hypothermia
   · Burns
   · Pregnancy greater than 20 weeks
   · Prehospital care provider judgment of high-risk condition

survey performed simultaneously. This principle is discussed in the Patient Assessment and Management chapter.

5. Provide Appropriate Airway Management While Maintaining Cervical Spine Stabilization as Indicated

After establishing scene safety and controlling exsanguinating hemorrhage, management of the airway is the highest priority in the treatment of critically injured patients. All prehospital care providers must be able to perform the "essential skills" of airway management with ease: head and neck immobilization, manual clearing of the airway, manual maneuvers to open the airway (jaw thrust and chin lift), suctioning, and the use of oropharyngeal and nasopharyngeal airways. This principle is discussed most directly in the Airway and Ventilation chapter, but it is also a key consideration in the Head Trauma and the Spinal Trauma chapters.

6. Support Ventilation and Deliver Oxygen to Maintain an SpO$_2$ ≥ 94%

Assessment and management of ventilation is another key aspect in the management of the critically injured patient. Prehospital care providers must recognize a ventilatory rate that is too slow (bradypnea) or too fast (tachypnea) and assist ventilations with a bag-mask device connected to supplemental oxygen. Trauma patients with obvious or suspected life-threatening conditions also need supplemental oxygen management. This principle is discussed in detail in the Airway and Ventilation chapter, and it is put into action in the Head Trauma chapter.

7. Control Any Significant External Hemorrhage

In the trauma patient, significant external hemorrhage is a finding that requires immediate attention. While measures aimed at resuscitation are often the immediate priority in patient care, attempted resuscitation will never be successful in the presence of ongoing external hemorrhage. Because blood is not available for administration in the prehospital setting, hemorrhage control becomes a paramount concern for prehospital care providers in order to maintain a sufficient number of circulating RBCs; *every red blood cell counts*. Bleeding control is a recurring topic throughout this text and is particularly relevant in the Shock: Pathophysiology of Life and Death, Abdominal Trauma, Musculoskeletal Trauma, Wilderness Trauma Care, and Civilian Tactical Emergency Medical Support chapters.

8. Provide Basic Shock Therapy, Including Appropriately Splinting Musculoskeletal Injuries and Restoring and Maintaining Normal Body Temperature

Once significant external blood loss has been controlled, the prehospital care provider must consider other causes and complications relating to shock. A fracture, for example, can produce internal bleeding that cannot be observed visually and cannot be stopped through bandaging or pressure; realignment of the fractured limb may be the only means of controlling this blood loss in the prehospital setting. Severe hypothermia can ensue if the patient's body temperature is not maintained. Hypothermia drastically impairs the ability of the body's blood clotting system to achieve hemostasis. Therefore, it is important to maintain body heat through the use of blankets and restore it with resuscitation and a warmed environment inside the ambulance. The Musculoskeletal Trauma chapter discusses methods of splinting extremity injuries. Measures for keeping the patient warm and avoiding hypothermia are discussed throughout the text, but particularly relevant discussions can be found in the Environmental Trauma I: Heat and Cold and the Wilderness Trauma Care chapters.

9. Maintain Manual Spinal Stabilization Until the Patient Is Immobilized

When contact with the trauma patient is made, manual stabilization of the cervical spine should be initiated and

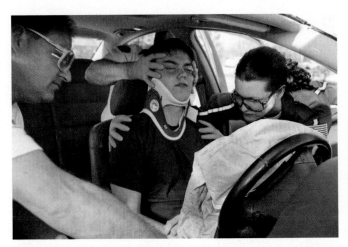

Figure 2-4 Maintain manual spinal immobilization until the patient is immobilized.
Courtesy of Rick Brady.

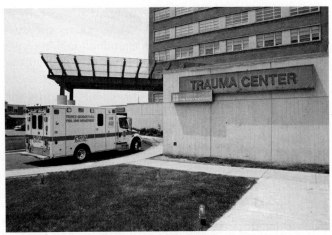

Figure 2-5 For critically injured trauma patients, initiate transport to the closest appropriate facility within 10 minutes of arrival on scene.
Courtesy of Rick Brady.

maintained until the patient is either (1) immobilized on an appropriate device or (2) deemed not to meet indications for spinal immobilization (**Figure 2-4**). See the Spinal Trauma chapter for a full discussion of the indications for and methods of spinal immobilization.

10. For Critically Injured Trauma Patients, Initiate Transport to the Closest Appropriate Facility as Soon as Possible After EMS Arrival on Scene

Patients who are critically injured (see Box 2-7) should be transported as soon as possible after EMS arrival on scene, ideally within 10 minutes, whenever possible—the "Platinum 10 Minutes" (**Figure 2-5**). Although prehospital care providers have become more proficient at airway management, ventilatory support, and administration of IV fluid therapy, most critically injured trauma patients are in hemorrhagic shock and are in need of two things that cannot be provided in the prehospital setting: (1) blood to carry oxygen and (2) plasma to provide internal clotting and control of internal hemorrhage. Prehospital care providers must keep in mind that the *closest* hospital may not be the *most appropriate* facility for many trauma patients; they must carefully consider the patient's needs and the receiving facility's capabilities to determine which destination will most promptly manage the patient's condition. Such decisions are discussed in the Patient Assessment and Management chapter. This principle applies to all trauma situations and is well illustrated in the Head Trauma and the Burn Injuries chapters.

11. Initiate Warmed Intravenous Fluid Replacement en Route to the Receiving Facility

Initiation of transport of a critically injured trauma patient should never be delayed simply to insert IV catheters and administer fluid therapy. Although crystalloid solutions do restore lost blood volume and improve perfusion, they do not transport oxygen. Additionally, restoring normal blood pressure may result in additional hemorrhage from clot disruption in damaged blood vessels that initially clotted off, thereby increasing patient mortality. Thus, the priority, as discussed in the preceding principle, is to deliver the patient to a facility that can meet his or her needs. Nonetheless, administration of crystalloid solution, preferably lactated Ringer solution, can be valuable. For example, warmed solution is given to aid in the prevention of hypothermia. While fluid administration can come into play in nearly any trauma scenario, the Shock: Pathophysiology of Life and Death and the Burn Injuries chapters demonstrate this principle in action.

12. Ascertain the Patient's Medical History and Perform a Secondary Survey When Life-Threatening Problems Have Been Satisfactorily Managed or Have Been Ruled Out

If life-threatening conditions are found in the primary survey, key interventions should be performed and the patient transported within the Platinum 10 Minutes.

However, if life-threatening conditions are not identified, a secondary survey is performed. The secondary survey is a systematic, head-to-toe physical examination that serves to identify all injuries. A SAMPLE history (**s**ymptoms, **a**llergies, **m**edications, **p**ast medical history, **l**ast meal, **e**vents preceding the injury) is also obtained during the secondary survey.

The patient's airway, respiratory, and circulatory status along with vital signs should be reassessed frequently because patients who initially present without life-threatening injuries may subsequently develop them. This principle is discussed in the Patient Assessment and Management chapter.

13. Provide Adequate Pain Relief

Patients who have sustained serious injury typically will experience significant pain. It was once thought that providing pain relief would mask the patient's symptoms and impair the ability of the trauma team to adequately assess the patient after arrival to the hospital. Numerous studies have shown that this is, in fact, not the case. Prehospital care providers should provide analgesics to relieve pain as long as no contraindications exist. The principle of pain management is discussed in the Patient Assessment and Management chapter, and it is applied in nearly every chapter of this text. As discussed in the Pediatric Trauma and the Geriatric Trauma chapters, although pain management is different in some patient populations, it should not be withheld on the basis of the patient's age.

14. Provide Thorough and Accurate Communication Regarding the Patient and the Circumstances of the Injury to the Receiving Facility

Communication about a trauma patient with the receiving hospital involves three components:

- Prearrival warning
- Verbal report upon arrival
- Written documentation of the encounter in the patient care report (PCR)

Care of the trauma patient is a team effort. The response to a critical trauma patient begins with the prehospital care provider and continues in the hospital. Delivering information from the prehospital setting to the receiving hospital allows for notification and mobilization of appropriate hospital resources to ensure an optimal reception of the patient. Methods of ensuring effective communication with the receiving facility are discussed in the Patient Assessment and Management chapter and apply to all patient care encounters.

Research

While historically there has been a lack of meaningful research specific to prehospital care, in recent years, that has started to change. Many of the established prehospital standards of care are being challenged by evidence-based research. For example, tourniquets are no longer considered a tool of last resort, and advanced airways are increasingly contraindicated in the prehospital setting. While some of the literature is controversial, prehospital care is ever-changing secondary to evidence-based medicine for the best interest of the patient. Throughout this text, the evidence from these studies is described and discussed to enable you to make the best choices for your patients based on your knowledge, training, skills, and resources.

Reading the EMS Literature

A major goal of PHTLS has been to ensure that the practice recommendations presented in this text accurately represent the best medical evidence available at the time of publication. PHTLS began this process with the sixth edition and has continued it with subsequent editions. We continue to add, as References and Suggested Readings, those manuscripts, sources, and resources that are fundamental to the topics covered and the recommendations made in each chapter. (See the Suggested Readings at the end of this chapter for further information on evaluating EMS literature.) Every medical practitioner and health care provider should obtain, read, and critically evaluate the publications and sources that make up the basis for all of the components of daily practice.

To make optimal use of available reference material, an understanding of exactly what constitutes medical literature and of how to interpret the various sources of information is essential. In many cases the first source that is accessed for information about a particular topic is a medical textbook. As our level of interest and sophistication grows, a search is undertaken to find the specific references that represent the source of the information communicated in those textbook chapters or to find what, if any, primary research studies have been performed and published. Then, after reviewing and analyzing the various sources, a decision can be made about the quality and strength of the evidence that will guide our decision making and patient care interventions.

Types of Evidence

There are a number of different systems for rating the quality and strength of medical evidence. Regardless of the exact rating system used, several common assessments can be found among them. The process of evaluation begins by reading the "methods" section of the article to determine what study type is being reported. The study type alone has important implications in terms of the strength of the recommendations in the conclusion of the study.

The highest quality source that leads to the strongest recommendation about the treatment under study is the randomized, double-blinded controlled trial. Studies of this type are usually referred to as Class I evidence. This type of study is considered the best type of study because (1) all patients entered into the study are randomized (meaning each patient has an equal chance of assignment to whatever type of treatment is being studied) and (2) neither the researchers nor the patients know which type of treatment the subject is receiving (double blinding). These factors minimize the chances of any bias affecting the results or interpretation of the results.

Class II evidence generally includes the other types of studies that can be found in the medical literature, including nonrandomized, nonblinded studies, retrospective case-control series, and cohort studies.

Finally, Class III evidence consists of case studies, case reports, consensus documents, textbook material, and medical opinion. Class III evidence is the weakest source of evidence, although often the easiest to obtain.

Unfortunately, if the literature related to prehospital care is critically reviewed, the majority of the published research qualifies as Class III evidence. There has been remarkably little research that would qualify as Class I. Much of the practice of medicine that has been applied to the prehospital setting has been adopted from and adapted to the out-of-hospital environment from the in-hospital delivery of emergency care. The result is that most of the prehospital care provided today is based on Class III evidence. However, more and more Class I and II studies related to prehospital care are being conducted. Class I studies are limited by rigid informed-consent regulations. Specifically, with few exceptions, the medical practice of prehospital care is based on "expert" opinion usually found in textbook chapters. The credentials and qualifications of the individual offering that opinion vary.

Recently, consensus has been building to use a formal system for grading the quality of evidence and the strength of a resulting clinical practice recommendation.[16-18] Several different grading systems have been developed; however, no one has been shown to be better than another.

Steps in Evaluation

Every medical practitioner should read medical literature and critically evaluate every study published that might alter treatment decisions in order to distinguish useful information and therapy from that which is useless or potentially even harmful. How, then, do you go about reading and critically evaluating medical literature?

The first step in this process is to develop a list of journals that will form the foundation of a regular medical literature review. This list should comprise not only those journals with the desired specialty in their name but also those publications that address related specialties or topics

and have a high likelihood of also publishing applicable studies (**Box 2-8**).

An alternative to reviewing multiple journals is to perform a computerized medical literature search if there is a particular topic of interest. The use of computerized search engines such as PubMed or Ovid allows the computer to search a massive database of many medical journals and automatically develop a list of suggested studies and publications (**Box 2-9**).

Narrow the Selection

The next step is to review the title of every article in the table of contents of each of the selected journals to narrow down the article choices to those that clearly relate to the topic of interest. It would be impossible to read each of the selected journals from cover to cover; nor is it necessary.

Box 2-8 Suggested Journals for Review

- *Academic Emergency Medicine*
- *American Journal of Emergency Medicine*
- *Annals of Emergency Medicine*
- *Journal of Emergency Medicine*
- *Journal of Special Operations Medicine*
- *Journal of Trauma and Acute Care Surgery*
- *Prehospital Emergency Care*

Box 2-9 Performing a Computerized Literature Search

PubMed can be accessed through the National Library of Medicine website at the following address: www.ncbi.nlm.nih.gov/pubmed. To perform a journal search for articles and studies, it is necessary to enter search terms (also known as keywords) into PubMed to find appropriate articles. The more specific you can be with the terms, the more likely you are to find articles that will meet your needs. However, being too specific can occasionally exclude articles that might be of interest to you. Therefore, a good strategy is to first conduct a search using very specific terms and then do a follow-up search with more generic terms. For example, if you are interested in finding articles about cricothyroidotomy in the prehospital setting, the initial search you perform might be done using the terms "cricothyroidotomy" and "prehospital." The next search might be performed using the terms "airway management" and "emergency medical services," recognizing that "airway management" may yield articles that include not only cricothyroidotomy but other forms of airway management as well.

By reviewing the table of contents, articles that are of no interest can be immediately dismissed.

Once the selection has been narrowed, there are still a number of preliminary actions to take before reading the text of the article. Look at the article's list of authors to see if any are already known for their work in this area. Next, read the summary or abstract of the article to see if this overview of the article fulfills the expectations generated when the title was first reviewed. Then, review the site where the study was conducted to assess the similarities, differences, and applicability to the setting in which the results of the study may subsequently be applied. Reading an abstract alone is not enough. It serves only as the window to determine whether or not to read the full article.

Read and Assess

Once these initial points have been evaluated, read the full text of the article and critically evaluate it. In doing so, consider several specific issues. The first issue is to determine the study design. You should understand whether the study is a randomized controlled trial, a cohort design, or some other study design.

Next, determine the patient population entered into the study to understand the similarities or differences to the patient population you are interested in treating. To do so, adequate information must be provided in the text describing the clinical and sociodemographic makeup of the study population. Ideally, studies that will be used to alter the care provided in the prehospital setting should have been performed in the prehospital setting.

The next issue for consideration is the outcome measure selected. All outcomes that are clinically relevant should have been considered and reported in the study. For example, cardiac arrest studies may describe such endpoints as cardiac rhythm conversion, return of spontaneous circulation, survival to hospital admission, or survival to discharge from the hospital.

Analysis of the results section also requires critical review. Just as it is important to evaluate the study population and inclusion criteria, it is equally important to see if all patients entered into the study at the beginning are accounted for at the end of the study. Specifically, the authors should describe any criteria used to exclude patients from the study analysis. Simple calculation by the reader of the various treatment groups or subgroups will quickly confirm if all patients were accounted for. The authors should also describe occurrences that might introduce bias into the results. For example, the authors should report mishaps such as control patients accidentally receiving the treatment or study patients receiving other diagnostics or interventions.

In addition, the clinical, as well as the statistical, significance of the results are important to consider. Although the statistical analyses may be difficult to understand, a basic comprehension of statistical test selection and utilization will validate the statistical tests performed. Equal to and perhaps more important than the statistical significance of a result is the clinical significance of the reported result. For example, in evaluating the effect of a new antihypertensive medication, the statistical analysis may show that the new drug causes a statistically significant decrease in blood pressure of 4 mm Hg. Clinically, however, the reported decrease is unimportant. Thus, the prehospital care provider must evaluate not only the statistical significance of the result but also its clinical importance.

If all of the prior issues have been answered satisfactorily, the last issue relates to the implementation of the study results and conclusion in the reader's health care system. To determine the practicality of applying the therapy, the authors need to describe the treatment in sufficient detail, the intervention or therapy must be available for use, and it must be clinically sensible in the planned setting.

Some differences exist in the evaluation of consensus statements, overviews, and textbook chapters. Ideally, the statement or overview should address a specific, focused question. The authors should describe the criteria used to select the articles included as references, and the reader will determine the appropriateness of these criteria. This in turn will help determine the likelihood that important studies were included and not missed. In addition, the reference list should be reviewed for known studies that should have been included.

A high-quality overview or consensus statement will include a discussion of the process by which the validity of the included studies was appraised. The validity assessment should be reproducible regardless of who actually performed the appraisal. Also, multiple studies with similar results help support the conclusions and ultimate decision about whether or not to change current practice.

Similar to the review of individual studies, the review and assessment of consensus statements, overviews, and textbook chapters include a determination of whether all clinically relevant outcomes were considered and discussed and whether the results can be applied to the reader's patient population. This determination also includes an analysis of the benefits versus the potential risks and harm.

Determine the Impact

The final step in evaluation is to determine when a publication should cause a change in daily medical practice. Ideally, any change in medical practice will result from studies of the highest quality, specifically a meta-analysis of randomized, controlled, double-blinded studies. The conclusion of that analysis will be based on results that have been critically evaluated, have both statistical and clinical significance, and have been reviewed and judged to be valid. The analysis should be the best information currently available on the issue. In addition, the change in practice must be feasible for the system planning to make the change, and the benefit of making the change must outweigh the risks.

SUMMARY

- Principles (or the *science* of medicine) define the duties required of the prehospital care provider in optimizing patient survival and outcome.
- Preferences (or the *art* of medicine) are the methods of achieving the principle. Considerations for choosing the method include the following:
  - Situation that currently exists
  - Condition of the patient
  - Knowledge and experience
  - Equipment available
- Critical thinking in medicine is a process in which the health care provider assesses the situation, the patient, and the resources. This information is rapidly analyzed and combined to provide the best care possible to the patient.
- There are four principles of biomedical ethics (autonomy, nonmaleficence, beneficence, and justice). Prehospital professionals must develop ethical reasoning skills necessary to manage ethical conflict in the prehospital environment.
- The following are the Golden Principles of prehospital trauma care:
  1. Ensure the safety of the prehospital care providers and the patient.
  2. Assess the scene situation to determine the need for additional resources.
  3. Recognize the physics of trauma that produced the injuries.
  4. Use the primary survey approach to identify life-threatening conditions.
  5. Provide appropriate airway management while maintaining cervical spine stabilization as indicated.
  6. Support ventilation and deliver oxygen to maintain an SpO_2 greater than or equal to 94%.
  7. Control any significant external hemorrhage.
  8. Provide basic shock therapy, including appropriately splinting musculoskeletal injuries and restoring and maintaining normal body temperature.
  9. Maintain manual spinal stabilization until the patient is immobilized or it is clear that spinal immobilization is not necessary.
  10. For critically injured trauma patients, initiate transport to the closest appropriate facility as soon as possible after EMS arrival on scene.
  11. Initiate warmed intravenous fluid replacement en route to the receiving facility.
  12. Ascertain the patient's medical history and perform a secondary survey when life-threatening problems have been satisfactorily managed or have been ruled out.
  13. Provide adequate pain relief.
  14. Provide thorough and accurate communication regarding the patient and the circumstances of the injury to the receiving facility.
- Research provides the foundation and basis for all medical practice, including prehospital care.
- The quality of research and the strength of the conclusions and recommendations vary depending on the type of study.
- Everyone who reads medical literature should know how to assess the type and quality of the study being read.

SCENARIO RECAP

You and your partner arrive at the scene of a two-vehicle T-bone collision. You are currently the only available unit. In a pickup truck, there is a young unrestrained male driver who smells strongly of alcohol and has an obvious forearm deformity. The truck struck the passenger's side front door of a small passenger sedan, with significant intrusion into the passenger compartment. There is an elderly female in the front passenger seat who does not appear to be breathing; the windshield is starred directly in front of her. The female driver of the sedan is also injured but conscious and extremely anxious. In the rear seats, there are two children restrained in car seats. The child on the passenger side appears to be approximately 3 years old and is unconscious and slumped over in the car seat. On the driver's side, a restrained 5-year-old boy is crying hysterically in a booster seat and appears to be uninjured.

(continued)

SCENARIO RECAP (CONTINUED)

The driver of the pickup truck is obviously injured with an open arm fracture, but he is belligerent and verbally abusive and is refusing treatment. Meanwhile, the driver of the sedan is frantically inquiring about her children and her mother.

- How would you manage this multiple-patient incident?
- Which of these patients is of highest priority?
- What would you tell the mother of the two children about their condition?
- How would you deal with the apparently intoxicated driver of the other vehicle?
- Would you allow the apparently intoxicated driver to refuse care?

SCENARIO SOLUTION

In this five-victim scenario, your ambulance crew, having no assistance available, faces a triage situation with the patients outnumbering the prehospital care providers. It is in this type of triage situation that the concept of justice becomes immediately applicable. Your available resources—two providers—are limited and must be distributed in a manner that will do the greatest good for the greatest number of people. This involves deciding who is treated first and by which provider.

In this scenario, a rapid decision must be made regarding whether to treat the older woman or the unconscious child first. Frequently a child has a higher likelihood of survival than an older adult when both patients have suffered similar traumatic injuries. However, additional assessment and medical history may change the clinical picture and the appropriateness of triaging decisions. For example, the mother may report that the unconscious minor child has a terminal condition, so making a triage decision based solely on age may not be the *just* action in this instance. While triage protocols generally provide direction in such situations and are based on concepts of justice, triage protocols cannot account for every unique situation encountered. Therefore, a basic understanding of the principle of justice can be helpful for situations in which "in the moment" triage decisions need to be made.

The appearance of the driver and his truck may lead to stereotyping behaviors and judgments on the part of the prehospital care providers. Stereotypes are inaccurate, simplistic generalizations or beliefs about a group of people that allow others to categorize the people and treat them based on those beliefs. Preconceived notions about a patient's appearance and behaviors can interfere with fair and equitable treatment.

While there is a duty to treat patients in a fair and consistent manner, prehospital care providers are a valuable resource and have no obligation to put themselves at undue risk. Providers have the right not only to protect themselves but also to protect their ability to care for others.

In addition to justice concerns, there are several challenges to autonomy raised by this scenario. You must assess the decision-making capacity of both the driver of the pickup truck and the female driver of the car. Both drivers are injured and emotionally distraught, and the male driver is potentially impaired by an intoxicant. Furthermore, the female driver may be asked to make medical decisions for herself and to act as a surrogate decision maker for her two children and her mother. If, upon assessing the decision-making capacity of the two drivers, you were to determine that either of the drivers is incapacitated, then you would proceed with providing emergency medical care based on established clinical protocols and the best interests of the patients.

The balancing of risks and benefits is an important part of medical decision making. In this case, the female driver is requesting information about her mother and children. While you have an obligation to tell the truth, both to establish patient–provider trust and to help the driver to make informed consent decisions for the incapacitated occupants of her vehicle, you must bear in mind that this patient may be injured and is likely traumatized, with the possibility of impairment and lack of capacity to make decisions. A full and truthful disclosure about the conditions of her mother and unconscious child may further traumatize her or cause harm.

SCENARIO SOLUTION (CONTINUED)

Her potential reactions to such information may further impair her decision-making capacity and could be upsetting to her 5-year-old child, who is conscious and already hysterical. Depending on the potential level of harm or burden that an action may cause—in this case, telling the female driver about the conditions of her loved ones—the principles of nonmaleficence and beneficence may allow you to postpone full disclosure until the patient is in a more stable environment.

As is clear in this scenario, ethics rarely gives black-and-white solutions to difficult situations. Rather, ethics can provide a framework, such as the four principles discussed in this chapter—autonomy, nonmaleficence, beneficence, and justice—in which to consider and reason through ethically difficult situations in an attempt to do the right thing.

References

1. Hendricson WD, Andrieu SC, Chadwick DG, et al. Educational strategies associated with development of problem-solving, critical thinking, and self-directed learning. *J Dent Educ.* 2006;70(9):925-936.
2. Cotter AJ. Developing critical-thinking skills. *EMS Mag.* 2007;36(7):86.
3. Carroll RT. *Becoming a Critical Thinker: A Guide for the New Millennium.* 2nd ed. Boston, MA: Pearson Custom Publishing; 2005.
4. Beauchamp TL, Childress JF. *Principles of Biomedical Ethics.* 6th ed. New York, NY: Oxford University Press; 2009.
5. Banning M. Measures that can be used to instill critical-thinking skills in nurse prescribers. *Nurse Educ Pract.* 2006;6(2):98-105.
6. Bamonti A, Heilicser B, Stotts K. To treat or not to treat: identifying ethical dilemmas in EMS. *JEMS.* 2001;26(3):100-107.
7. Derse AR. Autonomy and informed consent. In: Iserson KV, Sanders AB, Mathieu D, eds. *Ethics in Emergency Medicine.* 2nd ed. Tucson, AZ: Galen Press; 1995:99-105.
8. Post LF, Bluestein J, Dubler NN. *Handbook for Health Care Ethics Committees.* Baltimore, MD: The Johns Hopkins University Press; 2007.
9. New York State Department of Health. Medical orders for life-sustaining treatment (MOLST): frequently asked questions (FAQs). http://www.compassionandsupport.org/pdfs/professionals/training/Newest_MOLST_FAQs.pdf. Published December 2008. Accessed October 26, 2017.
10. Daniels N. *Just Health Care.* New York, NY: Cambridge University Press; 1985.
11. University of Maryland Medical Center. History of the Shock Trauma Center: tribute to R Adams Cowley, MD. http://umm.edu/programs/shock-trauma/about/history. Updated December 16, 2013. Accessed October 26, 2017.
12. Lerner EB, Moscati RM. The Golden Hour: scientific fact or medical "urban legend"? *Acad Emerg Med.* 2001; 8:758.
13. Tsybuliak GN, Pavlenko EP. Cause of death in the early post-traumatic period. *Vestn Khir Im I I Grek.* 1975;114(5):75.
14. Gunst M, Ghaemmaghami V, Gruszecki A, Urban J, Frankel H, Shafi S. Changing epidemiology of trauma deaths leads to a bimodal distribution. *Proc (Bayl Univ Med Cent).* 2010;23(4):349-354.
15. Sobrino J, Shafi S. Timing and causes of death after injuries. *Proc (Bayl Univ Med Cent).* 2013;26(2):120-123.
16. Guyatt GH, Oxman AD, Vist G, et al. Rating quality of evidence and strength of recommendations GRADE: an emerging consensus on rating quality of evidence and strength of recommendations. *BMJ.* 2008;336:924.
17. Spaite D. Prehospital evidence-based guidelines (presentation). From Evidence to EMS Practice: Building the National Model, a Consensus-Building Conference sponsored by the National Highway Traffic Safety Administration, the Federal Interagency Committee on EMS and the National EMS Advisory Council. September 2008.
18. Atkins D, Best D, Briss PA, et al. Grading quality of evidence and strength of recommendations (GRADE). *BMJ.* 2004;328:1490.

Suggested Reading

Adams JG, Arnold R, Siminoff L, Wolfson AB. Ethical conflicts in the prehospital setting. *Ann Emerg Med.* 1992;21(10):1259.

Beauchamp TL, Childress JF. *Principles of Biomedical Ethics.* 7th ed. New York, NY: Oxford University Press; 2013.

Buchanan AE, Brock DW. *Deciding for Others: The Ethics of Surrogate Decision Making.* New York, NY: Cambridge University Press; 1990.

Fitzgerald DJ, Milzman DP, Sulmasy DP. Creating a dignified option: ethical consideration in the formulation of prehospital DNR protocol. *Am J Emerg Med.* 1995;13(2):223.

Iverson KV. Foregoing prehospital care: should ambulance staff always resuscitate? *J Med Ethics.* 1991;17:19.

Iverson KV. Withholding and withdrawing medical treatment: an emergency medicine perspective. *Ann Emerg Med.* 1996;28(1):51.

Marco CA, Schears RM. Prehospital resuscitation practices: a survey of prehospital providers. *Ethics Emerg Med.* 2003;24(1):101.

Mohr M, Kettler D. Ethical aspects of prehospital CPR. *Acta Anaesthesiol Scand Suppl.* 1997;111:298-301.

Sandman L, Nordmark A. Ethical conflict in prehospital emergency care. *Nurs Ethics.* 2006;13(6):592.

Travers DA, Mears G. Physicians' experiences with prehospital do-not-resuscitate orders in North Carolina. *Prehosp Disaster Med.* 1996;11(2):91.

Van Vleet LM. Between black and white. The gray area of ethics in EMS. *JEMS.* 2006;31(10):55-56, 58-63; quiz 64-65.

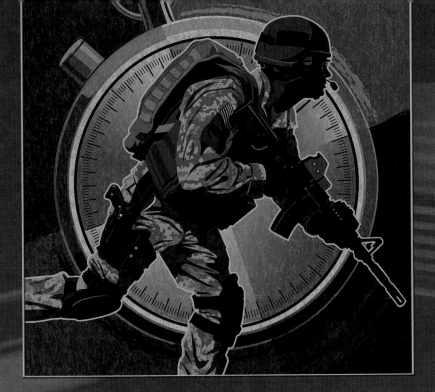

DIVISION **2**

Assessment and Management

CHAPTER 3

Shock: Pathophysiology of Life and Death

Lead Editors:
Craig Manifold, DO, FACEP, FAAEM
Heidi Abraham, MD, EMT-B, EMT-T, FAEMS

CHAPTER OBJECTIVES

At the completion of this chapter, you will be able to do the following:

- Define shock.
- Explain how preload, afterload, and contractility affect cardiac output.
- Classify shock on an etiologic basis.
- Explain the pathophysiology of shock and its progression through phases.
- Relate shock to acid–base status, energy production, etiology, prevention, and treatment.
- Describe the physical findings in shock.
- Clinically differentiate the types of shock.

- Discuss the limitations of the field management of shock.
- Recognize the need for rapid transport and early definitive management in various forms of shock.
- Apply principles of management of shock in the trauma patient.
- Describe the Fick principle.
- Discuss limitations of anaerobic metabolism in meeting cellular demands.

SCENARIO

You and your partner are dispatched to a 65-year-old man who fell approximately 8 feet (2.4 m) while working on his outdoor patio. Upon your arrival, you find the patient lying supine on the ground in moderate distress with chief complaints of lower back, sacral, and left hip pain.

Physical examination of the patient shows pale skin color, diaphoresis, decreased peripheral pulses and an unstable pelvis. The patient is alert and oriented. His vital signs are as follows: pulse 100 beats/minute, blood pressure 78/56 millimeters of mercury (mm Hg), oxygen saturation (SpO_2) 92% on room air, and respiratory rate 20 breaths/minute, regular and clear bilaterally.

- What possible injuries do you expect to see after this type of fall?
- How would you manage these injuries in the field?
- What are the major pathologic processes occurring in this patient?
- How will you correct the pathophysiology causing this patient's presentation?
- You are working for a rural EMS system approximately 30 to 45 minutes from the nearest trauma center. How does this factor alter your management plans?

INTRODUCTION

Shock was described by 19th-century doctor John Collins Warren as "a momentary pause in the act of death."[1] In 1872, it was described by surgeon Samuel Gross as a "rude unhinging of the machinery of life."[2] Though it has not always been discussed in the most concrete medical terms, shock following trauma has been recognized for more than three centuries and continues to play a central role in the causes of major morbidity and mortality in the trauma patient. Prompt diagnosis, resuscitation, and definitive management of shock resulting from trauma are essential in determining patient outcome.

Life depends on the complex interrelationship and interdependence of several body systems working together to ensure the necessary elements to sustain cellular energy production and vital metabolic processes are supplied and delivered to every cell in every organ of the body. The respiratory system, beginning with the airway and progressing to the alveoli of the lungs, and the circulatory system are crucial systems that function together to provide and distribute the crucial component of cellular energy production: oxygen. Anything that interferes with the ability of the body to provide oxygen to the red blood cells of the circulatory system or that affects the delivery of oxygenated red blood cells to the tissues of the body will lead to cell death and ultimately patient death if not corrected promptly.

The assessment and management of the trauma patient begin with the primary survey, which is focused on the identification and correction of problems affecting or interfering with the critical function of the delivery of oxygen to every cell in the body. Thus, an understanding of the physiology of life and pathophysiology that can lead to death is essential for the prehospital care provider if abnormalities are to be identified and addressed.

In the prehospital setting, the therapeutic challenge posed by the patient in shock is compounded by the need to assess and manage such patients in a relatively austere, and sometimes dangerous, environment in which sophisticated diagnostic and management tools are either unavailable or impractical to apply. This chapter focuses on the causes of traumatic shock and describes the pathophysiologic changes present to help direct management strategies.

Physiology of Shock

Metabolism

Cells maintain their normal metabolic functions by producing and using energy in the form of adenosine triphosphate (ATP). The most efficient method of generating this needed energy is via *aerobic metabolism*. The cells take in oxygen and glucose and metabolize them through a complicated physiologic process that produces energy, along with the by-products of water and carbon dioxide.

Anaerobic metabolism, in contrast to aerobic metabolism, occurs without the use of oxygen. It is the backup power system in the body and uses stored body fat as its energy source. Unfortunately, anaerobic metabolism can run only for a short time, it produces significantly less energy, it produces by-products such as lactic acid that are harmful to the body, and it may ultimately become irreversible. However, it may afford enough energy to power the cells for long enough to allow the body to restore its normal metabolism, with the assistance of the prehospital care provider.

If anaerobic metabolism is not reversed quickly, cells cannot continue to function and will die. If a sufficient number of cells in any one organ die, the entire organ ceases to function. When organs die, the patient eventually may die.

The sensitivity of cells to the lack of oxygen varies from organ system to organ system. This sensitivity is called ischemic (lack of oxygen) sensitivity, and it is greatest in the brain, heart, and lungs. It may take only 4 to 6 minutes of anaerobic metabolism before one or more of these vital organs are injured beyond repair. Skin and muscle tissue have a significantly longer ischemic sensitivity—as long as 4 to 6 hours. The abdominal organs generally fall between these two groups and are able to survive 45 to 90 minutes of anaerobic metabolism (**Table 3-1**).

Maintenance of normal function of the cells depends on the crucial relationship and interaction of several body systems. The patient's airway must be patent, and respirations must be of adequate volume and depth (see the Airway and Ventilation chapter). The heart must be functioning and pumping normally. The circulatory system must have enough red blood cells (RBCs) available to deliver adequate amounts of oxygen to tissue cells throughout the body, so these cells can produce energy.

Prehospital assessment and treatment of the trauma patient are directed at preventing or reversing anaerobic metabolism, thus avoiding cellular death and, ultimately, patient death. Ensuring that critical systems of the body are working together correctly—namely, that the patient's

Table 3-1 Organ Tolerance to Ischemia	
Organ	**Warm Ischemia Time**
Heart, brain, lungs	4–6 minutes
Kidneys, liver, gastrointestinal tract	45–90 minutes
Muscle, bone, skin	4–6 hours

Source: Modified from American College of Surgeons (ACS) Committee on Trauma. *Advanced Trauma Life Support for Doctors: Student Course Manual.* 7th ed. Chicago, IL: ACS; 2004.

airway is patent and that breathing and circulation are adequate—is the major emphasis of the primary survey. These functions are managed in the trauma patient by the following actions:

- Maintaining an adequate airway and ventilation, thus providing adequate oxygen to the RBCs (see the Airway and Ventilation chapter)
- Assisting ventilation with judicious use of supplemental oxygen
- Maintaining adequate circulation, thus perfusing tissue cells with oxygenated blood

Definition of Shock

The major complication of disruption of the normal physiology of life is known as *shock*. Shock is a state of change in cellular function from aerobic metabolism to anaerobic metabolism secondary to hypoperfusion of the tissue cells. As a result, the delivery of oxygen at the cellular level is inadequate to meet the body's metabolic needs. Shock is not defined as low blood pressure, rapid pulse rate, or cool, clammy skin; these are merely systemic manifestations of the entire pathologic process called shock. The correct definition of shock is insufficient tissue perfusion (oxygenation) at the cellular level, leading to anaerobic metabolism and loss of energy production needed to support life. Based on this definition, shock can be classified in terms of cellular perfusion and oxygenation. Understanding the cellular changes arising from this state of hypoperfusion, as well as the endocrine, microvascular, cardiovascular, tissue, and end-organ effects, will assist in directing treatment strategies.

Understanding this process is key to assisting the body in restoring aerobic metabolism and energy production. If the prehospital care provider is to understand this abnormal condition and be able to develop a treatment plan to prevent or reverse shock, it is important that he or she knows and understands what is happening to the body at a cellular level. The normal physiologic responses that the body uses to protect itself from the development of shock must be understood, recognized, and interpreted. Only then can a rational approach for managing the problems of the patient in shock be developed.

Shock can kill a patient in the field, the emergency department (ED), the operating room (OR), or the intensive care unit. Although actual physical death may be delayed for several hours or even several weeks, the most common cause of death is the failure of early and adequate resuscitation from shock. The lack of perfusion of cells by oxygenated blood results in anaerobic metabolism, the death of cells, and decreased energy production. Even when some cells in an organ are initially spared, death can occur later, because the remaining cells are unable to carry out the organ's functions indefinitely. The following section explains this phenomenon. Understanding this process is key to assisting the body in restoring aerobic metabolism and energy production.

Physiology of Shock

Metabolism: The Human Motor

The human body consists of over 100 million cells. Each one of these cells requires energy to function and glucose and oxygen to produce that energy. The cells take in oxygen and metabolize it through a complicated physiologic process, producing energy. At the same time, the metabolism of the cell requires energy, and cells must have fuel—glucose—to carry out this process. Each molecule of glucose yields 38 energy-storing ATP molecules when oxygen is available. As in any combustion event, a by-product is also produced. In the body, oxygen and glucose are metabolized to produce energy, with water and carbon dioxide as by-products.

The cellular metabolic process is similar to what occurs in a motor vehicle engine when gasoline and air are mixed and burned to produce energy and carbon monoxide is created as the by-product. The motor moves the car, the heater warms the driver, and the electricity generated is used for the headlights, all powered by the burning gasoline and air mixture in the vehicle's engine.

The same is true of the human motor. Aerobic metabolism is the main "driving" system, with anaerobic metabolism as the backup system. Unfortunately, it is not a strong backup. It produces much less energy than aerobic metabolism, and it cannot produce energy for a long period of time. In fact, anaerobic metabolism produces only two ATP molecules, a 19-fold decrease in energy. However, it can assist with survival for a short time while the body repairs itself with the assistance of the prehospital care provider.

As a comparison, alternate fuel sources are available in hybrid motor vehicles; it is possible to drive a hybrid car powered only by its battery and electric starting motor if air and gasoline are not available. The hybrid car will move as long as the energy stored in the battery lasts. This movement is slower and less efficient than that powered by gasoline and air; however, the battery is able to keep the car running until it is quickly drained of its power by running all of the systems in the car, a task it was not designed to do for long periods.

In the body, the problems with using anaerobic metabolism to provide power are similar to the disadvantages of solely using a battery to run an automobile: It can run only for a short time, it does not produce as much energy, it produces by-products that are harmful to the body, and it may ultimately be irreversible.

The major by-product of anaerobic metabolism is excessive amounts of acid. If anaerobic metabolism is not reversed quickly, cells cannot continue to function in the increasingly acidic environment, and without adequate energy, they will die. If a sufficient number of cells in any one organ die, the entire organ ceases to function. If a large number of cells in an organ die, the organ's function will be significantly reduced, and the remaining cells in that organ will have to work even harder to keep the organ functioning. These overworked cells may or may not be able to continue to support the function of the entire organ, and the organ may still die.

A classic example is a patient who has suffered a heart attack. Blood flow and oxygen are cut off to one portion of the myocardium (heart muscle), and some cells of the heart die. The loss of these cells impairs cardiac function, thus decreasing cardiac output and the oxygen supply to the rest of the heart. This in turn causes a further reduction in the oxygenation of the remaining heart cells. If not enough cells remain viable or if the remaining cells are not strong enough to ensure the heart can continue to meet the body's blood flow needs, then heart failure can result. Unless major improvement in cardiac output occurs, the patient will not survive.

Another example of this deadly process occurs in the kidneys. When the kidneys are injured or are deprived of adequate oxygenated blood, some of the kidney cells begin to die and kidney function decreases. Other cells may be compromised yet continue to function for a while before they, too, die. If enough kidney cells die, the decreased level of kidney function results in the inadequate elimination of the toxic by-products of metabolism. The increased level of toxins further exacerbates cell death throughout the body. If this systemic deterioration continues, more cells and organs will die, and eventually the entire organism (the human) dies.

Depending on the organ initially involved, the progression from cell death to organism death can be rapid or delayed. It can take as little as 4 to 6 minutes or as long as 2 or 3 weeks before the damage caused by hypoxia or hypoperfusion in the first minutes post trauma results in the patient's death. The effectiveness of the prehospital care provider's actions to reverse or prevent hypoxia and hypoperfusion in the critical prehospital period may not be immediately apparent. However, these resuscitation measures are unquestionably necessary if the patient is to ultimately survive. These initial actions are a critical component of the Golden Hour of trauma care described by R Adams Cowley, MD, and now often called the Golden Period because we know that the literal time frame within which critical abnormalities can be corrected is more variable than that conveyed by the figurative concept of the Golden Hour.

Long-term survival of the individual organs and the body as a whole requires delivery of the two most important nutrients (oxygen and glucose) to the tissue cells. Other nutrients are important, but because the resupply of these other materials is not a component of the prehospital emergency medical services (EMS) system, they are not discussed here. Although these factors are important, they are beyond the scope of the prehospital care provider's practice and resources. The most important supply item is oxygen.

The Fick Principle

The Fick principle is a description of the components necessary for oxygenation of the cells in the body. Simply stated, these three components are as follows:

1. On-loading of oxygen to RBCs in the lung
2. Delivery of RBCs to tissue cells
3. Off-loading of oxygen from RBCs to tissue cells

A crucial part of this process is that the patient must have enough RBCs available to deliver adequate amounts of oxygen to tissue cells throughout the body so cells can produce energy. Additionally, the patient's airway must be patent, and respirations must be of adequate volume and depth for oxygen to reach the lungs and RBCs. (See the Airway and Ventilation chapter.)

This process is influenced by the acid–base status of the patient at the time of treatment. You may have a patient adequately ventilating and on supplemental oxygen with good saturation who is nonetheless deteriorating secondary to inability to off-load oxygen at the cellular level because of hypothermia. The prehospital treatment of shock is directed at ensuring that critical components of the Fick principle are maintained, with the goal of preventing or reversing anaerobic metabolism, and thus avoiding cellular death and, ultimately, organ death leading to patient death. These components are the major emphasis of the primary survey performed by the prehospital care provider and are implemented in the management of the trauma patient by the following actions:

- Controlling exsanguinating extremity hemorrhage
- Maintaining an adequate airway and ventilation, thus providing adequate oxygen to the RBCs
- Using supplemental oxygen as part of ventilating the patient
- Keeping patient warm to facilitate oxygen off-loading that might be hindered in a hypothermic state
- Maintaining adequate circulation, thus perfusing tissue cells with oxygenated blood
  - Stopping loss of additional blood to maintain as many RBCs as possible to carry oxygen

The first component of the Fick principle is oxygenation of the lungs and RBCs. This is covered in detail in the Airway and Ventilation chapter. The second component involves perfusion, which is the delivery of blood to the tissue cells. A helpful analogy to use in describing perfusion is to think of the RBCs as transport vans, the lungs as oxygen warehouses, the blood vessels as roads and highways, and the body tissue cells as the oxygen's destination. An insufficient number of transport vans, obstructions along the roads and highways, and/or slow transport vans can all contribute to decreased oxygen delivery and the eventual starvation of the tissue cells.

The fluid component of the circulatory system—blood—contains not only RBCs but also infection-fighting factors (white blood cells and antibodies), platelets and coagulation factors to support clotting in hemorrhage, protein for cellular rebuilding, nutrition in the form of glucose, and other substances necessary for metabolism and survival.

Cellular Perfusion and Shock

The prime determinants of cellular perfusion are the heart (acting as the pump or the motor of the system), fluid volume (acting as the hydraulic fluid), the blood vessels (serving as the conduits or plumbing), and, finally, the cells of the body. Based on these components of the perfusion system, shock may be classified into the following categories:

1. Hypovolemic—primarily hemorrhagic in the trauma patient, related to loss of circulating blood cells and fluid volume with oxygen-carrying capacity. This is the most common cause of shock in the trauma patient.
2. Distributive (or vasogenic)—related to abnormality in vascular tone arising from several different causes, including spinal cord injury and anaphylaxis.
3. Cardiogenic—related to interference with the pump action of the heart, often occurring after a heart attack.

By far the most common cause of shock in the trauma patient is hypovolemic, resulting from hemorrhage, and the safest approach in managing the trauma patient in shock is to consider the cause of the shock as hemorrhagic until proven otherwise.

Anatomy and Pathophysiology of Shock

Cardiovascular Response

Heart

The heart consists of two receiving chambers (atria) and two major pumping chambers (ventricles). The function of the atria is to accumulate and store blood so the ventricles can fill rapidly, minimizing delay in the pumping cycle. The right atrium receives deoxygenated blood from the veins of the body and pumps it to the right ventricle. With each contraction of the right ventricle (**Figure 3-1**), blood is pumped through the lungs for on-loading of

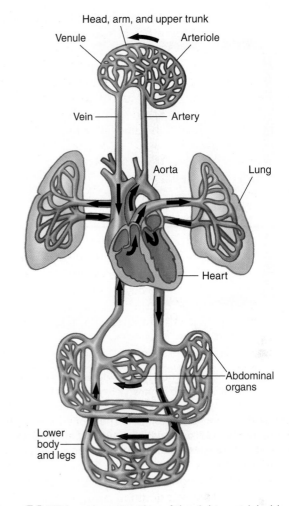

Figure 3-1 With each contraction of the right ventricle, blood is pumped through the lungs. Blood from the lungs enters the left side of the heart, and the left ventricle pumps it into the systemic vascular system. Blood returning from the lungs is pumped out of the heart and through the aorta to the rest of the body by left ventricular contraction.

oxygen to the RBCs. The oxygenated blood from the lungs is returned to the left atrium and is pumped into the left ventricle. Then, by the contraction of the left ventricle, the RBCs are pumped throughout the arteries of the body to the tissue cells.

Although it is one organ, the heart actually has two subsystems. The right atrium, which receives blood from the body, and the right ventricle, which pumps blood to the lungs, are referred to as the right heart. The left atrium, which receives oxygenated blood from the lungs, and the left ventricle, which pumps blood to the body, are referred to as the left heart (**Figure 3-2**). **Preload** (volume of blood entering into the heart) and **afterload** (pressure against which the blood has to push when it is squeezed out of the ventricle) of the right heart (pulmonary) and left heart (systemic) pumping systems are important concepts to understand.

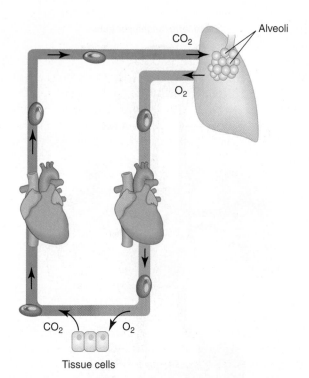

CO₂

Alveoli

O₂

CO₂   O₂

Tissue cells

Figure 3-2 Although the heart is considered to be one organ, it functions as if it were two organs. Deoxygenated blood is received into the right heart from the superior and inferior venae cavae and pumped through the pulmonary artery into the lungs. The blood is oxygenated in the lungs, flows back into the heart through the pulmonary vein, and is pumped out of the left ventricle.

© National Association of Emergency Medical Technicians (NAEMT).

Blood is forced through the circulatory system by the contraction of the left ventricle. This sudden pressure increase produces a pulse wave to push blood through the blood vessels. The peak of the pressure increase is the systolic blood pressure, and it represents the force of the pulse wave produced by ventricular contraction (systole). The resting pressure in the vessels between ventricular contractions is the diastolic blood pressure, and it represents the force that remains in the blood vessels that continues to move blood through the vessels while the ventricle is refilling for the next pulse of blood (**diastole**). The difference between the systolic and diastolic pressures is called **pulse pressure**. Pulse pressure is the pressure of the blood as it is being pushed out into the circulation. It is the pressure felt against the prehospital care provider's fingertip as the patient's pulse is checked.

Another term used in the discussion of blood pressure and shock but often not emphasized enough in the prehospital setting is **mean arterial pressure (MAP)**. This number gives a more realistic assessment of the overall pressure to produce blood flow than either the systolic or the diastolic pressures alone, and, in effect, it provides a numerical representation of end-organ perfusion. The

MAP is the average pressure in the vascular system and is calculated as follows:

MAP = Diastolic pressure + 1/3 Pulse pressure

For example, the MAP of a patient with a blood pressure of 120/80 mm Hg is calculated as follows:

$$\begin{aligned} \textbf{MAP} &= \textbf{80 + ([120 − 80]/3)} \\ &= \textbf{80 + (40/3)} \\ &= \textbf{80 + 13.3} \\ &= \textbf{93.3, rounded to 93} \end{aligned}$$

Many automatic noninvasive blood pressure (NIBP) devices automatically calculate and report the MAP in addition to the systolic and diastolic pressures. This is extremely helpful in guiding your treatment of trauma patients with permissive hypotension strategies. Permissive hypotension strategies are covered in greater detail in the Managing Volume Resuscitation section of this chapter. A normal MAP is considered to be 70 to 100 mm Hg.

The volume of fluid pumped into the circulatory system with each contraction of the ventricle is called the **stroke volume**, and the volume of blood pumped into the system over 1 minute is called the **cardiac output**. The formula for cardiac output is as follows:

Cardiac output (CO) = Heart rate (HR) × Stroke volume (SV)
Normal CO = 5-6 l/min

Cardiac output is reported in liters per minute (lpm or l/min). Cardiac output is not measured in the prehospital environment. However, understanding cardiac output and its relationship to stroke volume is important in understanding shock. For the heart to work effectively, an adequate volume of blood must be present in the venae cavae and pulmonary veins to fill the ventricles.

Starling's law is an important concept that helps to explain how this relationship works. This pressure fills the heart (preload) and stretches the myocardial muscle fibers. The more the ventricles fill, the greater the stretch of the cardiac muscle fibers and the greater the strength of the contraction of the heart, until the point of overstretching. Significant hemorrhage or relative hypovolemia decreases cardiac preload, so a reduced volume of blood is present and the fibers are not stretched as much, resulting in a lower stroke volume; therefore, blood pressure will fall. If the filling pressure of the heart is too great, the cardiac muscle fibers become overstretched and can fail to deliver a satisfactory stroke volume, and again blood pressure will decrease.

The resistance to blood flow that the left ventricle must overcome to pump blood out into the arterial system is called afterload, or **systemic vascular resistance**. As peripheral arterial vasoconstriction increases, the resistance to blood flow increases and the heart has to generate a greater force to pump blood into the arterial system. Conversely, widespread peripheral vasodilation decreases afterload.

The systemic circulation contains more capillaries and a greater length of blood vessels than the pulmonary circulation. Therefore, the left (or left-sided) heart system works at a higher pressure and bears a greater workload than the right (or right-sided) heart system. Anatomically, the muscle of the left ventricle is much thicker and stronger than that of the right ventricle.

Blood Vessels

The blood vessels contain the blood and route it to the various areas and cells of the body. They are the "highways" of the physiologic process of circulation. The aorta splits into multiple arteries of decreasing size, the smallest of which are the capillaries (**Figure 3-3**). A capillary may be only one cell wide; therefore, oxygen and nutrients carried by RBCs and plasma are able to diffuse easily through the walls of the capillary into the surrounding tissue cells (**Figure 3-4**). Each cell has a membranous covering called the cell membrane. Interstitial fluid is located between the cell membrane and the capillary wall. The amount of interstitial fluid varies tremendously. If little interstitial fluid is present, the cell membrane and the capillary wall are closer together, and oxygen can easily diffuse between them. When there is extra fluid (edema) forced into this space (such as occurs in over-resuscitation with crystalloid fluids), the cells move farther away from the capillaries, making transfer of oxygen and nutrients less efficient.

The size of the vascular "container" is controlled by smooth muscles in the walls of the arteries and arterioles and, to a lesser extent, by muscles in the walls of the venules and veins. These muscles respond to signals from the brain via the sympathetic nervous system, to the circulating hormones epinephrine and norepinephrine, and to other chemicals, such as nitric oxide. Depending on whether they are being stimulated to contract or allowed to relax, these muscle fibers in the walls of the vessels result in either the constriction or dilation of the blood vessels, thus changing the size of the container component of the cardiovascular system and thereby affecting the patient's blood pressure.

There are three fluid compartments: intravascular fluid (fluid inside the vessels), intracellular fluid (fluid inside the cells), and interstitial fluid (fluid between the cells and the vessels). When interstitial fluid is present in excess of normal amounts, it produces edema and causes the spongy, boggy feeling when the skin is compressed with a finger.

Hemodynamic Response

Blood

The fluid component of the circulatory system—the blood—contains (1) RBCs to carry oxygen, (2) infection-fighting factors (**white blood cells** [WBCs] and antibodies), and

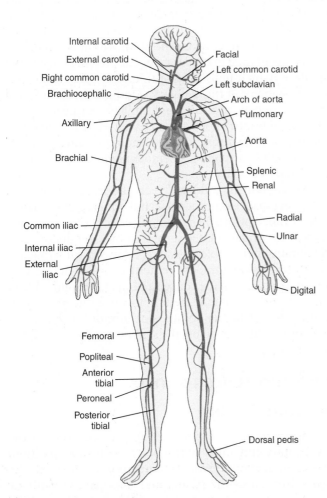

Figure 3-3 Principal arteries of the body.
© National Association of Emergency Medical Technicians (NAEMT).

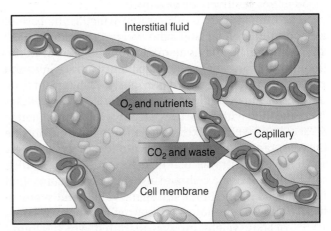

Figure 3-4 Oxygen from the RBCs and nutrients diffuse through the capillary wall, the interstitial fluid, and the cell membrane into the cell. Carbon dioxide and cellular waste products travel through the circulatory system to be eliminated by the lungs. By way of the buffer system of the body, this acid is converted into carbon dioxide and travels in the plasma along with the RBCs to be eliminated from the circulatory system by the lungs.
© National Association of Emergency Medical Technicians (NAEMT).

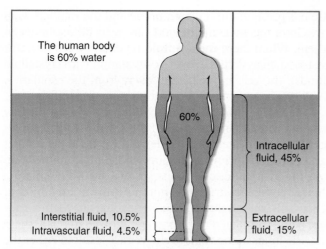

Figure 3-5 Body water represents 60% of body weight. This water is divided into intracellular and extracellular fluid. The extracellular fluid is further divided into interstitial and intravascular fluid.

© National Association of Emergency Medical Technicians (NAEMT).

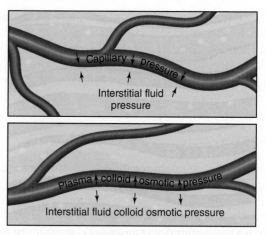

Figure 3-6 Forces governing fluid flux across capillaries.

© National Association of Emergency Medical Technicians (NAEMT).

(3) platelets and clotting factors essential for blood clotting at times of vascular injury, protein for cellular rebuilding, nutrients such as glucose, and other substances necessary for metabolism and survival. The various proteins and minerals provide a high **oncotic pressure** to help keep water from leaking out through the walls of the vessels. The volume of fluid within the vascular system must equal the capacity of the blood vessels if it is to adequately fill the container and maintain perfusion. Any variance in the volume of the vascular system container compared to the volume of blood in that container will affect the flow of blood either positively or negatively.

The human body is 60% water, which is the base of all body fluids. A person who weighs 154 pounds (70 kilograms [kg]) contains approximately 40 liters of water. Body water is present in two components: intracellular and extracellular fluid. As noted previously, each type of fluid has specific important properties (**Figure 3-5**). **Intracellular fluid**, the fluid within the cells, accounts for approximately 45% of body weight. **Extracellular fluid**, the fluid outside the cells, can be further classified into two subtypes: interstitial fluid and intravascular fluid. **Interstitial fluid**, which surrounds the tissue cells and also includes cerebrospinal fluid (found in the brain and spinal canal) and synovial fluid (found in the joints), accounts for approximately 10.5% of body weight. Intravascular fluid, which is found in the vessels and carries the formed components of blood as well as oxygen and other vital nutrients, accounts for approximately 4.5% of body weight.

A review of some key concepts is helpful in this discussion of how fluids move throughout the body. In addition to movement of fluid through the vascular system, there are two major types of fluid movements: (1) movement between the plasma and interstitial fluid (across capillaries) and (2) movement between the intracellular and interstitial fluid compartments (across cell membranes).

The movement of fluid through the capillary walls is determined by (1) the difference between the hydrostatic pressure within the capillary (which tends to push fluid out) and the hydrostatic pressure outside the capillary (which tends to push fluid in), (2) the difference in the oncotic pressure from protein concentration within the capillary (which keeps fluid in) and the oncotic pressure outside the capillary (which pulls fluid out), and (3) the "leakiness" or permeability of the capillary (**Figure 3-6**). Hydrostatic pressure, oncotic pressure, and capillary permeability are all affected by the shock state, as well as by the type and volume of fluid resuscitation, leading to alterations in circulating blood volume, hemodynamics, and tissue or pulmonary edema.

Movement of fluid between the intracellular and interstitial space occurs across cellular membranes, which is determined primarily by osmotic effects. **Osmosis** is the process by which solutes separated by a semipermeable membrane (permeable to water, relatively impermeable to solutes) govern the movement of water across that membrane based on the concentration of the solute. Water moves from the compartment of lower solute concentration to that of higher solute concentration to maintain osmotic equilibrium across the semipermeable membrane (**Figure 3-7**).

Endocrine Response

Nervous System

The **autonomic nervous system** directs and controls the involuntary functions of the body, such as respiration, digestion, and cardiovascular function. It is divided into two subsystems—the sympathetic and parasympathetic nervous systems. These systems oppose each other to keep vital body systems in balance.

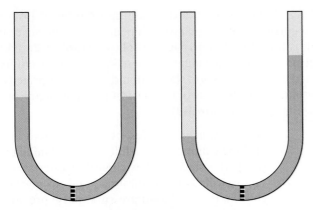

Figure 3-7 A U-tube, in which the two halves are separated by a semipermeable membrane, contains equal amounts of water and solid particles. If a solute that cannot diffuse through the semipermeable membrane is added to one side but not to the other, fluid will flow across the membrane to dilute the added particles. The pressure difference of the height of the fluid in the U-tube is known as osmotic pressure.

© National Association of Emergency Medical Technicians (NAEMT).

The **sympathetic nervous system** produces the fight-or-flight response. This response simultaneously causes the heart to beat faster and stronger, increases the ventilatory rate, and constricts the blood vessels to nonessential organs (skin and gastrointestinal tract) while dilating vessels and improving blood flow to muscles. The goal of this response system is to maintain sufficient amounts of oxygenated blood to critical tissues so an individual can respond to an emergency situation while shunting blood away from nonessential areas. In contrast, the **parasympathetic nervous system** slows the heart rate, decreases the ventilatory rate, and increases gastrointestinal activity.

In patients who are hemorrhaging after sustaining trauma, the body attempts to compensate for the blood loss and to maintain energy production. The cardiovascular system is regulated by the vasomotor center in the medulla. In response to a transient fall in blood pressure, stimuli travel to the brain via cranial nerves IX and X from stretch receptors in the carotid sinus and the aortic arch. These stimuli lead to increased sympathetic nervous system activity, with increased peripheral vascular resistance resulting from arteriolar constriction and increased cardiac output from an increased rate and force of cardiac contraction. Increased venous tone enhances circulatory blood volume. Blood is diverted from the extremities, bowel, and kidney to more vital areas—the heart and brain—in which vessels constrict very little under intense sympathetic stimulation. These responses result in cold, cyanotic extremities, decreased urine output, and decreased bowel perfusion.

A decrease in the left atrial filling pressure, a fall in blood pressure, and changes in plasma osmolality (the total concentration of all of the chemicals in blood) cause release of antidiuretic hormone (ADH) from the pituitary gland and aldosterone from the adrenal glands, which enhances retention of sodium and water by the kidneys. This process helps to expand the intravascular volume; however, many hours are required for this mechanism to make a clinical difference.

Classification of Traumatic Shock

The prime determinants of cellular perfusion are the heart (acting as the pump or the motor of the system), fluid volume (acting as the hydraulic fluid), the blood vessels (serving as the conduits or plumbing), and, finally, the cells of the body. Based on these components of the perfusion system, shock may be classified into the following categories (**Box 3-1**):

1. Hypovolemic shock is primarily hemorrhagic in the trauma patient, and it is related to loss of circulating blood cells with oxygen-carrying capacity and fluid volume. This is the most common cause of shock in the trauma patient.
2. Distributive (or vasogenic) shock is related to abnormality in vascular tone arising from various causes.
3. Cardiogenic shock is related to interference with the pump action of the heart.

Types of Traumatic Shock

Hypovolemic Shock

Acute loss of blood volume from hemorrhage (loss of plasma and RBCs) causes an imbalance in the relationship of fluid volume to the size of the container. The container retains its normal size, but the fluid volume is decreased. Hypovolemic shock is the most common cause of shock encountered in the prehospital environment, and blood

---

Box 3-1 Types of Traumatic Shock

The common types of shock seen after trauma in the prehospital setting include:

- Hypovolemic shock
  - Vascular volume smaller than normal vascular size
  - Result of blood and fluid loss
    - Hemorrhagic shock
- Distributive shock
  - Vascular space larger than normal
    - Neurogenic "shock" (hypotension)
- Cardiogenic shock
  - Heart not pumping adequately
  - Result of cardiac injury

loss is by far the most common cause of shock in trauma patients and the most dangerous for the patient.

When blood is lost from the circulation, the heart is stimulated to increase cardiac output by increasing the strength and rate of contractions. This stimulus results from the release of **epinephrine** from the adrenal glands. At the same time, the sympathetic nervous system releases **norepinephrine** to constrict blood vessels to reduce the size of the container and bring it more into proportion with the volume of remaining fluid. Vasoconstriction results in closing of the peripheral capillaries, which reduces oxygen delivery to those affected cells and forces the switch from aerobic to anaerobic metabolism at the cellular level.

These compensatory defense mechanisms work well up to a point and will temporarily help maintain the patient's vital signs. A patient who has signs of compensation such as tachycardia is already in shock, not "going into shock." When the defense mechanisms can no longer compensate for the amount of blood lost, a patient's blood pressure will drop. This decrease in blood pressure marks the switch from compensated to decompensated shock—a sign of impending death. Unless aggressive resuscitation occurs, the patient who enters decompensated shock has only one more stage of decline left—irreversible shock, leading to death.

Hemorrhagic Shock

The average 150-pound (70-kg) adult human has approximately 5 liters of circulating blood volume. Hemorrhagic shock (hypovolemic shock resulting from blood loss) is categorized into four classes, depending on the severity and amount of hemorrhage, as follows (**Table 3-2**), with the proviso that the values and descriptions for the criteria listed for these classes of shock should not be interpreted as absolute determinants of the class of shock, as significant overlap exists (**Figure 3-8**):

1. *Class I hemorrhage* represents a loss of up to 15% of blood volume in the adult (up to 750 milliliters [ml]). This stage has few clinical manifestations. Tachycardia is often minimal, and no measurable changes in blood pressure, pulse pressure, or ventilatory rate occur. Most healthy patients sustaining this amount of hemorrhage require only maintenance fluid as long as no further blood loss occurs. The body's compensatory mechanisms restore the intravascular container–fluid volume ratio and assist in the maintenance of blood pressure.

2. *Class II hemorrhage* represents a loss of 15% to 30% of blood volume (750 to 1,500 ml). Most adults are capable of compensating for this amount of blood loss by activation of the sympathetic nervous system, which will maintain their blood pressure. Clinical findings include increased ventilatory rate, tachycardia, and a narrowed pulse pressure. The clinical clues to this phase are tachycardia, tachypnea, and

Table 3-2 Classification of Hemorrhagic Shock				
	Class I	**Class II**	**Class III**	**Class IV**
Blood loss (ml)	< 750	750–1,500	1,500–2,000	> 2,000
Blood loss (% blood volume)	< 15%	15–30%	30–40%	> 40%
Pulse rate	< 100	100–120	120–140	> 140
Blood pressure	Normal	Normal	Decreased	Decreased
Pulse pressure (mm Hg)	Normal or increased	Decreased	Decreased	Decreased
Ventilatory rate	14–20	20–30	30–40	> 35
Central nervous system/ mental status	Slightly anxious	Mildly anxious	Anxious, confused	Confused, lethargic
Fluid replacement	Crystalloid	Crystalloid	Crystalloid and blood	Crystalloid and blood

Note: The values and descriptions for the criteria listed for these classes of shock should not be interpreted as absolute determinants of the class of shock, as significant overlap exists.

Source: From American College of Surgeons (ACS) Committee on Trauma. *Advanced Trauma Life Support for Doctors: Student Course Manual.* 8th ed. Chicago, IL: ACS; 2008.

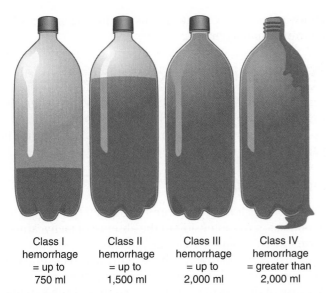

Class I
hemorrhage
= up to
750 ml

Class II
hemorrhage
= up to
1,500 ml

Class III
hemorrhage
= up to
2,000 ml

Class IV
hemorrhage
= greater than
2,000 ml

Figure 3-8 The approximate amount of blood loss for Class I, II, III, and IV hemorrhages.

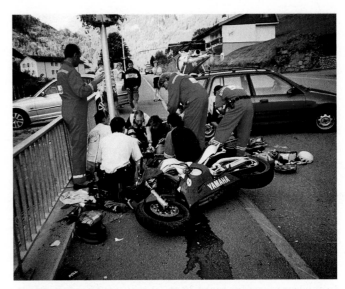

Figure 3-9 Massive blood loss, such as that sustained by the victim in this motorcycle crash, can rapidly lead to the onset of shock.

Photograph provided courtesy of Air Glaciers, Switzerland.

normal systolic blood pressure. Because the blood pressure is normal, this is called "compensated shock"; that is, the patient is in shock but is able to compensate for the time being. The patient often demonstrates anxiety or fright. Although not usually measured in the field, urine output drops slightly to between 20 and 30 ml/hour in an adult in the body's effort to preserve fluid. On occasion, these patients may require blood transfusion in the hospital; however, most will respond well to crystalloid infusion if hemorrhage is controlled at this point.

3. *Class III hemorrhage* represents a loss of 30% to 40% of blood volume (1,500 to 2,000 ml). When blood loss reaches this point, most patients are no longer able to compensate for the volume loss, and hypotension occurs. The classic findings of shock are obvious and include tachycardia (heart rate greater than 120 to 140 beats/minute), tachypnea (ventilatory rate of 30 to 40 breaths/minute), and severe anxiety or confusion. Urine output falls to 5 to 15 ml/hour. Many of these patients will require blood transfusion and surgical intervention for adequate resuscitation and control of hemorrhage.

4. *Class IV hemorrhage* represents a loss of more than 40% of blood volume (greater than 2,000 ml). This stage of severe shock is characterized by marked tachycardia (heart rate greater than 120 to 140 beats/minute), tachypnea (ventilatory rate greater than 35 breaths/minute), profound confusion or lethargy, and greatly decreased

systolic blood pressure, typically in the range of 60 mm Hg. These patients truly have only minutes to live (**Figure 3-9**). Survival depends on immediate control of hemorrhage (surgery for internal hemorrhage) and aggressive resuscitation, including blood and plasma transfusions with minimal crystalloid.

The rapidity with which a patient develops shock depends on how fast blood is lost from the circulation. A trauma patient who has lost blood needs to have the source of blood loss stopped, and, if significant blood loss has occurred, blood replacement needs to be accomplished. The fluid lost is whole blood containing all of its various components, including RBCs with oxygen-carrying capacity, clotting factors, and proteins to maintain oncotic pressure.

Whole blood replacement, or even component therapy, is usually not available in the prehospital environment; therefore, in the field, when treating trauma patients with hemorrhagic shock, providers must take measures to control external blood loss, provide minimal intravenous (IV) electrolyte solution (plasma when available), and transport rapidly to the hospital, where blood, plasma, and clotting factors are available and emergent interventions to control blood loss can be performed, as necessary (**Box 3-2**). Tranexamic acid (TXA) is a clot-stabilizing medication that has been used for years to control bleeding and has started to make its way into the prehospital environment. TXA works by binding to plasminogen and preventing it from becoming plasmin, thereby preventing the breakdown of fibrin in a clot. Ongoing studies will assist in determining the appropriate prehospital role for TXA.

> **Box 3-2** Lyophilized Plasma
>
> Lyophilized (freeze-dried) plasma and whole blood products are being used in the field in several countries. They are currently under study in the United States for use by EMS and are being used by a few EMS systems and air medical services in the United States.

Prior shock research recommended a replacement ratio with electrolyte solution of 3 liters of replacement for each liter of blood lost.[3] This high ratio of replacement fluid was thought to be necessary because only about one-fourth to one-third of the volume of an isotonic crystalloid solution such as normal saline or lactated Ringer solution remains in the intravascular space 30 to 60 minutes after infusing it.

More recent shock research has focused on the understanding that the administration of a limited volume of electrolyte solution before blood replacement is the correct approach while en route to the hospital. The result of administering too much crystalloid is increased interstitial fluid (edema), which potentially impairs oxygen transfer to the remaining RBCs and into the tissue cells. The goal is not to raise the blood pressure to normal levels but to provide only enough fluid to maintain perfusion and continue to provide oxygenated RBCs to the heart, brain, and lungs. Raising the blood pressure to normal levels may only serve to dilute clotting factors, disrupt any clot that has formed, and increase hemorrhage.

The commonly preferred crystalloid solution for treating hemorrhagic shock is lactated Ringer solution. Normal saline is another isotonic crystalloid solution used for volume replacement, but its use may produce hyperchloremia (marked increase in the blood chloride level), leading to acidosis in large volume resuscitation. Normosol and Plasma-Lyte are examples of balanced salt solutions that more closely match plasma concentrations of electrolytes, but they may also increase cost.

With significant blood loss, the optimal replacement fluid is ideally as near to whole blood as possible.[4,5] The first step is administration of packed RBCs and plasma at a ratio of 1:1 or 1:2. Platelets, cryoprecipitate, and other clotting factors are added as needed. Plasma contains a large number of the clotting factors and other components needed to control blood loss from small vessels. There are 13 identified factors in the coagulation cascade (**Figure 3-10**). In patients with massive blood loss requiring large volumes of blood replacement, most of the factors have been lost. Plasma transfusion is a reliable source of most of these factors. If major blood loss has occurred, the control of hemorrhage from large vessels requires operative management or, in some cases, endovascular placement of coils or clotting sponges for definitive management.

Distributive (Vasogenic) Shock

Distributive shock, or vasogenic shock, occurs when the vascular container enlarges without a proportional increase in fluid volume. After trauma, this is typically found in patients who have sustained a spinal cord injury.

Neurogenic "Shock"

Neurogenic "shock," or, more appropriately, neurogenic hypotension (hypotension in the absence of tachycardia), occurs when a spinal cord injury interrupts the sympathetic nervous system pathway. This usually involves injury to the lower cervical, thoracolumbar, and thoracic levels. Because of the loss of sympathetic control of the vascular system, which controls the smooth muscles in the walls of the blood vessels, the peripheral vessels dilate below the level of injury. The marked decrease in systemic vascular resistance and peripheral vasodilation occurs as the container for the blood volume increases results in relative hypovolemia. The patient is not really hypovolemic—the normal blood volume is simply insufficient to fill an expanded container.

Tissue oxygenation usually remains adequate (MAP > 65) in the neurogenic form of shock, and blood flow remains normal although the blood pressure is low (neurogenic hypotension). In addition, energy production remains adequate in neurogenic hypotension. Therefore, this decrease in blood pressure is not shock, because energy production remains unaffected. However, because there is less resistance to blood flow, the systolic and diastolic pressures are lower.

Decompensated hypovolemic shock and neurogenic shock both produce a decreased systolic blood pressure. However, the other vital and clinical signs, as well as the treatment for each condition, are different (**Table 3-3**). Hypovolemic shock is characterized by decreased systolic and diastolic pressures and a narrow pulse pressure. Neurogenic shock also displays decreased systolic and diastolic pressures, but the pulse pressure remains normal or is widened. Hypovolemia produces cold, clammy, pale, or cyanotic skin and delayed capillary refilling time. In neurogenic shock the patient has warm, dry skin, especially below the area of injury. The pulse in patients with hypovolemic shock is weak, thready, and rapid. In neurogenic shock, because of unopposed parasympathetic activity on the heart, bradycardia is typically seen rather than tachycardia, but the pulse quality may be weak. Hypovolemia produces a decreased level of consciousness (LOC), or, at least, anxiety and often combativeness. In the absence of a traumatic brain injury (TBI), the patient with neurogenic

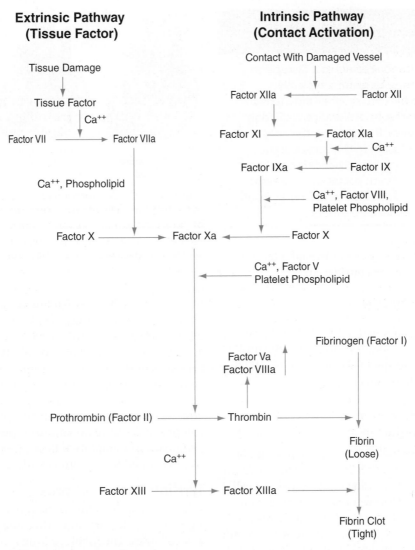

Figure 3-10 Clotting cascade.
© National Association of Emergency Medical Technicians (NAEMT).

Table 3-3 Signs Associated With Types of Shock			
Vital Sign	**Hypovolemic**	**Neurogenic**	**Cardiogenic**
Skin temperature/quality	Cool, clammy	Warm, dry	Cool, clammy
Skin color	Pale, cyanotic	Pink	Pale, cyanotic
Blood pressure	Drops	Drops	Drops
Level of consciousness	Altered	Lucid	Altered
Capillary refilling time	Slowed	Normal	Slowed

shock is usually alert, oriented, and lucid when in the supine position (**Box 3-3**).

Patients with neurogenic shock frequently have associated injuries that produce significant hemorrhage. Therefore, a patient who has neurogenic shock and potential physical signs of hypovolemia should first be treated as if blood loss is present. Stabilization of blood pressure with vasopressors may be helpful, but only after confirmation of adequate

The term *neurogenic shock* refers to a disruption of the sympathetic nervous system, typically from injury to the spinal cord or a hemodynamic phenomenon, which results in significant dilation of the peripheral arteries. If untreated, this may result in impaired perfusion to the body's tissues. Although typically lumped together, this condition should not be confused with spinal shock, a term that refers to an injury to the spinal cord that results in temporary loss of spinal cord function.

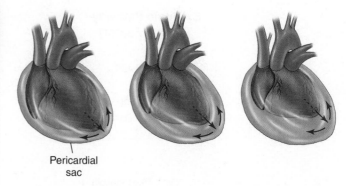

Pericardial sac

Figure 3-11 Cardiac tamponade. As blood courses from a hole in the heart muscle into the pericardial space, it limits expansion of the ventricle. Therefore, the ventricle cannot fill completely. As more blood accumulates in the pericardial space, less ventricular space is available, and cardiac output is reduced.
© National Association of Emergency Medical Technicians (NAEMT).

fluid resuscitation to address any hemorrhagic component of hypotension should this be considered.

Cardiogenic Shock

Cardiogenic shock, or failure of the heart's pumping activity, results from causes categorized as either intrinsic (a result of direct damage to the heart) or extrinsic (related to a problem outside the heart).

Intrinsic Causes

Heart Muscle Damage

Any injury that damages the cardiac muscle may affect its output. The damage may result from a direct bruise to the heart muscle (as in a blunt cardiac injury causing cardiac contusion). A recurring cycle will ensue: Decreased oxygenation causes decreased contractility, which results in decreased cardiac output and, therefore, decreased systemic perfusion. Decreased perfusion results in a continuing decrease in oxygenation and, thus, a continuation of the cycle. As with any muscle, the cardiac muscle does not work as efficiently when it becomes bruised or damaged.

Valvular Disruption

A sudden, forceful compressing blow to the chest or abdomen may damage the valves of the heart. Severe valvular injury results in acute valvular regurgitation, in which a significant amount of blood leaks back into the chamber from which it was just pumped. These patients often rapidly develop congestive heart failure, manifested by pulmonary edema and cardiogenic shock. The presence of a new heart murmur is an important clue in making this diagnosis.

Extrinsic Causes

Cardiac Tamponade

Fluid in the pericardial sac will prevent the heart from refilling completely during the diastolic (relaxation) phase of the cardiac cycle. In the case of trauma, blood leaks into the pericardial sac from a hole in the cardiac muscle. The blood accumulates, occupies space, and prevents the walls

of the ventricle from expanding fully. This has two negative effects on cardiac output: (1) Less volume is available for each contraction because the ventricle cannot expand fully, and (2) inadequate filling reduces the stretch of the cardiac muscle and results in diminished strength of the cardiac contraction. Additionally, more blood is forced out of the ventricle through the cardiac wound with each contraction and occupies more space in the pericardial sac, further compromising cardiac output (**Figure 3-11**). Severe shock and death may rapidly follow. (See the Thoracic Trauma chapter for additional information.)

Tension Pneumothorax

When either side of the thoracic cavity becomes filled with air that is under pressure, the lung becomes compressed and collapses. The involved lung is unable to refill with air from the outside through the nasopharynx. This produces at least four problems: (1) The tidal volume with each breath is reduced, (2) the collapsed alveoli are not available for oxygen transfer into the RBCs, (3) the pulmonary blood vessels are collapsed, reducing blood flow into the lung and heart, and (4) a greater force of cardiac contraction is required to force blood through the pulmonary vessels (pulmonary hypertension). If the volume of air and pressure inside the injured chest is great enough, the mediastinum is pushed away from the side of the injury. As the mediastinum shifts, the opposite lung becomes compressed, and compression and kinking of the superior and inferior venae cavae further impede venous return to the heart, producing a significant drop in preload (**Figure 3-12**). All of these factors reduce cardiac output, and shock rapidly ensues. (See the Thoracic Trauma chapter for additional information.)

Assessment

The assessment for the presence of shock must include looking for the subtle early evidence of hypoperfusion. In the prehospital setting, this requires the assessment of

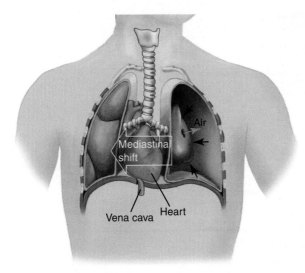

Figure 3-12 Tension pneumothorax. If the amount of air trapped in the pleural space continues to increase, not only is does the lung on the affected side collapse, but the mediastinum shifts to the opposite side. The mediastinal shift impairs blood return to the heart through the inferior vena cava, thus affecting cardiac output, while at the same time compressing the opposite lung.

© National Association of Emergency Medical Technicians (NAEMT).

organs and systems that are immediately accessible. Signs of hypoperfusion manifest as malfunction of these accessible organs or systems. Such systems are the brain and central nervous system (CNS), heart and cardiovascular system, respiratory system, skin and extremities, and kidneys. The signs of decreased perfusion and energy production and the body's response include the following:

- Decreased LOC, anxiety, disorientation, bizarre behavior (brain and CNS)
- Tachycardia, decreased systolic and pulse pressure (heart and cardiovascular system)
- Rapid, shallow breathing (respiratory system)
- Cold, pale, clammy, diaphoretic or even cyanotic skin with decreased capillary refilling time (skin and extremities)
- Decreased urine output (kidneys), identified rarely in the prehospital setting in situations of prolonged or delayed transport when a urinary catheter is present

Because hemorrhage is the most common cause of shock in the trauma patient, all shock in a trauma patient should be considered to be from hemorrhage until proven otherwise. The first priority is to examine for external sources of hemorrhage and control them as quickly and completely as possible. Controlling hemorrhage may involve such techniques as application of direct pressure, pressure dressings, tourniquets, or splinting of extremity fractures.

If there is no evidence of external hemorrhage, internal hemorrhage should be suspected. Although definitive management of internal hemorrhage is not practical in the prehospital setting, identification of an internal source of bleeding mandates rapid transport to the definitive care institution. Internal hemorrhage can occur in the chest,

abdomen, pelvis, or retroperitoneum. Evidence of blunt or penetrating chest injury with decreased breath sounds would suggest a thoracic source. The abdomen, pelvis, and retroperitoneum can be a source of bleeding with evidence of blunt trauma (e.g., ecchymosis) or penetrating trauma. This includes abdominal distension or tenderness, pelvic instability, leg-length inequality, pain in the pelvic area aggravated by movement, perineal ecchymosis, and blood at the urethral meatus.

As a general rule, patients who meet National Trauma Triage Protocol criteria 1 or 2 (or both) need rapid transport to the nearest appropriate trauma center (**Figure 3-13**).

If the assessment does not suggest hemorrhage as the cause of the shock, nonhemorrhagic causes should be suspected. These include cardiac tamponade and tension pneumothorax (both evident by distended neck veins versus collapsed neck veins in hemorrhagic shock) or neurogenic hypotension. Decreased breath sounds on the side of the chest injury, subcutaneous emphysema, respiratory distress (tachypnea), and tracheal deviation (a late finding rarely seen in the field) suggest tension pneumothorax. Presence of these signs suggests the need for immediate needle decompression of the involved side of the chest.

Different sources of cardiogenic shock are suspected with blunt or penetrating chest trauma, muffled heart sounds suggesting cardiac tamponade (difficult to detect in the noisy prehospital environment), dysrhythmias, and neurogenic hypotension with signs of spinal trauma, bradycardia, and warm extremities. Most, if not all, of these features can be detected by the astute prehospital care provider, who can determine the cause of the shock and the need for appropriate intervention when feasible in the field.

Areas of patient evaluation include status of the airway, ventilation, perfusion, skin color and temperature, capillary refilling time, and blood pressure. Each one is presented separately here in the context of both the primary survey and the secondary survey. Simultaneous evaluation is an important part of patient assessment to gather and process information from different sources expeditiously.

Primary Survey

One of the first steps in patient assessment is to get an initial observation of the patient's condition as quickly as possible. The following signs identify the need for suspicion of life-threatening conditions:

- Mild anxiety, progressing to confusion or altered LOC
- Mild tachypnea, leading to rapid, labored ventilations
- Mild tachycardia, progressing to marked tachycardia
- Weakened radial pulse, progressing to an absent radial pulse
- Pale or cyanotic skin color
- Prolonged capillary refilling time
- Loss of pulses in the extremities
- Hypothermia
- Sensation of thirst

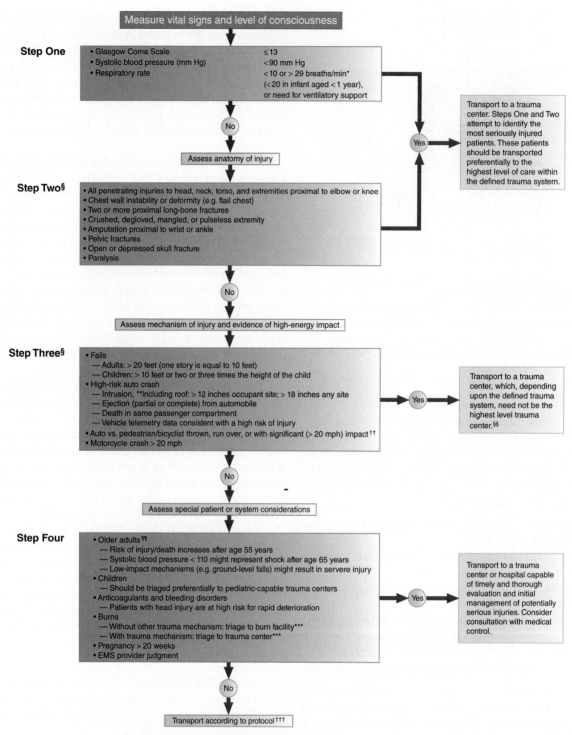

Measure vital signs and level of consciousness

Step One
- Glasgow Coma Scale — ≤13
- Systolic blood pressure (mm Hg) — <90 mm Hg
- Respiratory rate — <10 or >29 breaths/min*
  (<20 in infant aged <1 year),
  or need for ventilatory support

No ↓   **Yes →**

Transport to a trauma center. Steps One and Two attempt to identify the most seriously injured patients. These patients should be transported preferentially to the highest level of care within the defined trauma system.

Assess anatomy of injury

Step Two§
- All penetrating injuries to head, neck, torso, and extremities proximal to elbow or knee
- Chest wall instability or deformity (e.g. flail chest)
- Two or more proximal long-bone fractures
- Crushed, degloved, mangled, or pulseless extremity
- Amputation proximal to wrist or ankle
- Pelvic fractures
- Open or depressed skull fracture
- Paralysis

No ↓

Assess mechanism of injury and evidence of high-energy impact

Step Three§
- Falls
  — Adults: > 20 feet (one story is equal to 10 feet)
  — Children: > 10 feet or two or three times the height of the child
- High-risk auto crash
  — Intrusion, **including roof: > 12 inches occupant site; > 18 inches any site
  — Ejection (partial or complete) from automobile
  — Death in same passenger compartment
  — Vehicle telemetry data consistent with a high risk of injury
- Auto vs. pedestrian/bicyclist thrown, run over, or with significant (> 20 mph) impact††
- Motorcycle crash > 20 mph

Yes →

Transport to a trauma center, which, depending upon the defined trauma system, need not be the highest level trauma center.§§

No ↓

Assess special patient or system considerations

Step Four
- Older adults¶¶
  — Risk of injury/death increases after age 55 years
  — Systolic blood pressure < 110 might represent shock after age 65 years
  — Low-impact mechanisms (e.g. ground-level falls) might result in severe injury
- Children
  — Should be triaged preferentially to pediatric-capable trauma centers
- Anticoagulants and bleeding disorders
  — Patients with head injury are at high risk for rapid deterioration
- Burns
  — Without other trauma mechanism: triage to burn facility***
  — With trauma mechanism: triage to trauma center***
- Pregnancy > 20 weeks
- EMS provider judgment

Yes →

Transport to a trauma center or hospital capable of timely and thorough evaluation and initial management of potentially serious injuries. Consider consultation with medical control.

No ↓

Transport according to protocol†††

When in doubt, transport to a trauma center

Abbreviation: EMS = emergency medical services.
* The upper limit of respiratory rate in infants is > 29 breaths per minute to maintain a higher level of overtriage for infants.
§ Any injury noted in Step Two or mechanism identified in Step Three triggers a "yes" response.
¶ Age < 15 years.
** Intrusion refers to interior compartment intrusion, as opposed to deformation, which refers to exterior damage.
†† Includes pedestrians or bicyclists thrown or run over by a motor vehicle or those with estimated impact > 20 mph with a motor vehicle.
§§ Local or regional protocols should be used to determine the most appropriate level of trauma center within the defined trauma system; need not be the highest level trauma center.
¶¶ Age > 55 years.
*** Patients with both burns and concomitant trauma for whom the burn injury poses the greatest risk for morbidity and mortality should be transferred to a burn center.
  If the nonburn trauma presents a greater immediate risk, the patient may be stabilized in a trauma center and then transferred to a burn center.
††† Patients who do not meet any of the triage criteria in Steps One through Four should be transported to the most appropriate medical facility as outlined in local EMS protocols.

Figure 3-13 2011 Guidelines for Field Triage of Injured Patients.

Adapted from Centers for Disease Control and Prevention, *Morbidity and Mortality Weekly Report (MMWR)*, January 13, 2012.

Box 3-4 XABCDE

The primary survey of the trauma patient now emphasizes control of life-threatening external bleeding as the first step in the sequence. While the steps of the primary survey are taught and displayed in a sequential manner, many of the steps can, and should, be performed simultaneously. The steps can be remembered using the mnemonic XABCDE:

- **X**—Control of severe external (exsanguinating) bleeding
- **A**—Airway management and cervical spine stabilization
- **B**—Breathing (ventilation and oxygenation)
- **C**—Circulation (perfusion and other hemorrhage)
- **D**—Disability
- **E**—Expose/environment

Any compromise or failure of the airway, breathing, or circulatory system must be managed before proceeding. The following steps are described in an ordered series; however, all of these assessments are carried out more or less simultaneously (**Box 3-4** and **Box 3-5**).

Exsanguinating Hemorrhage

Exsanguinating hemorrhage can kill a patient faster than most other trauma mechanisms. It is possible to bleed to death in a few minutes from a significant arterial injury, and therefore this type of bleeding must be controlled immediately. The patient may be lying on the major source of the hemorrhage, or it may be hidden by the patient's clothes. The patient can lose a significant volume of blood from scalp lacerations because of the high concentration of blood vessels or from wounds that damage major blood vessels (subclavian, axillary, brachial, radial, ulnar, carotid, femoral, or popliteal). Rapidly scan the patient for any signs of severe bleeding from a major vessel, and initiate appropriate interventions such as a tourniquet on a limb, pressure dressing on a scalp or packing of a wound that is not amenable to any other therapy.

Airway

The airway should be evaluated quickly in all patients. A patent airway is a component in ensuring delivery of adequate amounts of oxygen to the cells of the body. Patients in need of immediate management of their airway include those with the following conditions, in order of importance:

1. Patients who are not breathing
2. Patients who have obvious airway compromise
3. Patients who have ventilatory rates greater than 20 breaths/minute
4. Patients who have noisy sounds of ventilation

Box 3-5 MARCH

MARCH is an alternative patient assessment acronym to XABCDE that is used by EMS practitioners working in trauma and tactical situations. MARCH stands for:

- **M**—Massive bleeding: Control the bleeding of a life-threatening hemorrhage with a tourniquet, hemostatic dressing, or conventional pressure dressing.
- **A**—Airway: Assess for obstruction, and secure the casualty's airway with body positioning, nasopharyngeal airway, advanced airways, or surgical airway.
- **R**—Respirations: Assess and treat for penetrating chest wounds, sucking chest wounds, and tension pneumothoraces.
- **C**—Circulation: Assess for shock. Establish intravenous or intraosseous access, and initiate fluid resuscitation if medically indicated.
- **H**—Head/hypothermia: Protect the casualty from hypothermia. Heat, chemical, or toxic exposures may also be risk factors. Splint any major fracture, and provide spinal motion restriction for patients at risk.

The MARCH approach aligns closely with the XABCDE approach, which is the patient assessment acronym for trauma patients used by EMS practitioners. A side-by-side comparison shows the following parallel features:

Massive hemorrhage	e**X**sanguinating hemorrhage
Airway	**A**irway
Respirations	**B**reathing
Circulation	**C**irculation
Head/hypothermia	**D**isability
	Expose/environment

Breathing

The anaerobic metabolism associated with decreased cellular oxygenation produces an increase in lactic acid. The hydrogen ions produced from the acidosis are converted by the buffer system in the body into water and carbon dioxide. The brain's sensing system detects this abnormal increase in the amount of carbon dioxide and stimulates the respiratory center to increase the rate and depth of ventilation to remove the carbon dioxide. Thus, tachypnea is frequently one of the earliest signs of anaerobic metabolism and shock, even earlier than increased pulse rate. In the primary survey, time is not taken to measure a ventilatory rate. Instead, ventilations should be estimated to be slow, normal, fast, or very fast. A slow ventilatory rate, in conjunction with shock, generally indicates a patient is in profound shock and may be moments away from cardiac arrest. A fast ventilatory rate is a concern and should serve as an impetus to search for the cause of shock. It could also be a sign of a purely respiratory problem, such as a simple pneumothorax or early cardiac tamponade.

A patient who tries to remove an oxygen mask, particularly when such action is associated with anxiety and confusion, is displaying another sign of cerebral ischemia. This patient has "air hunger" and feels the need for more ventilation. The presence of a mask over the nose and mouth creates a psychological feeling of ventilatory restriction. This action should be a clue that the patient is not receiving enough oxygen and is hypoxic.

Decreased oxygen saturation (SpO_2), as measured by the pulse oximeter, will confirm this suspicion. Any pulse oximeter reading below 94% (at sea level) is worrisome and should serve as a stimulus to identify the cause of hypoxia. Measurement and continuous monitoring of end-tidal carbon dioxide ($ETCO_2$) is a routine practice in EMS patients whose airway has been managed with procedures such as endotracheal intubation. While the correlation between the $ETCO_2$ and the partial pressure of carbon dioxide in arterial blood ($PaCO_2$) is good in the patient who has adequate perfusion, the correlation is poor in the patient in shock, thus limiting its utility to guide respirations. Monitoring $ETCO_2$ may still help to detect changes and trends in perfusion. It is always important to remember to evaluate readings from machines in the context of the patient's appearance. If the appearance of the patient suggests hypoxia, treat the patient for hypoxia even if the machine would suggest otherwise. Classical thinking suggests the clinical situation is always more important than the reading given by any device.

For example, note that peripheral pulse oximetry measurements are not reliable when patients are in decompensated shock. Either a central pulse oximetry measurement should be used or the prehospital care provider should examine the oximeter waveform to determine the reliability of the reading. The waveform should be consistent with each pulse.

Circulation

The two components in the assessment of circulation are as follows:

- Hemorrhage and the amount of blood loss
- Perfusion with oxygenated blood
  - Total body
  - Regional

The data accumulated during the circulatory assessment help to make a quick initial determination of the patient's total blood volume and perfusion status and, secondarily,

provide a similar assessment of specific regions of the body. For example, when checking the capillary refilling time, the pulse, skin color, and temperature of a lower extremity may show compromised perfusion while the same signs may be normal in the upper extremity. This discrepancy does not mean the signs are inaccurate, only that one part is different from another. The immediate question to be answered is "Why?" It is important to check for the following circulatory and perfusion findings in more than one part of the body and to remember that the assessment of the total body condition should not be based on a single part.

Hemorrhage

Efforts at restoring perfusion will be less effective or completely ineffective in the face of ongoing hemorrhage. Severe external hemorrhage should already be controlled at this point. The prehospital care provider should now go back and reassess to ensure major bleeding remains under control and look for any additional sources of bleeding.

Loss of blood means loss of RBCs and a resulting loss of oxygen-carrying capacity. Thus, while a patient who has been bleeding may have an SpO_2 that is "normal" because what blood the patient does have is fully saturated with oxygen, the patient, in fact, has diminished total oxygen because there is just not enough blood to carry the amount of oxygen needed to supply all of the cells of the body.

Pulse

The next important assessment point for perfusion is the pulse. Initial evaluation of the pulse determines whether it is palpable at the artery being examined. In general, loss of a radial pulse indicates severe hypovolemia (or vascular damage to the arm), especially when a central pulse, such as the carotid or femoral artery, is weak, thready, and extremely fast, indicating the status of the total body circulatory system. If the pulse is palpable, its character and strength should be noted, as follows:

- Is the pulse rate strong, or is it weak and thready?
- Is the pulse rate normal, too fast, or too slow?
- Is the pulse rate regular or irregular?

Although many prehospital care providers involved in the management of trauma patients focus on the patient's blood pressure, precious time should not be spent during the primary survey to obtain a blood pressure reading. The exact level of the blood pressure is much less important in the primary survey than other, earlier signs of shock. Significant information can be determined from the pulse rate and its character. In one series of trauma patients, a radial pulse characterized by providers as "weak" was associated with blood pressure that averaged 26 mm Hg lower than a pulse thought to be "normal." More importantly, trauma patients with a weak radial pulse were 15 times more likely to die than were patients with a normal pulse.[6] Although generally obtained at the beginning of the secondary survey, blood pressure can be palpated or auscultated earlier in the patient assessment if sufficient assistance is present, or once the primary survey has been completed and life-threatening issues are being addressed during transport.

Level of Consciousness

Mental status is part of the disability evaluation, but altered mental status can represent impaired cerebral oxygenation resulting from decreased perfusion. Assessment of mental status represents an assessment of end-organ perfusion and function. An anxious, confused patient should be assumed to have cerebral ischemia and anaerobic metabolism until another cause is identified. Drug and alcohol overdose and cerebral contusion are conditions that cannot be treated rapidly, but cerebral ischemia can be treated. Therefore, all patients in whom cerebral ischemia might be present should be managed as if it were present.

In addition to the concerns of the presence of hypoxia and poor perfusion, altered mental status also suggests TBI. The combination of hypoxia or decreased blood pressure and TBI has a profound negative impact on patient survival; therefore, hypoxia and hypotension must be corrected if present and prevented from developing if not present.

Skin Color

Pink skin color generally indicates a well-oxygenated patient without anaerobic metabolism. Blue (cyanotic) or mottled skin indicates unoxygenated hemoglobin and a lack of adequate oxygenation to the periphery. Pale, mottled, or cyanotic skin has inadequate blood flow resulting from one of the following three causes:

1. Peripheral vasoconstriction (most often associated with hypovolemia)
2. Decreased supply of RBCs (acute anemia)
3. Interruption of blood supply to that portion of the body, such as might be found with a fracture or injury of a blood vessel supplying that part of the body

Pale skin may be a localized or generalized finding with different implications. Other findings, such as tachycardia, should be used to resolve these differences and to determine whether the pale skin is a localized, regional, or systemic condition. Also, cyanosis may not develop in hypoxic patients who have lost a significant number of their RBCs from hemorrhage. In patients with dark-pigmented skin, cyanosis may be difficult to detect in the skin, but it can be noted in the lips, gums, and palms.

Skin Temperature

As the body shunts blood away from the skin to more important parts of the body, skin temperature decreases. Skin that is cool to the touch indicates vasoconstriction, decreased cutaneous perfusion, and decreased energy production and,

therefore, shock. Because a significant amount of heat can be lost during the assessment phase, steps should be taken to preserve the patient's body temperature.

The environmental conditions in which the determination of body temperature is made can affect the results, as can an isolated injury that affects perfusion; therefore, the results of this assessment must be evaluated in the context of the entire situation.

Skin Quality

In addition to skin color and temperature, the skin is evaluated for dryness or moistness. The trauma patient in shock from hypovolemia typically has clammy (moist, diaphoretic) skin. In contrast, the patient with hypotension from a spinal cord injury usually has dry skin.

Capillary Refilling Time

The ability of the cardiovascular system to refill the capillaries after blood has been "removed" represents an important support system. Analyzing this support system's level of function by compressing capillaries to remove the blood and then measuring the refilling time provides insight into perfusion of the capillary bed being assessed. Generally, the body shuts down circulation in the most distal parts first and restores this circulation last. Evaluation of the nail bed of the big toe or thumb provides the earliest indication hypoperfusion is developing. Additionally, it provides a strong indication as to when resuscitation is complete. However, as with many other signs a patient may exhibit, several conditions—both environmental and physiologic—can alter the results. A test of the capillary refilling time is a measurement of the time required to reperfuse the skin and, therefore, an indirect measurement of the actual perfusion of that part of the body. It is not a diagnostic test of any specific disease process or injury.

Capillary refilling time has been described as a poor test of shock. However, it is not a test of shock but rather a test of perfusion of the capillary bed being analyzed. Used along with other tests and components of the assessment, it is a good indicator of perfusion and suggestive of shock, but it must be interpreted in the context of the current situation and circumstances.

Shock may be the cause of poor perfusion and delayed capillary refilling, but there are other causes, such as arterial interruption from a fracture, a vessel wounded by penetrating trauma (e.g., gunshot wound), hypothermia, and even arteriosclerosis. Another cause of poor capillary refilling is decreased cardiac output resulting from hypovolemia (other than from hemorrhage).

Capillary refilling time is a helpful diagnostic sign used to monitor the progress of resuscitation. If the resuscitation of the patient is progressing in a positive manner and the patient's condition is improving, the capillary refilling time will also show improvement.

Disability

One regional body system that can be readily evaluated in the field is brain function. At least six conditions can produce an altered LOC or change in behavior (combativeness or belligerence) in trauma patients:

1. Hypoxia
2. Stroke
3. Shock with impaired cerebral perfusion
4. TBI
5. Intoxication with alcohol or drugs
6. Metabolic processes such as diabetes, seizures, and eclampsia

Of these six conditions, the easiest to treat—and the one that will kill the patient most quickly if not treated—is hypoxia. Any patient with an altered LOC should be treated as if decreased cerebral oxygenation is the cause. An altered LOC is usually one of the first visible signs of shock.

TBI may be considered primary (caused by direct trauma to brain tissue) or secondary (caused by the effects of hypoxia, hypoperfusion, edema, loss of energy production, etc.). There is no effective treatment in the prehospital setting for the primary brain injury, but secondary brain injury can essentially be prevented or significantly reduced by maintaining oxygenation and perfusion.

The brain's ability to function decreases as perfusion and oxygenation drop and ischemia develops. This decreased function evolves through various stages as different areas of the brain become affected. Anxiety and belligerent behavior are usually the first signs, followed by a slowing of the thought processes and a decrease of the body's motor and sensory functions. The level of cerebral function is an important and measurable prehospital sign of shock. A belligerent, combative, anxious patient or one with a decreased LOC should be assumed to have a hypoxic, hypoperfused brain until another cause can be identified. Hypoperfusion and cerebral hypoxia frequently accompany brain injury and make the long-term result even worse. Even brief episodes of hypoxia and shock may worsen the original brain injury and result in poorer outcomes.

Expose/Environment

The patient's body is exposed to assess for less obvious sites of external blood loss and for clues indicating internal hemorrhage. The possibility of hypothermia is also considered. This exposure may be best performed in the heated patient compartment of the ambulance in order to protect the patient from the environment.

Secondary Survey

In some cases, the patient's injuries may be too severe for an adequate secondary survey to be completed in the field. If time permits, the secondary survey can be done while en route to the hospital if no other issues need to be addressed.

Vital Signs

Measurement of an accurate set of vital signs is one of the first steps in the secondary survey or, after reassessing the primary survey, when a few minutes are available during transport.

Ventilatory Rate

The normal ventilatory rate for an adult is 12 to 20 breaths/minute. This rate will vary depending on age. (See the Pediatric Trauma chapter.) A rate of 20 to 30 breaths/minute indicates a borderline abnormal rate; it suggests the onset of shock and the need for supplemental oxygen. A rate greater than 30 breaths/minute indicates a late stage of shock and the need for assisted ventilation. The physiologic drive for the increased ventilatory rate is the acidosis caused by shock, but it is usually associated with a decreased tidal volume. Both of these ventilatory rates indicate the need to look for the potential sources of impaired perfusion. An accurate ventilatory rate is most often obtained via $ETCO_2$ monitoring.

Pulse

In the secondary survey, the pulse rate is determined more precisely. The normal pulse range for an adult is 60 to 100 beats/minute. With lower rates, except in athletic individuals, an ischemic heart, medications, or a pathologic condition such as complete heart block should be considered. A pulse in the range of 100 to 120 beats/minute identifies a patient who has early shock, with an initial cardiac response of tachycardia. A pulse above 120 beats/minute is a definite sign of shock unless it is caused by pain or fear, and a pulse over 140 beats/minute is considered critical.

Blood Pressure

Blood pressure is one of the least sensitive signs of shock. Blood pressure does not begin to drop until a patient is profoundly hypovolemic (from either true fluid loss or container-enlarged relative hypovolemia). Decreased blood pressure indicates the patient can no longer compensate for the hypovolemia and hypoperfusion. In otherwise healthy patients, blood loss may exceed 30% of blood volume before the patient's compensatory mechanisms fail and systolic blood pressure drops below 90 mm Hg. For this reason, ventilatory rate, pulse rate and character, capillary refilling time, and LOC are more sensitive indicators of hypovolemia than is blood pressure.

When the patient's blood pressure has begun to drop, an extremely critical situation exists, and rapid intervention is required. In the prehospital environment, a patient who is found to be hypotensive has already lost a significant volume of blood, and ongoing blood loss is likely. The development of hypotension as a first sign of shock means that earlier signs may have been overlooked.

The severity of the situation and the appropriate type of intervention vary based on the cause of the condition. For example, low blood pressure associated with neurogenic shock is not nearly as critical as low blood pressure from hypovolemic shock. **Table 3-4** presents the signs used to assess compensated and decompensated hypovolemic shock.

An important pitfall to avoid involves equating systolic blood pressure with cardiac output and tissue perfusion. As previously emphasized, significant blood loss is typically required before the patient becomes hypotensive (Class III hemorrhage). Thus, patients will have decreased cardiac output and impaired tissue oxygenation when they have lost 15% to 30% of their blood volume, despite having a normal systolic blood pressure. Ideally, shock will be recognized and treated in the earlier stages before decompensation occurs.

Another possible source of error involves obtaining a single hypotensive blood pressure measurement and not believing it. The blood pressure is repeated and may return to normal (as a part of compensation). Additionally, a blood pressure may be obtained/attempted, and the non-invasive cuff is unable to produce a reading after multiple repeated attempts are cycled. Both of these issues should be concerning until proven otherwise. Do not ignore these potentially ominous signs.

Brain injuries do not cause hypotension until the brain begins to herniate. Therefore, a patient with a brain injury and hypotension should be assumed to have hypovolemia (usually blood loss) from other injuries and not from the brain injury. Young infants (less than 6 months of age) are the exception to this rule because they may bleed enough inside their head to produce hypovolemic shock as a result of open sutures and fontanelles that can spread apart and accommodate large amounts of blood.

Future Monitoring Capabilities

Current research is identifying physiologic monitoring capabilities to assist in managing the acutely injured patient. These advances are expected to enhance our abilities, not replace our physical examination skills. Ultrasound to identify volume status, tissue oxygenation monitoring, shock index monitoring, and compensatory reserve index monitoring are methods that may evolve to assist providers in the prehospital environment.

The shock index (SI) is a tool sometimes used to help predict a trauma patient's course. SI is calculated as heart rate divided by systolic blood pressure. Normal SI is 0.5 to 0.7. The higher the SI, the more likely the patient is to require a blood transfusion. An abnormal SI should raise concern for major injury, but the index is not sensitive enough to use as a reliable screening tool at this time.

The compensatory reserve index (CRI) is a method to noninvasively measure the body's capacity to compensate for blood loss. Compensatory reserve measurement devices are able to monitor the patient's arterial pressure waveform each time the heart contracts and trend changes in those values to predict the body's impending decompensation. These devices have been shown to have greater sensitivity than changes in heart rate, blood pressure, SI, or SpO_2. Research suggests that the CRI provides an early and accurate method to assess for shock in the trauma patient, as it provides the early warning signs of the patient's volume status.

Musculoskeletal Injuries

Significant internal hemorrhage can occur with fractures (**Table 3-5**). Fractures of the femur and pelvis are of greatest

Table 3-4 Shock Assessment in Compensated and Decompensated Hypovolemic Shock		
Vital Sign	**Compensated**	**Decompensated**
Pulse	Increased; tachycardia	Greatly increased; marked tachycardia that can progress to bradycardia
Skin	Pale, cool, moist	White, cold, waxy
Blood pressure range	Normal	Decreased
Level of consciousness	Unaltered	Altered, ranging from disoriented to coma

Table 3-5 Approximate Internal Blood Loss Associated With Fractures	
Type of Fracture	**Internal Blood Loss (ml)**
Rib	125
Radius or ulna	250–500
Humerus	500–750
Tibia or fibula	500–1,000
Femur	1,000–2,000
Pelvis	1,000–massive

concern. A single femoral fracture may be associated with up to 2 to 4 units (1,000 to 2,000 ml) of blood loss into a thigh. This injury alone could potentially result in the loss of 30% to 40% of an adult's blood volume, resulting in decompensated hypovolemic shock. Pelvic fractures, especially those resulting from significant falls or crushing mechanisms, can be associated with massive internal hemorrhage into the retroperitoneal space. A victim of blunt trauma can have multiple fractures and Class III or IV shock but no evidence of external blood loss, hemothoraces, intra-abdominal bleeding, or pelvic fracture. For example, an adult pedestrian struck by a vehicle and sustaining four rib fractures, a humerus fracture, a femur fracture, and bilateral tibia/fibula fractures may experience internal bleeding of 3,000 to 5,500 ml of blood. This potential blood loss is enough for the patient to die from shock if it is unrecognized and inadequately treated.

Confounding Factors

Numerous factors can confound the assessment of the trauma patient, obscuring or blunting the usual signs of shock. These factors may mislead the unwary prehospital care provider into thinking a trauma patient is stable when in fact he or she is not.

Age

Patients at the extremes of life—the very young (neonates) and the elderly—have diminished capability to compensate for acute blood loss and other shock states. A relatively minor injury that would be tolerated without difficulty in a healthy adult may produce decompensated shock in these individuals. In contrast, children and young adults have a tremendous ability to compensate for blood loss and may appear relatively normal on a quick scan. They often appear to be doing well until they suddenly deteriorate into decompensated shock. A closer look may reveal subtle signs of shock, such as mild tachycardia and tachypnea, pale skin with delayed capillary refilling time, and anxiety. Because of their powerful compensatory mechanisms, children found in decompensated shock represent dire emergencies. Elderly individuals may be more prone to certain complications of prolonged shock, such as acute renal failure.

Athletic Status

Well-conditioned athletes often have enhanced compensatory capabilities. Many have resting heart rates in the range of 40 to 50 beats/minute. A heart rate of 100 to 110 beats/minute or hypotension may a be warning sign indicating significant hemorrhage in a well-conditioned athlete.

Pregnancy

During pregnancy, a woman's blood volume may increase by 45% to 50%. Heart rate and cardiac output during pregnancy are also increased. Thus, a pregnant female may not demonstrate signs of shock until her blood loss exceeds 30% to 35% of her total blood volume. Also, well before a pregnant woman demonstrates signs of hypoperfusion, the fetus may be adversely affected because the placental circulation is more sensitive to the vasoconstrictive effects of catecholamines released in response to the shock state. During the third trimester, the gravid uterus may compress the inferior vena cava, greatly diminishing venous return to the heart and resulting in hypotension. Elevation of the pregnant patient's right side once she has been immobilized to a long backboard may alleviate this compression. Hypotension in a pregnant female persisting after performing this maneuver typically represents life-threatening blood loss.

Preexisting Medical Conditions

Patients with serious preexisting medical conditions, such as coronary artery disease, congestive heart failure, and chronic obstructive pulmonary disease, are typically less able to compensate for hemorrhage and shock. These patients may experience angina as their heart rate increases in an effort to maintain their blood pressure. Patients with implanted fixed-rate pacemakers are typically unable to develop the compensatory tachycardia necessary to maintain blood pressure. Patients with diabetes often have longer hospital and intensive care unit stays and more complications than patients without the underlying disease. Their blood vessels may be less compliant due to the long-term effects of hyperglycemia, and they also have decreased sensitivity and ability to respond to hemodynamic changes.

Medications

Numerous medications may interfere with the body's compensatory mechanisms. Beta-adrenergic blocking agents and calcium channel blockers used to treat hypertension may prevent an individual from developing a compensatory tachycardia to maintain blood pressure. Additionally, nonsteroidal anti-inflammatory drugs (NSAIDs), used in the treatment of arthritis and musculoskeletal pain, may impair platelet activity and blood clotting and may result in increased hemorrhage. Newer anticoagulant medications may prevent clotting for several days, and there are no prehospital antidotes to reverse the clotting abnormality. Antiplatelet agents and anticoagulants ("blood thinners") may alter your choice of trauma center destination. If a history of medication use can be obtained from the patient or family members, this is important information to relay to the receiving trauma team.

Time Between Injury and Treatment

In situations in which the EMS response time has been brief, patients may be encountered who have life-threatening internal injury but have not yet lost enough blood to manifest severe shock (Class III or IV hemorrhage). Even patients with penetrating wounds to their aorta, venae cavae, or iliac vessels may arrive at the receiving facility with a normal systolic blood pressure if the EMS response, scene, and transport times are brief. The assumption that patients are not bleeding internally just because they "look good" is frequently wrong. The patient may "look good" because he or she is in compensated shock or because not enough time has elapsed for the signs of shock to manifest. Patients should be thoroughly assessed for even the subtlest signs of shock, and internal hemorrhage should be assumed to be present until it is definitively ruled out. The possibility of late-presenting internal hemorrhage is one reason why continued reassessment of trauma patients is essential.

Management

Steps in the management of shock are as follows:

1. Control any external severe hemorrhage.
2. Ensure oxygenation (adequate airway and ventilation).
3. Identify any hemorrhaging. (Control external bleeding, and recognize the likelihood of internal hemorrhage.)
4. Transport the patient to definitive care.
5. Administer fluid or blood therapy when appropriate.

In addition to securing the airway and providing ventilation to maintain oxygenation, the prime goals of shock treatment include identifying the source or cause, treating the cause as specifically as possible, and supporting the circulation. By maintaining perfusion and oxygen delivery to the cells, energy production is supported and cellular function can be ensured.

In the prehospital setting, external sources of bleeding should be identified and directly controlled immediately. Internal causes of shock usually cannot be definitively treated in the prehospital setting; therefore, the approach is to transport the patient to the definitive care setting while supporting the circulation in the best way possible. Resuscitation in the prehospital setting includes the following:

- Control both external hemorrhage and internal hemorrhage to the extent possible in the prehospital setting. Every red blood cell counts.
- Improve oxygenation of the RBCs in the lungs through:
  - Appropriate airway management
  - Providing ventilatory support with a bag-mask device and delivering a high concentration of supplemental oxygen (fraction of inspired oxygen [F_{IO_2}] greater than 0.85)
- Improve circulation to deliver the oxygenated RBCs more efficiently to the systemic tissues, and improve oxygenation and energy production at the cellular level.

- Maintain body heat by all means possible.
- Reach definitive care as soon as possible for hemorrhage control and replacement of lost RBCs, plasma, coagulation factors, and platelets.

Without appropriate measures, a patient will continue to deteriorate rapidly until he or she reaches the ultimate "stable" condition—death.

The following four questions need to be addressed when deciding what treatment to provide for a patient in shock:

1. What is the cause of the patient's shock?
2. What is the definitive care for the patient's shock?
3. Where can the patient best receive definitive care?
4. What interim steps can be taken to support the patient and manage the condition while the patient is being transported to definitive care?

Although the first question may be difficult to answer accurately in the field, identification of the possible source of the shock assists in defining which facility is best suited to meeting the patient's needs and what measures may be necessary during transport to improve the patient's chances of survival.

Exsanguinating Hemorrhage

Major hemorrhage must be controlled rapidly. A number of different tourniquets are available for use on extremity or junctional hemorrhage, as well as several types of wound packing/clot-promoting materials. Life-threatening hemorrhage must be treated promptly and aggressively.

Hemorrhage Control

Control of obvious major external hemorrhage immediately precedes securing the airway and initiating oxygen therapy and ventilatory support, or it is performed simultaneously with these steps if sufficient assistance is present. When the hemorrhage is clearly life threatening, then efforts to control the hemorrhage take priority. Early recognition and control of external bleeding in the trauma patient help preserve the patient's blood volume and RBCs and ensure continued perfusion of tissues. Even a small trickle of blood can add up to substantial blood loss if it is ignored for a long enough time. Thus, in the multisystem trauma patient, no bleeding is minor, and every RBC counts toward ensuring continued perfusion of the body's tissues.

The steps in the field management of external hemorrhage include:

- Hand-held direct pressure
- Compression dressings
- Wound packing
- Elastic wrap
- Tourniquet
- Hemostatic agent
- Junctional tourniquets when indicated

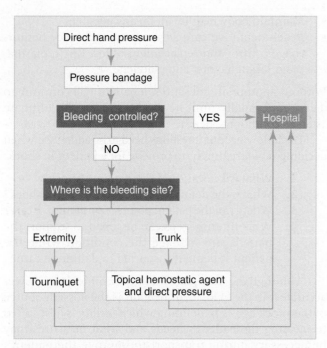

Figure 3-14 Hemorrhage control in the field.

© National Association of Emergency Medical Technicians (NAEMT).

Control of external hemorrhage should proceed in a stepwise fashion, escalating if initial measures fail to control bleeding (**Figure 3-14**). Some tactical situations may identify the need for tourniquet placement as the initial hemorrhage control maneuver.

Direct Pressure

Direct hand pressure or a pressure dressing, applied directly over a bleeding site, is the initial technique employed to control external hemorrhage. This application of pressure is based upon Bernoulli's principle and involves a number of considerations:

Fluid leak = Transmural pressure × Size of hole in vessel wall

Transmural pressure is the difference between the pressure within the vessel and the pressure outside the vessel. The pressure exerted against the inside of the blood vessel walls by the intravascular fluids and blood pressure cycle is called the **intramural (intraluminal) pressure**. The force exerted against the wall of the blood vessel from the outside (such as by a hand or a dressing) is called the **extramural (extraluminal) pressure**. To illustrate this relationship:

Transmural pressure = Intramural pressure − Extramural pressure

The higher the pressure inside the vessel, the faster that blood is forced out of the hole. The more pressure that the prehospital care provider applies, the more slowly that blood will leak out. Direct pressure on the wound increases the extramural pressure, thus slowing the leak.

The ability of the body to respond to and control bleeding from a lacerated vessel is a function of the following:

- The size of the vessel
- The pressure within the vessel
- The presence of clotting factors
- The ability of the injured vessel to go into spasm and reduce the size of the hole and blood flow at the injury site
- The pressure of the surrounding tissue on the vessel at the injury site and any additional pressure provided by the prehospital care provider from the outside

Blood vessels, especially arteries, that are completely transected often retract and go into spasm. There is often less hemorrhage from the stump of an extremity with a complete amputation than from an extremity with severe trauma in which blood vessels are damaged but not completely transected.

Direct pressure over the site of hemorrhage increases the extraluminal pressure and, therefore, reduces the transmural pressure, helping to slow or stop bleeding. Direct pressure also serves a second and equally important function. Compressing the sides of the torn vessel reduces the size (area) of the opening and further reduces blood flow out of the vessel. Even if blood loss is not completely stemmed, it may be diminished to the point that the blood-clotting system can stop the hemorrhage. This is why direct pressure is almost always successful at controlling bleeding. Multiple studies involving hemorrhage from femoral artery puncture sites after cardiac catheterization have documented that direct pressure is an effective technique.[6,7-9]

Following a leaky pipe analogy, if there is a small hole in the pipe, simply putting one's finger over the hole will stop the leak temporarily. Tape can then be wrapped around the pipe for a short-term fix of the leak. The same concept applies to the hemorrhaging patient. Direct pressure on the open wound is followed by a pressure dressing. However, for the pressure dressing to be most effective, the pressure must be placed directly on the injury in the vessel. A simple dressing placed on the skin over the wound does not impart any direct pressure on the bleeding site itself.

To achieve the most effective use of a pressure dressing, the dressing material must be packed tightly down into the wound and the elastic bandage placed on the outside. Packing of a wound may be accomplished with the use of a hemostatic agent such as Combat Gauze or Celox or may be performed using a plain gauze roll. The key is to place the packing material into the base of the wound, directly onto the bleeding site and then pack the entire roll into the wound. Then direct pressure over the wound should be placed for a minimum of 3 minutes or per the manufacturer's instructions and for 10 minutes if using plain gauze.

From a vascular and patient perspective, this means the MAP (intraluminal pressure) and the pressure in the tissue surrounding the vessel (extraluminal pressure) have a direct relationship in controlling the rate of blood loss from the vessel as well as the size of the hole in the vessel. Of note, when a patient's blood pressure has been reduced by blood loss, it is appropriate not to increase it to back to normal levels; rather, blood loss should be stopped and blood pressure maintained at a level sufficient to perfuse vital organs. This level generally occurs when the patient's systolic blood pressure is between 80 and 90 mm Hg. This means avoiding overinfusion of IV fluids into the patient and maintaining a modest degree of hypotension. Raising the blood pressure back to normal levels by administering large volumes of IV crystalloid fluids produces the exact opposite of the desired effect, increasing hemorrhage as a result of "popping" any clot that has formed over an opening in a blood vessel.

Therefore, the steps in managing hemorrhage are to (1) increase external pressure (hand-pressure dressing), which decreases the size of the hole in the lumen of the blood vessel and decreases the differential between internal and external pressure, both of which contribute to retarding blood flow out of the injured vessel, and (2) use the technique of hypotensive resuscitation to ensure that the intraluminal pressure is not raised extensively.

THREE CRITICAL POINTS

Three additional points about direct pressure should be emphasized. First, when managing a wound with an impaled object, pressure should be applied on either side of the object rather than over the object. Impaled objects should not be removed in the field because the object may have damaged a vessel, and the object itself could be tamponading the bleeding. Removal of the object could result in uncontrolled internal hemorrhage.

Second, if hands are required to perform other lifesaving tasks, a pressure (compression) dressing can be created using gauze pads and an elastic roller bandage or a blood pressure cuff inflated until hemorrhage stops. This dressing is placed directly over the bleeding site.

Third, applying direct pressure to exsanguinating hemorrhage takes precedence over insertion of IV lines and fluid resuscitation. It would be a serious error to deliver a well-packaged trauma victim to the receiving facility with two IV lines inserted and neatly taped in place but who is dying from the hemorrhage of a wound that only has trauma dressings taped in place with no direct pressure applied.

Tourniquets

If external bleeding from an extremity cannot be controlled by pressure, application of a tourniquet is the reasonable next step in hemorrhage control. Tourniquets had fallen out of favor because of concern about potential complications, including damage to nerves and blood vessels and potential loss of the limb if the tourniquet is left on too long. None of these concerns has been proven; in fact, data from the Iraq and Afghanistan wars have demonstrated just the opposite.[10,11] There have been no limbs lost as a result of tourniquet placement by the U.S. military. Data from the military experience suggest that appropriately applied tourniquets could potentially have prevented 7 out of every 100 combat deaths.[12,13]

Tourniquet control of exsanguinating limb hemorrhage is 80% or better.[14,15] In addition, tourniquets occluding arterial inflow have been widely used in the OR by surgeons for many years with satisfactory results. Used properly, tourniquets are not only safe but also lifesaving.[16]

A study from the military in Iraq and Afghanistan showed a marked difference in survival when the tourniquet was applied before the patient decompensated into shock compared to when it was applied after blood pressure had dropped.[17] When the tourniquet was applied before the patient went into shock, survival was 96%; when it was placed after the patient developed shock, survival was 4%.

For hemorrhage from locations not amenable to placement of a tourniquet, such as on the abdomen or groin, it is reasonable to use hemostatic agents. Currently, the U.S. Army Institute of Surgical Research recommends Combat Gauze as the preferred third-generation product. This recommendation may change over time; please visit the NAEMT website for the latest information.

DEVICE OPTIONS

Because of the U.S. military's interest in an effective, easy-to-use tourniquet (especially one that a soldier could apply quickly with one hand should the other arm be injured), many commercial tourniquets have been developed and marketed. In a laboratory study, three products were 100% effective in occluding distal arterial blood flow: Combat Application Tourniquet (C-A-T; North American Rescue), the Emergency & Military Tourniquet (EMT; Delfi Medical Innovations), and the Special Operations Force Tactical Tourniquet (SOFT-T; Tactical Medical Solutions) (**Figure 3-15**).[18-20] Of these, the Committee on Tactical Combat Casualty Care (CoTCCC) currently recommends use of the C-A-T and the SOFT-T. Again, this recommendation may change over time, and the latest updates from the CoTCCC and PHTLS will appear on the NAEMT website.

APPLICATION SITE

A tourniquet should be applied in the groin or axilla. If one tourniquet does not completely stop the hemorrhage, then another one should be applied just proximal to the first. By placing two tourniquets side by side, the area of compression is doubled and successful control of hemorrhage is more likely. Once applied, the tourniquet site should not be covered so it can be easily seen and monitored.

APPLICATION TIGHTNESS

A tourniquet should be applied tight enough to block arterial flow and occlude the distal pulse. A device that occludes only venous outflow from a limb will actually

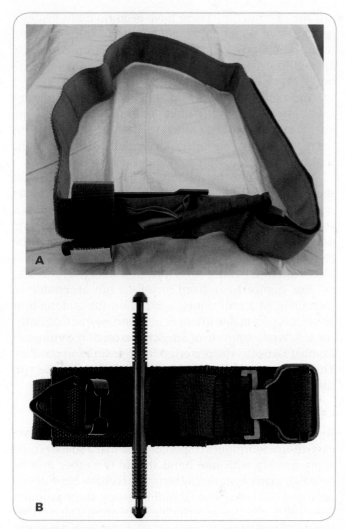

Figure 3-15 **A.** A C-A-T tourniquet. **B.** A SOF-T tourniquet.

A. Courtesy of Peter T. Pons, MD, FACEP. **B.** Courtesy of TacMed Solutions.

increase hemorrhage from a wound. A direct relationship exists between the amount of pressure required to control hemorrhage and the size of the limb. Thus, on average, a tourniquet will need to be placed more tightly on a leg to achieve hemorrhage control than on an arm.

TIME LIMIT

Arterial tourniquets have been used safely for up to 120 to 150 minutes in the OR without significant nerve or muscle damage. Even in suburban or rural settings, most EMS transport times are significantly less than this period. In general, a tourniquet placed in the prehospital setting should remain in place until the patient reaches definitive care at the closest appropriate hospital. U.S. military use has not shown significant deterioration with prolonged application times.[10] If application of a tourniquet is required, the patient will most likely need emergency surgery to control the hemorrhage. Thus, the ideal receiving facility for such a patient is one with surgical capabilities.

In the past, it was often recommended that a tourniquet be loosened every 10 to 15 minutes to allow for some blood flow back into the injured extremity with the thought being that this blood flow would help preserve the limb and prevent subsequent amputation. This practice serves only to increase the blood loss sustained by the patient and does nothing for the limb itself. Once applied, the tourniquet should be left in place until no longer needed.

A tourniquet can be painful for a conscious patient to tolerate, and pain management should be considered. **Box 3-6** provides a sample protocol for tourniquet application.

Hemostatic Agents

The U.S. Food and Drug Administration (FDA) has approved a number of topical hemostatic agents for use. Hemostatic agents are designed to be placed or packed into a wound to enhance clotting and promote control of life-threatening hemorrhage that cannot be stopped with direct pressure alone in areas of the body that are not amenable to tourniquet placement. These agents generally come in the form of a gauze impregnated with the hemostatic material that is applied to or packed into the wound (**Figure 3-16**).

It is important to note that these agents require packing the hemostatic dressing directly into the wound, not merely applying the dressing as a cover to the open injury. Also, a minimum of 3 minutes of direct pressure must be

---

Box 3-6 Protocol for Tourniquet Application

Tourniquets should be used if controlling the hemorrhage with direct pressure or pressure dressing is not possible or fails. The steps in applying a tourniquet are as follows:

1. Apply a commercially manufactured tourniquet to the extremity at the level of the groin for the lower extremity or the axilla for the upper extremity.
2. Tighten the tourniquet until hemorrhage ceases, and then secure it in place.
3. Write the time of tourniquet application on a piece of tape, and secure it to the tourniquet. For example, "TK 2145" indicates that the tourniquet was applied at 2145 hours.
4. Leave the tourniquet uncovered so the site can be seen and monitored. If bleeding continues after application and tightening of the initial tourniquet, a second tourniquet can be applied just above the first.
5. Anticipate the need for pain management.
6. Transport the patient, ideally to a facility that has surgical capability.

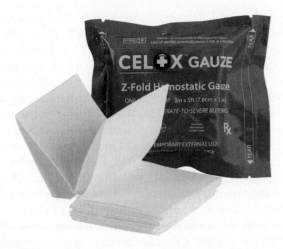

Figure 3-16 Hemostatic agents are designed to be placed or packed in areas of the body that are not amenable to tourniquet placement.

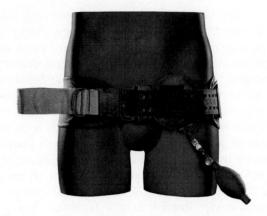

Figure 3-17 Junctional tourniquets have been used by the U.S. military in combat theaters to control severe bleeding.

applied to the wound site for most of the available agents. At least one manufacturer has recently offered a hemostatic product that they report does not require the application of direct pressure after the placement of the product in the wound.

Combat Gauze was the product recommended for use by the CoTCCC based on research done by both the U.S. Navy and U.S. Army research labs. Again, this recommendation may change over time, and the latest updates from the CoTCCC and PHTLS will appear on the PHTLS website.

One study that compared a number of different hemostatic agents to plain gauze packing demonstrated no difference in blood loss or animal survival between the hemostatic agents and the plain gauze material.[21] This finding strongly suggests that, while the hemostatic agent aids in promoting clotting, the primary factor controlling hemorrhage is likely the proper packing of the dressing into the wound with the application of direct pressure onto the bleeding site.

Junctional Hemorrhage Control

Wounds located in the so-called junctional areas of the body, locations where the extremities and head join the trunk (groin, axilla and shoulder, and neck), may injure major blood vessels that can bleed profusely. In particular, wounds of the lower extremities from improvised explosive devices (IEDs) often result in high amputations and wounds that cannot accommodate tourniquet placement. The CoTCCC has recommended a number of devices designed to control bleeding from wounds such as these (**Figure 3-17**). These devices include the Combat Ready Clamp (CRoC; Combat Medical Systems), the Junctional Emergency Treatment Tool (JETT; North American Rescue

Products, LLC), and the SAM Junctional Tourniquet (SJT; SAM Medical Products). Some of these devices have been vetted by the U.S. military for use in combat theaters. The role and utility of these devices in the civilian setting have not been well studied or defined.

Elevation and Pressure Points

In the past, emphasis was placed on elevation of an extremity and compression on a pressure point (proximal to the bleeding site) as intermediate steps in hemorrhage control. No research has been published on whether elevation of a bleeding extremity slows hemorrhage. If a bone in the extremity is fractured, this maneuver could potentially result in converting a closed fracture to an open one or in causing increased internal hemorrhage. Similarly, the use of pressure points for hemorrhage control has not been studied. Thus, in the absence of compelling data, these interventions are no longer recommended for situations in which direct pressure or a pressure dressing has failed to control hemorrhage.

Airway

Advanced techniques for securing the airway and maintaining ventilation may be required in the prehospital setting. (See the Airway and Ventilation chapter.) The importance of essential airway skills, especially when transport times are brief, should not be underestimated.

Breathing

Once a patent airway is ensured, patients in shock or those at risk for developing shock (almost all trauma patients) should initially receive supplemental oxygen in a concentration as close to 100% (FIO_2 of 1.0) as possible. This level of oxygenation can be achieved only with a device with a reservoir attached to the oxygen source. Nasal prongs, a nasal cannula, or a simple face mask do not meet this requirement. Spo_2 should be monitored by pulse oximetry in virtually all trauma patients and maintained at or above 94% (at sea level) and correlated with the patient's condition.

A nonbreathing patient, or one who is breathing without an adequate depth and rate, needs ventilatory assistance by opening the airway and adjunct airway devices such as oropharyngeal and nasopharyngeal airways. If there is no response to these maneuvers, use a bag-mask device immediately. It is critical to pay close attention to the quality of your assisted ventilations. Hyperventilation during assisted ventilation produces a negative physiologic response, especially in the patient with hypovolemic shock or with TBI. Ventilating too deeply or too quickly can make the patient alkalotic. This chemical response increases the affinity of hemoglobin for oxygen, resulting in decreased oxygen delivery to the tissue. In addition, hyperventilation may increase the intrathoracic pressure, leading to impaired venous return to the heart and hypotension. Data from animal experiments using a hypovolemic shock model suggest normal or higher ventilatory rates in animals with even moderate hemorrhage-impaired hemodynamic functioning, as exhibited by lower systolic blood pressure and cardiac output.[20,21] The increase in intrathoracic pressure could result either from large tidal volumes (10 to 12 ml/kg body weight) or from the creation of "auto-PEEP" (positive end-expiratory pressure) when ventilated too quickly (inadequate exhalation leads to air trapping in the lungs). In the patient with TBI, inadvertent hyperventilation will lead to cerebral vasoconstriction and decreased cerebral blood flow. This will exacerbate the secondary injury occurring in the brain. For an adult patient, giving a reasonable tidal volume (350 to 500 ml) at a rate of 10 ventilations/ minute is probably sufficient.

$ETCO_2$ monitoring is often used in conjunction with pulse oximetry to maintain the patient in a **eucapnic state** (normal blood carbon dioxide level) with satisfactory oxygenation; however, in the patient with compromised perfusion, the correlation of $ETCO_2$ with $Paco_2$ may be altered and cannot be relied upon to accurately judge ventilation.

Internal Hemorrhage

Internal hemorrhage from fracture sites should also be considered. Rough handling of an injured extremity not only may convert a closed fracture to an open one but also may significantly increase internal bleeding from bone ends, adjacent muscle tissue, or damaged vessels. All suspected extremity fractures should be immobilized in an effort to minimize this hemorrhage. Time may be taken to splint several fractures individually if the patient has no evidence of life-threatening conditions. If the primary survey identifies threats to the patient's life, however, the patient should be immobilized rapidly on an appropriate device such as a long backboard or vacuum mattress, thereby immobilizing all of the extremities in an anatomic manner, and transported to a medical facility. Pelvic binders have been shown to splint and approximate the fractures of the pelvic bone, and while no studies have been done to show any change in outcome if used in the prehospital setting, there is good reason to believe that judicious early use of pelvic binders can limit hemorrhage from pelvic fractures and potentially limit mortality. There is no evidence that use of such devices in the prehospital setting or elsewhere is at all dangerous. Current CoTCCC recommendations support the application of pelvic binders.

Disability

There are no unique, specific interventions for altered mental status in the shock patient. If the patient's abnormal neurologic status is the result of cerebral hypoxia and poor perfusion, efforts to correct hypoxia and restore perfusion throughout the body should result in improved mental status. In assessing a patient's prognosis after TBI, an "initial" Glasgow Coma Scale (GCS) score is typically considered to be the score established following adequate resuscitation and restoration of cerebral perfusion. Assessing a patient's GCS score while still in shock may result in an overly grim prognosis.

Expose/Environment

Maintaining the patient's body temperature within a normal range is critically important. Hypothermia results from exposure to colder environments by convection, conduction, and other physical means (see the Environmental Trauma I: Heat and Cold chapter) and from loss of energy production with anaerobic metabolism. The greatest concern regarding hypothermia is its effect on blood clotting. As the body cools, clotting is impaired. In addition, hypothermia worsens coagulopathy, myocardial dysfunction, hyperkalemia, vasoconstriction, and a host of other problems that negatively affect a patient's chance of survival.[22] Although cold temperatures preserve tissue for a short time, the temperature drop must be very rapid and very low for preservation to occur. Such a rapid change has not been proven effective for the patient in shock after trauma.

In the prehospital setting, increasing the core temperature once hypothermia has developed can be difficult; therefore, all steps that can be taken in the field to preserve normal body temperature should be initiated. Once exposed and examined, the patient must be protected from the environment and body temperature maintained. Any wet clothing, including that saturated with blood, is removed from the patient because wet clothing increases heat loss. The patient is covered with warm blankets. The need for warming the patient can be anticipated and blankets placed near heater vents in the ambulance en route to the call. An alternative to blankets involves covering the patient with plastic sheets, such as heavy, thick garbage bags. They are inexpensive, easily stored, disposable, and effective devices for heat retention. Heated, humidified oxygen, if available, may help preserve body heat, especially in intubated patients.

Once assessed and packaged, the patient in shock is moved into the warmed patient compartment of the ambulance. Ideally, the patient compartment of an ambulance is kept at 85°F (29°C) or more when transporting a severely injured trauma patient. The patient's rate of heat loss into a cold compartment is very high. The conditions must be ideal for the patient, not for the prehospital care providers, because the patient is the most important person in any emergency. A good general rule is that if the provider is comfortable in the patient compartment, it is too cold for the patient.

Patient Transport

Effective treatment of a patient in severe hemorrhagic shock requires emergent evaluation and access to a trauma center with an OR and blood products. Because neither is routinely available in the prehospital trauma setting, rapid transport to a facility capable of managing the patient's injuries is important. Rapid transport does not mean doing the old-fashioned "scoop and run" and disregarding or neglecting the treatment modalities that are important in patient care. Diesel is not an appropriate therapeutic maneuver, as is often mentioned in the prehospital social setting. The prehospital care provider must quickly institute critical, potentially lifesaving measures, such as hemorrhage control, airway management, and ventilatory support. Time must not be wasted on an inappropriate assessment or with unnecessary immobilization maneuvers. When caring for a critically injured patient, many steps, such as warming the patient, starting intravascular therapy, and even performing the secondary survey, are accomplished in the ambulance while en route to the appropriate trauma facility.

Patient Positioning

In general, trauma patients who are in shock may typically be transported in the supine position. Special positioning, such as the Trendelenburg position (placed on an incline with the feet elevated above the head) or the "shock" position (head and torso supine with legs elevated), although used for 150 years, has not been proven to be effective. The

Trendelenburg position may aggravate already impaired ventilatory function, may present an aspiration/airway obstruction risk, and may increase intracranial pressure in patients with TBI. More important, patients who are in severe hypovolemic shock are, generally, maximally vasoconstricted.[23,24] Patients with isolated TBI should typically be transported with the head of the bed elevated to 30 degrees. This position facilitates improvement in cerebral perfusion pressure and decreases intracranial pressure. Additionally, if a patient is intubated, there is a benefit to elevating the head of the bed to 30 degrees to decrease risk of aspiration and later stage ventilator-associated pneumonia.

Vascular Access

Intravenous Route

Intravascular access is obtained in a trauma patient who has known or suspected serious injuries so the prehospital care provider can initiate resuscitation if appropriate. Except in unusual circumstances, such as a patient undergoing extrication from a vehicle or providers awaiting the arrival of a helicopter, IV access should be obtained after the patient has been placed in the ambulance and transport has been initiated to the closest appropriate facility. Gaining IV access should not delay transport to the hospital for the severely injured patient.

Although volume resuscitation of a trauma patient in shock makes empiric sense, no research has demonstrated improved survival rates of critically injured trauma patients when IV fluid therapy was initiated in the prehospital setting. Transport of the trauma patient should never be delayed to initiate IV lines.

One study demonstrated there was no benefit from the use of IV fluids before hemorrhage was controlled.[25] Unfortunately, there have been no good studies that randomized the use of fluid resuscitation in patients with only uncontrolled hemorrhage as opposed to including patients with controlled hemorrhage. All of the studies that have been done mix both types of patients. Until such a study is done, the use of anecdotal and mixed studies must be the basis for the recommended practice.

For patients in shock or with potentially serious injuries, one or preferably two large-bore (18-gauge), short (1-inch [25 mm]) IV catheters should be inserted by percutaneous puncture as time permits. The rate of fluid administration is directly proportional to the fourth power of the radius of the catheter and inversely proportional to its length (meaning more fluid will rapidly flow through a shorter, larger diameter catheter than through a longer, smaller diameter catheter). The preferred site for percutaneous access is a vein of the forearm. Alternative sites for IV access are the veins of the antecubital fossa, the hand, and the upper arm (cephalic vein).

Intraosseous Route

An alternative for vascular access in adults is the intraosseous route.[26,27] The intraosseous route of giving IV fluids is not new and was described by Dr. Walter E. Lee in 1941. This method of vascular access can be accomplished in a number of ways. It is most commonly established in sites such as the distal femur, humeral head, or proximal or distal tibia. Studies show best flow rates are through the humeral head and distal femur sites. It can also be established via the sternal technique, using appropriately designed devices (**Figure 3-18** and **Figure 3-19**).[28,29] These techniques are commonly used in the prehospital setting, but the focus should be on rapid transport rather than IV fluid administration. For delayed or prolonged transport to definitive care, intraosseous vascular access may have a role in adult trauma patients. Fluid administration via the interosseous route in an awake patient may be quite painful. Appropriate analgesia should be administered in accordance with local policy.

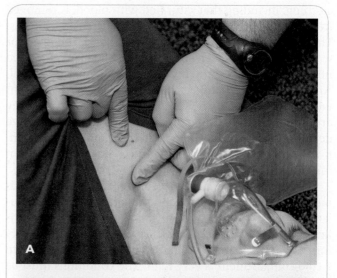

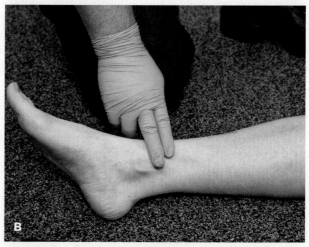

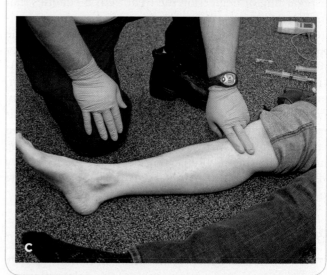

Figure 3-19 A. Sternal insertion site in the manubrium below the suprasternal notch. Note that the EZ-IO device cannot be used at the sternal site. **B.** Distal tibia insertion site above the ankle. **C.** Proximal tibia insertion site below the knee.

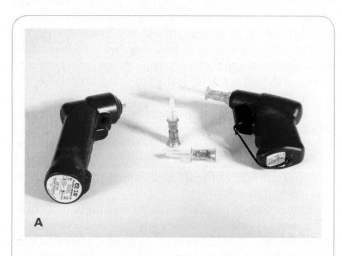

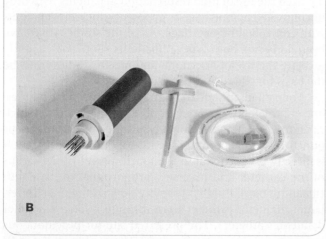

Figure 3-18 A. IO needles and IO gun for manual insertion (various sizes shown). **B.** IO sternal driver.

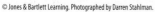

Volume Resuscitation

There are two general categories of fluid resuscitation products that have been used in the past 50 years for the management of trauma patients—blood and IV solutions. These products can be further subdivided as follows:

- Blood
  - Packed red blood cells (PRBCs)
  - Whole blood
  - Reconstituted whole blood as blood products
  - Plasma
  - Additional blood component therapy
- IV solutions
  - Crystalloid solutions
  - Hypertonic fluid
    - 7% saline
    - 3% saline
  - Colloid solutions
  - Hypotensive or restricted fluid strategies
  - Blood substitutes

Each of these products has advantages and disadvantages.

Blood

Because of its ability to transport oxygen, blood or various blood products remain the fluid of choice for the resuscitation of a patient in severe hemorrhagic shock. Experience gained by the U.S. military as a result of the Iraq and Afghanistan wars has demonstrated the importance of administration of whole blood, packed RBCs, and plasma to the survival of injured soldiers. This "reconstituted" blood replaces the lost oxygen-carrying capacity, clotting factors, and proteins needed to maintain oncotic pressure to prevent fluid loss from the vascular system. Unfortunately, blood, for the most part, is impractical for use in the civilian prehospital setting primarily because blood and its subcomponents are perishable if not kept refrigerated or frozen until the moment of use.

Currently, lyophilized plasma is being used in the field in several countries. Lyophilized plasma is human plasma that has been freeze dried. It has a stable shelf life of approximately 2 years, does not require refrigeration, and must be reconstituted prior to use. Liquid plasma is being carried by a few EMS and HEMS (helicopter EMS) systems in the United States, and research is under way to evaluate the use of plasma in the civilian prehospital setting for the resuscitation of trauma patients. Additional investigations using whole blood transfusion are in the initial stages as well.

Intravenous Solutions

Alternative solutions for volume resuscitation fall into one of four categories: (1) isotonic crystalloids, (2) hypertonic crystalloids, (3) synthetic (artificial) colloids, and (4) blood substitutes.

Isotonic Crystalloid Solutions

Isotonic crystalloids are balanced salt solutions comprised of electrolytes (substances that separate into charged ions when dissolved in solutions). They act as effective volume expanders for a short time, but they possess no oxygen-carrying capacity. Immediately after infusion, crystalloids fill the vascular space depleted by blood loss, improving preload and cardiac output. **Lactated Ringer solution** remains the isotonic crystalloid solution of choice for the management of shock because its composition is most similar to the electrolyte composition of blood plasma. It contains specific amounts of sodium, potassium, calcium, chloride, and lactate ions. **Normal saline** (0.9% sodium chloride [NaCl] solution) remains an acceptable alternative, although hyperchloremia (a marked increase in the blood chloride level) may occur with massive volume resuscitation with normal saline administration. Normosol and Plasma-Lyte are another option as more "balanced" acid–base solutions than normal saline. Solutions of dextrose in water (e.g., D_5W) are not effective volume expanders and have no place in the resuscitation of trauma patients. In fact, administration of glucose-containing fluids serves only to increase the patient's blood glucose level, which then has a diuretic effect and will actually increase fluid loss via the kidneys.

Unfortunately, within 30 to 60 minutes after administration of a crystalloid solution, only about one-fourth to one-third of the administered volume remains in the cardiovascular system. The rest has shifted into the interstitial space because both the water and the electrolytes in the solution can freely cross the capillary membranes. The lost fluid becomes edema in the soft tissues and organs of the body. This extra fluid causes difficulties with the on-loading and off-loading of oxygen to the RBCs.

If possible, IV fluids should be warmed to about 102°F (39°C) before infusion. Infusion of large amounts of room-temperature or cold IV fluid contributes to hypothermia and increased hemorrhage.

Hypertonic Crystalloid Solutions

Hypertonic crystalloid solutions have extremely high concentrations of electrolytes compared to blood plasma. The most commonly used experimental model is **hypertonic saline**, a 7.5% NaCl solution, which is more than eight times the concentration of NaCl in normal saline. This is an effective plasma expander, especially in that a small, 250-ml infusion often produces the same effect as infusing 2 to 3 liters of isotonic crystalloid solution.[30,31] An analysis of several studies of hypertonic saline failed, however, to demonstrate improved survival rates over the use of isotonic crystalloids.[32] This solution is not FDA approved for patient care in the United States. Lesser concentrations, such as 3.0%, are approved for patient care and are frequently used in intensive care units.

Synthetic Colloid Solutions

Proteins are large molecules produced by the body that are comprised of amino acids. They have countless functions. One type of protein found in the blood, albumin, helps maintain fluid in the intravascular space. Intravenous administration of human albumin is costly and has been associated with the transmission of infectious diseases, such as hepatitis. When administered to a patient in hemorrhagic shock, synthetic colloid solutions draw fluid from the interstitial and intracellular spaces into the intravascular space, thereby producing expansion of the blood volume. As with crystalloids, colloid plasma expanders do not transport oxygen.

Gelofusine is a 4% gelatin solution produced from bovine protein, and it is occasionally used in Europe and Australia for fluid resuscitation. It is moderately expensive and carries a risk of severe allergic reactions. A small infusion of gelofusine produces expansion of the intravascular volume for several hours.

Hetastarch (Hespan, Hextend) and dextran (Gentran) are synthetic colloids that have been created by linking numerous starch (amylopectin) or dextrose molecules together until they are similar in size to an albumin molecule. These solutions are moderately expensive compared to crystalloids and have been associated with allergic reactions and impairment of blood typing. Two recent meta-analyses of the literature related to the use of hetastarch have raised concerns about an increased incidence of acute kidney injury and increased mortality related to administration of these compounds.[33,34]

The use of crystalloids versus colloids has caused a long-standing debate in the management of trauma patients.[35] A study of almost 7,000 patients admitted to intensive care units demonstrated no difference in outcome when patients were resuscitated with colloid (albumin) versus normal saline.[36] A subsequent meta-analysis echoed this finding.[34] A single study presented at the 2009 American Association for the Surgery of Trauma (AAST) meeting identified a greater survival with Hextend than with normal saline; however, more information is needed before its routine use can be recommended. Hextend is a colloid solution that has been used in military situations as a volume expander. The benefits are that it is a smaller and lighter (although more expensive) package, which is more easily carried; it improves perfusion without overloading the patient with crystalloid; and it appears to be effective. However, a recent meta-analysis raises the question about possible increased mortality from acute kidney injury from this type of product.[33]

Virtually no research involving the use of these synthetic colloid solutions in the civilian prehospital setting has been published, and no data exist from their use in hospitals that shows them to be superior to crystalloid solutions. These products are not recommended for the prehospital management of shock.

Blood Substitutes

Blood transfusion has several limitations and undesirable qualities, including the need to type and crossmatch, a short shelf life, perishability when not refrigerated, a potential for transmission of infectious disease, and an increasing shortage of donated units that limits its use in the prehospital setting. This has led to intense research in blood substitutes during the past two to three decades. The U.S. military has played a central role in this research because a blood substitute that does not need refrigeration and does not require blood typing could be carried to a wounded soldier on the battlefield and infused rapidly to treat shock.

Perfluorocarbons (PFCs) are synthetic compounds that have high oxygen solubility. These inert materials can dissolve approximately 50 times more oxygen than blood plasma can. PFCs contain no hemoglobin or protein; they are completely free of biologic materials, thereby greatly reducing the threat of infectious agents being found in them; and oxygen is transported by dissolving in the plasma portion. First-generation PFCs were of limited use because of numerous problems, including a short half-life and the need for a concurrent high-F_{IO_2} administration. Newer PFCs have fewer disadvantages, but their role as oxygen carriers remains undetermined.

Most hemoglobin-based oxygen carriers (HBOCs) use the same oxygen-carrying molecule (hemoglobin) found in human, bovine, or porcine blood cells. The major difference between HBOCs and human blood is that the hemoglobin in HBOCs is not contained within a cell membrane. This removes the need for conducting type and crossmatch studies because the antigen–antibody risk is removed when the hemoglobin is extracted from the cell. Additionally, many of these HBOCs can be stored for long periods, making them the ideal solution for mass-casualty incidents. Early problems with hemoglobin-based oxygen-carrying solutions included toxicity from hemoglobin. To date, none of those experimental solutions has been found to be safe or effective in humans.

Warming Intravenous Fluids

Any IV fluid given to a patient in shock should be warm, not room temperature or cold. The ideal temperature for such fluids is 102°F (39°C). Wrapping heat packs around the bag can warm fluid. Commercially available fluid-warmer units for the patient care compartment provide an easy and reliable means to keep fluids at the correct temperature. These units are costly but justifiable for prolonged transports. Innovative solutions for warming fluids should be undertaken to prevent hypothermia in the trauma patient.

Managing Volume Resuscitation

As noted earlier, significant controversy surrounds pre-hospital fluid administration for a trauma patient who is in shock. When Prehospital Trauma Life Support (PHTLS) was first introduced in the United States, prehospital care providers adopted the approach used by emergency physicians and surgeons in most trauma centers: Administer an IV crystalloid solution until the vital signs return to normal (typically, pulse less than 100 beats/minute and systolic blood pressure greater than 100 mm Hg). When sufficient crystalloid solution is infused to restore vital signs to normal, the patient's perfusion should be improved. At the time, experts believed such rapid intervention would clear lactic acid and restore energy production in the cells of the body and decrease the risk of developing irreversible shock and kidney failure. However, no study of trauma patients in the prehospital setting has shown that the administration of IV fluid actually does decrease complications and death.

A major contribution of PHTLS over the past two decades has been to establish the conceptual change that, in the critically injured trauma patient, transport should never be delayed while IV lines are placed and fluid is infused. These actions can be performed in the back of the ambulance en route to the closest appropriate facility. The critically injured trauma patient who is in shock generally requires blood transfusion and intervention to control internal hemorrhage, neither of which can be accomplished in the field. Almost nothing should delay the bleeding patient en route to an operating room or emergency department where the hemorrhage can be controlled.

Research, primarily in experimental models of shock, has shown that resuscitation using crystalloid fluids may have detrimental side effects when administered before surgical control of the source of hemorrhage. In experimental animals, internal hemorrhage often continues until the animal is hypotensive, at which point bleeding slows and a blood clot (thrombus) typically forms at the site of the injury. In one sense, this hypotension is protective, in that it is associated with a dramatic slowing or cessation of internal hemorrhage. When aggressive IV fluids were administered to the animals in an attempt to restore perfusion and blood pressure, internal hemorrhage started again, and the thrombus was disrupted.

In addition, crystalloid infusions may dilute coagulation factors. The experimental animals often had a worse outcome compared with animals after surgical control of the injury site.[37-39] In a similar animal model, improved survival was noted with "hypotensive resuscitation," in which the blood pressure was purposefully kept low until hemorrhage was controlled, and then resuscitation took place.[40-42]

Clearly, these studies have potential implications on fluid resuscitation in the prehospital setting. Aggressive volume resuscitation can return the blood pressure to normal. This, in turn, may dislodge blood clots formed at bleeding sites in the peritoneal cavity or elsewhere and may result in renewed hemorrhage that cannot be controlled until the patient reaches the OR. On the other hand, withholding IV fluid from a patient in profound shock only leads to further tissue hypoxia and failure of energy production. A single clinical study conducted in an urban prehospital setting demonstrated a worse outcome in trauma patients who received crystalloid solutions before control of internal hemorrhage (survival rate of 62% versus 70% in the delayed-treatment group).[22] The findings of this single study have not been replicated in other prehospital systems, and the findings cannot be generalized to rural EMS systems. In a survey of trauma surgeons, fewer than 4% opted for an approach that involved withholding IV fluid from a patient in Class III shock. However, almost two-thirds of the surgeons recommended that such a patient be maintained in a relatively hypotensive state during transport.[43]

Prehospital volume resuscitation should be tailored to the clinical situation, as described in the following discussion (**Figure 3-20**).

Uncontrolled Hemorrhage

For patients with suspected internal hemorrhage in the chest, abdomen, or retroperitoneum (pelvis), sufficient IV crystalloid solution should be titrated to maintain a systolic blood pressure in the range of 80 to 90 mm Hg, which will provide a MAP of 60 to 65 mm Hg. This blood pressure level should maintain adequate perfusion to the kidneys with less risk of worsening internal hemorrhage. A fluid bolus should not be administered because this may "overshoot" the target blood pressure range, resulting in recurrent intrathoracic, intra-abdominal, or retroperitoneal bleeding.

The current philosophy of restricted crystalloid administration in the prehospital setting and during initial hospital care has been called by several names, including permissive hypotension, hypotensive resuscitation, and "balanced" resuscitation, meaning that a balance must be struck between the amount of fluid administered and the degree of blood pressure elevation. Once the patient arrives at the hospital, fluid administration continues by giving plasma and blood (1:1 ratio) until the hemorrhage is controlled. Blood pressure is then returned to normal values with ongoing 1:1 (plasma to blood) transfusion with restricted crystalloid administration in most trauma centers. Studies on permissive hypotension were all done using crystalloid as the resuscitative fluid. We may find that when using blood, it is actually better to aim for normal blood pressure. Answers to these questions are yet to be determined.

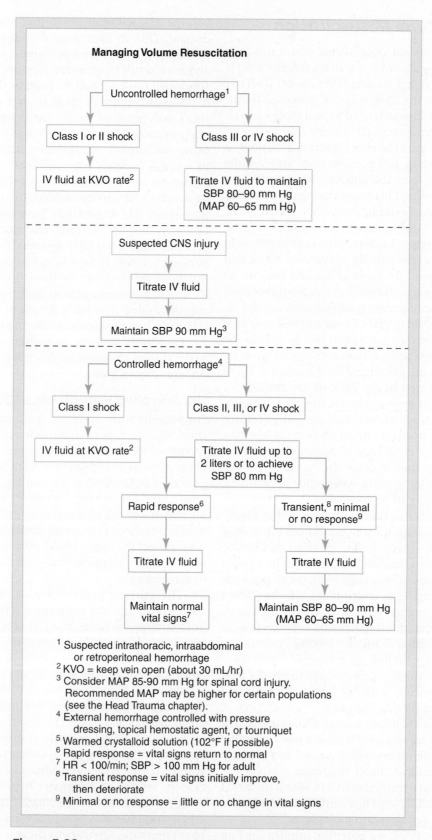

Figure 3-20 A. Algorithm for managing volume resuscitation.

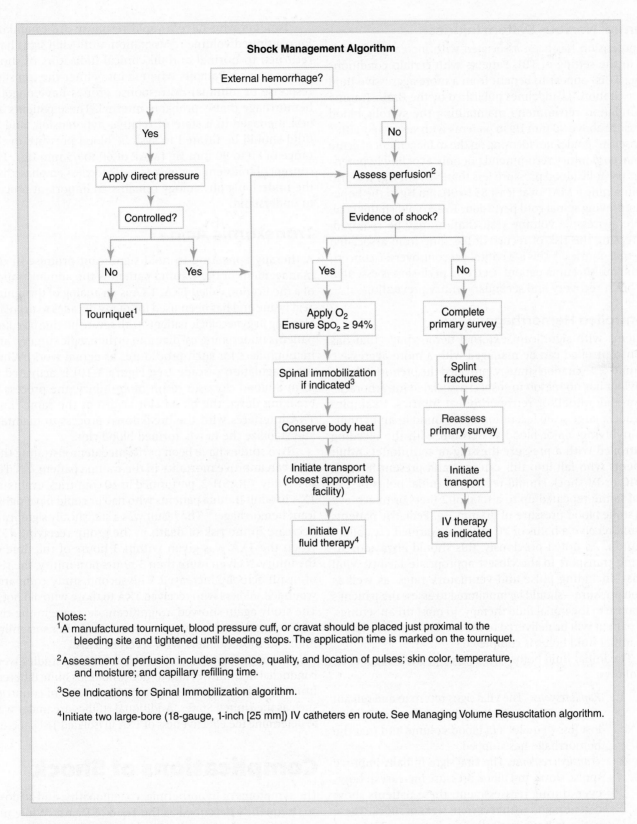

Figure 3-20 B. Algorithm for managing shock.

Notes:

[1] A manufactured tourniquet, blood pressure cuff, or cravat should be placed just proximal to the bleeding site and tightened until bleeding stops. The application time is marked on the tourniquet.

[2] Assessment of perfusion includes presence, quality, and location of pulses; skin color, temperature, and moisture; and capillary refilling time.

[3] See Indications for Spinal Immobilization algorithm.

[4] Initiate two large-bore (18-gauge, 1-inch [25 mm]) IV catheters en route. See Managing Volume Resuscitation algorithm.

Central Nervous System Injuries

Hypotension has been associated with increased mortality in the setting of TBI. Patients with certain conditions (e.g., TBIs) appear to benefit from a more aggressive fluid resuscitation.[44] Guidelines published by the Brain Trauma Foundation recommend maintaining the systolic blood pressure above 90 mm Hg in patients with suspected TBI.[45] Consensus guidelines focusing on the management of acute spinal cord injury recommend not only avoiding hypotension (systolic blood pressure less than 90 mm Hg) but also maintaining a MAP of at least 85 to 90 mm Hg in the hopes of improving spinal cord perfusion. To accomplish this goal, more aggressive volume resuscitation may be required, increasing the risk of recurrent bleeding from associated internal injuries.[46] This is a critical yet controversial concern in the multitrauma patient. Cerebral perfusion is essential for brain recovery and secondary injury prevention.

Controlled Hemorrhage

Patients with significant external hemorrhage that has been controlled can be managed with a more aggressive volume resuscitation strategy, provided the prehospital care provider has no reason to suspect associated intrathoracic, intra-abdominal, or retroperitoneal injuries. Examples include a large scalp laceration or a wound in an extremity involving major blood vessels but with the bleeding controlled with a pressure dressing or tourniquet. Adult patients who fall into this category and present in Class II, III, or IV shock should receive an initial bolus of 250 cc of saline repeated up to a total of 2 liters or to achieve a systolic blood pressure of 80 mm Hg. Pediatric patients should receive a bolus of 20 ml/kg of warmed crystalloid solution. As noted previously, this should always occur during transport to the closest appropriate facility. Vital signs—including pulse and ventilatory rates, as well as blood pressure—should be monitored to assess the patient's response to the initial fluid therapy. In most urban settings, the patient will be delivered to the receiving facility before the initial fluid bolus is completed.

The initial fluid bolus elicits three possible responses, as follows:

1. *Rapid response.* The vital signs return to and remain normal. This typically indicates the patient has lost less than 20% of blood volume and that the hemorrhage has stopped.
2. *Transient response.* The vital signs initially improve (pulse slows and blood pressure increases); however, during reassessment, these patients show deterioration with recurrent signs of shock. These patients have typically lost between 20% and 40% of their blood volume.
3. *Minimal or no response.* These patients show virtually no change in the profound signs of shock after a 1- to 2-liter bolus.

Patients who have a rapid response are candidates for continued volume resuscitation, until vital signs have returned to normal and all clinical indicators of shock have resolved. Patients who fall into either the transient response or minimal/no response groups have ongoing hemorrhage that is probably internal. These patients are best managed in a state of relative hypotension, and IV fluid should be titrated to systolic blood pressure in the range of 80 to 90 mm Hg (MAP of 60 to 65 mm Hg). The concept of transient response is receiving less emphasis, but the underlying physiology remains an important process to understand.

Tranexamic Acid

A therapy appearing to hold significant promise in the management of the trauma patient is the administration of a medication called TXA. TXA is an analog of the amino acid lysine and has been used for many decades to decrease bleeding in gynecologic patients with severe uterine bleeding, patients undergoing cardiac and orthopaedic surgery, and hemophiliacs for such procedures as dental work. When the coagulation cascade (see Figure 3-10) is activated to form a blood clot as a result of an injury, the process of breaking down the blood clot begins at the same time. TXA interferes with the breakdown process to maintain and stabilize the newly formed blood clot.

Two studies have been performed demonstrating that TXA can improve mortality in the trauma patient.[47,48] The first study, CRASH-2, performed in 40 countries, evaluated TXA in adult trauma patients who had or could have significant hemorrhage.[47] The result was a statistically significant decrease in the risk of death in the group receiving TXA when the TXA was given within 3 hours of the time of the injury. If given more than 3 hours post injury, the risk of death actually increased. The second study compared wounded soldiers who received TXA to those who did not.[48] The study again showed a significant decrease in the risk of death and need for massive transfusion after sustaining injury in those soldiers who received TXA.

It is important to note that both of these studies were conducted in countries and under conditions quite different from the urban, rapid response EMS systems of countries such as the United States. Additional studies are under way to determine the effectiveness of TXA in isolated TBI patients.

Complications of Shock

The symptoms of hypothermia, coagulopathy, and acidosis are frequently described as the Triad of Death. While not actually causes of death, they are symptoms indicating impending death. They are markers of anaerobic metabolism and loss of energy production, and they are an indicator of the interventions needed to reverse anaerobic metabolism that must be provided quickly. Several complications may result in patients with persistent or inadequately resuscitated shock, which is why early recognition and aggressive management of shock are essential. The quality of care delivered in the prehospital setting can affect a patient's hospital course and outcome. Recognizing shock and initiating proper treatment in the prehospital setting may shorten the patient's hospital length of stay and improve his or her chances for survival. The following complications of shock are not often seen in the prehospital setting, but they are a result of shock both in the field and in the ED. In addition, they may be encountered when transferring patients between facilities. Knowing the outcome of the process of shock helps in the understanding of the severity of the condition, the importance of rapid hemorrhage control, and appropriate fluid replacement.

Acute Renal Failure

Impaired circulation to the kidneys changes the aerobic metabolism in the kidney to anaerobic metabolism. The reduced energy production leads to renal cellular swelling, which decreases renal perfusion, thus causing additional anaerobic metabolism. The cells that make up the renal tubules are sensitive to ischemia and may die if their oxygen delivery is impaired for more than 45 to 60 minutes. This condition, referred to as **acute tubular necrosis (ATN)** or acute renal failure, reduces the filtration process of the renal tubules. The result is decreased renal output and reduced clearing of toxic products and electrolytes. Because the kidneys are no longer functioning, excess fluid is not excreted, and volume overload may result. Also, the kidneys lose their ability to excrete metabolic acids and electrolytes, leading to a metabolic acidosis and hyperkalemia (increased blood potassium). These patients often require dialysis for several weeks or months. Most patients who develop ATN resulting from shock eventually recover normal renal function.

Acute Respiratory Distress Syndrome

Acute respiratory distress syndrome (ARDS) results from damage to the alveolar cells of the lung and decreased energy production to maintain the metabolism of these cells. This injury, combined with fluid overload produced by too much crystalloid administration during resuscitation, leads to leakage of fluid into the interstitial spaces and alveoli of the lungs, making it much more difficult for oxygen to diffuse across the alveolar walls and into the capillaries and bind with the RBCs. This problem was first described during World War II but was formally recognized during the Vietnam War where it was called Da Nang lung (after the location of the hospital that saw many of these cases). Although these patients do have pulmonary edema, it is not the result of impaired cardiac function, as in congestive heart failure (cardiogenic pulmonary edema). ARDS represents a noncardiogenic pulmonary edema. The change of the resuscitative process to restricted crystalloid, permissive hypertension, and damage control resuscitation (RBCs-to-plasma ratio of 1:1) has significantly reduced ARDS in the immediate trauma period (24 to 72 hours).

Hematologic Failure

The term **coagulopathy** refers to impairment in the normal clotting capabilities of blood. This abnormality may result from hypothermia (decreased body temperature), dilution of clotting factors from administration of fluids, or depletion of the clotting substances as they are used up in an effort to control bleeding (consumptive coagulopathy). The normal blood-clotting cascade involves several enzymes and factors that eventually result in the creation of fibrin molecules that serve as a matrix to trap platelets and form a plug in a vessel wall to stop bleeding (**Figure 3-21**). This process functions best within a narrow temperature range (i.e., near-normal body temperature). As the core temperature of the body falls (even just a few degrees) and energy production lessens, blood clotting is compromised, leading to continued hemorrhage. The blood-clotting factors may also be used up as they form blood clots in an effort to slow and control hemorrhage. The decreased body temperature worsens the clotting problems, which exacerbates hemorrhage, which further reduces the ability of the body to maintain its temperature. With inadequate resuscitation, this becomes an ever-worsening cycle. Several studies have reported fewer difficulties with coagulopathy since the increase in the use of plasma for resuscitation.[3,4]

Hepatic Failure

Severe damage to the liver may occur, although it is a less common result of prolonged shock. Evidence of damage to the liver from shock typically does not become manifest for several days, until laboratory results document elevated liver function tests. Liver failure is manifested by persistent hypoglycemia (low blood sugar), persistent lactic acidosis, and jaundice. Because the liver produces many of the clotting factors necessary for hemostasis, a coagulopathy may accompany liver failure.

Overwhelming Infection

There is increased risk of infection associated with severe shock. This increased risk is attributed to the following causes:

- Marked decrease in the number of WBCs, predisposing the shock patient to infection, is another manifestation of hematologic failure.
- Ischemia and reduction in energy production in the cells of the shock patient's bowel wall may allow bacteria to leak out into the bloodstream.

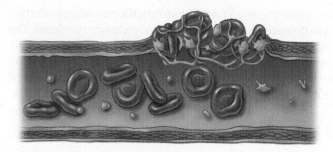

Figure 3-21 Blood clotting involves several enzymes and factors that eventually result in the creation of fibrin molecules that serve as a matrix to trap platelets and form a plug in a vessel wall to stop bleeding.

- Decreased function of the immune system in the face of ischemia and loss of energy production.
- Increased permeability of the capillary membranes in the lung secondary to ischemic injury and to circulating inflammatory factors leads to fluid buildup in the alveoli. This leads to respiratory insufficiency and need for intubation. The combination of these factors predisposes shock patients to pneumonia episodes, which can cause systemic sepsis.
- Most important, multiple procedures, vascular intrusion, and indwelling catheters increase the risk of infections in the critically injured patient.

Multiple Organ Failure

Shock, if not successfully treated, can lead to dysfunction first in one organ, then in several other organs simultaneously, with sepsis as a common accompaniment, leading to multiple organ dysfunction syndrome.

Failure of one major body system (e.g., lungs, kidneys, blood-clotting cascade, liver) is associated with a mortality rate of about 40%. Cardiovascular failure, in the form of cardiogenic and septic shock, can only occasionally be reversed. By the time four organ systems fail, the mortality rate is essentially 100%.[49]

Prolonged Transport

During prolonged transport of a trauma patient in shock, it is important to maintain perfusion to the vital organs. Airway management should be optimized before a long transport and endotracheal intubation performed if there is any question regarding airway patency. Ventilatory support is provided, with care taken to ensure ventilations are of a reasonable tidal volume and rate (maintaining minute volume) so as not to compromise a patient with already tenuous perfusion. Pulse oximetry should be monitored continuously. Capnography provides information regarding the position of the endotracheal tube, as well as information on the patient's perfusion status. A marked drop in $ETco_2$ indicates that the airway has become dislodged or the patient has experienced a significant drop in perfusion. Additional considerations such as tension pneumothorax should be evaluated and interventions performed in appropriate patients.

Direct pressure by hand is impractical during a long transport, so significant external hemorrhage should be controlled with pressure dressings. If these efforts fail, a tourniquet should be applied. In situations in which a tourniquet has been applied and transport time is expected to exceed 4 hours, attempts should be considered to remove the tourniquet after more aggressive attempts at local hemorrhage control. The tourniquet should be slowly loosened while observing the dressing for signs of hemorrhage. If bleeding does not reoccur, the tourniquet is completely loosened but left in place in case hemorrhage recurs. Conversion of a tourniquet back to a dressing should not be attempted in the following situations: (1) presence of Class III or IV shock, (2) complete amputation, (3) inability to observe the patient for reoccurrence of bleeding, and (4) tourniquet in place longer than 6 hours.[12] Internal hemorrhage control should be optimized by splinting all fractures.

Techniques for maintaining normal body temperature, as previously described, are even more important in the case of prolonged transport time. In addition to a warmed patient compartment, the patient should be covered with blankets or materials that preserve body heat; even large, plastic garbage bags help prevent loss of heat. Intravenous fluids should be warmed before administration. Room-temperature intravenous fluids in the trauma patient can lead to hypothermia, which, in turn, can affect the patient's natural clotting factors.

In prolonged transport circumstances, vascular access for fluid administration may be needed, and two large-bore IV lines should be established. For both children and adults, inability to obtain peripheral vascular access may necessitate use of the intraosseous route, as described previously.

For patients with suspected ongoing hemorrhage, maintaining systolic blood pressure in the range of 80 to 90 mm Hg or MAP of 60 to 65 mm Hg can usually accomplish the goal of maintaining perfusion to vital organs with less risk of renewing internal hemorrhage. Patients with suspected TBIs or spinal cord injuries should have systolic blood pressure maintained above 90 to 100 mm Hg.

Vital signs should be reassessed frequently to monitor response to resuscitation. The following should be documented at serial intervals: ventilation rate, pulse rate, blood pressure, skin color and temperature, capillary refill, GCS score, Spo_2, and $ETco_2$, if available.

Although insertion of a urinary catheter is not usually required in rapid transport circumstances, monitoring urine output is an important tool to help guide decisions regarding the need for additional fluid therapy during prolonged transport. Insertion of a urinary catheter, if local protocols permit, should be considered so urine output can be monitored. Adequate urine outputs include 0.5 ml/kg/hour for adults, 1 ml/kg/hour for pediatric patients, and 2 ml/kg/hour for infants younger than 1 year. Urine output of less than these amounts may be a key indicator that the patient requires further volume infusion.

If time and local protocols permit during prolonged transport, placement of a nasogastric catheter should be considered for intubated patients. If midfacial fractures are present, placement of an orogastric catheter instead should be considered. Gastric distension may cause unexplained hypotension and dysrhythmias, especially in children. Placement of a nasogastric or orogastric tube may also decrease the risk of vomiting and aspiration.

SUMMARY

- In the trauma patient, hemorrhage is the most common cause of shock.
- Humans produce the energy needed to sustain life via a complex system, called "aerobic metabolism," using glucose and oxygen. This entire process depends on the respiratory system to provide adequate amounts of oxygen to the circulatory system, which must be able to deliver the oxygen to the cells of the body.
- The backup system to aerobic metabolism is called anaerobic metabolism. It does not require oxygen, but it is inefficient and only creates a small amount of energy.
- Shock is a state of generalized change in cellular function from aerobic metabolism to anaerobic metabolism secondary to hypoperfusion of the tissue cells, in which the delivery of oxygen at the cellular level is inadequate to meet metabolic needs. As a result, cellular energy production falls, and, over a relatively short period of time, cellular functions become impaired, eventually leading to cell death.
- Shock may be classified into the following categories:
  - Hypovolemic—primarily hemorrhagic in the trauma patient, related to loss of circulating blood cells and fluid volume with oxygen-carrying capacity (the most common cause of shock in the trauma patient)
  - Distributive (or vasogenic)—related to abnormality in vascular tone
  - Cardiogenic—related to interference with the pump action of the heart, often occurring after a heart attack

- Care of the patient in shock, or one who may go into shock, begins with an assessment of the patient, beginning with a history of the event and a quick visual examination of the patient looking for obvious signs of shock and blood loss.
- Steps in the management of shock are as follows:
  1. Control any arterial hemorrhage.
  2. Ensure oxygenation.
  3. Identify any hemorrhaging.
  4. Transport to definitive care.
  5. Administer fluid or blood therapy when appropriate. External hemorrhage should be controlled with direct pressure, followed by application of a pressure dressing. If this is not rapidly effective, a tourniquet should be applied to the extremity at the level of the groin or axilla. A topical hemostatic agent may also provide additional hemorrhage control.
- In some cases, nonhemorrhagic sources of shock in the trauma patient (e.g., tension pneumothorax) can be rapidly corrected.
- All trauma patients in shock, in addition to maintenance of adequate oxygenation, require rapid extrication and expeditious transport to a definitive care institution where the cause of the shock can be specifically identified and treated.
- Transport should not be delayed for measures such as IV access and volume infusion. These interventions should be done in the ambulance during transport.
- Overaggressive fluid infusion should be avoided to minimize further bleeding and edema formation in the patient with hemorrhagic shock after trauma.

SCENARIO RECAP

You and your partner are dispatched to a 65-year-old man who fell approximately 8 feet (2.4 m) while working on his outdoor patio. Upon your arrival, you find the patient lying supine on the ground in moderate distress with chief complaints of lower back, sacral, and left hip pain.

Physical examination of the patient shows pale skin color, diaphoresis, decreased peripheral pulses, and an unstable pelvis. The patient is alert and oriented. His vital signs are as follows: pulse 100 beats/minute, blood pressure 78/56 mm Hg, SpO_2 92% on room air, and respiratory rate 20 breaths/minute regular and clear bilaterally.

- What possible injuries do you expect to see after this type of fall?
- How would you manage these injuries in the field?
- What are the major pathologic processes occurring in this patient?
- How will you correct the pathophysiology causing this patient's presentation?
- You are working for a rural EMS system approximately 30 to 45 minutes from the nearest trauma center. How does this factor alter your management plans?

SCENARIO SOLUTION

You recognize the patient is showing the signs of hypovolemia (increased heart rate, decreased blood pressure, and increased ventilatory rate). You are concerned about internal hemorrhage secondary to pelvic fracture. You perform spinal motion restriction, immediately apply a commercial pelvic binder, transfer him to the ambulance, and begin transport to the closest trauma center.

While en route, you apply oxygen at 2 l/min via $ETCO_2$ NC and initiate two 18-gauge IV lines, giving only enough fluid to maintain a MAP of > 60 mm Hg. Due to the patient's hemodynamics and the potential for internal hemorrhage, you note the patient is a candidate for TXA administration. Additionally, you warm the fluids that are administered and prevent heat loss of the patient by apply appropriate environmental controls such as turning up the heat in the patient compartment and layering blankets. En route to the trauma center, you provide your report via radio. You identified that the patient takes anticoagulants. Upon arrival at the receiving facility, the patient is transferred to trauma staff with no change in condition.

References

1. Thal AP. *Shock: A Physiologic Basis for Treatment.* Chicago, IL: Yearbook Medical Publishers; 1971.
2. Gross SD. *A System of Surgery: Pathological, Diagnostic, Therapeutic, and Operative.* Philadelphia, PA: Blanchard and Lea; 1859.
3. McClelland RN, Shires GT, Baxter CR, et al. Balanced salt solutions in the treatment of hemorrhagic shock. *JAMA.* 1967;199:830.
4. Duchesne JC, Hunt JP, Wahl G, et al. Review of current blood transfusions strategies in a mature level I trauma center: were we wrong for the last 60 years? *J Trauma.* 2008;65(2):272-276; discussion 276-278.
5. Holcomb JB, Jenkins D, Rhee P, et al. Damage control resuscitation: directly addressing the early coagulopathy of trauma. *J Trauma.* 2007;62(2):307-310.
6. Koreny M, Riedmuller E, Nikfardjam M, et al. Arterial puncture closing devices compared with standard manual compression after cardiac catheterization: systematic review and meta analysis. *JAMA.* 2004;291:350.
7. Pepe PE, Raedler C, Lurie KG, et al. Emergency ventilatory management in hemorrhagic states: elemental or detrimental? *J Trauma.* 2003;54:1048.
8. Pepe PE, Roppolo LP, Fowler RL. The detrimental effects of ventilation during low-blood-flow states. *Curr Opin Crit Care.* 2005;11:212.
9. Walker SB, Cleary S, Higgins M. Comparison of the FemoStop device and manual pressure in reducing groin puncture site complications following coronary angioplasty and coronary stent placement. *Int J Nurs Pract.* 2001;7:366.

10. Simon A, Baumgarner B, Clark K, et al. Manual versus mechanical compression for femoral artery hemostasis after cardiac catheterization. *Am J Crit Care*. 1998;7:308.

11. Lehmann KG, Heath-Lange SJ, Ferris ST. Randomized comparison of hemostasis techniques after invasive cardiovascular procedures. *Am Heart J*. 1999;138:1118.

12. Beekley AC, Sebesta JA, Blackbourne LH, et al. Prehospital tourniquet use in Operation Iraqi Freedom: effect on hemorrhage control and outcomes. *J Trauma*. 2008;64(2):S28-S37.

13. Kragh JF Jr, Walters TJ, Baer DG, et al. Practical use of emergency tourniquets to stop bleeding in major limb trauma. *J Trauma*. 2008;64(2):S38-S50.

14. Bellamy RF. The causes of death in conventional land warfare: implications for combat casualty care research. *Mil Med*. 1984;149:55.

15. Mabry RL, Holcomb JB, Baker AM, et al. United States Army Rangers in Somalia: an analysis of combat casualties on an urban battlefield. *J Trauma*. 2000;49:515.

16. Lakstein D, Blumenfeld A, Sokolov T, et al. Tourniquets for hemorrhage control on the battlefield: a 4-year accumulated experience. *J Trauma*. 2003;54:S221-S225.

17. Kragh JF, Walters TJ, Baer DG, et al. Survival with emergency tourniquet use to stop bleeding in major limb trauma. *Ann Surg*. 2009;249(1):1-7.

18. Walters TJ, Mabry RL. Use of tourniquets on the battlefield: a consensus panel report. *Mil Med*. 2005;170:770.

19. Kragh JF Jr, Littrel ML, Jones JA, et al. Battle casualty survival with emergency tourniquet use to stop limb bleeding. *J Emerg Med*. 2011;41:590-597.

20. Walters TL, Wenke JC, Kauvar DS, et al. Effectiveness of self-applied tourniquets in human volunteers. *Prehosp Emerg Care*. 2005;9:416-422.

21. Littlejohn LF, Devlin JJ, Kircher SS, Lueken R, Melia MR, Johnson AS. Comparison of Celox-A, ChitoFlex, Wound Stat, and combat gauze hemostatic agents versus standard gauze dressing in control of hemorrhage in a swine model of penetrating trauma. *Acad Emerg Med*. 2011;18(4):340-350.

22. Gentilello LM. Advances in the management of hypothermia. *Surg Clin North Am*. 1995;75:2.

23. Marino PL. *The ICU Book*. 2nd ed. Baltimore, MD: Williams & Wilkins; 1998.

24. Johnson S, Henderson SO, Myth L. The Trendelenburg position improves circulation in cases of shock. *Can J Emerg Med*. 2004;6:48.

25. Bickell WH, Wall MJ Jr, Pepe PE, et al. Immediate versus delayed fluid resuscitation for hypotensive patients with penetrating torso injuries. *N Engl J Med*. 1994;331:1105.

26. Deboer S, Seaver M, Morissette C. Intraosseous infusion: not just for kids anymore. *J Emerg Med Serv*. 2005;34:54.

27. Glaeser PW, Hellmich TR, Szewczuga D, et al. Five-year experience in prehospital intraosseous infusions in children and adults. *Ann Emerg Med*. 1993;22:1119.

28. Sawyer RW, Bodai BI, Blaisdell FW, et al. The current status of intraosseous infusion. *J Am Coll Surg*. 1994;179:353.

29. Macnab A, Christenson J, Findlay J, et al. A new system for sternal intraosseous infusion in adults. *Prehosp Emerg Care*. 2000;4:173.

30. Vassar MJ, Fischer RP, Obrien PE, et al. A multicenter trial of resuscitation of injured patients with 7.5% sodium chloride: the effect of added dextran 70. *Arch Surg*. 1993;128:1003.

31. Vassar MJ, Perry CA, Holcroft JW. Prehospital resuscitation of hypotensive trauma patients with 7.5% NaCl versus 7.5% NaCl with added dextran: a controlled trial. *J Trauma*. 1993;34:622.

32. Wade CE, Kramer GC, Grady JJ. Efficacy of hypertonic 7.5% saline and 6% dextran in treating trauma: a meta-analysis of controlled clinical trials. *Surgery*. 1997;122:609.

33. Zarychanski R, Abou-Setta AM, Turgeon AF, et al. Association of hydroxyethyl starch with mortality and acute kidney injury in critically ill patients requiring volume resuscitation. *JAMA*. 2013;309:678-688.

34. Perel P, Roberts I, Ker K. Are colloids more effective than crystalloids in reducing death in people who are critically ill or injured? The Cochrane Library, 2013. http://www.cochrane.org/CD000567/INJ_are-colloids-more-effective-than-crystalloids-in-reducing-death-in-people-who-are-critically-ill-or-injured. Accessed July 31, 2017.

35. Rizoli SB. Crystalloids and colloids in trauma resuscitation: a brief overview of the current debate. *J Trauma*. 2003;54:S82.

36. SAFE Study Investigators. A comparison of albumin and saline for fluid resuscitation in the intensive care unit. *N Engl J Med*. 2004;350:2247.

37. Solomonov E, Hirsh M, Yahiya A, et al. The effect of vigorous fluid resuscitation in uncontrolled hemorrhagic shock after massive splenic injury. *Crit Care Med*. 2000;28:749.

38. Krausz MM, Horn Y, Gross D. The combined effect of small volume hypertonic saline and normal saline solutions in uncontrolled hemorrhagic shock. *Surg Gynecol Obstet*. 1992;174:363.

39. Bickell WH, Bruttig SP, Millnamow, et al. The detrimental effects of intravenous crystalloid after aortotomy in swine. *Surgery*. 1991;110:529.

40. Kowalenko T, Stern S, Dronen SC, et al. Improved outcome with hypotensive resuscitation of uncontrolled hemorrhagic shock in a swine model. *J Trauma*. 1992;33:349.

41. Sindlinger JF, Soucy DM, Greene SP, et al. The effects of isotonic saline volume resuscitation in uncontrolled hemorrhage. *Surg Gynecol Obstet*. 1993;177:545.

42. Capone AC, Safar P, Stezoski W, et al. Improved outcome with fluid restriction in treatment of uncontrolled hemorrhagic shock. *J Am Coll Surg*. 1995;180:49.

43. Salomone JP, Ustin JS, McSwain NE, et al. Opinions of trauma practitioners regarding prehospital interventions for critically injured patients. *J Trauma*. 2005;58:509.

44. York J, Abenamar A, Graham R, et al. Fluid resuscitation of patients with multiple injuries and severe closed head injury: experience with an aggressive fluid resuscitation strategy. *J Trauma*. 2000;48(3):376.

45. Brain Trauma Foundation. *Guidelines for Prehospital Management of Traumatic Brain Injury*. New York, NY: BTF; 2000.

46. American Association of Neurological Surgeons and Congress of Neurological Surgeons Joint Section on Disorders of the Spine and Peripheral Nerves. Blood pressure management after acute spinal cord injury. *Neurosurgery*. 2002;50:S58.

47. The CRASH-2 Collaborators. Effects of tranexamic acid on death, vascular occlusive events, and blood transfusion in

trauma patients with significant haemorrhage (CRASH-2): a randomised, placebo-controlled trial. *Lancet*. 2010;376:23-32.

48. Morrison JJ, Dubose JJ, Rasmussen TE, Midwinter MJ. Military Application of Tranexamic Acid in Trauma Emergency Resuscitation (MATTERs) Study. *Arch Surg*. 2012;147:113-119.

49. Marshall JC, Cook DJ, Christou NV, et al. The multiple organ dysfunction score: a reliable descriptor of a complex clinical syndrome. *Crit Care Med*. 1995;23:1638.

Suggested Reading

Allison KP, Gosling P, Jones S, et al. Randomized trial of hydroxyethyl starch versus gelatine for trauma resuscitation. *J Trauma*. 1999;47:1114.

American College of Surgeons (ACS) Committee on Trauma. Shock. In: *Advanced Trauma Life Support for Doctors, Student Course Manual*. 10th ed. Chicago, IL: ACS; 2017.

Hypoperfusion. In: Bledsoe B, Porter RS, Cherry RA, eds. *Essentials of Paramedic Care*. 2nd ed. Upper Saddle River, NJ: Brady-Pearson Education; 2011:257-265.

Moore EE. Blood substitutes: the future is now. *J Am Coll Surg*. 2003;196:1.

Novak L, Shackford SR, Bourgenignon P, et al. Comparison of standard and alternative prehospital resuscitation in uncontrolled hemorrhagic shock and head injury. *J Trauma*. 1999;47(5):834.

Otero RM, Nguyen HB, Rivers EP. Approach to the patient in shock. In: Tintinalli J, ed. *Emergency Medicine: A Comprehensive Study Guide*. New York, NY: McGraw-Hill; 2011:165-172.

Proctor KG. Blood substitutes and experimental models of trauma. *J Trauma*. 2003;54:S106.

Revell M, Greaves I, Porter K. Endpoints for fluid resuscitation in hemorrhagic shock. *J Trauma*. 2003;54:S637.

Shock. In: Bledsoe B, Porter RS, Cherry RA, eds. *Essentials of Paramedic Care*. 2nd ed. Upper Saddle River, NJ: Brady-Pearson Education; 2011:837-849.

Shock overview. In: Chapleau W, Burba AC, Pons PT, Page D, eds. *The Paramedic*. Updated ed. New York, NY: McGraw-Hill; 2012:259-273.

Trunkey DD. Prehospital fluid resuscitation of the trauma patient: an analysis and review. *Emerg Med*. 2001;30(5):93.

SPECIFIC SKILLS

Intraosseous Vascular Access

Principle: To establish a vascular access site for fluids and medications when traditional IV access is unobtainable.

This technique may be performed in both adult and pediatric patients, using a variety of commercially available devices.

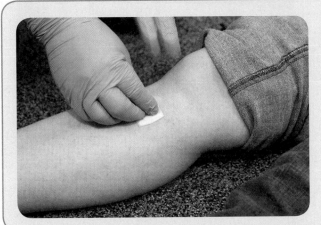

1 Assemble the equipment, which includes an intraosseous infusion needle, syringe filled with at least 5 ml of sterile saline, antiseptic, IV fluid and tubing, and tape. Ensure proper body substance isolation (BSI). Place the patient in a supine position.

The choice of insertion site may be the humeral head, distal femur, tibia, or sternum. For pediatric patients, a common insertion site is the anterior-medial proximal tibia just below the tibial tuberosity. The prehospital care provider identifies the tibia is the insertion site; the lower extremity is stabilized by another provider. Clean the insertion site area with an antiseptic.

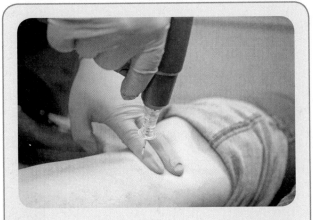

2 Holding the drill and needle at a 90-degree angle to the selected bone, activate the drill and insert the rotating needle through the skin and into the bone cortex. A "pop" will be felt upon entering the bone cortex.

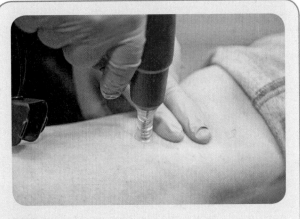

3 When you feel a lack of resistance against the needle, release the trigger of the drill. While holding the needle, remove the drill from the needle.

(continued)

Intraosseous Vascular Access (continued)

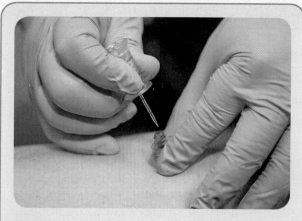

4   Release and remove the trocar from the center of the needle.

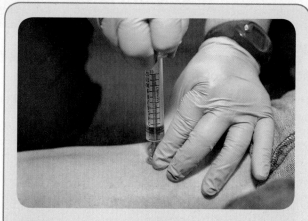

5   Attach the syringe with saline to the needle hub. Draw back with the syringe plunger slightly, looking for fluid from the marrow cavity to mix with the saline. "Dry" taps are not uncommon.

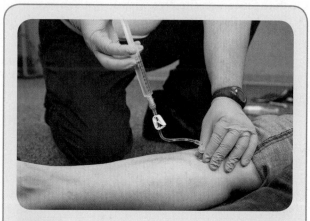

6   Next, inject 5 ml of the saline, observing for signs of infiltration. If there are no signs of infiltration, remove the syringe from the needle hub, attach the IV tubing, and set the flow rate. Secure the needle and IV tubing.

Tourniquet Application

The Combat Application Tourniquet (C-A-T) is demonstrated in these photos. Any approved tourniquet may be used.

Note: A patient with bleeding severe enough to warrant tourniquet application is at risk for lightheadedness and loss of consciousness; therefore, should be placed in a supine position rapidly. In this example, the model is sitting upright to facilitate demonstration of the tourniquet application procedure.

C-A-T Application to an Upper Extremity

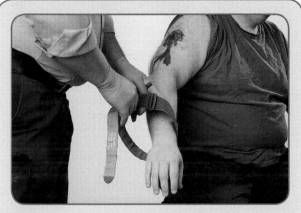

1 Insert the wounded extremity through the loop of the self-adhering band.

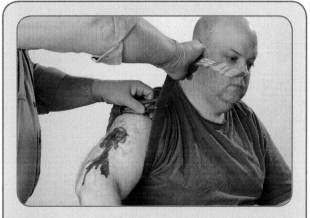

2 Pull the self-adhering band tight, and securely fasten it back on itself.

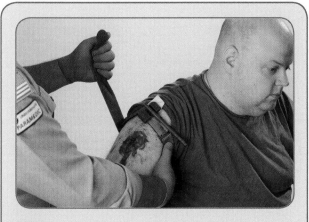

3 Adhere the band around the arm. Do not adhere the band past the clip.

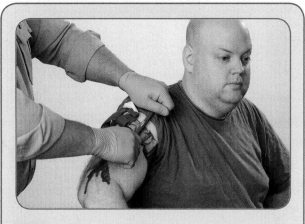

4 Twist the windlass rod until the bleeding stops (usually no more than three 180-degree turns).

(continued)

Tourniquet Application (continued)

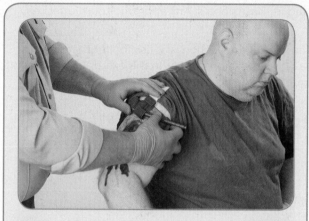

5   Lock the rod in place with the windlass clip.

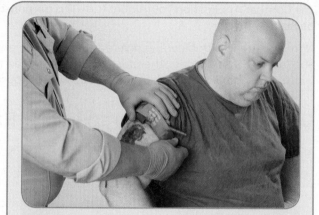

6   Adhere the band over the windlass rod. For small extremities, continue to adhere the band around the extremity.

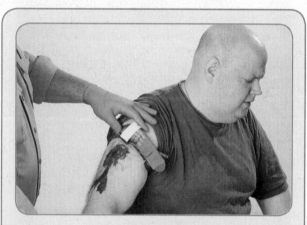

7   Secure the rod and band with the windlass strap. Grasp the strap, pull it tight, and adhere it to the opposite hook on the windlass clip.

Tourniquet Application (continued)

C-A-T Application to a Lower Extremity

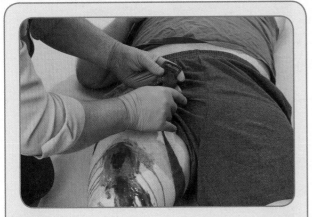

1 Place the tourniquet at the most proximal possible location on the thigh.

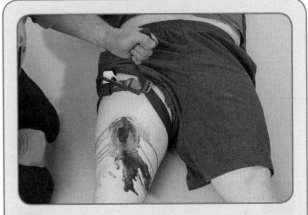

2 Pass the band through the outside slit of the friction adapter buckle, which will lock the band in place.

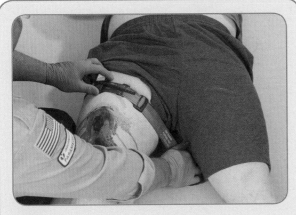

3 Pull the self-adhering band tight, and securely fasten it back on itself.

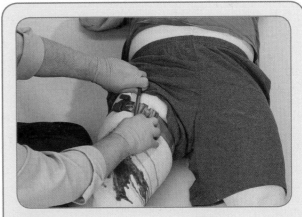

4 Twist the windlass rod until the bleeding stops (usually no more than three 180-degree turns).

(continued)

Tourniquet Application (continued)

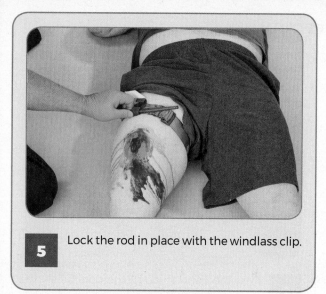

5 Lock the rod in place with the windlass clip.

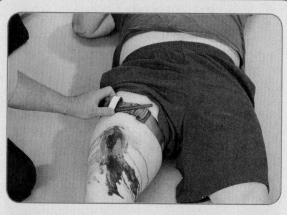

6 Secure the rod with the windlass strap. Grasp the strap, pull it tight, and adhere it to the opposite hook on the windlass clip.

On occasion, multiple tourniquets may be required to manage hemorrhage. Place the additional tourniquet immediately adjacent (just proximal, if possible) the previous application.

Wound Packing With Topical Hemostatic Dressing or Plain Gauze

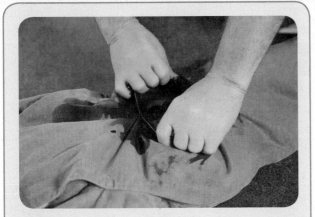

1 Expose the wound.

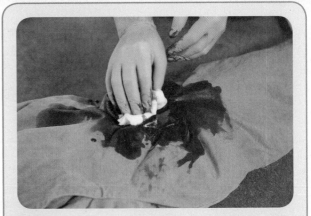

2 Gently remove excess blood from the wound site while trying to preserve any clots that have formed. Locate the source of active bleeding in the wound (often at the base of the wound).

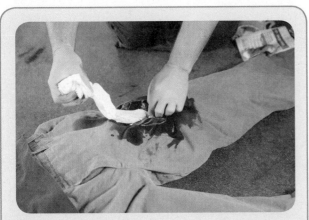

3 Remove the selected dressing from its packaging, and pack the entire dressing tightly into the wound, directly over the most active point of bleeding.

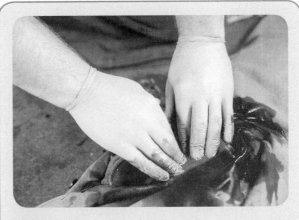

4 Apply direct pressure onto the wound and packing for a minimum of 3 minutes (if using a hemostatic agent and per the manufacturer's instructions) or 10 minutes if using plain gauze.

(continued)

Wound Packing With Topical Hemostatic Dressing or Plain Gauze (continued)

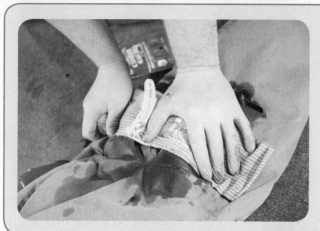

5 Reassess to ensure that bleeding has stopped. Wound may be repacked or a second dressing inserted into the wound if needed to control continued bleeding. If bleeding is controlled, leave packing in place and apply a compression wrap around the wound to secure the dressing.

Pressure Dressing Using Israeli Trauma Bandage

Principle: To provide mechanical circumferential pressure and dressing to an open wound of an extremity with uncontrolled hemorrhage.

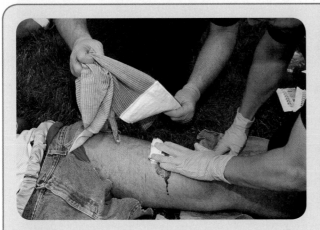
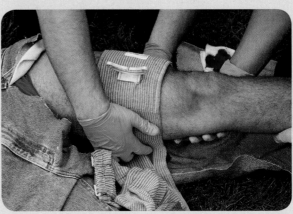

1 Ensure proper BSI, and place the dressing pad over the wound.

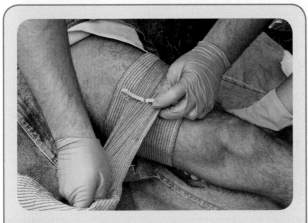

2 Wrap the elastic bandage around the extremity at least once.

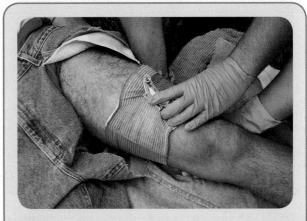

3 Loop the elastic bandage through the bar.

(continued)

Pressure Dressing Using Israeli Trauma Bandage (continued)

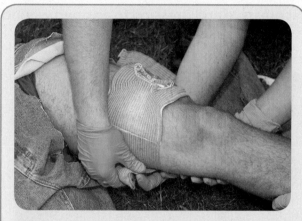

4 Wrap the bandage tightly around the wounded extremity in the opposite direction, applying enough pressure to control the bleeding.

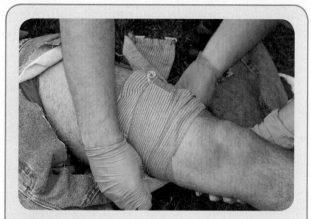

5 Continue wrapping the bandage around the extremity.

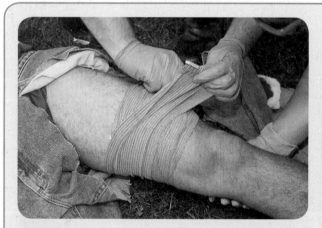

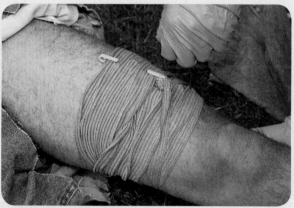

6 Secure the distal end of the bandage to maintain continued pressure to control the hemorrhage.

CHAPTER 4

The Physics of Trauma

Lead Editors:
Andrew Schmidt, MD
Lauren MacCormick, MD

CHAPTER OBJECTIVES

At the completion of this chapter, you will be able to do the following:

- Define energy in the context of producing injury.
- Explain the association between the laws of motion, energy, and the physics of trauma.
- Describe the relationship of injury and energy exchange to speed.
- Discuss energy exchange and cavitation.
- Given the description of a motor vehicle crash, use the physics of trauma to predict the likely injury pattern for an unrestrained occupant.
- Describe the specific injuries and their causes as related to interior and exterior vehicle damage.
- Discuss the function of restraint systems for vehicle occupants.
- Relate the laws of motion and energy to mechanisms other than motor vehicle crashes (e.g., blasts, falls).
- Define the five phases of blast injury and the injuries produced in each phase.
- Explain the differences in the production of injury with low-, medium-, and high-energy weapons.
- Discuss the relationship of the frontal surface of an impacting object to energy exchange and injury production.
- Integrate principles of the physics of trauma into trauma patient assessment.

SCENARIO

Before first light on a cold winter morning, you and your partner are dispatched to a single-vehicle crash. On arrival, you find a single vehicle that has crashed into a tree on a rural road. The front end of the vehicle appears to have impacted the tree, and the car has spun around the tree and backed into a drainage ditch on the side of the road. The driver appears to be the only occupant. The air bag has deployed and the driver is moaning, still restrained by his seat belt. You note damage to the front end of the car where it impacted the tree as well as rear-end damage from spinning around and going into the ditch backward.

- What is the potential for injury for this patient based on the physics of trauma of this event?
- How would you describe the patient's condition based on the physics of trauma?
- What injuries do you expect to find?

INTRODUCTION

In the United States, 35,092 people were killed in vehicle crashes in 2015. This total marked an increase of more than 7% from 2014, the largest single-year increase in nearly 50 years.[1] The World Health Organization (WHO) reports that nearly 1.25 million people are killed annually in car crashes around the world. From 2007 to 2013, the worldwide rate of deaths from road traffic accidents has remained fairly constant, despite a 16% rise in the number of vehicles on the world's roads from 2012 to 2015. In their 2015 publication, *Global Status Report on Road Safety*,[2] WHO reports that road crashes have remained the leading cause of death globally for individuals aged 15 to 29 years. More than 90% of these deaths occur in low-income and middle-income countries.[2]

In the United States, firearms are a major cause of death, accounting for 33,594 deaths in 2014. The two primary causes of firearm-related death were suicide, accounting for nearly two-thirds of the deaths, and homicide.[3] Blast injuries are a major cause of injuries in many countries, whereas penetrating injuries from knives are prominent in others.

Successful management of trauma patients depends on the identification of both obvious and hidden injuries, and it demands the use of good assessment skills. It is difficult in the prehospital setting to determine the exact injury produced in a given setting, but understanding the potential for injury and the potential for significant blood loss will allow the prehospital care provider to use his or her critical-thinking skills to recognize this likelihood and make appropriate triage, management, and transport decisions.

The management of any patient begins (after initial resuscitation) with the history of the patient's injury. In trauma, the history is the story of the impact and the energy exchange that resulted from this impact.[4] An understanding of the energy exchange process allows prehospital care providers to anticipate a high percentage of potential injuries encountered.

The physics of trauma deals with the motion of objects without reference to the forces that cause the motion.[4] Any injury that results from a force applied to the body is related directly to the interaction between the host and a moving object that impacts the host. When the prehospital care provider, at any level of care, does not understand the principles of the physics of trauma or the mechanisms involved, injuries may be missed. An understanding of these principles will increase the level of suspicion for certain injuries that are likely to be encountered given a specific mechanism. This information and the suspected injuries can be used to properly assess the patient on the scene and can be transmitted to the physicians and nurses in the emergency department (ED). At the scene and en route, these suspected injuries can be managed to provide the most appropriate patient care and "do no further harm."

Injuries that are not obvious but still severe can be fatal if they are not recognized at the scene and communicated to the medical team on arrival at the trauma center or appropriate hospital. Knowing where to look and how to assess for injuries is as important as knowing what to do after finding injuries. A complete, accurate history of a traumatic incident and proper interpretation of these data will provide this information. Many of a patient's injuries can be predicted by a proper survey of the scene, even before examining the patient.

This chapter discusses the general principles of understanding the physics of trauma. The general principles begin with the laws of mechanics that govern energy exchange and the general effects of the energy exchange. Mechanical principles address the interaction of the human body with the components of a crash. A crash is the interaction that occurs when an object with energy, usually something solid, impacts another. Though we often associate the word *crash* with a motor vehicle impact, it can also refer to the crash of a falling body onto the pavement, the impact of a bullet on the external and internal tissues of the body, and the overpressure and debris of a blast. All of these events involve energy exchange, all result in injury, all can result in potentially life-threatening conditions, and all require correct treatment by a knowledgeable and insightful prehospital care provider.

General Principles

A traumatic event can be divided into three phases: pre-event, event, and postevent. Simply stated, the *pre-event* phase is the prevention phase (**Box 4-1**). The *event* phase is that portion of the traumatic event that involves the exchange of energy or the physics of trauma (mechanics of energy). Last, the *postevent* is the patient care phase.

Whether the injury results from a car crash, a weapon, a fall, or a building collapse, energy is transformed into injury when it is absorbed into the body.

Box 4-1 Trauma Prevention

The most efficient and effective method to combat injury is to prevent it from happening in the first place. Health care providers at all levels play an active role in injury prevention to achieve the best results not only for the community at large but also for themselves. EMS systems are transforming themselves from a solely reactionary discipline to a broader, more effective discipline that includes aspects such as community paramedicine and places more emphasis on prevention. The Injury Prevention chapter details the role prehospital care providers have in preventing trauma.

Pre-event

The *pre-event phase* includes all of the events that preceded the incident. Conditions that were present before the incident occurred and that are important in the management of the patient's injuries are assessed as part of the pre-event history. These considerations include the patient's acute or preexisting medical conditions (and medications to treat those conditions), ingestion of recreational substances (illegal and prescription drugs, alcohol, etc.), and the patient's state of mind.

Typically, young trauma patients do not have chronic illnesses. With older patients, however, medical conditions that are present before the trauma event can cause serious complications in the prehospital assessment and management of the patient and can significantly influence the outcome. For example, a 75-year-old driver of a vehicle that has struck a utility pole may have chest pain indicative of a myocardial infarction (heart attack). Did the driver hit the utility pole and have a heart attack, or did he have a heart attack and then strike the utility pole? Does the driver take medication (e.g., beta blocker) that will prevent elevation of the pulse in shock? Most of these conditions not only directly influence the assessment and management strategies (discussed in the Scene Assessment and the Patient Assessment and Management chapters) but also are important in overall patient care, even if they do not necessarily influence the physics of trauma of the crash.

Event

The *event phase* begins at the time of impact between one moving object and a second object. The second object can be moving or stationary and can be either an object or a person. Using a vehicle crash as an example, three impacts occur in most vehicular crashes:

1. The impact of the two objects
2. The impact of the occupants into the vehicle
3. The impact of the vital organs inside the occupants

For example, when a vehicle strikes a tree, the first impact is the collision of the vehicle with the tree. The second impact is the occupant of the vehicle striking the steering wheel or windshield. If the occupant is restrained, an impact occurs between the occupant and the seat belt. The third impact is between the occupant's internal organs and his or her chest wall, abdominal wall, or skull.

While the term *crash* typically brings to mind a motor vehicle incident, it does not necessarily refer to a vehicular crash. The impact of a vehicle into a pedestrian, a missile (bullet) into the abdomen, and a construction worker onto asphalt after a fall are all examples of a crash. Note that in a fall, only the second and third types of impacts are involved.

In all crashes, energy is exchanged between a moving object and the tissue of the human body or between the moving human body and a stationary object. The direction in which the energy exchange occurs, the amount of energy that is exchanged, and the effect that these forces have on the patient are all important considerations as assessment begins.

Postevent

During the *postevent phase*, the information gathered about the crash and pre-event phase is used to assess and manage a patient. This phase begins as soon as the energy from the crash is absorbed. The onset of the complications from life-threatening trauma can be slow or fast (or these complications can be prevented or significantly reduced), depending in part on the care provided at the scene and en route to the hospital. In the postevent phase, the understanding of the physics of trauma, the index of suspicion regarding injuries, and strong assessment skills all become crucial to the provider's ability to influence patient outcome.

To understand the effects of the forces that produce bodily injury, the prehospital care provider first needs to understand two components—energy exchange and human anatomy. For example, in a motor vehicle collision (MVC), what does the scene look like? Who hit what and at what speed? How long was the stopping time? Were the occupants using appropriate restraint devices such as seat belts? Did the air bag deploy? Were the children restrained properly in child seats, or were they unrestrained and thrown about the vehicle? Were occupants thrown from the vehicle? Did they strike objects? If so, how many objects and what was the nature of those objects? These and many other questions must be answered if the prehospital care provider is to understand the exchange of forces that took place and translate this information into a prediction of injuries and appropriate patient care.

The astute prehospital care provider will use his or her knowledge of the physics of trauma in the process of surveying the scene to determine what forces and motion were involved and what injuries might have resulted from those forces. Because the physics of trauma is based on fundamental principles of physics, an understanding of the pertinent laws of physics is necessary.

Energy

The initial steps in obtaining a history include evaluating the events that occurred at the time of the crash (**Figure 4-1**), estimating the energy that was exchanged with the human body, and making a gross approximation of the specific conditions that resulted.

Laws of Energy and Motion

Newton's first law of motion states that a body at rest will remain at rest and a body in motion will remain in motion unless acted on by an outside force. In **Figure 4-2**, the skier

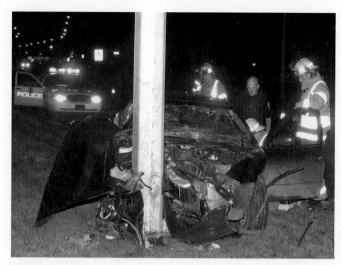

Figure 4-1 Evaluating the scene of an incident is critical. Information such as direction of impact, passenger-compartment intrusion, and amount of energy exchange provides insight into the possible injuries of the occupants.

© Jack Dagley Photography/Shutterstock.

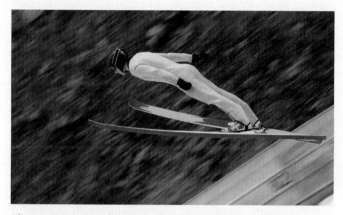

Figure 4-2 The skier was stationary until the energy from gravity moved him down the slope. Once in motion, although he leaves the ground, the momentum will keep him in motion until he hits something or returns to the ground, and the transfer of energy (friction or a collision) causes him to come to a stop.

© technotr/iStock/Getty Images.

was stationary until the energy from gravity moved him down the slope. Once in motion, although he leaves the ground, he will remain in motion until he hits something or returns to the ground and comes to a stop.

As previously mentioned, in any collision, when the body of the potential patient is in motion, there are three collisions:

1. The vehicle of the crash hitting an object, moving or stationary
2. The potential patient hitting the inside of the vehicle, crashing into an object, or being struck by energy in an explosion
3. The internal organs interacting with the walls of a compartment of the body or being torn loose from their supporting structures

An example is an occupant sitting in the front seat of a vehicle who is not wearing any restraint devices. When the vehicle hits a tree and stops, the unrestrained occupant continues in motion—at the same rate of speed—until he or she hits the steering column, dashboard, and windshield. The impact with these objects stops the forward motion of the torso or head, but the internal organs of the occupant remain in motion until the organs hit the inside of the chest wall, abdominal wall, or skull, halting the forward motion.

As described by the **law of conservation of energy** and **Newton's second law of motion**, energy can neither be created nor destroyed but can be changed in form. The motion of the vehicle is a form of energy. To start the vehicle, energy from the engine is transferred by a set of gears to the wheels, which grasp the road as they turn and impart motion to the vehicle. To stop the vehicle, the energy of its motion must be changed to another form, such as by heating up the brakes or crashing into an object and bending the frame. When a driver applies the brakes, the energy of motion is converted into the heat of friction (thermal energy) by the brake pads on the brake drums/discs and by the tires on the roadway. The vehicle thus decelerates.

Newton's third law of motion is perhaps the most well-known of Newton's three laws. It states that for every action or force there is an equal and opposite reaction. As we walk across the ground, the earth is exerting a force against us equal to the force we are applying upon the earth. Those who have fired a shotgun have felt the third law as the impact of the butt of the gun against their shoulder.

Just as the mechanical energy of a vehicle that crashes into a wall is dissipated by the bending of the frame or other parts of the vehicle (**Figure 4-3**), the energy of motion of the organs and the structures inside the body must be dissipated as these organs stop their forward motion. The same concepts apply to the human body when it is

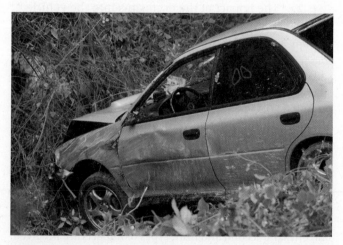

Figure 4-3 Energy is dissipated by deformation of the vehicle frame.

© Peter Seyfferth/image/age footstock.

stationary and comes into contact and interacts with an object in motion such as a knife, a bullet, or a baseball bat.

Kinetic energy is a function of an object's mass and velocity. Although they are not technically the same, a victim's weight may be used to represent his or her mass. Likewise, speed is used to represent velocity (which really is speed and direction). The relationship between weight and speed as it affects kinetic energy is as follows:

Kinetic energy = One-half the mass times the velocity squared

$$KE = 1/2 \ (mv^2)$$

Thus, the kinetic energy involved when a 150-pound (lb) (68-kilogram [kg]) person travels at 30 miles per hour (mph) (48 kilometers per hour [km/hr]) is calculated as follows:

$$KE = 150/2 \times 30^2 = 67,500 \text{ units}$$

For the purpose of this discussion, no specific physical unit of measure (e.g., foot-pounds, joules) is used. The units are used merely to illustrate how this formula affects the change in the amount of energy. As just shown, a 150-lb (68-kg) person traveling at 30 mph (48 km/hr) would have 67,500 units of energy that must be converted to another form when he or she stops. This change takes the form of damage to the vehicle and injury to the person in it unless the energy dissipation can take some less harmful form, such as on a seat belt or into an air bag.

Which factor in the formula, however, has the greatest effect on the amount of kinetic energy produced: mass or velocity? Consider adding 10 lb (4.5 kg) to the 150-lb (68-kg) person traveling at 30 mph (48 km/hr) in the prior example, making the mass equal to 160 lb (73 kg):

$$KE = 160/2 \times 30^2 = 72,000 \text{ units}$$

This 10-lb increase has resulted in a 4,500-unit increase in kinetic energy. Using the initial example of a 150-lb (68-kg) person once again, let's now see how increasing the velocity by 10 mph (16 km/hr) affects the kinetic energy:

$$KE = 150/2 \times 40^2 = 120,000 \text{ units}$$

This velocity increase has resulted in a 52,500-unit increase in kinetic energy.

These calculations demonstrate that increasing the velocity (speed) increases the kinetic energy much more than does increasing the mass. Much more energy exchange will occur (and, therefore, produce greater injury to either the occupant, the vehicle, or both) in a high-speed crash than in a crash at a slower speed. The velocity is exponential and the mass is linear, making velocity the more critical factor even when there is a great mass disparity between two objects.

In anticipating the injuries sustained during a high-speed crash, it can be helpful to bear in mind that the force involved in initiating an event is equal to the force transferred or dissipated at the end of that event.

Mass × Acceleration = Force = Mass × Deceleration

Force (energy) is required to put a structure into motion. This force (energy) is required to create a specific speed. The speed imparted is dependent on the weight (mass) of the structure. Once this energy is passed on to the structure and it is placed in motion, the structure will remain in motion until the energy is given up (Newton's first law of motion). This loss of energy will place other components in motion (tissue particles) or be lost as heat (dissipated into the brake discs on the wheels). An example of this process is gun-related trauma. In the chamber of a gun is a cartridge that contains gunpowder. When this gunpowder is ignited, it burns rapidly, creating energy that pushes the bullet out of the barrel at a great speed. This speed is equivalent to the weight of the bullet and the amount of energy produced by the burning of the gunpowder or force. To slow down (Newton's first law of motion), the bullet must give up its energy into the structure that it hits. This transfer of energy will produce an explosion in the tissue that is equal to the explosion that occurred in the chamber of the gun when the initial speed was given to the bullet. The same phenomenon occurs in the moving automobile, the patient falling from a building, or the explosion of an improvised explosive device (IED).

Another important factor in a crash is the **stopping distance**. The shorter the stopping distance and the quicker the rate of that stop, the more energy is transferred to the occupant and the more damage or injury is done to the patient. Consider a vehicle that stops against a brick wall versus one that stops when the brakes are applied. Both dissipate the same amount of energy, just in a different manner. The rate of energy exchange (into the vehicle body or into the brake discs) is different and occurs over a different distance and time. In the first instance, the energy is absorbed in a very short distance and amount of time by the bending of the vehicle's frame. In the latter case, the energy is absorbed over a longer distance and period of time by the heat of the brakes. The forward motion of the occupant of the vehicle (energy) is absorbed in the first instance by damage to the soft tissue and bones of the occupant. In the second instance, the energy is dissipated, along with the energy of the vehicle, into the brakes.

This inverse relationship between stopping distance and injury also applies to falls. A person has a better chance of surviving a fall if he or she lands on a compressible surface, such as deep powder snow. A fall from the same height terminating on a hard surface, such as concrete, can produce more severe injuries. The compressible material (i.e., the snow) increases the stopping distance and absorbs at least some of the energy rather than allowing all of the energy to be absorbed by the body. The result is decreased injury and damage to the body. This principle also applies

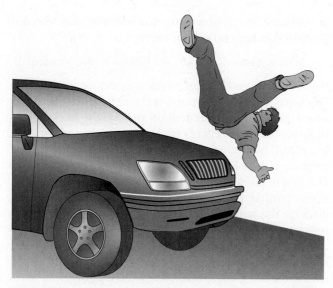

Figure 4-4 The energy exchange from a moving vehicle to a pedestrian crushes tissue and imparts speed and energy to the pedestrian, knocking the victim away from the point of impact. Injury to the victim can occur as the pedestrian is hit by the vehicle and as the pedestrian is thrown to the ground or into another vehicle.

© National Association of Emergency Medical Technicians (NAEMT).

to other types of crashes. An unrestrained driver will be more severely injured than a restrained driver because the restraint system, rather than the body, absorbs a significant portion of the energy transfer.

Therefore, once an object is in motion and has energy in the form of motion, in order for it to come to a complete rest, the object must lose all of its energy by converting the energy to another form or transferring it to another object. For example, if a vehicle strikes a pedestrian, the pedestrian is knocked away from the vehicle (**Figure 4-4**). Although the vehicle is somewhat slowed by the impact, the greater force of the vehicle imparts much more acceleration to the lighter-weight pedestrian than it loses in speed because of the mass difference between the two. The softer body parts of the pedestrian versus the harder body parts of the vehicle also means more damage to the pedestrian than to the vehicle.

Energy Exchange Between a Solid Object and the Human Body

When the human body collides with a solid object, or vice versa, the number of body tissue particles that are impacted by the solid object determines the amount of energy exchange that takes place. This transfer of energy produces the amount of damage (injury) that occurs to the patient. The number of tissue particles affected is determined by (1) the density (particles per volume) of the tissue and (2) the size of the contact area of the impact.

Density

The denser the tissue (measured in particles per volume), the greater the number of particles that will be impacted by a moving object and, therefore, the greater the rate and the total amount of energy exchanged. Driving a fist into a feather pillow and driving a fist at the same speed into a brick wall will produce different effects on the hand. The fist absorbs more energy colliding with the dense brick wall than with the less dense feather pillow, thus leading to more significant injury to the hand (**Figure 4-5**).

Simplistically, the body has three different types of tissue densities: **air density** (much of the lung and some portions of the intestine), **water density** (muscle and most solid organs; e.g., liver, spleen), and **solid density** (bone). Therefore, the amount of energy exchange (with resultant injury) will depend on which type of tissue is impacted.

Contact Area

Wind exerts pressure on a hand when it is extended out of the window of a moving vehicle. When the palm of the hand is horizontal and parallel to the direction of the flow through the wind, some backward pressure is exerted on the front of the hand (fingers) as the particles of air strike the hand. Rotating the hand 90 degrees to a vertical position places a larger surface area into the wind; thus, more air particles make contact with the hand, increasing the amount of force on it.

For trauma events, the energy imparted and the resulting damage can be modified by any change in the size of the impact surface area. Examples of this effect on the human

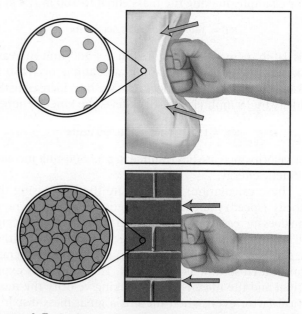

Figure 4-5 The fist absorbs more energy colliding with the dense brick wall than with the less dense feather pillow, which dissipates the force.

© National Association of Emergency Medical Technicians (NAEMT).

body include the front of an automobile, a baseball bat, or a rifle bullet. The automobile's front surface contacts a large portion of the victim, a baseball bat contacts a smaller area, and a bullet contacts a very small area. The amount of energy exchange that would produce damage to the patient depends on the energy of the object and the density of the tissue in the pathway of the energy exchange.

If all of the impact energy is in a small area and this force exceeds the resistance of the skin, the object is forced through the skin. Consider the difference between striking a wooden table with a hammer and striking a nail held to the surface of the table with that same hammer. When you strike the table with the hammer, the force of the hammer striking the table is spread out across the surface of the table and the entire head of the hammer, limiting penetration and creating only a dent. In contrast, striking the head of a nail with the hammer using the same amount of force drives the nail into the wood as all of that force is applied over a very small area. When the force is spread out over a larger area and the skin is not penetrated (like the hammer striking the table), the injury is defined as **blunt trauma**. If the force is applied over a small area and the object penetrates the skin and underlying tissues (like the hammer driving the nail through the table), the injury is defined as **penetrating trauma**. In either instance, a cavity in the patient is created by the force of the impacting object.

Even with an object such as a bullet, the impact surface area can be different based on such factors as bullet size, its motion (tumble) within the body, deformation ("mushroom"), and fragmentation. These factors are discussed later in this chapter.

Cavitation

The basic mechanics of energy exchange are relatively simple. The impact on the tissue particles accelerates those tissue particles away from the point of impact. These tissues then become moving objects themselves and crash into other tissue particles, producing a "falling domino" effect. Similarly, when a solid object strikes the human body or when the human body is in motion and strikes a stationary object, the tissue particles of the human body are knocked out of their normal position, creating a hole or cavity. Thus, this process is called **cavitation**. A common example that provides a visual illustration of cavitation is the game of pool (i.e., billiards).

The cue ball is driven down the length of a pool table by the force of the muscles in the arm. The cue ball crashes into the racked balls at the other end of the table. The energy from the arm into the cue ball is thus transferred onto each of the racked balls (**Figure 4-6**). The cue ball gives up its energy to the other balls. The other balls begin to move while the cue ball, which has lost its

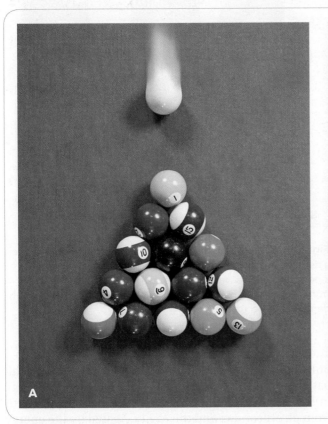
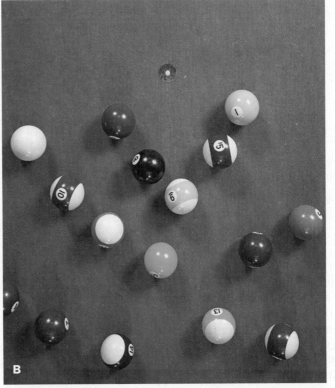

Figure 4-6 A. The energy of a cue ball is transferred to each of the other balls. **B.** The energy exchange pushes the balls apart to create a cavity.

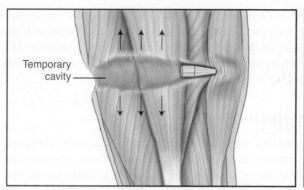
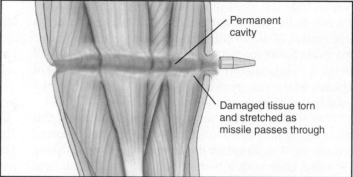

Figure 4-7 Damage to tissue is greater than the permanent cavity that remains from a missile injury. The faster or heavier the missile, the larger the temporary cavity and the greater the zone of tissue damage.

© National Association of Emergency Medical Technicians (NAEMT).

energy, slows or even stops. The other balls take on this energy as motion and move away from the impact point. A cavity has been created where the rack of balls once was. The same kind of energy exchange occurs when a bowling ball rolls down the alley, hitting the set of pins at the other end. The result of this energy exchange is a cavity. This same type of energy exchange occurs in both blunt and penetrating trauma.

Two types of cavities are created:

- A *temporary cavity* is caused by the stretching of the tissues that occurs at the time of impact. Because of the elastic properties of the body's tissues, some or all of the contents of the temporary cavity return to their previous position. The size, shape, and portions of the cavity that become part of the permanent damage depend on the tissue type, the elasticity of the tissue, and how much rebound of tissue occurs. The extent of this cavity usually is not visible when the prehospital care or hospital provider examines the patient, even seconds after the impact.

- A *permanent cavity* is left after the temporary cavity collapses and is the visible part of the tissue destruction. In addition, a crush cavity is produced by the direct impact of the object on the tissue. Both of these cavities can be seen when the patient is examined (**Figure 4-7**).[5]

The amount of the temporary cavity that remains as a permanent cavity is related to the elasticity (stretch ability) of the tissue involved. For example, forcefully swinging a baseball bat into a steel drum leaves a dent, or cavity, in its side. Swinging the same baseball bat with the same force into a mass of foam rubber of similar size and shape will leave no dent once the bat is removed (**Figure 4-8**). The difference is **elasticity**. The foam rubber is more elastic than the steel drum. The human body is more like the foam rubber than the steel drum. If a person punches another person's abdomen, he or she would feel the fist go in. However, when the person

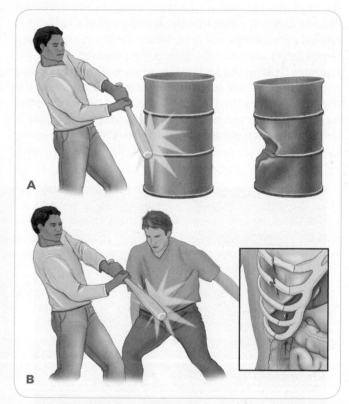

Figure 4-8 A. Swinging a baseball bat into a steel drum leaves a dent, or cavity, in its side. **B.** Swinging a baseball bat into a person usually leaves no visible cavity; the elasticity of the trunk usually returns the body to its normal shape even though damage has occurred.

© National Association of Emergency Medical Technicians (NAEMT).

pulls the fist away, no dent is left. Similarly, a baseball bat swung into the chest will leave no obvious cavity in the thoracic wall, but it would cause damage, both from direct contact and the cavity created by the energy exchange. The history of the incident and the interpretation of energy transfer will provide the information

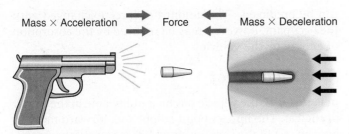

Figure 4-9 As a bullet travels through tissue, its kinetic energy is transferred to the tissue with which it comes in contact, accelerating the tissue away from the bullet.

© National Association of Emergency Medical Technicians (NAEMT).

needed to determine the potential size of the temporary cavity at the time of impact. The organs or the structures involved predict injuries.

When the trigger of a loaded gun is pulled, the firing pin strikes the cap and produces an explosion in the cartridge. The energy created by this explosion is applied to the bullet, which speeds from the muzzle of the weapon. The bullet now has energy, or force (acceleration × mass = force). Once such force is imparted, the bullet cannot slow down until acted on by an outside force (Newton's first law of motion). For the bullet to stop inside the human body, an explosion must occur within the tissues that is equivalent to the explosion in the weapon (acceleration × mass = force = mass × deceleration) (**Figure 4-9**). This explosion is the result of energy exchange accelerating the tissue particles out of their normal position, creating a cavity.

Blunt and Penetrating Trauma

Trauma is generally classified as either blunt or penetrating. However, the energy exchanged and the injuries produced are similar in both types of trauma. Cavitation occurs in both; only the type and direction are different. The only real difference is penetration of the skin. If an object's entire energy is concentrated on one small area of skin, the skin likely will tear, and the object will enter the body and create a more concentrated energy exchange along its pathway. This can result in greater destructive power to one area. A larger object whose energy is dispersed over a larger area of skin may not penetrate the skin. The damage will be distributed over a larger area of the body, and the injury pattern will be less localized. An example is the difference in the impact of a large truck into a pedestrian versus a gunshot impact (**Figure 4-10**).

The cavitation in blunt trauma is frequently only a temporary cavity and is directed away from the point of impact. Penetrating trauma creates both a permanent and a temporary cavity. The temporary cavity that is created will spread away from the pathway of this missile in both frontal and lateral directions.

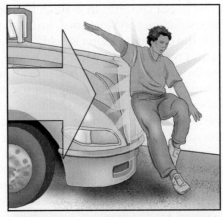

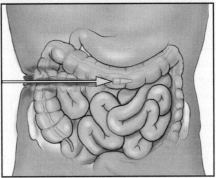

Figure 4-10 The force from the collision of a vehicle with a person is generally distributed over a large area, whereas the force of a collision between a bullet and a person is localized to a small area and results in penetration of the body and underlying structures.

© National Association of Emergency Medical Technicians (NAEMT).

Blunt Trauma

The on-scene observations of the probable circumstances that led to a crash resulting in blunt trauma provide clues as to the severity of the injuries and the potential organs involved. The factors to assess are (1) direction of the impact, (2) external damage to the vehicle (type and severity), (3) internal damage (e.g., occupant compartment intrusion, steering wheel/column bending, fracture in the windshield, mirror damage, dashboard–knee impacts), (4) location of occupants within the vehicle, and (5) restraint devises employed or deployed at the time of the crash.

In blunt trauma, two forces are involved in the impact—**shear** and **compression**—both of which may result in cavitation. *Shear* is the result of one organ or structure (or part of an organ or structure) changing speed faster than another organ or structure (or part of an organ or structure). This difference in acceleration (or deceleration) causes the parts to separate and tear. A classic example of shear force is the rupture of the thoracic aorta. The ascending aorta and aortic arch are loosely held in place within the mediastinum, whereas the descending aorta is tightly bound to the spinal column. In a sudden deceleration incident, the ascending aorta and aortic arch can continue moving while the descending aorta is held in place, leading to shearing and rupture of the aorta (see Figure 4-14).

Compression is the result of an organ or structure (or part of an organ or structure) being directly squeezed between other organs or structures. A common example of compression involves the bowel being compressed between the spinal column and the inside of the anterior abdominal wall in a patient wearing only a seat belt (see Figure 4-28). Injury can result from any type of impact, such as MVCs (vehicle or motorcycle), pedestrian collisions with vehicles, falls, sports injuries, or blast injuries. All of these mechanisms are discussed separately, followed by the results of this energy exchange on the specific anatomy in each of the body regions.

As discussed previously in this chapter, three collisions occur in blunt trauma. The first is the collision of the vehicle into another object. The second is the collision that occurs when the occupant strikes the inside of the vehicular passenger compartment, strikes the ground at the end of a fall, or is struck by the force created in an explosion. The third is when the structures within the various regions of the body (head, chest, abdomen, etc.) strike the wall of that region or are torn (shear force) from their attachment within this compartment. The first of these collisions will be discussed as it relates to MVCs, falls, and explosions. The latter two will be discussed in the specific regions involved.

Motor Vehicle Crashes

Many forms of blunt trauma occur, but MVCs (including motorcycle crashes) are the most common.[6] In 2015 in the United States, 36,092 people died and an estimated 2.6 million people were injured in MVCs. While the majority of the injuries were to occupants of the vehicles, over 230,000 of the injuries were to motorcyclists, over 460,000 were to bicyclists, and over 180,000 were to pedestrians.[6]

MVCs can be divided into the following five types:

1. Frontal impact
2. Rear impact
3. Lateral impact
4. Rotational impact
5. Rollover[6]

Although each pattern has variations, accurate identification of the five patterns can provide insight into other, similar types of crashes.

One method to estimate the potential for injury to the occupant is to look at the vehicle and determine which of the five types of collisions occurred, the energy exchange involved, and the direction of the impact. The occupant is vulnerable to the same type of force as the vehicle from the same direction as the vehicle, and the potential injuries

can be predicted.[6] The amount of force exchanged with the occupant, however, may be reduced by the absorption of energy by the vehicle.

Frontal Impact

In **Figure 4-11**, the vehicle has hit a utility pole in the center of the car. The impact point stopped its forward motion, but the rest of the car continued forward until the energy was absorbed by the bending of the car. The same type of motion occurs to the driver, resulting in injury. The stable steering column is impacted by the chest, perhaps in the center of the sternum. Just as the car continued in forward motion, significantly deforming the front of the vehicle, so too did the driver's chest. As the sternum stops forward motion against the dash, the posterior thoracic wall continues until the energy is absorbed by the bending and possible fracture of the ribs. This process may also crush the heart and the lungs, which are trapped between the sternum and the vertebral column and the posterior thoracic wall.

The amount of damage to the vehicle is related to the approximate speed of the vehicle at the time of impact. The greater the intrusion into the body of the vehicle, the greater the likely speed at the time of impact. The greater the vehicle speed, the greater the energy exchange and the more likely the occupants are to be injured.

Although the vehicle suddenly ceases to move forward in a frontal impact, the occupant continues to move and

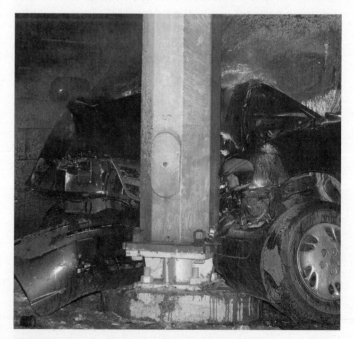

Figure 4-11 As a vehicle impacts a utility pole, the front of the car stops, but the rear portion of the vehicle continues traveling forward, causing deformation of the vehicle.

© Jack Dagley Photography/Shutterstock.

will follow one of two possible paths: up and over or down and under.

The use of a seat belt and the deployment of an air bag or restraint system will absorb some or most of the energy, thus reducing the injury to the victim. For clarity and simplicity of discussion, the occupant in these examples is assumed to be unrestrained.

Up-and-Over Path

In this sequence, the body's forward motion carries it up and over the steering wheel (**Figure 4-12**). The head is usually the lead body portion striking the windshield, windshield frame, or roof. The head then stops its forward motion. The torso continues in motion until its energy/force is absorbed along the spine. The cervical spine is the least protected segment of the spine. The chest or abdomen then collides with the steering column, depending on the position of the torso. The impact of the chest into the steering column produces thoracic cage, cardiac, lung, and aortic injuries (see the Regional Effects of Blunt Trauma section). The impact of the abdomen into the steering column can compress and crush the solid organs, produce overpressure injuries (especially to the diaphragm), and rupture the hollow organs.

The kidneys, spleen, and liver are also subject to shear injury as the abdomen strikes the steering wheel and abruptly stops. An organ may be torn from its normal

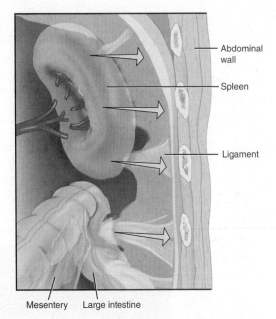

Figure 4-13 Organs can tear away from their point of attachment to the abdominal wall. The spleen, kidney, and small intestine are particularly susceptible to these types of shear forces.

© National Association of Emergency Medical Technicians (NAEMT).

anatomic restraints and supporting tissues (**Figure 4-13**). For example, the continued forward motion of the kidneys after the vertebral column has stopped moving produces shear along the attachment of the organs at their blood supply. The aorta and vena cava are tethered tightly to the posterior abdominal wall and vertebral column. The continued forward motion of the kidneys can stretch the renal vessels to the point of rupture. A similar action may tear the aorta in the chest at the point where the unattached arch becomes the tightly adhered descending aorta (**Figure 4-14**).

Down-and-Under Path

In a down-and-under path, the occupant moves forward, downward, and out of the seat into the dashboard (**Figure 4-15**). The importance of understanding the physics of trauma is illustrated by the injuries produced to the lower extremity in this pathway. Because many of the injuries are difficult to identify, an understanding of the mechanism of injury is important.

The foot, if planted on the floor panel or on the brake pedal with a straight knee, can twist as the continued torso motion angulates and fractures the ankle joint. More often, however, the knees are already bent, and the force is not directed to the ankle. Therefore, the knees strike the dashboard.

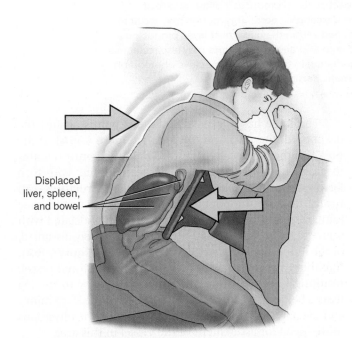

Figure 4-12 Configuration of the seat and position of the occupant can direct the initial force on the upper torso, with the head following the up-and-over path.

© National Association of Emergency Medical Technicians (NAEMT).

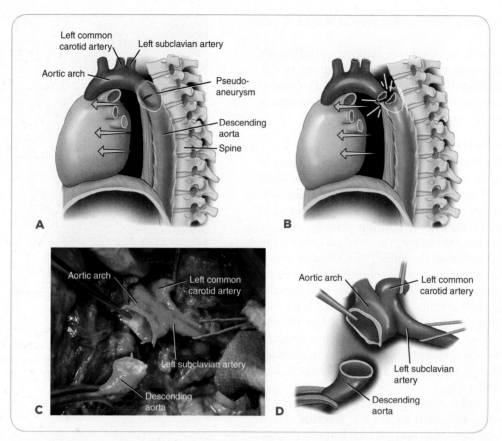

Figure 4-14 A. The descending aorta is a fixed structure that moves with the thoracic spine. The arch, aorta, and heart are freely mobile. Acceleration of the torso in a lateral-impact collision or rapid deceleration of the torso in a frontal-impact collision produces a different rate of motion between the arch–heart complex and the descending aorta. This motion may result in a tear of the inner lining of the aorta that is contained within the outermost layer, producing a pseudo-aneurysm. **B.** Tears at the junction of the arch and descending aorta may also result in a complete rupture, leading to immediate exsanguination in the chest. **C.** Operative photograph of a traumatic aortic tear. **D.** Illustration of a traumatic aortic tear.

A and B: © National Association of Emergency Medical Technicians (NAEMT); **C and D:** Courtesy of Norman McSwain, MD, FACS, NREMT-P.

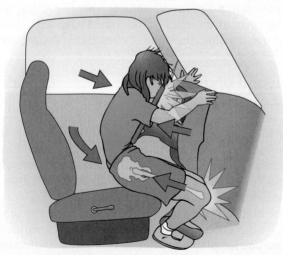

Figure 4-15 The occupant and the vehicle travel forward together. The vehicle stops, and the unrestrained occupant continues forward until something stops that motion.

© National Association of Emergency Medical Technicians (NAEMT).

The knee has two possible impact points against the dashboard, the tibia and the femur (**Figure 4-16A**). If the tibia hits the dashboard and stops first, the femur remains in motion and overrides it. A dislocated knee, with torn ligaments, tendons, and other supporting structures, can result. Because the popliteal artery lies close to the knee joint, dislocation of the joint is frequently associated with injury to this vessel.[7] The artery can be completely disrupted, or the lining alone (*intima*) may be damaged (**Figure 4-16B**). In either case, a blood clot may form in the injured vessel, resulting in significantly decreased blood flow to the leg tissues below the knee. Early recognition of the knee injury and the potential for vascular injury will alert the physicians to the need for assessment of the vessel in this area.

Early identification and treatment of such a popliteal artery injury significantly decrease the complications of distal limb ischemia. Perfusion to this tissue needs to be reestablished within about 6 hours. Delays could occur because the prehospital care provider failed to consider the

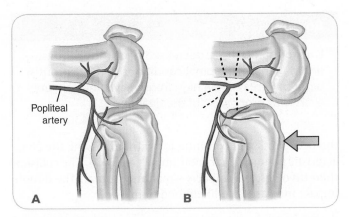

Figure 4-16 **A.** The knee has two possible impact points in a motor vehicle crash: the tibia and the femur. **B.** The popliteal artery lies close to the joint, tightly tied to the femur above and tibia below. Separation of these two bones stretches, kinks, and tears the artery.

© National Association of Emergency Medical Technicians (NAEMT).

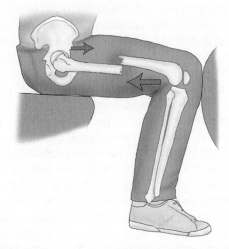

Figure 4-18 When the femur is the point of impact, the energy is absorbed by the femoral shaft, which can then break.

© National Association of Emergency Medical Technicians (NAEMT).

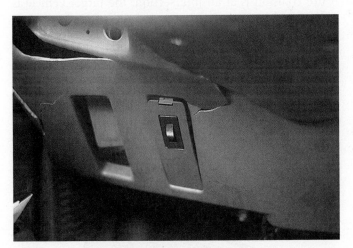

Figure 4-17 An imprint on the dashboard where the knee impacted is a key indicator that significant energy was focused on this joint and adjacent structures.

Courtesy of Norman McSwain, MD, FACS, NREMT-P.

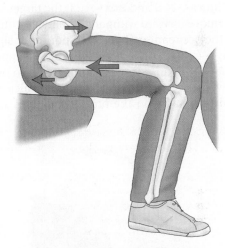

Figure 4-19 The continued forward motion of the pelvis relative to the femur can result in a posterior dislocation of the hip joint.

© National Association of Emergency Medical Technicians (NAEMT).

physics of trauma of the injury or overlooked important clues during assessment of the patient.

Although most of these patients have evidence of injury to the knee, an imprint on the dashboard where the knee impacted is a key indicator that significant energy was focused on this joint and adjacent structures (**Figure 4-17**). Further investigation is needed in the hospital to better define the possible injuries.

When the femur is the point of impact, the energy is absorbed by the shaft of the bone, which can then break (**Figure 4-18**). If the femur remains intact, the continued forward motion of the pelvis onto the femur can dislocate the femoral head from the acetabulum (**Figure 4-19**).

After the knees and legs stop their forward motion, the upper body will bend forward into the steering column or dashboard. The unrestrained occupant may then sustain many of the same injuries described previously for the up-and-over pathway.

Recognizing these potential injuries and relaying the information to the ED physicians can result in long-term benefits to the patient.

Rear Impact

Rear-impact collisions occur when a slower-moving or stationary vehicle is struck from behind by a vehicle moving at a faster speed. For ease of understanding, the more rapidly moving vehicle is called the "bullet vehicle," and the slower-moving or stopped object is called the "target vehicle." In such collisions, the energy of the bullet vehicle at the moment of impact is converted to acceleration of the target vehicle, and damage results to both vehicles. The greater the difference in the momentum of the two vehicles, the greater the force of the initial impact and the more energy is available to create damage and acceleration.

During a rear-impact collision, the target vehicle (in front) is accelerated forward. Everything that is attached to the frame will move forward at the same speed. This includes the seats in which the occupants are riding. The unattached objects in the vehicle, including the occupants, will begin forward motion only after something in contact with the frame begins to transmit the energy of the forward motion to them. As an example, the torso is accelerated by the back of the seat after some of the energy has been absorbed by the springs in the seats. If the headrest is improperly positioned behind and below the occiput of the head, the head will begin its forward motion after the torso, resulting in hyperextension of the neck. Shear and stretching of the ligaments and other support structures, especially in the anterior part of the neck, can result in injury (**Figure 4-20A**).

If the headrest is properly positioned, the head moves at approximately the same time as the torso without hyperextension (**Figure 4-20B** and **Box 4-2**). If the target vehicle is allowed to move forward without interference until it slows to a stop, the occupant will probably not suffer significant injury because most of the body's motion is supported by the seat, similar to an astronaut launching into orbit.

However, if the vehicle strikes another vehicle or object or if the driver slams on the brakes and stops suddenly,

Box 4-2 Headrests
Due to osteoporosis, decreased neck muscle mass, and degenerative spinal conditions such as arthritis, older patients have a high frequency of neck injury, even with proper use of the headrest.[8]

the occupants will continue forward, following the characteristic pattern of a frontal-impact collision. The collision then involves two impacts—rear and frontal. The double impact increases the likelihood of injury.

Lateral Impact

Lateral-impact mechanisms come into play when the vehicle is involved in an intersection (T-bone) collision or when the vehicle veers off the road and impacts sideways into a utility pole, tree, or other obstacle on the roadside. If the collision is at an intersection, the target vehicle is accelerated from the impact in the direction away from the force created by the bullet vehicle. The side of the vehicle or the door that is struck is thrust against the side of the occupant. The occupants may be injured as they are accelerated laterally (**Figure 4-21**) or as the passenger compartment is bent inward by the door's projection (**Figure 4-22**). Injury caused by the vehicle's movement is less severe if the occupant is restrained and moves with the initial motion of the vehicle.[9]

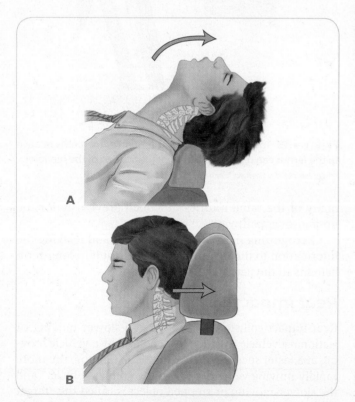

Figure 4-20 A. A rear-impact collision forces the torso forward. If the headrest is improperly positioned, the head is hyperextended over the top of the headrest. **B.** If the headrest is up, the head moves with the torso, and neck injury is prevented or reduced.

© National Association of Emergency Medical Technicians (NAEMT).

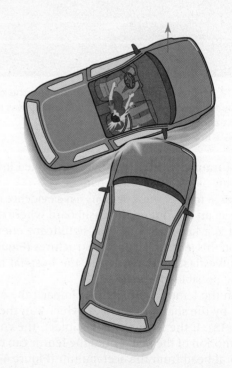

Figure 4-21 Lateral impact of the vehicle pushes the entire vehicle into the unrestrained passenger. A restrained passenger moves laterally with the vehicle.

© National Association of Emergency Medical Technicians (NAEMT).

Five body regions can sustain injury in a lateral impact:

- *Clavicle*. The clavicle can be compressed and fractured if the force is against the shoulder (**Figure 4-23A**).
- *Chest*. Compression of the thoracic wall inward can result in fractured ribs, pulmonary contusion, or compression injury of the solid organs beneath the rib cage, as well as overpressure injuries (e.g., pneumothorax) (**Figure 4-23B**). Shear injuries of the aorta

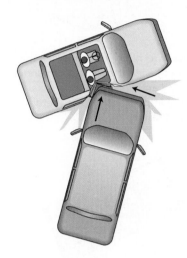

Figure 4-22 Intrusion of the side panels into the passenger compartment provides another source of injury.

© National Association of Emergency Medical Technicians (NAEMT).

can result from the lateral acceleration (25% of aortic shear injuries occur in lateral-impact collisions).[10,11]

- *Abdomen and pelvis*. The intrusion compresses and fractures the pelvis and pushes the head of the femur through the acetabulum (**Figure 4-23C**). Occupants on the driver's side are vulnerable to spleen injuries because the spleen is on the left side of the body, whereas occupants on the passenger side are more likely to receive an injury to the liver.
- *Neck*. The torso can move out from under the head in lateral collisions as well as in rear impacts. The attachment point of the head is posterior and inferior to the center of gravity of the head. Therefore, the motion of the head in relationship to the neck is lateral flexion and rotation. The contralateral side of the spine will be opened (distraction) and the ipsilateral side compressed. This motion can fracture the vertebrae, or more likely, produce jumped (dislocated) facets and possible dislocation as well as spinal cord injury (**Figure 4-24**).
- *Head*. The head can impact the frame of the door and the side window. Near-side impacts produce more injuries than far-side impacts.

Rotational Impact

Rotational-impact collisions occur when one corner of a vehicle strikes an immovable object, the corner of another vehicle, or a vehicle moving slower or in the opposite

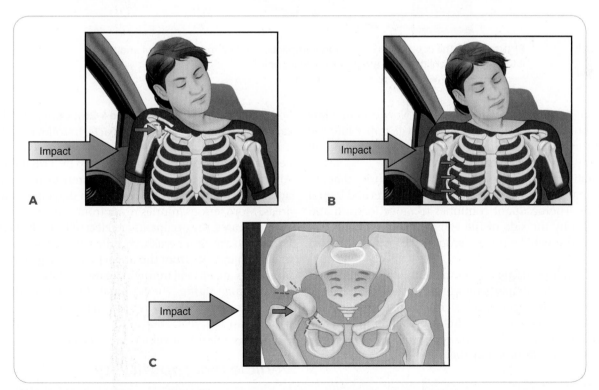

Figure 4-23 A. Compression of the shoulder against the clavicle produces midshaft fractures of this bone. **B.** Compression against the lateral chest and abdominal wall can fracture ribs and injure the underlying spleen, liver, and kidney. **C.** Lateral impact on the femur pushes the head through the acetabulum or fractures the pelvis.

© National Association of Emergency Medical Technicians (NAEMT).

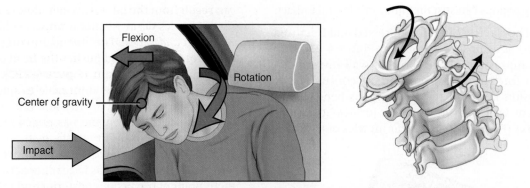

Figure 4-24 The center of gravity of the skull is anterior and superior to its pivot point between the skull and cervical spine. During a lateral impact, when the torso is rapidly accelerated out from under the head, the head turns toward the point of impact, in both lateral and anterior–posterior angles. Such motion separates the vertebral bodies from the side opposite the impact and rotates them apart. Jumped facets, ligament tears, and lateral compression fractures result.
© National Association of Emergency Medical Technicians (NAEMT).

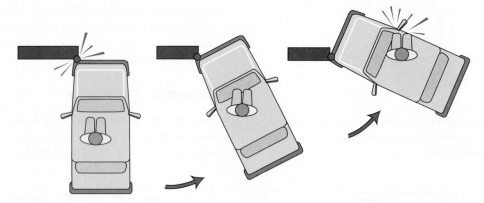

Figure 4-25 The occupant in a rotational-impact crash first moves forward and then laterally as the vehicle pivots around the impact point.
© National Association of Emergency Medical Technicians (NAEMT).

direction of the first vehicle. Following Newton's first law of motion, this corner of the vehicle will stop while the rest of the vehicle continues its forward motion until all its energy is completely transformed.

Rotational-impact collisions result in injuries that are a combination of those seen in frontal impacts and lateral collisions. The occupant continues to move forward and then is hit by the side of the vehicle (as in a lateral collision) as the vehicle rotates around the point of impact (**Figure 4-25**).

With multiple occupants, the patient closest to the point of impact will likely have the worst injuries because all of the energy of the impact is transferred into his or her body. Additional occupants may benefit from the deformation and rotation of the vehicle, which use up some of the energy before it can be absorbed by their bodies.

Rollover

During a rollover, a vehicle may undergo several impacts at many different angles, as may the unrestrained occupant's body and internal organs (**Figure 4-26**). Injury and damage can occur with each of these impacts. In rollover collisions, a restrained occupant is at risk for shearing-type injuries because of the significant forces created by a rolling vehicle. Although the occupants are held securely by restraints, the internal organs still move and can tear at the connecting tissue areas. More serious injuries result from being unrestrained. In many cases, the occupants are ejected from the vehicle as it rolls and are either crushed as the vehicle rolls over them or sustain injuries from the impact with the ground. If the occupants are ejected onto the roadway, they can be struck by oncoming traffic. The National Highway Traffic Safety Administration (NHTSA) reports that in crashes involving fatalities in the year 2008, 77% of occupants who were totally ejected from a vehicle were killed.[12]

Vehicle Incompatibility

The types of vehicles involved in the crash play a significant role in the potential for injury and death to the occupants. For example, in a lateral impact between two cars that

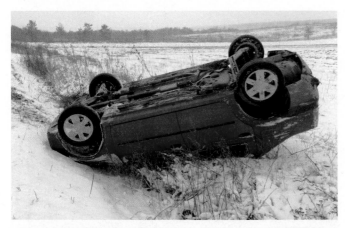

Figure 4-26 During a rollover, the unrestrained occupant can be wholly or partially ejected from the vehicle or can bounce around inside the vehicle. This action produces multiple and somewhat unpredictable injuries that are often severe.

© Rechitan Sorin/Shutterstock.

lack air bags, the occupants of the car struck on its lateral aspect are more likely to die than are the occupants in the vehicle that strikes the car. This disproportionate risk to the occupants of the struck vehicle can be explained largely by the relative lack of protection on the side of a car. In comparison, a large amount of deformation can occur to the front end of a vehicle before there is intrusion into the passenger compartment. When the vehicle that is struck in a lateral collision (by a car) is a sport utility vehicle (SUV), van, or pickup truck rather than a car, the risk of death to occupants in both vehicles is almost the same. This is because the passenger compartments of SUVs, vans, and pickup trucks sits higher off the ground than does that of a car, meaning the occupants sustain less of a direct blow in a lateral impact.

More serious injuries and a greatly increased risk of death to vehicle occupants have been documented when a car is struck on its lateral aspect by a van, SUV, or pickup. In a lateral-impact collision between a van and a car, the occupants of the car struck broadside are more likely to die than are those in the van. If the striking vehicle is a pickup truck or SUV, the occupants of the car struck broadside are more likely to die than are those in the pickup truck or SUV. This tremendous disparity results from the higher center of gravity and increased mass of the van, SUV, or pickup truck. Knowledge of vehicle types in which occupants were located in a crash may lead the prehospital care provider to have a higher index of suspicion for serious injury.

Occupant Protective and Restraining Systems

Seat Belts

In the injury patterns described previously, the occupants were assumed to be unrestrained. The NHTSA has reported a steady increase in seat belt use since 2000, and only 9.9% of passengers were unrestrained in 2016.[13] Ejection from vehicles accounted for approximately 25% of the 44,000 vehicular deaths in 2002.[12] About 77% of passenger vehicle occupants who were totally ejected were killed; 1 in 13 ejection victims sustained a spine fracture.[12] After ejection from a vehicle, the body is subjected to a second impact as the body strikes the ground (or another object) outside the vehicle. This second impact can result in injuries that are even more severe than the initial impact. The risk of death for ejected victims is six times greater than for those who are not ejected. Clearly, seat belts save lives.[14]

The NHTSA reports that 49 states and the District of Columbia have seat belt legislation for both adults and minors. The only exception is New Hampshire, which has regulations for minors but not adults. Research has found that seat belts, when used, reduce the risk of fatal injury to front-seat car occupants by 45% and the risk of serious injury by 50%. In 2014 alone, seat belts saved an estimated 12,802 lives.[13]

While the Centers for Disease Control and Prevention (CDC) and NHTSA report that in 2011, 86% of motor vehicle occupants were restrained, that still leaves one in seven adults who do not wear seat belts on every trip.[15]

What occurs when the occupants are restrained? If a seat belt is positioned properly, the pressure of the impact is absorbed by the pelvis and the chest, resulting a decreased risk of serious injuries (**Figure 4-27**). The proper use of restraints transfers the force of the impact from the occupant's body to the restraint belts and restraint system. With restraints, the chance of receiving life-threatening injuries is greatly reduced.[14,16,17]

Seat belts must be worn properly to be effective. An improperly worn belt may not protect against injury in the event of a crash, and it may even cause injury. When lap belts are worn loosely or are strapped above the pelvis, compression injuries of the soft abdominal organs can occur. Injuries of the soft intra-abdominal organs (spleen, liver, and pancreas) result from compression between the seat belt and the posterior abdominal wall or spinal column (**Figure 4-28**). Increased intra-abdominal pressure can cause diaphragmatic rupture and herniation of abdominal organs. Lap belts should be worn in combination with a shoulder restraint. Anterior compression fractures of the lumbar spine can occur as the upper and lower parts of the torso pivot over the lap belt and the restrained twelfth thoracic (T12), first lumbar (L1), and second lumbar (L2) vertebrae. Occasionally vehicle occupants place the diagonal strap under the arm and not over the shoulder, decreasing its effectiveness.

With the passage and enforcement of mandatory laws on seat belt use in the United States, the overall severity of injuries has decreased, and the number of fatal crashes has been significantly reduced.

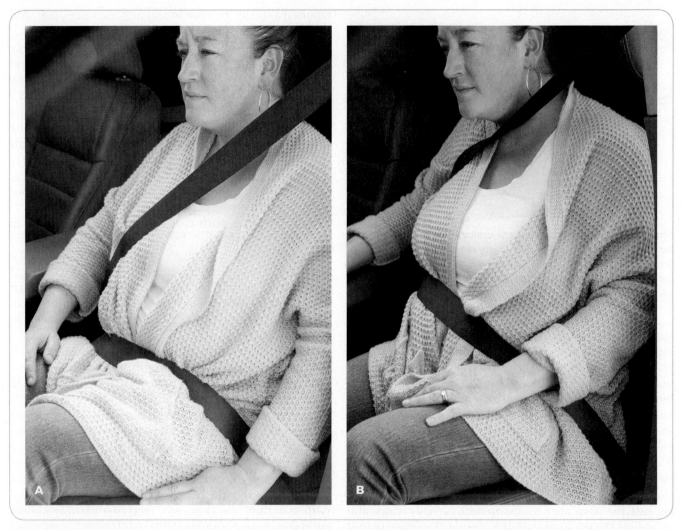

Figure 4-27 A. A properly positioned seat belt is located below the anterior-superior iliac spine on each side, above the femur, and is tight enough to remain in this position. The bowl-shaped pelvis protects the soft intra-abdominal organs. **B.** Improperly placed restraints can result in significant injury in the event of a crash.

© Jones & Bartlett Learning. Photographed by Darren Stahlman.

Air Bags

Air bags (in addition to seat belts) provide supplemental protection to the vehicle occupant. Originally, front-seat driver and passenger air bag systems were designed to cushion the forward motion of only the front-seat occupants. The air bags absorb energy slowly by increasing the body's stopping distance. They are extremely effective in the first collision of frontal and near-frontal impacts (the 65% to 70% of crashes that occur within 30 degrees of the headlights). However, air bags deflate immediately after the impact and, therefore, are not effective in multiple-impact or rear-impact collisions. An air bag deploys and deflates within 0.5 second. As the vehicle veers into the path of an oncoming vehicle or off the road into a tree after the initial impact, no air bag protection is left. Side air bags do add to the protection of occupants.

When air bags deploy, they can produce minor but noticeable injuries that the prehospital care provider needs to identify (**Box 4-3**). These injuries include abrasions of the arms, chest, and face (**Figure 4-29**); foreign bodies to the face and eyes; and injuries caused by the occupant's eyeglasses (**Figure 4-30**).

Air bags that do not deploy can still be dangerous to both the patient and the prehospital care provider. Air bags can be deactivated by an extrication specialist trained to do so properly and safely. Such deactivation should not delay patient care or extrication of the critical patient.

Air bags pose a significant hazard to infants and children if the child is either unrestrained or placed in a rear-facing child seat in the front-passenger compartment.

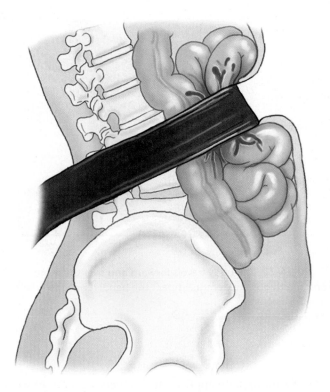

Figure 4-28 A seat belt that is incorrectly positioned above the brim of the pelvis allows the abdominal organs to be trapped between the moving posterior spinal column and the belt. Injuries to the pancreas and other retroperitoneal organs result, as well as blowout ruptures of the small intestine and colon.

© National Association of Emergency Medical Technicians (NAEMT).

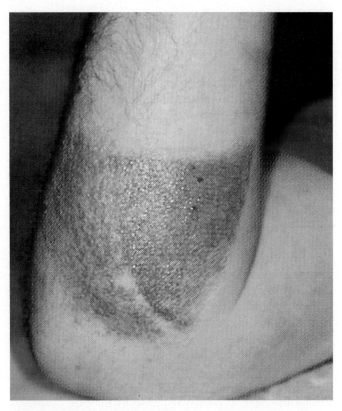

Figure 4-29 Abrasions of the forearm are secondary to rapid expansion of the air bag when the hands are tight against the steering wheel.

Courtesy of Norman McSwain, MD, FACS, NREMT-P.

Box 4-3 Air Bag Hazards

Front-seat passenger air bags have been shown to be dangerous to children and small adults, especially when children are placed in incorrect positions in the front seat or in incorrectly installed child seats. Children 12 years of age and younger should always be in the proper restraint device for their size and should be in the back seat. It is estimated that 46% of all car seats and booster seats are used incorrectly in one or more ways. By seat type, misuse of forward-facing car seats is 61%, rear-facing infant car seats is 49%, rear-facing convertible car seats is 44%, backless belt-positioning boosters is 24%, and high-back belt-positioning boosters is 16%.[18]

Drivers should always be at least 10 inches (25 centimeters [cm]) from the air bag cover, and front-seat passengers should be at least 18 inches (45 cm) away. In most cases, when the proper seating arrangements and distances are used, air bag injuries are limited to simple abrasions.

Many vehicles now have air bags in the sides and tops of the doors.

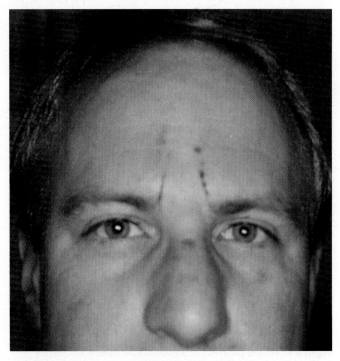

Figure 4-30 Expansion of the air bag into eyeglasses produces abrasions.

Courtesy of Norman E. McSwain Jr., MD, FACS, NREMT-P.

Motorcycle Crashes

Motorcycle crashes account for a significant number of the motor vehicle deaths each year. While the laws of physics for motorcycle crashes are the same, the mechanism of injury varies from automobile and truck crashes. This variance occurs in each of the following types of impacts: head on, angular, and ejection. An additional factor that leads to increased death, disability, and injury is the lack of structural framework around the rider that is present in other motor vehicles.

Head-on Impact

A head-on collision into a solid object stops the forward motion of a motorcycle (**Figure 4-31**). Because the motorcycle's center of gravity is above and behind the front axle, which often becomes a pivot point in such a collision, the motorcycle will tip forward, and the rider may crash into the handlebars. The rider may receive injuries to the head, chest, abdomen, or pelvis, depending on which part of the anatomy impacts with the handlebars or another object first. If the rider's feet remain on the pegs of the motorcycle and the thighs hit the handlebars, the forward motion may be absorbed by the midshaft of the femur, sometimes resulting in bilateral femoral fractures (**Figure 4-32**). The interaction between the rider's pelvis and the handlebars can result in various combinations of bone or ligament injuries that may disrupt the anterior pubic symphysis while the posterior pelvic ring opens like the hinge of a book (thus the term *open-book* pelvis injuries). Such injuries may result in life-threatening intra-pelvic hemorrhage,

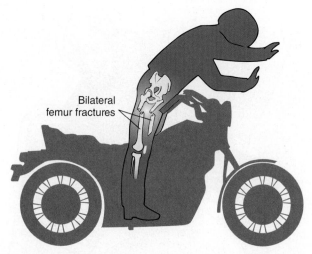

Figure 4-32 The body travels forward and over the motorcycle, and the thighs and femurs impact the handlebars. The rider can also be ejected.
© National Association of Emergency Medical Technicians (NAEMT).

and the immediate application of a pelvic binder of some sort could be a lifesaving measure. This is a great example of the application of kinematic assessment leading to a potentially lifesaving intervention in the field.

Angular Impact

In an angular-impact collision, the motorcycle hits an object at an angle. The motorcycle will then collapse on the rider or cause the rider to be crushed between the motorcycle and the object that was struck. Injuries to the upper or lower extremities can occur, resulting in fractures and extensive soft-tissue injury (**Figure 4-33**). Injuries can also occur to organs of the abdominal cavity as a result of energy exchange.

Ejection Impact

Because of the lack of restraints, the rider is susceptible to ejection. The rider will continue in flight until the head, arms, chest, abdomen, or legs strike another object, such as a motor vehicle, a telephone pole, or the road. Injury will occur at the point of impact and will radiate to the rest of the body as the energy is absorbed.[19]

Injury Prevention

Many motorcycle riders do not use proper protection. Protection for motorcyclists includes boots, leather clothing, and helmets. Of the three, the helmet affords the best protection. It is built similarly to the skull: strong and supportive externally and energy-absorbent internally. The helmet's structure absorbs much of the impact, thereby decreasing injury to the face, skull, and

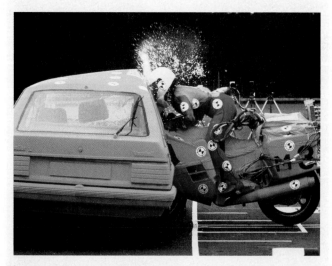

Figure 4-31 The position of a motorcycle rider is above the pivot point of the front wheel as the motorcycle impacts an object head on.
© TRL Ltd./Science Photo Library/Getty Images.

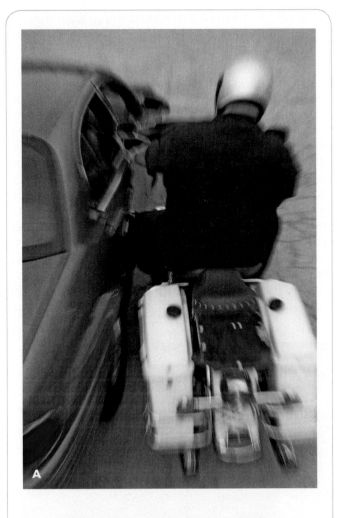

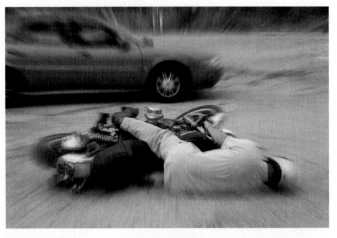

Figure 4-34 To prevent being trapped between two pieces of steel (motorcycle and vehicle), the rider "lays the bike down" to dissipate the injury. This tactic often causes abrasions ("road rash") as the rider's speed is slowed on the asphalt.
© National Association of Emergency Medical Technicians (NAEMT).

brain. The helmet provides only minimal protection for the neck but does not cause neck injuries. Mandatory helmet laws are effective. Most states that have passed mandatory helmet legislation have found an associated reduction in motorcycle incidents.

"Laying the bike down" is a protective maneuver used by riders to separate themselves from the motorcycle in an impending crash (**Figure 4-34**). The rider turns the motorcycle sideways and drags the inside leg on the ground. This action slows the rider more than the motorcycle so that the motorcycle moves out from under the rider. The rider will slide along on the pavement but will not be trapped between the motorcycle and any object it hits. Using this maneuver, riders usually receive abrasions ("road rash") and minor fractures but generally avoid the severe injuries associated with the other types of impacts, unless they directly strike another object (**Figure 4-35**).

Pedestrian Injuries

One common scenario in collisions in which motor vehicles impact pedestrians involves three separate phases, each with its own injury pattern, as follows:

1. The initial impact is to the legs and sometimes the hips (**Figure 4-36A**).
2. The torso rolls onto the hood of the vehicle (and may strike the windshield) (**Figure 4-36B**).
3. The pedestrian then falls off the vehicle and onto the ground, usually headfirst, with possible cervical spine trauma (**Figure 4-36C**).

The injuries produced in pedestrian crashes vary according to the height of the pedestrian and the height

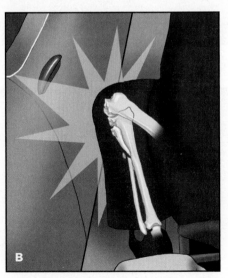

Figure 4-33 A. If the motorcycle does not hit an object head-on, it collapses like a pair of scissors. **B.** This collapse traps the rider's lower extremity between the object that was impacted and the motorcycle.
© National Association of Emergency Medical Technicians (NAEMT).

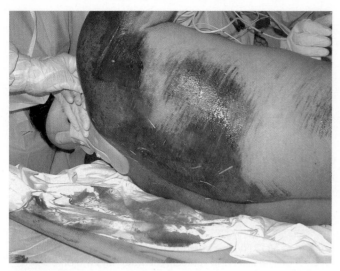

Figure 4-35 Road "burns" (abrasions) after a motorcycle crash without protective clothing.
Courtesy of Dr. Jeffrey Guy.

of the vehicle (**Figure 4-37**). A child and an adult standing in front of a vehicle present different anatomic impact points to the vehicle.

Adults are usually struck first by the vehicle's bumper in the lower legs, fracturing the tibia and fibula. As the pedestrian is impacted by the front of the vehicle's hood, depending on the height of the hood, the abdomen and thorax are struck by the top of the hood and the windshield. This substantial second strike can result in fractures of the upper femur, pelvis, ribs, and spine, producing intra-abdominal or intrathoracic crush and shear. If the victim's head strikes the hood or if the victim continues to move up the hood so that the head strikes the windshield, injury to the face, head, and cervical and thoracic spine can occur. If the vehicle has a large frontal area (such as with trucks and SUVs), the entire pedestrian is hit simultaneously.

The third impact occurs as the victim is thrown off the vehicle and strikes the pavement. The victim can

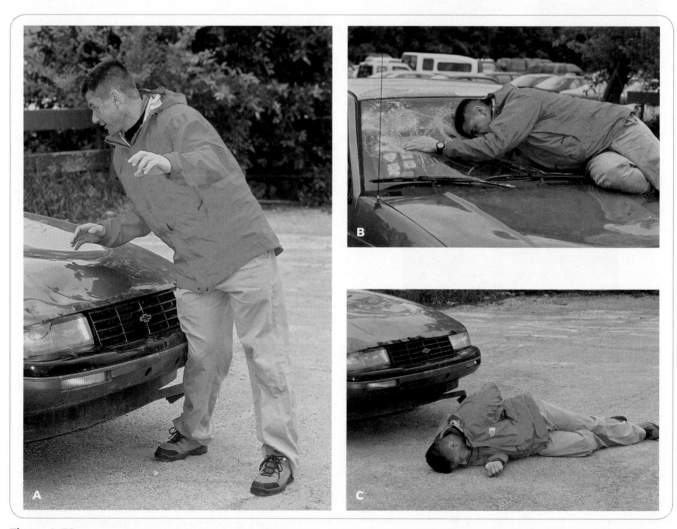

Figure 4-36 Phases of vehicle–pedestrian crashes. **A.** Phase 1: Initial impact is to the legs and sometimes to the hips. **B.** Phase 2: The torso of the pedestrian rolls onto the hood of the vehicle. **C.** Phase 3: The pedestrian falls off the vehicle and hits the ground.
© National Association of Emergency Medical Technicians (NAEMT).

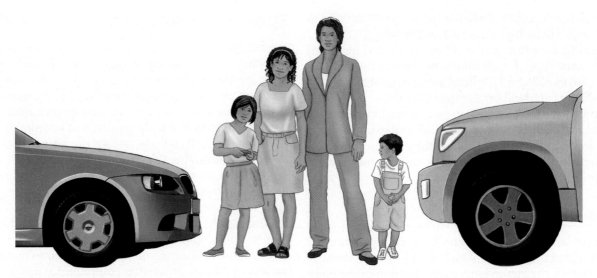

Figure 4-37 The injuries resulting from vehicle–pedestrian crashes vary according to the height of the pedestrian and the height of the vehicle.

© National Association of Emergency Medical Technicians (NAEMT).

receive a significant blow on one side of the body, injuring the hip, shoulder, and head. Head injury often occurs when the pedestrian strikes either the vehicle or the pavement. Similarly, because all three impacts produce sudden, violent movement of the torso, neck, and head, an unstable spine fracture may result. After falling, the victim may be struck by a second vehicle traveling next to or behind the first.

Because they are shorter, children are initially struck higher on the body than adults (**Figure 4-38A**). The first impact generally occurs when the bumper strikes the child's legs (above the knees) or pelvis, damaging the femur or pelvic girdle. The second impact occurs almost instantly afterward as the front of the vehicle's hood continues forward and strikes the child's thorax. Then, the head and face strike the front or top of the vehicle's hood (**Figure 4-38B**). Because of the child's smaller size and weight, the child may not be thrown clear of the vehicle, as usually occurs with an adult. Instead, the child may be dragged by the vehicle while partially under the vehicle's front end. If the child falls to the side, the lower limbs may also be run over by a front wheel (**Figure 4-38C**). If the child falls backward, ending up completely under the vehicle, almost any injury can occur (e.g., being dragged, struck by projections, or run over by a wheel).

If the foot is planted on the ground at the time of impact, the child will receive energy exchange at the upper leg, hip, and abdomen. This will force the hips and abdomen away from the impact. The upper part of the torso will come along later, as will the planted foot. The energy exchange moving the torso but not the feet will fracture the pelvis and shear the femur, producing severe angulation at the point of impact and possible spine injury as well.

To complicate these injuries further, a child will likely turn toward the car out of curiosity, exposing the anterior

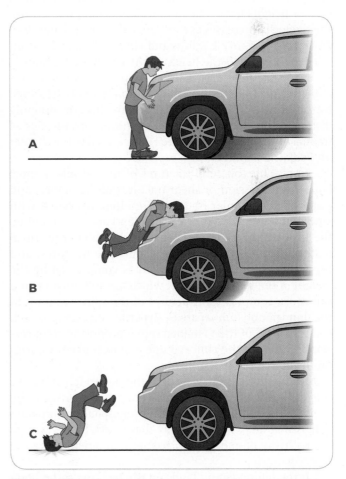

Figure 4-38 A. The initial impact with a child occurs when the vehicle strikes the child's upper leg or pelvis. **B.** The second impact occurs when the child's head and face strike the front or top of the vehicle's hood. **C.** A child may be thrown clear of a vehicle, as shown here, but also may be trapped and dragged by the vehicle.

© National Association of Emergency Medical Technicians (NAEMT).

body and face to injuries, whereas an adult will attempt to escape and will be hit in the back or the side.

As with an adult, any child struck by a vehicle can receive some type of head injury. Because of the sudden, violent forces acting on the head, neck, and torso, cervical spine injuries are high on the suspicion list.

Knowing the specific sequence of multiple impacts in a vehicle–pedestrian collision and understanding the multiple underlying injuries that they can produce are keys to making an initial assessment and determining the appropriate management of a patient.

Falls

Victims of falls can sustain injury from multiple impacts. The estimated height from which the victim fell, the surface on which the victim landed, and the part of the body impacted first are important factors to determine because they indicate the level of energy involved and, thus, the energy exchange that occurred. Victims who fall from greater heights have a higher incidence of injury because their velocity increases as they fall. Falls from greater than 20 feet (ft; [6.1 m]) in adults and 10 ft (3.0 m) in children (two to three times the height of the child) are frequently severe.[20] The type of surface on which the victim lands and its degree of **compressibility** (ability to be deformed by the transfer of energy) also have an effect on stopping distance. Information about the unique the physics of trauma of fall injuries in children is presented in the chapter on Pediatric Trauma.

In real life, bilateral fractures of the calcaneus (heel bone), compression or shear fractures of the ankles, and distal tibial or fibular fractures are often associated with landing on the feet. After the feet land and stop moving, the legs are the next body part to absorb energy. Tibial plateau fractures of the knee, long-bone fractures, and hip fractures can result. The body is compressed by the weight of the head and torso, which are still moving, and can cause compression fractures of the spinal column in the thoracic and lumbar areas. Hyperflexion occurs at each concave bend of the S-shaped spine, producing compression injuries on the concave side and distraction injuries on the convex side.

If a victim falls forward onto the outstretched hands, the result can be fractures of one or both the wrists. If the victim did not land on the feet, the prehospital care provider will assess the part of the body that struck first, evaluate the pathway of energy displacement, and determine the injury pattern.

If the falling victim lands on the head with the body almost inline, as often occurs in shallow-water diving injuries, the entire weight and force of the moving torso, pelvis, and legs compress the head and cervical spine. A fracture of the cervical spine may be a result, as with the up-and-over pathway of the frontal-impact vehicle collision.

Sports Injuries

Severe injury can occur during many sports or recreational activities, such as skiing, diving, baseball, and football. These injuries can be caused by sudden deceleration forces or by excessive compression, twisting, hyperextension, or hyperflexion. In recent years, various sports activities have become available to a wide spectrum of occasional, recreational participants who often lack the necessary training and conditioning or the proper protective equipment. Recreational sports and activities include participants of all ages. Sports such as downhill skiing, waterskiing, bicycling, and skateboarding are all potentially high-velocity activities. Other sports, such as trail biking, all-terrain vehicle riding, and snowmobiling, can produce velocity deceleration, collisions, and impacts similar to motorcycle crashes or MVCs. Protective equipment worn in sports can provide some protection but may have the potential to create injury, such as when a helmeted football player drives his head into another player.

The potential injuries of a victim who is in a high-speed collision and then ejected from a skateboard, snowmobile, or bicycle are similar to those sustained when an occupant is ejected from an automobile at the same speed because the amount of energy is the same. (See the specific mechanisms of MVCs and motorcycle crashes described earlier.)

The potential mechanisms associated with each sport are too numerous to list in detail. However, the general principles are the same as for MVCs. While assessing the mechanism of injury, the prehospital care provider considers the following questions to assist in the identification of injuries:

- What forces acted on the victim and how?
- What are the apparent injuries?
- To what object or part of the body was the energy transmitted?
- What other injuries are likely to have been produced by this energy transfer?
- Was protective gear worn?
- Was there sudden compression, deceleration, or acceleration?
- What injury-producing movements occurred (e.g., hyperflexion, hyperextension, compression, excessive lateral bending)?

When the mechanism of injury involves a high-speed collision between two participants, as in a crash between two skiers, reconstruction of the exact sequence of events from eyewitness accounts is often difficult. In such crashes, the injuries sustained by one skier are often guidelines for examination of the other. In general, knowing which part of one victim struck which part of the other victim, and what injury resulted from the energy transfer, is important. For example, if one victim sustains an impact fracture of the hip, a part of the other skier's body must have been struck with substantial force and, therefore, may have sustained a similar high-impact injury. If the second skier's head struck the first skier's hip, the prehospital care provider will suspect potentially serious head injury and an unstable spinal injury for the second skier.

Broken or damaged equipment is also an important indicator of injury and must be included in the evaluation of the mechanism of injury. A broken sports helmet is evidence of the magnitude of the force involved. Because skis are made of highly durable material, a broken ski indicates that extreme localized force came to bear, even when the mechanism of injury may appear unimpressive. A snowmobile with a severely dented front end indicates the force with which it struck a tree. The presence of a broken stick after an ice hockey skirmish raises the questions of whether it was broken as a result of a fight or whether it broke as a result of normal hockey.

Victims of significant crashes who do not complain of injury must be thoroughly assessed, as severe yet occult injuries may exist. The steps are as follows:

1. Evaluate the patient for life-threatening injury.
2. Evaluate the patient for mechanism of injury. (What happened and exactly how did it happen?)
3. Determine how the forces that produced injury in one victim may have affected any other person.
4. Determine whether any protective gear was worn. (It may have already been removed.)
5. Assess damage to the protective equipment. (What are the implications of this damage relative to the patient's body?)
6. Assess whether the damage was caused by this incident or whether it was preexisting and worsened.
7. Thoroughly assess the patient for possible associated injuries.

High-speed falls, collisions, and falls from heights without serious injury are common in many contact sports. The ability of athletes to experience incredible collisions and falls and sustain only minor injury—largely as a result of impact-absorbing equipment—may be confusing. The potential for injury in sports participants may be overlooked. The principles of the physics of trauma and careful consideration of the exact sequence and mechanism of injury provide insight into sports collisions in which greater forces than usual came to bear. The physics of trauma is an essential tool in identifying possible underlying injuries and determining which patients require further evaluation and treatment at a medical facility.

Regional Effects of Blunt Trauma

The body can be divided into several regions: head, neck, thorax, abdomen, pelvis, and extremities. Each body region is subdivided into (1) the external part of the body, usually composed of skin, bone, soft tissue, vessels, and nerves,

and (2) the internal part of the body, usually vital internal organs. The injuries produced as a result of shear, cavitation, and compression forces are used to provide an overview in each component and region for potential injuries.

Head

The only external indication that compression and shear injuries have occurred to the patient's head may be a soft-tissue injury to the scalp, a contusion of the scalp, or a bull's-eye fracture of the windshield (**Figure 4-39**).

Compression

When the body is traveling forward with the head leading the way, as in a frontal vehicular crash or a headfirst fall, the head is the first structure to receive the impact and the energy exchange. The continued momentum of the torso then compresses the head. The initial energy exchange occurs on the scalp and the skull. The skull can be compressed and fractured, pushing the broken, bony segments of the skull into the brain (**Figure 4-40**).

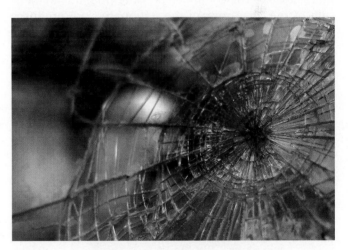

Figure 4-39 A bull's-eye fracture of the windshield is a major indication of skull impact and energy exchange to both the skull and the cervical spine.

© Kristin Smith/Shutterstock.

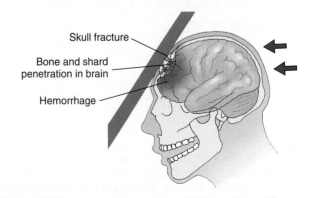

Skull fracture

Bone and shard penetration in brain

Hemorrhage

Figure 4-40 As the skull impacts an object, pieces of bone may be fractured and pushed into the brain.

© National Association of Emergency Medical Technicians (NAEMT).

Shear

After the skull stops its forward motion, the brain continues to move forward, compressing against the intact or fractured skull with resultant concussion, contusions, or lacerations. The brain is soft and compressible; therefore, its length is shortened. The posterior part of the brain can continue forward, pulling away from the skull, which has already stopped moving. As the brain separates from the skull, stretching or breaking (shearing) of brain tissue itself or any blood vessels in the area occurs (**Figure 4-41**). Hemorrhage into the epidural, subdural, or subarachnoid space can result, as well as diffuse axonal injury of the brain. If the brain separates from the spinal cord, it will most likely occur at the brain stem.

Neck

Compression

The dome of the skull is fairly strong and can absorb the impact of a collision; however, the cervical spine is much more flexible. The continued pressure from the momentum of the torso toward the stationary skull produces angulation or compression (**Figure 4-42**). Hyperextension or hyperflexion of the neck may result in fracture or dislocation of one or more vertebrae and injury to the spinal cord. The result can be jumped facets, fractures, spinal cord compression, or soft-tissue (ligament) injuries (**Figure 4-43**). Direct inline compression crushes the bony

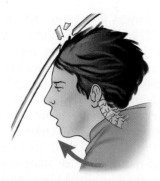

Figure 4-42 The skull frequently stops its forward motion, but the torso does not. The torso continues its forward motion until its energy is absorbed. The weakest point of this forward motion is the cervical spine.

© National Association of Emergency Medical Technicians (NAEMT).

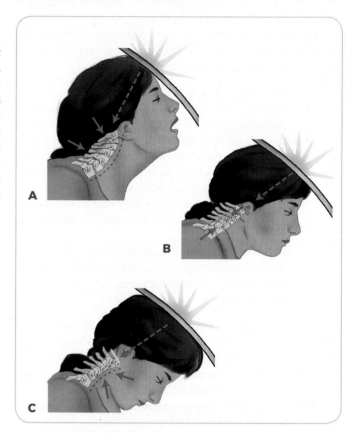

Figure 4-43 The spine can be compressed directly along its own axis or angled in hyperextension or hyperflexion.

© National Association of Emergency Medical Technicians (NAEMT).

vertebral bodies. Both angulation and inline compression can result in an unstable spine.

Shear

The skull's center of gravity is anterior and cephalad to the point at which the skull attaches to the bony spine. Therefore, a lateral impact on the torso when the neck is unrestrained will produce lateral flexion and rotation of the neck (see Figure 4-24). Extreme flexion

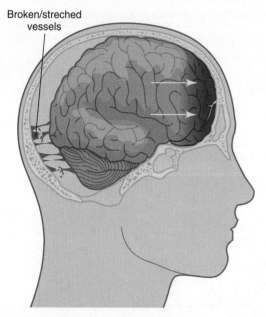

Broken/streched vessels

Figure 4-41 As the skull stops its forward motion, the brain continues to move forward. The part of the brain nearest the impact is compressed, bruised, and perhaps even lacerated. The portion farthest from the impact is separated from the skull, with tearing and lacerations of the vessels involved.

© National Association of Emergency Medical Technicians (NAEMT).

or hyperextension may also cause stretching injuries to the soft tissues of the neck.

Thorax

Compression

If the impact of a collision is centered on the anterior part of the chest, the sternum will receive the initial energy exchange. When the sternum stops moving, the posterior thoracic wall (muscles and thoracic spine) and the organs in the thoracic cavity continue to move forward until the organs strike and are compressed against the sternum.

The continued forward motion of the posterior thorax bends the ribs. If the tensile strength of the ribs is exceeded, fractured ribs and a flail chest can develop (**Figure 4-44**). Flexion injury with resultant compression or burst fracture to the thoracolumbar spine can occur. This injury is similar to what happens when a vehicle stops suddenly against a dirt embankment (see Figure 4-3). The frame of the vehicle bends, which absorbs some of the energy. The rear of the vehicle continues to move forward until the bending of the frame absorbs all the energy. In the same way, the posterior thoracic wall continues to move until the ribs absorb all the energy.

Compression of the chest wall is common with frontal and lateral impacts and produces an interesting phenomenon called the "paper bag effect," which may result in a pneumothorax. A victim instinctively takes a deep breath and holds it just before impact. This closes the glottis, effectively sealing off the lungs. With a significant energy exchange on impact and compression of the chest wall, the lungs may then burst, like a paper bag full of air that is popped (**Figure 4-45**). The lungs can also become compressed and contused, compromising ventilation.

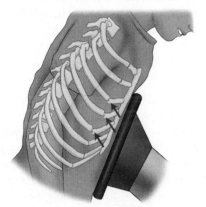
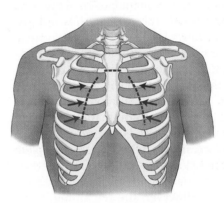

Figure 4-44 Ribs forced into the thoracic cavity by external compression usually fracture in multiple places, sometimes producing the clinical condition known as flail chest.
© National Association of Emergency Medical Technicians (NAEMT).

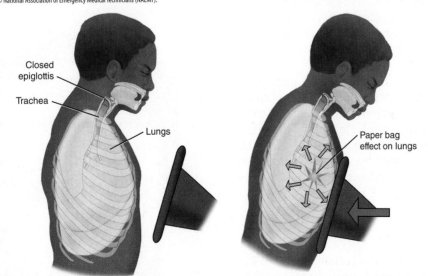

Closed epiglottis

Trachea

Lungs

Paper bag effect on lungs

Figure 4-45 Compression of the lung against a closed glottis, by impact on either the anterior or the lateral chest wall, produces an effect similar to compressing a paper bag when the opening is closed tightly by the hands. The paper bag ruptures, as does the lung.
© National Association of Emergency Medical Technicians (NAEMT).

Compression injuries of the internal structures of the thorax may include cardiac contusion, which occurs as the heart is compressed between the sternum and the spine and can result in significant dysrhythmias. Perhaps a more frequent injury is compression of the lungs leading to pulmonary contusion. Although the clinical consequences may develop over time, the patient may immediately lose the ability to properly ventilate. Pulmonary contusion can have consequences in the field for the prehospital care provider and for the physicians during resuscitation after arrival in the hospital. In situations in which long transport times are required, this condition can play a role en route.

Shear

The heart, ascending aorta, and aortic arch are relatively unrestrained within the thorax. The descending aorta, however, is tightly adherent to the posterior thoracic wall and the vertebral column. The resultant motion of the aorta is similar to holding the flexible tubes of a stethoscope just below where the rigid tubes from the earpiece end and swinging the acoustic head of the stethoscope from side to side. As the skeletal frame stops abruptly in a collision, the heart and the initial segment of the aorta continue their forward motion. The shear forces produced can tear the aorta at the junction of the portion that moves freely with the tightly bound portion (see Figure 4-14).

An aortic tear may result in an immediate, complete transection of the aorta followed by rapid exsanguination. Some aortic tears are partial, where one or more layers of tissue remain intact. However, the remaining layers are under great pressure, and a traumatic aneurysm can develop, similar to a bubble that forms on a weak part of a tire. The aneurysm can eventually rupture within minutes, hours, or days after the original injury. It is important that the prehospital care provider recognize the potential for such injuries and relay this information to the hospital personnel.

Shear injury can occur to the thoracolumbar spine resulting in fractures and fracture-dislocations that can be associated with neurologic compromise and may place the patient at risk for secondary neurologic injury with further motion. Similarly, excess extension anywhere along the thoracolumbar spine can produce unstable fracture or dislocation with potential neurologic injury.

Abdomen

Compression

Internal organs compressed by the vertebral column into the steering wheel or dashboard during a frontal collision may rupture. The effect of this sudden increase in pressure is similar to the effect of placing the internal organ on an anvil and striking it with a hammer. Solid organs frequently injured in this manner include the spleen, liver, and kidneys.

Injury may also result from overpressure within the abdomen. The diaphragm is a ¼-inch-thick (5-mm-thick) muscle located across the top of the abdomen that separates the abdominal cavity from the thoracic cavity. Its contraction causes the pleural cavity to expand for ventilation. The anterior abdominal wall comprises two layers of fascia and one very strong muscle. Laterally, there are three muscle layers with associated fascia, and the lumbar spine and its associated muscles provide strength to the posterior abdominal wall. The diaphragm is the weakest of all the walls and structures surrounding the abdominal cavity. It may be torn or ruptured as the intra-abdominal pressure increases (**Figure 4-46**). This injury has the following four common consequences:

- The "bellows" effect that is usually created by the diaphragm is lost, and ventilation is impaired.
- The abdominal organs can enter the thoracic cavity and reduce the space available for lung expansion.
- The displaced organs can become ischemic from compression of their blood supply.
- If intra-abdominal hemorrhage is present, the blood can also cause a hemothorax.

Another injury caused by increased abdominal pressure is from sudden retrograde blood flow up the aorta and against the aortic valve. This force against the valve can rupture it. This injury is rare but can occur when a collision with the steering wheel or involvement in another type of incident (e.g., ditch or tunnel cave-in) has produced a rapid increase in intra-abdominal pressure. This rapid pressure increase results in a sudden increase of aortic blood pressure. Blood is pushed back (retrograde) against

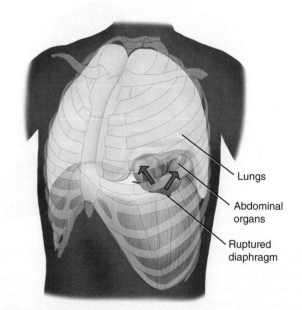

Figure 4-46 With increased pressure inside the abdomen, the diaphragm can rupture.

the aortic valve with enough pressure to cause rupture of the valve cusps.

Shear

Injury to the abdominal organs occurs at their points of attachment to the mesentery. During a collision, the forward motion of the body stops, but the organs continue to move forward, causing tears at the points where the organs attach to the abdominal wall. If the organ is attached by a pedicle (a stalk of tissue), the tear can occur where the pedicle attaches to the organ, where it attaches to the abdominal wall, or anywhere along the length of the pedicle (see Figure 4-13). Organs that can shear in this manner are the kidneys, small intestine, large intestine, and spleen.

Another type of injury that often occurs during deceleration is laceration of the liver caused by its impact with the *ligamentum teres*. The liver is suspended from the diaphragm but is only minimally attached to the posterior abdomen near the lumbar vertebrae. The ligamentum teres attaches to the anterior abdominal wall at the umbilicus and to the left lobe of the liver in the midline of the body. (The liver is not a midline structure; it lies more on the right than on the left.) A down-and-under pathway in a frontal impact or a feet-first fall causes the liver to bring the diaphragm with it as it descends into the ligamentum teres (**Figure 4-47**). The ligamentum teres will fracture or transect the liver, analogous to pushing a cheese-cutting wire into a block of cheese.

Pelvic fractures are the result of damage to the external abdomen and may cause injury to the bladder or lacerations of the blood vessels in the pelvic cavity. Between

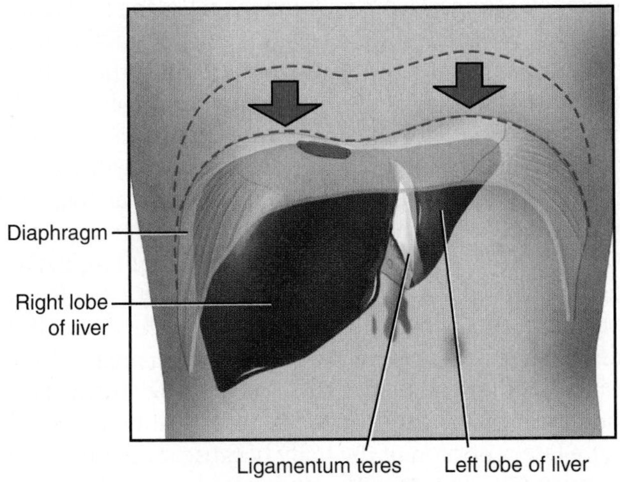

Figure 4-47 The liver is not supported by any fixed structure. Its major support is from the diaphragm, which moves freely. As the body travels in the down-and-under pathway, so does the liver. When the torso stops but the liver does not, the liver continues downward onto the ligamentum teres, tearing the liver. This is much like pushing a cheese-cutting wire into a block of cheese.

© National Association of Emergency Medical Technicians (NAEMT).

4% and 15% of patients with pelvic fractures also have a genitourinary injury.[21]

Pelvic fractures resulting from compression from the side, usually due to a lateral-impact collision, have two components. One is the compression of the proximal femur into the pelvis, which pushes the head of the femur into the acetabulum. This frequently produces fractures that involve the hip joint. Further compression of the femur and/or of the lateral walls of the pelvis produce compression fractures of the pelvic bones or the ring of the pelvis. Because a ring generally cannot be fractured in only one place, usually two fractures to the ring occur, although some of the fractures may involve the acetabulum.

The other type of compression fracture occurs anteriorly when the compression force is directly over the symphysis pubis. This force will either break the symphysis by pushing in on both sides or break one side and push it back toward the sacroiliac joint. This latter mechanism opens the joint, producing the so-called open-book.

Shear fractures usually involve the ilium and the sacral area. This shearing force tears the joint open. Because joints in a ring, such as the pelvis, generally must be fractured in two places, frequently there will be a fracture somewhere else along the pelvic ring.

For more detailed information about pelvic fractures, Andrew Burgess and his coauthors have discussed these mechanisms of injury.[22]

Penetrating Trauma
Physics of Penetrating Trauma

The principles of physics discussed earlier are equally important when dealing with penetrating injuries. Again, the kinetic energy that a striking object transfers to body tissue is represented by the following formula:

$$KE = 1/2 \ (mv^2)$$

Energy can neither be created nor destroyed, but it can be transformed. This principle is important in understanding penetrating trauma. For example, although a lead bullet is in the brass cartridge casing that is filled with explosive powder, the bullet has no force. However, when the primer explodes, the powder burns, producing rapidly expanding gases that are transformed into force. The bullet then moves out of the gun and toward its target.

According to Newton's first law of motion, after this force has acted on the missile, the bullet will remain at that speed and force until it is acted on by an outside force. When the bullet hits something, such as a human body, it strikes the individual tissue cells. The energy (speed and mass) of the bullet's motion is exchanged for the energy that crushes these cells and moves them away (cavitation) from the path of the bullet:

$$Mass \times Acceleration = Force = Mass \times Deceleration$$

Factors That Affect the Size of the Frontal Area

The larger the frontal surface area of the moving missile, the greater the number of particles that will be hit—therefore, the greater the energy exchange that occurs and the larger the cavity that is created. The size of the frontal surface area of a projectile is influenced by three factors: profile, tumble, and fragmentation. Energy exchange or potential energy exchange can be analyzed based on these factors.

Profile

Profile describes an object's initial size and whether that size changes at the time of impact. The profile, or frontal area, of an ice pick is much smaller than that of a baseball bat, which, in turn, is much smaller than that of a truck. A hollow-point bullet flattens and spreads on impact (**Box 4-4**). This change enlarges the frontal area so that it hits more tissue particles and produces greater energy exchange. As a result, a larger cavity forms and more injury occurs.

In general, a bullet should remain aerodynamic as it travels through the air en route to the target. Low resistance while passing through the air (hitting as few air particles as possible) is a good thing. It allows the bullet to maintain most of its speed. To avoid resistance, the frontal area is kept small in a conical shape. A lot of drag (resistance to travel) is a bad thing. A good bullet design would have little drag while passing through the air but much more drag when passing through the body's tissues. If that missile strikes the skin and becomes deformed, covering a larger area and creating much more drag, then a much greater energy exchange will occur. Therefore, the ideal bullet is designed to keep its shape while in the air and deform only on impact.

Tumble

Tumble describes whether the object turns over and over and assumes a different angle inside the body than the angle it assumed as it entered the body, thus creating more drag inside the body than in the air. A wedge-shaped

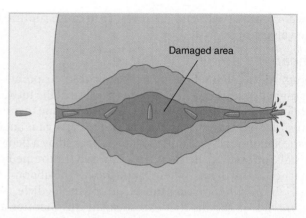

Figure 4-48 The tumble motion of a missile maximizes its damage at 90 degrees.

© National Association of Emergency Medical Technicians (NAEMT).

bullet's center of gravity is located nearer to the base than to the nose of the bullet. When the nose of the bullet strikes something, it slows rapidly. Momentum continues to carry the base of the bullet forward, with the center of gravity seeking to become the leading point of the bullet. A slightly asymmetrical shape causes an end-over-end motion, or tumble. As the bullet tumbles, the normally horizontal sides of the bullet become its leading edges, and strike many more particles than when the bullet was in the air (**Figure 4-48**). More energy exchange is produced, and therefore, greater tissue damage occurs.

Fragmentation

Fragmentation describes whether the object breaks up to produce multiple parts or rubble and, therefore, more drag and more energy exchange. There are two types of fragmentation rounds: (1) fragmentation on leaving the weapon (e.g., shotgun pellets) (**Figure 4-49**) and (2) fragmentation after entering the body. Fragmentation inside the body can be active or passive. Active fragmentation involves a bullet that has an explosive inside it that detonates inside the body. In contrast, bullets with soft noses or vertical cuts in the nose and safety slugs that contain many small fragments to increase body damage by breaking apart on impact are examples of passive fragmentation. The resulting mass of fragments creates a larger frontal area than a single solid bullet, and energy is dispersed rapidly into the tissue. If the missile shatters, it will spread out over a wider area, with two results: (1) more tissue particles will be struck by the larger frontal projection, and (2) the injuries will be distributed over a larger portion of the body because more organs will be struck (**Figure 4-50**). The multiple pieces of shot from a shotgun blast produce similar results. Shotgun wounds are an excellent example of the fragmentation injury pattern.

Damage and Energy Levels

Knowing the energy capacity of a penetrating object helps to predict the damage caused in a penetrating injury. Weapons

---

Box 4-4 Expanding Bullets

A munitions factory in Dum Dum, India, manufactured a bullet that expanded when it hit the skin. Ballistic experts recognized this design as one that would cause more damage than is necessary in war; therefore, these bullets were prohibited in military conflicts. The Petersburg Declaration of 1868 and the Hague Convention of 1899 affirmed this principle, denouncing these "Dum-Dum" projectiles and other expanding missiles, such as silver-tipped bullets, hollow-point bullets, scored-lead cartridges or jackets, and partially jacketed bullets, and outlawing their use in war.

that cause penetrating injuries can be categorized by their energy capacity as low-, medium-, and high-energy weapons.

Low-Energy Weapons

Low-energy weapons include hand-driven weapons such as a knife or an ice pick. These weapons produce damage only with their sharp points or cutting edges. Because these are low-velocity injuries, they are usually associated with less secondary trauma (i.e., less cavitation will occur). Injury in these patients can be predicted by tracing the path of the weapon into the body. If the weapon has been removed, the prehospital care provider should try to identify the type of weapon used, if time permits.

The gender of the attacker is an important factor in determining the trajectory of a knife. Men tend to thrust with the blade on the thumb side of the hand and with an upward or inward motion, whereas women tend to hold the blade on the little finger side and stab downward (**Figure 4-51**).

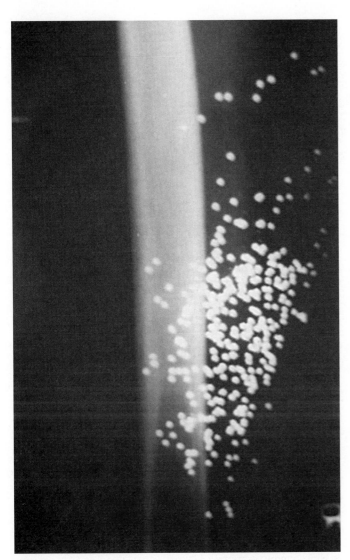

Figure 4-49 Maximum fragmentation damage is caused by a shotgun.

© National Association of Emergency Medical Technicians (NAEMT).

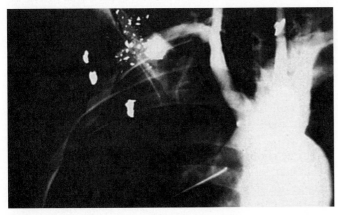

Figure 4-50 When the missile breaks up into smaller particles, this fragmentation increases its frontal area and increases the energy distribution.

Courtesy of Norman McSwain, MD, FACS, NREMT-P.

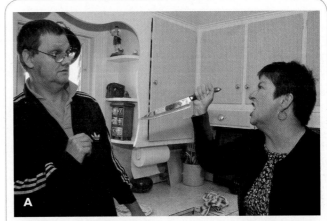

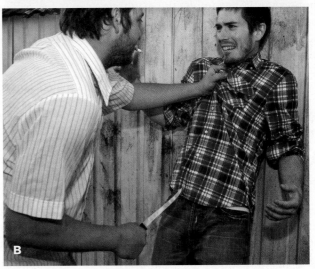

Figure 4-51 The gender of an attacker often determines the trajectory of the wound in stabbing incidents. Male attackers tend to stab upward, whereas female attackers tend to stab downward.

© National Association of Emergency Medical Technicians (NAEMT).

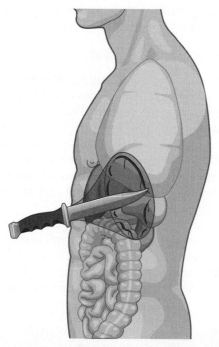

Figure 4-52 Damage produced by a knife depends on the movement of the blade inside the victim.

© National Association of Emergency Medical Technicians (NAEMT).

An attacker may stab a victim and then move the knife around inside the body. A simple-appearing entrance wound may produce a false sense of security. The entrance wound may be small, but the damage inside may be extensive. The potential scope of the movement of the inserted blade is an area of possible damage (**Figure 4-52**).

Evaluation of the patient for associated injury is important. For example, the diaphragm can reach as high as the nipple line on deep expiration. A stab wound to the lower chest can injure intra-abdominal as well as intra-thoracic structures, and a wound of the upper abdomen may involve the lower chest.

Penetrating trauma can result from impaled objects such as fence posts and street signs in vehicle crashes and falls, ski poles in snow sports, and handlebar injuries in bicycling.

Medium-Energy and High-Energy Weapons

Firearms fall into two groups: medium energy and high energy. Medium-energy weapons include handguns and some rifles whose muzzle velocity is 1,000 feet per second (ft/sec) (305 m/sec). The temporary cavity created by this weapon is three to five times the caliber of the bullet. High-energy weapons have muzzle velocity in excess of 2,000 ft/sec (610 m/sec) and significantly greater muzzle energy. They create a temporary cavity that is 25 or more times the caliber of the bullet. As the amount of gunpowder

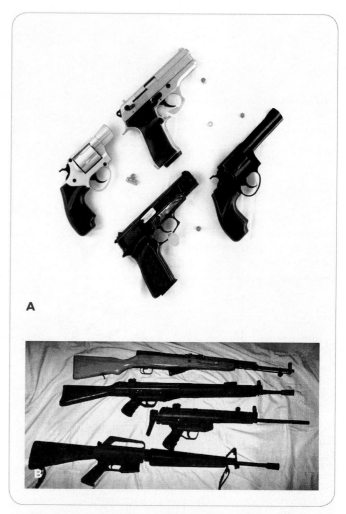

Figure 4-53 A. Medium-energy weapons are usually guns that have short barrels and contain cartridges with less power. **B.** High-energy weapons.

A. © RaidenV/Shutterstock. **B.** Courtesy of Norman Mc Swain, MD, FACS, NREMT-P.

in the cartridge increases and the size of the bullet increases, the speed and mass of the bullet and, therefore, its kinetic energy increase (**Figure 4-53**). The mass of the bullet is an important, but smaller, contributor to the kinetic energy imparted than is the velocity (KE = ½[mv²]).

However, the bullet mass should not be discounted. In the American Civil War, the Kentucky long rifle 0.55-caliber Minie ball had almost the same muzzle energy as the modern M16 rifle. The mass of the missile becomes more important when considering the damage produced by a 12-gauge shotgun at close range or an IED.

In general, medium-energy and high-energy weapons damage not only the tissue directly in the path of the missile but also the tissue involved in the temporary cavity on each side of the missile's path. The variables of missile profile, tumble, and fragmentation influence the rapidity of the energy exchange and, therefore, the extent and direction of the injury. The force of the tissue particles moved out

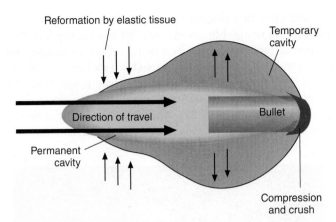

Figure 4-54 A bullet crushes tissues directly in its path. A cavity is created in the wake of the bullet. The crushed part is permanent. The temporary expansion also produces injury.

© National Association of Emergency Medical Technicians (NAEMT).

of the direct path of the missile compresses and stretches the surrounding tissue (**Figure 4-54**).

High-energy weapons discharge high-velocity missiles (**Figure 4-55**). Tissue damage is much more extensive with a high-energy penetrating object than it is from a medium-energy penetrating object. The vacuum created in the cavity created by a high-speed missile can pull clothing, bacteria, and other debris from the surface into the wound.

A consideration in predicting the damage from a gunshot wound is the range or distance from which the gun (either medium or high energy) is fired. Air resistance slows the bullet; therefore, increasing the distance decreases the energy at the time of impact and will result in less injury. Most shootings with handguns are done at close range, so the probability of serious injury is related to both the anatomy involved and the energy of the weapon rather than loss of kinetic energy.

High-Energy Weapons

Cavitation

The unusual injury pattern of an AK-47 is described Fackler and Malinowski. Because of its eccentricity, the bullet tumbles and travels at almost a right angle to the area of entrance. During this tumbling action, the rotation carries it over and over so that there are two or sometimes even three (depending on how long the bullet stays in the body) cavitations.[23] The very high energy exchange produces the cavitation and a significant amount of damage.

The size of the permanent cavity is associated with the elasticity in the tissue struck by the missile. For example, if the same bullet going the same speed penetrates muscle or the liver, the result is very different. Muscle has much more elasticity and will expand and return to a relatively small permanent cavity. The liver, however, has little

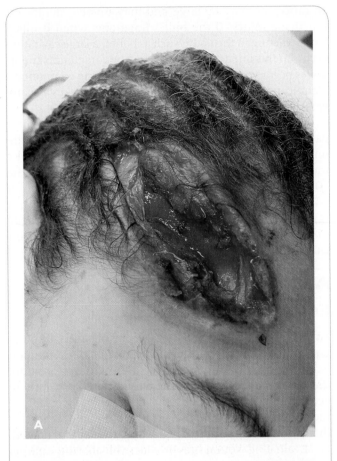

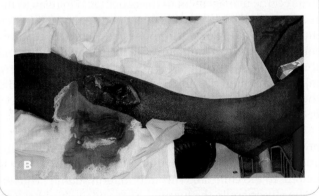

Figure 4-55 A. Graze wound to the scalp created by a projectile from a high-velocity weapon. The skull was not fractured. **B.** High-velocity gunshot wound to the leg demonstrating the large, permanent cavity.

Courtesy of Norman McSwain, MD, FACS, NREMT-P.

elasticity; it develops fracture lines and a much larger permanent cavity than is produced by the same energy exchange in muscle.[24,25]

Fragmentation

The combination of a high-energy weapon with fragmentation can produce significant damage. If the high-energy missile fragments on impact (many do not), the initial entrance site may be large and may involve significant soft-tissue injury. If the bullet fragments when it hits a hard structure in the body (such as bone), a large cavitation occurs at this impact point, and the bony fragments themselves become part of the damage-producing component. Significant destruction to the bone and nearby organs and vessels may result.[23]

Emil Theodor Kocher, a surgeon living in the latter part of the 19th century, was extremely active in the understanding of ballistics and the damage produced by the weapons. He was a strong advocate of not using the "Dum-Dum" bullet.[26] The St. Petersburg Declaration of 1868 outlawed explosive projectiles less than 400 grams (g) in weight. This measure was followed by the Hague Convention of 1899, which outlawed the use of Dum-Dum bullets in war.

Anatomy

Entrance and Exit Wounds

Tissue damage occurs at the site of missile entry into the body, along the path of the penetrating object, and upon exit from the body. Knowledge of the victim's position, the attacker's position, and the weapon used is helpful in determining the path of injury. If the entrance wound and the exit wound can be related, the anatomic structures that would likely be in this pathway can be approximated.

Evaluating wound sites provides valuable information to direct the management of the patient and to relay to the receiving facility. Do two holes in the victim's abdomen indicate that a single missile entered and exited or that two missiles entered and are both still inside the patient? Did the missile cross the midline (usually causing more severe injury) or remain on the same side? In what direction did the missile travel? What internal organs are likely to have been in its path?

Entrance and exit wounds usually, but not always, produce identifiable injury patterns to soft tissue. Evaluation of the apparent trajectory of a penetrating object is helpful to the clinician. This information should be given to the physicians in the hospital. That said, prehospital care providers (and most physicians) do not have the experience or the expertise of a forensic pathologist; therefore, the assessment of which wound is an entrance wound and which is an exit wound is fraught with uncertainty. Such information is solely to assist in patient care to try to gauge the trajectory of the missile and not for legal purposes to determine specifics about the incident. These two issues should not be confused. The prehospital care provider must have as much information as possible to determine the potential injuries sustained by the patient and to best decide how the patient should be managed. The legal issues related to the specifics of entrance and exit wounds are best left to others.

An entrance wound from a gunshot lies against the underlying tissue, but an exit wound has no support. The former is typically a round or oval wound, depending on the entry path, and the latter is usually a **stellate (starburst) wound** (**Figure 4-56**). Because the missile is spinning as it enters the skin, it leaves a small, pink area of abrasion (1 to 2 mm in size) (**Figure 4-57**). Abrasion is not present on the exit side. If the muzzle was placed directly against the skin

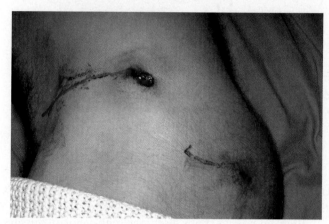

Figure 4-56 An entrance wound is round or oval in shape, and an exit wound is often stellate or linear.
© Mediscan/Alamy Stock Photo.

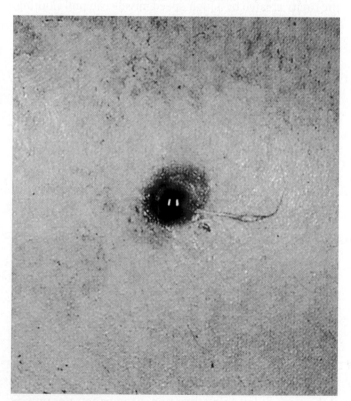

Figure 4-57 The abraded edge indicates that the bullet traveled from top right to bottom left.
Courtesy of Norman McSwain, MD, FACS, NREMT-P.

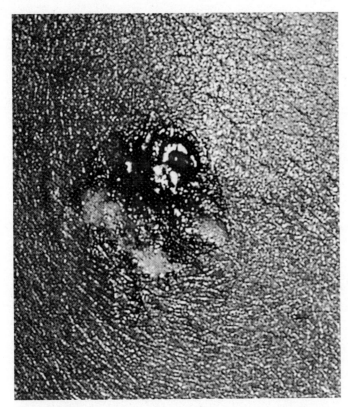

Figure 4-58 Hot gases coming from the end of a muzzle held in proximity to the skin produce partial-thickness and full-thickness burns on the skin.

Courtesy of Norman McSwain, MD, FACS, NREMT-P.

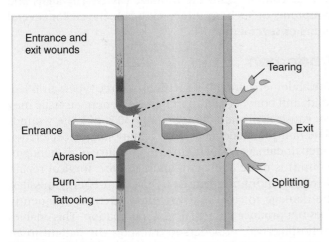

Figure 4-59 Spin and compression of the bullet on entrance produce round or oval holes. On exit, the wound is pressed open.

© National Association of Emergency Medical Technicians (NAEMT).

at the time of discharge, the expanding gases will enter the tissue and produce crepitus on examination (**Figure 4-58**). If the muzzle is within 2 to 3 inches (5 to 7 cm), the hot gases that exit will burn the skin; at 2 to 6 inches (5 to 15 cm) the smoke will adhere to the skin; and inside 10 inches (25 cm) the burning cordite particles will tattoo the skin with small (1- to 2-mm) burned areas (**Figure 4-59**).

Regional Effects of Penetrating Trauma

This section discusses the injuries sustained by various parts of the body during penetrating trauma.

Head

After a missile penetrates the skull, its energy is distributed within a closed space. Particles accelerating away from the missile are forced against the unyielding skull, which cannot expand as can skin, muscle, or even the abdomen. Thus, the brain tissue is compressed against the inside of the skull, producing more injury than would otherwise occur if it could expand freely. It is similar to putting a firecracker in an apple and then placing the apple in a metal can. When the firecracker explodes, the apple will be destroyed against the wall of the can. In the case of a missile penetrating the skull, if the forces are strong enough, the skull may explode from the inside out (**Figure 4-60**).

A bullet may follow the curvature of the interior of the skull if it enters at an angle and has insufficient force to exit the skull. This path can produce significant damage (**Figure 4-61**). Because of this characteristic, small-caliber, medium-velocity weapons, such as the 0.22-caliber or

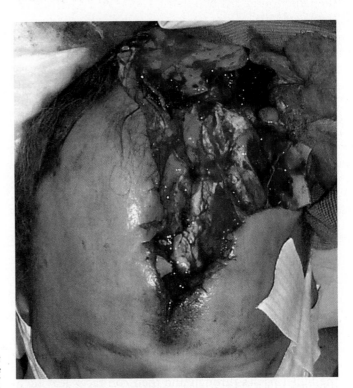

Figure 4-60 After a missile penetrates the skull, its energy is distributed within a closed space. It is like putting a firecracker in a closed container. If the forces are strong enough, the container (the skull) may explode from the inside out.

Courtesy of Norman McSwain, MD, FACS, NREMT-P.

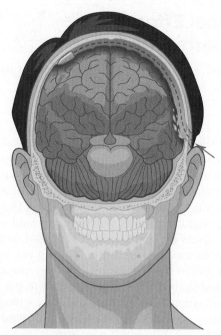

Figure 4-61 The bullet may follow the curvature of the skull.
© National Association of Emergency Medical Technicians (NAEMT).

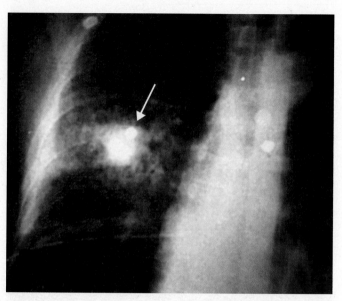

Figure 4-62 Lung damage produced by the cavity at a distance from the point of impact. The arrow shows a bullet fragment.
Courtesy of Norman McSwain, MD, FACS, NREMT-P.

0.25-caliber pistol, have been called the "assassin's weapon." They go in and exchange all of their energy into the brain.

Thorax

Three major groups of structures are inside the thoracic cavity: the pulmonary system, vascular system, and gastrointestinal tract. The bones and muscles of the chest wall and spine make up the outer structure of the thorax. One or more of the anatomic structures of these systems may be injured by a penetrating object.

Pulmonary System

Lung tissue is less dense than blood, solid organs, or bone; therefore, a penetrating object will hit fewer particles, exchange less energy, and do less damage to lung tissue. Damage to the lungs can be clinically significant (**Figure 4-62**), but fewer than 15% of patients will require surgical exploration.[27]

Vascular System

Smaller vessels that are not attached to the chest wall may be pushed aside without significant damage. However, larger vessels, such as the aorta and venae cavae, are less mobile because they are tethered to the spine or the heart. They cannot move aside easily and are more susceptible to damage.

The myocardium (almost totally muscle) stretches as the bullet passes through and then contracts, leaving a smaller defect. The thickness of the muscle may control the bleeding from a low-energy penetration, such as by a knife, or even a small, medium-energy 0.22-caliber bullet. This closure can prevent immediate exsanguination and allow time to transport the victim to an appropriate facility.

Gastrointestinal Tract

The **esophagus**, the part of the gastrointestinal tract that traverses the thoracic cavity, can be penetrated and can leak its contents into the thoracic cavity. The signs and symptoms of such an injury may be delayed for several hours or several days.

Abdomen

The abdomen contains structures of three types: air filled, solid, and bony. Penetration by a low-energy missile may not cause significant damage; only 30% of knife wounds penetrating the abdominal cavity require surgical exploration to repair damage. A medium-energy injury (e.g., handgun wound) is more damaging; most require surgical repair. However, in injuries caused by medium-energy missiles, the damage to solid and vascular structures frequently does not produce immediate exsanguination. This enables prehospital care providers to transport the patient to an appropriate facility in time for effective surgical intervention.

Extremities

Penetrating injuries to the extremities can include damage to bones, muscles, nerves, or vessels. When bones are hit, bony fragments become secondary missiles, lacerating surrounding tissue (**Figure 4-63**). Muscles often expand away from the path of the missile, causing hemorrhage. The missile may penetrate blood vessels, or a near miss may damage the lining of a blood vessel, causing clotting and obstruction of the vessel within minutes or hours.

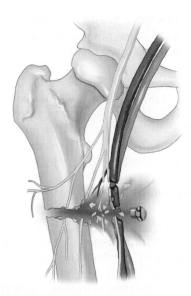

Figure 4-63 Bone fragments become secondary missiles themselves, producing damage by the same mechanism as the original penetrating object.

© National Association of Emergency Medical Technicians (NAEMT).

Shotgun Wounds

Although shotguns are not high-velocity weapons, they are high-energy weapons, and, at close range, they can be more lethal than some of the highest energy rifles. Handguns and rifles predominantly use **rifling** (grooves) on the inside of the barrel to spin a single missile in a flight pattern toward the target. In contrast, most shotguns possess a smooth, cylindrical-tube barrel that directs a load of missiles in the direction of the target. Devices known as **chokes** and **diverters** can be attached to the end of a shotgun barrel to shape and form the column of missiles into specific patterns (e.g., cylindrical or rectangular). Regardless, when a shotgun is fired, a large number of missiles are ejected in a **spread**, or **spray**, pattern. The barrels may be shortened ("sawed off") to prematurely widen the trajectory of the missiles.

Although shotguns may use various types of ammunition, the structure of most shotgun shells is similar. A typical shotgun shell contains gunpowder, wadding, and projectiles. When discharged, all of these components are propelled from the muzzle and can inflict injury on the victim. Certain types of gunpowder can **stipple** ("tattoo") the skin in close-range injuries. Wadding, which is usually lubricated paper, fibers, or plastic used to separate the shot (missiles) from the charge of gunpowder, can provide another source of infection in the wound if not removed. The missiles can vary in size, weight, and composition. A wide variety of missiles are available, from compressed metal powders to *birdshot* (small metal pellets), *buckshot* (larger metal pellets), *slugs* (a single metal missile), and, more recently, plastic and rubber alternatives. The average

shell is loaded with 1 to 1.5 ounces (28 to 43 g) of shot. Fillers that are placed within the shot (polyethylene or polypropylene granules) can become embedded in the superficial layers of the skin.

An average birdshot shell may contain 200 to 2,000 pellets, whereas a buckshot shell may contain 6 to 20 pellets (**Figure 4-64**). It is important to note that as the size of the pellets increases, they approach the wounding

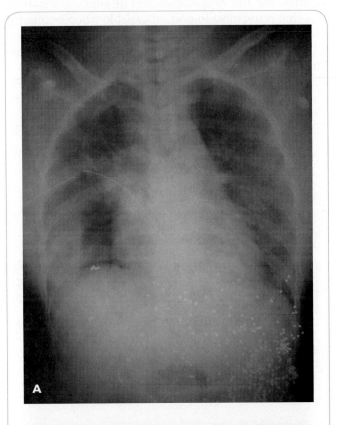

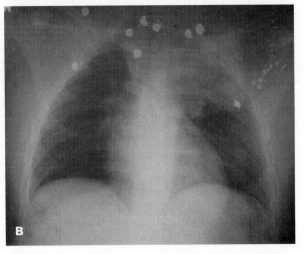

Figure 4-64 **A.** An average birdshot shell may contain 200 to 2,000 pellets. **B.** A buckshot shell may contain 6 to 20 pellets.

Courtesy of Norman McSwain, MD, FACS, NREMT-P.

characteristics of 0.22-caliber missiles in regard to effective range and energy transfer characteristics. Larger or *magnum* shells are also available. These shells may contain more shot and a larger charge of gunpowder or only the larger powder charge to boost the muzzle velocity.

Categories of Shotgun Wounds

The type of ammunition used is important in gauging injuries, but the range (distance) at which the patient was shot is the most important variable when evaluating the shotgun-injury victim (**Figure 4-65**). Shotguns eject a large number of missiles, most of which are spherical. These projectiles are especially susceptible to the effects of air resistance, quickly slowing once they exit the muzzle. The effect of air resistance on the projectiles decreases the effective range of the weapon and changes the basic characteristics of the wounds that it generates. Consequently,

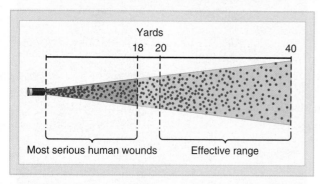

Figure 4-65 The diameter of the spread of a shot column expands as range increases.

Modified from DeMuth WE. The mechanism of gunshot wounds. *J Trauma*. 1971;11:219. Modified from Sherman RT, Parrish RA. Management of shotgun injuries: a review of 152 cases. *J Trauma*. 1978;18:236.

shotgun wounds have been classified into four major categories: contact, close-range, intermediate-range, and long-range wounds (**Figure 4-66**).

Contact Wounds

Contact wounds occur when the muzzle is touching the victim at the time the weapon is discharged. Discharge at this range typically results in circular entrance wounds, which may or may not have soot or an imprint of the muzzle (see Figure 4-58). Searing or burning of the wound edges is common, secondary to the high temperatures and the expansion of hot gases as the missiles exit the muzzle. Some contact wounds may be more stellate in appearance, caused by the superheated gases from the barrel escaping from the tissue. Contact wounds usually result in widespread tissue damage and are associated with high mortality. The length of a standard shotgun barrel makes it difficult to commit suicide with this weapon because it is difficult to reach and pull the trigger. Such attempts usually result in a split face without the shot reaching the brain.

Close-Range Wounds

Close-range wounds (less than 6 ft [1.8 m]), although still typically characterized by circular entrance wounds, will likely have more evidence of soot, gunpowder, or filler stippling around the wound margins than contact wounds. Additionally, abrasions and markings from the impact of the wadding that coincide with the wounds from the missiles may be found. Close-range wounds create significant damage in the patient; missiles fired from this range retain sufficient energy to penetrate deep structures and exhibit a slightly wider spread pattern. This pattern increases the extent of injury as missiles travel through soft tissue.

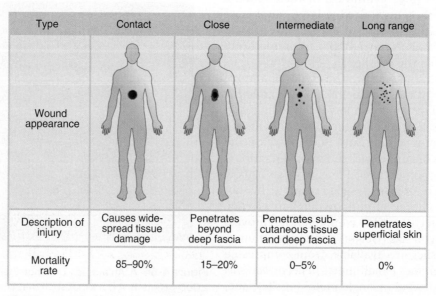

Type	Contact	Close	Intermediate	Long range
Wound appearance				
Description of injury	Causes widespread tissue damage	Penetrates beyond deep fascia	Penetrates subcutaneous tissue and deep fascia	Penetrates superficial skin
Mortality rate	85–90%	15–20%	0–5%	0%

Figure 4-66 Patterns of shotgun injury.

Intermediate-Range Wounds

Intermediate-range wounds are characterized by the appearance of satellite pellet holes emerging from the border around a central entrance wound. This pattern is a result of individual pellets spreading from the main column of shot and generally occurs at a range of 6 to 18 ft (1.8 to 5.5 m). These injuries are a mixture of deep, penetrating wounds and superficial wounds and abrasions. Because of the deep, penetrating components of this injury, however, victims may still have a relatively high mortality rate.

Long-Range Wounds

Long-range wounds are rarely lethal. These wounds are typically characterized by the classic spread of scattered pellet wounds and result from a range of greater than 18 ft (5.5 m). However, even at these slower velocities, the pellets can cause significant damage to certain sensitive tissues (e.g., eyes). In addition, larger buckshot pellets can retain sufficient velocity to inflict damage to deep structures, even at long range. The prehospital care provider needs to consider the cumulative effects of many small missile wounds and their locations, focusing on sensitive tissues. *Adequate exposure* is essential when examining patients involved in trauma, and shotgun injuries are no exception.

Assessment of Shotgun Wounds

These varying characteristics need to be taken into account when evaluating injury patterns in patients with shotgun injuries. For example, a single circular shotgun wound could represent a contact or close-range injury with birdshot or buckshot in which the missiles have retained a tight column or grouping. Conversely, this may represent an intermediate-range to long-range injury with a slug or solitary missile. Only detailed examination of the wound will allow differentiation of these injuries that can involve significant damage to internal structures despite strikingly different missile characteristics.

Contact and close-range wounds to the chest may result in a large, visually impressive wound resulting in an open pneumothorax, and bowel may eviscerate from such wounds to the abdomen. On occasion, a single pellet from an intermediate-range wound may penetrate deep enough to perforate the bowel, leading eventually to peritonitis, or may damage a major artery, resulting in vascular compromise to an extremity or organ. Alternatively, a patient who exhibits multiple small wounds in a spread pattern may have dozens of entrance wounds. However, none of the missiles may have retained enough energy to penetrate through fascia, let alone produce significant damage to internal structures.

Although immediate patient care must always remain the priority, any information (e.g., shell type, suspected range of the patient from the weapon, number of shots fired) that prehospital care providers can gather from the scene and relay to the receiving facility can assist with appropriate diagnostic evaluation and treatment of the shotgun-injured patient. Furthermore, recognition of various wound types can aid providers in maintaining a high index of suspicion for internal injury regardless of the initial impression of the injury.

Blast Injuries

Injury From Explosions

Explosive devices are the most frequently used weapons in combat and by terrorists. Explosive devices cause human injury by multiple mechanisms, some of which are exceedingly complex. The greatest challenges for clinicians at all levels of care in the aftermath of an explosion are the large numbers of casualties and the presence of multiple penetrating injuries (**Figure 4-67**).[28]

Physics of Blast

Explosions are physical, chemical, or nuclear reactions that result in the almost instantaneous release of large amounts of energy in the form of heat and rapidly expanding, highly compressed gas, capable of projecting fragments at extremely high velocities. The energy associated with an explosion can take multiple forms: kinetic and heat energy in the **blast wave**, kinetic energy of fragments formed by the breakup of the weapon casing and surrounding debris, and electromagnetic energy.

Blast waves can travel at greater than 16,400 ft/sec (5,000 m/sec) and are composed of static and dynamic components. The static component (**blast overpressure**) surrounds objects in the flow field of the explosion, loading them on all sides with a discontinuous rise in pressure called the **shock front** or **shock wave**, up to a **peak overpressure value**. Following the shock front, the overpressure drops down to ambient pressure, and then a partial vacuum is often formed as a

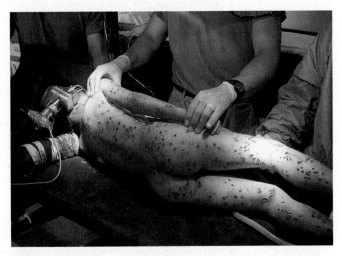

Figure 4-67 Patient with multiple fragment wounds from a bomb blast.

result of air being sucked back (**Figure 4-68**). The dynamic component (**dynamic pressure**) is directional and is experienced as a **blast wind**. The primary significance of the blast wind is that it propels fragments at speeds in excess of several thousand meters per second (faster than standard ballistic weapons such as bullets and shells).[29] Whereas the effective range of both the static and dynamic pressure is measured in tens of feet, the fragments accelerated by the dynamic pressure will quickly outpace the blast wave to become the dominant cause of injury out to ranges of thousands of feet.

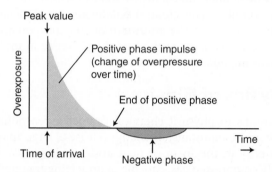

Figure 4-68 Pressure–time history of a blast wave. This graph shows the sudden massive increase in pressure (blast overpressure) following the decrease in pressure and negative pressure phase.

From EXPLOSIVE BLAST 4 T - Federal Emergency Management Agency: www.fema.gov/pdf/plan/prevent/rms/428/fema428_ch4.pdf.

Interaction of Blast Waves With the Body

Blast waves interact with the body and other structures by transmitting energy from the blast wave into the structure. This energy causes the structure to deform in a manner dependent on the strength and the natural period of oscillation of the structure being affected. Changing density interfaces within a structure cause complex re-formations, convergences, and couplings of the transmitted blast waves. Such interactions can be seen particularly in large-density interfaces such as solid tissue to air or liquid (e.g., lung, heart, liver, and bowel).

Explosion-Related Injuries

Injuries from explosions are generally classified as primary, secondary, tertiary, quaternary, and quinary after the injury taxonomy described in Department of Defense Directive 6025.21E24 (**Table 4-1**). Detonation of an explosive device sets off a chain of interactions in the objects and people in its path.[27] If an individual is close enough, the initial blast wave increases pressure in the body, causing stress and shear, particularly in gas-filled organs such as the ears, lungs, and (rarely) bowels. Morbidity and mortality associated with primary blast injury decrease as the distance from the blast location increases and is proportionate to the magnitude of

Table 4-1 Blast Injury Categories		
Category	**Definition**	**Typical Injuries**
Primary	■ Produced by contact of blast shock wave with body ■ Stress and shear waves occur in tissues ■ Waves reinforced/reflected at tissue density interfaces ■ Gas-filled organs (lungs, ears, etc.) at particular risk	■ Tympanic membrane rupture ■ Blast lung ■ Eye injuries ■ Concussion

Secondary	■ Ballistic wounds produced by:
	  · Primary fragments (pieces of exploding weapon)
	  · Secondary fragments (environmental fragments [e.g., glass])
	■ Threat of fragment injury extends farther than that from blast wave
		■ Penetrating injuries
		■ Traumatic amputations
		■ Lacerations

Tertiary	■ Blast wave propels individuals onto surfaces/objects or objects onto individuals, causing whole body translocation ■ Crush injuries caused by structural damage and building collapse	■ Blunt injuries ■ Crush syndrome ■ Compartment syndrome
Quaternary	■ Other explosion-related injuries, illnesses, or diseases	■ Burns ■ Toxic gas and other inhalation injury ■ Injury or infection from environmental contamination
Quinary	■ Injuries resulting from specific additives such as bacteria and radiation ("dirty bombs")	

Data from National Association of Emergency Medical Technicians (NAEMT). *PHTLS: Prehospital Trauma Life Support.* Military 8th ed. Burlington, MA: Jones & Bartlett Learning; 2015.

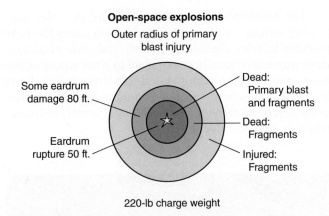

Open-space explosions

Outer radius of primary blast injury

Some eardrum damage 80 ft.

Dead: Primary blast and fragments

Dead: Fragments

Injured: Fragments

Eardrum rupture 50 ft.

220-lb charge weight

Figure 4-69 Morbidity and mortality as a function of distance from open-space detonation of a 220-lb (100-kg) explosive.
© National Association of Emergency Medical Technicians (NAEMT).

the explosive force (**Figure 4-69**). These primary blast injuries are more prevalent when the explosion occurs in an enclosed space because the blast wave bounces off surfaces, thus enhancing the destructive potential of the pressure waves.[30]

Immediate death from pulmonary barotrauma (blast lung) occurs more often in enclosed-space than in open-air bombings.[26-33] Most (95%) blast injuries in Iraq and Afghanistan have resulted from open-space explosions.[34]

The most common form of primary blast injury is tympanic membrane rupture.[35,36] Tympanic membrane rupture, which may occur at pressures as low as 5 pounds per square inch (psi; 35 kilopascals [kPa]),[35-37] is often the only significant overpressure injury experienced. The next major injury occurs at less than 40 psi (276 kPa), a threshold known to be associated with pulmonary injuries, including pneumothorax, air embolism, interstitial and subcutaneous emphysema, and pneumomediastinum.[38] Data from burned soldiers from Operation Iraqi Freedom confirm that tympanic membrane rupture is not predictive of lung injury.

The shock front of the blast wave quickly dissipates and is followed by the blast wind, which propels fragments to create multiple penetrating injuries. Although these injuries are termed *secondary*, they are usually the predominant wounding agent.[38] The blast wind also propels large objects into people or people onto hard surfaces (whole or partial body translocation), creating blunt (tertiary blast) injuries. This category of injury includes crush injuries caused by structural collapse.[38] Heat, flames, gas, and smoke generated during explosions cause quaternary injuries that include burns, inhalation injury, and asphyxiation.[39] Quinary injuries are produced when bacteria, chemicals, or radioactive materials are added to the explosive device and released upon detonation.

Injury From Fragments

Conventional explosive weapons are designed to maximize damage caused by fragments. With initial velocities of many thousands of feet per second, the distance that fragments may be thrown for a 50-lb (23-kg) bomb will be well over 1,000 ft (0.3 km), whereas the lethal radius of the blast

overpressure is approximately 50 ft (15 m). The developers of both military and terrorist weapons, therefore, design weapons to maximize fragmentation injury to significantly increase the damage radius of a free-field explosive.

Few explosive devices cause injury solely by blast overpressure, and serious primary blast injury is relatively rare compared to the predominant numbers of secondary and tertiary injuries. Thus, few patients have injuries dominated by primary blast effects. The entire array of explosion-related injuries is often referred to en masse as "blast injuries," leading to major confusion regarding what constitutes a blast injury. Because energy from the blast wave dissipates rapidly, most explosive devices are constructed to cause damage primarily from fragments. These may be primary fragments generated through the breakup of the casing surrounding the explosive device or secondary fragments created from debris in the surrounding environment. Regardless of whether the fragments are created from shattered munitions casing, flying debris, or embedded objects that terrorists often pack into homemade bombs, they exponentially increase the range and lethality of explosives and are the primary cause of explosion-related injury.

Multi-etiology Injury

In addition to the direct effects of an explosion, prehospital care providers must be mindful of the other causes of injury from attacks with explosions. For instance, an IED that targets a vehicle may result in minimal initial damage to the vehicle occupants. However, the vehicle itself may be displaced vertically or vectored off course resulting in occupant blunt trauma from collision, from flipping upside down as part of the vertical displacement process, or from rollover, for instance, down an embankment or culvert. In these circumstances, occupants sustain injury based on the mechanisms previously described for blunt trauma.

In the military setting, a vehicle's occupants may be afforded some protection from blunt injury by virtue of their body armor. Furthermore, the occupants of a vehicle that is disabled following an IED attack are subject to ambush and may be attacked with gunfire as they exit the vehicle, thus potentially becoming victims of penetrating injury.

Using the Physics of Trauma in Assessment

The assessment of a trauma patient must involve knowledge of the physics of trauma. For example, a driver who hits the steering wheel (blunt trauma) will have a large cavity in the anterior chest at the time of impact; however, the chest rapidly returns to, or near to, its original shape as the driver rebounds from the steering wheel. If two prehospital care providers examine the patient separately—one who understands the physics of trauma and another who does not—the one without knowledge of the physics of trauma will be concerned only with the bruise visible on the patient's chest. The provider who understands the physics of trauma will recognize that a large cavity was present at the time of impact, that the ribs had to bend in for the cavity to form, and that the heart, lungs, and great vessels were compressed by the formation of the cavity. Therefore, the knowledgeable provider will suspect injury to the heart, lungs, great vessels, and chest wall. The other provider will not be aware of these possibilities.

The knowledgeable prehospital care provider, suspecting serious intrathoracic injuries, will assess for these potential injuries, manage the patient, and initiate transport more aggressively, rather than react to what would otherwise appear to be a minor closed soft-tissue injury. Early identification, adequate understanding, and appropriate treatment of underlying injury will significantly influence whether a patient lives or dies.

SUMMARY

- Integrating the principles of the physics of trauma into the assessment of the trauma patient is key to discovering the potential for severe or life-threatening injuries.
- Up to 95% of injuries can be anticipated by understanding the energy exchange that occurs with the human body at the time of a collision. Knowledge of the physics of trauma allows for injuries that are not immediately apparent to be identified and treated appropriately. Left unsuspected, undetected, and therefore untreated, these injuries contribute significantly to morbidity and mortality resulting from trauma.
- Energy can be neither created nor destroyed, only changed in form. The kinetic energy of an object, expressed as a function of both velocity (speed) and mass (weight), is transferred to another object on contact.
- Damage to the object or body tissue impacted is not only a function of the amount of kinetic energy applied to it but also a function of the tissue's ability to tolerate the forces applied to it.

Blunt Trauma

- The direction of the impact determines the pattern of and potential for injury: frontal, lateral, rear, rotational, rollover, or angular.
- Ejection from a car reduces the protection on impact afforded by the vehicle.
- Energy-absorbing protective devices are important. These devices include seat belts, air bags, drop-down engines, and energy-absorbing auto parts, such as bumpers, collapsible steering wheels, dashboards, and helmets. The damage to the vehicles and the direction of the impact will indicate which occupants are most likely to have been more severely injured.
- Pedestrian injuries vary according to the height of the victim and which part of the patient had direct contact with the vehicle.

Falls

- The distance traveled before impact affects the severity of the injury sustained.
- The energy-absorbing capability of the surface at the end of the fall (e.g., concrete versus soft snow) affects the severity of the injury.
- The victim body parts that hit the surface and progression of the energy exchange through the victim's body are important.

Penetrating Trauma

- The energy varies depending on the primary injuring agent:
  - Low energy—hand-driven cutting devices
  - Medium energy—most handguns
  - High energy—high-powered rifles, assault weapons, etc.
- The distance of the victim to the perpetrator and the objects that the bullet might have struck affect the amount of energy at the time of impact with the body and, therefore, the available energy to be dissipated into the patient to produce damage to the body parts.
- Organs in proximity to the pathway of the penetrating object determine the potential life-threatening conditions.
- The pathway of the penetrating trauma is determined by the wound of entrance and the wound of exit.

Blasts

- There are five types of injuries in a blast:
  - Primary—blast shock wave
  - Secondary—projectiles (the most common source of injury from blasts)
  - Tertiary—propulsion of the body into another object
  - Quaternary—heat and flames
  - Quinary—radiation, chemicals, bacteria

SCENARIO RECAP

Before first light on a cold winter morning, you and your partner are dispatched to a single-vehicle crash. On arrival, you find a single vehicle that has crashed into a tree on a rural road. The front end of the vehicle appears to have impacted the tree, and the car has spun around the tree and backed into a drainage ditch on the side of the road. The driver appears to be the only occupant. The air bag has deployed and the driver is moaning, still restrained by his seat belt. You note damage to the front end of the car where it impacted the tree as well as rear-end damage from spinning around and going into the ditch backward.

- What is the potential for injury for this patient based on the physics of trauma of this event?
- How would you describe the patient's condition based on the physics of trauma?
- What injuries do you expect to find?

SCENARIO SOLUTION

As you approach the patient, your understanding of the physics of trauma of this event leads you to be concerned about the potential for head, neck, chest, and abdominal injuries. The patient is responsive, but his speech is slurred and he smells of alcohol. While providing manual immobilization of his head and neck, you note a small laceration on the bridge of his nose as you continue to assess him for injury. He admits that he has been drinking and is unsure of the time of day or where he was going.

Releasing the seat belt and shoulder harness, you note tenderness and an abrasion over his left clavicle. He also complains of some tenderness of his face, neck, anterior chest, and mid-abdomen. Due to his admitted alcohol use, slurred speech, and confusion, you cannot rule out more serious injuries, so you provide spinal immobilization as you remove him from the vehicle.

Continuing your exam en route to the trauma center, you note that the patient has significant tenderness to both lower abdominal quadrants, and you are concerned that there may be hollow organ injury.

References

1. U.S. Department of Transportation, National Highway Traffic Safety Administration. 2015 motor vehicle crashes overview. https://crashstats.nhtsa.dot.gov/Api/Public/ViewPublication/812318. Published August 2016. Accessed September 27, 2017.
2. World Health Organization. *Global Status Report on Road Safety: Time for Action*. http://whqlibdoc.who.int/publications/2009/9789241563840_eng.pdf. Published 2015. Accessed May 6, 2017.
3. Centers for Disease Control and Prevention/National Center for Health Statistics. All injuries. https://www.cdc.gov/nchs/fastats/injury.htm. Updated May 3, 2017. Accessed September 27, 2017.
4. Hunt JP, Marr AB, Stuke LE. Kinematics. In: Mattox KL, Moore EE, Feliciano DV, eds. *Trauma*. 7th ed. New York, NY: McGraw-Hill; 2013.
5. Hollerman JJ, Fackler ML, Coldwell DM, et al. Gunshot wounds: 1. Bullets, ballistics, and mechanisms of injury. *Am J Roentgenol*. 1990;155(4):685-690.
6. Centers for Disease Control and Prevention. Leading causes of death. https://www.cdc.gov/injury/wisqars/index.html. Updated April 20, 2017. Accessed May 30, 2017.
7. Boyce RH, Singh K, Obremskey WT. Acute management of traumatic knee dislocations for the generalist. *J Am Acad Orthop Surg*. 2015 Dec;23(12):761-768.
8. Hernandez IA, Fyfe KR, Heo G, et al. Kinematics of head movement in simulated low velocity rear-end impacts. *Clin Biomech*. 2005;20(10):1011-1018.
9. Kumaresan S, Sances A, Carlin F, et al. Biomechanics of side-impact injuries: evaluation of seat belt restraint system, occupant kinematics, and injury potential. *Conf Proc IEEE Eng Med Biol Soc*. 2006;1:87-90.
10. Siegel JH, Yang KH, Smith JA, et al. Computer simulation and validation of the Archimedes lever hypothesis as a mechanism for aortic isthmus disruption in a case of lateral impact motor vehicle crash: a Crash Injury Research Engineering Network (CIREN) study. *J Trauma*. 2006;60(5):1072-1082.
11. Horton TG, Cohn SM, Heid MP, et al. Identification of trauma patients at risk of thoracic aortic tear by mechanism of injury. *J Trauma*. 2000;48(6):1008-1013; discussion 1013-1014.
12. National Highway Traffic Safety Administration, National Center for Statistics and Analysis. Traffic safety facts: 2008 data. https://crashstats.nhtsa.dot.gov/Api/Public/ViewPublication/811162. Accessed September 28, 2017.

13. U.S. Department of Transportation, National Highway Traffic Safety Administration. Seat belt use in 2016. *Traffic Safety Facts*. https://crashstats.nhtsa.dot.gov/Api/Public/ViewPublication/812351. Published November 2016. Accessed May 30, 2017.

14. U.S. Department of Transportation, National Highway Traffic Safety Administration. 2011 motor vehicle crashes: overview. http://www-nrd.nhtsa.dot.gov/Pubs/811701.pdf. Published December 2012. Accessed September 29, 2017.

15. Centers for Disease Control and Prevention. Adult seat belt use in the U.S. *Vital Signs*. http://www.cdc.gov/VitalSigns/SeatBelt Use/. Updated January 4, 2011. Accessed September 29, 2017.

16. U.S. Department of Transportation, National Highway Traffic Safety Administration. Lives saved in 2008 by restraint use and minimum drinking age laws. *Traffic Safety Facts*. https://crashstats.nhtsa.dot.gov/Api/Public/ViewPublication/811153. Published May 2010. Accessed September 29, 2017.

17. U.S. Department of Transportation, National Highway Traffic Safety Administration. Seat belt use in 2008: use rates in the states and territories. *Traffic Safety Facts*. https://crashstats.nhtsa.dot.gov/Api/Public/ViewPublication/811106. Published April 2009. Accessed September 29, 2017.

18. Greenwell NK. *Results of the national child restraint use special study* (Report No. DOT HS 812 142). Washington, DC: National Highway Traffic Safety Administration; May 2015.

19. Rogers CD, Pagliarello G, McLellan BA, et al. Mechanism of injury influences the pattern of injuries sustained by patients involved in vehicular trauma. *Can J Surg*. 1991;34(3):283-286.

20. Centers for Disease Control and Prevention. Guidelines for field triage of injured patients: recommendations of the National Expert Panel on Field Triage. *MMWR*. 2012;61:1-20.

21. Pedersen A, Stinner DJ, McLaughlin HC, Bailey JR, Walter JR, Hsu JR. Characteristics of genitourinary injuries associated with pelvic fractures during Operation Iraqi Freedom and Operation Enduring Freedom. AMSUS website. http://militarymedicine.amsus.org/doi/full/10.7205/MILMED-D-14-00410. Published March 2015. Accessed September 28, 2017.

22. Burgess AR, Eastridge BJ, Young JW, et al. Pelvic ring disruptions: effective classification system and treatment protocols. *J Trauma*. 1990;30(7):848-856.

23. Fackler ML, Malinowski JA. Internal deformation of the AK-74: a possible cause for its erratic path in tissue. *J Trauma*. 1998;28(suppl 1):S72-S75.

24. Fackler ML, Surinchak JS, Malinowski JA, et al. Wounding potential of the Russian AK-74 assault rifle. *J Trauma*. 1984;24(3):263-266.

25. Fackler ML, Surinchak JS, Malinowski JA, et al. Bullet fragmentation: a major cause of tissue disruption. *J Trauma*. 1984;24(1):35-39.

26. Fackler ML, Dougherty PJ. Theodor Kocher and the Scientific Foundation of Wound Ballistics. *Surg Gynecol Obstet*. 1991;172(2):153-160.

27. American College of Surgeons (ACS) Committee on Trauma. *Advanced Trauma Life Support Course*. Chicago, IL: ACS; 2002.

28. Wade CE, Ritenour AE, Eastridge BJ, et al. Explosion injuries treated at combat support hospitals in the Global War on Terrorism. In: Elsayed N, Atkins J, eds. *Explosion and Blast-Related Injuries*. Burlington, MA: Elsevier; 2008.

29. Department of Defense. Directive Number 6025:21E: Medical Research for Prevention, Mitigation, and Treatment of Blast Injuries. http://www.dtic.mil/whs/directives/corres/pdf/602521p.pdf. Published July 5, 2006. Accessed October 18, 2013.

30. Leibovici D, Gofrit ON, Stein M, et al. Blast injuries: bus versus open-air bombings—a comparative study of injuries in survivors of open-air versus confined-space explosions. *J Trauma*. 1996;41:1030-1035.

31. Gutierrez de Ceballos JP, Turégano-Fuentes F, Perez-Diaz D, et al. The terrorist bomb explosions in Madrid, Spain—an analysis of the logistics, injuries sustained, and clinical management of casualties treated at the closest hospital. *Crit Care Med*. 2005;9:104-111.

32. Gutierrez de Ceballos JP, Turégano Fuentes F, Perez Diaz D, et al. Casualties treated at the closest hospital in the Madrid, March 11, terrorist bombings. *Crit Care Med*. 2005;33(suppl 1):S107-S112.

33. Avidan V, Hersch M, Armon Y, et al. Blast lung injury: clinical manifestations, treatment, and outcome. *Am J Surg*. 2005;190:927-931.

34. Ritenour AE, Blackbourne LH, Kelly JF, et al. Incidence of primary blast injury in U.S. military overseas contingency operations: a retrospective study. *Ann Surg*. 2010;251(6):1140-1144.

35. Ritenour AE, Wickley A, Ritenour JS, et al. Tympanic membrane perforation and hearing loss from blast overpressure in Operation Enduring Freedom and Operation Iraqi Freedom wounded. *J Trauma*. 2008;64:S174-S178.

36. Zalewski T. Experimentelle Untersuchungen uber die Resistenzfahigkeit des Trommelfells. *Z Ohrenheilkd*. 1906;52:109.

37. Helling ER. Otologic blast injuries due to the Kenya embassy bombing. *Mil Med*. 2004;169:872-876.

38. Nixon RG, Stewart C. When things go boom: blast injuries. *Fire Engineering*. May 1, 2004.

39. National Association of Emergency Medical Technicians. Injuries from explosives. In: Butler FK, Callaway DW, Champion H, et al., eds. *PHTLS: Prehospital Trauma Life Support*. Military 7th ed. St. Louis, MO: Mosby JEMS Elsevier; 2011.

Suggested Reading

Alderman B, Anderson A. Possible effect of air bag inflation on a standing child. In: *Proceedings of 18th American Association of Automotive Medicine*. Barrington, IL: American Association of Automotive Medicine; 1974.

American College of Surgeons (ACS) Committee on Trauma. *Advanced Trauma Life Support Course*. Chicago, IL: ACS; 2018.

Anderson PA, Henley MB, Rivara P, et al. Flexion distraction and chance injuries to the thoracolumbar spine. *J Orthop Trauma*. 1991;5(2):153.

Anderson PA, Rivara FP, Maier RV, et al. The epidemiology of seatbelt-associated injuries. *J Trauma*. 1991;31(1):60.

Bartlett CS. Gunshot wound ballistics. *Clin Orthop*. 2003;408:28.

DePalma RG, Burris DG, Champion HR, et al. Current concepts: blast injuries. *N Engl J Med*. 2005;352:1335.

Di Maio VJM. *Gunshot Wounds: Practical Aspects of Firearms, Ballistics and Forensic Techniques*. Boca Raton, FL: CRC Press; 1999.

Garrett JW, Braunstein PW. The seat belt syndrome. *J Trauma*. 1962;2:220.

Huelke DF, Mackay GM, Morris A. Vertebral column injuries and lap-shoulder belts. *J Trauma*. 1995;38:547.

Huelke DF, Moore JL, Ostrom M. Air bag injuries and occupant protection. *J Trauma*. 1992;33(6):894.

Hunt JP, Marr AB, Stuke LE. Kinematics. In: Mattox KL, Moore EE, Feliciano DV, eds. *Trauma*. 7th ed. New York, NY: McGraw-Hill; 2013.

Joksch H, Massie D, Pichler R. *Vehicle Aggressivity: Fleet Characterization Using Traffic Collision Data*. Washington, DC: Department of Transportation; 1998.

McSwain NE Jr, Brent CR. Trauma rounds: lipstick sign. *Emerg Med*. 1998;21:46.

McSwain NE Jr, Paturas JL. *The Basic EMT: Comprehensive Prehospital Patient Care*. 2nd ed. St. Louis, MO: Mosby; 2001.

Ordog GJ, Wasserberger JN, Balasubramaniam S. Shotgun wound ballistics. *J Trauma*. 1922;28:624.

Oreskovich MR, Howard JD, Compass MK, et al. Geriatric trauma: injury patterns and outcome. *J Trauma*. 1984;24:565.

Rutledge R, Thomason M, Oller D, et al. The spectrum of abdominal injuries associated with the use of seat belts. *J Trauma*. 1991;31(6):820.

States JD, Annechiarico RP, Good RG, et al. A time comparison study of the New York State Safety Belt Use Law utilizing hospital admission and police accident report information. *Accid Anal Prev*. 1990;22(6):509.

Swierzewski MJ, Feliciano DV, Lillis RP, et al. Deaths from motor vehicle crashes: patterns of injury in restrained and unrestrained victims. *J Trauma*. 1994;37(3):404.

Sykes LN, Champion HR, Fouty WJ. Dum-dums, hollowpoints, and devastators: techniques designed to increase wounding potential of bullets. *J Trauma*. 1988;28:618.

CHAPTER 5

Scene Management

Lead Editors:
Blaine Enderson, MD, MBA, FACS, FCCM
Catherine L. McKnight, MD

CHAPTER OBJECTIVES

At the completion of this chapter, you will be able to do the following:

- Identify potential threats to the safety of the patient, bystanders, and emergency personnel that are common to all emergency scenes.
- Discuss potential threats that are unique to a given scenario.
- Integrate analysis of scene safety, scene situation, and the physics of trauma into assessment of the trauma patient to make patient care decisions.

- Describe appropriate steps that need to be taken to mitigate potential threats to safety.
- Given a mass-casualty incident (MCI) scenario (hazardous materials incident, weapons of mass destruction), discuss the use of a triage system in managing the scene, and make triage decisions based on assessment findings.

SCENARIO

You are dispatched to the scene of a domestic altercation. It is 0245 hours on a hot summer night. As you arrive on the scene of a single-family dwelling, you can hear a man and woman arguing loudly and the sounds of children crying in the background. Police have been dispatched to this call but have not yet arrived to the location.

- What are your concerns about the scene?
- What considerations are important before you contact the patient?

INTRODUCTION

There are a number of concerns that the prehospital care provider must consider when responding to a call and arriving at a scene:

1. The potential hazards associated with the call should be considered when receiving the assignment. Preliminary assessment of scene safety is initiated while en route based on information from the dispatcher. This assessment takes into consideration the need for other public safety emergency responders, such as police and fire fighters.

2. The first priority for everyone arriving at a trauma incident is overall assessment of the scene. This assessment involves (1) establishing that the scene is safe enough for emergency medical services (EMS) to enter, (2) ensuring provider and patient safety, and (3) determining alterations in patient care based on the current conditions. Any issues identified in this evaluation must be addressed before beginning the assessment of individual patients. In some situations, such as combat or hazardous materials exposures, this evaluation process becomes even more critical and can alter the methods of providing patient care.

   Scene assessment is not a one-time event. Continuous attention must be paid to what is going on around the emergency responders. A scene initially deemed safe for entry can change rapidly, and all emergency responders must be prepared to take appropriate steps to ensure their continued safety, should the conditions change.

3. After performing the scene assessment, the next priority is evaluating individual patients. (See the Patient Assessment and Management chapter.) The overall scene assessment will indicate whether the incident involves a single patient or multiple patients. If the scene involves more than one patient, the situation is classified as either a multiple-patient incident or a mass-casualty incident (MCI). MCIs are discussed further in the Disaster Management chapter. In an MCI, the number of patients exceeds available resources and the priority shifts from focusing all resources on the most injured patient to saving the maximum number of patients. An initial abbreviated form of triage (discussed in the final section of this chapter) identifies the patients to be treated first when there are multiple victims. The prioritization of patient management is (a) conditions that may result in the loss of life, (b) conditions that may result in the loss of limb, and (c) all other conditions that do not threaten life or limb.

Scene Assessment

Scene and patient assessment begins when dispatch either gathers and processes information by questioning the caller or records information provided by other public safety units already on the scene. Dispatch then relays the initial information about the incident and the patient to the responding EMS unit.

While traveling to the scene, taking the time to prepare and practicing good communication skills may be the difference between a well-managed scene and a chaotic scene. Good observation, perception, and communication skills are the best tools.

The on-scene information-gathering process for the prehospital care provider begins immediately upon arrival at the incident. Before making contact with the patient, the provider should evaluate the scene by:

1. Obtaining a general impression of the situation for scene safety
2. Looking at the cause and results of the incident
3. Observing family members and bystanders

The scene's appearance creates an impression that influences the entire assessment. A wealth of information is gathered by simply looking, listening, and cataloguing as much information as possible, including the mechanisms of injury, the present situation, and the overall degree of safety.

Just as the patient's condition can improve or deteriorate, so can the condition of the scene. Evaluating the scene initially and then failing to reassess how the scene may change can result in serious consequences to the prehospital care providers and the patient.

Scene assessment includes the following two major components: safety and situation.

Safety

The primary consideration when approaching any scene is the safety of *all* emergency responders. Rescue efforts should not be attempted by those without training. When EMS personnel become victims, they can no longer assist other injured people, and they add to the number of patients. Patient care may need to wait until the scene is safe enough that EMS can enter without undue risk. Safety concerns vary from commonplace events, such as exposure to body fluids, to rare events, such as exposure to chemical weapons used in warfare. Clues to potential risks and hazards on scene include not only the obvious, such as the sound of gunshots or the presence of blood and other body fluids, but also more subtle findings, such as odors or smoke.

Scene safety involves both emergency responder safety and patient safety. In general, patients in a hazardous situation should be moved to a safe area before assessment and treatment begin. Conditions that pose a threat to patient or emergency responder safety include fire, downed electrical lines, explosives, hazardous materials (including body fluids, traffic, floodwater, and weapons), and environmental conditions. Also, an assailant may still be on the scene and may intervene to harm the patient, emergency responders, or bystanders. However, it has been recognized that in situations involving an active shooter, having EMS work in a coordinated fashion with law enforcement to enter a scene as soon as possible improves patient survival.

Situation

Assessment of the situation follows the safety assessment. The situational survey includes both issues that may affect how the prehospital care provider manages the patient as well as incident-specific concerns related to the patient directly. Questions that providers should consider when assessing the issues posed by a given situation include the following:

- What really happened at the scene? What were the circumstances that led to the injury? Was it intentional or unintentional?
- Why was help summoned, and who summoned it?
- What was the mechanism of injury? (See The Physics of Trauma chapter.) The majority of patient injuries can be predicted based on evaluating and understanding the physics of trauma involved in the incident.
- How many people are involved, and what are their ages?
- Are additional EMS units needed for scene management, patient treatment, or transport?
- Are any other personnel or resources needed (e.g., law enforcement, fire department, power company)?
- Is special extrication or rescue equipment needed?
- Is helicopter transport necessary?
- Is a physician needed to assist with triage or on-scene medical care issues?
- Could a medical problem be the instigating factor that led to the trauma (e.g., a vehicle collision that resulted from the driver's heart attack or stroke)?

Issues related to safety and situation have significant overlap; many safety topics are also specific to certain situations, and certain situations pose serious safety hazards. These issues are discussed in further detail in the following sections.

Safety Issues

Traffic Safety

The majority of EMS personnel who are killed or injured each year were involved in motor vehicle–related incidents (**Figure 5-1**).[1] Although most of these fatalities and injuries are related to direct ambulance collisions during the response phase, a subset occurs while working on the

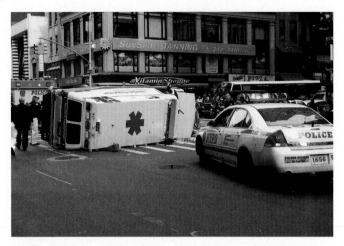

Figure 5-1 The majority of EMS personnel who are killed or injured each year were involved in motor vehicle–related incidents.
© Robert Brenner/PhotoEdit.

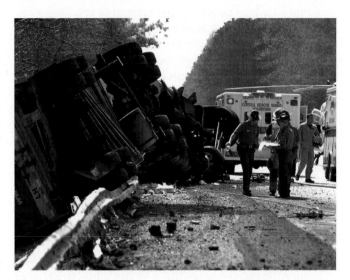

Figure 5-2 A significant number of prehospital care providers who are injured or killed were working at the scene of an MVC.
© Jeff Thrower/Shutterstock.

scene of a motor vehicle crash (MVC). Many factors can result in prehospital care providers being injured or killed on the scene of an MVC (**Figure 5-2**). Some factors, such as weather conditions or road design, cannot be changed; however, the provider can be aware that these conditions exist and act appropriately to mitigate the dangers present at these situations.

Weather/Light Conditions

Many prehospital care responses to MVCs take place in adverse weather conditions and at night. Prehospital care providers may need to deal with ice and snow during the winter months. Other weather conditions that may pose risks include fog, rainstorms, or sandstorms in which oncoming traffic may not see or be able to stop in time to avoid emergency vehicles or EMS personnel parked on the scene.

Highway Design

High-speed, limited-access highways have made moving large amounts of traffic efficient, but when a crash occurs, the resulting traffic backup and "rubbernecking" by drivers create dangerous situations for all emergency responders. Elevated roadways and overpasses may limit an oncoming driver's vision of what lies ahead, and the driver may suddenly encounter stopped vehicles and emergency responders on the road upon reaching the apex of the overpass. Law enforcement is usually reluctant to shut down a limited-access highway and strives to keep the flow of traffic moving. Although this approach may appear to produce further danger to emergency responders, it may prevent additional rear-end collisions caused by the backup of vehicles.

Rural roads present other problems. Although the volume of traffic is much less than on urban roadways, the winding, narrow, and hilly nature of these roads prevents drivers from seeing the scene of an MVC until they are dangerously close to it. Additionally, rural roads may not be as well maintained as those in urban areas, resulting in slippery conditions long after a storm has passed and catching unsuspecting drivers off guard. Isolated areas of snow, ice, or fog that caused the original MVC may still be present, may hinder EMS arrival, and may result in suboptimal conditions for oncoming drivers.

Risk Mitigation Strategies

Because prehospital care providers must respond at all times of day and in any weather condition, steps must be taken to reduce the risks of becoming a victim while working at the scene of an MVC. The best way is to limit the number of responders, particularly on limited-access highways. The number of people on the scene should be only what is needed to accomplish the tasks at hand. For example, having three ambulances and a supervisor's vehicle at a scene that has one patient dramatically increases the risk of a provider being hit by a passing vehicle. Although many dispatch protocols require multiple-ambulance response to limited-access highways, *all but the initial ambulance should be staged at a convenient access point nearby unless immediately needed.*

The location of equipment in the ambulance also plays a role in safety. Equipment should be placed so that it can be gathered without stepping into traffic. The passenger's side of the ambulance is often toward the guardrails, and placing the equipment most often used at MVCs in these compartments will keep prehospital care providers out of the flow of traffic.

Reflective Clothing

In most cases when prehospital care providers are hit by oncoming vehicles, drivers state that they did not see the provider in the road. To enhance visibility, reflective clothing should be worn at all MVC scenes. Both the National Fire Protection Association (NFPA) and the Occupational Safety and Health Administration (OSHA) have standards for reflective warning garments to be worn when working on highways. OSHA has three levels of protection for workers on highways, with the highest level (level 3) to be used at night on high-speed roadways. The Federal Highway Administration has mandated that all workers, including all emergency responders, wear American National Standards Institute (ANSI) Class 2 or Class 3 reflective vests when responding to an incident on a highway funded by federal aid. The ANSI standards can be met either by affixing reflective material to the outer jacket or by wearing an approved reflective vest.

Vehicle Positioning and Warning Devices

Vehicle positioning at the scene of an MVC is of the utmost importance. The incident commander or the safety officer should ensure that responding vehicles are placed in the best positions to protect prehospital care providers. It is important for the first-arriving emergency vehicles to "take the lane" of the accident (**Figure 5-3**). Although placement of the ambulance behind the scene will not facilitate the loading of the patient, it will protect providers and patient(s) from oncoming traffic. As additional emergency vehicles arrive, they should generally be placed on the same side of the road as the incident. These vehicles should be placed farther from the incident to give increased warning time to oncoming drivers.

Headlights, especially high beams, should be turned off to avoid blinding approaching drivers unless needed to illuminate the scene. The number of warning lights at the scene should be evaluated; too many lights may only serve to confuse oncoming drivers. Many departments use warning signs stating "accident ahead" to give ample

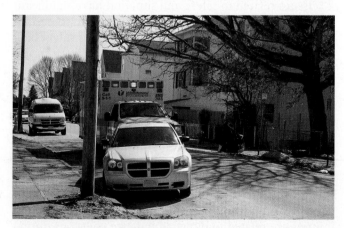

Figure 5-3 The correct positioning of an emergency vehicle.
© Jones & Bartlett Learning. Photographed by Darren Stahlman.

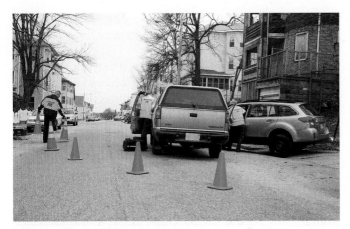

Figure 5-4 The placement of traffic delineation devices.
© Jones & Bartlett Learning. Photographed by Darren Stahlman.

warning for drivers. Flares may be arranged to warn and direct traffic flow; however, care should be used in dry conditions to prevent grass fires. Reflective cones can serve to direct traffic flow away from the lane taken up by the emergency (**Figure 5-4**).

If traffic needs to be directed, law enforcement or personnel with special training in traffic control should handle this task so that EMS can focus on patient management. Confusing or contradicting instructions given to drivers create additional safety risks. The best situations are created when traffic is not impeded and normal flow can be maintained around the emergency.

Traffic Safety Education

Several educational programs are available that are designed to educate emergency responders about safe operations at the scene of an MVC. Each organization should check with its state EMS agency, the National Highway Traffic Safety Administration (NHTSA), or OSHA about the local availability of these programs and incorporate them into their annual required training programs. NAEMT's EMS Safety course prepares emergency responders to respond to and operate safely at the scene of MVCs.

Violence

Each call has the potential to take the prehospital care provider into an emotionally charged environment. Some EMS agencies have a policy that requires the presence of law enforcement before providers enter a scene of violence. Even a scene that appears benign has the potential to deteriorate into violence; therefore, providers must always be alert to subtle clues that suggest a changing situation. The patient, family, or bystanders on the scene may not be able to perceive the situation rationally. These individuals may think the response time was too long, may be overly sensitive to words or actions, and may misunderstand the "usual" approach to patient assessment. Maintaining a confident and professional manner while demonstrating

respect and concern is important to gaining the patient's trust and achieving control of the scene.

It is important that EMS personnel train themselves to *observe* the scene. EMS personnel must learn to notice the numbers and locations of individuals when arriving on the scene, the movement of bystanders into or out of the scene, any indicators of stress or tension, unexpected or unusual reactions to EMS presence, or other "gut" feelings that may develop. Watch the patient's and bystanders' hands. Look for unusual bulges in waistbands, clothing that is worn out of season, or oversized clothing that could easily hide a weapon. If a developing threat is perceived, immediately prepare to leave the scene. An assessment or a procedure may need to be completed in the ambulance. The safety of prehospital care providers is the first priority.

Consider the following situation: You and your partner are in the living room of a patient's home. While your partner is checking the patient's blood pressure, an apparently intoxicated individual enters the room from the back of the house. He looks angry, and you notice what appears to be the handle of a gun sticking out of the waistband of his pants. Your partner does not see or hear this person enter the room because he is focused on the patient. The suspicious person begins to question your presence and is extremely agitated about your uniform and your badge. His hands repeatedly move toward, then away from, his waist. He begins to pace and mumble. How can you and your partner prepare for this sort of situation?

Managing the Violent Scene

Partners need to discuss and agree on methods to handle a violent patient or bystander. Attempting to develop a process during the event is prone to failure. Partners can use a hands-on/hands-off approach, as well as predetermined code words and hand signals, for emergencies.

- The role of the *hands-on* prehospital care provider is to take charge of the patient assessment, giving necessary attention to the patient. The *hands-off* provider stands back to observe the scene, interact with family or bystanders, collect necessary information, and create better access and egress. In essence, the hands-off provider is monitoring the scene and "covering" his or her partner's back.
- A predetermined *code word* and *hand signals* allow partners to communicate a threat without alerting others of their concerns.

If both prehospital care providers have all of their attention focused on the patient, the scene can quickly become threatening, and early clues may be missed. In many situations, patient, family, and bystander tension and anxiety are immediately reduced when one attentive provider begins interacting with and assessing the patient, while the other provider observes the scene.

There are various methods for dealing with a scene that has become dangerous, including the following:

1. *Don't be there.* When responding to a known violent scene, stage at a safe location until the scene has been rendered safe by law enforcement and clearance to respond has been given.

2. *Retreat.* If threats are presented when approaching the scene, tactfully retreat to the vehicle and leave the scene. Stage at a safe location and notify appropriate personnel.

3. *Defuse.* If a scene becomes threatening during patient care, use verbal skills to reduce tension and aggression (while preparing to leave the scene).

4. *Defend.* As a last resort, prehospital care providers may find it necessary to defend themselves. It is important that such efforts are to "disengage and get away." Do not attempt to chase or subdue an aggressive party. Ensure that law enforcement personnel have been notified and are en route. Again, the safety of the providers is the priority.

The Active Shooter

Situations involving an active shooter have become all too frequent. To improve patient outcomes from injuries sustained in these incidents there is a growing trend for EMS agencies to partner with law enforcement colleagues to enter these scenes much earlier than would normally occur. In these cases, a contact team of officers enters the scene to engage and neutralize the threat. A joint EMS and law enforcement team follows the contact team to identify and begin treating victims quickly. (See the Civilian Tactical Emergency Medical Support chapter for more information.)

Hazardous Materials

Understanding the prehospital care provider's risk of exposure to hazardous materials is not as simple as recognizing environments that have obvious potential for hazardous material exposure. Hazardous materials are widespread in the modern world; vehicles, buildings, and even homes can contain hazardous materials. In addition to hazardous materials, this discussion applies equally to weapons of mass destruction. Because these dangers exist in such varied forms, all providers must obtain a minimum of awareness-level hazardous materials training. Note that you will sometimes encounter the term hazardous materials abbreviated *HazMat*.

There are four levels of hazardous materials training:

- **Awareness:** This is the first of four levels of training available to emergency responders, and it is designed to provide a basic level of knowledge on hazardous materials incidents.

- **Operations:** Whereas awareness represents the minimum level of training, operations-level training is helpful for all emergency responders, as it provides the training and knowledge to help control the hazardous

materials event. These emergency responders are trained to set up perimeters and safety zones, limiting the spread of the event.

- **Technician:** Technicians are trained to work within the hazardous area and stop the release of hazardous materials.

- **Specialist:** This advanced level allows the emergency responder to provide command and support skills at a hazardous materials event.

Scene Safety

Because the first priority at any scene is the safety of prehospital care providers, an important first step is to evaluate the site for the potential of hazardous materials exposure. The information given by dispatch may establish a high index of suspicion of hazardous materials. A call that involves a large number of patients who are presenting with similar symptoms should raise the possibility of a hazardous material exposure. Additional information can be requested while en route if providers have any concerns or questions related to the scene.

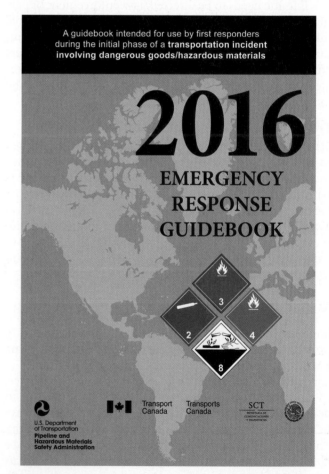

Figure 5-5 The *Emergency Response Guidebook* produced by the U.S. Department of Transportation provides critical information at the scene of a potential hazardous materials incident. The *ERG* is also available as an app for smartphones.

Courtesy of United States Department of Transportation, PHMSA.

Once a scene has been determined to involve a hazardous material, the focus must shift to securing the scene and summoning appropriate help to safely isolate the involved area and remove and decontaminate exposed patients and individuals. The general rule is, "If the scene is not safe, make it safe." If the prehospital care provider cannot make the scene safe, help should be summoned. The *Emergency Response Guidebook* (*ERG*), produced by the U.S. Department of Transportation, or contact with an organization such as CHEMTREC, is useful to identify potential hazards (**Figure 5-5**). The guidebook uses a simple system that allows identification of a material by its name or identification placard number. The text then refers the reader to a page that provides basic information about safe distances for emergency responders, life and fire hazards, and the patient's likely complaints. CHEMTREC is available 24 hours a day, 7 days a week, and can be contacted for assistance by telephone (1-800-424-9300).

Use binoculars to read labels from a distance; if labels can be read without the use of viewing devices, the prehospital care provider is too close and likely to be exposed. A good rule is that if your extended thumb held at arm's length does not cover the entire incident scene, then you are too close.

At a hazardous materials scene, security of the site must be ensured: "Nobody in, nobody out." The staging area should be established upwind and upgrade at a safe distance from the hazard. Entry into and exit from the scene should be denied until the arrival of hazardous materials specialists. In most cases, patient care begins when a decontaminated patient is delivered to the prehospital care provider.

It is important for the prehospital care provider to understand the command system and structure of the work zones in a hazardous materials operation (**Figure 5-6**). The scene of an incident involving a weapon of mass destruction or hazardous material is generally divided into hot, warm, and cold zones. For a description of the functions of each zone, see the Explosions and Weapons of Mass Destruction chapter.

Situation Issues

There are a number of situation issues that can profoundly affect the medical care that prehospital providers are able to offer a patient.

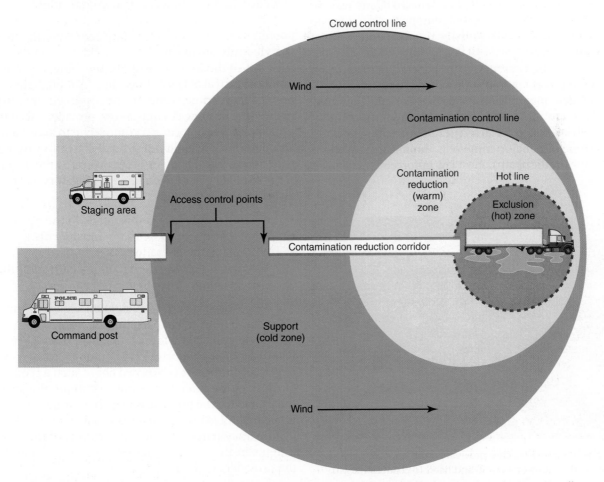

Crowd control line

Wind ⟶

Contamination control line

Contamination reduction (warm) zone

Hot line

Exclusion (hot) zone

Access control points

Staging area

Command post

Contamination reduction corridor

Support (cold zone)

Wind ⟶

Figure 5-6 The scene of an incident involving a weapon of mass destruction or hazardous material is generally divided into hot, warm, and cold zones.

© National Association of Emergency Medical Technicians (NAEMT).

Crime Scenes

Unfortunately, a sizable percentage of trauma patients encountered by prehospital care providers are injured intentionally. In addition to shootings and stabbings, patients may be victims of assaults with fists, blunt objects, or attempted strangulation. In other cases, victims may have been intentionally struck by a vehicle or pushed off of a structure or out of a moving vehicle, resulting in significant injury. Even an MVC can be considered a crime scene if one of the drivers is thought to have been driving under the influence of alcohol or drugs, driving recklessly, speeding, or texting while driving.

When managing these types of patients, prehospital care personnel often interact with law enforcement personnel (**Figure 5-7**). Although both EMS and law enforcement share the goal of preserving life, these parties occasionally find that their duties at a crime scene come into conflict. EMS personnel focus on the need to assess a victim for signs of life and viability, whereas law enforcement personnel are concerned with preserving evidence at a crime scene or bringing a perpetrator to justice. Law enforcement and criminal investigation should never preclude proper patient care. Should the scene need to be disrupted in any way for patient assessment or care, documentation and follow-up communication with the investigating law enforcement agency are imperative.

By developing awareness of the general approach taken by law enforcement personnel at a crime scene, prehospital care providers may not only aid their patient, they may also cooperate more effectively with law enforcement personnel, leading to the arrest of their patient's assailant. At the scene of a major crime (e.g., homicide, suspicious death, rape, traffic death), most law enforcement agencies

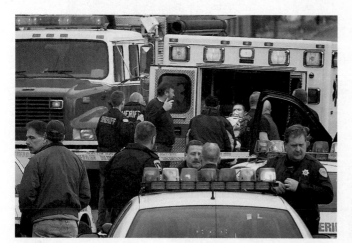

Figure 5-7 Prehospital care providers often have to manage patients at the scene of a crime and need to collaborate with law enforcement to preserve evidence.
© Jason Hunt/*The Coeur d'Alene Press*/AP Images.

collect and process evidence. Law enforcement personnel typically perform the following duties:

- Canvass the scene to identify all evidence, including weapons and shell casings.
- Photograph the scene.
- Sketch the scene.
- Create a log of everyone who has entered the scene.
- Conduct a more thorough search of the entire scene, looking for all potential evidence.
- Look for and collect trace evidence, ranging from fingerprints to items that may contain DNA evidence (e.g., cigarette butts, strands of hair, fibers).

Police investigators believe that everyone who enters a crime scene brings some type of evidence into a scene and, unknowingly, removes some evidence from the scene. To solve the crime, a detective's goal is to identify the evidence deposited and removed by the perpetrator. To accomplish this, the investigators have to account for any evidence left or removed by other law enforcement officers, EMS personnel, citizens, and anyone else who may have entered the scene. Careless behavior by prehospital care personnel at a crime scene may disrupt, destroy, or contaminate vital evidence, hampering a criminal investigation.

On occasion, prehospital care providers arrive at a potential crime scene before law enforcement officers. If the victim is obviously dead, providers should carefully back out of the location without touching any items and await the arrival of law enforcement. Although they would prefer that a crime scene not be disturbed, investigators realize that in some circumstances, providers need to turn a body or move objects at a crime scene to access a patient and determine viability. If providers need to transport a patient or move a body or other objects in the area before the arrival of law enforcement, investigators will typically ascertain the following:

- When were the alterations made to the scene?
- What was the purpose of the movement?
- Who made the alterations?
- At what time was the victim's death identified by EMS personnel?

If prehospital care providers entered a crime scene before law enforcement personnel, investigators may want to interview and take a formal statement from the providers regarding their actions or observations. Providers should never be alarmed or concerned about such a request. The purpose of the interview is not to critique the actions of the providers; the purpose is to gain information that may prove helpful to the investigator in solving the case. Investigators may request to take fingerprints of the providers if items in the crime scene were touched or handled by the providers without gloves.

Proper handling of a patient's clothing may preserve valuable evidence. If a patient's clothing needs to be removed, law enforcement officers and medical examiners prefer that prehospital care providers refrain from cutting through bullet or knife holes in the clothing. If the clothing is cut, investigators may ask what alterations were made to the clothing, who made the alterations, and the reason for alterations. Any clothing that is removed should be placed in a paper (not plastic) bag and turned over to investigators.

One final important issue involving victims of violent crimes is the value of any statements made by the patient while under the care of prehospital care providers. Some patients, realizing the critical nature of their injuries, may tell providers who inflicted their injuries. This information should be documented and passed on to investigators. If possible, providers should inform officers of the critical nature of a patient's injuries so that a sworn officer can be present if the patient is capable of providing any information regarding the perpetrator. This is called a "dying declaration."

Weapons of Mass Destruction

The response to a scene involving a weapon of mass destruction (WMD) has safety and other concerns similar to the response to a scene involving hazardous materials, as discussed earlier.

Every scene that involves multiple victims, especially if they complain of similar symptoms or findings, or that was reported to have resulted from an explosion should trigger two questions: (1) Was a WMD involved? (2) Could there be a secondary device intended to harm emergency responders? (See the Explosions and Weapons of Mass Destruction chapter for greater detail.)

To avoid becoming a victim, the prehospital care provider needs to approach such scenes with extreme caution and resist the urge to rush in to care for the victims. Instead, the provider should approach the scene from an upwind position and take a moment to stop, look, and listen for clues indicating the possible presence of a WMD. Obvious spills of wet or dry material, visible vapors, and smoke should be avoided until the nature of the material has been ascertained. Enclosed or confined spaces should never be entered without the appropriate training and personal protective equipment (PPE). (See the Explosions and Weapons of Mass Destruction chapter for greater detail about PPE for hazardous materials and WMD incidents.)

Once a WMD has been included as a possible cause, the prehospital care provider needs to take all appropriate steps for self-protection and protection of other responders arriving at the scene. These steps include the use of PPE appropriate to the function and level of training of the individual provider. For example, emergency responders responsible for entering the hot zone must wear the highest level of skin and respiratory protection; in the cold zone, standard precautions will suffice in most instances.

Information that this may be a WMD incident should be relayed back to dispatch to alert incoming emergency responders from all services. Staging areas for additional equipment, emergency responders, and helicopters should be established upwind and at a safe distance from the site.

The scene should be secured, and zones indicating hot, warm, and cold areas should be designated. Sites for decontamination should also be established. Once the nature of the agent has been determined (chemical, biologic, or radiologic), specific requests for antidote or antibiotics can be made.

Scene Control Zones

Just as was done at the scene of a hazardous materials incident to limit the spread of the hazardous material, the designation and use of control zones is essential at a WMD incident. Adherence to these principles reduces the likelihood of spread of contamination and injury to emergency responders and bystanders. **Table 5-1** lists safe evacuation distances for bomb threats.

While these zones are typically illustrated as three concentric circles (see Figure 5-6), in reality, at most scenes, these zones will likely be irregularly shaped depending on the geography and wind conditions. If a patient is delivered to the hospital or aid station from a hazardous materials or WMD scene, it is most prudent to reevaluate whether that patient has been decontaminated and to mimic the concepts of these zones.

Decontamination

Whether the incident involves a hazardous material or a WMD, decontamination of an exposed individual is often required. **Decontamination** is the reduction or removal of hazardous chemical, biologic, or radiologic agents. The first priority is ensuring personal safety if there is any question of a continued exposure. Decontamination of the patient by appropriately trained hazardous materials technician-level personnel is the next priority. This will minimize the exposure risk to the prehospital care provider during assessment and treatment of the patient and will prevent contamination of equipment and vehicles.

OSHA provides regulatory guidelines for PPE used by prehospital care providers during the emergency care of victims in a potentially hazardous environment. Individuals providing medical care within environments of an unknown hazard must have a minimum level of appropriate training and be supplied and trained with level B protection. Level B protection consists of splash-protective, chemical-resistant clothing and self-contained breathing sources. Training in advance of the need to use this level of PPE is required. (See the Explosions and Weapons of Mass Destruction chapter for greater detail about PPE for hazardous materials and WMD incidents.)

Table 5-1 Bomb Threats: Safe Evacuation Distances

Threat Description	Explosives Capacity (TNT Capacity)	Building Evacuation Distance	Outdoor Evacuation Distance
Pipe bomb	5 lb (2.3 kg)	70 ft (21.3 m)	1,200 ft (365.8 m)
Briefcase/suitcase bomb	50 lb (22.7 kg)	150 ft (45.7 m)	1,850 ft (564 m)
Car	500 lb (227 kg)	320 ft (97.5 m)	1,500 ft (457 m)
SUV/van	1,000 lb (454 kg)	400 ft (122 m)	2,400 ft (731.5 m)
Small moving van, delivery truck	4,000 lb (1,814 kg)	640 ft (195 m)	3,800 ft (1,158 m)
Moving van, small tank truck	10,000 lb (4,536 kg)	860 ft (262 m)	5,100 ft (1,554.5 m)
Semitrailer	60,000 lb (27,216 kg)	1,570 ft (479 m)	9,300 ft (2,835 m)

Note: lb = pounds; kg = kilograms; ft = feet; m = meters.
Data from U.S. Department of Homeland Security.

If the patient is conscious and able to assist, it is best to enlist the patient's cooperation and have the patient perform as much of the decontamination as possible to reduce the likelihood of cross-contamination to prehospital care providers. In performing or overseeing patient decontamination, providers need to ensure not only that the hazardous product is safely removed from the patient but that it is controlled and cannot further contaminate the scene. For a detailed review of the decontamination process, see the Burn Injuries chapter.

Secondary Devices

Within months after the bombing at the 1996 Atlanta Summer Olympics, the metropolitan area of Atlanta, Georgia, experienced two additional bombings. These bombings, at an abortion clinic and a nightclub, had secondary bombs planted and represented the first time in 17 years in the United States that secondary bombs had been planted, presumably to kill or injure rescuers responding to the scene of the first blast. Unfortunately, the secondary device at the abortion clinic was not detected prior to its detonation, and there were six casualties. Secondary devices have been used with regularity by terrorists in many countries. All prehospital care personnel need to be mindful of the potential presence of a secondary device.

After these incidents, the Georgia Emergency Management Agency developed the following guidelines for rescuers and prehospital care personnel responding to the scene of a bombing at which a secondary bomb might be planted:

1. *Refrain from use of electronic devices.* Sound waves from cell phones and radios may cause a secondary device to detonate, especially if used close to the bomb. Equipment used by the news media may also trigger a detonation.
2. *Ensure sufficient standoff distance for the scene.* The hot zone should extend 1,000 feet (ft; 305 meters [m]) in all directions (including vertically) from the original blast site. As more powerful bombs are created, shrapnel may travel farther. The initial bomb blast may damage infrastructure, including gas lines and power lines, which may further jeopardize the safety of emergency responders. Access to and exit from the hot zone should be carefully controlled.
3. *Provide rapid evacuation of victims from the scene and hot zone.* An EMS command post should be established 2,000 to 4,000 ft (610 to 1219 m) from the scene of the initial bombing. Emergency responders can rapidly evacuate victims from the bombing site with minimal interventions until victims and emergency responders are out of the hot zone.
4. *Collaborate with law enforcement personnel on preserving and recovering evidence.* Bombing sites

constitute a crime scene, and emergency responders should disrupt the scene only as necessary to evacuate victims. Any potential evidence that is inadvertently removed from the scene with a victim should be documented and turned over to law enforcement personnel to ensure proper chain of custody. Prehospital care personnel can document exactly where they were in the scene and which items they touched.

Command Structure

An ambulance responding to a call will typically have one prehospital care provider in charge (the incident commander) and another assisting in a rudimentary incident command structure. As an incident grows larger and more emergency responders from other agencies respond to the scene, the need for a formal system and structure to oversee and control the response becomes increasingly important.

Incident Command

The **incident command system (ICS)** has developed over the years as an outgrowth of planning systems used by firefighting services for multiple-service responses to major fire situations. In 1987, the NFPA published NFPA Standard 1561, *Standard on Fire Department Incident Command Management System*. NFPA 1561 was later revised as the *Standard on Emergency Services Incident Management System and Command Safety*. This version can be implemented and adjusted to any type or size of event by any agency managing an incident. In the 1990s, the National Fire Incident Management System (IMS) was created, which further refined the single-incident management approach.

Dealing with any incident, large or small, is enhanced by the precise command structure afforded by the ICS. At the core of the ICS is the establishment of centralized command at the scene and the subsequent buildup of divisional responsibilities. The first-arriving unit establishes the command center, and communications are established through command for the buildup of the response. The five key elements of the ICS are:

1. *Command* provides overall control of the event and the communications that will coordinate the movement of resources in and patients out of the incident scene.
2. *Operations* includes divisions to handle the tactical needs of the event. Fire suppression, EMS, and rescue are examples of operational branches.
3. *Planning* is a continuous process of evaluating immediate and potential needs of the incident and planning the response. Throughout the event, this element will be used to evaluate the effectiveness of operations and to make suggested alterations in the response and tactical approach.

4. *Logistics* handles the task of acquiring resources identified by the planning section and moving them to where they are needed. These resources include personnel, shelter, vehicles, and equipment.

5. *Finance* tracks the money. Response personnel from all involved agencies as well as contractors, personnel, and vendors brought into service in the incident are tracked so that the cost of the event can be determined and these groups can be paid for goods, supplies, equipment, and services.

Unified Command

An expansion of the ICS is the unified command system. This expansion takes into account the need to coordinate numerous agencies that cross jurisdictional boundaries. The technical aspects of bringing resources to bear from multiple communities, counties, and states are covered by this additional coordinating structure.

National Incident Management System

On February 28, 2003, President George W. Bush directed the secretary of Homeland Security through Presidential Directive HSPD-5 to produce a National Incident Management System (NIMS). The goal of this directive is to establish a consistent, nationwide approach for federal, state, and local governments to work effectively together to prepare for, respond to, and recover from domestic incidents regardless of cause, size, or complexity. The Department of Homeland Security authorized NIMS on March 1, 2004, after collaborating with detailed working groups consisting of state and local government officials and representatives of the National Association of Emergency Medical Technicians (NAEMT), Fraternal Order of Police (FOP), International Association of Fire Chiefs (IAFC), and International Association of Emergency Managers (IAEM), as well as a wide range of other public safety organizations.[2]

NIMS focuses on the following incident management characteristics:

- Common terminology
- Modular organization
- Management by objectives
- Reliance on an incident action plan
- Manageable span of control
- Predesignated "incident mobilization center" locations and facilities
- Comprehensive resource management
- Integrated communications
- Establishment of transfer of command
- Chain of command and unity of command
- Unified command
- Accountability of resources and personnel
- Deployment
- Information and intelligence management

The key components of NIMS are as follows:

1. Preparedness
2. Communications and information management
3. Resource management
4. Command and management
5. Ongoing management and maintenance

Command

Command comprises the **incident commander (IC)** and command staff. Every incident should have an identified commander who oversees the response. Command staff positions to assist the IC are assigned as appropriate to the size and nature of the event and may include public information officer, safety officer, and liaison officer. Other positions can be created as deemed necessary by the IC.

As described earlier, unified command is an enhancement to incident command in situations involving multiple jurisdictions. In a single-command situation, the IC is solely responsible for the incident management. In a unified command structure, individuals representing various jurisdictions jointly determine objectives, plans, and priorities. The unified command system seeks to solve problems involving differences in communications and operational standards (**Figure 5-8**).

One element not included in the ICS that is added with unified command and NIMS is *intelligence*. Based on the size of the event, intelligence and information gathering related to national security may include risk-management assessment, medical intelligence, weather information, structural design of buildings, and information on toxic containment. Although these functions are typically handled in the planning section, the IC may separate information gathering from planning in certain situations.

In NIMS, the IC can assign intelligence and information gathering as follows:

- Within the command staff
- As a unit of the planning section
- As a branch of operations
- As a separate general staff function

Incident Action Plans

Incident action plans (IAPs) include overall incident objectives and strategies established by the IC or unified command personnel. The planning section develops and documents the IAP. The IAP addresses the tactical objectives and support activities for a designated operational period, which is generally 12 to 24 hours. The planning section provides an ongoing critique, or "lessons learned" process, to ensure the response meets the needs of the event.

In very large incidents, multiple ICS organizations may be established. Area command may be established to manage multiple ICS organizations. Area command does

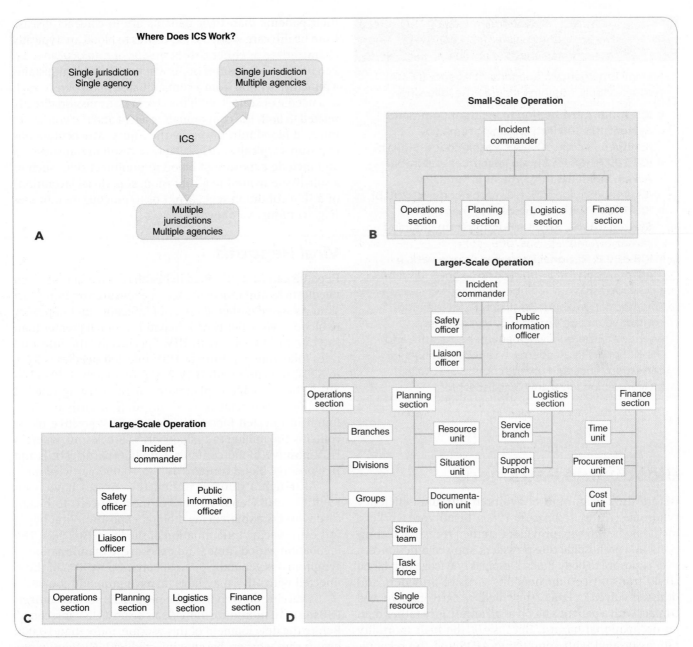

Figure 5-8 The incident command structure is flexible and can be expanded or decreased based on the number of patients and the complexity of the event. The operational functions of each of the sections under incident command are the branches. The Medical Services Branch is the operational component responsible for coordinating and providing medical services needed to meet the tactical objectives of the incident. These services include equipment and personnel management, triage, communications with medical facilities, and transport.

© National Association of Emergency Medical Technicians (NAEMT).

not have operational responsibilities; however, it performs the following duties:

- Sets overall incident-related priorities for the agency
- Allocates critical resources according to established priorities
- Ensures that incidents are managed properly
- Ensures effective communications
- Ensures that incident management objectives are met and do not conflict with each other or with agency policies

- Identifies critical resource needs and reports to the Emergency Operations Center(s)
- Ensures that short-term emergency recovery is coordinated to assist in the transition to full-recovery operations
- Provides for personnel accountability and safe operating environments

Detailed information and training programs regarding the ICS and NIMS can be found on the Federal Emergency Management Agency's website (**Box 5-1**).

Bloodborne Pathogens

Before the recognition of acquired immunodeficiency syndrome (AIDS) in the early 1980s, health care workers, including health care providers, sterile processing technicians, and prehospital care providers, showed little concern over exposure to body fluids. Despite knowledge that blood could transmit certain hepatitis viruses, providers and others involved in emergency medical care often viewed contact with a patient's blood as an annoyance rather than an occupational hazard. Because of the high mortality rate associated with contracting AIDS and the recognition that the human immunodeficiency virus (HIV)—the causative agent of AIDS—could be transmitted in blood, health care workers became much more concerned about the patient as a vector of disease. Federal agencies, such as the Centers for Disease Control and Prevention (CDC) and OSHA, developed guidelines and mandates for health care workers to minimize exposure to bloodborne pathogens, including HIV and hepatitis. The primary infectious agents transmitted through blood include the hepatitis B virus (HBV), hepatitis C virus (HCV), and HIV. Although this issue became a concern because of HIV, it is important to note that hepatitis infection occurs much more easily and requires much less inoculum than does HIV infection.

Epidemiologic data demonstrate that health care workers are much more likely to contract bloodborne illness from their patients than their patients are to contract disease from health care workers. Exposures to blood are typically characterized as either **percutaneous** or **mucocutaneous**. Percutaneous exposures occur when an individual sustains a puncture wound from a contaminated sharp object, such as a needle or scalpel, with the risk of transmission directly related to both the contaminating agent and the volume of infected blood introduced by the injury. Mucocutaneous exposures typically are less likely to result in transmission and include exposure of blood to nonintact skin, such as a soft-tissue wound (e.g., abrasion, superficial laceration) or a skin condition (e.g., acne) or to mucous membranes (e.g., conjunctiva of eye).

Viral Hepatitis

Hepatitis can be transmitted to health care workers through needlesticks and mucocutaneous exposures on nonintact skin. As stated earlier, the rate of infection after exposure to blood from patients with hepatitis is much greater than the rate of infection with HIV. Specifically, the infection rates following exposure to HBV-infected needles is 37% to 62%. Infection with HCV is approximately 1.8% (1 in 50).[3] The probable explanation for the varying rates of infection is the relative concentration of virus particles found in infected blood. In general, HBV-positive blood contains 100 million to 1 billion virus particles/ml, whereas HCV-positive blood contains 1 million particles/ml, and HIV-positive blood contains 100 to 10,000 particles/ml.

Although a number of hepatitis viruses have been identified, HBV and HCV are of most concern to health care workers experiencing a blood exposure. Viral hepatitis causes acute inflammation of the liver (**Box 5-2**). The incubation period (time from exposure to manifestation of symptoms) is generally 60 to 90 days. Up to 30% of those infected with HBV may have an asymptomatic course.[3]

A vaccine derived from the hepatitis B surface antigen (HBsAg) can immunize individuals against HBV infection.[6] Before the development of this vaccine, more than 10,000 health care workers became infected with HBV annually, and several hundred died each year from either severe hepatitis or complications of chronic HBV infection.[7] OSHA now requires employers to offer HBV vaccine to health care workers in high-risk environments. All prehospital care providers should be immunized against HBV infection. Almost everyone who completes the series of three vaccines will develop antibody (Ab) to HBsAg, and immunity can be determined by testing the health care worker's blood for the presence of HBsAb. If a health care worker is exposed to blood from a patient who is potentially infected with HBV before the health care worker has developed immunity (i.e., before completing the vaccine series), passive protection from HBV can be conferred to the health care worker by the administration of hepatitis B immune globulin (HBIG).

Box 5-2 Hepatitis

The clinical manifestations of viral hepatitis are right upper-quadrant pain, fatigue, loss of appetite, nausea, vomiting, and alteration in liver function. Jaundice, a yellowish coloration of the skin, results from an increased level of bilirubin in the bloodstream. Although most individuals with hepatitis recover without serious problems, a small percentage of patients develop acute fulminant hepatic failure and may die. A significant number of those who recover develop a carrier state in which their blood can transmit the virus.

As with HBV infection, infection with HCV can range from a mild, asymptomatic course to liver failure and death. The incubation period for hepatitis C is somewhat shorter than for hepatitis B, typically 6 to 9 weeks. Chronic infections with HCV are much more common than with HBV, and about 75% to 85% of those who contract HCV will develop persistently abnormal liver function, predisposing them to hepatocellular carcinoma.[4] Hepatitis C is primarily transmitted through blood, whereas hepatitis B can be transmitted through blood or sexual contact. The risk of intravenous drug abusers becoming infected with HCV increases with the duration of intravenous drug use.[5] Before routine testing of donated blood for the presence of HBV and HCV, blood transfusion was the primary reason patients contracted hepatitis.

Box 5-3 Human Immunodeficiency Virus

Two serotypes of HIV have been identified. HIV-1 accounts for virtually all AIDS in the United States and equatorial Africa, and HIV-2 is found almost exclusively in Western Africa. Although early victims of HIV were male homosexuals, intravenous drug users, or hemophiliacs, HIV disease is now found in many teenage and adult heterosexual populations, with the fastest growing numbers in minority communities. The screening test for HIV is very sensitive, but false-positive tests occasionally occur. All positive screening tests should be confirmed with a more specific technique (e.g., Western blot electrophoresis).

After infection with HIV, when patients develop one of the characteristic opportunistic infections or cancers, they transition from being considered HIV positive to having AIDS. In the past decade, significant advances have been made in the treatment of HIV disease, primarily in developing new drugs to combat its effects. This progress has enabled many individuals with HIV infection to lead fairly normal lives because the progression of the disease is slowed dramatically.

Although health care workers typically are more concerned about contracting HIV because of the stigma of its disease transmission modalities and its fatal prognosis if untreated, they are at greater risk of contracting HBV or HCV.

At present, no immune globulin or vaccine is available to protect health care workers from exposure to HCV, emphasizing the need for using standard precautions. Direct-acting oral agents are capable of curing HCV infection. These drugs were approved in the United States in 2011. The treatment regimen depends on the genotype, viral load, and level of cirrhosis. The cost of these new agents limits universal accessibility.

Human Immunodeficiency Virus

After infection, HIV targets the immune system of its new host. Over time, the number of certain types of white blood cells falls dramatically, leaving the individual prone to developing unusual infections or cancers (**Box 5-3**).

Only about 0.3% (about 1 in 300) of needlestick exposures to HIV-positive blood lead to infection.[4] The risk of infection appears higher with exposure to a larger quantity of blood, exposure to blood from a patient with a more advanced stage of disease, a deep percutaneous injury, or an injury from a hollow-bore, blood-filled needle. HIV is primarily transmitted through infected blood or semen, but vaginal secretions and pericardial, peritoneal, pleural, amniotic, and cerebrospinal fluids are all considered potentially infected. Unless obvious blood is present, tears, urine, sweat, feces, and saliva are generally considered noninfectious. Prophylactic treatment in the context of high-risk exposure has been shown to reduce the risk of seroconversion and chronic infection. Immediate referral to a local needlestick and exposure hotline or your service's infection control officer is therefore warranted in the context of occupational exposure.

Standard Precautions

Because clinical examination cannot reliably identify all patients who pose a potential infection threat to health care workers, standard precautions were developed to prevent health care workers from coming into direct contact with any patient's body fluid. At the same time, these precautions help protect the patient from infections the prehospital care provider may have. OSHA has developed regulations that mandate that employers and their employees follow standard precautions in the workplace. Standard precautions consist of both physical barriers to blood and body fluid and exposure as well as safe-handling practices for needles and other "sharps." Because trauma patients often have external hemorrhage and because blood is an extremely high-risk body fluid, appropriate protective devices should be worn by providers while caring for patients.

Physical Barriers

Gloves

Gloves should be worn when touching nonintact skin, mucous membranes, or areas contaminated by gross blood or other body fluids. Because perforations may readily occur in gloves while caring for a patient, gloves should be examined regularly for defects and changed immediately if a problem is noted (**Figure 5-9**). Gloves should also be changed between contact with each patient at a multiple-casualty incident.

Masks and Face Shields

Masks serve to protect the health care worker's oral and nasal mucous membranes from exposure to infectious agents, especially in situations in which airborne pathogens are known or suspected. Masks and face shields should be changed immediately if they become wet or soiled.

Eye Protection

Eye protection must be worn in circumstances in which droplets of potentially infected fluid or blood may be splattered, such as while providing airway management to a patient with blood in the oropharynx or when dealing with any open wounds.

Gowns

Disposable gowns with impervious plastic liners offer the best protection, but they may be extremely uncomfortable and impractical in the prehospital environment. Gowns or clothing should be changed immediately if significant soilage occurs.

Resuscitation Equipment

Health care workers should have access to bag-mask devices or mouthpieces to protect them from direct contact with a patient's saliva, blood, and vomit.

Hand Washing

Hand washing is a fundamental principle of infection control. Hands should be washed with soap and running water if gross contamination with blood or body fluid occurs. Alcohol-based hand antiseptics are useful toward preventing transmission of many infectious agents but are not appropriate for situations in which obvious soiling has occurred; however, they can provide some cleansing and protective effect in situations in which running water and soap are not available. After removal of gloves, hands should be cleansed with either soap and water or an alcohol-based antiseptic.

Preventing Sharps Injuries

As noted earlier, percutaneous exposure to a patient's blood or body fluid constitutes a significant manner in which viral infections could be transmitted to health care workers. Many percutaneous exposures are caused by injuries from needlesticks with contaminated needles or other sharps. Eliminate unnecessary needles and sharps, never recap a used needle, and implement safety devices such as needleless intravenous systems when possible (**Box 5-4**).

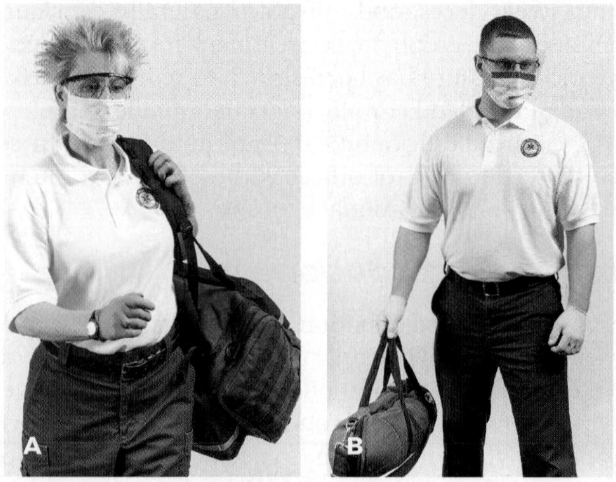

Figure 5-9 At a minimum, PPE for prehospital care providers should consist of gloves, mask, and eye protection. **A.** Goggles, face mask, and gloves. **B.** Face shield, face mask, and gloves.
© Jones & Bartlett Learning. Photographed by Darren Strahlman.

Box 5-4 Preventing Sharps Injuries

Prehospital care providers are at significant risk for injury from needles and other sharps. Strategies for reducing sharps injuries include the following:

- Use safety devices, such as shielded or retracting needles and scalpels and automatically retracting lancets.
- Use "needleless" systems that allow injection of medication at ports without needles.
- Refrain from recapping needles and other sharps.
- Immediately dispose of contaminated needles into rigid sharps containers rather than setting them down or handing them to someone else for disposal.
- Use prefilled medication syringes rather than drawing medication from an ampule.
- Provide a written exposure control plan, and ensure that all employees are aware of the plan.
- Maintain a sharps injury log.

Management of Occupational Exposure

In the United States, OSHA mandates that every organization providing health care have a control plan for managing occupational exposures of its employees to blood and body fluids. Each exposure should be thoroughly documented, including the type of injury and estimation of the volume of inoculate. If a health care worker has a mucocutaneous or percutaneous exposure to blood or sustains an injury from a contaminated sharp, efforts are taken to prevent bacterial infection, including tetanus, HBV, and HIV infection. No prophylactic therapy to prevent HCV infection is currently approved or available. **Box 5-5** describes a typical blood and body-fluid exposure protocol.

Patient Assessment and Triage

Once all the preceding issues have been addressed, the actual process of assessing and treating patients can begin. The greatest challenge occurs when the prehospital care provider is faced with multiple victims.

Triage is a French word meaning "to sort." Triage is a process that is used to assign priority for treatment and transport. In the prehospital environment, triage is used in two different contexts:

1. *Sufficient resources are available to manage all patients.* In this triage situation, the most severely injured patients are treated and transported first, and those with lesser injuries are treated and transported later.
2. *The number of patients exceeds the immediate capacity of on-scene resources.* The objective in such triage situations is to ensure survival of the largest possible number of injured patients. Patients are sorted into categories, and care must be rationed because the number of patients exceeds the available resources. Relatively few prehospital care providers ever experience an MCI with 50 to 100 or more simultaneously injured patients, but many will be involved in MCIs with 10 to 20 patients, and most providers have managed an incident with 2 to 10 patients.

Incidents that involve sufficient emergency responders and medical resources allow for the treatment and transport of the most severely injured patients first. In a large-scale MCI, limited resources require that patient treatment and transport be prioritized to salvage the victims with the greatest chance of survival. These victims are prioritized for treatment and transport (**Figure 5-10**).

The goal of patient management at the MCI scene is to do the most good for the most patients with the resources available. It is the responsibility of the prehospital care provider to make decisions about who should be managed first. The usual rules about saving lives are different

---

Box 5-5 Sample Exposure Protocol

After a percutaneous or mucocutaneous exposure to blood or other potentially infected body fluids, taking the appropriate actions and instituting appropriate postexposure prophylaxis (PEP) can help minimize the potential for acquiring viral hepatitis or HIV infection. Appropriate steps include:

1. Prevent bacterial infection.
   - Cleanse exposed skin thoroughly with germicidal soap and water; exposed mucous membranes should be irrigated with *copious* amounts of water.
   - Administer a tetanus toxoid booster, if not received in the previous 5 years.
2. Perform baseline laboratory studies on both the exposed health care worker and the source patient, if known.
   - Health care worker: Hepatitis B surface antibody (HBsAb), HCV, and HIV tests.
   - Source patient: Hepatitis B and C serology and HIV test.
3. Prevent HBV infection.
   - If the health care worker has not been immunized against hepatitis B, the first dose of HBV vaccine is administered along with HBIG.
   - If the health care worker has begun but not yet completed the HBV vaccine series or if the health care worker has completed all HBV immunizations, HBIG is given if the HBsAb test fails to show the presence of protective antibodies and the source patient's tests demonstrate active infection with HBV. HBIG may be administered up to 7 days after an exposure and still be effective.
4. Prevent HIV infection.
   - PEP depends upon the route of exposure and the likelihood and severity of HIV infection in the source patient. If the source patient is known to be negative, PEP is not indicated regardless of exposure route. In the past, when recommended, PEP has generally involved a two-drug regimen. With the development of numerous antiretroviral medications, the number of drug regimen combinations has increased. In addition, three-drug treatment is warranted in specific cases involving high risk of transmission. Therefore, it is recommended that an expert evaluate an exposed prehospital care provider to determine the most appropriate PEP regimen, given the circumstances of the particular exposure.

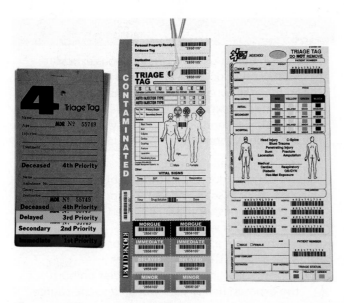

Figure 5-10 Examples of triage tags.

© File of Life Foundation, Inc.

in MCIs. The decision is always to save the most lives; however, when the available resources are not sufficient for the needs of all of the injured patients present, these resources should be used for the patients who have the best chance of surviving. In a choice between a patient with a catastrophic injury, such as severe brain trauma, and a patient with acute intra-abdominal hemorrhage, the proper course of action in an MCI is to manage first the salvageable patient—the patient with the abdominal hemorrhage. Treating the patient with severe head trauma first will probably result in the loss of both patients.

In a triage MCI situation, the catastrophically injured patient may need to be considered "lower priority," with treatment delayed until more help and equipment become available. These are difficult decisions and circumstances, but a prehospital care provider must respond quickly and properly. EMS personnel should not make efforts to resuscitate a traumatic cardiac arrest patient with little or no chance of survival while three other patients die because of airway compromise or external hemorrhage. The "sorting scheme" most often used divides patients into five categories based on need of care and chance of survival:

1. *Immediate*—Patients whose injuries are critical but who require only minimal time or equipment to manage and who have a good prognosis for survival. An example is the patient with a compromised airway or massive external hemorrhage.
2. *Delayed*—Patients whose injuries are debilitating but who do not require immediate management to salvage life or limb. An example is the patient with a long-bone fracture.
3. *Minor*—Patients, often called the "walking wounded," who have minor injuries that can wait for treatment

or who may even assist in the interim by comforting other patients or helping as litter bearers.

4. *Expectant*—Patients whose injuries are so severe that they have a minimal chance of survival. An example is the patient with a 90% full-thickness burn and thermal pulmonary injury.
5. *Dead*—Patients who are unresponsive, pulseless, and breathless. In a disaster, resources rarely allow for attempted resuscitation of cardiac arrest patients.

Box 5-6, **Figure 5-11**, and **Figure 5-12** describe a commonly used triage scheme known as START, which uses only four categories: immediate, delayed, minor, and dead.

Box 5-6 START Triage

In 1983, medical personnel from Hoag Memorial Hospital and fire fighter–paramedics from the Newport Beach Fire Department created a triage process for emergency medical responders called Simple Triage and Rapid Treatment (START) (see Figure 5-11). This triage process was designed to identify critically injured patients easily and quickly. START does not establish a medical diagnosis but instead provides a rapid and simple sorting process. START uses three simple assessments to identify those victims most at risk to die from their injuries. Typically, the process takes 30 to 60 seconds per victim. START requires no tools, specialized medical equipment, or special knowledge.

How Does START Work?

The first step is to direct anyone who can walk to a designated safe area. If the victims can walk and follow commands, their condition is categorized as minor, and they will be further triaged and tagged when more rescuers arrive. This initial sorting leads to a smaller group of presumably more seriously injured victims remaining to triage. The mnemonic "30-2-can do" is used as the START triage prompt (see Figure 5-12). The "30" refers to the victim's respiratory rate, the "2" refers to capillary refilling time, and the "can do" refers to the ability of the victim to follow commands. Any victim with respirations fewer than 30 per minute, capillary refilling time of less than 2 seconds, and the ability to follow verbal commands and to walk is categorized as minor. When victims meet these criteria but cannot walk, they are categorized as delayed. Victims who are unconscious or have rapid breathing, or who have delayed capillary refilling time or absent radial pulse are categorized as immediate.

(continued)

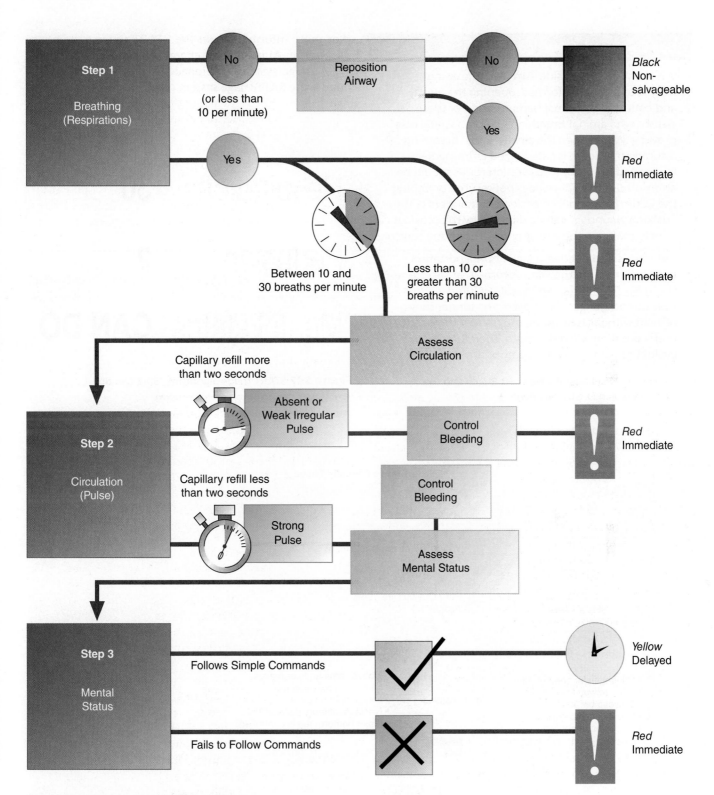

Figure 5-11 START triage algorithm: decision map.

Courtesy of Hoag Hospital Newport Beach and the Newport Beach Fire Department.

Box 5-6 START Triage (*continued*)

While at the victim's side, two basic lifesaving measures can be performed: opening the airway and controlling external hemorrhage. For those victims who are not breathing, the prehospital care provider should open the airway, and if breathing resumes, the victim is categorized as immediate. No cardiopulmonary resuscitation (CPR) should be attempted. If the victim does not resume breathing, the victim is categorized as dead. Bystanders or the "walking wounded" can be directed by the provider to help maintain the airway and hemorrhage control.

Retriage is also needed if lack of transportation prolongs the time the victims remain at the scene. Using START criteria, significantly injured victims may be categorized as delayed. The longer they remain without treatment, the greater the chance their condition will deteriorate. Therefore, repeat evaluation and triage are appropriate over time.

Courtesy of Hoag Hospital Newport Beach and the Newport Beach Fire Department.

(For more information on the START triage system, see the Disaster Management chapter.)

A triage system developed specifically with MCIs in mind is the SALT triage system (**Box 5-7** and **Figure 5-13**).[8]

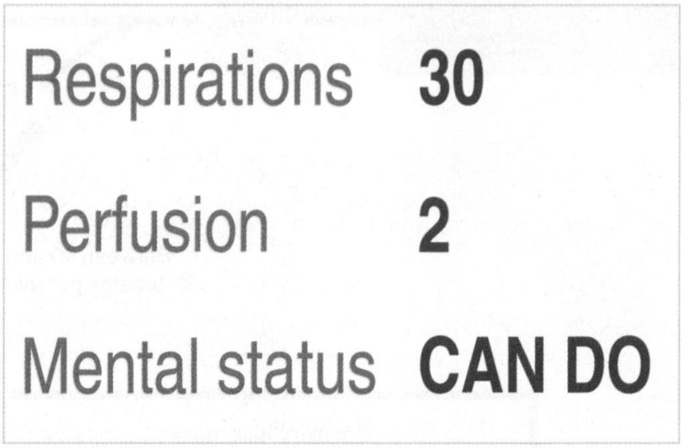

Respirations **30**

Perfusion **2**

Mental status **CAN DO**

Figure 5-12 START triage algorithm: "30-2-can do."

Courtesy of Hoag Hospital Newport Beach and the Newport Beach Fire Department.

SALT Mass Casualty Triage

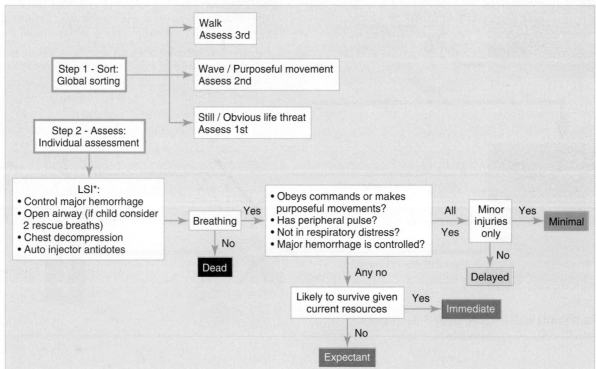

*Note: LSI stands for lifesaving interventions.

Figure 5-13 SALT triage algorithm.

Chemical Hazards Emergency Medical Management, U.S. Department of Health and Human Services. http://chemm.nlm.nih.gov/chemmimages/salt.png. Accessed October 16, 2017.

Box 5-7 SALT Triage

The CDC, in conjunction with an expert panel representing a large constituency of medical organizations, developed the SALT triage scheme. The intent of the project was to develop a triage methodology that would serve as a basis for a nationally agreed-upon triage system. This system begins by using a global sorting process: asking victims to walk or wave (follow commands). Those victims who do not respond are then assessed for life threats and subsequently categorized into immediate, delayed, minimal, or dead (see Figure 5-13).

SUMMARY

- As a part of assessing the scene for safety in each and every patient contact, it is important to assess for hazards of all types. Hazards include traffic issues, environmental concerns, violence, bloodborne pathogens, and hazardous materials.
- Assessing the scene will assure that EMS personnel and equipment are not compromised and unavailable for others and ensure that other emergency responders are protected from hazards that are not isolated or removed.
- Sometimes hazards will be ruled out quickly, but if they are not looked for, they will not be seen.
- Prehospital care providers should have a plan in place to mitigate risk at potentially dangerous scenes. For example, they should wear reflective clothing and park strategically at motor vehicle crashes; at a scene that involves a hostile person, partners should have a plan in place to prevent violence.

- Certain situations, such as crime scenes or intentional acts, including the use of weapons of mass destruction, will affect how the prehospital care provider responds to the scene and the patients at that scene.
- Incidents are managed using an incident command system structure, and EMS is one of the components in that structure. Prehospital care providers must know and understand the ICS and their role within that system.
- Prehospital care providers must take precautionary steps to avoid contamination by bloodborne pathogens, including hepatitis viruses and HIV. Key considerations include using standard precautions, employing physical barriers, washing hands, and preventing sharps injury.
- Prehospital care providers faced with multiple victims must be prepared to triage patients based on the severity of their condition and resources available.

SCENARIO RECAP

You are dispatched to the scene of a domestic altercation. It is 0245 hours on a hot summer night. As you arrive on the scene of a single-family dwelling, you can hear a man and woman arguing loudly and the sounds of children crying in the background. Police have been dispatched to this call but have not yet arrived at the location.

- What are your concerns about the scene?
- What considerations are important before you contact the patient?

SCENARIO SOLUTION

Assessment of the scene reveals several potential hazards. Domestic violence incidents are among the most hazardous to emergency responders. These incidents often escalate and can lead to assault of emergency responders. Therefore, the presence of law enforcement should be considered prior to entering the scene. As with all trauma cases, a bloody patient exposes prehospital care providers to the risks of bloodborne infections, and the providers should wear physical barriers, including gloves, masks, and eye protection.

In this case, you wait until the police arrive before entering the home. Upon entering the house, you note that the female has obvious multiple bruises on her face and a small laceration over one cheek. The officers take the male into custody. You perform your primary survey, which reveals no life threats. The secondary survey does not reveal any additional injuries. You transport the patient to the closest hospital without incident.

References

1. Reichard A, Marsh S, Moore P. Fatal and nonfatal injuries among emergency medical technicians and paramedics. *Prehosp Emerg Care*. 2011;15(4):511-517.
2. National Incident Management System. U.S. Department of Homeland Security. *National Incident Management System*. December 2008. https://www.fema.gov/pdf/emergency/nims/NIMS_core.pdf. Accessed October 16, 2017.
3. Centers for Disease Control and Prevention. Updated U.S. Public Health Service guidelines for the management of occupational exposures to HBV, HCV, and HIV and recommendations for postexposure prophylaxis. *MMWR*. June 29, 2001;50(RR11):1-42.
4. Chen SL, Morgan TR. The natural history of hepatitis C virus (HCV) infection. *Int J Med Sci*. 2006;3(2):47-52.
5. Bell J, Batey RG, Farrell GC, Crewe EB, Cunningham AL, Byth K. Hepatitis C virus in intravenous drug users. *Med J Aust*. 1990 Sep 3;153(5):274-276.
6. Poland GA, Jacobson RM. Prevention of hepatitis B with the hepatitis B vaccine. *N Engl J Med*. 2004;351:2832.
7. U.S. Department of Health and Human Services, Centers for Disease Control and Prevention. Exposure to blood: what healthcare personnel need to know. July 2003. https://www.cdc.gov/hai/pdfs/bbp/exp_to_blood.pdf. Accessed October 16, 2017.
8. Lerner EB, Schwartz RB, Coule PL, et al. Mass casualty triage: an evaluation of the data and development of a proposed national guideline. *Disaster Med Pub Health Prep*. 2008;2:S25-S34.

Suggested Reading

Centers for Disease Control and Prevention: See website for information on standard precautions and postexposure prophylaxis, http://www.cdc.gov.

Rinnert KJ. A review of infection control practices, risk reduction, and legislative regulations for blood-borne disease: applications for emergency medical services. *Prehosp Emerg Care*. 1998;2(1):70.

Rinnert KJ, O'Connor RE, Delbridge T. Risk reduction for exposure to blood-borne pathogens in EMS: National Association of EMS Physicians. *Prehosp Emerg Care*. 1998;2(1):62.

CHAPTER 6

Patient Assessment and Management

Lead Editors:
Vince Mosesso, MD, FACEP
Michael Holtz, MD

CHAPTER OBJECTIVES

At the completion of this chapter, you will be able to do the following:

- Relate the significance of patient assessment in the context of overall management of the trauma patient.
- Explain how to perform a rapid primary survey, as well as how assessment and management are integrated during the primary survey.

- Describe the components of the secondary survey and when it is used in the assessment of the trauma patient.
- Utilize the Field Triage Decision Scheme to determine the destination for a trauma patient.

SCENARIO

It is a Saturday morning in early November. The weather is clear, with an outside temperature of 42°F (5.5°C). Your squad is dispatched to a residential area for a person who has fallen from the roof of a two-story building. Upon arrival at the scene, you are met by an adult family member who leads you around the house to the backyard. The family member states the patient was cleaning leaves from the rain gutters with a leaf blower when he lost his balance and fell approximately 12 feet (ft; 3.6 meters [m]) from the roof, landing on his back. The patient initially lost consciousness for a "brief period" but was conscious by the time the family member called 9-1-1.

Approaching the patient, you observe an approximately 40-year-old man lying supine on the ground with two bystanders kneeling by his side. The patient is conscious and talking with the bystanders. You do not see any signs of severe bleeding. As your partner provides manual stabilization to the patient's head and neck, you ask the patient where he hurts. The patient states both his upper and lower back hurt the most.

Your initial questioning serves the multiple purposes of obtaining the patient's chief complaint, determining his initial level of consciousness, and assessing his ventilatory effort. Detecting no shortness of breath, you proceed with the patient assessment. The patient answers your questions appropriately to establish that he is oriented to person, place, and time.

- Based on the physics of trauma as they relate to this incident, what potential injuries do you anticipate finding during your assessment?
- What are your next priorities?
- How will you proceed with this patient?

INTRODUCTION

Assessment is the cornerstone of all patient care. For the trauma patient, as for other critically ill patients, assessment is the foundation on which all management and transport decisions are based. An overall impression of a patient's status is developed, and baseline values for the status of the patient's respiratory, circulatory, and neurologic systems are established. When life-threatening conditions are identified, immediate intervention and resuscitation are initiated. If time and the patient's condition allow, a secondary survey is conducted for injuries that are not life or limb threatening. Often this secondary survey occurs during patient transport.

All of these steps are performed quickly and efficiently with a goal of minimizing time spent on the scene. Critical patients should not remain in the field for care other than to manage immediate life threats, unless they are trapped or other complications exist that prevent early transport. By applying the principles learned in this course, on-scene delay can be minimized, and patients can be moved rapidly to an appropriate medical facility. Successful assessment and intervention require a strong knowledge base of trauma physiology and a well-developed plan of management that is carried out quickly and effectively.

The trauma management literature frequently mentions the need to transport the trauma patient to definitive surgical care within a minimum amount of time after the onset of the injury. This urgency is because a critical trauma patient who does not respond to initial therapy may be bleeding internally. This blood loss will continue until the hemorrhage is controlled. Definitive hemorrhage control for most serious bleeding is best accomplished in the hospital setting.

The primary concerns for assessment and management of the trauma patient are (1) major hemorrhage control, (2) airway, (3) oxygenation, (4) ventilation, (5) perfusion, and (6) neurologic function. This sequence protects both the ability of the body to oxygenate and the ability of the red blood cells (RBCs) to deliver oxygen to the tissues.

R Adams Cowley, MD, developed the concept of the "Golden Hour" of trauma. He believed that the time between injury occurrence and definitive care was critical. During this period, when bleeding is uncontrolled and inadequate tissue oxygenation is occurring because of decreased perfusion, damage occurs throughout the body. Dr. Cowley believed that if bleeding was not controlled and tissue oxygenation was not restored rapidly after injury, the patient's chances of survival dramatically decreased.

The Golden Hour is now referred to as the "Golden Period" because this critical period of time is not literally 1 hour. Some patients have less than an hour in which to receive care, whereas others have more time. The prehospital care provider is responsible for recognizing the urgency of a given situation and transporting a patient as quickly as possible to a facility in which definitive care can be accomplished. To deliver the trauma patient to definitive care, the seriousness of the patient's life-threatening injuries must be quickly identified; only essential, lifesaving care provided at the scene; and rapid transport initiated to an appropriate medical facility. In many urban prehospital systems, the average time between activation of emergency services and arrival to the scene is 8 to 9 minutes, not including the time between the injury and the call to the public safety answering point. Usually another 8 to 9 minutes are spent transporting the patient. If the providers spend only 10 minutes on the scene, over 30 minutes of time will have already passed by the time a patient arrives at the receiving facility. Every additional minute spent on the scene is additional time that the patient is bleeding, and valuable time is ticking away from the Golden Hour, or Period.

To address this critical trauma management issue, rapid, efficient evaluation and management of the patient are the ultimate objectives. Scene time should be minimized, and while the "platinum 10 minutes" is not directly supported by research, there is evidence that correlates scene time with mortality.[1]

The longer the patient is kept on scene, the greater the potential for blood loss and death. Extended scene times should occur only for extenuating circumstances, such as prolonged extrication, scene hazards, and other unexpected situations. Almost nothing should impede the progress of the bleeding trauma patient in moving toward the operating room.

This chapter covers the essentials of patient assessment and initial management in the field and is based on the approach taught to physicians in the Advanced Trauma Life Support (ATLS) program.[2] In addition, the approach taught in Prehospital Trauma Life Support (PHTLS) reflects the differences in prehospital care versus the in-hospital care taught in ATLS. The principles described are identical to those learned in initial basic- or advanced-provider training programs, although different terminology may occasionally be used. For example, the phrase *primary survey* is used in the ATLS program to describe the patient assessment activity known as *primary assessment* in the National EMS Education Standards. For the most part, the activities performed in this phase are exactly the same; various courses simply use different terminology.

Establishing Priorities

There are three immediate priorities on arrival to a scene:

1. The first priority for everyone involved at a trauma incident is assessment of the scene and scene safety. Personal protective equipment (PPE)

appropriate to the situation should be donned, and standard precautions (for protection from blood and body fluids) should be followed. The Scene Assessment chapter discusses this topic in detail.

2. Responders must recognize the existence of multiple-patient incidents and mass-casualty incidents (MCIs). In an MCI, the priority shifts from focusing all resources on the most injured patient to saving the maximum number of patients (providing the greatest good to the greatest number). Factors that may impact the triage decisions when there are multiple patients include severity of the injuries and the resources (manpower and equipment) available to care for the patients. The Scene Management chapter and the Disaster Management chapter also discuss triage.

3. Once a brief scene assessment has been performed and pertinent needs addressed, attention can be turned to evaluating individual patients. The assessment and management process begins by focusing on the patient or patients who have been identified as most critical, as resources allow. Emphasis is placed on the following, in this order: (a) conditions that may result in the loss of life, (b) conditions that may result in the loss of limb, and (c) all other conditions that do not threaten life or limb. Depending on the severity of the injury, the number of injured patients, and the proximity to the receiving facility, conditions that do not threaten life or limb may never be addressed at the scene.

Most of this chapter focuses on the critical-thinking skills required to conduct a proper assessment, interpret the findings, and set priorities for proper patient care. This process will allow for the appropriate provision of needed interventions.

Primary Survey

In the critical multisystem trauma patient, the priority for care is the rapid identification and management of life-threatening conditions (**Box 6-1**). The overwhelming majority of trauma patients have injuries that involve only one system (e.g., an isolated limb fracture). For these single-system trauma patients, there is more often time to be thorough in both the primary and the secondary surveys. For the critically injured patient, the prehospital care provider may not be able to conduct more than just a primary survey. In these critical patients, the emphasis is on rapid evaluation, initiation of resuscitation, and transport to an appropriate medical facility. The emphasis on rapid transport does not eliminate the need for prehospital treatment. Rather, treatment should be done faster

> **Box 6-1** Multisystem Versus Single-System Trauma Patient
>
> - A **multisystem trauma patient** has injuries involving more than one body system, including the pulmonary, circulatory, neurologic, gastrointestinal, musculoskeletal, and integumentary systems. An example would be a patient involved in a motor vehicle crash who has a traumatic brain injury (TBI), pulmonary contusions, a splenic injury with shock, and a femur fracture.
> - A **single-system trauma patient** has injury to only one body system. An example would be a patient with an isolated ankle fracture and no evidence of blood loss or shock. Patients often have more than one injury within that single system.

and more efficiently and possibly started en route to the receiving facility.

Quick establishment of priorities and the initial evaluation and recognition of life-threatening injuries must become ingrained in the prehospital care provider. Therefore, the components of the primary and secondary surveys need to be memorized and the logical progression of priority-based assessment and treatment understood and performed the same way every time, regardless of the severity of the injury. The provider must think about the pathophysiology of a patient's injuries and conditions.

One of the most common life-threatening conditions in trauma is lack of adequate tissue oxygenation (shock), which leads to anaerobic (without oxygen) metabolism. Metabolism is the mechanism by which cells produce energy. Four steps are necessary for normal metabolism: (1) an adequate amount of RBCs, (2) oxygenation of RBCs in the lungs, (3) delivery of RBCs to the cells throughout the body, and (4) off-loading of oxygen to these cells. The activities involved in the primary survey are aimed at identifying and correcting problems with these steps.

General Impression

The primary survey begins with a rapid global overview of the status of a patient's respiratory, circulatory, and neurologic systems to identify obvious threats to life or limb, such as evidence of severe compressible hemorrhage; airway, breathing, or circulation compromise; or gross deformities. When initially approaching a patient, the prehospital care provider looks for severe compressible hemorrhage and observes whether the patient appears to be moving air effectively, is awake or unresponsive, and is moving spontaneously. Once at the patient's side, the provider introduces him- or herself to the patient and asks the patient's name. A reasonable next step is to ask the patient, "What happened to you?" If the patient appears comfortable and answers with a coherent explanation in complete sentences, the provider can conclude that the patient has a **patent airway**, sufficient respiratory function to support speech, adequate cerebral perfusion, and reasonable neurologic functioning; that is, there are probably no immediate threats to this patient's life.

If a patient is unable to provide such an answer or appears in distress, a detailed primary survey to identify life-threatening problems is begun. Within a few seconds, a general impression of the patient's overall condition has been obtained. By rapidly assessing vital functions, the primary survey serves to establish whether the patient is presently or imminently in a critical condition.

Sequence of Primary Survey

The primary survey must proceed rapidly and in a logical order. If the prehospital care provider is alone, some key interventions may be performed as life-threatening conditions are identified. If the problem is easily correctable, such as suctioning an airway or placing a tourniquet, the provider may opt to address the issue before moving on to the next step. Conversely, if the problem cannot be quickly addressed at the scene, such as shock resulting from suspected internal hemorrhage, the remainder of the primary survey is expeditiously completed. If more than one provider is present, one provider may complete the primary survey while others initiate care for the problems identified. When several critical conditions are identified, the primary survey allows the provider to establish treatment priorities. In general, compressible external hemorrhage is managed first, an airway issue is managed before a breathing problem, and so forth.

The same primary survey approach is utilized regardless of the patient type. All patients, including elderly, pediatric, or pregnant patients, are assessed in a similar fashion to ensure that all components of the assessment are covered and that no significant pathology is missed.

Similar to ACLS, in which the priority of the primary survey has changed from ABC to CAB, the primary survey of the trauma patient now emphasizes control of life-threatening external bleeding as the first step in the sequence. While the steps of the primary survey are taught and displayed in a sequential manner, many of the steps can, and should, be performed simultaneously. The steps can be remembered using the mnemonic XABCDE:

- X—Exsanguinating hemorrhage (control of severe external bleeding)
- A—Airway management and cervical spine stabilization
- B—Breathing (ventilation and oxygenation)
- C—Circulation (perfusion and other hemorrhage)
- D—Disability
- E—Expose/environment

X—Exsanguinating Hemorrhage (Control of Severe External Bleeding)

In the primary survey of a trauma patient, life-threatening external hemorrhage must be immediately identified and managed. If exsanguinating external hemorrhage is present, it must be controlled even before assessing the airway (or simultaneously, if adequate assistance is present at the scene) or performing other interventions, such as spinal immobilization. This type of bleeding typically involves arterial bleeding from an extremity but may also occur from the scalp or at the junction of an extremity with the trunk (junctional bleeding) and other sites.

Exsanguinating arterial hemorrhage from an extremity is best managed by immediately placing a tourniquet as proximal as possible (i.e., near the groin or axilla) on the affected extremity. Other bleeding control measures, such as direct pressure and hemostatic agents, may also be used but should not delay or take the place of tourniquet placement in such cases. Direct pressure and hemostatic packing and dressings should be applied in cases of nonarterial severe bleeding in extremities and severe bleeding from truncal sites. Occasionally, bleeding from distal or smaller arteries can be controlled with focal direct compression of the artery. However, this should only be performed if such bleeding can be controlled with a rapidly applied pressure dressing or if sufficient personnel are present on scene such that one prehospital care provider can maintain manual direct pressure. If not, a tourniquet should be applied to the affected extremity. Severe bleeding from junctional areas may be managed by placing an appropriate junctional tourniquet, if available, or packing with hemostatic gauze and placing pressure dressing (**Box 6-2**).

Hemorrhage Control

External hemorrhage is identified and controlled in the primary survey because if severe bleeding is not controlled as soon as possible, the potential for the patient's death increases dramatically. The three types of external hemorrhage are capillary, venous, and arterial, which are described as follows:

1. *Capillary bleeding* is caused by abrasions that have scraped open the tiny capillaries just below the skin's surface. Capillary bleeding is generally not life threatening and may have slowed or even stopped before the arrival of prehospital care providers.
2. *Venous bleeding* is caused by laceration or other injury to a vein, which leads to steady flow of dark red blood from the wound. This type of bleeding is usually controllable with direct pressure.

Box 6-2 Severe Bleeding at Junctional Locations

Junctional hemorrhage is defined as bleeding that occurs where two anatomically distinct zones come together. Examples of junctional areas include the lower abdomen, groin, axillae, and proximal extremities (**Figure 6-1**). The use of a tourniquet or pressure dressing in these areas is often both impractical and ineffective.

The key treatment for junctional hemorrhage is direct compression of the large vessels that span the area proximal to the injury. In the prehospital setting, a significant amount of direct pressure to the femoral, iliac, or axillary arteries may be necessary to slow the bleeding. This is often combined with the use of externally applied hemostatic agents and pressure dressings. Additionally, evidence supports the empiric application of a pelvic binder in the patient with traumatic amputation of the lower extremity above the level of the knee to aid in bleeding control.[3] The significant forces encountered in these traumatic injuries often damage the adjoining structures, such as the pelvic and shoulder girdle; thus stabilization of these areas should also be considered.

The Committee on Tactical Combat Casualty Care (CoTCCC) recommends three tourniquets purpose-built for use at junctional hemorrhage sites. These include the Combat Ready Clamp (CRoC), Junctional Emergency Treatment Tool (JETT), and SAM Junctional Tourniquet (SJT). Various advantages and disadvantages have been identified in studies comparing these devices in the laboratory setting, all of which should be taken into consideration when choosing a device with which to equip field personnel.[3-7]

The most important concepts to consider when attempting to control bleeding at junctional sites are (1) that a large amount of direct pressure and compression to the blood vessels spanning the area will be necessary, and (2) a direct pressure dressing, ideally with a hemostatic agent, should be placed on the open surface of the wound. When these two techniques are combined, they offer increased chances for survival in what is otherwise often a fatal traumatic injury.[8] The bottom line is: You need to get a pressure dressing on the injury and pressure on bleeding arterial points as soon as possible.

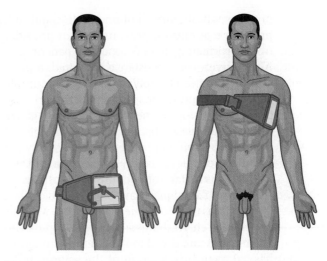

Figure 6-1 The junctional areas at the axillae and inguinal regions.

Venous bleeding is usually not life threatening unless bleeding is prolonged or a large vein is involved.

3. *Arterial bleeding* is caused by an injury that has lacerated an artery. This is the most important and most difficult type of blood loss to control. It is generally characterized by spurting blood that is bright red in color. However, arterial bleeding may also present as blood that rapidly "pours out" of a wound if a deep artery is injured. Even a small, deep arterial puncture wound can produce life-threatening blood loss.

Rapid control of bleeding is one of the most important goals in the care of a trauma patient. The primary survey cannot advance unless external hemorrhage is controlled. Hemorrhage can be controlled in the following ways:

1. *Direct pressure*. Direct pressure is exactly what the name implies—applying pressure to the site of bleeding. This is accomplished by placing a dressing (e.g., hemostatic gauze is preferred) directly over the site of bleeding (if it can be identified) and applying pressure. Pressure should be applied as precisely and focally as possible. A finger on a visible compressible artery is very effective. Pressure should be applied continuously for at a minimum of 3 minutes or per the manufacturer's instructions and for 10 minutes if using plain gauze; prehospital care providers should avoid the temptation to remove pressure to check if the wound is bleeding before that time period. The application and maintenance of direct

pressure will require all of one prehospital care provider's attention, preventing that provider from participating in other aspects of patient care. Alternatively, or if assistance is limited, a pressure dressing can be applied. There are multiple commercial options (e.g., Israeli bandage), or a pressure dressing can be fashioned out of gauze pads and an elastic bandage. If bleeding is not controlled, it will not matter how much oxygen or fluid the patient receives; perfusion will not improve in the face of ongoing hemorrhage.

2. *Tourniquets.* Tourniquets have often been described in the past as the technique of last resort. Military experience in Afghanistan and Iraq, plus the routine and safe use of tourniquets by surgeons, has led to reconsideration of this approach.[9-11] Tourniquets are very effective in controlling severe hemorrhage and should be used if direct pressure or a pressure dressing fails to control hemorrhage from an extremity or if sufficient personnel are not available on scene to perform other bleeding control methods. (See the Shock: Pathophysiology of Life and Death chapter.) The use of "elevation" and pressure on "pressure points" is no longer recommended because of insufficient data supporting their effectiveness.[12,13] As noted previously, in the case of life-threatening or exsanguinating hemorrhage, a tourniquet should be applied instead of, or concurrent with, other bleeding control measures (i.e., as a first-line treatment for this type of bleeding) Also note that improvised tourniquets may have more limited effectiveness than commercially available verisons.[14]

A—Airway Management and Cervical Spine Stabilization

Airway

The patient's airway is quickly checked to ensure that it is **patent** (open and clear) and that no danger of obstruction exists. If the airway is compromised, it will have to be opened, initially using manual methods (trauma chin lift or trauma jaw thrust), and cleared of blood, body substances, and foreign bodies, if necessary (**Figure 6-2**). Eventually, as equipment and time become available, airway management can advance to include suction and mechanical means (oral airway, nasal airway, supraglottic airways, and endotracheal intubation or transtracheal methods). Numerous factors play a role in determining the method of airway management, including available equipment, the skill level of the prehospital care provider, and the distance from the trauma center. Some airway injuries, such as a laryngeal fracture or incomplete airway transection, can be aggravated by attempts at endotracheal intubation.

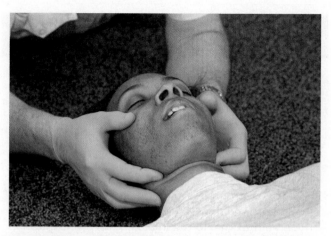

Figure 6-2 If the airway appears compromised, it must be opened while continuing to protect the spine.
© National Association of Emergency Medical Technicians (NAEMT).

Airway management is discussed in detail in the Airway and Ventilation chapter.

Cervical Spine Stabilization

Every trauma patient with a significant blunt mechanism of injury is suspected of spinal injury until spinal injury is conclusively ruled out. It is particularly important to maintain a high index of suspicion for spinal injury in elderly or chronically debilitated patients, even with more minor mechanisms of injury. (See the Spinal Trauma chapter for a complete list of indications for spinal immobilization.) Therefore, when establishing an open airway, the possibility of cervical spine injury must always be considered. Excessive movement in any direction could either produce or aggravate neurologic damage because bony compression of the spinal cord may occur in the presence of a fractured spine. The solution is to ensure that the patient's head and neck are manually maintained (stabilized) in the neutral position during the entire assessment process, especially when opening the airway and administering necessary ventilation. This need for stabilization does not mean that necessary airway maintenance procedures cannot be applied. Instead, it means that the procedures will be performed while protecting the patient's spine from unnecessary movement. If spinal immobilization devices that were placed need to be removed in order to reassess the patient or perform some necessary intervention, manual stabilization of the head and neck is employed until the patient can again be placed in spinal immobilization.

B—Breathing (Ventilation and Oxygenation)

Breathing functions to effectively deliver oxygen to a patient's lungs to help maintain the aerobic metabolic process. Hypoxia can result from inadequate ventilation of the lungs and leads to lack of oxygenation of the patient's tissues. Once the patient's airway is open, the quality and quantity of the patient's breathing (ventilation) can be evaluated as follows:

1. Check to see if the patient is breathing by looking for chest motion and feeling for air movement from the mouth or nose. If uncertain, auscultate both sides of the chest to evaluate for spontaneous air movement.

2. If the patient is not breathing (i.e., is **apneic**), immediately begin assisting ventilations (while maintaining cervical spine stabilization in a neutral position, when indicated) with a bag-mask device with supplemental oxygen before continuing the assessment.

3. Ensure that the patient's airway is patent, continue assisted ventilation, and prepare to insert an oral, nasal (if no severe facial trauma), or supraglottic airway (if no signs of severe oropharyngeal trauma); intubate; or provide other means of mechanical airway protection. Be prepared to suction blood, vomitus, or other fluids from the airway.

4. Although commonly referred to as the "respiratory rate," a more correct term for how fast a patient is breathing is "ventilatory rate." Ventilation refers to the process of inhalation and exhalation, whereas respiration best describes the physiologic process of gas exchange between the capillaries and the alveoli. This text uses the term *ventilatory rate* rather than respiratory rate. If the patient is breathing, estimate the adequacy of the ventilatory rate and depth to determine whether the patient is moving enough air (recall that minute ventilation is rate × depth). (See the Airway and Ventilation chapter.)

5. Ensure that the patient is not hypoxic and that the oxygen saturation is greater than or equal to 94%. Supplemental oxygen (and assisted ventilation) is provided as needed to maintain an adequate oxygen saturation.

6. If the patient is conscious, listen to the patient talk to assess whether he or she can speak a full sentence without difficulty.

The ventilatory rate can be divided into the following five categories:

1. *Apneic.* The patient is not breathing. This includes occasional agonal gasps, which do not effectively result in air exchange.

2. *Slow.* A very slow ventilatory rate, below 10 breaths/minute (**bradypnea**), may indicate severe injury to or ischemia (decreased supply of oxygen) of the brain. In these cases, the provider must assure adequate volume of air exchange is occurring. Often it will be necessary to either assist or completely take over the patient's breathing with a bag-mask device. Assisted or total ventilatory support with

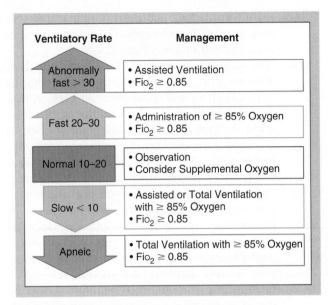

Figure 6-3 Airway management based on spontaneous ventilation rate.

the bag-mask device should include supplemental oxygen to ensure an oxygen saturation greater than or equal to 94% (**Figure 6-3**).

3. *Normal.* If the ventilatory rate is between 10 and 20 breaths/minute (**eupnea**, a normal rate for an adult), the prehospital care provider watches the patient closely. Although the patient may appear stable, supplemental oxygen should be considered.

4. *Fast.* If the ventilatory rate is between 20 and 30 breaths/minute (**tachypnea**), the patient must be watched closely to see whether he or she is improving or deteriorating. The drive for increasing the ventilatory rate is increased accumulation of carbon dioxide in the blood or a decreased level of blood oxygen (due to hypoxia or anemia). When a patient displays an abnormal ventilatory rate, the cause must be investigated. A rapid rate may indicate that not enough oxygen is reaching the body tissue. This lack of oxygen initiates anaerobic metabolism (see Shock: Pathophysiology of Life and Death chapter) and, ultimately, an increase in the carbon dioxide level in the blood leading to metabolic acidosis. The body's detection system recognizes this increased level of carbon dioxide and tells the ventilatory system to increase depth and volume to eliminate this excess. Therefore, an increased ventilatory rate may indicate that the patient needs better perfusion or oxygenation, or both. Administration of supplemental oxygen to achieve an oxygen saturation of 94% or greater is indicated for this patient—at least until the patient's overall status is determined. The prehospital care provider must

remain concerned about the patient's ability to maintain adequate ventilation and alert for any deterioration in overall condition.

5. *Extremely fast.* A ventilatory rate greater than 30 breaths/minute (severe tachypnea) indicates hypoxia, anaerobic metabolism, or both, with a resultant **acidosis**. A search for the cause of the rapid ventilatory rate should begin at once to ascertain if the etiology is a primary ventilatory problem or an RBC delivery problem. Injuries that can produce major impairment in oxygenation and ventilation include tension pneumothorax, flail chest with pulmonary contusion, massive hemothorax, and open pneumothorax. Once the cause is identified, the intervention must occur immediately to correct the problem. (See the Thoracic Trauma chapter.) Patients with ventilatory rates greater than 30 breaths/minute should be placed on oxygen. Carefully monitor these patients for fatigue or signs of inadequate ventilation such as decreasing mental status, elevation of end-tidal carbon dioxide levels, or low oxygen saturation, and assist ventilations with a bag-mask device as needed to obtain adequate oxygen saturation.

In the patient with abnormal ventilation, the chest must be exposed, observed, and palpated rapidly. Then, auscultation of the lungs will identify abnormal, diminished, or absent breath sounds. Injuries that may impede ventilation include tension pneumothorax, flail chest, spinal cord injuries, and TBIs. These injuries should be identified or suspected during the primary survey and require that ventilatory support be initiated at once. Needle decompression should be performed immediately if tension pneumothorax is suspected.

When assessing the trauma patient's ventilatory status, the ventilatory *depth* as well as the rate is assessed. A patient can be breathing at a normal ventilatory rate of 16 breaths/minute but have a greatly decreased ventilatory depth. Conversely, a patient can have a normal ventilatory depth but an increased or decreased ventilatory rate. The tidal volume is multiplied by the ventilatory rate to calculate the patient's minute ventilation volume. (See the Airway and Ventilation chapter.)

In some circumstances, it may be difficult for even experienced prehospital care providers to differentiate an airway problem from a breathing problem. In such cases, an attempt may be made to establish a secure airway. If the problem persists after management of the airway, it is most likely a breathing problem that is impairing ventilation.

C—Circulation and Bleeding (Perfusion and Internal Hemorrhage)

Assessing for circulatory system compromise or failure is the next step in caring for the trauma patient. Oxygenation of the RBCs without delivery to the tissue cells is of no benefit to the patient. In the first step of the sequence, life-threatening bleeding was identified and controlled. After subsequently assessing the patient's airway and breathing status, the prehospital care provider can obtain an adequate overall estimate of the patient's cardiac output and perfusion status. Hemorrhage—either external or internal—is the most common cause of preventable death from trauma.

Perfusion

The patient's overall circulatory status can be determined by checking peripheral pulses and evaluating skin color, temperature, and moisture (**Box 6-3**). Assessment of perfusion may be challenging in elderly or pediatric patients or in those who are well conditioned or on certain medications. Shock in trauma patients is almost always due to hemorrhage. (Refer to the Shock: Pathophysiology of Life and Death chapter.)

The potential sites of massive internal hemorrhage include the chest (both pleural cavities), the abdomen (peritoneal cavity), the pelvis, the retroperitoneal space, and the extremities (primarily the thighs). If internal hemorrhage is suspected, the thorax, abdomen, pelvis, and thighs are exposed to quickly inspect and palpate for signs of injury. Hemorrhage in these areas is not easy to control outside the hospital. If available, a pelvic binder should be applied rapidly to prevent potential "open book" pelvic injuries. The goal is rapid delivery of the patient to a facility equipped and appropriately staffed for rapid control of hemorrhage in the operating room (i.e., the highest level trauma center available).

Box 6-3 Capillary Refilling Time

The capillary refilling time is checked by pressing over the nail beds and then releasing the pressure. This downward pressure removes the blood from the visible capillary bed. The rate of return of blood to the nail beds after releasing pressure (refilling time) is a tool for estimating blood flow through this most distal part of the circulation. A capillary refilling time of greater than 2 seconds may indicate that the capillary beds are not receiving adequate perfusion. However, capillary refilling time by itself is a poor indicator of shock because it is influenced by many other factors. For example, peripheral vascular disease (arteriosclerosis), cold temperatures, the use of pharmacologic vasodilators or constrictors, or the presence of neurogenic shock can skew the results. Measuring the capillary refilling time becomes a less useful check of cardiovascular function in these cases. Capillary refilling time has a place in the evaluation of circulatory adequacy, but it should always be used in conjunction with other physical examination findings (e.g., blood pressure).

Pulse

The pulse is evaluated for presence, quality, and regularity. A quick check of the pulse reveals whether the patient has tachycardia, bradycardia, or an irregular rhythm. In the past, the presence of a radial pulse has been thought to indicate a systolic blood pressure of at least 80 mm Hg, with the presence of a femoral pulse indicating blood pressure of at least 70 mm Hg, and the presence of only a carotid pulse indicating blood pressure of 60 mm Hg. Evidence has shown this theory to be inaccurate and to actually overestimate blood pressures.[15] While the absence of peripheral pulses in the presence of central pulses likely represents profound hypotension, the presence of peripheral pulses should not be overly reassuring regarding the patient's blood pressure.

In the primary survey, determination of an exact pulse rate is not necessary. Instead, a rough estimate is rapidly obtained, and the actual pulse rate is obtained later in the process. In trauma patients, it is important to consider treatable causes of abnormal vital signs and physical findings. For example, the combination of compromised perfusion and impaired breathing should prompt the prehospital care provider to consider the presence of a tension pneumothorax. If clinical signs are present, needle decompression can be lifesaving. (See the Thoracic Trauma chapter.)

Skin

The skin examination can reveal a great deal about a patient's circulatory status.

- *Color.* Adequate perfusion produces a pinkish hue to the skin. Skin becomes pale when blood is shunted away from an area. Pale coloration is associated with poor perfusion. Bluish coloration indicates poor oxygenation. The bluish color is caused by perfusion with deoxygenated blood to that region of the body. Skin pigmentation can often make this determination difficult. In patients with deeply pigmented skin, examination of the color of nail beds, palms/soles, and mucous membranes helps overcome this challenge because changes in color usually first appear in the lips, gums, or fingertips due to relative lack of pigmentation in these areas.
- *Temperature.* As with overall skin evaluation, skin temperature is influenced by environmental conditions. Cool skin indicates decreased perfusion, regardless of the cause. Skin temperature can be assessed with a simple touch of the patient's skin with the back of the hand. Normal skin temperature is warm to the touch, neither cool nor hot.
- *Condition.* Under normal circumstances, skin is usually dry. Moist, cool skin can occur in patients with poor perfusion due to sympathetic stimulation (diaphoresis). However, it is important to consider ambient conditions when evaluating skin findings. A patient in a hot or humid environment may have moist skin at baseline, regardless of severity of injury.

D—Disability

After evaluating and correcting, to the extent possible, the factors involved in delivering oxygen to the lungs and circulating it throughout the body, the next step in the primary survey is assessment of cerebral function, which is an indirect measurement of cerebral oxygenation. This begins with determining the patient's level of consciousness (LOC).

The prehospital care provider should assume that a confused, belligerent, combative, or uncooperative patient is hypoxic or has suffered a TBI until proved otherwise. Most patients want help when their lives are medically threatened. If a patient refuses help, the reason must be questioned. Does the patient feel threatened by the presence of a provider on the scene? If so, further attempts to establish rapport will often help to gain the patient's trust. If nothing in the situation seems to be threatening, the source of the behavior should be considered physiologic and reversible conditions identified and treated. During the assessment, the history can help determine whether the patient lost consciousness at any time since the injury occurred, whether toxic substances might be involved (and what they might be), and whether the patient has any preexisting conditions that may produce a decreased LOC or aberrant behavior. Careful observation of the scene can provide invaluable information in this regard.

A decreased LOC alerts a prehospital care provider to the following possibilities:

1. Decreased cerebral oxygenation (caused by hypoxia/hypoperfusion) or severe hypoventilation (carbon dioxide narcosis)
2. Central nervous system (CNS) injury (e.g., TBI)
3. Drug or alcohol overdose or toxin exposure
4. Metabolic derangement (e.g., caused by diabetes, seizure, or cardiac arrest)

A more in-depth discussion about altered mental status can be found in the Head Injury chapter, including a thorough explanation of the Glasgow Coma Scale (GCS). Recent research found that using only the Motor component of the GCS, and specifically if this component is less than 6 (meaning the patient does not follow commands), is just as predictive for severe injury as using the whole GCS. So, at this point in the primary survey it would be sufficiently informative to simply determine whether the patient follows commands or not.[16]

The GCS score is a tool used for determining LOC and is preferred over the AVPU classification (**Box 6-4**).[17] It is a quick, simple method for determining cerebral function and is predictive of patient outcome, especially the best motor response. It also provides a baseline of cerebral function for serial neurologic evaluations. The GCS score is divided into three sections: (1) *eye* opening, (2) *verbal* response, and (3) *motor* response. The patient is assigned a score according to the *best* response to each component of

Box 6-4 The AVPU System

The mnemonic AVPU is often used to describe the patient's LOC. In this system, A stands for *alert*, V for responds to *verbal* stimulus, P for responds to *painful* stimulus, and U for *unresponsive*. This approach, although simple, fails to provide information regarding specifically *how* the patient responds to verbal or painful stimuli. In other words, if the patient responds to verbal questioning, is the patient oriented, confused, or mumbling incomprehensibly? Likewise, when the patient responds to painful stimulus, does the patient localize, withdraw, or demonstrate decorticate or decerebrate posturing? Because of its lack of precision, the use of AVPU has fallen out of favor.

Eye Opening	**Points**
Spontaneous eye opening	4
Eye opening on command	3
Eye opening to pressure	2
No eye opening	1
Best Verbal Response	
Answers appropriately (oriented)	5
Gives confused answers	4
Inappropriate words	3
Makes unintelligible noises	2
Makes no verbal response	1
Best Motor Response	
Follows command	6
Localizes	5
Normal flexion response	4
Abnormal flexion response	3
Extension response	2
Gives no motor response	1
Total	

Figure 6-4 Glasgow Coma Scale (GCS).

the GCS (**Figure 6-4**). For example, if a patient's right eye is so severely swollen that the patient cannot open it, but the left eye opens spontaneously, the patient receives a 4 for the best eye movement. If a patient lacks spontaneous eye opening, the prehospital care provider should use a verbal command (e.g., "Open your eyes"). If the patient does not respond to a verbal stimulus, a painful stimulus, such as pressing the nail bed with a pen or squeezing the axillary tissue, can be applied.

The patient's verbal response is determined by using a question such as, "What happened to you?" If fully oriented, the patient will supply a coherent answer. Otherwise, the patient's verbal response is scored as confused, inappropriate, unintelligible, or absent. If a patient is intubated, the GCS score includes a 1 to reflect the lack of a verbal response, the eye and motor scales are calculated and added, and the letter T is added to note the inability to assess the verbal response (e.g., 8T).

The third component of the GCS is the motor score. A simple, unambiguous command, such as, "Hold up two fingers" or "Show me a thumbs-up," is given to the patient. If the patient complies with the command, the highest score of 6 is given. A patient who squeezes or grasps the finger of a prehospital care provider may simply be demonstrating a grasping reflex and not purposefully following a command. If the patient fails to follow a command, a painful stimulus, as noted previously, should be used, and the patient's best motor response should be scored. A patient who attempts to push away a painful stimulus is considered to be *localizing*. Other possible responses to pain include withdrawal from the stimulus, abnormal flexion (*decorticate posturing*) or extension (*decerebrate posturing*) of the upper extremities, or absence of motor function.

The maximum GCS score is 15, indicating a patient with no disability. The lowest score of 3 is generally an ominous sign. A score of less than 8 indicates a major injury, 9 to 12 a moderate injury, and 13 to 15 a minor injury. A GCS score of 8 or less is an indication for considering active airway management of the patient. The prehospital care provider can easily calculate and relate the individual components of the score and should include them in the verbal report to the receiving facility as well as in the patient care report. Often, it is preferable to communicate individual components of the GCS scale rather than just the total score, as specific changes can then be documented. A patient care report that states that "the patient is E4, V4, M6" indicates that the patient is confused but follows commands.

Although the GCS score is almost ubiquitous in the evaluation of trauma patients, there are several issues that may limit its usefulness in the prehospital setting. For example, it has poor interrater reliability, meaning providers may score the same patient differently and thus provide different management.[18-20] Also, as noted previously, scores are skewed in intubated patients. Therefore, there has been a search for a simpler scoring system that still has predictive value for patient severity and outcomes. Evidence suggests that the motor component of the GCS alone is essentially as useful in evaluating a patient as the entire score.[21] It has been shown to accurately predict outcomes such as a patient's need for intubation and survival to hospital discharge.[22] One study even suggests that whether a patient can follow commands (i.e., has a motor score of 6) or not predicts severity of injury as well as total GCS score.[16]

If a patient is not awake, oriented, or able to follow commands, the prehospital care provider can quickly assess spontaneous extremity movement as well as the patient's pupils. Are the pupils equal and round, reactive to light (PERRLA)? Are the pupils equal to each other? Is each pupil round and of normal appearance, and does it appropriately react to light by constricting, or is it unresponsive and dilated? A GCS score of less than 14 in combination with an abnormal pupil examination can indicate the presence of a life-threatening TBI.

E—Expose/Environment

An early step in the assessment process is to remove a patient's clothes because exposure of the trauma patient is critical to finding all injuries (**Figure 6-5**). The saying, "The one part of the body that is not exposed will be the most severely injured part," may not always be true, but it is true often enough to warrant a total body examination. Also, blood can collect in and be absorbed by clothing and go unnoticed. After seeing the patient's entire body, the prehospital care provider can then cover the patient again to conserve body heat.

Although it is important to expose a trauma patient's body to complete an effective assessment, **hypothermia** is a serious problem in the management of a trauma patient. Only what is necessary should be exposed to the outside environment. Once the patient has been moved inside the warm emergency medical services (EMS) unit, the complete examination can be accomplished and the patient covered again as quickly as possible.

The amount of the patient's clothing that should be removed during an assessment varies depending on the conditions or injuries found. A general rule is to remove as much clothing as necessary to determine the presence or absence of a suspected condition or injury. If a patient has normal mental status and an isolated injury, only the area around the injury generally needs to be exposed. Patients with a serious mechanism of injury or altered mental

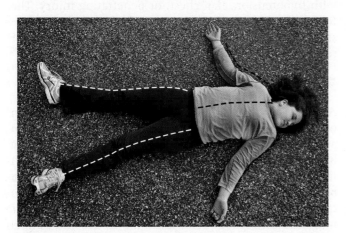

Figure 6-5 Clothing can be quickly removed by cutting, as indicated by the dotted lines.
© National Association of Emergency Medical Technicians (NAEMT).

Unfortunately, some trauma patients are victims of violent crimes. In these situations, it is important to do everything possible to preserve evidence for law enforcement personnel. When cutting clothing from a crime victim, care should be taken not to cut through holes in the clothing made by bullets (projectiles), knives, or other objects because this can compromise valuable forensic evidence. If clothing is removed from a victim of a potential crime, it should be placed in a paper (not plastic) bag and turned over to law enforcement personnel on scene before patient transport. Any weapons, drugs, or personal belongings found during patient assessment should also be turned over to law enforcement personnel. If the patient's condition warrants transport before the arrival of law enforcement, these items should be brought with the patient to the hospital. The local law enforcement agency should be notified of the destination facility. Document the turnover of the patient's belongings to law enforcement or the hospital per local protocols. Note, however, that patient care always comes first. No procedure or intervention should be delayed or altered in the name of a pending criminal investigation.

status should be fully exposed to evaluate for injuries. The prehospital care provider need not be afraid to remove clothing if it is the only way to complete the assessment and treatment properly. On occasion, patients can sustain multiple mechanisms of injury, such as experiencing a motor vehicle crash after being shot. Life-threatening injuries may be missed if the patient is inadequately examined. Injuries cannot be treated if they are not identified.

Special care should be taken when cutting and removing clothing from a victim of a crime so as not to inadvertently destroy evidence (**Box 6-5**).

To maintain body temperature and prevent hypothermia, the patient should be covered as soon as practical after assessment and treatment. In cold environments, prehospital care providers should consider using thermal blankets. Once in the ambulance, providers should adjust the vehicle heater to adequately warm the patient compartment, even though this may feel uncomfortably hot to providers.

Simultaneous Evaluation and Management

As mentioned earlier in this chapter, while the primary survey is presented and taught in a stepwise fashion, many steps can be assessed simultaneously. By asking questions such as, "Where do you hurt?," airway patency is assessed and respiratory function observed. This questioning can occur while the prehospital care provider is palpating the radial pulse and feeling the temperature and moistness of the skin. The patient's LOC and mentation can be determined by the appropriateness of the patient's verbal responses. Then the provider can rapidly scan the patient from head to foot looking for signs of hemorrhage or other injury. The second provider could be directed to apply direct pressure or a tourniquet to an external hemorrhage while the first provider continues to assess the patient's airway and breathing. By using this approach, a rapid evaluation for life-threatening injuries is achieved. The primary survey should be repeated frequently, especially in patients with serious injury.

Adjuncts to Primary Survey

Several adjuncts may be useful in monitoring the patient's condition, including the following:

- *Pulse oximetry.* A pulse oximeter should be applied during the primary survey (or at its completion). Oxygen can then be titrated to maintain oxygen saturation (SpO_2) of greater than or equal to 94%. A pulse oximeter also alerts the prehospital care provider to the patient's heart rate. Any drop in SpO_2 should prompt a repeat of the primary survey to identify the underlying cause. It is important to remember that pulse oximetry is subject to a "lag time" between the true blood oxygen saturation and what is displayed on the monitor because the signal is averaged, generally over 5 to 30 seconds. In patients with poor peripheral perfusion or peripheral vasoconstriction, the latency period becomes significantly longer, up to 120 seconds or more.[23] Therefore, a patient can (temporarily, at least) have a normal oximetry reading without adequate oxygenation, and vice versa. Other factors, such as carbon monoxide, can also affect the reliability of pulse oximetry readings.
- *End-tidal carbon dioxide ($ETCO_2$) monitoring.* Monitoring the $ETCO_2$ can be useful in confirming proper placement of an endotracheal tube and supraglottic airway as well as indirectly measuring the patient's arterial carbon dioxide level ($PaCO_2$).[24] While $ETCO_2$ may not always correlate well with the patient's $PaCO_2$, especially in multisystem trauma patients, trending of $ETCO_2$ may be useful in guiding ventilatory rate.
- *Electrocardiographic (ECG) monitoring.* ECG monitoring is less useful than monitoring pulse oximetry, as the presence of an organized cardiac electrical pattern on the monitor does not always correlate with adequate perfusion. Monitoring of the pulse and/or blood pressure is still required to assess for perfusion. An audible signal can alert the prehospital care provider of a change in the patient's heart rate or rhythm.
- *Automated blood pressure monitoring.* In general, obtaining blood pressure is not part of the primary survey; however, in a critically injured patient whose condition does not permit a more thorough secondary survey, application of an automated blood pressure monitor during transport can provide additional information regarding the patient's degree of shock. Whenever time permits, the provider should attempt to obtain a blood pressure reading by auscultation rather than by automated means. Automated blood pressure measurements are less accurate than manual readings in trauma.[25]

Resuscitation

Resuscitation describes treatment steps taken to correct life-threatening problems as identified in the primary survey. PHTLS assessment is based on a "treat as you go" philosophy, in which treatment is initiated as each threat to life is identified or at the earliest possible moment (**Figure 6-6**).

Transport

If life-threatening conditions are identified during the primary survey, the patient should be rapidly packaged after initiating limited field intervention. Transport of critically injured trauma patients to the closest appropriate facility should be initiated as soon as possible (**Box 6-6**). Unless complicating circumstances exist, scene time should be as short as possible for these patients. Limited scene time and initiation of rapid transport to the closest appropriate facility—preferably a trauma center—are fundamental aspects of prehospital trauma resuscitation.

Recent research found that worse outcomes occurred in severely injured trauma patients when the on-scene time was extended compared to the response and transport intervals. This finding was particularly true for patients with hypotension, flail chest, or penetrating injury. The finding further supports the concept that time on scene should be as short as possible, with only interventions for reversible life-threatening conditions performed on scene.[26]

Fluid Therapy

Another important step in resuscitation is the restoration of the perfusing volume within the cardiovascular system as quickly as possible. This step does not involve restoring blood pressure to normal but rather providing enough fluid to ensure that vital organs are perfused. Because blood is usually only available in the prehospital setting on critical care and helicopter EMS units, lactated Ringer or normal saline solution is most commonly used for trauma resuscitation. In addition to sodium and chloride, lactated Ringer solution contains small amounts of potassium, calcium, and lactate, making it less acidotic than saline.

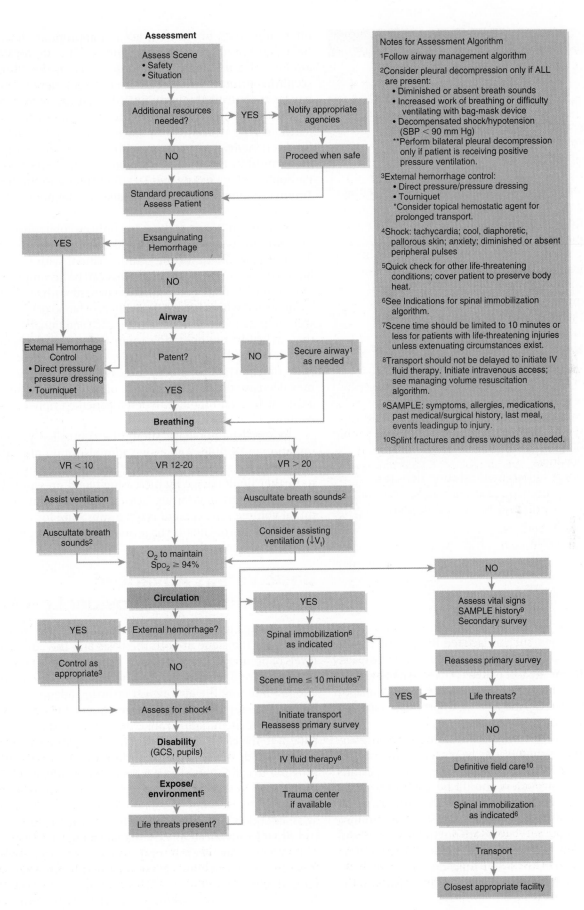

Figure 6-6 Assessment algorithm.

© National Association of Emergency Medical Technicians (NAEMT).

Box 6-6 Critical Trauma Patient

Keep scene time as brief as possible (ideally 10 minutes or less) when any of the following life-threatening conditions is present:

1. Inadequate or threatened airway
2. Impaired ventilation, as demonstrated by the following:
   · Abnormally fast or slow ventilatory rate
   · Hypoxia (Spo$_2$ < 94% even with supplemental oxygen)
   · Dyspnea
   · Open pneumothorax or flail chest
   · Suspected closed or tension pneumothorax
3. Significant external hemorrhage or suspected internal hemorrhage
4. Abnormal neurologic status
   · GCS score ≤ 13 or Motor component < 6
   · Seizure activity
   · Sensory or motor deficit
5. Penetrating trauma to the head, neck, or torso or proximal to the elbow or knee in the extremities
6. Amputation or near-amputation proximal to the fingers or toes
7. Any significant trauma in the presence of the following:
   · History of serious medical conditions (e.g., coronary artery disease, chronic obstructive pulmonary disease, bleeding disorder)
   · Age > 55 years
   · Hypothermia
   · Burns
   · Pregnancy

Crystalloid solutions, such as lactated Ringer and normal saline, however, do not replace the oxygen-carrying capacity of the lost RBCs or the lost platelets that are necessary for clotting and bleeding control. Therefore, rapid transport of a severely injured patient to an appropriate facility is an absolute necessity.

En route to the receiving facility, one or two 18-gauge intravenous (IV) catheters may be placed in the patient's forearm or antecubital veins, if possible, as time permits. Prehospital care providers should be cognizant of the increased risk of needlestick injury while starting an IV in a moving ambulance and should take steps to minimize this risk. If attempts at IV access are not quickly successful, intraosseous (IO) access should be initiated. The proximal humerus site allows for faster fluid flow rates than the proximal tibia.[27] In general, central IV lines (subclavian, internal jugular, or femoral) are not appropriate for the field management of trauma patients. The appropriate amount of fluid administration depends on the clinical scenario, primarily whether the patient's hemorrhage has been controlled when the IV fluid is initiated, if the patient is hypotensive, or whether the patient has evidence of TBI. A recent study suggests that prehospital IV fluid is beneficial for patients with hypotension but may be harmful in those without hypotension.[28] The Shock: Pathophysiology of Life and Death chapter and the Head Trauma chapter provide more detailed guidelines for fluid resuscitation.

Starting an IV line at the scene only prolongs on-scene time and delays transport. As addressed previously, the definitive treatment for the trauma patient with internal hemorrhage or significant blood loss can be accomplished only in the hospital. For example, a patient with an injury to the spleen who is losing 50 milliliters of blood per minute will continue to bleed at that rate for each additional minute that arrival in the operating room (OR) or angiography suite is delayed. Initiating IV lines on the scene instead of early transport will not only increase blood loss but also may decrease the patient's chance of survival. Exceptions exist, such as entrapment, when a patient simply cannot be moved immediately.

External hemorrhage should be controlled prior to initiation of IV fluid. Aggressive administration of IV fluids should be avoided as it may "pop the clot" and lead to further hemorrhage by increasing blood pressure and diluting platelets and clotting factors. More important, continual volume replacement is not a substitute for manual control of external hemorrhage and initiation of transport for internal hemorrhage.

Basic Versus Advanced Prehospital Care Provider Levels

The key steps in resuscitating a critically injured trauma patient are the same at both the basic and the advanced levels of prehospital care provider. They include (1) immediately controlling major external hemorrhage, (2) opening and maintaining the airway, (3) ensuring adequate ventilation, (4) rapidly packaging the patient for transport, and (5) quickly initiating rapid, but safe, transport of the patient to the closest appropriate facility. If transport time is prolonged, it may be appropriate for the basic-level provider to call for assistance from a nearby advanced life support (ALS) service that can rendezvous with the basic unit en route. Helicopter evacuation to a trauma center is another option. Both the ALS service and the flight service can provide advanced airway management and IV fluid replacement. Air medical services may also carry blood, fresh frozen plasma, and other therapies beyond typical ground ALS.

Secondary Survey

The secondary survey is a more detailed head-to-toe evaluation of a patient. It is performed only after the primary survey is completed, all identified life-threatening injuries have been treated, and resuscitation has been initiated. The objective of the secondary survey is to identify injuries or problems that were not identified during the primary survey. Because a well-performed primary survey will identify all immediately life-threatening conditions, the secondary survey, by definition, deals with less serious problems. Therefore, a critical trauma patient is transported as soon as possible after conclusion of the primary survey and not held in the field for either IV initiation or a secondary survey.

The secondary survey uses a "look, listen, and feel" approach to evaluate the patient. The provider identifies injuries and correlates physical findings region by region, beginning at the head and proceeding through the neck, chest, and abdomen to the extremities, concluding with a detailed neurologic examination. The following phrases capture the essence of the entire assessment process:

- *See*, don't just look.
- *Hear*, don't just listen.
- *Feel*, don't just touch (**Figure 6-7**).

While examining the patient, all available information is used to formulate a patient care plan.

See

- Examine all of the skin of each region.
- Be attentive for external hemorrhage or signs of internal hemorrhage, such as distension of the abdomen, swollen and tense extremity, or an expanding hematoma.
- Note soft-tissue injuries, including abrasions, burns, contusions, hematomas, lacerations, and puncture wounds.
- Note any masses or swelling or deformation of bones (deformities).
- Note abnormal indentations on the skin and the skin's color.
- Note anything that does not "look right."

Hear

- Note any unusual sounds when the patient inhales or exhales. Normal breathing is quiet.
- Note any abnormal sounds when auscultating the chest.
- Check whether the breath sounds are equal in both lung fields (**Figure 6-8**).
- Auscultate over the carotid arteries, and note any unusual sounds (bruits) over the vessels that would indicate vascular damage (often not realistic on a trauma scene).

Feel

- Firmly palpate all parts of the region, including bones. Note whether anything moves that should not, whether there is any crepitus or subcutaneous emphysema, whether the patient complains of tenderness, whether all pulses are present (and where they are felt), and whether pulsations are felt that should not be present.
- Carefully move each joint in the region. Note any resulting crepitus, pain, or limitation of range of motion, or unusual movement, such as laxity.

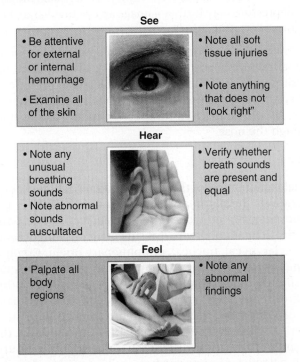

See

- Be attentive for external or internal hemorrhage
- Examine all of the skin

- Note all soft tissue injuries
- Note anything that does not "look right"

Hear

- Note any unusual breathing sounds
- Note abnormal sounds auscultated

- Verify whether breath sounds are present and equal

Feel

- Palpate all body regions

- Note any abnormal findings

Figure 6-7 The physical assessment of a trauma patient involves careful observation, auscultation, and palpation.

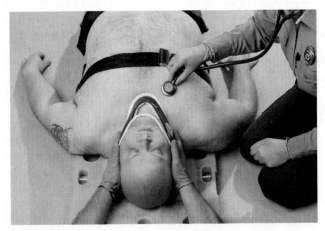

Figure 6-8 Check whether the breath sounds are equal in both lung fields.

Vital Signs

The first step of the secondary survey is measuring the vital signs. The rate and quality of the pulse, rate and depth of ventilation, and the other components of the primary survey are continually reevaluated and compared to previous findings because significant changes can occur rapidly. Depending on the situation, a second prehospital care provider may obtain vital signs while the first provider completes the primary survey, to avoid further delay. However, exact "numbers" for pulse rate, ventilatory rate, and blood pressure are not critical in the initial management of the patient with severe multisystem trauma. Therefore, the measurement of the exact numbers can be delayed until completion of the essential steps of resuscitation and stabilization.

A set of complete vital signs includes blood pressure, pulse rate and quality, ventilatory rate and depth, oxygen saturation (pulse oximetry), and skin color and temperature (skin temperature and body temperature). For the critical trauma patient, a complete set of vital signs are evaluated and recorded every 3 to 5 minutes, if possible, and at the time of any change in condition or a medical problem. Even if an automated, noninvasive blood pressure device is available, the initial blood pressure should be taken manually. Automated blood pressure devices may be inaccurate when the patient is significantly hypotensive; therefore, in these patients, all blood pressure measurements should be obtained manually, or at least confirm correlation of an automated reading with a manual reading.

SAMPLE History

A quick history is obtained on the patient. This information should be documented on the patient care report and passed on to the medical personnel at the receiving facility. The mnemonic SAMPLE serves as a reminder of the key components:

- *Symptoms.* What does the patient complain of? Pain? Trouble breathing? Numbness? Tingling?
- *Allergies.* Does the patient have any known allergies, particularly to medications?
- *Medications.* What prescription or nonprescription drugs (including vitamins, supplements, and other over-the-counter medications) does the patient regularly take? What recreational substance does he or she use regularly and, in particular, today?
- *Past medical and surgical history.* Does the patient have any significant medical problems requiring ongoing medical care? Has the patient undergone any prior surgeries?
- *Last meal/last menstrual period.* How long has it been since the patient last ate? Many trauma patients will require surgery, and recent food intake increases the

risk of aspiration during induction of anesthesia. For female patients of childbearing age, when was their last menstrual period? Is there a possibility of pregnancy?
- *Events.* What events preceded the injury? Immersion in water (drowning or hypothermia) and exposure to hazardous materials should be included.

Assessing Anatomic Regions

Head

Visual examination of the head and face will reveal contusions, abrasions, lacerations, bone asymmetry, hemorrhage, bony defects of the face and supportive skull, and abnormalities of the eye, eyelid, external ear, mouth, and mandible. The following steps are included during a head examination:

- Search thoroughly through the patient's hair for any soft-tissue injuries.
- Check pupil size for reactivity to light, equality, accommodation, roundness, and irregular shape.
- Carefully palpate the bones of the face and skull to identify focal tenderness, crepitus, deviation, depression, or abnormal mobility. (This is extremely important in the nonradiographic evaluation for head injury.) **Figure 6-9** reviews the bony anatomy of the skull.
- Care should be exercised when attempting to open and examine the eyes of an unconscious trauma patient who has evidence of facial injury. Even small amounts of pressure may further damage an eye that has a blunt or penetrating injury.

Fractures of the bones of the midface are often associated with a fracture of the portion of the skull base called the cribriform plate. If the patient has midface trauma (e.g., injury between the upper lip and orbits), a gastric tube, if used, should be inserted through the mouth rather than through the nose.

Neck

Visual examination of the neck for contusions, abrasions, lacerations, hematomas, and deformities will alert the prehospital care provider to the possibility of underlying injuries. Palpation may reveal subcutaneous emphysema from a laryngeal, tracheal, or pulmonary origin. Crepitus of the larynx, hoarseness, and subcutaneous emphysema constitute a triad classically indicative of laryngeal fracture. Lack of tenderness of the cervical spine may help rule out cervical spine fractures (when combined with strict criteria), whereas tenderness may frequently indicate the presence of a fracture, dislocation, or ligamentous injury. Such palpation is performed carefully, ensuring that the cervical spine remains in a neutral, in-line position. Absence of a neurologic deficit does not exclude the possibility of an unstable cervical spine injury. Reevaluation may reveal

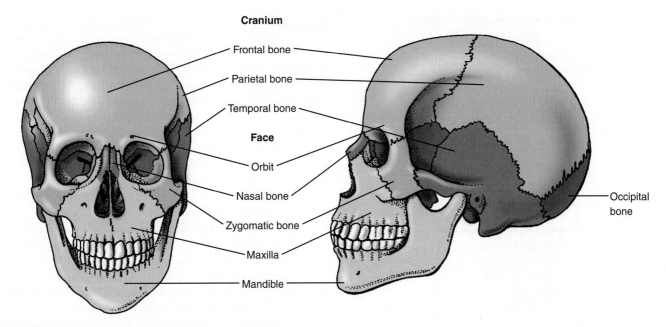

Cranium
- Frontal bone
- Parietal bone
- Temporal bone

Face
- Orbit
- Nasal bone
- Zygomatic bone
- Maxilla
- Mandible
- Occipital bone

Figure 6-9 Normal anatomic structure of the face and skull.
© National Association of Emergency Medical Technicians (NAEMT).

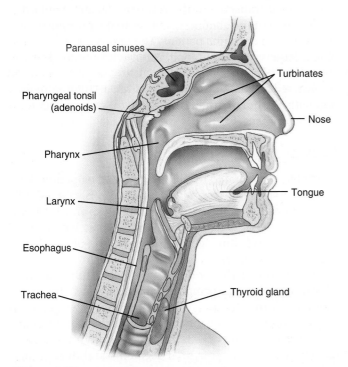

- Paranasal sinuses
- Pharyngeal tonsil (adenoids)
- Pharynx
- Larynx
- Esophagus
- Trachea
- Turbinates
- Nose
- Tongue
- Thyroid gland

Figure 6-10 Normal anatomy of the neck.
© National Association of Emergency Medical Technicians (NAEMT).

expansion of a previously identified hematoma or shifting of the trachea. **Figure 6-10** reviews the normal anatomic structure of the neck.

Chest

Because the thorax is strong, resilient, and elastic, it can absorb a significant amount of trauma. Close visual examination of the chest for deformities, areas of para-doxical movement, contusions, and abrasions is necessary to identify underlying injuries. Other signs for which the prehospital care provider should watch closely include splinting and guarding, unequal bilateral chest excursion, and intercostal, suprasternal, or supraclavicular bulging or retraction.

A contusion over the sternum may be the only indication of an underlying cardiac injury. Penetrating wounds may affect body areas remote from the entry site. It is important to understand the relationship between the body surface and underlying organs, such as the diaphragm and its variable position during exhalation and inhalation. A line traced from the fourth intercostal space anteriorly to the sixth intercostal space laterally and to the eighth intercostal space posteriorly defines the upward excursion of the diaphragm at full expiration (**Figure 6-11**). A penetrating injury that occurs below this line (which is about the level of the nipples) or with a path that may have taken it below this line should be considered to have traversed both the thoracic and abdominal cavities.

Auscultation with a stethoscope is an essential part of the chest examination. A patient will most often be in a supine position so that only the anterior and lateral chest is available for auscultation. It is important to recognize normal and decreased breath sounds with a patient in this position. Diminished or absent breath sounds indi-cate a possible pneumothorax, tension pneumothorax, or hemothorax. Crackles heard posteriorly (when the patient is logrolled) or laterally may indicate pulmonary contu-sion. Cardiac tamponade is characterized by distant heart

Lateral View of Diaphragm Position

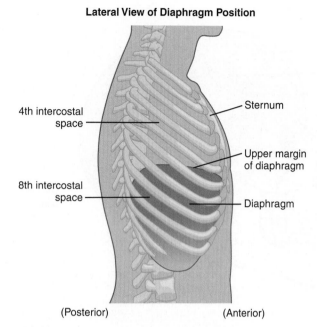

Figure 6-11 Lateral view of diaphragm position at full expiration.

© National Association of Emergency Medical Technicians (NAEMT).

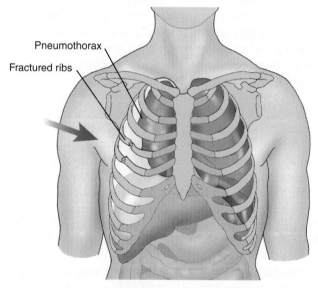

Figure 6-12 Compression injury to the chest can result in rib fracture and subsequent pneumothorax.

© National Association of Emergency Medical Technicians (NAEMT).

sounds; however, these may be difficult to ascertain given the commotion at the scene or road noise during transport.

A small area of rib fractures may indicate a severe underlying pulmonary contusion. Any type of compression injury to the chest can result in a pneumothorax (**Figure 6-12**). The thorax is palpated for the presence of subcutaneous emphysema (air in the soft tissue).

Abdomen

The abdominal examination begins, as with the other parts of the body, by visual evaluation. Abrasions and ecchymosis indicate the possibility of underlying injury; in particular, periumbilical and flank ecchymosis is associated with retroperitoneal bleeding. In the case of a motor vehicle collision, the abdomen should be examined carefully for a telltale transverse contusion, which suggests that a seat belt may have caused underlying injury. A significant portion of patients with this sign will have underlying injury, most frequently small bowel injury.[29-31] Lumbar spine fractures may also be associated with the "seat belt sign."

Examination of the abdomen also includes palpation of each quadrant to evaluate for tenderness, abdominal muscle guarding, and masses. When palpating, the prehospital care provider notes whether the abdomen is soft or whether rigidity or guarding is present. There is no need to continue palpating after discovering abdominal tenderness or pain. Additional information will not alter prehospital management, and the only outcomes of a continued abdominal examination are further discomfort to the patient and delayed transport to the receiving facility. Similarly, auscultation of the abdomen adds virtually nothing to the assessment of a trauma patient. The peritoneal cavity can hide a large volume of blood, often with minimal or no abdominal distension.

Altered mental status resulting from a TBI or intoxication with alcohol or other drugs often obscures evaluation of the abdomen.

Pelvis

The pelvis is evaluated by observation and palpation. The pelvis is first visually examined for abrasions, contusions, hematomas, lacerations, open fractures, and signs of distension. Pelvic fractures can produce massive internal hemorrhage, resulting in rapid deterioration of a patient's hemodynamic status.

Palpation of the pelvis in the prehospital setting provides minimal information that will affect the management of the patient. When examined, the pelvis is palpated only once for tenderness and instability as part of the secondary survey. Because palpation of the unstable pelvis can move fractured segments and disrupt any clot that has formed, thus aggravating hemorrhage, this examination step should be performed only once and not repeated. Palpation is accomplished by gently applying anterior-to-posterior pressure with the heels of the hands on the symphysis pubis and then medial pressure to the iliac crests bilaterally, evaluating for pain and abnormal movement. Any evidence of instability should preclude further palpation of the pelvis and prompt placement of a pelvic binder, if available.

Genitals

In general, genitalia are not examined in detail in the prehospital setting. However, note should be made of bleeding from the external genitalia, obvious blood at the urethral meatus, or presence of priapism in males. Additionally, clear fluid noted in the pants of a pregnant patient may represent amniotic fluid from rupture of the amniotic membranes.

Back

The back should be examined for evidence of injury. This is best accomplished when logrolling the patient for placement onto or removal from the long backboard. Breath sounds should be auscultated over the posterior thorax; the back should be observed for contusions, abrasions, and deformities; and the spine should be palpated for tenderness.

Extremities

The examination of the extremities begins at the clavicle in the upper extremity and the pelvis in the lower extremity and then proceeds toward the most distal portion of each extremity. Each individual bone and joint is evaluated by visual inspection for deformity, hematoma, or ecchymosis and by palpation to determine the presence of crepitus, pain, tenderness, or unusual movements. Any suspected fracture should be immobilized. Circulation and motor and sensory nerve function at the distal end of each extremity are also checked. If an extremity is immobilized, pulses, movement, and sensation should be checked both before and after splinting.

Neurologic Examination

As with the other regional examinations described, the neurologic examination in the secondary survey is conducted in much greater detail than in the primary survey. Calculation of the GCS score, evaluation of motor and sensory function, and observation of pupillary response are all included. A gross examination of sensory capability and motor response will determine the presence or absence of weakness or loss of sensation in the extremities, suggesting brain or spinal cord injury, and will identify areas that require further examination. When examining a patient's pupils, equality of response in addition to equality of size are evaluated. A small but significant portion of the population has pupils of differing sizes (*anisocoria*) as a normal condition. Even in these patients, however, the pupils should react to light in a similar manner. Pupils that react at differing speeds to the introduction of light are considered to be unequal. Unequal pupils in an unconscious trauma patient may indicate increased intracranial pressure or pressure on the third cranial nerve, caused by either cerebral edema or a

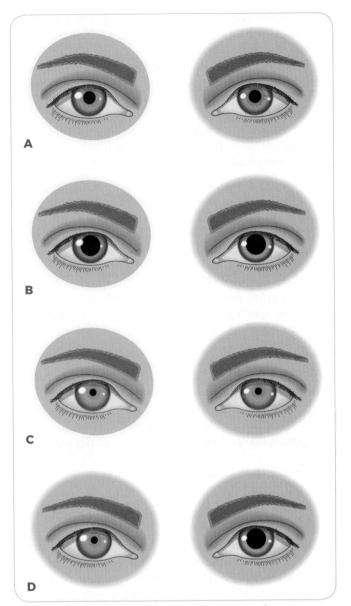

Figure 6-13 **A.** Normal pupils. **B.** Pupil dilation. **C.** Pupil constriction. **D.** Unequal pupils.

rapidly expanding intracranial hematoma (**Figure 6-13**). Direct eye injury can also cause unequal pupils.

Definitive Care in the Field

Definitive care is an intervention that completely corrects a particular condition. The following are examples of definitive care:

- For a patient with cardiac arrest in ventricular fibrillation, definitive care is defibrillation resulting in return of spontaneous circulation (ROSC).

- For a patient in a diabetic hypoglycemic coma, definitive care is glucose administration and a return to normal blood glucose levels.
- For a patient with an obstructed airway, definitive care is relief of the obstruction, which may be accomplished by a maneuver as simple as the trauma jaw thrust and assisted ventilation.
- For the patient with severe bleeding, definitive care is hemorrhage control by surgical repair or vascular occlusion and resuscitation from shock.

In general, while definitive care for some of the problems encountered in the prehospital setting can be provided in the field, definitive care for many of the injuries sustained by the critical trauma patient can be provided only in the hospital setting. Anything that delays the administration of that definitive care will decrease the patient's chance of survival. Furthermore, while one injury or condition may be definitively treated in the field, most major trauma patients will have others that must be treated in the hospital.

Preparation for Transport

As discussed previously, spinal injury should be suspected in all trauma patients with significant mechanism of injury. Therefore, when indicated, stabilization of the spine should be an integral component of packaging the trauma patient.

If time is available, the following measures are accomplished:

- Careful stabilization of extremity fractures using specific splints
- If the patient is in critical condition, rapid immobilization of all fractures as the patient is stabilized on a long backboard ("trauma" board) for transport
- Bandaging of major wounds as necessary and appropriate (i.e., wounds with active hemorrhage, abdominal evisceration)

Transport

Transport should begin as soon as the patient is loaded and immediate life threats are addressed. As discussed previously, delay at the scene to start an IV line or to complete the secondary survey only extends the period before the receiving facility can administer blood and control hemorrhage. Continued evaluation and further resuscitation occur en route to the receiving facility. *For some critically injured trauma patients, initiation of transport is the single most important aspect of definitive care in the field.*

A patient whose condition is not critical can receive attention for individual injuries before transport, but even this patient should be transported rapidly before a hidden condition becomes critical.

Field Triage of Injured Patients

Selection of the proper destination facility for a critically injured patient can be every bit as important as other life-saving interventions provided in the prehospital setting, and it is based on the assessment of the patient's injuries or suspected injuries (**Box 6-7**). For more than 40 years, numerous articles published in the medical literature have documented that facilities that have made the commitment to be prepared to care for injured patients—i.e., trauma centers—have better outcomes.[32-36] A study funded by the Centers for Disease Control and Prevention (CDC), published in 2006, demonstrated that patients were 25% more likely to survive their injuries if they received care

---

Box 6-7 CDC Guidelines for Field Triage of Injured Patients

At first glance, the Centers for Disease Control (CDC) Guidelines for Field Triage of Injured Patients may appear highly technical. To simplify, it may be helpful to break the flowchart down into three distinct questions:

1. Does the patient have unstable vital signs and/or serious injuries that warrant transport to the highest level trauma center?
2. Does the mechanism of injury warrant evaluation at a trauma center (not necessarily the highest level)?
3. Does the patient have extenuating circumstances that need to be considered for evaluation at a trauma center (not necessarily the highest level)?

Patients with concerning vital signs and/or apparent serious injuries warrant immediate stabilization and transport to the highest available trauma center in the region. In patients who have clinically stable vital signs, the presence of significant mechanism of injury may warrant evaluation at a trauma center, although it does not necessarily have to be the highest level available in the region. Patients who do not fall under the first two questions but who have extenuating circumstances (such as geriatric, pediatric, and pregnant patients and patients with burns) may warrant consideration for trauma center evaluation. The best destination for these patients is based on their extenuating circumstances and consultation with medical control, if needed.

The CDC recommends that, when in doubt, transport to a trauma center. It is better to overtriage rather than undertriage, although both should be avoided if possible.[43]

at a level I trauma center than if they were cared for in a nontrauma center.[37] Although 82.1% of the population lives within 60 minutes of a trauma center, slightly more than half of all persons injured did not receive their care from a designated trauma center, including 36% of major trauma victims.[38-40] The data seem clear: The mortality rate from injury can be significantly reduced by transporting injured patients to designated trauma centers.

One of the more challenging decisions faced by a prehospital care provider involves determining which injured patients are best cared for in trauma centers. Proper selection of which patients to transport to a trauma center involves a balance between "overtriage" and "undertriage." Transporting all trauma patients to trauma centers may result in overtriage, meaning that a significant number of these injured patients will not need the specialized services offered by these facilities. Overtriage could result in worse care to the more seriously injured patients, as the trauma center's resources are overwhelmed by those having less serious injuries. At the opposite end of the spectrum is undertriage, where a seriously injured patient is taken to a nontrauma center. Undertriage can also result in worse patient outcomes, as the facility may lack the capabilities to properly care for the patient. Some degree of undertriage seems inevitable, as some life-threatening conditions may not be identifiable in the prehospital setting. To minimize undertriage, experts estimate that an overtriage rate of 30% to 50% is necessary, meaning that 30% to 50% of injured patients transported to a trauma center will not need the specialized care available there.[41]

The commonly recognized definition for a "major trauma patient" is a patient with an Injury Severity Score (ISS) of 16 or higher (**Box 6-8**). Unfortunately, an ISS can be calculated only once all of the patient's injuries are diagnosed, including those found through advanced imaging (e.g., computed tomography) or surgery. Thus, the patient's ISS cannot be calculated in the prehospital setting. Alternative definitions that have been proposed include trauma patients who (1) die in the emergency department or within 24 hours of admission, (2) need massive transfusion of blood products, (3) need admission to an intensive care unit, (4) require urgent surgery for their injuries, or (5) require control of internal hemorrhage using interventional angiography. While all of these definitions are useful for research purposes, they cannot be identified by prehospital care providers.

In an effort to identify patients who would most benefit from transport to and care at a trauma center, the CDC published a report called "Guidelines for Field Triage of Injured Patients: Recommendations of the National Expert Panel." Most recently updated in 2011, this document provides evidence-based guidelines to assist EMS providers in making appropriate decisions about the transport destination of individual trauma patients. This 2011 revision appears in **Figure 6-14**, and it was also published in the CDC's *Morbidity and Mortality Weekly Report* (*MMWR*).[42]

Box 6-8 ISS Assessment

Various scoring systems are used to analyze and categorize patients who suffer traumatic injury in the hospital setting. Scoring systems may also be used to predict patient outcomes based on the severity of their traumatic injury. These scoring systems generally are not calculated until the patient has been fully evaluated at the trauma center. They offer limited use in the initial triage of injured patients in the field, but they do have significant value in the overall quality assessment and quality improvement (QA/QI) process of trauma care delivery.

One of the most commonly discussed scoring systems is the **Injury Severity Score (ISS)**. The ISS categorizes injuries into six anatomically distinct body regions:

1. Head and neck
2. Face
3. Chest
4. Abdomen
5. Extremities
6. External

Only the most severe injury in any one region is taken into account. After the most severe injuries in all six regions have been identified, they are assigned a value from 1 to 6 using the **Abbreviated Injury Scale (AIS)**:

1. Minor
2. Moderate
3. Serious
4. Severe
5. Critical
6. Unsurvivable

The highest three values are then squared to give additional weight to the highest scores and minimize the lowest scores. These values are then added together to calculate the final ISS.[44]

Higher ISS scores correlate linearly with mortality, morbidity, length of stay in the hospital, and other measures of severity. The major limitations of the ISS are that AIS scoring errors are amplified when calculated into the ISS, and there is no consideration given to the fact that injuries to certain areas of the body may inherently be more severe than injuries to other areas. While of limited use in the field triage of trauma patients, an understanding of how injury severity scores are calculated is highly valuable for the EMS provider when reading research articles and practice updates.

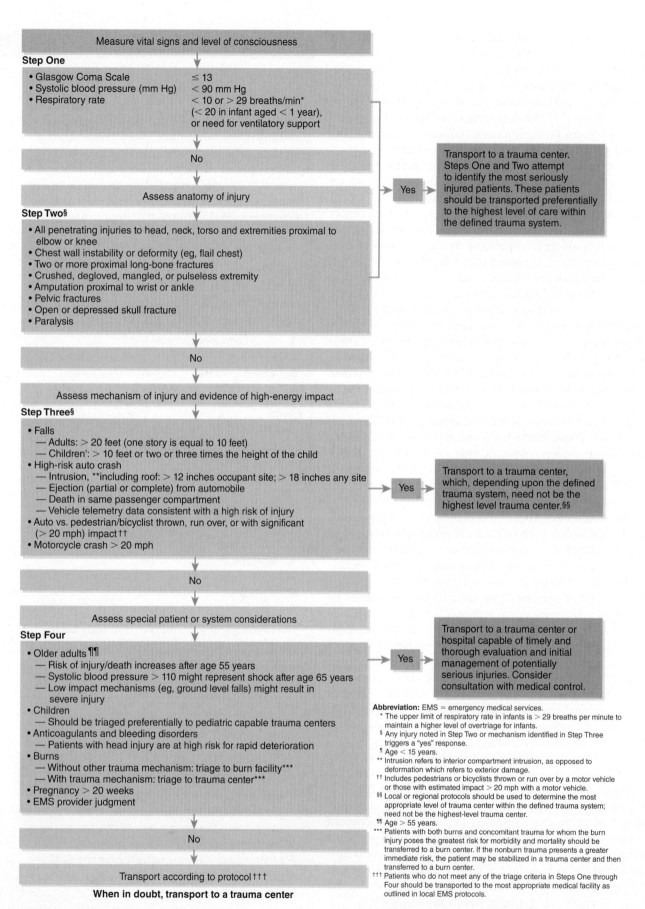

Figure 6-14 Deciding where to transport a patient is critical, requiring consideration of the type and location of available facilities. Situations that will most likely require an in-house trauma team are detailed in the Field Triage Guidelines.

Adapted from Centers for Disease Control and Prevention, *Morbidity and Mortality Weekly Report (MMWR)*, January 13, 2012.

The Field Triage Guidelines are broken down into four sections:

- *Step I: Physiologic criteria.* This section includes alteration in mental status (GCS < 14), hypotension (systolic blood pressure [SBP] < 90), and respiratory abnormalities (ventilation rate [VR] < 10 or > 29 or need for ventilator support).
- *Step II: Anatomic criteria.* If response times are brief, patients may not yet have developed significant alterations in physiology despite the presence of life-threatening injuries. This section lists anatomic findings that may be associated with severe injury.
- *Step III: Mechanism of injury criteria.* These criteria identify additional patients who may have occult injury not manifested with physiologic derangement or obvious external injury.
- *Step IV: Special considerations.* These criteria identify how factors such as age, use of anticoagulants, or the presence of burns or pregnancy may affect the decision to transport to a trauma center.

Patients who meet either physiologic or anatomic injury criteria should be transported to the highest level of trauma care available in a given region. Patients who meet mechanism of injury criteria should be transported to a trauma center, but not necessarily to the highest level of trauma care in the region. Patients who meet the special considerations criteria of step IV may be transported to a trauma center or another capable hospital, based on clinical judgment and possible discussion with online medical control. As with any decision tool, however, it should be used as guidance and not as a replacement for good judgment. When in doubt, transportation to a trauma center is recommended.

Duration of Transport

As discussed previously, the prehospital care provider should choose a receiving facility according to the severity of the patient's injury. In simple terms, the patient should be transported to the closest appropriate facility (i.e., the closest facility most capable of managing the patient's problems). If the patient's injuries are severe or indicate the possibility of continuing hemorrhage, the provider should take the patient to a facility that will provide definitive care as quickly as possible (i.e., a trauma center, if available).

For example, an ambulance responds to a call in 8 minutes, and the prehospital team spends 6 minutes on the scene to package and load the patient into the transporting unit. So far 14 minutes have passed. The closest hospital is 5 minutes away, and the trauma center is 14 minutes away. In scenario 1, the patient is taken to the trauma center. On arrival, the surgeon is in the emergency department (ED) with the emergency physician and the entire trauma team. The OR is staffed and ready. After 10 minutes in the ED for resuscitation, necessary radiographs, and blood work, the patient is taken to the OR. The total time since the incident is now 38 minutes. In scenario 2, the patient is taken to the closest hospital, which is 9 minutes closer than the trauma center. It has an available emergency physician, but the surgeon and OR team are out of the hospital. The patient's 10 minutes in the ED for resuscitation could stretch to 45 minutes by the time the surgeon arrives and examines the patient. Another 30 minutes could elapse while waiting for the OR team to arrive once the surgeon has examined the patient and decided to operate. The total time for scenario 2 is 94 minutes, or 2½ times longer than the trauma center scenario. The 9 minutes saved by the shorter ambulance ride to the closest hospital actually cost 56 minutes, during which time operative management could have been started and hemorrhage control achieved at the trauma center.

In a rural community, the transport time to an awaiting trauma team may be 45 to 60 minutes or even longer. In this situation, the closest hospital with an on-call trauma team is the appropriate receiving facility.

Another consideration is that many nontrauma centers do not provide definitive care for severely injured patients and so will transfer these patients to a trauma center. If such were the case in scenario 2, the delay to definitive care would be even longer in many instances.

Method of Transport

Another aspect of the patient assessment and transport decision is the transportation method. Some systems have air transport available. Air medical services may offer a higher level of care than ground units for critically injured trauma victims. Air transport may also be quicker and smoother than ground transport in some circumstances. As previously mentioned, if air transport is available in a community and is appropriate for the specific situation, the earlier in the assessment process that the decision is made to call for air transport, the greater the likely benefit to the patient. Helicopter EMS should be considered for those patients meeting guideline criteria for transport to the hospital with the highest level of care in the region.

Monitoring and Reassessment (Ongoing Assessment)

After the primary survey and initial care are complete, the patient must be continuously monitored, the vital signs reassessed, and the primary survey repeated several times while en route to the receiving facility or at the scene if transport is delayed. Continuous reassessment of the components of the primary survey will help ensure that vital functions do not deteriorate or are immediately corrected if they do. The provider should pay particular attention to any significant change in a patient's condition and reconsider management options if such a change is noted. Furthermore, the continued monitoring of a patient helps reveal conditions or problems that were overlooked during the primary survey or that are only now presenting. Often the patient's condition will not be obvious, and looking at and listening to the patient provides much information. How the information is gathered is not as important as ensuring that all the information is gathered. Reassessment should be conducted as quickly and thoroughly as possible. Monitoring during a prolonged transport situation is described later.

Communication

Communication between prehospital providers and hospital personnel is a critical part of quality patient care and consists of multiple components: prearrival notification, verbal report on arrival at bedside, and the formal written patient care report. Communication with the receiving facility should be undertaken as soon as possible. Early communication allows the facility to assemble the appropriate personnel and equipment necessary to best care for the patient, often by way of a trauma alerting system. During transport, a member of the prehospital care team should provide a brief patient care report to the receiving facility that includes the following information:

- Patient gender and exact or estimated age
- Mechanism of injury
- Life-threatening injuries, conditions identified, and anatomic location of injuries
- Current vital signs
- Interventions that have been performed, including the patient's response to treatment
- Estimated time of arrival (ETA)

If time permits, additional information can be included, such as pertinent medical conditions and medications, other non-life-threatening injuries, characteristics of the scene including protective gear used by the patient (seat belt, helmet, etc.), and information about additional patients. Otherwise this can be given at the bedside.

The prehospital care provider also verbally transfers responsibility for a patient (often called "sign off," "report off," or "transfer over") to the physician or nurse who takes over the patient's care at the receiving facility. This verbal report is typically more detailed than the radio report but less detailed than the written PCR, providing an overview of the significant history of the incident, the action taken by the providers, and the patient's response to this action. Both the verbal and written reports must highlight any

significant changes in the patient's condition that have taken place since transmitting the radio report. Transfer of important prehospital information further emphasizes the team concept of patient care.

Some trauma centers have formalized this process to avoid miscommunication and misunderstandings between prehospital and hospital personnel. Upon arrival of the patient in the trauma bay, the trauma team leader will do a rapid primary survey to assure the patient is breathing and has a pulse and then pause to listen to a "20-second shout-out" from the EMS team leader. This verbal report should include the following elements:

1. Age, gender, mechanism of injury, and time of event
2. Prehospital vital signs, including any instance of SBP < 90 mm Hg
3. Injuries identified
4. Prehospital interventions
5. Changes in patient status, particularly neurologic or hemodynamic
6. Patient medical history, allergies and medications, particularly blood thinners

For severely injured patients, the trauma team will not be able to hold their assessment for longer than this 20- to 30-second period, and additional information can be given to a nurse or other member of the trauma team not involved in direct assessment or procedures with the patient.

Also important is the written **patient care report (PCR)**. A good PCR is valuable for the following two reasons:

1. It gives the receiving facility staff a thorough understanding of the events that occurred and of the patient's condition should any questions arise after the prehospital care providers have left.
2. It helps ensure quality control throughout the prehospital system by making case review possible.

For these reasons, it is important that the prehospital care provider fill out the PCR accurately and completely and provide it to the receiving facility. The PCR should stay with the patient; it is of little use if it does not arrive until hours or days after the patient arrives. If an agency uses an electronic record program, a written summary of key information can be left at bedside, and the full record should be transmitted to the hospital when complete.

The PCR is a part of the patient's medical record. It is a legal record of what was found and what was done and can be used as part of a legal action. The report is considered to be the official record of the injuries found and the actions taken. As such, it should be thorough and accurate. Another important reason for providing a copy of the PCR to the receiving facility is that most trauma centers maintain a "trauma registry," a database of all trauma patients admitted to their facility. The prehospital information is an important aspect of this database and may aid in valuable research.

Special Considerations

Traumatic Cardiopulmonary Arrest

Cardiopulmonary arrest resulting from trauma differs from that caused by medical problems in several significant ways. First, medical cardiac arrest is generally the result of either a respiratory problem (e.g., foreign body airway obstruction) or a cardiac dysrhythmia. These are best managed with attempts at resuscitation at the scene. Traumatic cardiac arrest is most often due to exsanguination or TBI or other CNS injury. These patients generally cannot be appropriately resuscitated in the field. Survival from traumatic cardiac arrest is poor, with less than 4% overall survival and less than 2% surviving with good neurologic status.[45]

The decisions regarding the management of traumatic cardiac arrest in the prehospital setting are often complex and must take a variety of factors into consideration. Guidelines and position statements developed by the National Association of EMS Physicians (NAEMSP) and ACS-COT, as well as the European Resuscitation Council represent the best understanding of the available evidence. However, this evidence is not always clear or complete and local factors must be taken into account, and so some local protocols may deviate from these guidelines.

General Principles

Unless obvious signs of death (e.g., exposed brain matter) are immediately apparent or the patient clearly meets the criteria for withholding resuscitation described in the next section, resuscitation should be initiated while performing further assessment and preparing for transport. External hemorrhage should be immediately controlled. While many protocols include the use of closed chest compressions in algorithms for the management of traumatic cardiopulmonary arrest, the effectiveness of cardiopulmonary resuscitation (CPR) in the setting of severe trauma/exsanguination is questionable. Despite this reservation, it is reasonable to attempt CPR in patients who may be salvageable while prioritizing management of reversible causes of traumatic arrest. As with all CPR attempts, prehospital care providers should limit interruptions to compressions.[46]

If an ALS provider is available, ALS is provided while maintaining basic life support (BLS) techniques. The airway is secured with an appropriate airway device (while maintaining in-line stabilization of the cervical spine), such as

an endotracheal tube or supraglottic device. Breath sounds should be auscultated, and tension pneumothorax should be considered if a decrease in breath sounds or inadequate chest excursion during ventilation is noted. If any doubt exists that the patient may have a tension pneumothorax, chest decompression should be performed. Appropriate venous access is obtained and isotonic crystalloid solution is delivered through a wide-open line. ECG monitoring is performed and cardiac rhythm assessed.

In general, patients with severe trauma are best served by short scene times and rapid transport to a trauma center. However, for patients in traumatic cardiac arrest, the decision on when to transport (or whether to transport at all) is much more complex. If a patient does not respond to resuscitation efforts on scene, the time frame in which hospital-based interventions might be effective is relatively short, making the transport time to an appropriate receiving facility the most important consideration for the transport of a traumatic cardiac arrest patient. Aeromedical services may be able to provide more advanced capabilities on scene, such as blood transfusion, and their speed may allow them to reach a hospital faster than ground transportation. However, many aeromedical services do not transport patients who are in cardiac arrest.

If cardiac arrest is witnessed by EMS personnel, or if prehospital care providers have reason to believe that cardiac arrest has occurred within several minutes prior to their arrival on scene, and the patient can be transported to an appropriate receiving facility within 10 to 15 minutes, consider immediate transport with further treatment and resuscitation efforts performed en route. If the patient cannot arrive at an appropriate hospital, preferably a trauma center, within this time frame, providers may consider providing resuscitation efforts on scene followed by termination of resuscitation, if appropriate.

Withholding Resuscitation

Resuscitation attempts in patients who are extremely unlikely to survive, aside from demonstrating very low success rates, put prehospital care providers at risk from exposure to blood and body fluids as well as injuries sustained in motor vehicle crashes during transport. Such unsuccessful attempts at resuscitation may also divert resources away from patients who are viable and have a greater likelihood of survival. For these reasons, good judgment needs to be exercised regarding the decision to initiate resuscitation attempts for victims of traumatic cardiopulmonary arrest.

The NAEMSP collaborated with the ACS-COT to develop guidelines for withholding or terminating resuscitation in the prehospital setting.[47] Victims of drowning, lightning strike, or hypothermia, as well as pediatric or pregnant patients deserve special consideration before a decision is made to withhold or terminate resuscitation. A patient found in cardiopulmonary arrest at the scene of a traumatic event may have experienced the arrest because of a medical problem (e.g., myocardial infarction), especially if the patient is elderly or evidence of injury is minimal. In such patients, for whom a medical cause of cardiac arrest is deemed more likely than a traumatic cause, standard guidelines for out-of-hospital cardiac arrest should be followed.

For patients with traumatic injuries that are believed to be the most likely cause of cardiac arrest and who meet the following criteria, resuscitation may be withheld and the patient declared dead[47]:

- Presence of an obviously fatal injury (e.g., decapitation, exposed brain matter) or when evidence of irreversibility exists (dependent lividity, rigor mortis, or decomposition).
- For victims of blunt trauma, resuscitation efforts may be withheld if the patient is pulseless and apneic and without organized electrocardiographic activity on arrival of prehospital care providers.
- For victims of penetrating trauma, resuscitation efforts may be withheld if the patient is pulseless, apneic, and there are no other signs of life (no pupillary reflexes, no spontaneous movement, no organized electrocardiographic activity) on the arrival of prehospital providers.

Extreme caution must be exercised when assessing a potentially dead victim, as the decision to withhold resuscitation is medically justifiable only when proper assessment has been performed. Several times each year, a story hits the press of a trauma patient who was incorrectly presumed to be deceased only to later be discovered to have vital signs. Virtually all of these patients go on to succumb to their injuries, but such incidents can be embarrassing to both the prehospital care providers and their agencies. In the excitement of a scene with multiple patients, a provider may not adequately assess for presence of a pulse. Dying trauma patients may be profoundly bradycardic and hypotensive, thus contributing to the difficulty in identifying a preterminal condition. Prior to making the decision to withhold resuscitation in a patient without obvious signs of death, the EMS provider must perform adequate assessment, including palpating for a pulse (preferably at multiple sites), evaluation of the patient's neurologic status (e.g., pupillary reflexes, assessing for spontaneous movement or response to painful stimuli, etc.), and application of an EKG monitor.

Terminating Resuscitation

The NAEMSP and the ACS-COT have published revised guidelines for termination of resuscitation in the prehospital setting.[48] Termination of resuscitation for trauma patients should be considered when there are no signs of life and no ROSC despite appropriate field EMS treatment that includes minimally interrupted CPR and treatment of reversible causes of arrest (**Table 6-1**). The appropriate duration of resuscitation of a patient in traumatic cardiac arrest before termination of that resuscitation should be considered is still unclear. A reasonable guideline is 15 minutes of resuscitative efforts; however, local protocols may dictate different periods of time. Termination of resuscitation is generally not feasible after transport has been initiated. Considerations for choosing to withhold resuscitation in traumatic cardiac arrest are presented in **Table 6-2**.

Pain Management

Pain management (*analgesia*) is often used in the prehospital setting for pain caused by angina or myocardial infarction. Traditionally, pain management has had a limited role in the management of trauma patients, primarily because of the concern that side effects (decreased ventilatory drive and vasodilatation) of narcotics may aggravate preexisting hypoxia and hypotension. This concern has resulted in pain relief being denied to some patients with appropriate indications, such as an isolated limb injury or spinal fracture. The prehospital care provider may consider pain management in such patients, particularly if prolonged transport occurs, provided that signs of ventilatory impairment or shock are not present.

The Musculoskeletal Trauma chapter devotes a section to pain management as it relates to isolated extremity injuries and fractures. Fentanyl is typically the agent of choice, as it has minimal effect on hemodynamics and is short acting. Alternative medications for analgesia include morphine sulfate, hydromorphone, and nonopioids such as acetaminophen, nonsteroidal anti-inflammatory drugs (NSAIDs), ketamine, and nitrous oxide. Local therapies such as ice and immobilization and verbal calming also greatly reduce pain.

Pulse oximetry and serial vital signs must be monitored if any narcotics are administered to a trauma patient. Sedation with an agent such as a benzodiazepine should be reserved for exceptional circumstances, such as a combative intubated patient, because the combination of a narcotic and benzodiazepine may result in respiratory arrest. Prehospital care providers should collaborate with their medical control to develop appropriate protocols.

Injury Due to Interpersonal Abuse

A prehospital care provider is often the first person on the scene, allowing him or her to assess for a potentially abusive situation. The provider inside a house can observe and relay the details at the scene to the receiving facility

Table 6-1 Considerations for Terminating Resuscitation in Traumatic Cardiac Arrest (TCA)

Consideration	Presentation	Recommendation
Signs of life are present	■ Spontaneous respirations, movement, a pulse, or measurable blood pressure is present	Do not terminate resuscitation **GO**
PEA with organized ECG activity is present	■ Narrow-complex PEA with normal or tachycardic rhythm (more likely to survive) ■ Wide-complex PEA with bradycardic rhythm (less likely to survive)	Do not terminate resuscitation **GO**
The patient may benefit from EDT	■ Penetrating chest trauma with witnessed signs of life ■ Narrow-complex PEA with normal or tachycardic rate on ECG	Do not terminate resuscitation **GO**
The patient is progressing into less-favorable ECG activity despite effective CPR	■ Narrow-complex PEA with a normal rate decompensates into wide-complex PEA with a bradycardic rate	Consider terminating resuscitation **STOP**
The duration of resuscitation is consistent with poor prognosis	■ Generally accepted to be no longer than 15 minutes ■ Certain patient considerations may extend this 15-minute duration	Consider terminating resuscitation **STOP**

Note: CPR, cardiopulmonary resuscitation; ECG, electrocardiogram; EDT, emergency department thoracotomy; PEA, pulseless electrical activity.

so that the appropriate social services in the area can be alerted of the concern for abuse. The provider is often the only medically trained person to be in a position to observe, suspect, and relay information about this silent danger. Note that some states may have legislation that mandates EMS providers to report potential abuse to the appropriate law enforcement agency, even if they notify hospital personnel of their concern.

Anyone at any age can be a potential victim of abuse or an abuser. A pregnant woman, infant, toddler, child, adolescent, young adult, middle-aged adult, and older adult are all at risk for abuse. Several different types of abuse exist, including physical, psychological (emotional), and financial. Abuse may occur by **commission**, in which a purposeful act results in an injury (i.e., physical abuse or sexual abuse), or by **omission** (e.g., neglectful care

of a dependent). This section does not discuss types of abuse and only introduces the general characteristics and heightens a prehospital care provider's awareness and suspicion of abuse.

General characteristics of a potential abuser include dishonesty, the "story" not correlating with the injuries, a negative attitude, abrasiveness with prehospital care providers, or (in the case of a young patient) lack of interest of the parent and/or not wanting to answer any questions. General characteristics of the abused patient include quietness, reluctance to elaborate on details of the incident, constant eye contact or lack of eye contact with someone at the scene, and minimization of personal injuries. Abuse, abusers, and the abused can take many different forms, and providers need to keep their level of suspicion high if the scene and the story do not correlate.

Table 6-2 Considerations for Choosing to Withhold Resuscitation in TCA

Consideration	Presentation	Recommendation
Death is the most likely outcome even when resuscitation is initiated.	▪ The patient is pulseless, apneic, lacks organized ECG activity, and has no spontaneous movement or pupillary reflexes	Withhold resuscitation STOP
The injuries present are not compatible with life.	▪ Decapitation ▪ Traumatic separation of the torso (hemicorporectomy)	Withhold resuscitation STOP
There is evidence of prolonged cardiac arrest.	▪ Rigor mortis ▪ Dependent lividity ▪ Evidence of decay	Withhold resuscitation STOP
There is evidence of a nontraumatic cause of arrest.*	▪ Minor vehicle damage with a patient who appears uninjured ▪ A fall from an otherwise nonfatal height without evidence of significant injury	Initiate resuscitation GO

*These are patients in whom there is suspicion that the traumatic event was a result of preceding cardiac arrest and not the cause of the cardiac arrest (e.g., falling from a ladder after suffering a major heart attack, crashing a vehicle after suffering a stroke, etc.).

Prolonged Transport and Interfacility Transfers

Although most urban or suburban EMS transports take 30 minutes or less, transport times may be prolonged as a result of weather conditions, traffic congestion, trains that block a crossing, or bridges that may be up to allow a ship to pass. These sorts of delays should be documented on the patient care report to explain prolonged return times to the trauma center. Many prehospital care providers in rural and frontier settings routinely manage patients for much longer periods of time during transport. Additionally, providers are called on to manage patients during transfer from one medical facility to another, either by ground or air. These transfers may take up to several hours.

Special preparations need to be taken when prehospital care providers are involved in the prolonged transport of a trauma patient, particularly interfacility transfers. The issues that must be considered before undertaking such a transport can be divided into those dealing with the patient, the prehospital crew, and the equipment.

Patient Issues

Of preeminent importance is providing a safe, warm, and secure environment in which the patient is transported. The gurney should be appropriately secured to the ambulance and the patient properly secured to the gurney. As emphasized throughout this text, hypothermia is a potentially deadly complication in a trauma patient, and the patient compartment must be sufficiently warm. If you, as a fully clothed prehospital care provider, are comfortable with the temperature in the patient compartment, it is likely too cold for the patient who has been exposed.

The patient should be secured in a position that allows maximum access to the patient, especially the injured areas. Before transport, the security of any airway devices placed must be confirmed, and equipment (e.g., monitors, oxygen tanks) should be placed and secured so that they do not become projectiles in the event that the ambulance has to swerve in an evasive action or is involved in a motor vehicle crash. Equipment should not rest on the patient because pressure ulcers might be created during a prolonged transport. During transport, all IV lines and catheters must be securely fastened to prevent loss of the venous access. If prolonged transport time is anticipated and a backboard was used to transfer the patient to the gurney, consider removing the patient from the backboard prior to transport by carefully logrolling the patient off of the board while maintaining appropriate spinal immobilization. This will increase patient comfort and decrease the risk of decubitus ulcer formation associated with prolonged immobilization on a hard surface.

The patient should undergo serial assessments of the primary survey and vital signs at frequent intervals. Pulse oximetry and ECG are monitored continuously for virtually all seriously injured patients, as well as ETCO$_2$, if available. Note that for nonintubated patients, capnography can be obtained using the naso-oral cannula. The prehospital care providers accompanying the patient should be trained at a level appropriate to the anticipated needs of the patient. Critically injured patients should generally be managed by providers with advanced training. If the patient is anticipated to require blood transfusion during transport, an individual should be in attendance whose scope of practice allows this procedure; in the United States, this generally requires a critical care trained provider, registered nurse, advanced care practitioner, or physician.

Two management plans should be devised. The first, a medical plan, is developed to manage either anticipated or unexpected problems with the patient during transport. Necessary equipment, medications, and supplies should be readily available. The second plan involves identifying the most expeditious route to the receiving hospital. Weather conditions, road conditions (e.g., construction), and traffic concerns should be identified and anticipated. Additionally, the prehospital care providers should be knowledgeable about the medical facilities along the transport route in case a problem arises that cannot be managed en route to the primary destination.

Adjuncts to the care of the patient during prolonged transport, or performed at the referring facility prior to transfer, may include the following:

- *Gastric tube*. If trained in proper insertion, a nasogastric or orogastric tube can be inserted into the patient's stomach. Suctioning out gastric contents can decrease abdominal distension and potentially decrease the risk of vomiting and aspiration.

- *Urinary catheter*. If trained on proper insertion, a urinary catheter may be inserted into the patient's bladder. Urine output can be a sensitive measure of the patient's renal perfusion and a marker of the patient's volume status.

- *Arterial or venous blood gas monitoring via point-of-care testing*. While the pulse oximeter gives valuable information regarding the oxyhemoglobin saturation, a blood gas reading may give useful information regarding the patient's partial pressure of carbon dioxide (PCO$_2$) and the base deficit, an indicator of the severity of shock.

Crew Issues

The safety of the prehospital care crew is as important as that of the patient. The prehospital care crew should be adequately rested and fed, particularly for long-duration transfers. A recent evidence-based review recommends a number of fatigue management strategies, including use of caffeinated drinks, napping, and avoidance of shifts that are 24 hours or longer in duration.[49] The crew should have and use appropriate safety devices, including seat belts in both the driver and patient compartments. The prehospital care crew members must use standard precautions and ensure that sufficient gloves and other PPE to avoid body fluids, blood, and other possible exposures are available for the trip.

Equipment Issues

Equipment issues during prolonged transport involve the ambulance, supplies, medications, monitors, and communications. The ambulance must be in good working order, including an adequate amount of fuel. The prehospital care crew must make sure sufficient supplies and medications are available and accessible for the transport, including gauze and pads for reinforcing dressings, IV fluids, oxygen, and pain medications. Medication supplies are based on anticipated patient needs and include sedatives, paralytic agents, analgesics, and antibiotics. A good general rule is to stock the ambulance with about 50% more supplies and medications than the anticipated need in case a significant delay is encountered. Patient care equipment must be in good working order, including monitors (with functioning alarms), oxygen regulators, ventilators, and suction devices. Also, success of a prolonged transport may depend on functional communications, including the ability to communicate with other crew members, medical control, and the destination facility.

The management of specific injuries during prolonged transport is discussed in the subsequent corresponding chapters of this text.

SUMMARY

- The likelihood of survival for a patient with traumatic injuries depends on the immediate identification and mitigation of conditions that interfere with tissue perfusion.
- The identification of these conditions requires a systematic, prioritized, logical process of collecting information and acting on it. This process is referred to as patient assessment.
- Patient assessment begins with assessment of the scene including a safety evaluation and includes the formation of a general impression of the patient, a primary survey, and, when the patient's condition and availability of additional EMS personnel permit, a secondary survey.
- The information obtained through this assessment process is analyzed and used as the basis for patient care and transport decisions.
- In the care of the trauma patient, a missed problem is a missed opportunity to potentially aid in an individual's survival.
- After the simultaneous determination of scene safety and general impression of the situation, providers initiate the primary survey, following the XABCDE format:
  - X—Exsanguinating hemorrhage (control of severe external bleeding)
  - A—Airway management and cervical spine stabilization

  - B—Breathing (ventilation and oxygenation)
  - C—Circulation (perfusion and other hemorrhage)
  - D—Disability
  - E—Expose/environment
- Despite the sequential presentation of this mnemonic, the actions of the primary survey occur essentially at the same time.
- Immediate threats to the patient's life are quickly corrected in a "find and fix" manner. Once the prehospital care provider controls exsanguinating hemorrhage and manages the patient's airway and breathing, he or she packages the patient and begins transport without additional treatment at the scene. The limitations of field management of trauma require the safe, expedient delivery of the patient to definitive care.
- The primary and secondary surveys should be repeated frequently to identify any changes in the patient's condition and new problems that demand prompt intervention.
- The patient's outcome can be greatly improved when the prehospital care provider selects the most appropriate destination for the patient, communicates with the receiving facility, and thoroughly documents the patient's condition and the actions performed in the prehospital setting.

SCENARIO RECAP

It is a Saturday morning in early November. The weather is clear, with an outside temperature of 42°F (5.5°C). Your squad is dispatched to a residential area for a person who has fallen from the roof of a two-story building. Upon arrival at the scene, you are met by an adult family member who leads you around the house to the backyard. The family member states the patient was cleaning leaves from the rain gutters with a leaf blower when he lost his balance and fell approximately 12 ft (3.6 m) from the roof, landing on his back. The patient initially lost consciousness for a "brief period" but was conscious by the time the family member called 9-1-1.

Approaching the patient, you observe an approximately 40-year-old man lying supine on the ground with two bystanders kneeling by his side. The patient is conscious and talking with the bystanders. You do not see any signs of severe bleeding. As your partner provides manual stabilization to the patient's head and neck, you ask the patient where he hurts. The patient states both his upper and lower back hurt the most.

Your initial questioning serves the multiple purposes of obtaining the patient's chief complaint, determining his initial level of consciousness, and assessing his ventilatory effort. Detecting no shortness of breath, you proceed with the patient assessment. The patient answers your questions appropriately to establish that he is oriented to person, place, and time.

- Based on physics of trauma as they relate to this incident, what potential injuries do you anticipate finding during your assessment?
- What are your next priorities?
- How will you proceed with this patient?

SCENARIO SOLUTION

You have been on the scene for 1 minute, yet you have obtained much important information to guide further assessment and treatment of the patient. In the first 15 seconds of patient contact, you have developed a general impression of the patient, determining that resuscitation is not necessary. With a few simple actions, you have evaluated the X, A, B, C, and D of the primary survey. There was no severe external bleeding. The patient spoke to you without difficulty, indicating that his airway is open and he is breathing with no signs of distress. At the same time, with an awareness of the mechanism of injury, you have stabilized the cervical spine. Your partner has assessed the radial pulse, and you have observed the patient's skin color, temperature, and moisture. These findings indicate no immediate threats to the patient's circulatory status. Additionally, you have simultaneously found no initial evidence of disability because the patient is awake and alert, answers questions appropriately, and can move all extremities. This information, along with information about the fall, will help you determine the need for additional resources, the type of transport indicated, and the type of facility to which you should deliver the patient.

Now that you have completed these steps and no immediate lifesaving intervention is necessary, you will proceed with step E of the primary survey early in the evaluation process and then obtain vital signs. You will expose the patient to look for additional injuries and bleeding that may have been concealed by clothing and then cover the patient to protect him from the environment. During this process, you will perform a more detailed examination, noting less serious injuries.

The next steps you will take are packaging the patient, including splinting the entire spine and extremity injuries and bandaging wounds, if time allows; initiating transport; and communicating with medical direction and the receiving facility. During the trip to the hospital, you will continue to reevaluate and monitor the patient. Your knowledge of the physics of trauma and the patient's witnessed loss of consciousness will generate a high index of suspicion for TBI, lower extremity injuries, and injuries to the spine. IV access will be established en route to the receiving facility.

References

1. Brown JB, Rosengart MR, Forsythe RM, et al. Not all pre-hospital time is equal: influence of scene time on mortality. *J Trauma Acute Care Surg.* 2016;81:93-100.

2. Advanced Trauma Life Support (ATLS) Subcommittee, Committee on Trauma. Initial assessment and management. In: *Advanced Trauma Life Support Course for Doctors, Student Course Manual.* 10th ed. Chicago, IL: American College of Surgeons; 2018.

3. Kotwal RS, Butler FK, Gross KR, et al. Management of junctional hemorrhage in Tactical Combat Casualty Care: TCCC guidelines–Proposed Change 13-03. *J Spec Oper Med.* 2013;13:85-93.

4. Kragh JF Jr, Mann-Salinas EA, Kotwal RS, et al. Laboratory assessment of out-of-hospital interventions to control junctional bleeding from the groin in a manikin model. *Am J Emerg Med.* 2013;31:1276-1278.

5. Kragh JF Jr, Parsons DL, Kotwal RS, et al. Testing of junctional tourniquets by military medics to control simulated groin hemorrhage. *J Spec Oper Med.* 2014;14:58-63.

6. Kragh JF, Kotwal RS, Cap AP, et al. Performance of junctional tourniquets in normal human volunteers. *Prehosp Emerg Care.* 2015;19:391-398.

7. Chen J, Benov A, Nadler R, et al. Testing of junctional tourniquets by medics of the Israeli Defense Force in control of simulated groin hemorrhage. *J Spec Oper Med.* 2016;16:36-42.

8. Bulger EM, Snyder D, Schoelles K, et al. An evidence-based prehospital guideline for external hemorrhage control: American College of Surgeons Committee on Trauma. *Prehosp Emerg Care.* 2014;18(2):163-173.

9. Kragh JF, Littrel ML, Jones JA, et al. Battle casualty survival with emergency tourniquet use to stop limb bleeding. *J Emerg Med.* 2011;41:590-597.

10. Beekley AC, Sebesta JA, Blackbourne LH, et al. Prehospital tourniquet use in Operation Iraqi Freedom: effect on hemorrhage control and outcomes. *J Trauma.* 2008;64:S28-S37.

11. Doyle GS, Taillac PP. Tourniquets: a review of current use with proposals for expanded prehospital use. *Prehosp Emerg Care.* 2008;12:241-256.

12. First Aid Science Advisory Board. First aid. *Circulation.* 2005;112(III):115.

13. Swan KG Jr, Wright DS, Barbagiovanni SS, et al. Tourniquets revisited. *J Trauma.* 2009;66:672-675.

14. King DR, Larentzakis A, Ramly EP; Boston Trauma Collaborative. Tourniquet use at the Boston Marathon bombing: lost in translation. *J Trauma Acute Care Surg.* 2015;78(3):594-599.

15. Deakin CD, Low JL. Accuracy of the advanced trauma life support guidelines for predicting systolic blood pressure using carotid, femoral, and radial pulses: observational study. *Br Med J.* 2000;321(7262):673-674.

16. Kupas DF, Melnychuk EM, Young AJ. Glasgow Coma Scale motor component ("patient does not follow commands") performs similarly to total Glasgow Coma Scale in predicting severe injury in trauma patients. *Ann Emerg Med.* 2016; 68(6):744-750.

17. Teasdale G, Jennett B. Assessment of coma and impaired consciousness: a practical scale. *Lancet.* 1974;2:81.

18. Bledsoe B, Casey M, Feldman J, et al. Glasgow Coma Scale scoring is often inaccurate. *Prehosp Disaster Med.* 2015;30(1): 46-53.

19. Gill MR, Reiley DG, Green SM. Interrater reliability of Glasgow Coma Scale scores in the emergency department. *Ann Emerg Med.* 2004;43(2):215-223.

20. Kerby JD, Maclennan PA, Burton JN, Mcgwin G, Rue LW. Agreement between prehospital and emergency department Glasgow Coma scores. *J Trauma.* 2007;63(5):1026-1031.

21. Healey C, Osler TM, Rogers FB, et al. Improving the Glasgow Coma Scale score: motor score alone is a better predictor. *J Trauma.* 2003;54:671.

22. Beskind DL, Stolz U, Gross A, et al. A comparison of the prehospital motor component of the Glasgow Coma Scale (mGCS) to the prehospital total GCS (tGCS) as a prehospital risk adjustment measure for trauma patients. *Prehosp Emerg Care.* 2014;18(1):68-75.

23. Aguilar SA, Davis DP. Latency of pulse oximetry signal with use of digital probes associated with inappropriate extubation during prehospital rapid sequence intubation in head injury patients: case examples. *J Emerg Med.* 2012;42(4):424-428.

24. Vithalani VD, Vlk S, Davis SQ, Richmond NJ. Unrecognized failed airway management using a supraglottic airway device. *Resuscitation.* 2017;119:1-4.

25. Davis JW, Davis IC, Bennink LD, Bilello JF, Kaups KL, Parks SN. Are automated blood pressure measurements accurate in trauma patients? *J Trauma.* 2003;55(5):860-863.

26. Brown JB, Rosengart MR, Forsythe RM, et al. Not all prehospital time is equal: influence of scene time on mortality. *J Trauma Acute Care Surg.* 2016;81:93-100.

27. Pasley J, Miller CH, Dubose JJ, et al. Intraosseous infusion rates under high pressure: a cadaveric comparison of anatomic sites. *J Trauma Acute Care Surg.* 2015;78(2):295-299.

28. Brown JB, Cohen MJ, Minei JP, et al. Goal directed resuscitation in the prehospital setting: a propensity adjusted analysis. *J Trauma Acute Care Surg.* 2013;74(5):1207-1214.

29. Biswas S, Adileh M, Almogy G, Bala M. Abdominal injury patterns in patients with seatbelt signs requiring laparotomy. *J Emerg Trauma Shock.* 2014;7(4):295-300.

30. Bansal V, Conroy C, Tominaga GT, Coimbra R. The utility of seat belt signs to predict intra-abdominal injury following motor vehicle crashes. *Traffic Inj Prev.* 2009;10(6):567-572.

31. Chandler CF, Lane JS, Waxman KS. Seatbelt sign following blunt trauma is associated with increased incidence of abdominal injury. *Am Surg.* 1997;63(10):885-888.

32. Moylan JA, Detmer DE, Rose J, Schulz R. Evaluation of the quality of hospital care for major trauma. *J Trauma.* 1976;16(7):517-523.

33. West JG, Trunkey DD, Lim RC. Systems of trauma care. A study of two counties. *Arch Surg.* 1979;114(4):455-460.

34. West JG, Cales RH, Gazzaniga AB. Impact of regionalization. The Orange County experience. *Arch Surg.* 1983;118(6):740-744.

35. Shackford SR, Hollingworth-Fridlund P, Cooper GF, Eastman AB. The effect of regionalization upon the quality of trauma care as assessed by concurrent audit before and after institution of a trauma system: a preliminary report. *J Trauma.* 1986;26(9):812-820.

36. Waddell TK, Kalman PG, Goodman SJ, Girotti MJ. Is outcome worse in a small volume Canadian trauma centre? *J Trauma.* 1991;31(7):958-961.

37. MacKenzie EJ, Rivara FP, Jurkovich GJ, et al. A national evaluation of the effect of trauma-center care on mortality. *N Engl J Med.* 2006;354(4):366-378.

38. Branas CC, MacKenzie EJ, Williams JC, et al. Access to trauma centers in the United States. *JAMA.* 2005;293(21):2626-2633.

39. Nathens AB, Jurkovich GJ, Rivara FP, Maier RV. Effectiveness of state trauma systems in reducing injury-related mortality: a national evaluation. *J Trauma.* 2000;48(1):25-30; discussion 30-31.

40. Report Card Task Force Members, American College of Emergency Physicians (ACEP) Staff. America's emergency care environment, a state-by-state report card: 2014 edition. *Ann Emerg Med.* 2014;63(2):97-242.

41. American College of Surgeons. *Resources for the Optimal Care of the Injured Patient.* 6th ed. Chicago, IL: American College of Surgeons; 2014.

42. Centers for Disease Control and Prevention. Guidelines for field triage of injured patients: recommendations of the national expert panel on field triage 2011. *Morb Mortal Wkly Rep.* 2012;61:1-21.

43. McCoy CE, Chakravarthy B, Lotfipour S. Guidelines for Field Triage of Injured Patients: In conjunction with the *Morbidity and Mortality Weekly Report* published by the Centers for Disease Control and Prevention. *West J Emerg Med.* 2013;14(1):69-76.

44. Baker SP, O'Neill B, Haddon W Jr, Long WB. The injury severity score: a method for describing patients with multiple injuries and evaluating emergency care. *J Trauma.* 1974;14(3):187-196.

45. Truhlář A, Deakin CD, Soar J, et al. European Resuscitation Council Guidelines for Resuscitation 2015: Section 4. Cardiac arrest in special circumstances. *Resuscitation.* 2015;95:148-201.

46. American Heart Association. 2015 guidelines for cardiopulmonary resuscitation and emergency cardiovascular care. *Circulation.* 2015;132:S313-S314.

47. National Association of EMS Physicians and American College of Surgeons Committee on Trauma. NAEMSP position statement: withholding of resuscitation for adult traumatic cardiopulmonary arrest. *Prehosp Emerg Care.* 2013;17:291.

48. The National Association of EMS Physicians (NAEMSP) and the American College of Surgeons Committee on Trauma (ACS-COT). Termination of resuscitation for adult traumatic cardiopulmonary arrest. *Prehosp Emerg Care.* 2012;16(4):571.

49. Patterson DP, Higgins JS, Van Dongen HPA, et al. Evidence-based guidelines for fatigue risk management in emergency medical services. *Prehosp Emerg Care.* 2018;22:(1):89-101.

Suggested Reading

American Heart Association. 2015 guidelines for cardiopulmonary resuscitation and emergency cardiovascular care. *Circulation.* 2015;132:S313-S314.

CHAPTER **7**

Airway and Ventilation

Lead Editors:
Jean-Cyrille Pitteloud, MD
Bruno Goulesque, MD

CHAPTER OBJECTIVES

At the completion of this chapter, you will be able to do the following:

- Integrate the principles of ventilation and gas exchange with the pathophysiology of trauma to identify patients with inadequate perfusion.
- Relate the concepts of minute volume and oxygenation to the pathophysiology of trauma.
- Understand the difference between ventilation and respiration.
- Explain the mechanisms by which supplemental oxygen and ventilatory support are beneficial to the trauma patient.
- Given a scenario that involves a trauma patient, select the most effective means of providing a patent airway to suit the patient's needs.

- Presented with a scenario that involves a patient who requires ventilatory support, discuss the most effective means available to suit the trauma patient's needs.
- Given situations that involve various trauma patients, formulate a plan for airway management and ventilation.
- Presented with current research, understand the risks versus benefits when discussing new invasive procedures.
- Discuss the indications and limitations of end-tidal carbon monoxide ($ETCO_2$) monitoring in the trauma patient.

SCENARIO

You are called to the scene of a motorcycle crash on a busy freeway. As you arrive on scene, you see the patient lying supine about 50 feet (ft) from a destroyed motorcycle. The patient is a 20-year-old male who still has his helmet on. He is not moving, and you see from a distance that he is breathing quickly with small and paradoxical thorax movements. As you approach the patient, you see a pool of blood around his head, and you notice that his breathing is noisy, with snoring and gurgling sounds.

You are 15 minutes from a trauma center, and the dispatch center informs you that the helicopter emergency medical services (HEMS) cannot fly due to bad weather.

- What indicators of airway compromise are evident in this patient?
- What other information, if any, would you seek from witnesses or the emergency medical responders?
- Describe the sequence of actions you would take to manage this patient before and during transport.

INTRODUCTION

Two of the most important prehospital maneuvers are those that provide and maintain airway patency and pulmonary ventilation. The failure to adequately ventilate a trauma patient and maintain oxygenation of organs sensitive to ischemia such as the brain and heart causes additional damage, including secondary brain injury, which compounds the primary brain injury produced by the initial trauma. Ensuring patency of the airway and maintaining the patient's oxygenation and supporting ventilation, when necessary, are critical steps in minimizing the overall burden of injury and improving the likelihood of good outcome. To be clear on the use of terminology: *oxygenation* refers to the process by which oxygen concentration increases within a tissue, and *ventilation* refers to the mechanical exchange of air between the outside environment and the alveoli of the lungs.

Cerebral oxygenation and oxygen delivery to other parts of the body maintained by adequate airway management and ventilation remain among the most important components of prehospital patient care. Because techniques and adjunct devices are changing and will continue to change, keeping abreast of these changes is important. These techniques may require active ventilation or passive observation of the patient's breathing.

The respiratory system serves two primary functions:

1. Provides oxygen to the red blood cells, which carry the oxygen to all of the body's cells
2. Removes carbon dioxide from the body

The inability of the respiratory system to provide oxygen to the cells or the inability of the cells to use the oxygen supplied results in anaerobic metabolism and can quickly lead to death. Failure to eliminate carbon dioxide can lead to coma and acidosis.

Anatomy

The respiratory system comprises the upper airway and the lower airway, including the lungs (**Figure 7-1**). Each part of the respiratory system plays an important role in ensuring gas exchange—the process by which oxygen enters the bloodstream and carbon dioxide is removed.

Upper Airway

The upper airway consists of the nasal cavity and the oral cavity (**Figure 7-2**). Air entering the nasal cavity is warmed, humidified, and filtered to remove impurities. Beyond these cavities is the area known as the **pharynx**, which runs from the back of the soft palate to the upper end of the esophagus. The pharynx is composed of muscle lined with mucous membranes. The pharynx is divided into three discrete sections: the **nasopharynx** (upper portion), the

oropharynx (middle portion), and the **hypopharynx** (lower or distal end of the pharynx). Below the pharynx is the **esophagus**, which leads to the stomach, and the trachea, at which point the lower airway begins. Above the trachea is the **larynx** (**Figure 7-3**), which contains the vocal cords and the muscles that make them work, housed in a strong cartilaginous box. The vocal cords are folds of tissue that meet in the midline. The false cords, or **vestibular folds**, direct the airflow through the vocal cords. Supporting the cords posteriorly is the arytenoid cartilage. Directly above the larynx is a leaf-shaped structure called the **epiglottis**. Acting as a gate or flapper valve, the epiglottis directs air into the trachea and solids and liquids into the esophagus.

Lower Airway

The lower airway consists of the trachea, its branches, and the lungs. On inspiration, air travels through the upper airway and into the lower airway before reaching the alveoli, where the actual gas exchange occurs. The trachea divides into the right and left main bronchi. The right main bronchus is shorter, wider, and more vertical than the left. The right main bronchus comes off the trachea at approximately a 25-degree angle, whereas the left has a 45-degree angulation. (This difference explains why right main bronchus placement of an endotracheal tube is a common complication of intubation.)

Each of the main bronchi subdivides into several primary bronchi and then into bronchioles. **Bronchioles** (very small bronchial tubes) terminate at the **alveoli**, which are tiny air sacs surrounded by capillaries. The alveoli are the site of gas exchange where the respiratory and circulatory systems meet.

Physiology

The airway is a pathway that leads atmospheric air through the nose, mouth, pharynx, trachea, and bronchi to the alveoli (as discussed in the Shock: Pathophysiology of Life and Death chapter). With each breath, the average 150-pound (lb) (70-kilogram [kg]) adult takes in approximately 500 milliliters (ml) of air. The airway system holds up to 150 ml of air that never actually reaches the alveoli to participate in the critical gas-exchange process. The space in which this air is held is known as *dead space*. The air inside this dead space is not available to the body to be used for oxygenation because it never reaches the alveoli.

With each breath, air is drawn into the lungs. The movement of air into and out of the alveolus results from changes in intrathoracic pressure generated by the contraction and relaxation of specific muscle groups. The primary muscle of breathing is the **diaphragm**. Normally, the muscle fibers of the diaphragm shorten when a stimulus is received from the brain. In addition to the diaphragm, the

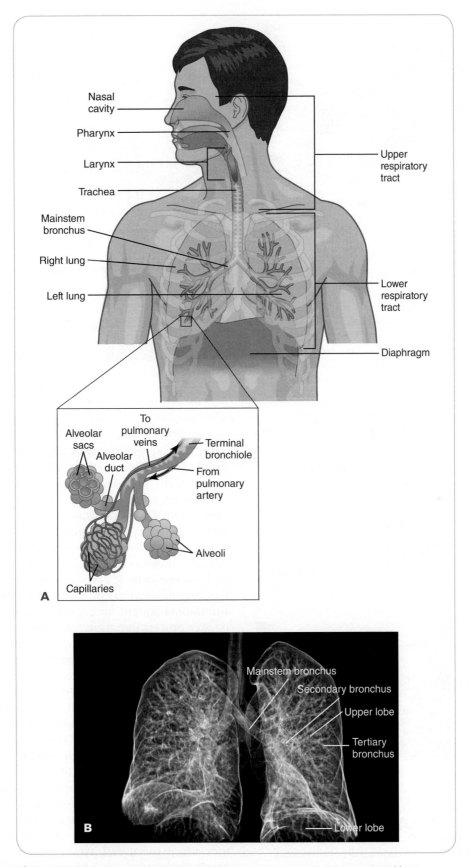

Figure 7-1 A. Organs of the respiratory system: upper respiratory tract and lower respiratory tract. **B.** Cross-section of the lower respiratory tract.

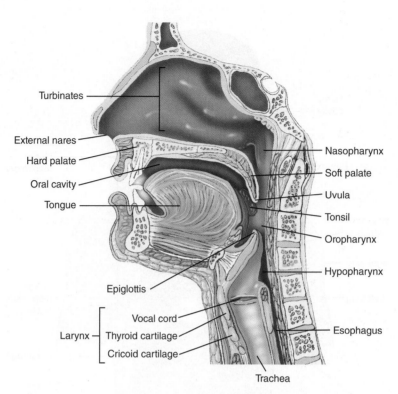

Figure 7-2 Sagittal section through the nasal cavity and pharynx viewed from the medial side.

© National Association of Emergency Medical Technicians (NAEMT).

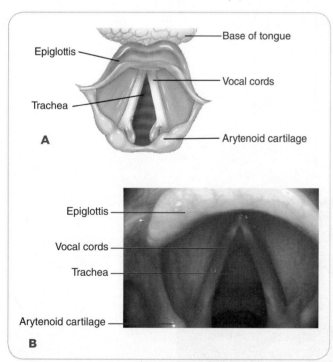

Figure 7-3 Vocal cords viewed from above, showing their relationship to the paired cartilages of the larynx and the epiglottis. Unlike the upper part of the airway, which is all teeth and muscles, the larynx is made up of a thin mucosa and delicate cartilage that won't withstand rough treatment.

A: © National Association of Emergency Medical Technicians (NAEMT); **B:** Courtesy of James P. Thomas, M.D., www.voicedoctor.net.

external intercostal muscles help pull the ribs forward and upward. This flattening of the diaphragm along with the action of the intercostal muscles is an active movement that creates a negative pressure inside the thoracic cavity. This negative pressure causes atmospheric air to enter the intact pulmonary tree (**Figure 7-4**). Other muscles attached to the chest wall can also contribute to the creation of this negative pressure; these include the sternocleidomastoid and scalene muscles. The use of these secondary muscles will be seen as the work of breathing increases in the trauma patient. In contrast, exhalation is normally a passive process in nature, caused by the relaxation of the diaphragm and chest wall muscles and the elastic recoil of these structures. However, exhalation can become active as the work of breathing increases.

Generating this negative pressure during inspiration requires an intact chest wall. For example, in the trauma patient, a wound that creates an open pathway between the outside atmosphere and the thoracic cavity can result in air being pulled in through the open wound rather than into the lungs. In addition, damage to the bony structure of the chest wall may compromise the patient's ability to generate the needed negative pressure required for adequate ventilation. (See the Thoracic Trauma chapter.)

When atmospheric air reaches the alveoli, oxygen moves from the alveoli, across the alveolar–capillary membrane, and into the red blood cells (RBCs) (**Figure 7-5**). The circulatory system then delivers the oxygen-carrying

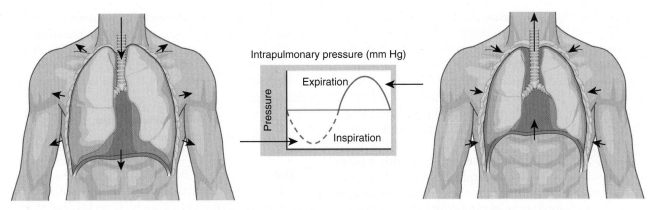

Figure 7-4 This graph shows the relationship of intrapulmonary pressure during the phases of ventilation.

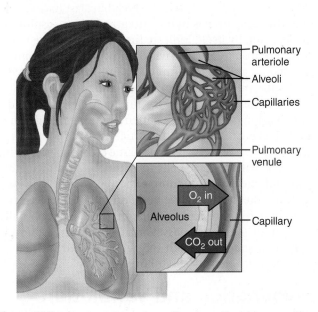

Figure 7-5 Diffusion of oxygen and carbon dioxide across the alveolar–capillary membrane of the alveoli in the lungs.

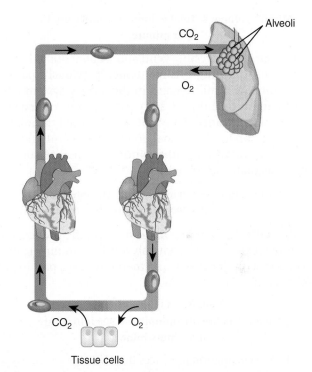

Figure 7-6 Oxygen (O_2) moves into the red blood cells from the alveoli. The O_2 is transferred to the tissue cell on the hemoglobin molecule. After leaving the hemoglobin molecule, the O_2 travels into the tissue cell. Carbon dioxide (CO_2) travels in the reverse direction, but not on the hemoglobin molecule. It travels in the plasma as CO_2.

© National Association of Emergency Medical Technicians (NAEMT).

RBCs to the body tissues, where oxygen is used as fuel for metabolism. As oxygen is transferred from inside the alveoli across the cell wall and capillary endothelium, through the plasma, and into the RBCs, carbon dioxide is exchanged in the opposite direction, from the blood to the alveoli. Carbon dioxide, which is carried dissolved in the plasma (approximately 10%), bound to proteins (mostly hemoglobin in the RBCs [approximately 20%]), and as bicarbonate (approximately 70%), moves from the bloodstream, across the alveolar–capillary membrane, and into the alveoli, where it is eliminated during exhalation (**Figure 7-6**). On completion of this exchange, the oxygenated RBCs and plasma with a low carbon dioxide level return to the left side of the heart to be pumped to all the cells in the body.

Once at the cell, the oxygenated RBCs deliver their oxygen, which the cells then use for aerobic metabolism. (See the Shock: Pathophysiology of Life and Death chapter.) Carbon dioxide, a by-product of aerobic metabolism, is released into the blood plasma. Deoxygenated blood returns to the right side of the heart. The blood is pumped to the lungs, where it is again supplied with oxygen, and the carbon dioxide is eliminated by diffusion. The oxygen is transported mostly by hemoglobin in the RBCs themselves, whereas the carbon dioxide is transported in the three ways previously mentioned: in the plasma, bound to proteins such as hemoglobin, and buffered as bicarbonate.

It is important to remember that while CO_2 is transported dissolved in the plasma, or as bicarbonate, 97% of O_2 is transported bound to hemoglobin in the RBCs; thus, O_2 depends on the amount of RBCs for transport, even in the face of perfect lung function.

Alveoli must be constantly replenished with a fresh supply of air that contains an adequate amount of oxygen. This replenishment of air, known as *ventilation*, is also essential for the elimination of carbon dioxide. Ventilation is measurable. The size of each breath, called the tidal volume, multiplied by the ventilatory rate for 1 minute equals the **minute volume**:

Minute volume = Tidal volume × Ventilatory rate per minute

During normal resting ventilation, about 500 ml of air is taken into the lungs. As mentioned previously, part of this volume, 150 ml, remains in the airway system (the trachea and bronchi) as dead space and does not participate in gas exchange. Only 350 ml is actually available for gas exchange. If the tidal volume is 500 ml and the ventilatory rate is 14 breaths/minute, the minute volume can be calculated as follows:

Minute volume = 500 ml × 14 breaths/minute
= 7,000 ml/minute, or 7 liters/minute

However, by factoring in dead space, the prehospital care provider will realize that only 4.9 liters/minute comes in contact with the alveoli and therefore takes part in gas exchange. That is:

500 ml − 150 ml = 350 ml
350 ml × 14 breaths/minute = 4,900 ml/minute,
or 4.9 liters/minute

This second calculation produces the **effective ventilation**, which is total minute ventilation minus dead space ventilation. It has important consequences when speaking of ventilation in the trauma patient.

If the minute volume falls below normal, the patient has inadequate ventilation, a condition called *hypoventilation*. Hypoventilation leads to a buildup of carbon dioxide in the body. Hypoventilation is common when head or chest trauma causes an altered breathing pattern or an inability to move the chest wall adequately.

For example, a patient with rib fractures who is breathing quickly and shallowly because of the pain of the injury may have a tidal volume of 200 ml and a ventilatory rate of 30 breaths/minute. This patient's minute volume can be calculated as follows:

Minute volume = 200 ml × 30 breaths/minute
= 6,000 ml/minute, or 6 liters/minute

If 7 liters/minute is necessary for adequate gas exchange in a nontraumatized person at rest, 6 liters/minute is less than the body requires to eliminate carbon dioxide effectively, indicating hypoventilation. Furthermore, calculating the effective minute ventilation reveals the true severity of the patient's condition:

200 ml − 150 ml = 50 ml
50 ml × 30 breaths/minute = 1,500 ml/minute,
or 1.5 liters/minute

Almost no oxygenated air will reach the alveoli; the air will get only as far as the trachea and bronchi. If left untreated, this hypoventilation will quickly lead to severe respiratory distress and, ultimately, death.

In the previous example, the patient with rib fractures is hypoventilating even though the ventilatory rate is 30 breaths/minute. This patient is breathing fast (tachypneic) but at the same time is hypoventilating. Thus, respiratory rate does not, by itself, indicate the adequacy of the ventilation. Prehospital care providers must take tidal volume into account and never simply assume that a patient with a fast ventilatory rate is hyperventilating.

Assessment of ventilatory function always includes an evaluation of how well a patient is taking in, diffusing, and delivering oxygen to the tissue cells. Without proper intake, delivery of oxygen to the tissue cells, and processing of oxygen within these cells to maintain aerobic metabolism and energy production, anaerobic metabolism will begin. In addition, effective ventilation must be ensured. A patient may accomplish ventilation completely, partially, or not at all. Aggressive assessment and management of these inadequacies in both oxygenation and ventilation are paramount to a successful outcome.

Oxygenation and Ventilation of the Trauma Patient

The oxygenation process within the human body involves the following three phases:

1. *External respiration* is the transfer of oxygen molecules from air to the blood. Air contains oxygen (20.95%), nitrogen (78.1%), argon (0.93%), and carbon dioxide (0.031%), but for practical purposes, the content of air is oxygen 21% and nitrogen 79%. All alveolar oxygen exists as free gas; therefore, each oxygen molecule exerts pressure. Increasing the percentage of oxygen in the inspired atmosphere will increase alveolar oxygen pressure or tension. When supplemental oxygen is provided, the ratio of oxygen in each inspiration increases, causing an increase in the amount of oxygen in each alveolus. This, in turn, will increase the amount of gas that gets transferred to blood because the amount of gas that will enter a liquid is directly related to the

pressure it exerts. The greater the pressure of the gas, the greater the amount of that gas that will be absorbed into the fluid.

2. *Oxygen delivery* is the result of oxygen transfer from the atmosphere to the RBCs during ventilation and the transportation of these RBCs to the tissues via the cardiovascular system. The volume of oxygen consumed by the body in 1 minute in order to maintain energy production is known as oxygen consumption and depends on adequate cardiac output and the delivery of oxygen to the cells by RBCs. The RBCs could be described as the body's "oxygen tankers." These oxygen tankers move along the vascular system "highways" to "off-load" their oxygen supply at the body's distribution points, the capillary beds.

3. *Internal (cellular) respiration* is the movement, or diffusion, of oxygen from the RBCs into the tissue cells. Metabolism normally occurs through glycolysis and the Krebs cycle to produce energy. While understanding the specific details of these processes is not necessary, it is important to have a general understanding of their role in energy production. Because the actual exchange of oxygen between the RBCs and the tissues occurs in the thin-walled capillaries, any factor that interrupts a supply of oxygen will disrupt this cycle. A major factor in this regard is the amount of fluid (or edema) located between the alveolar walls, the capillary walls, and the wall of the tissue cells (also known as the interstitial space). Overhydration of the vascular space with crystalloid, which leaks out of the vascular system into the interstitial space within 30 to 45 minutes after administration, is a major problem during resuscitation. Supplemental oxygen can help overcome some of these factors. The tissues and cells cannot consume adequate amounts of oxygen if adequate amounts are not available.

Adequate oxygenation depends on all three of these phases. Although the ability to assess tissue oxygenation in prehospital situations is improving rapidly, appropriate ventilatory support for all trauma patients begins by providing supplemental oxygen to help ensure that hypoxia is corrected or averted entirely.

Pathophysiology

Trauma can affect the respiratory system's ability to adequately provide oxygen and eliminate carbon dioxide in the following ways:

- Diminished oxygen uptake due to hypoventilation
  - Obstructed airway
  - Hypoventilation due to rib fractures, pneumothorax, or flail chest
  - Diminished oxygen uptake due to lung contusion
- Diminished oxygen transport due to shock. (See the Shock: Pathophysiology of Life and Death chapter.)
- Diminished oxygen unloading due to vascular compromise or to systemic factors (cyanide intoxication)

Hypoventilation results from the reduction of minute volume. If left untreated, hypoventilation results in carbon dioxide buildup, acidosis, and eventually death. Management involves improving the patient's ventilatory rate and depth by correcting existing airway problems and assisting ventilation as appropriate.

Hyperventilation, on the other hand, can cause vasoconstriction, which can be especially detrimental in the management of the traumatic brain-injured patient, and large tidal volumes can reduce venous return, which can be especially detrimental in patients who are in shock.

Causes and Sites of Airway Obstruction in the Trauma Patient

Decreased minute volume can be caused by two clinical conditions: mechanical obstruction of the upper airway and a decreased level of consciousness (LOC), with both conditions frequently occurring together.

When you look at it externally, the upper airway extends from the tip of the nose down to the sternal notch. Anything that happens in the front part of that region can cause or become an airway problem. A general good rule is that the more distal an obstruction occurs, the more challenging it is to correct.

The most common cause of upper airway obstruction is the tongue falling rearward and obstructing the hypopharynx. The tongue may become an obstruction when an unconscious patient loses muscle tone; when, following bilateral fracture of the mandible, the tongue is no longer attached to the mandible; or following extensive maxillofacial trauma (**Figure 7-7**). This condition causes airway obstruction along with snoring and abnormal thorax excursions, and in the trauma patient is often further complicated by blood and secretions accumulating in the upper airway.

This condition can be corrected by positioning and simple airway maneuvers, such as the trauma jaw thrust or chin lift.

Another common cause is accumulation of secretions, blood, and debris in the hypopharynx whenever the patient is unable to clear his or her airway due to decreased LOC or to extensive trauma. A gurgling respiration is a sure sign that the patient is unable to clear his or her airway and is at risk of aspiration and/or airway obstruction with the very next breath. This condition can

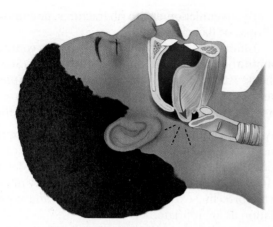

Figure 7-7 In an unconscious patient, the tongue has lost its muscle tone and falls back into the hypopharynx, occluding the airway and preventing passage of oxygen into the trachea and lungs.

© National Association of Emergency Medical Technicians (NAEMT).

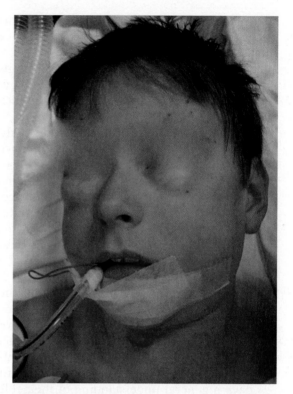

Figure 7-8 A patient who sustained trauma to the anterior neck, causing rupture of the trachea and subcutaneous emphysema of the neck and face. If you look just in the patient's mouth, you are likely to miss a vital piece of information.

Photograph provided courtesy of J.C. Pitteloud, M.D., Switzerland.

be corrected, at least temporarily, by drainage or suction of the upper airway.

The third most common place of upper airway obstruction is the larynx, where obstruction can be caused either by direct trauma to the laryngeal cartilage or by inhalation burns with swelling of the mucosa (**Figure 7-8**). This condition will manifest with hoarseness and stridor and usually will require an advanced airway (**endotracheal (ET) tube** or surgical airway).

A decreased LOC, from traumatic brain injury (TBI) or associated issues such as alcohol or drug use, will also affect ventilatory drive and may reduce the rate of ventilation, the volume of ventilation, or both. This reduction in minute volume may be temporary or permanent.

Assessment of the Airway and Ventilation

The ability to assess the airway is required in order to effectively manage it. Prehospital care providers perform many aspects of assessing the airway automatically. A patient who is alert and talking with a normal voice as the provider walks through the door has an open and patent airway. But when the patient's LOC is decreased, it is essential to thoroughly assess the airway prior to moving to other, lower priority injuries. When examining the airway during the primary survey, the following items need to be assessed:

- Position of the airway and patient
- Any sounds emanating from the upper airway
- Airway obstructions
- Chest rise

Position of the Airway and Patient

As you make visual contact with the patient, observe the patient's position. Patients in a supine position with a decreased LOC are at risk for airway obstruction from the tongue falling back into the airway. Most trauma patients will be placed in the supine position on a backboard for spinal immobilization. Any patient exhibiting signs of decreased LOC will need constant reexamination for airway obstruction and the placement of an adjunctive device to ensure an open airway may be necessary. Patients who present with an open airway while lying on their side may obstruct their airways when placed supine on a backboard. Patients with massive facial trauma and active bleeding may need to be maintained in the position in which they are found if they are maintaining their own airway. In some cases, this may mean allowing the patient to sit in an upright position as long as the airway is being maintained. Placing these patients supine on a backboard may cause obstruction to the airway and possible aspiration of blood. In such cases, if the patients are maintaining their own airways, the best course of action may be to let them continue. Suction should be available if needed to remove blood and secretions. If necessary, stabilization of the cervical spine can be accomplished by manually holding the head in the position needed to allow for maintenance of an open airway. Stabilization of the thoracolumbar spine is harder to accomplish in this position, but if the choice is between increased protection of the thoracolumbar spine versus inability to maintain an open airway in a patient who was found in an upright position, maintaining airway patency must take priority.

Upper Airway Sounds

Noise coming from the upper airway is never a good sign. These noises can often be heard as you approach the patient. They are usually a result of a partial airway obstruction caused by the tongue, blood, or foreign bodies in the upper airway.

The type of sound you hear can give you some clues as to the cause and location of upper airway obstruction. Snoring is caused by the base of the tongue and the soft palate falling backward and obstructing the upper airway. Gurgling occurs when blood, vomit, or secretions are present in the pharynx; it signals that the patient is unable to clear and protect his or her airway. Stridor comes from the vocal cords and signals a problem at that level, especially when inspiratory, caused by an obstruction at the level of the larynx. Stridor is typically caused by direct trauma, foreign body, or swelling of the mucosa, as in inhalation burns. Swelling is a challenging situation because it occurs at the narrowest point of the upper airway. An edematous airway is an emergent situation that demands quick action to prevent total airway obstruction. Steps must be taken immediately to alleviate the obstructions and maintain an open airway.

Examine the Airway for Obstructions

Because the upper airway extends from the tip of the nose to the sternal notch, simply looking in the mouth is not enough. Look in the mouth for any obvious foreign matter, such as vomit, blood, or debris or any gross anatomic malformations, such as hematoma or swelling in the mouth, and then look along the anterior neck down to the jugulum. A thorough evaluation of the airway is important because some especially dangerous airway obstructions are situated in the anterior neck. Remove any foreign bodies found.

Look for Chest Rise

Limited chest rise can be a sign of an obstructed airway. Additional signs, like the use of accessory muscles and the appearance of increased work of breathing, should lead to a high index of suspicion of airway compromise.

When a patient is working hard to move air across an obstructed airway, negative pressure will build up in the chest, and retractions will be observed between the ribs and at the jugular notch when muscle and tissues are pulled into the chest. These retractions are especially visible in children.

When the airway becomes even more obstructed, "seesaw breathing" or "rocking boat breathing" is likely to occur. As the patient attempts to breathe through the obstructed airway, the diaphragm descends, causing the abdomen to lift (as in normal inspiration) and the chest to sink (not normal). The reverse happens as the diaphragm relaxes. Prehospital care providers observing this pattern of breathing should suspect an airway obstruction.

Management
Airway Control

After controlling any severe hemorrhage, ensuring a patent airway is the next priority of trauma management and resuscitation, and no action is more crucial in airway management than appropriate assessment of the airway. Ideally, the airway of the trauma patient should be both open for air entry and protected against aspiration and occlusion through swelling, which can be achieved by endotracheal intubation. However, ensuring an open airway is the first priority, and most of the time it can be accomplished quickly with no equipment other than the prehospital care provider's hands. Regardless of how the airway is managed, a cervical spine injury must be considered if the mechanism of injury suggests the potential for cervical spine injury. The use of any of these methods of airway control requires simultaneous manual stabilization of the cervical spine in a neutral position until the patient has been completely immobilized. (See the Spinal Trauma chapter.) The exception to this rule is penetrating trauma. Data have shown that spinal immobilization is usually not necessary in these patients. (See the Spinal Trauma chapter.)

Essential Skills

Management of the airway in trauma patients is a primary consideration, because without an adequate airway, a positive outcome cannot be achieved. Management of the airway can be challenging, but in most patients, manual or simple procedures may be sufficient initially.[1] Even prehospital care providers who have been trained in more complex airway techniques need to maintain their ability to perform these simple and essential manual skills, because as these methods, depending on the situation, that can be applied immediately without any material other than the provider's hands and lead to a better patient outcome than more complex techniques, which require increased time, personnel, and equipment. Providers always need to weigh the risk versus the benefit of performing highly invasive, complex procedures. Such procedures require a high degree of skill proficiency and close oversight by the medical director. They should not be initiated unnecessarily.

Airway maintenance skills can be broken into three different levels. The application of these skills, as long as they are within the prehospital care provider's scope of practice, should be patient driven, dependent on the situation and the severity of the patient.

Categories for Airway Adjuncts and Procedures

Manual

Manual methods of opening the airway are the easiest to use and require no equipment other than the prehospital care provider's hands. The airway can be maintained with these methods, even if the patient has a gag reflex. There are no contraindications for the use of manual techniques in airway management of the trauma patient. Examples of this type of airway management include the **trauma chin lift** and the **trauma jaw thrust**. Positioning and manual clearing of the airway also fall into this category (**Figure 7-9**).

Simple

Simple airway management involves the use of adjunctive devices that require only one piece of equipment, and the technique for inserting the device necessitates minimal training. The risks associated with placement of these types of airway devices are extremely low compared to the potential benefit of maintaining a patent airway. If the airway is improperly placed, it is easily recognizable and correctable. Examples of these airways include oropharyngeal and nasopharyngeal airways (**Figure 7-10**).

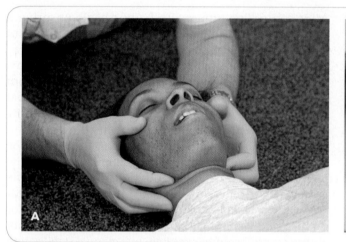
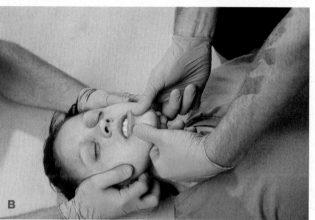

Figure 7-9 A. Trauma jaw thrust. The thumb is placed on each zygoma, with the index and long fingers at the angle of the mandible. The mandible is lifted superiorly. **B.** Trauma chin lift. The chin lift performs a function similar to that of the trauma jaw thrust. It moves the mandible forward by moving the tongue.

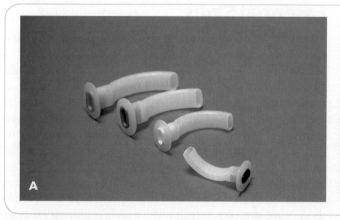
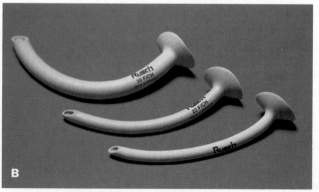

Figure 7-10 A. Oropharyngeal airways. **B.** Nasopharyngeal airways.

Complex

Complex airways include airway adjuncts that require significant initial training and then ongoing training to ensure continuing proficiency. While complex airways provide greater airway protection compared to basic techniques, their use in the field requires more time and personnel. Adjuncts that fall into this category require multiple pieces of equipment and the possible use of pharmaceuticals as well as multiple steps to insert the airway and, in some cases, direct visualization of the tracheal opening. In addition, surgical airway techniques such as cricothyrotomy (both needle and surgical) fall into this category. The penalty for failure when using complex airways is high and may include a less than optimal outcome for the patient. Continuous monitoring of oxygen saturation and ETCO$_2$ is also highly recommended when using this group of airways, adding to the complexity of their use. Examples of these airways include endotracheal tubes and supraglottic airways (**Figure 7-11**).

See **Box 7-1** for a breakdown of the three methods of airway management.

Manual Clearing of the Airway

The first step in airway management is a quick visual inspection of the oropharyngeal cavity. Foreign material (e.g., pieces of food) or broken teeth or dentures and blood may be found in the mouth of a trauma patient. These objects are swept out of the mouth using a gloved finger plus a mechanical block for protection or, in the case of blood or vomitus, may be suctioned away. In addition, positioning of the patient on his or her side or in a sitting position, when not contraindicated by possible spinal trauma, will allow for gravity-assisted clearing of secretions, blood, and vomitus, especially if there are large amounts. If spinal trauma is suspected, the patient can be logrolled onto his or her side to allow clearing of blood and vomit.

Manual Maneuvers

In unresponsive patients, the tongue becomes flaccid, falling back and blocking the hypopharynx (see Figure 7-7). The tongue is the most common cause of airway obstruction. Manual methods to clear this type of obstruction can easily be accomplished because the tongue is attached to the mandible (jaw) and moves forward with it. Any maneuver that moves the mandible forward will pull the tongue away from the back of the hypopharynx:

- *Trauma jaw thrust.* In patients with suspected head, neck, or facial trauma, the cervical spine is maintained in a neutral in-line position. The trauma jaw thrust maneuver allows the prehospital care provider to open the airway with little or no movement of the head and cervical spine (see Figure 7-9). The mandible is thrust forward by placing the thumbs on each zygoma (cheekbone), placing the index and long fingers on the mandible, and at the same angle, pushing the mandible forward. This maneuver can be applied from the head or from the front position by a single provider.

- *Trauma chin lift.* The trauma chin lift maneuver is used to relieve a variety of anatomic airway obstructions in patients who are breathing spontaneously (see Figure 7-9). The chin and, if necessary, the lower incisors are grasped and then lifted to pull the mandible forward. The prehospital care provider wears gloves to avoid body fluid contamination. This technique requires two providers; one performs the chin lift while the other stabilizes the head. It should be used with caution if the patient is reactive and can bite the provider's thumb.

Both of these techniques result in movement of the lower mandible anteriorly (upward) and slightly caudal (toward the feet), pulling the tongue forward, away from the posterior airway, and opening the mouth. The trauma jaw thrust pushes the mandible forward, whereas the trauma chin lift pulls the mandible. The trauma jaw thrust and the trauma chin lift are modifications of the conventional jaw thrust and chin lift. The modifications provide protection to the patient's cervical spine while opening the airway by displacing the tongue from the posterior pharynx.

Suctioning

A trauma patient may not be capable of effectively clearing the buildup of secretions, vomitus, blood, or foreign objects from the trachea. Providing suction is an important part of maintaining a patent airway.

The trauma patient whose airway has not yet been managed may require aggressive suctioning of the upper airway. Large amounts of blood and vomit may have already accumulated in the airway before the arrival of emergency medical services (EMS) providers, and this may have already compromised ventilation and oxygen transport into the alveoli. This accumulation may be more than a simple suction unit can quickly clear. If so, the patient may be logrolled onto his or her side while maintaining cervical spine stabilization; gravity will assist in clearing the airway. A rigid large-bore suction device is preferred to clear the oropharynx.

The best technique to suction the mouth and the pharynx is to insert the suction catheter via the side of the mouth lateral to the teeth. This approach is less stimulating and can be accomplished even if the patient is clenching his or her teeth (**Figure 7-12**).

The most significant complication of suctioning is that suctioning for prolonged periods will produce hypoxemia, which produces significant detrimental effects at the tissue level in many organs. The most obvious clinical sign that the patient is becoming hypoxic is a cardiac abnormality (e.g., tachycardia or dysrhythmias). Preoxygenation of the trauma patient by providing supplemental oxygen will help

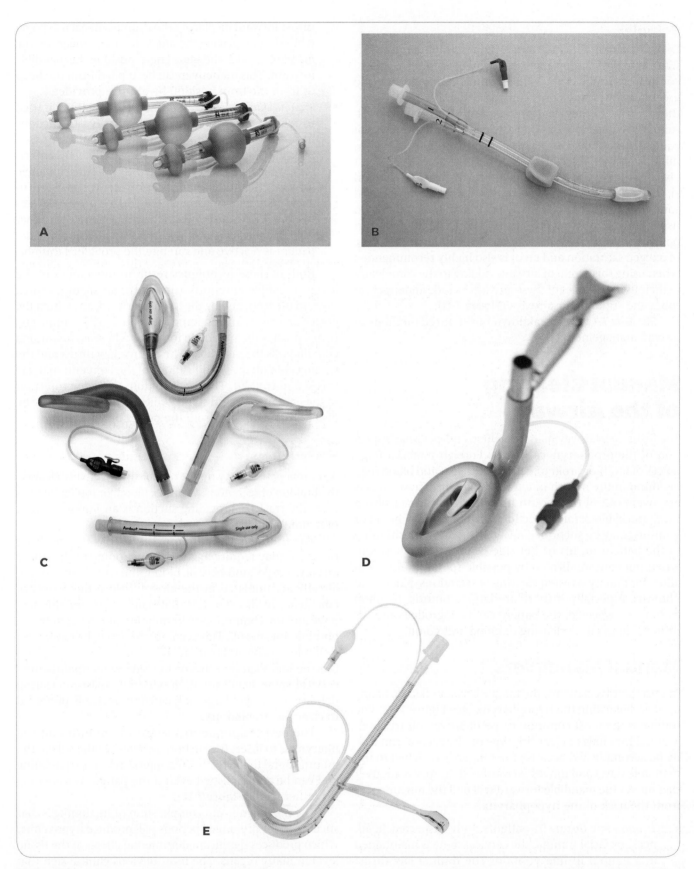

Figure 7-11 A. King laryngotracheal airway. **B.** Combitube. **C.** Laryngeal mask airway (LMA). **D.** Intubating LMA. **E.** Intubating LMA with ET tube in place.

A, B, C: Courtesy of Ambu, Inc. D and E: Courtesy of Teleflex, Inc.

Box 7-1 Methods of Airway Management

Manual
- Hands only

Simple
- Oropharyngeal airway
- Nasopharyngeal airway

Complex
- Endotracheal intubation
- Supraglottic airways
- Pharmacologically assisted/rapid-sequence intubation/delayed-sequence intubation
- Percutaneous airway
- Surgical airway

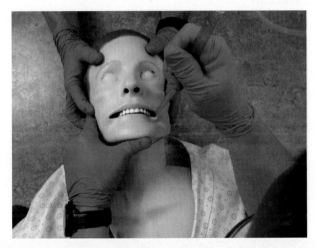

Figure 7-12 Using a rigid suction catheter while maintaining cervical spine alignment.

Photograph provided courtesy of J.C. Pitteloud M.D., Switzerland.

prevent hypoxemia. In addition, when suctioning close to or below the larynx (i.e., when suctioning an endotracheal tube), the suction catheter may stimulate either the internal branch of the superior laryngeal nerve or the recurrent laryngeal nerve that supplies the larynx above and below the cords, both of which are vagal in origin. Vagal stimulation may lead to profound bradycardia and hypotension.

Although hypoxia can result from prolonged suctioning, a totally obstructed airway will provide no air exchange. Aggressive suctioning and patient positioning are continued until the airway is at least partially clear. At that point, hyperoxygenation followed by repeated suctioning can be performed. Hyperoxygenation, like preoxygenation, may be accomplished with either a nonrebreathing mask on a high flow of oxygen or a bag-mask device running at 15 liters/minute. The goal when hyperoxygenating is to maintain an oxygen saturation at or above 95% at sea level.

Suctioning intubated patients requires additional precautions, which will be discussed later in the chapter.

Selection of Adjunctive Device

Problems found with the airway during the primary survey require immediate action to establish and maintain a patent airway. These initial steps are the manual maneuvers, such as a trauma jaw thrust or chin lift. Once opened, the airway must be maintained. The particular device should be selected based on the prehospital care provider's level of training and proficiency with that particular device and a risk–benefit analysis for the use of various types of devices and techniques that relate to the particular patient. (See the Golden Principles, Preferences, and Critical Thinking chapter.) The choice of the airway adjunct should be patient driven: "What is the best airway for this particular patient in this particular situation?"

During initial training as well as during ongoing continuing education, prehospital care providers at various levels are exposed to a range of adjunctive devices to help maintain an open airway. The amount of training directly relates to the difficulty in placement of the device. At the emergency medical responder level, providers are trained to place oropharyngeal airways. At the other end of the spectrum, advanced providers have been trained to use complex airway devices, with some protocols allowing surgical airway procedures.

With complex skills such as intubation or surgical cricothyrotomy, the more times a skill is performed, the better the chance for a successful outcome. A new paramedic who has performed these procedures only in the classroom setting has less of a chance of intubating a difficult patient successfully compared to a 10-year veteran who has performed these interventions numerous times during his or her career. The more steps there are in a procedure, the more difficult the procedure is to learn and master. These complex skills also lend themselves to a greater probability of failure as greater knowledge is required and more steps are involved in completing the intervention. As a skill increases in difficulty, so do the educational requirements, both in initial training and ongoing skill maintenance. Generally the more difficult a procedure is to perform, the greater the penalty to the patient for failure or error. This is particularly true with airway procedures.

There are several types of airway devices that may be selected depending on the needs or potential needs of the patient (**Box 7-2** and **Box 7-3**):

- Simple adjuncts
  - Devices that lift the tongue from the back of the pharynx only
    - Oral airway
    - Nasal airway
  - To ventilate requires a mask (usually with bag-mask device)

- Complex airways
  - Devices that occlude the oral pharynx
    - Supraglottic airways
      - Combitube
      - Laryngeal mask airway
      - Laryngeal tubes (LTs; e.g., King LT)
  - Devices that isolate the trachea from the esophagus
    - ET tube
    - Surgical airway
  - No mask required to ventilate

Box 7-2 Factors in Selecting Airway Adjuncts

The prehospital care provider should choose from any of the adjuncts available in the airway toolbox based on the situation. Factors influencing the decision include, but are not limited to, the following:

- Training
- Available assistance
- Transport time
- Perceived difficulty
- Ability to maintain the patient's airway with a simple adjunct

---

Simple Adjuncts

When manual airway maneuvers are unsuccessful or when continued maintenance of an open airway is necessary, the use of an artificial airway is the next step (**Figure 7-13**). After placement of a simple adjunctive device, a decision to escalate to a complex airway may be appropriate, depending on the particular patient and situation. The simple airway adjuncts are discussed next.

Oropharyngeal Airway

The most frequently used artificial airway is the **oropharyngeal airway (OPA)** (see Figure 7-10). The OPA is inserted in either a direct or an inverted manner.

Indications
- Patient who is unable to maintain his or her airway
- To prevent an intubated patient from biting an ET tube

Contraindications
- Patient who is conscious or semiconscious
- Patient with a gag reflex

Complications
- Because it stimulates the gag reflex, use of the OPA may lead to gagging, vomiting, and laryngospasm in patients who are conscious

---

Box 7-3 Airway Technique Synopsis

Basic Airway Techniques
Principle: In the normal state the upper airway is open and the esophagus is closed. Basic life support (BLS) airway maneuvers maintain the upper airway open so that air flows through the larynx into the lungs.

Specific Skills
- Positioning
- Suctioning
- Trauma chin lift, trauma jaw thrust
- Oropharyngeal airway (OPA), nasopharyngeal airway (NPA)

Can be used in a patient with a gag reflex (except OPA)

No airway protection against aspiration

Advanced Airway Techniques
Principle: Opens the airway while separating it from the digestive tract so that air goes selectively through the larynx into the lungs

Specific Skills
Supraglottic airway devices (LMA, King Airway)
Occludes the esophagus while opening the airway

- Requires an unconscious patient
- Offers only a little protection against aspiration

Endotracheal intubation
Tube goes through the larynx into the trachea

- Requires a deeply anesthetized and relaxed patient
- Protects the airway against both bronchoaspiration and occlusion through swelling

Surgical airway
Tube goes through the cricothyroid membrane into the trachea

- Because it bypasses the pharynx and the glottis, it can be done in a conscious patient with local anesthesia or no anesthesia at all
- Protects the airway against bronchoaspiration

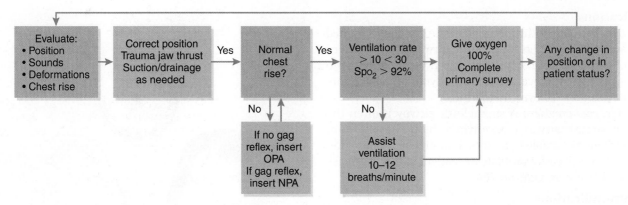

Figure 7-13 Basic airway management algorithm.

Nasopharyngeal Airway

The **nasopharyngeal airway (NPA)** is a soft, rubberlike device that is inserted through one of the nares and then along the curvature of the posterior wall of the nasopharynx and oropharynx (see Figure 7-10).

Indications
- Patient who is unable to maintain his or her airway

Contraindications
- No need for an airway adjunct
- Although we know of a case report of intracranial insertion of an NPA, evidence has not supported the claim that facial/basilar skull fractures are a contraindication to placement of an NPA if one is needed.[1] Correct insertion technique should minimize the risks.[1,2]

Complications
- Bleeding caused by insertion may be a complication

Complex Airways

Complex airway adjuncts and management techniques are appropriate when simple airway maneuvers and devices are inadequate to maintain a patent airway. Any time a complex airway device is considered for placement in a patient, the prehospital care provider must consider the possibility that the procedure will be unsuccessful and have a backup plan in mind, including the possibility to go back to a more basic technique. Alternate methods of managing the airway should be considered and the necessary equipment prepared in the event the first choice of intervention proves unsuccessful.

In most trauma patients, the cervical spine should remain immobilized during the process of airway management. A properly sized cervical collar will add to the difficulty of airway management by limiting mouth opening. This difficulty can be overcome by opening the cervical collar while a second provider stabilizes from the front. When

---

> **Box 7-4** Common Supraglottic Airways
>
> - King LT airway
> - Combitube
> - Laryngeal mask airway
> - Intubating LMA

done correctly, this method will stabilize the cervical spine without limiting mouth opening.

Supraglottic Airways

Supraglottic airways offer a functional alternative airway to endotracheal intubation (**Box 7-4**; see Figure 7-11). Many jurisdictions allow the use of these devices because minimal training is required to achieve and retain competency. These devices are inserted without direct visualization of the vocal cords. They are also a useful backup airway when endotracheal intubation attempts are unsuccessful, even when rapid-sequence intubation has been attempted, or when, after careful evaluation of the airway, the prehospital care provider feels that the chance for successful placement is higher than for endotracheal intubation. The primary advantage of supraglottic airways is that they may be inserted independent of the patient's position, which may be especially important in trauma patients with access and extrication difficulties or a high suspicion of cervical injury. They can be useful if it is difficult to obtain a tight mask seal.

When placed into a patient, supraglottic airways are designed to isolate the trachea from the esophagus. However, none of these devices provides a complete seal of the trachea; therefore, while the risk of aspiration is lowered, it is not completely eliminated.

Some manufacturers have developed supraglottic airways in pediatric sizes. Prehospital care providers should ensure proper sizing according to the manufacturer's specifications if using these types of airways on pediatric patients.

Indications

- *Basic providers*. If the prehospital care provider is trained and authorized, a supraglottic airway is an efficient airway device for an unconscious trauma patient who lacks a gag reflex and is apneic or ventilating at a rate of less than 10 breaths/minute.
- *Advanced providers*. A supraglottic airway is often the alternative airway device when the prehospital care provider is unable to perform endotracheal intubation and cannot easily ventilate the patient with a bag-mask device and an OPA or NPA.

Contraindications

- Intact gag reflex
- Nonfasting (recent meal) (*Note:* While this caveat can be found in the user's manual of most of these devices, it applies to the operating room [OR] setting and not to the trauma patient in the field, who is unlikely to be fasting. Still, it should be a reminder that this airway does not provide complete protection from aspiration should vomiting occur.)
- Known esophageal disease (This contraindication is especially relevant for the Combitube and the King LT airways; the risk is reduced with the LMA because it does not enter the esophagus.)
- Recent ingestion of caustic substances

Complications

- Gagging and vomiting (if gag reflex is intact)
- Aspiration
- Damage to the esophagus
- Hypoxia if ventilated using the incorrect lumen

Laryngeal Mask Airway

The **laryngeal mask airway (LMA)** is another alternative for unconscious or seriously obtunded adult and pediatric patients. The device comprises an inflatable silicone ring attached diagonally to a silicone tube (**Figure 7-14**). When inserted, the ring creates a low-pressure seal between the LMA and the glottic opening, without direct insertion of the device into the larynx itself (**Figure 7-15**).

Different brands and designs of LMAs are available, including some models with a rigid, anatomically curved conduit. The I-gel LMA is made from a medical-grade thermoplastic elastomer. It has been designed to create a noninflatable, anatomic seal of the pharyngeal, laryngeal, and perilaryngeal structures while avoiding compression trauma. All of these models are available in different sizes, including pediatric models.

Advantages of the LMA include the following:

- The LMA is designed for blind insertion. Direct visualization of the trachea and vocal cords is unnecessary.
- With proper cleaning and storage, some LMAs can be reused multiple times.
- Disposable LMAs are now available.
- The LMA is available in a range of sizes to accommodate both pediatric and adult patient groups.

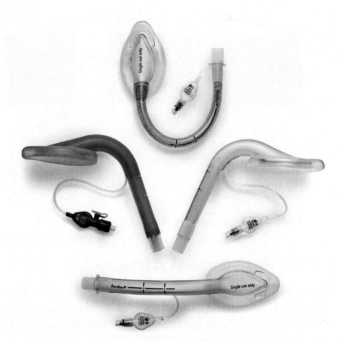

Figure 7-14 Laryngeal mask airway.
Courtesy of Ambu, Inc.

Prehospital use of the LMA thus far has been more prevalent in Europe than in North America. A recent development is the introduction of an "intubating LMA." This device is inserted similarly to the original LMA, but a flexible ET tube is then passed though the LMA, intubating the trachea. The success rate is up to 90% in difficult intubations. This approach secures the airway without the need to visualize the vocal cords. As an added bonus, it will allow ventilation and oxygenation, even if intubation is impossible.

Indications

- As a primary airway device in some EMS systems
- When unable to perform endotracheal intubation and the patient cannot be ventilated using a bag-mask device

Contraindications

- When endotracheal intubation can be performed
- Insufficient training

Complications

- Aspiration, because the LMA does not completely prevent regurgitation and protect the trachea
- Laryngospasm

Endotracheal Intubation

Traditionally, endotracheal intubation has been the preferred method for achieving maximum control of the airway in trauma patients who are apneic, are unable to maintain/protect their airway, or require assisted ventilation (**Figure 7-16** and **Box 7-5**). Studies, however, have shown that in an urban environment, critically injured trauma patients with endotracheal intubation had no better

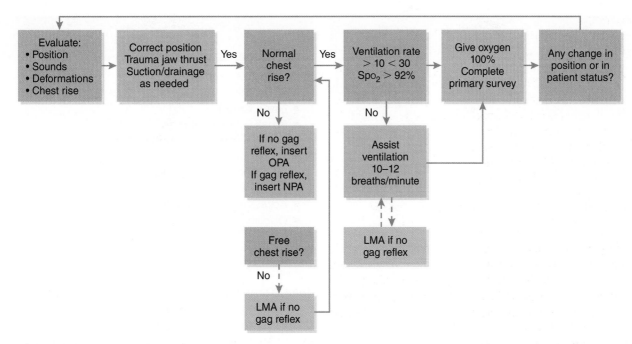

Figure 7-15 LMA in the airway management algorithm.

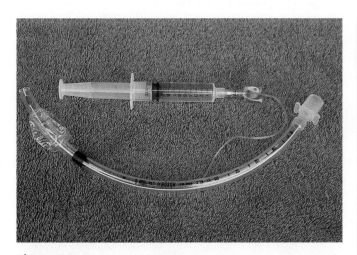

Figure 7-16 Endotracheal tube.
Courtesy of Ambu, Inc.

outcome than those transported with a bag-mask device and OPA.[3] As a result, the role of endotracheal intubation has increasingly come under question. Few studies have demonstrated any benefit to the technique.[4] The decision to perform endotracheal intubation or to use an alternative device should be made after assessment of the airway has helped define the difficulty of the intubation. The risk of hypoxia from prolonged intubation attempts for a patient who has a difficult airway needs to be weighed against the need to insert the ET tube in the field. Consideration should be given to the effect of the increase in scene time necessary to perform the procedure.

Intubation in the field will always be more difficult than in the hospital, no matter how skilled the crew is, so

Box 7-5 Equipment for Endotracheal Intubation

As with any advanced life support (ALS) skill, prehospital care providers need to have the proper equipment. The standard components of an intubation kit should include the following (Figure 7-17):

■ Laryngoscope with adult- and pediatric-sized straight and curved blades
■ Extra batteries and spare lightbulbs

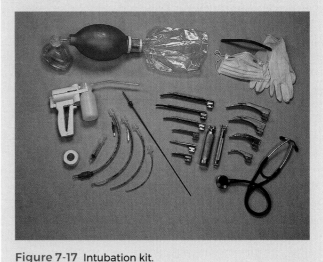

Figure 7-17 Intubation kit.
© National Association of Emergency Medical Technicians (NAEMT).

(*continued*)

Box 7-5 Equipment for Endotracheal
              Intubation (*continued*)

- Suction equipment including rigid and flexible catheters
- Adult- and pediatric-sized ET tubes
- Stylet
- Gum elastic bougie
- 10-ml syringe
- Water-soluble lubricant
- Magill forceps
- End-tidal carbon dioxide detection device for ETCO$_2$ detection
- Waveform capnography
- Tube-securing device

Box 7-6 Factors That Contribute to
              Difficult Intubation

- Receding chin
- Short neck
- Large tongue
- Small mouth opening
- Cervical immobilization or stiff neck
- Facial trauma
- Bleeding into the airway
- Active vomiting
- Access to the patient
- Obesity

---

while there might be good reasons to intubate a patient for a 30-minute flight to the hospital, those reasons are less compelling if the patient is 5 minutes from a well-equipped and well-staffed emergency room.

Prediction of Potentially Difficult Endotracheal Intubation

It is imperative that prior to performing endotracheal intubation an assessment of the difficulty of the intubation be done. Many factors can result in a difficult intubation of the trauma patient (**Box 7-6**). Some of these are directly related to the trauma that they have sustained; others are due to anatomic anomalies of the face and upper airway; others to positioning of the patient.

The mnemonic LEMON has been developed to assist in the assessment of the relative difficulty that will be involved in a particular intubation (**Box 7-7**). Although not all components of the LEMON mnemonic may be applied to the trauma patient in the field, an understanding of the

---

Box 7-7 LEMON Assessment for Difficult Intubation

L = **Look externally:** Look for characteristics that are known to cause difficult intubation or ventilation.

E = **Evaluate the 3-3-2 rule:** To allow for alignment of the pharyngeal, laryngeal, and oral axes, and therefore simple intubation, the following relationships should be observed (**Figure 7-18**):
- The distance between the patient's upper and lower incisor teeth should be at least 3 fingerbreadths
- The distance between the hyoid bone and the chin should be at least 3 fingerbreadths
- The distance between the thyroid notch and floor of the mouth should be at least 2 fingerbreadths

M = **Mallampati:** The hypopharynx should be visualized adequately. This has been done traditionally by assessing the Mallampati classification (**Figure 7-19**).
- When possible, the patient is asked to sit upright, open the mouth fully, and protrude the tongue as far as possible. The examiner then looks into the mouth with a light to assess the degree of hypopharynx visible. In supine patients, the Mallampati score can be estimated by asking the

patient to open the mouth fully and protrude the tongue; a laryngoscopy light is then shone into the hypopharynx from above.

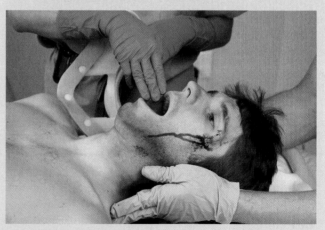

Figure 7-18 The 3-3-2 rule enables alignment of the pharyngeal, laryngeal, and oral axes and, therefore, simple intubation. The following relationships should be observed: **A.** The distance between the patient's incisor teeth should be at least 3 fingerbreadths.

© National Association of Emergency Medical Technicians (NAEMT).

Box 7-7 LEMON Assessment for Difficult Intubation (*continued*)

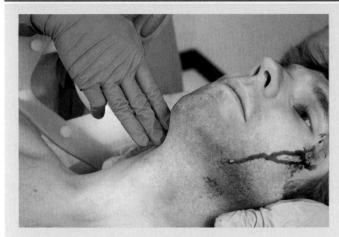

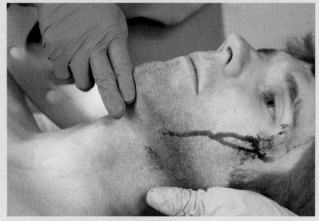

Figure 7-18 **B.** The distance between the hyoid bone and the chin should be at least 3 fingerbreadths.
© National Association of Emergency Medical Technicians (NAEMT).

Figure 7-18 **C.** The distance between the thyroid notch and the floor of the mouth should be at least 2 fingerbreadths.
© National Association of Emergency Medical Technicians (NAEMT).

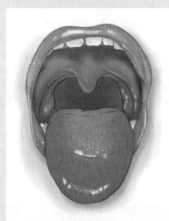 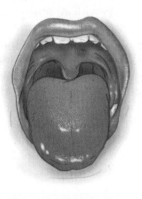 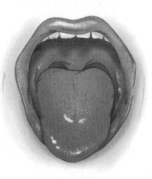 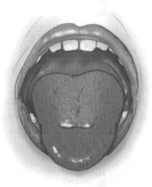

Class I
Entire posterior pharynx is fully exposed

Class II
Posterior pharynx is partially exposed

Class III
Posterior pharynx cannot be seen; base of the uvula is exposed

Class IV
No posterior pharyngeal structures can be seen

Figure 7-19 Mallampati classifications are used to visualize the hypopharynx. Class I: soft palate, uvula, fauces, pillars visible. Class II: soft palate, uvula, fauces visible. Class III: soft palate, base of uvula visible. Class IV: hard palate only visible.

O = Obstruction: Any condition that can cause obstruction of the airway will make laryngoscopy and ventilation difficult. Such conditions include epiglottitis, peritonsillar abscess, and trauma.

N = Neck mobility: This is normally an important requirement for successful intubation. It can be assessed easily by asking the patient to place his or her chin onto the chest and then extending the neck so that he or she is looking toward the ceiling. Patients in a hard collar neck immobilizer obviously have no neck movement and limited mouth opening and are, therefore, more difficult to intubate.

Modified with permission from Reed MJ, Dunn MJG, McKeown DW. Can an airway assessment score predict difficulty at intubation in the emergency department? *Emerg Med J.* 2005;22:99-102. (In: *Advanced Trauma Life Support.* Chicago: American College of Surgeons; 2008.)

components can help the prehospital care provider to prepare for the difficult intubation. Other procedures or devices may be selected if the difficulty of the procedure is deemed high. The standard LEMON examination is often impossible in a combative and uncooperative patient. However, even in this situation, neck thickness, mouth opening, and size of the upper incisors can be quickly assessed.

HEAVEN is a new set of criteria to predict difficult intubation that seems to be better adapted to trauma patients in the prehospital environment (**Box 7-8**).[5]

HEAVEN is a new set of criteria to predict difficult intubation, which seems to be better adapted to trauma patients in the prehospital environment.[5]

- Hypoxemia: oxygen saturation value ≤ 93% at the time of initial laryngoscopy
- Extremes of size: pediatric patient ≤ 8 years of age or clinical obesity
- Anatomic challenge: includes trauma, mass, swelling, foreign body, or other structural abnormality limiting laryngoscopic view
- Vomit/blood/fluid: clinically significant fluid present in the pharynx/hypopharynx at the time of laryngoscopy
- Exsanguination: suspected anemia that could potentially accelerate desaturation during rapid-sequence intubation–associated apnea
- Neck: limited cervical range of motion

Transport time may also be a factor when deciding on the appropriate modality; an example may be a patient who is being maintained effectively with an OPA and bag-mask device with a short transport time to the trauma center. The prehospital care provider may elect not to intubate but rather transport while maintaining the airway using simple airway techniques. Providers need to assess the risks versus the benefits when making the decision to perform complex airway procedures.

Despite the potential challenges of this procedure, endotracheal intubation remains the preferred method of airway control because it does the following:

- Isolates the airway
- Allows for ventilation with 100% oxygen (Fio_2 of 1.0)
- Eliminates the need to maintain an adequate mask-to-face seal
- Significantly decreases the risk of aspiration (vomitus, foreign material, blood)
- Facilitates deep tracheal suctioning
- Prevents gastric insufflation

Indications, Contraindications, and Complications

Indications
- Patient who is unable to protect his or her airway
- Patient with significant oxygenation problem, requiring administration of high concentrations of oxygen
- Patient with significant ventilatory impairment requiring assisted ventilation

Contraindications
- Lack of training or maintenance of training in technique
- Lack of proper indications

- Proximity to receiving facility (relative contraindication)
- High probability of failed airway

Complications
- Hypoxemia from prolonged intubation attempts
- Hypercarbia from prolonged intubation attempts
- Vagal stimulation causing bradycardia
- Increased intracranial pressure
- Trauma to the airway with resultant hemorrhage and edema
- Right main bronchus intubation
- Esophageal intubation
- Vomiting leading to aspiration
- Loose or broken teeth
- Injury to the vocal cords
- Conversion of a cervical spine injury without neurologic deficit to one with neurologic deficit
- Conversion of a simple pneumothorax to a tension pneumothorax due to positive-pressure ventilation
- Circulatory collapse due to the effect of sedative medications combined with positive-pressure ventilation

As with all procedures, the prehospital care provider, along with the medical director, makes a risk–benefit judgment when employing any complex procedures. Performing procedures simply because "the protocols allow it" is inappropriate. Think of the possible benefits and the possible risks, and form a plan based on the best interest of the patient in a given situation. Situations differ dramatically based on transport time, location (urban vs. rural), and the provider's level of comfort in performing a given procedure (**Box 7-9**). Keep in mind that the success

Research studies have shown that practice increases the likelihood of success when intubating. Although no correlation was found between success rate and length of time as a paramedic, there was a correlation between the number of patients intubated by the paramedic and the success rate. Experience with the procedure increases the likelihood of successful performance.[7] One hospital study has shown that it takes operators in the OR 70 intubations to achieve a 90% success rate. In the prehospital trauma setting, in a patient with immobilized cervical spine, this number is likely to be even higher.[2]

In assessing success rate, speed and number of attempts are important considerations; both factors have been shown to correlate significantly with morbidity and mortality.[6] Prehospital care providers must keep in mind that the patient's oxygenation and perfusion, not the kind of airway used, will determine the outcome.

rate is not the only aspect, because speed and number of attempts have been shown to correlate significantly with morbidity and mortality.[6]

Methods of Endotracheal Intubation

Several alternative methods are available for performing endotracheal intubation. The method of choice depends on such factors as the patient's needs, the level of urgency (orotracheal vs. nasotracheal, intubation with intubating laryngeal mask vs. video laryngoscope), patient positioning (face to face), or training and scope of practice (pharmacologically assisted intubation). Regardless of the method selected, the patient's head and neck should be stabilized in a neutral position during the procedure and until spinal immobilization is completed. In general, if intubation is not successful after three attempts, consider trying another method of airway control. Going back to a more basic method often is the best option. It is better to bring a well-oxygenated patient into the emergency department (ED) without an ET tube than a intubated patient with additional brain damage after multiple prolonged episodes of hypoxia.

Orotracheal Intubation

Orotracheal intubation involves placing an ET tube into the trachea through the mouth. The nontrauma patient is often placed in a "sniffing" position to facilitate intubation. Because this position hyperextends the cervical spine at C1–C2 (the second most common site for cervical spine fractures) and hyperflexes it at C5–C6 (the most common site for cervical spine fractures), it should not be used for patients with blunt trauma (**Figure 7-20**). It is useful to remember that orotracheal intubation with cervical spine protection has become much easier with video laryngoscopes.

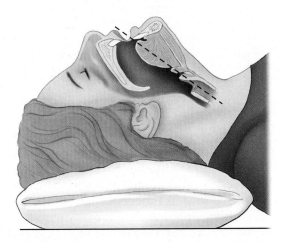

Figure 7-20 Placing the patient's head in the "sniffing" position provides ideal visualization of the larynx through the mouth. However, such positioning hyperextends the patient's neck at C1 and C2 and hyperflexes it at C5 and C6. These are the two most common points of fracture of the cervical spine.

© National Association of Emergency Medical Technicians (NAEMT).

Nasotracheal Intubation

In conscious trauma patients or in those with an intact gag reflex, endotracheal intubation may be difficult to accomplish. If spontaneous ventilations are present, **blind nasotracheal intubation (BNTI)** may be attempted if the benefit outweighs the risk. Although nasotracheal intubation is often more difficult to perform than direct visualization and oral intubation, a high success rate has been reported in traumatized patients. During BNTI, the patient must be breathing to ensure that the ET tube is passed through the vocal cords. Many texts suggest that BNTI is contraindicated in the presence of midface trauma or fractures, but an exhaustive literature search reveals no documentation of an ET tube entering the cranial vault. Apnea is a contraindication specific to BNTI. In addition, no stylet is used when BNTI is performed.

Face-to-Face Intubation

Face-to-face intubation is indicated when standard trauma intubation techniques cannot be used because of the inability of the prehospital care provider to assume the standard position at the head of the trauma patient. These situations include but are not limited to the following:

- Vehicle entrapment
- Pinning of the patient in rubble

Intubation With Intubating Laryngeal Mask (ILMA)

The ILMA is a modified version of the LMA and is designed to allow the passage of an ET tube. It is a rigid, anatomically curved tube that is wide enough to accept an ET tube and short enough that the end of the ET tube enters the trachea (**Figure 7-21**). Several studies have shown a high success rate in difficult intubation cases[8] (i.e., patients in whom intubation by direct laryngoscopy had failed). Added benefits of the ILMA include that it is possible to ventilate the patient intermittently during intubation attempts and that a backup plan is already in place if the intubation fails.

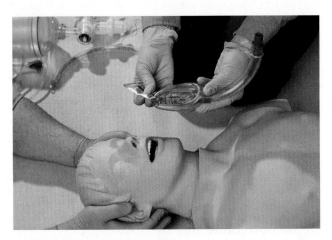

Figure 7-21 Intubating laryngeal mask.

© Jones & Bartlett Learning. Photographer by Darren Stahlman.

Intubation With Video Laryngoscope

Video laryngoscopes are new devices that allow for indirect visualization of the larynx, which can prove useful when direct laryngoscopy is difficult (**Figure 7-22**). Although studies show that their use can improve intubation success rates, especially in trauma patients where cervical spine alignment must be maintained, blood and secretions can obscure the provider's vision through the video channel. Furthermore, the video screen can be difficult to see in bright sunlight.

Video laryngoscopes are either unchanneled or channeled. With unchanneled video laryngoscopes (C-MAC, McGrath, GlideScope), the ET tube has to be brought into the field of view freehand, whereas with the channeled type, the ET tube is inserted into the laryngoscope blade and advanced through the channel once good visualization of the larynx is obtained (Airtraq, King Vision, Upsher-Scope). Unlike conventional laryngoscopes, which must displace the tissues to provide a clear line of sight, channeled video laryngoscopes can slide under the soft tissues until the lens and the intubating channel are aligned with the vocal cords.

Pharmacologically Assisted Intubation

Several studies have shown that pharmacologically assisted intubation increases the success rate of intubation. However, pharmacologic sedation and relaxation are not without risks, including the risk of respiratory depression, apnea, and circulatory collapse. In skilled hands, this technique can facilitate effective airway control when other methods fail or are otherwise not acceptable. To maximize the effectiveness of this procedure and ensure patient safety, prehospital care providers using medications to assist with intubation need to be familiar with applicable local protocols, medications, and indications for use of the technique. The use of medications to assist with intubation, particularly rapid-sequence intubation, does have risks above and beyond those of intubation alone. Intubation using medications falls into the following three categories:

1. *Intubation using sedatives or narcotics.* Medications such as diazepam, midazolam, fentanyl, or morphine are used alone or in combination, with the goal being to relax the patient enough to permit intubation but not to abolish protective reflexes or breathing. The effectiveness of a single pharmacologic agent, such as midazolam, has been well documented.[9] Ketamine is another excellent induction agent, especially when used in combination with midazolam. It causes far less circulatory depression than the other induction agents and has a strong analgesic effect.

2. **Rapid-sequence intubation (RSI)** *using paralytic agents* (**Figure 7-23**). The aim of RSI is to minimize the period at risk for aspiration. To that purpose, sedative medications and a fast-acting paralytic are given simultaneously, as opposed to the traditional sequence where sedation is given first. The aim of RSI is to smoothly and quickly render the patient unconscious and unresponsive and to induce muscle relaxation in only the time necessary for the medication to reach the brain in order to make intubation possible while maintaining stable cerebral perfusion pressure and cardiovascular hemodynamics. This method provides complete muscle paralysis, removes all protective reflexes, and causes apnea, making intubation much easier. However, this procedure is not without risk, since from the moment the patient's ventilation stops, there is definite risk of hypoxia if the patient cannot be intubated and/or ventilated.

   Studies of this method of airway management have demonstrated successful performance of the technique in the field, with intubation success rates reported in the mid-90% range. However, few studies have critically evaluated whether patient outcome is affected.[10] One center reported its experience with RSI in the field and documented that patients with TBI who underwent RSI had a poorer outcome than those who did not require RSI.[11] Subsequent analysis has shown that unrecognized hyperventilation leading to hypocarbia and unrecognized hypoxia were major contributors to the poor outcome.[12]

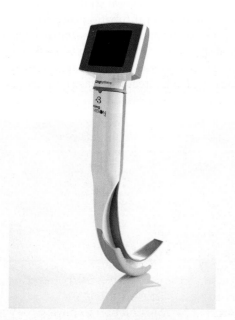

Figure 7-22 The King Vision laryngoscope.
© Ambu, Inc.

Rapid-Sequence Induction

The aim of RSI is to smoothly and quickly render the patient unconscious, unresponsive, and amnestic in one arm/heart/brain circulation time to make intubation possible while maintaining stable cerebral perfusion pressure and cardiovascular hemodynamics. The choice of drugs may vary according to local protocols. The following drug sequence is given as an example.

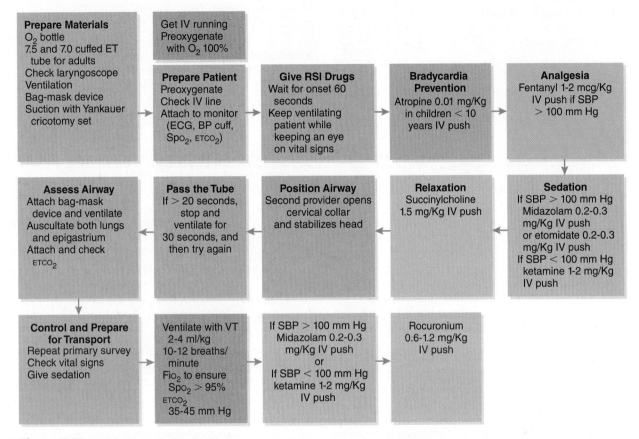

Figure 7-23 Rapid-sequence intubation.

Another study showed a better outcome at 6 months for patients with TBI who were intubated in the field when compared to those intubated in the hospital.[13] The final answer to the important question of whether long-term patient outcome is positively or negatively impacted by prehospital RSI has not yet been answered by the available research. What is certain is that this technique is for highly trained prehospital care providers only and that efficient ventilation and perfusion are the aim no matter what technique is used.

3. **Delayed-sequence intubation (DSI)**. DSI, a newer technique of medication-assisted intubation emphasizing preoxygenation with CPAP and apneic oxygenation during intubation, has shown some promising results (**Box 7-10** and **Figure 7-24**). The patient is preoxygenated under ketamine sedation, then muscle relaxant is administered and the patient is intubated, with a nasal canula providing apnea oxygenation (**Box 7-11** and **Box 7-12**).[14]

Box 7-10 Problems Identified in the Literature with Endotracheal Intubation

- Hypoxia during intubation attempts is frequent and often unrecognized, as SpO_2 signal is often lagging behind in patients with poor circulation.
- Hyperventilation occurs in spite of $ETCO_2$ monitoring, which is especially detrimental in TBI patients.
- Number of complications is proportional to number of attempts.
- Possible solutions:
  · Optimize oxygenation with preoxygenation and apneic oxygenation during intubation attempts.
  · Use video laryngoscopes to increase the chances of first-pass success.
  · Prevent hyperventilation by paying meticulous attention to proper rate and volume.

Delayed-Sequence Intubation

The delayed-sequence intubation (DSI) is a modified version of DAI that emphasizes the preoxygenation process to prevent hypoxemia during the intubation process. Ketamine is the drug of choice for this technique since its effect on spontaneous respiration is minimal.

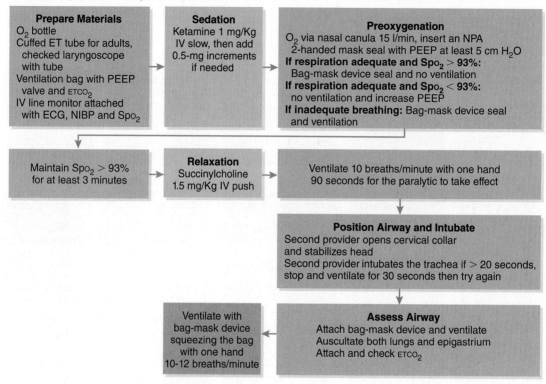

Figure 7-24 Delayed-sequence intubation.

Box 7-11 Apneic Oxygenation During Intubation

Although not a new concept, apneic oxygenation during intubation has experienced a revival in recent years. In the apnea patient, alveoli in the lung will continue to take up oxygen at about 250 ml/minute in the adult, while about 20 ml of CO_2 will be released at the same time. This will create a subatmospheric pressure in the lung, which will draw air from the pharynx into the lung. Giving oxygen via nasal canula at about 15 liters/minute will fill the pharynx and the upper airway, increasing the amount of oxygen flowing to the lungs. Although respiratory acidosis will begin to develop due to CO_2 retention, this technique has proven efficient to reduce the risk of desaturation during intubation attempts.

Pharmacologically assisted intubation of any type requires time to accomplish. For every trauma patient for whom this intubation is contemplated, the benefits of securing an airway are weighed against the additional time spent on the scene to perform the procedure.

Box 7-12 The Sellick Maneuver

The Sellick maneuver (cricoid pressure) has been gradually falling out of favor. While it has been considered to reduce the likelihood of aspiration from regurgitated stomach contents, there is little evidence that it, in fact, does so. Several studies show that the esophagus is located to the side of the trachea and that the Sellick maneuver does little to compress the esophagus.[15-18] In addition, cricoid pressure may obscure the view of the larynx and make intubation more difficult.

Indications

- A patient who requires a secure airway and is difficult to intubate because of uncooperative behavior (as induced by hypoxia, TBI, hypotension, or intoxication)

Relative Contraindications

- Availability of an alternative airway (e.g., supraglottic)
- Severe facial trauma that would impair or preclude successful intubation
- Neck deformity or swelling that complicates or precludes placement of a surgical airway

- Known allergies to indicated medications
- Medical problems that would preclude use of indicated medications

Absolute Contraindications
- Inability to intubate
- Inability to maintain airway with bag-mask device and OPA

Complications
- Inability to insert the ET tube in a sedated or paralyzed patient no longer able to protect his or her airway or breathe spontaneously; patients who are medicated and

then cannot be intubated require prolonged bag-mask ventilation until the medication wears off.
- Development of hypoxia or hypercarbia during prolonged intubation attempts
- Aspiration
- Hypotension—virtually all of the medications have the side effect of decreasing blood pressure.

Patients who are mildly or moderately hypovolemic but compensating may have a profound drop in blood pressure associated with the intravenous administration of many of these medications. Exercise caution whenever the use of medications for intubation is considered (**Table 7-1**).

Table 7-1 Common Drugs Used for Pharmacologically Assisted Intubation					
	Dosage (adult)	**Duration**	**Effect**	**Side Effects**	**Tricks of the Trade**
Sedation					
Midazolam	0.1–0.3 mg/Kg IV	1–2 hours	Long-acting sedation, amnesia	Respiratory depression, apnea, hypotension	Classic induction agent, the onset is somewhat slow (up to 3 minutes)
Etomidate	0.2–0.3 mg/Kg IV	3–10 minutes	Induced anesthesia	Apnea, hypotension, vomiting	Fast onset, causes only moderate hypotension. Suppression of the adrenal cortex
Ketamine	1–2 mg/Kg IV	10 minutes	Sedation, induced anesthesia, analgesia	Tachycardia, hypertension, increased intracranial pressure (?)	Provides both anesthesia and analgesia. Best choice in shock patient Caution is advised if SBP is above normal
Propofol	1–2 mg/Kg IV	5–10 minutes	Sedation, induced anesthesia	Apnea, hypotension	Very popular anesthetic but causes profound hypotension. Its use in the trauma patient is tricky even in experienced hands
Analgesia					
Fentanyl	2–3 mcg/Kg IV	20–30 minutes	Analgesia	Respiratory depression, apnea, hypotension	Classic analgesic for RSI, powerful and fast acting

(continued)

Table 7-1 Common Drugs Used for Pharmacologically Assisted Intubation (*continued*)

	Dosage (adult)	Duration	Effect	Side Effects	Tricks of the Trade
Morphine	0.01 mg/Kg IV	2–3 hours	Analgesia	Respiratory depression, apnea, hypotension	Not well adapted for rapid RSI because of its very slow onset (up to 5 minutes)
Ketamine*	0.1–0.3 mg/Kg	10 minutes		Hallucinations, especially at doses above 0.5 mg/kg	Ketamine is an "all in one" analgesic and anesthetic. In low doses, it provides excellent analgesia with normal muscle tone and without respiratory depression
Relaxation					
Succinylcholine	1–2 mg/Kg IV	3–5 minutes	Fast (30–60 seconds) and short-acting muscle relaxation	Hyperkalemia, muscle fasciculation	Quick, cheap, and efficient Contraindicated in patients with neuromuscular diseases
Rocuronium	0.6–1.2 mg/Kg IV	30 minutes	Fast and long-acting muscle relaxation		Quick and efficient. An antidote (sugamadex) is available.
Vecuronium	0.1 mg/Kg IV	30–40 minutes	Muscle relaxation	Slow onset	Its slow onset (up to 5 minutes) makes it second choice for RSI

*Caveat for tactical providers: *Never* give ketamine before the victim has been disarmed!

Note: IV, intravenous; kg, kilogram; mcg, microgram; mg, milligram; RSI, rapid-sequence intubation; SBP, systolic blood pressure.

Verification of Endotracheal Tube Placement

Once intubation has been performed, prehospital care providers must take specific measures to ensure that the ET tube has been properly placed in the trachea. Once a patient is intubated and relaxed, ventilation and oxygenation depend completely on the provider, so monitoring of ventilation, oxygenation, and vital signs must be meticulous. Inadvertent esophageal placement of an ET tube, if unrecognized for only a brief period, may result in profound hypoxia, with resultant brain injury (hypoxic encephalopathy) and even death. Therefore, it is important that proper placement be confirmed. Techniques to verify intubation include the use of both clinical assessments and adjunct devices.[16] Clinical assessments include the following:

- Direct visualization of the ET tube passing through the vocal cords
- Presence of bilateral breath sounds (auscultate laterally below the axilla) and absence of air sounds over the epigastrium
- Visualization of the chest rising and falling during ventilation
- Fogging (water vapor condensation) in the ET tube on expiration

Unfortunately, none of these techniques is 100% reliable *by itself* for verifying proper ET tube placement. Therefore, prudent practice involves assessing and documenting all of these clinical signs, if possible. On rare occasions, because of difficult anatomy, visualization of the ET tube passing through the vocal cords may not be possible. In a moving vehicle (ground or aeromedical), engine noise may make auscultation of breath sounds almost impossible. Obesity and chronic obstructive pulmonary disease may interfere with the ability to see chest movement during ventilation.

Monitoring devices include the following:

- $ETCO_2$ monitoring (capnography)
- Colorimetric carbon dioxide detector
- Pulse oximetry

In a patient with a perfusing rhythm, $ETCO_2$ monitoring (capnography) serves as the "gold standard" for confirming ET tube placement. This technique should be used in the prehospital setting whenever available. Patients in cardiopulmonary arrest may not exhale carbon dioxide, because too little CO_2 is transported to the lungs, even with CPR in progress. Therefore, colorimetric detectors or capnography are of limited use in patients who lack a perfusing cardiac rhythm.

Because *none* of these techniques is universally reliable, *all* the clinical assessments noted previously should be performed, unless impractical, followed by use of at least *one* of the monitoring devices. If any of the techniques used to verify proper placement suggests that the ET tube may not be properly positioned, the ET tube should be immediately removed and reinserted, with placement verified again. All of the techniques used to verify ET tube placement should be noted on the patient care report.

Securing an Endotracheal Tube

Once endotracheal intubation has been performed, the ET tube must be manually held in place and proper tube placement verified; the depth of tube insertion at the central incisors (front teeth) should be noted. Next, the ET tube is secured in place. Several commercially available products may serve to secure the ET tube adequately. A study identified that umbilical tape held the ET tube as effectively as commercial devices; however, it needs to be tied around the ET tube using appropriate knots and technique. Ideally, if sufficient EMS personnel are present, someone should be assigned the task of manually holding the ET tube in proper position to ensure that it does not move.

Continuous pulse oximetry should be considered necessary for all patients who require endotracheal intubation. Any decline in the pulse oximetry reading (i.e., oxygen saturation [Spo_2]) or development of cyanosis requires reverification of ET tube placement. Additionally, an ET tube may become dislodged during any movement of the patient. Reverify ET tube position after every move of a patient, such as logrolling to a long backboard, loading or unloading into or from the ambulance, or carrying the patient down a staircase.

Alternate Techniques

If endotracheal intubation has been unsuccessful after three attempts, consideration of airway management using the manual and simple skills described previously and ventilating with a bag-mask device is appropriate. If the receiving facility is reasonably close, these techniques may be the most prudent option for airway management when faced with a brief transport time. If the nearest appropriate facility is more distant, one of the following alternate techniques may be considered. Again, it is better to bring a well-oxygenated patient to the ED without an ET tube than an intubated patient with additional brain damage following a long episode of hypoxia. Remember, it is hypoxia that will further damage the injured brain, not the lack of an ET tube.

Needle Cricothyrotomy

In rare cases, a trauma patient's airway obstruction cannot be relieved using the methods previously discussed. In these patients, depending on your local protocols, a needle cricothyrotomy may be performed using a percutaneously placed needle or catheter. It has been shown that adequate oxygenation can be achieved using **percutaneous transtracheal ventilation (PTV)**.[19] This technique, while it provides for oxygenation, does not support adequate ventilation for any length of time. As a result, rising levels of carbon dioxide will occur, which can be tolerated for approximately 30 minutes, after which formal airway management must be accomplished to prevent profound respiratory acidosis from developing. This technique is a temporizing measure to maintain oxygenation until a definitive airway can be obtained to provide adequate ventilation.

However, needle cricothyrotomy is a very difficult technique to use in the prehospital environment, because even a slight movement of the head can kink or dislodge the catheter. What is more, it does not protect the trachea against aspiration. This makes needle cricothyrotomy second choice when compared to surgical cricothyrotomy.

The advantages of PTV include the following:

- Ease of access (landmarks usually easily recognized)
- Ease of insertion
- Minimal equipment required
- No incision necessary
- Minimal training required

Indications
- When all other alternative methods of airway management fail or are impractical and the patient cannot be ventilated with a bag-mask device

Contraindications
- Insufficient training
- Lack of proper equipment
- Ability to secure airway by another technique (as described previously) or ability to ventilate with a bag-mask device

Complications

- Hypercarbia from prolonged use (carbon dioxide elimination is not as effective as with other methods of ventilation)[13]
- Damage to surrounding structures, including the larynx, thyroid gland, carotid arteries, jugular veins, and esophagus
- Catheter displacement. The catheter can become easily kinked and/or dislodged if the head is moved, so good fixation not only of the catheter but of the head and neck are paramount.

Surgical Cricothyrotomy

Surgical cricothyrotomy involves the creation of a surgical opening in the *cricothyroid membrane*, which lies between the larynx (thyroid cartilage) and the cricoid cartilage. In most patients, the skin is very thin in this location, making it amenable to immediate access to the airway.[20] Consider this a technique of last resort in prehospital airway management (**Figure 7-25**).

There are a number of ways that surgical cricothyrotomy can be accomplished. The traditional method is to formally incise the skin and cricothyroid membrane using a scalpel. An alternative method is to use one of the several different types of commercially available cricothyrotomy kits. Learning to use these kits is easier than learning to perform a formal surgical cricothyrotomy, and generally they create an opening that is larger than that of a needle cricothyrotomy but smaller than the surgical technique.

The use of this surgical airway in the prehospital arena is controversial. Complications are common with this procedure.[21] Proficient endotracheal intubation skills should minimize the need even to consider its use. Surgical cricothyrotomy should *never* be the initial airway control method. Insufficient data exist at this time to support a recommendation that surgical cricothyrotomy be established as a national standard for routine use in prehospital airway management.

For this technique to be successful in actual field practice, training must be done on real tissue. Current mannequins and other simulation devices do not replicate actual human tissue and the feel of the anatomy in a patient. The prehospital care provider's first exposure to real tissue should not be a dying patient. In addition, this skill, perhaps more than other airway interventions, requires frequent practice in order to maintain the anatomic familiarity and skills needed to perform it correctly in only seconds during a true emergency. Usually there is no second chance to get it right. It must be done correctly the first time.

Indications

- Massive midface trauma precluding the use of a bag-mask device
- Inability to control the airway using less invasive maneuvers

Contraindications

- Any patient who can be safely intubated, either orally or nasally
- Patients with laryngotracheal injuries
- Children under 10 years of age

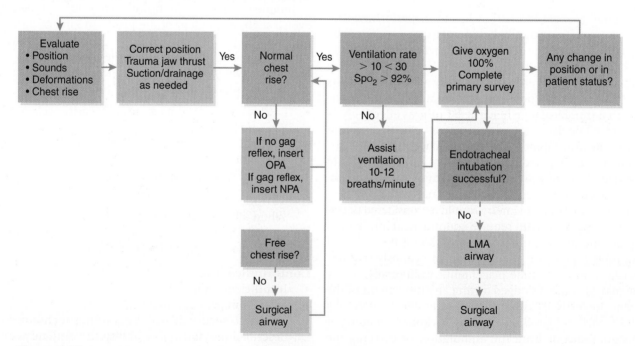

Figure 7-25 The surgical airway in the airway management algorithm.

- Patients with acute laryngeal disease of traumatic or infectious origin
- Insufficient training

Complications
- Prolonged procedure time
- Hemorrhage
- Aspiration
- Misplacement or false passage of the ET tube
- Injury to neck structures or vessels
- Perforation of the esophagus

Suctioning the Intubated Patient

When suctioning intubated patients through the ET tube, the suction catheter should be made of soft material to limit trauma to the tracheal mucosa and to minimize frictional resistance. It needs to be long enough to pass the tip of the artificial airway (20 to 22 inches, or 50 to 55 centimeters [cm]). The soft catheter will probably not be effective in suctioning copious amounts of foreign material or fluid from the pharynx of a trauma patient, in which case the device of choice will be one with a tonsil-tip or Yankauer design. Under no circumstances should a tonsil-tip or Yankauer rigid suction device be placed in the end of the ET tube.

When suctioning an intubated patient, aseptic procedures are vital. This technique includes the following steps:

1. Preoxygenate the trauma patient with 100% oxygen (fraction of inspired oxygen [Fio_2] of 1.0).
2. Prepare the equipment while maintaining sterility.
3. Insert the catheter without suction. Suctioning is then initiated and continued for up to 10 seconds while withdrawing the catheter.
4. Reoxygenate the patient, and ventilate for at least five assisted ventilations.
5. Repeat as necessary, allowing time for reoxygenation to take place between procedures.

Ventilatory Devices

All trauma patients receive appropriate ventilatory support with supplemental oxygen to ensure that hypoxia is corrected or averted entirely. In deciding which method or equipment to use, prehospital care providers should consider the following devices and their respective oxygen concentrations.

Pocket Masks

Regardless of which mask is chosen to support ventilation of the trauma patient, the ideal mask has the following characteristics:

1. Is a good fit
2. Is equipped with a one-way valve

3. Is made of a transparent material
4. Has a supplemental oxygen port
5. Is available in infant, pediatric, and adult sizes

Mouth-to-mask ventilation satisfactorily delivers adequate tidal volumes by ensuring a tight face seal even when performed by those who do not use this skill often. Pocket masks offer the added advantage of being small and easy to transport. However, even with oxygen supply, mouth-to-mask ventilation provides a maximal Fio_2 of only 50%.

Bag-Mask Device

The bag-mask device consists of a self-inflating bag and a nonrebreathing device; it can be used with simple (OPA, NPA) or complex (endotracheal, nasotracheal) airway devices. Most bag-mask devices have a volume of 1,600 ml and can deliver an oxygen concentration of 90% to 100%. Some models also have a built-in colorimetric carbon dioxide detector. However, a single prehospital care provider attempting to ventilate with a bag-mask device may create poor tidal volumes secondary to the inability both to create a tight face seal and to squeeze the bag adequately. Ongoing practice of this skill is necessary to ensure that the technique is effective and that the trauma patient receives adequate ventilatory support.

Positive-Pressure Ventilators

Positive-pressure volume ventilators during prolonged transport have long been used in the aeromedical environment. However, more ground units are now adopting the use of mechanical ventilation as a means of controlling rate, depth, and minute volume in trauma patients. Importantly, only volume ventilators with appropriate alarms and pressure control/relief should be used. These ventilators do not need to be as sophisticated as those used in the hospital and only have a few simple modes of ventilation, as described in the following sections.

Assist Control Ventilation

Assist control (A/C) ventilation is probably the most widely used mode of ventilation in prehospital transport from the scene to the ED. The A/C setting delivers ventilations at a preset rate and tidal volume. If patients initiate a breath on their own, an additional ventilation of the full tidal volume is delivered, which may lead to breath-stacking and overinflation of the lungs.

Intermittent Mandatory Ventilation

Intermittent mandatory ventilation (IMV) delivers a set rate and tidal volume to patients. If patients initiate their own breath, only the amount that they actually pull on their own will be delivered.

Positive End-Expiratory Pressure

Positive end-expiratory pressure (PEEP) provides an elevated level of pressure at the end of expiration, thus keeping the alveolar sacs and small airways open and filled with air for a longer time. This intervention provides greater oxygenation. However, by increasing the end-expiratory pressure and, therefore, the overall intrathoracic pressure, PEEP may decrease blood return to the heart. In hemodynamically unstable patients, PEEP may further decrease blood pressure. PEEP should also be avoided in patients with TBIs. The increase in thoracic pressure can cause an elevation in intracranial pressure.

Initial Settings for Mechanical Ventilations

Rate

The rate is set initially at between 10 and 12 breaths/minute on nonbreathing adult patients.

Tidal Volume

The tidal volume should be set using 5 to 7 ml/kg of the patient's ideal body weight. This should be used as a guide and may need to be adjusted in the trauma patient.

PEEP

PEEP should be set initially at 5 cm of water (cm H_2O). This setting will maintain what is known as physiologic PEEP, which is the amount of PEEP that is normally present in the airway prior to intubation. Once intubated, this positive pressure is taken away. Although increased levels of PEEP may be needed as the traumatic insult worsens, this rarely ever takes place in the first few hours following the traumatic event. The prehospital care provider may encounter patients requiring high levels of PEEP during a transfer of a patient from one hospital to another. The hospital staff prior to the transfer will have established these levels of PEEP. Normal physiologic PEEP values range from 5 to 10 cm H_2O. The more PEEP that is used, the greater the risk of untoward effects. Great care must be taken if PEEP is increased, as there can be adverse complications:

- Decreased blood pressure secondary to decreased venous return
- Increased intracranial pressure
- Increased intrathoracic pressure leading to pneumothorax or tension pneumothorax

Oxygen Concentration

The oxygen concentration should be set to maintain a saturation of 94% or greater at sea level in the trauma patient.

High-Pressure Alarm/Pop-Off

The high-pressure alarm and pressure relief pop-off should be set at no more than 10 cm H_2O above the pressure needed to normally ventilate the patient (peak inspiratory pressure). Care should be taken when setting the alarm above 40 cm H_2O. Levels above this have been shown to produce barotrauma and a higher possibility of a pneumothorax. Should more than 40 cm H_2O be needed to deliver the desired tidal volume, reassessment of the airway and preset tidal volume is required. Decreasing the tidal volume and increasing the rate to maintain the same alveolar minute ventilation may be the prudent action in this case.

As with any alarm, if the high-pressure alarm continues to activate for more than a few breaths, the patient should be removed from the ventilator and manually ventilated with a bag-mask device while the ventilator circuit and ET tube are evaluated. The patient should also be reevaluated for an increase in compliance. This increase in compliance or resistance may be caused by many factors. The most common, early in the care of the trauma patient, is either tension pneumothorax or an increasing LOC causing "bucking" on the ET tube. The tension pneumothorax should be treated with chest decompression as indicated. An increasing LOC should be treated with the administration of a sedative agent if available. Other potential problems include displacement or obstruction of the ET tube. In no case should the prehospital care provider simply continue to increase the upper pressure limit and alarm. A listing of basic ventilator settings can be found in **Box 7-13**.

Low-Pressure Alarm

The low-pressure alarm alerts the prehospital care provider if the connection between the patient and the ventilator is disconnected or is losing significant volume through a leak in the ventilator circuit, or if the airway device has been dislodged. In most transport ventilators, this alarm is preset and cannot be adjusted. See **Box 7-14** for ventilator troubleshooting.

Box 7-13 Basic Ventilator Settings

- Tidal volume: 5 to 7 ml/kg
- Ventilatory rate: 10 to 12 breaths/minute
- Fio_2: 100% initially, then reduce gradually to maintain $Spo_2 > 94\%$
- Peak pressure alarm: 28 cm H_2O
- Low pressure alarm: 5 cm H_2O below normal peak pressure to have an early warning of circuit disconnection

Box 7-14 Ventilator Troubleshooting

- *Check the patient first.* Disconnect the patient from the ventilator and ventilate manually. Then check:
  - ET tube position, depth, and permeability. Suction if needed.
  - Auscultate both lung fields to rule out tension pneumothorax. Check ETCO₂.
  - Check blood pressure and heart rate (high blood pressure can be a sign of insufficent sedation).
  - Check sedation level to avoid having the patient fighting the ventilator.
  - Check the ventilator setting.
- Remember the old saying that most problems involving a $30,000 ventilator can be solved with a $30 bag. Always check the patient first!

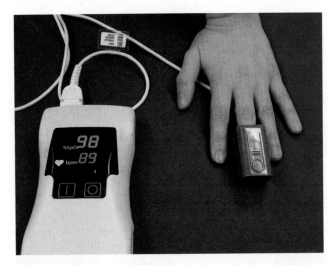

Figure 7-26 Pulse oximeter.

Evaluation

Pulse Oximetry

Over the past decades, the use of pulse oximetry has increased in the prehospital environment. Appropriate use of pulse oximetry devices allows early detection of pulmonary compromise or cardiovascular deterioration before physical signs are evident. **Pulse oximeters** are particularly useful in prehospital applications because of their high reliability, portability, ease of application, and applicability across all age ranges and races (**Figure 7-26**).

Pulse oximeters provide measurements of oxygen saturation (Sp_{O_2}) and pulse rate. Sp_{O_2} is determined by measuring the absorption ratio of red and infrared light passed through tissue. A small microprocessor correlates changes in light absorption caused by the pulsation of blood through vascular beds to determine arterial saturation and pulse rate. Normal Sp_{O_2} is greater than 94% at sea level. When Sp_{O_2} falls below 90%, oxygen delivery to the tissues is likely severely compromised. At higher altitudes, the acceptable levels of Sp_{O_2} are lower than at sea level. Prehospital care providers should know what Sp_{O_2} levels are acceptable at higher altitudes, if practicing in such settings.

To ensure accurate pulse oximetry readings, the following general guidelines should be followed:

1. Use the appropriate size and type of sensor.
2. Ensure proper alignment of sensor light.
3. Ensure that sources and photodetectors are clean, dry, and in good repair.
4. Avoid sensor placement on grossly edematous (swollen) sites.
5. Remove any nail polish that may be present.

Common problems that can produce inaccurate Sp_{O_2} measurement include the following:

- Excessive motion
- Moisture in Sp_{O_2} sensors
- Improper sensor application and placement
- Poor patient perfusion or vasoconstriction from hypothermia
- Anemia
- Carbon monoxide poisoning

In a critical trauma patient, pulse oximetry may be less than accurate because of poor capillary perfusion status. Therefore, pulse oximetry is a valuable addition to the prehospital care provider's "toolbox" only when combined with a thorough knowledge of trauma pathophysiology and strong assessment and intervention skills.

Capnography

Capnography, or end-tidal carbon dioxide (ETCO₂) monitoring, has been used in critical care units for many years. Recent advances in technology have allowed smaller, more durable units to be produced for prehospital use (**Figure 7-27**). Capnography measures the partial pressure of carbon dioxide (P_{CO_2}, or ETCO₂) in a sample of gas. If this sample is taken at the end of exhalation in a patient with good peripheral perfusion, it correlates closely to arterial P_{CO_2} (Pa_{CO_2}). However, in the multiple trauma patient with compromised perfusion, the correlation of ETCO₂ to arterial P_{CO_2} remains questionable.[22,23]

Most critical care units within the hospital setting use the mainstream technique. This technique places a sensor directly into the "mainstream" of the exhaled gas. In the patient being ventilated with a bag-mask device, the sensor is placed between the bag-mask device and the ET tube. In

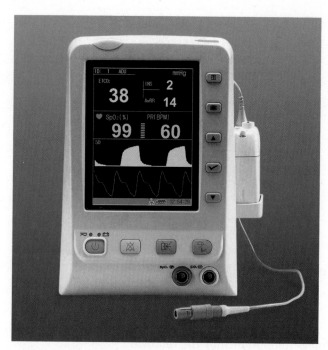

Figure 7-27 Handheld end-tidal carbon dioxide detector.
Courtesy of DRE Medical Equipment.

the critical patient, the $Paco_2$ is generally 2 to 5 millimeters of mercury (mm Hg) higher than the $ETCO_2$. (A normal $ETCO_2$ reading in a critical trauma patient is 30 to 40 mm Hg.) Although these readings may not totally reflect the patient's $Paco_2$, working to maintain the readings between normal levels will usually be beneficial to the patient.

Although capnography correlates closely with $Paco_2$, certain conditions will cause variations in accuracy. These conditions are often seen in the prehospital environment and include severe hypotension, high intrathoracic pressure, and any increase in dead space ventilation, as with pulmonary embolism. Therefore, following trends in $ETCO_2$ levels may be more important than focusing on specific readings.

Continuous capnography provides another tool in the prehospital management of a trauma patient and must be correlated with all other information about a patient. Initial transport decisions are based on physical and environmental conditions. For example, it would be inappropriate to take time at the scene to place the patient on monitors if the patient is losing blood. Instead, capnography should be applied en route to the hospital in such a situation. Remember, however, that capnography is the gold standard for monitoring proper tube placement, and a sudden drop in expired carbon dioxide, as may result either from dislodgment of the ET tube or from decreased perfusion, should prompt a reevaluation of patient status and ET tube position.[24] However, $ETCO_2$ is the ultimate means to determine whether air exchange with the lung is taking place. As a general rule, it is advisable to have a working CO_2 monitor when using an advanced airway.

Continuous Quality Improvement in Intubation

With the literature questioning the effectiveness of prehospital intubation of the trauma patient, it is important that the medical director or his or her designee individually review all out-of-hospital intubations or invasive airway techniques. This is even more imperative if medications have been used to facilitate the intubation attempt. Specific points include the following:

- Adherence to protocol and procedures
- Number of attempts
- Confirmation of tube placement and the procedures used for verification
- Outcome and complications
- Proper indications for the use of induction agents if used
- Proper documentation of medication dosage routes and monitoring of the patient during and after intubation
- Vital signs before, during, and after intubation

An effective continuous quality improvement (CQI) program for airway management must not be seen as a "punishment" but rather as an educational opportunity by the prehospital care providers, management, and the medical director. Because most CQI programs are self-reporting, any results that are used to discipline a particular provider may result in misreporting. CQI should be tied directly to the continuing education program within an organization. After identifying a problem in performance, an educational component should be developed that addresses those issues. Follow-up evaluations should take place to determine if the educational component has been effective.

Prolonged Transport

Airway management of a patient prior to and during a prolonged transport requires complex decision making on the part of the prehospital care provider. Interventions to control and secure the airway, especially using complex techniques, depend on numerous factors, including the patient's injuries, the clinical skills of the provider, the equipment available, and the distance and transport time to definitive care. Risks and benefits of all of the airway options available should be considered prior to making a final airway decision. Both a longer distance of transport and a longer transport time lower the threshold for securing the airway with endotracheal intubation. For transports of 15 to 20 minutes, essential skills, including an oral airway and bag-mask ventilation, may be sufficient. Use of air medical transport also lowers the threshold to perform endotracheal intubation, as a cramped, noisy environment makes ongoing airway assessment and management difficult.

Any patient requiring airway management or ventilatory support requires ongoing patient monitoring. Continuous pulse oximetry should be performed on all trauma patients during transport, and capnography should be considered mandatory for all intubated patients. Loss of ETCO$_2$ indicates that the ventilator circuit has become disconnected or, more important, the ET tube has been dislodged, or the patient's perfusion has decreased significantly. All of these possible causes require immediate action.

Serial vital signs should be recorded on patients requiring airway or ventilation interventions. Confirmation of endotracheal intubation, as described previously, should be performed each time the patient is moved or repositioned. It is also a good idea to frequently confirm the security of any airway device.

Any patient who requires increasing FiO$_2$ or PEEP in order to maintain oxygenation needs to be carefully reevaluated. Possible etiologies include the development of a pneumothorax or worsening of pulmonary contusions. Any known or suspected pneumothorax must be monitored closely for the development of a tension pneumothorax, and pleural decompression should be performed if hemodynamic compromise occurs. If the patient has had an open pneumothorax sealed, the dressing should be opened to release any pressure that may have accumulated. If the patient is receiving positive-pressure ventilation, the positive-pressure ventilation can convert a simple pneumothorax to a tension pneumothorax.

Burn patients should receive supplemental oxygen to maintain SpO$_2$ greater than 94%, whereas those with known or suspected carbon monoxide poisoning should receive 100% oxygen. (See the Burn Injuries chapter for more information.)

Table 7-2 Oxygen Tank Size and Duration

Flow Rate (liter/min)	Tank Size and Duration (in hours)				
	D	**E**	**M**	**G**	**H/K**
2	2.5	4.4	24.7	38.2	49.7
5	1	1.8	9.9	15.3	19.9
10	0.5	0.9	4.9	7.6	9.9
15	0.3	0.6	3.3	5.1	6.6

Note: This table shows the approximate duration in hours of various sizes of oxygen tanks and flow rates. The numbers are based on the assumption that the oxygen tank is completely full at 2,100 pounds per square inch (psi).

Prior to embarking on a prolonged transport of a patient, potential oxygen needs should be calculated, and sufficient amounts of oxygen should be made available for the transport (**Table 7-2**). A good general rule is to bring 50% more oxygen than the anticipated need.

Intubated patients should be sedated for the transport according to local protocols. Sedation may also decrease the work of breathing and any "fighting the ventilator" when mechanical ventilation is being used. If sedating the patient, small doses of benzodiazepines should be titrated intravenously. The use of neuromuscular blocking agents may be considered if the patient is significantly combative, the airway is secured with an ET tube, and prehospital care personnel are properly trained and credentialed. However, patients should *not* receive neuromuscular blocking agents without proper sedation.

SUMMARY

- Cerebral oxygenation and oxygen delivery to other parts of the body provided by adequate airway management and ventilation are the most important components of prehospital patient care.
- To properly care for the trauma patient, the provider must be able to integrate the principles of ventilation and gas exchange with the pathophysiology of trauma.
- Effective ventilation is defined as total minute ventilation minus dead space ventilation. When the minute volume falls below normal, the patient has inadequate ventilation, or *hypoventilation*.

- Decreased minute volume can be caused by either mechanical obstruction (usually the tongue) or a decreased level of consciousness, with both conditions frequently occurring together.
- Noise coming from the upper airway usually indicates a partial airway obstruction caused by the tongue, blood, or foreign bodies in the upper airway. Providers must listen and look for signs of obstruction.
- All trauma patients receive ventilatory support with supplemental oxygen to ensure that

(continued)

SUMMARY (CONTINUED)

hypoxia is corrected or averted entirely. Prehospital care providers must decide which method or equipment to use by considering the devices available and their respective oxygen concentrations.

- Categories for airway adjuncts and procedures include the following:
  - *Manual methods* are easiest to use and require no additional equipment; they include the trauma chin lift and the trauma jaw thrust.
  - *Simple airway management* involves the use of adjunctive devices that require only one piece of equipment, and the technique for inserting the device necessitates minimal training; they include oropharyngeal and nasopharyngeal airways.
  - *Complex airways* include airway adjuncts that require significant initial training and ongoing training to ensure continuing proficiency; they include endotracheal tubes and supraglottic airways.

- The decision to perform endotracheal intubation or to instead use an alternative device should be made after assessment of the airway has helped define the difficulty of the intubation. It constitutes a risk–benefit judgment that takes into account such factors as skill/experience of the provider and transport length to the nearest trauma center.
- End-tidal carbon dioxide ($ETCO_2$) monitoring (capnography) serves as the "gold standard" for confirming ET tube placement. This technique should be used in the prehospital setting whenever available.
- Managing the airway is not without risks. When applying certain skills and modalities, the risk has to be weighed against the potential benefit for that particular patient. What may be the best choice for one patient in a certain situation may not be for another with a similar presentation.
- Sound critical-thinking skills need to be in place to make the best judgments for the trauma patient.

SCENARIO RECAP

You are called to the scene of a motorcycle crash on a busy freeway. As you arrive on scene, you see the patient lying supine about 50 ft from a destroyed motorcycle. The patient is a 20-year-old male, who still has his helmet on. He is not moving, and you see from a distance that he is breathing quickly with small and paradoxical thorax movements. As you approach the patient, you see a pool of blood around his head, and you notice that his breathing is noisy, with snoring and gurgling sounds.

You are 20 minutes from a trauma center, and the dispatch center informs you that the HEMS cannot fly due to bad weather.

- What indicators of airway compromise are evident in this patient?
- What other information, if any, would you seek from witnesses or the emergency medical responders?
- Describe the sequence of actions you would take to manage this patient before and during transport.

SCENARIO SOLUTION

Bystanders confirm that the patient was alone, and while checking that traffic has been stopped, you observe that the patient is lying 50 ft from his destroyed motorcycle, which indicates a significant mechanism of injury. His breathing pattern, as well as the pool of blood around his head, are highly suggestive of an airway problem even from a distance. Snoring and gurgling sounds confirm your suspicion as you approach the patient.

You and your partner remove the helmet while maintaining cervical spine protection. The snoring sounds disappear once you apply a trauma jaw thrust and suction the airway; still, the breathing remains fast and

SCENARIO SOLUTION (CONTINUED)

superficial. Auscultation on both sides is normal, but SpO_2 is 80% so you decide to assist ventilation, which quickly brings the SpO_2 up to 94%. Your partner informs you that the pulse is fast and thready. His Glasgow Coma Scale (GCS) score is 7 without lateralizing signs. Because the patient still has a gag reflex, you choose to insert an NPA before putting on a cervical collar and fixing the patient on the board.

Because the HEMS is not available, you immediately start the transport to the hospital. During the ride, you ventilate the patient with 100% O_2 at a rate of 12 breaths/minute while your partner establishes an IV line and connects the patient to a monitor. The vital signs read SpO_2 95%, heart rate 100 beats/minute, and blood pressure 110/60 mm Hg as you hand over the patient to the trauma team 15 minutes later.

References

1. Roberts K, Whalley H, Bleetman A. The nasopharyngeal airway: dispelling myths and establishing the facts. *Emerg Med J.* 2005;22:394-396.

2. Buis ML, Maissan M, Hoeks SE, Klimek M, Stolker RJ. Defining the learning curve for endotracheal intubation using direct laryngoscopy: a systematic review. *Resuscitation.* February 2016;99:63-71.

3. Stockinger ZT, McSwain NE Jr. Prehospital endotracheal intubation for trauma does not improve survival over bag-mask ventilation. *J Trauma.* 2004;56(3):531.

4. Davis DP, Koprowicz KM, Newgard CD, et al. The relationship between out-of-hospital airway management and outcome among trauma patients with Glasgow Coma Scale scores of 8 or less. *Prehosp Emerg Care.* 2011;15(2):184-192.

5. Davis DP, Olvera DJ. HEAVEN criteria: derivation of a new difficult airway prediction tool. *Air Med J.* 2017;36(4):195-197.

6. Warner KJ, Sharar SR, Copass MK, Bulger EM. Prehospital management of a difficult airway: a prospective cohort study. *J Emerg Med.* 2008;36(3):257-265.

7. Garza AG, Gratton MC, Coontz D, et al. Effect of paramedic experience on orotracheal intubation success rates. *J Emerg Med.* 2003;25(3):251.

8. Tentillier E, Heydenreich C, Cros AM, Schmitt V, Dindart JM, Thicoïpé M. Use of the intubating laryngeal mask airway in emergency pre-hospital difficult intubation. *Resuscitation.* 2008 Apr;77(1):30-34.

9. Dickinson ET, Cohen JE, Mechem CC. The effectiveness of midazolam as a single pharmacologic agent to facilitate endotracheal intubation by paramedics. *Prehosp Emerg Care.* 1999;3(3):191.

10. Wang HE, Davis DP, O'Connor RE, et al. Drug-assisted intubation in the prehospital setting. *Prehosp Emerg Care.* 2006;10(2):261.

11. Davis DP, Hoyt DB, Ochs M, et al. The effect of paramedic rapid sequence intubation on an outcome in patients with severe trauma brain injury. *J Trauma.* 2003;54:444.

12. Davis DP, Dunford JV, Poste JC, et al. The impact of hypoxia and hyperventilation on outcome after paramedic rapid sequence intubation of severely head-injured patient. *J Trauma.* 2004;57:1.

13. Bernard SA, Nguyen V, Cameron P, et al. Prehospital rapid sequence intubation improves functional outcome for patients with severe traumatic brain injury: a randomized controlled trial. *Ann Surg.* 2010;252(6):959-965.

14. Weingart SD, Levitan RM. Preoxygenation and prevention of desaturation during emergency airway management. *Ann Emerg Med.* 2012;59(3):165-175.

15. Smith KJ, Dobranowski J, Yip G, Dauphin A, Choi PT. Cricoid pressure displaces the esophagus: an observational study using magnetic resonance imaging. *Anesthesiology.* 2003;99(1):60-64.

16. Werner SL, Smith CE, Goldstein JR, Jones RA, Cydulka RK. Pilot study to evaluate the accuracy of ultrasonography in confirming endotracheal tube placement. *Ann Emerg Med.* 2007;49(1):75-80.

17. Butler J, Sen A. Best evidence topic report. Cricoid pressure in emergency rapid sequence induction. *Emerg Med J.* Nov 2005;22(11):815-816.

18. O'Connor RE, Swor RA. Verification of endotracheal tube placement following intubation. *Prehosp Emerg Care.* 1999;3:248.

19. Frame SB, Simon JM, Kerstein MD, et al. Percutaneous transtracheal catheter ventilation (PTCV) in complete airway obstruction: a canine model. *J Trauma.* 1989;29:774.

20. American College of Surgeons (ACS) Committee on Trauma. Airway management and ventilation. In: *Advanced Trauma Life Support, Student Course Manual.* 10th ed. Chicago, IL: ACS; 2018.

21. Mabry RL, Frankfurt A. An analysis of battlefield cricothyrotomy in Iraq and Afghanistan. *J Spec Oper Med.* 2012;12(1):17-23.

22. Warner KJ, Cuschieri J, Garland B, et al. The utility of early end-tidal capnography in monitoring ventilation status after severe injury. *J Trauma.* 2009;66:26-31.

23. Cooper CJ, Kraatz JJ, Kubiak DS, Kessel JW, Barnes SL. Utility of prehospital quantitative end tidal CO_2? *Prehosp Disaster Med.* 2013;28(2):87-93.

24. Silvestri S, Ralis GA, Krauss B, et al. The effectiveness of out-of-hospital use of continuous end-tidal carbon dioxide monitoring on the rate of unrecognized misplaced intubations within a regional emergency medical services system. *Ann Emerg Med.* 2005;45:497.

Suggested Reading

American College of Surgeons Committee on Trauma. *Advanced Trauma Life Support, Student Course Manual*. 10th ed. Chicago, IL: American College of Surgeons; 2018.

Brainard C. Whose tube is it? *JEMS*. 2006;31:62.

Dunford JV, David DP, Ochs M, et al. The incidence of transient hypoxia and heart rate reactivity during paramedic rapid sequence intubation. *Ann Emerg Med*. 2003;42:721.

Soubani AO. Noninvasive monitoring of oxygen and carbon dioxide. *Am J Emerg Med*. 2001;19:141.

Walls RM, Murphy MF, eds. *Manual of Emergency Airway Management*. 4th ed. Philadelphia, PA: Lippincott Williams & Wilkins Publishers/Wolters Kluwer Health; 2012.

Weingart SD, Levitan RM. Preoxygenation and prevention of desaturation during emergency airway management. *Ann Emerg Med*. 2012;59:165-175.

Weitzel N, Kendal J, Pons P. Blind nasotracheal intubation for patients with penetrating neck trauma. *J Trauma*. 2004;56(5):1097.

Smith C, Como J. *Trauma Anesthesia*. 2nd ed. Cambridge, UK: Cambridge University Press; 2015.

SPECIFIC SKILLS

Airway Management and Ventilation Skills

Trauma Jaw Thrust

Principle: To open the airway without moving the cervical spine.

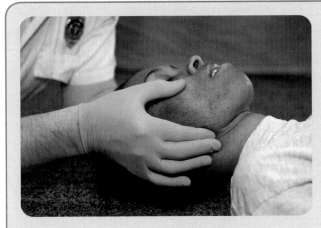

1 In both the trauma jaw thrust and the trauma chin lift, manual neutral in-line stabilization of the head and neck is maintained while the mandible is moved anteriorly (forward). This maneuver moves the tongue forward, away from the hypopharynx, and holds the mouth slightly open.

From a position above the patient's head, the prehospital care provider positions his or her hands on either side of the patient's head, fingers pointing **caudad** (toward the patient's feet).

Depending on the size of the prehospital care provider's hands, the fingers are spread across the face and around the angle of the patient's mandible.

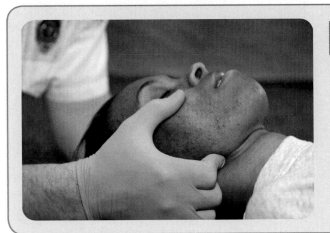

2 Gentle, equal pressure is applied with these digits to move the patient's mandible anteriorly (forward) and slightly downward (toward the patient's feet).

(continued)

Airway Management and Ventilation Skills (continued)

Alternate Trauma Jaw Thrust

Principle: To open the airway without moving the cervical spine.

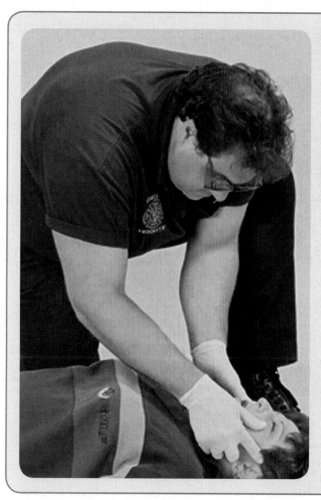

1 The trauma jaw thrust can also be performed while positioned beside the patient, facing the patient's head. The prehospital care provider's fingers point cephalad (toward the top of the patient's head). Depending on the size of the provider's hands, the fingers are spread across the face and around the angle of the patient's mandible.

2 Gentle, equal pressure is applied with these digits to move the patient's mandible anteriorly (forward) and slightly downward (toward the patient's feet).

Airway Management and Ventilation Skills *(continued)*

Trauma Chin Lift

Principle: To open the airway without moving the cervical spine.

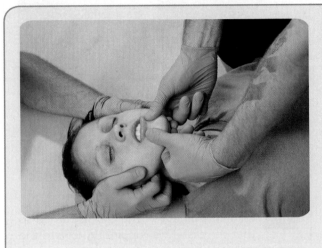

1 From a position above the patient's head, the patient's head and neck are moved into a neutral in-line position, and manual stabilization is maintained. The prehospital care provider is positioned at the patient's side between the patient's shoulders and hips, facing the patient's head. The provider grabs the patient's chin with both hands, with the index fingers hooked under the patient's chin and the thumbs on the patient's chin. The provider then opens the patient's mouth and pulls the mandible forward. For this move to be successful, it is essential to open the patient's mouth first.

This technique avoids insertion of the thumb into the patient's mouth, which can be dangerous should the patient bite or have a seizure.

Oropharyngeal Airway

Principle: An adjunct used to maintain an open airway mechanically in a patient without a gag reflex.

The oropharyngeal airway (OPA) is designed to hold the patient's tongue anteriorly out of the pharynx. The OPA is available in various sizes. Proper sizing to the patient is required to ensure a patent airway. Placement of an OPA in the hypopharynx is *contraindicated* in patients who have an intact gag reflex.

Two methods for insertion of the OPA are effective: the tongue jaw lift insertion method and the tongue blade insertion method. Regardless of which method is used, the first prehospital care provider stabilizes the patient's head and neck in a neutral in-line position, while the second provider measures and inserts the OPA.

(continued)

Airway Management and Ventilation Skills (continued)

Tongue Jaw Lift Insertion Method

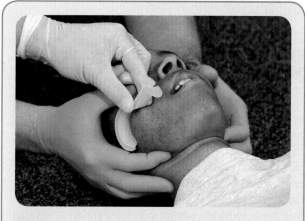

1 The first provider brings the patient's head and neck into a neutral in-line position and maintains stabilization while opening the patient's airway with a trauma jaw thrust maneuver. The second provider selects and measures for a properly sized OPA. The distance from the corner of the patient's mouth to the earlobe is a good estimate for proper size.

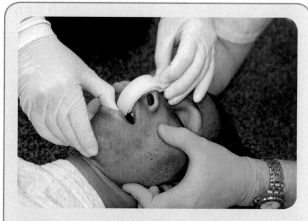

2 The patient's airway is opened with the chin lift maneuver. The OPA is turned so that the distal tip is pointing toward the top of the patient's head (flanged end pointing toward patient's head) and tilted toward the mouth opening.

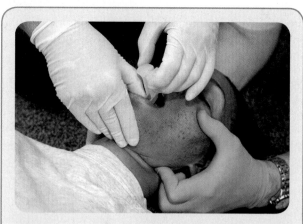

3 The OPA is inserted into the patient's mouth and rotated to fit the contours of the patient's anatomy.

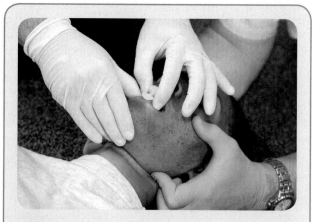

4 The OPA is rotated until the inside curve is resting against the tongue and holding it out of the posterior pharynx. The flanges of the OPA should be resting against the outside surface of the patient's teeth.

Airway Management and Ventilation Skills (continued)

Tongue Blade Insertion Method

The tongue blade insertion method is probably a safer method than the tongue jaw lift because it eliminates the possibility of accidental tearing or puncturing of gloves or skin by sharp, pointed, or broken teeth. This method also eliminates the possibility of being bitten if the patient's level of consciousness is not as deep as previously assessed or if seizure activity occurs.

As an added bonus, this method allows the provider to check with the tongue blade if some degree of gag reflex is still present. It also carries less risk of dislodging loose teeth in the case of facial trauma.

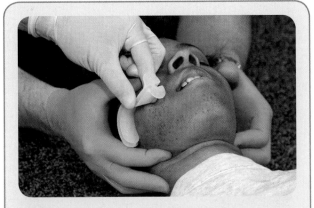

1 The first provider brings the patient's head and neck into a neutral in-line position and maintains stabilization while opening the patient's airway with the trauma jaw thrust maneuver. The second provider selects and measures for a properly sized OPA.

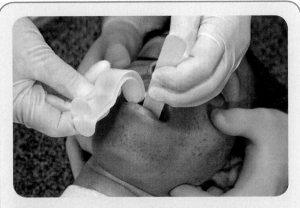

2 The second provider pulls the patient's mouth open by the chin and places a tongue blade into the patient's mouth to move the tongue forward in place and keep the airway open.

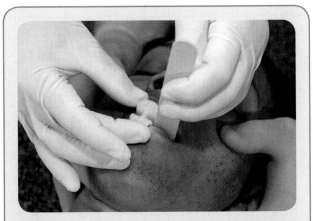

3 The device is inserted with the flanged end pointing toward the patient's feet and the distal tip pointing into the patient's mouth, following the curvature of the airway.

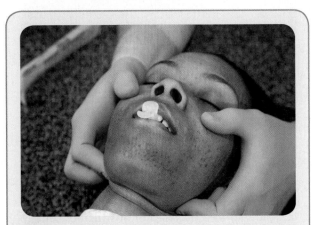

4 The OPA is advanced until the flanged end of the OPA rests against the outside surface of the patient's teeth.

(continued)

Airway Management and Ventilation Skills (continued)

Nasopharyngeal Airway

Principle: An adjunct used to maintain an open airway mechanically in a patient with or without a gag reflex or in a patient with clenched teeth.

The nasopharyngeal airway (NPA) is a simple airway adjunct that provides an effective way to maintain a patent airway in patients who may still have an intact gag reflex. Most patients will tolerate the NPA if properly sized. NPAs are available in a range of diameters (internal diameters of 5 to 9 mm), and the length varies appropriately with the size of the diameter. NPAs are usually made of a flexible, rubberlike material. Rigid NPAs are not recommended for field use.

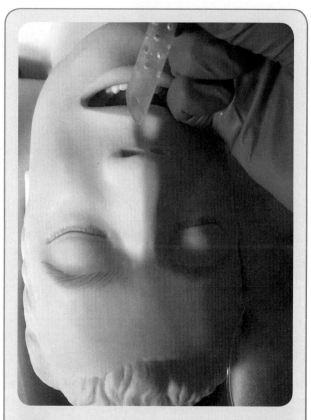

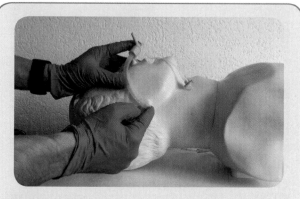

2 The length of the NPA is important. The NPA needs to be long enough to supply an air passage between the patient's tongue and the posterior pharynx. The distance from the patient's nose to the earlobe is a good estimate for proper size. (*Note:* The NPA must not be stretched out when measuring this distance.)

1 The first provider brings the patient's head and neck into a neutral in-line position and maintains stabilization while opening the patient's airway with the trauma jaw thrust maneuver. A second provider examines the patient's nostrils with a light and selects the one that is the largest and least deviated or obstructed (usually the right nostril). The second provider selects the appropriately sized NPA for the patient's nostril, a size slightly smaller in diameter than the size of the nostril opening (frequently the diameter of the patient's little finger).

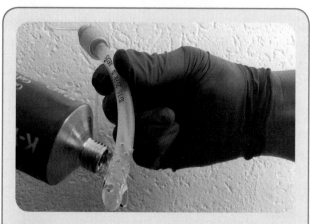

3 The distal tip (nonflanged end) of the NPA is lubricated liberally with a water-soluble jelly.

Airway Management and Ventilation Skills *(continued)*

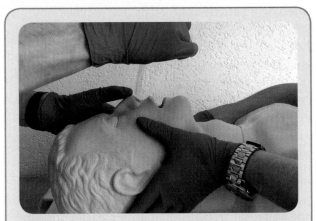

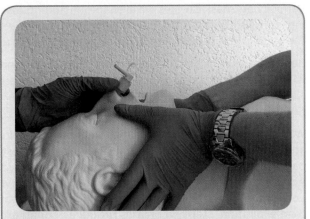

4 The NPA is slowly inserted into the nostril of choice. Insertion should be in an anterior-to-posterior direction along the floor of the nasal cavity, not in a superior-to-inferior direction. If resistance is met at the posterior end of the nostril, a gentle back-and-forth rotation of the NPA between the fingers will usually aid in passing it beyond the turbinate bones of the nasal cavity without damage. Should the NPA continue to meet with resistance, the NPA should not be forced past the obstruction but rather withdrawn, and the distal tip should be relubricated and inserted into the other nostril.

5 The second provider continues insertion until the flange end of the NPA is next to the anterior nares or until the patient gags. If the patient gags, or coughs, it can be a sign that the end of the NPA tube is in contact with the upper part of the larynx and has to be withdrawn slightly.

Photograph provided courtesy of J.C. Pitteloud M.D., Switzerland.

Bag-Mask Ventilation

Principle: The preferred method of providing assisted ventilation.

Ventilation using a bag-mask device has an advantage over other ventilatory support systems because it gives a prehospital care provider feedback by the feel of the bag (compliance). Positive feedback ensures the operator of successful ventilations; changes in the feedback indicate a loss of mask seal, the presence of a pathologic airway, or a thoracic problem interfering with the delivery of successful ventilations. This "feel" and the control it provides also make the bag-mask device suitable for assisting ventilations. The bag-mask device's portability and readiness for immediate use make it useful for immediate delivery of ventilations on identification of the need.

Without supplemental oxygen, however, a bag-mask device provides an oxygen concentration of only 21%, or a fraction of inspired oxygen (Fio_2) of 0.21; as soon as time allows, an oxygen reservoir and high-concentration supplemental oxygen should be connected to the bag-mask. When oxygen is connected without a reservoir, the Fio_2 is limited to 0.50 or less; with a reservoir, the Fio_2 is 0.85 or greater.

If the patient being ventilated is unconscious without a gag reflex, a properly sized OPA should be inserted before attempting to ventilate with the bag-mask device. If the patient has an intact gag reflex, a properly sized NPA should be inserted before attempting to assist ventilations.

(continued)

Airway Management and Ventilation Skills *(continued)*

Various bag-mask devices are available, including disposable single-patient-use models that are relatively inexpensive. Different brands have varying bag, valve, and reservoir designs. All of the parts used should be of the same model and brand because these parts are usually not safely interchangeable.

Bag-mask devices are available in adult, pediatric, and neonatal sizes. Although an adult bag can be used with the properly sized pediatric mask in an emergency, use of the correct bag size is recommended as a safe practice. Adequate ventilations of an adult patient are being delivered when there is normal chest rise achieved.

When ventilating with any positive-pressure device, inflation should stop once a normal tidal volume has been achieved. When using the bag-mask device, the chest should be visualized for maximum inflation and the bag felt to recognize any marked increased resistance in the bag when lung expansion is at its maximum. Adequate time for exhalation is needed (1:3 ratio between time for inhalation and time for exhalation). If enough time is not allowed, "stepped or stacked breaths" occur, providing a greater volume of inspiration than expiration. Stepped breaths produce poor air exchange and result in hyperinflation, increased pressure, opening of the esophagus, and gastric distension.

It is very important to pay attention to proper ventilation rate and to allow normal expiration.

Two-Provider Method

Assisting ventilation with a bag-mask device is easier with two or more prehospital care providers than with only one provider. The first provider can focus attention on maintaining an adequate mask seal, while the second provides good delivery volume by using both hands to squeeze (deflate) the bag.

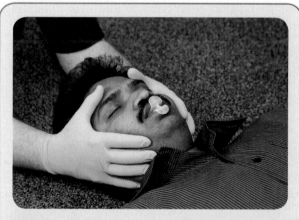

1 The first provider kneels above the patient's head and maintains manual stabilization of the patient's head and neck in a neutral in-line position.

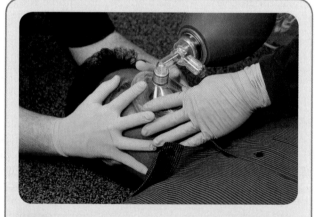

2 The face mask is placed over the patient's nose and mouth, and the mask is held in place with the thumbs on the lateral portion of the mask while pulling the mandible up into the mask. The other fingers provide the manual stabilization and maintain a patent airway.

Airway Management and Ventilation Skills *(continued)*

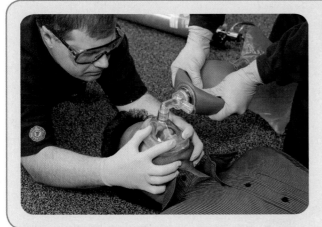

3 The second provider kneels at the side of the patient and squeezes the bag with both hands to inflate the lungs.

© National Association of Emergency Medical Technicians (NAEMT).

Supraglottic Airway

Note: The King airway is used in the following illustrations for demonstration purposes only. Other brands of supraglottic airways may be used according to local preference.

King LT Airway

Principle: A blindly inserted single-lumen airway used to provide ventilation of the trauma patient.

The King LT (laryngeal tube) may be used in patients over 4 ft (120 cm) in height and in whom the risk of aspiration is considered to be low. The King LT is a single-lumen tube with both a distal and oral (proximal) cuff. Unlike dual-lumen airways, there is only one ventilatory tube and one cuff-inflation port. This design simplifies the insertion procedure of this device. It should be noted that the King LT does not provide protection from aspiration. In fact, the manufacturer lists lack of fasting as a contraindication to its use as well as "situations where gastric contents may be present [that] include, but are not limited to . . . multiple or massive injury, acute abdominal or thoracic injury." While these contraindications apply to the OR setting, they should be a reminder that King LT provides only limited protection from aspiration in an emergency situation. Therefore, significant care must be taken to avoid aspiration when the King LT is used in these situations.

(continued)

Airway Management and Ventilation Skills (continued)

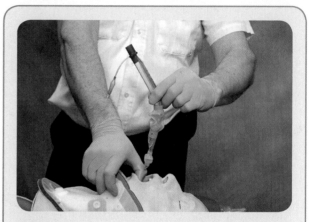

1 The prehospital provider chooses the correct King LT size, based on patient height. The cuff-inflation system is tested by injecting the maximum recommended volume of air into the cuff using a large syringe. The second provider preoxygenates the patient.

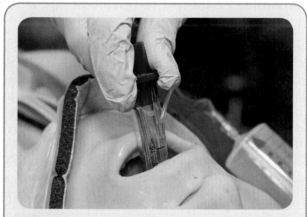

2 The first provider applies a water-based lubricant to the beveled distal tip and posterior aspect of the tube and holds the King LT with his or her dominant hand. With the nondominant hand, the first provider opens the patient's mouth and applies a chin lift. The second provider maintains cervical spine stabilization as necessary.

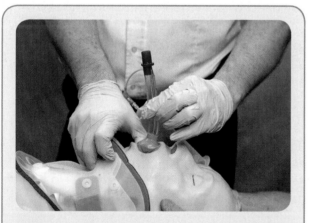

3 The first provider introduces the tip into the patient's mouth and advances it behind the base of the tongue. The first provider then rotates the tube back to the midline as the tip reaches the posterior wall of the pharynx.

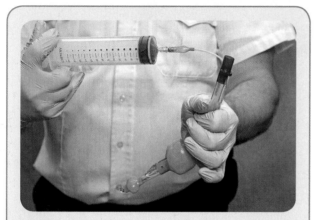

4 The first provider advances the King LT until the base of the connector is aligned with the patient's teeth.

Airway Management and Ventilation Skills (continued)

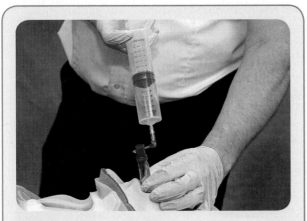

5 The first provider inflates the cuff with a large syringe. Typical inflation volumes are as follows:

- Size 3, 45 to 60 ml
- Size 4, 60 to 80 ml
- Size 5, 70 to 90 ml

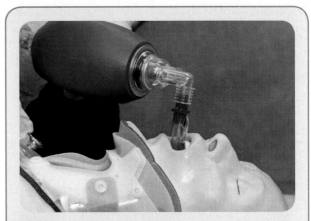

6 The first provider attaches a bag-mask device to the King LT. While gently ventilating the patient to assess ventilation, the first provider simultaneously withdraws the airway until ventilation is easy and free-flowing (large tidal volume with minimal airway pressure). Reference marks are provided at the proximal end of the King LT, which, when aligned with the upper teeth, give an indication of the depth of insertion.

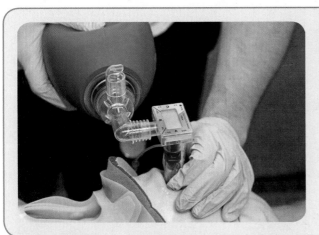

7 The first provider confirms proper position by auscultation, chest movement, and verification of carbon dioxide by capnography. The first provider readjusts the cuff inflation to 60 cm H_2O (or to seal volume). The first provider secures the King LT to the patient using tape or other accepted means. A bite block can also be used, if desired.

*Adapted from King LT manufacturer's instructions.

© National Association of Emergency Medical Technicians (NAEMT).

I-Gel Laryngeal Mask Airway

Principle: A mechanical device used to maintain an open airway without direct visualization of the airway.

The I-gel is an airway device that can be inserted by the prehospital care provider without the need for direct visualization of the vocal cords. This blind insertion technique has advantages over endotracheal intubation, as initial training requirements are less, and skill retention is easier to accomplish.

(continued)

Airway Management and Ventilation Skills (continued)

The objective of the I-gel is creation of a noninflatable seal of the pharyngeal, laryngeal, and perilaryngeal structures while avoiding compression trauma. The disadvantage of the I-gel is that although it forms a seal around the glottic opening, this seal is not as occlusive as that of an endotracheal tube cuff. Aspiration remains a potential problem. As with any airway in the trauma patient, cervical stabilization must be maintained for the duration of the procedure.

The I-gel LMA is available in a range of sizes to accommodate both pediatric and adult patient groups.

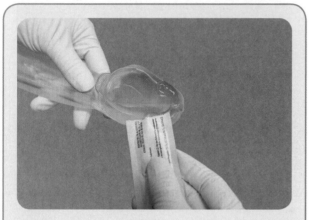

1 The prehospital care provider takes out the protective cradle and applies a water-soluble lubricant to the posterior surface. The I-gel is held along the bite block in the dominant hand. A second provider stabilizes the head from the front.

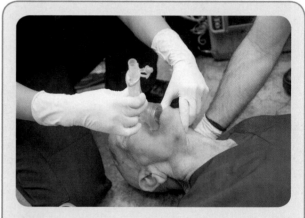

2 The first provider at the head gently presses the chin down, then introduces the leading soft tip into the mouth toward the hard palate.

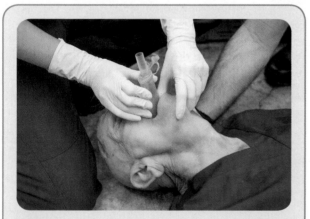

3 The first provider continues to advance the LMA into the hypopharynx until a definite resistance is felt. At this point, the tip is located in the upper esophagus and the cuff around the larynx. The incisors should be resting on the bite block.

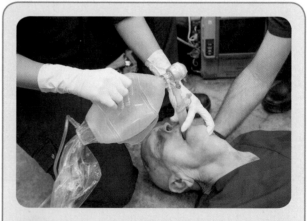

4 The first provider tapes the I-gel down on the patient's maxilla. The first provider attaches a bag-mask device to the LMA and confirms breath sounds while ventilating the patient.

Intubating Laryngeal Mask (ILMA)

Principle: A mechanical device used to maintain an open airway without direct visualization of the airway.

Once the laryngeal mask is positioned in front of the larynx, the ET tube is introduced into the ILMA and then down into the trachea.

As with any airway in the trauma patient, cervical stabilization must be maintained for the duration of the procedure.

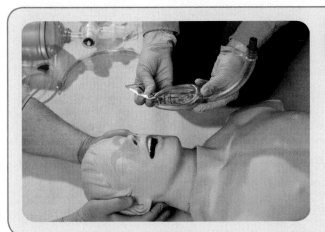

1 The first provider deflates the cuff and places water-soluble lubricant on the posterior surface of the ILMA.

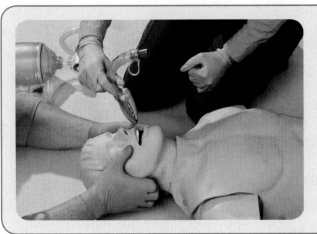

2 The second provider stabilizes the patient's head, while the first provider holds the ILMA between thumb and index finger, with the connector pointing downward toward the patient's chest and the tip of the distal end toward the hard palate.

(*continued*)

Airway Management and Ventilation Skills *(continued)*

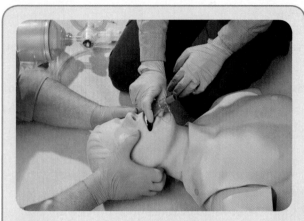

3 The first provider introduces the tip into the patient's mouth and while maintaining pressure, continues to rotate the mask downward in a circular motion, following the contour of the hard palate until a definite resistance is felt.

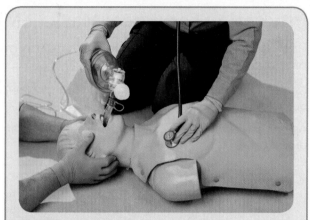

4 The first provider attaches a bag-mask device to the LMA and confirms breath sounds while ventilating the patient to ensure the mask is located in front of the tracheal opening.

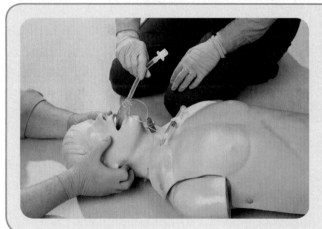

5 The first provider introduces the ET tube into the proximal opening of the ILMA up to the mark. The cuff is then inflated by the first provider. While the patient is ventilated via the ET tube, breath sounds are auscultated to confirm proper placement.

© Jones & Bartlett Learning. Photographed by Darren Stahlman.

Visualized Orotracheal Intubation of the Trauma Patient

Principle: To secure a definitive airway without manipulating the cervical spine.

Visualized orotracheal intubation of the trauma patient is done with the patient's head and neck stabilized in a neutral in-line position. Orotracheal intubation while maintaining manual in-line stabilization requires additional training and practice beyond that for intubation of nontrauma patients. As with all skills, training requires observation, critique, and certification initially and at least twice a year by the medical director or designee.

In hypoxic trauma patients who are not in cardiac arrest, intubation should not be the initial airway maneuver. The prehospital care provider should perform intubation only after he or she has preoxygenated the patient

Airway Management and Ventilation Skills *(continued)*

with a high concentration of oxygen using a simple airway adjunct or manual maneuver. Contact with the deep pharynx when intubating a severely hypoxic patient without preoxygenation can easily produce vagal stimulation, resulting in a dangerous bradycardia.

The prehospital care provider should not interrupt ventilation for more than 20 seconds when intubating the patient. Ventilation should never be interrupted for more than 30 seconds for any reason.

Visualized orotracheal intubation is extremely difficult in conscious patients or patients with an intact gag reflex. The prehospital care provider should consider use of topical anesthesia or paralytic agents after additional training, protocol development, and approval by the EMS medical director.

For the novice prehospital care provider, the use of a straight laryngoscope blade tends to produce less rotary force (pulling the patient's head toward a "sniffing" position) than that produced by the use of a curved blade. However, because the success rate of intubation is often related to the provider's comfort with a given design, the style of blade selection for the laryngoscope remains a matter of individual preference.

Note: The cervical collar will limit forward motion of the mandible and complete opening of the mouth. Therefore, after adequate spinal immobilization is ensured, the cervical collar is removed, manual stabilization of the cervical spine is held, and intubation is attempted. Once intubation is accomplished, the collar is reapplied.

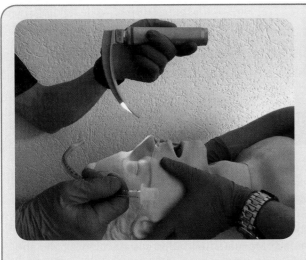

1 Before attempting intubation, the prehospital care providers should assemble and test all required equipment and follow standard precautions. The first provider kneels at the patient's head and ventilates the patient with a bag-mask device and high-concentration oxygen. The second provider, kneeling at the patient's side, provides manual stabilization of the patient's head and neck. The second provider holds the head with the thumb resting on the patient's cheekbones and the fingers behind the head. Improper hand positioning can block the mouth opening and make laryngoscopy impossible. After preoxygenation, the first provider stops ventilations and grasps the laryngoscope in the left hand and the ET tube (with syringe attached to pilot valve) in the right hand. If a stylet is used, this should have been inserted when the equipment was inspected and tested. The distal end of the stylet should be inserted just short of the ET tube's distal opening.

(continued)

Airway Management and Ventilation Skills *(continued)*

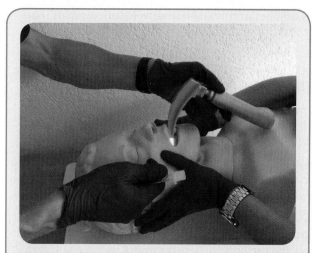

2 The laryngoscope blade is inserted into the right side of the patient's airway to the correct depth, sweeping toward the center of the airway while observing the desired landmarks.

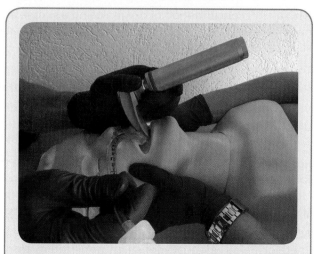

3 After identification of desired landmarks, the ET tube is inserted between the patient's vocal cords to the desired depth. The laryngoscope is then removed while holding the ET tube in place; the depth marking on the side of the ET tube is noted. If a malleable stylet has been used, it should be removed at this time.

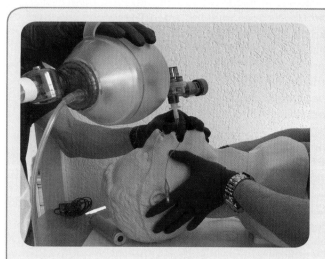

4 The pilot valve is inflated with enough air to complete the seal between the patient's trachea and the cuff of the ET tube (usually 5 ml of air), and the syringe is removed from the pilot valve. The first provider attaches the bag-valve system with a reservoir attached to the proximal end of the ET tube, and ventilation is resumed while observing the rise of the patient's chest with each delivered breath. Manual stabilization of the patient's head and neck is maintained throughout the process. Bilateral breath sounds and absence of air sounds over the epigastrium and other indications of proper ET tube placement, including waveform capnography, are checked (see the earlier discussion in this chapter, under Verification of Endotracheal Tube Placement). Once ET tube placement is confirmed, the ET tube is secured in place. Although the use of tape or other commercially available devices is adequate in controlled situations in which the patient is not moved, the *best* way to guard against displacement of the ET tube in the prehospital situation is to physically hold onto the tube at all times.

Photograph provided courtesy of J.C. Pitteloud M.D., Switzerland.

Airway Management and Ventilation Skills (continued)

Face-to-Face Orotracheal Intubation

Principle: An alternative method of securing a definitive airway when patient positioning limits use of traditional methods.

Situations may arise in the prehospital setting in which the prehospital care provider cannot take a position above the patient's head to initiate endotracheal intubation in a traditional manner. The face-to-face method for intubation is a viable option in these situations. The basic concepts of intubation still apply with face-to-face intubation: Preoxygenate the patient with a bag-mask device and high-concentration oxygen before attempting intubation, maintain manual stabilization of the patient's head and neck throughout the intubation, and do not interrupt ventilation for longer than 20 to 30 seconds at a time.

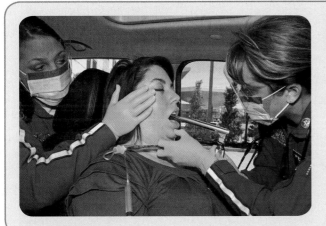

1 While manual stabilization of the patient's head and neck in a neutral in-line position is held, the prehospital care provider positions himself or herself in front of the patient, "face to face." The laryngoscope is held in the right hand with the blade on the patient's tongue. The blade moves the tongue down and out rather than up and out. The patient's mouth is opened with the left hand, and the laryngoscope is placed into the patient's airway. After the laryngoscope blade is placed in the patient's airway, the desired landmarks are found. Looking into the airway from a position above the open airway provides the best view.

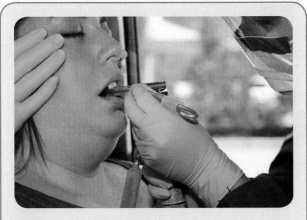

2 After identification of desired landmarks, the ET tube is passed between the patient's vocal cords to the desired depth with the left hand. The cuff is inflated with air to form the seal, and the syringe is removed. A bag-valve device is attached, and placement of the ET tube is confirmed.

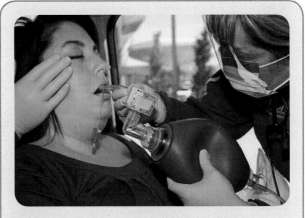

3 After confirmation of ET tube placement, the patient is ventilated while the prehospital care provider holds onto the ET tube and maintains manual stabilization of the patient's head and neck. The ET tube should then be secured in place.

(continued)

Airway Management and Ventilation Skills (continued)

Surgical Cricothyroidotomy

Principle: A method of securing an airway in a patient with an airway obstruction that cannot be relieved by simple means.

The role of a surgical airway in the civilian prehospital environment is still unclear. This management technique requires a high degree of skill since it carries a high risk of complications and there is no second chance to perform it correctly.

Although there are many devices on the market, the technique described here utilizes simple and inexpensive materials stored in the ambulance. The equipment includes a scalpel, a curved hemostat, and a 5.0-mm to 7.0-mm-diameter endotracheal tube or alternatively a commercial tracheostomy tube. Endotracheal tubes are second choice since they are too long and carry the risk of selective intubation. This technique is not recommended in children under 12 years.

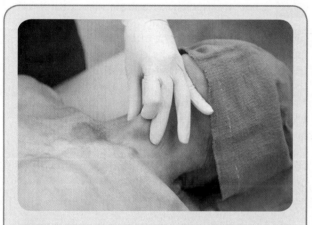

1 The cricothyroid membrane is located by palpation. The larynx is stabilized with two fingers, while the index fingers locate the cricothyroid membrane.

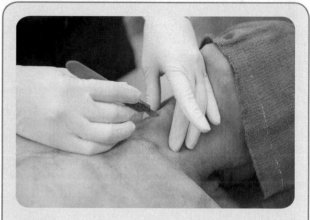

2 A 2- to 3-cm vertical incision is made over the cricothyroid membrane, and the cricothyroid membrane, is carefully incised transversely.

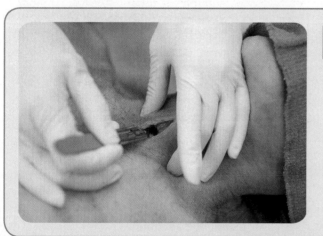

3 A curved hemostat is inserted into the incision and rotated 90° to open the incision (a scalpel handle can be used as an alternative).

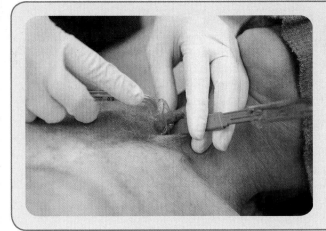

4 A proper sized cuffed tube is inserted into the trachea. The tube position is verified with auscultation and $ETCO_2$ monitoring.

Intubation With Airtraq Channeled Video Laryngoscope

Principle: The Airtraq device allows visualization of the glottis around the tongue and includes a channel to facilitate direction of the endotracheal tube through the vocal cords.

The Airtraq is available in four sizes, ranging from 0 (infant) to 3 (average-sized adult).

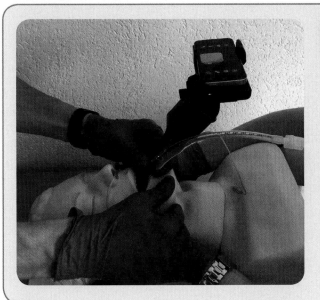

1 The second provider stabilizes the patient's head from the front while the first provider opens the cervical collar. The first provider turns on the light and slides the tube into the lateral channel of the Airtraq from the top, aligning the top with the end of the guiding channel. (*Warning:* Inserting the tube farther will obscure visualization.) While opening the mouth with the thumb of the nondominant hand, the first provider uses the dominant hand to facilitate insertion into the patient's mouth. The Aitraq is held with the fingers and not with the palm of the hand, and it is not held from the top.

(*continued*)

Airway Management and Ventilation Skills *(continued)*

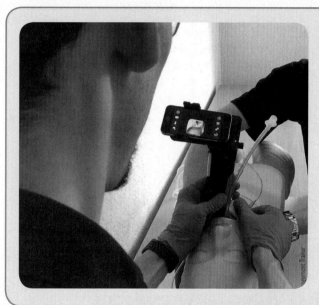

2 The first provider inserts the Airtraq into the midline of the patient's mouth, avoiding putting pressure on the upper teeth, until the tip has reached the back of the tongue. Once the Airtraq is inserted into the posterior oropharynx, the epiglottis, the arytenoids, and the vocal cords are identified.

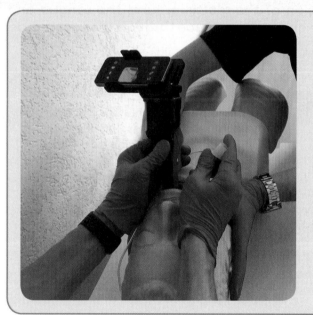

3 The first provider inserts the tube between the vocal cords by pushing it forward while keeping it inside the guiding channel. The first provider detaches the tube from the Airtraq by pulling the Airtraq laterally while holding the tube in position. The first provider confirms the correct position of the tube by auscultation and ETCO$_2$.

4 The first provider detaches the tube from the Airtraq by pulling the Airtraq laterally while holding the tube in position. The first providers confirms the correct positon of the tube by auscultation and ETCO$_2$.

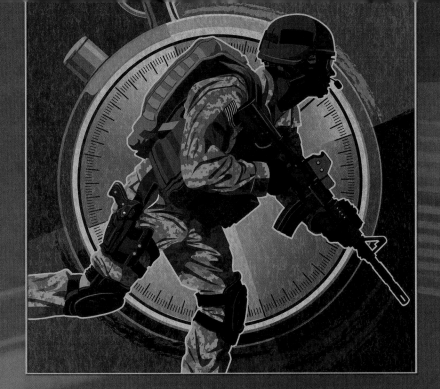

DIVISION **3**

Specific Injuries

CHAPTER 8

Head Trauma

Lead Editors:
Deborah Stein, MD
Christine Ramirez, MD

CHAPTER OBJECTIVES   At the completion of this chapter, you will be able to do the following:

- Relate the physics of trauma to the potential for traumatic brain injury (TBI).
- Incorporate the recognition of pathophysiologic manifestations and historical data significant for TBI into the assessment of the trauma patient to formulate a field impression.
- Discuss the importance of the motor portion of the Glasgow Coma Scale score in neurologic assessment.

- Formulate a plan of field intervention for both short and prolonged transport times for patients with TBI.
- Compare and contrast the pathophysiology, management, and potential consequences of specific types of primary TBIs and secondary brain injuries.
- Identify criteria for patient care decisions with regard to mode of transport, level of prehospital care, and hospital resources needed for the appropriate management of the TBI patient.

SCENARIO

On an 85°F (29°C) summer day, you and your partner are dispatched to the finish line of a marathon race for a 30-year-old man who fell 14 feet (ft; 4.3 meters [m]) off a ladder while attempting to secure the finish line banner. Upon your arrival, the patient is supine and unresponsive. A bystander is holding the patient's head and neck in-line.

You note an irregular breathing rate that increases and then decreases in depth. You also note that there is bloody fluid coming from both ears and both nostrils of the patient. The patient's airway is maintained with an oropharyngeal airway once absence of the gag reflex is noted. Your partner ventilates the patient with a bag-mask device at a rate of 12 breaths/minute. You notice that the patient's right pupil is dilated. The radial pulse is 54 and regular. Oxygen saturation (Spo_2) is 96%. The patient's skin is cool, dry, and pale. His Glasgow Coma Scale (GCS) score is calculated to be 7, with eyes = 2, verbal = 1, and motor = 4 (E2V1M4).

You rapidly prepare the patient for transport and place him into your ambulance to perform the secondary survey while en route to the hospital. Palpation of the occiput generates a painful moan from the patient.

(continued)

INTRODUCTION

Traumatic brain injury (TBI) is a worldwide public health problem that affects over 10 million people annually throughout the world. According to the World Health Organization (WHO), TBI will surpass many diseases as the major cause of death and disability by 2020. In the United States, approximately 2.8 million TBI-related events occur yearly, including deaths, hospitalizations, and emergency department (ED) visits. This total equates to one person sustaining a TBI every 21 seconds. TBI is the most frequent cause of death and disability among children in the United States, with more than 1 million children sustaining brain injuries yearly. Over 80% of all TBIs are mild, and the patients are discharged from the ED; however, approximately 282,000 patients are hospitalized, and each year 50,000 die from moderate to severe TBIs. Mortality rates for moderate and severe brain injuries are about 10% and 30%, respectively. Of those who survive moderate or severe brain injuries, 50% to 99% have some degree of permanent neurologic disability.[1,2]

Common causes of TBIs include motor vehicle collisions, falls, violence, and unintentional workplace or sports-related injuries (10%). Motor vehicle crashes are the leading cause of TBI in patients between the ages of 5 and 75 years of age, while falls are the leading cause of TBI in pediatric patients up to 4 years of age and in the older adult population.[1]

Patients with TBI can be some of the most challenging trauma patients to treat. They may be combative, and attempts to manage the airway can be extremely difficult because of clenched jaw muscles and vomiting. Assessment can be further hindered by the presence of shock from other injuries or drug and/or alcohol intoxication. Occasionally, serious intracranial injuries can be present with minimal or no external evidence of trauma. Skilled care in the prehospital setting focuses on ensuring the adequate delivery of oxygen and nutrients to the brain and rapidly identifying patients at risk for herniation and elevated intracranial pressure. This approach can not only decrease mortality from TBI, but it also reduces the incidence of permanent neurologic disability. Our goal when treating TBI is to allow no further harm to occur to even a single brain cell and to establish conditions optimal for healing and recovery.

Anatomy

Knowledge of head and brain anatomy is essential to understanding the pathophysiology of TBI. The scalp is the outermost covering of the head and offers some protection to the skull and brain. It is composed of several layers, including skin, connective tissue, the aponeurosis (or **galea aponeurotica**), and the periosteum of the skull bones. The galea is a layer of tough, thick fibrous tissue that provides structural support to the scalp, while the periosteum provides nutrition to the bone. The scalp and soft tissues overlying the head are highly vascular and can bleed profusely when lacerated.

The skull, or cranium, is composed of a number of bones that fuse into a single structure during childhood (see Figure 6-7). Several small openings (**foramina**) through the base of the skull provide pathways for blood vessels and cranial nerves. One large opening, the **foramen magnum**, is located at the base of the skull and serves as a passageway for the brain stem to the spinal cord (**Figure 8-1**). In infants, "soft spots" known as **fontanelles**, can be identified between the bones. The infant has no bony protection over these portions of the brain until the bones fuse, typically by 2 years of age. In addition, because the infant's skull is not fused, hemorrhage within the skull can cause the bones to spread apart, allowing more blood to accumulate within the cranium.

The cranium provides significant protection to the brain. It is made of two layers of compact cortical tissue, known as the outer and inner tables, which sandwich a layer of spongy cancellous bone. Most of the bones forming

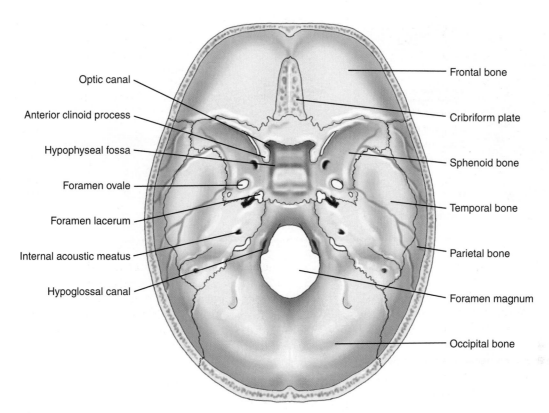

Figure 8-1 Internal view of the base of the skull.
© National Association of Emergency Medical Technicians (NAEMT).

the cranium are thick and strong. However, the skull is especially thin in the temporal and ethmoid regions and is therefore more prone to fracture in these regions. In addition, the interior surface of the skull base is rough and irregular (see Figure 8-1). When exposed to a blunt force, the brain may slide across these irregularities, producing cerebral contusions or lacerations.

The brain is covered by three separate membranes known as the **meninges**: the dura mater, arachnoid mater, and pia mater (**Figure 8-2**). The outermost layer, the **dura mater**, is composed of tough fibrous tissue and lines the inner table of the skull. Under normal circumstances, there is no space between the dura and the skull. However, this juncture is a potential space known as the **epidural space** that can develop if the dura is stripped away from the skull. For example, the middle meningeal arteries are located in grooves in the temporal bones on either side of the head, between the dura and the inner table. A temporal bone fracture can tear the middle meningeal artery, resulting in an **epidural hematoma**.

The **arachnoid mater** is deep to the dura mater and covers the brain and its blood vessels in a spiderweb appearance. The space between the dura mater and arachnoid mater is known as the subdural space. Unlike the epidural space, the subdural space is an actual space located beneath the dura mater. This space is spanned in places by bridging veins, which create a vascular communication between the skull and the brain. The traumatic rupture of these veins often creates **subdural hematomas**, which are often associated with additional injury to the brain tissue. Injury to these bridging veins accounts for the morbidity of subdural hematomas.

The deepest membrane is the **pia mater**. It is the final brain covering that is adherent to the brain. The space between the arachnoid mater and pia mater is known as the subarachnoid space. It is also an actual space that contains cerebral blood vessels, which emerge from the base of the brain and cover the brain. Their rupture (usually from trauma or a ruptured cerebral aneurysm) will result in bleeding into the subarachnoid space, causing a **subarachnoid hematoma**. Subarachnoid hematomas can be indicators of other serious concomitant brain injuries.

The brain occupies about 80% of the **cranial vault** and is divided into three main regions: the **cerebrum, cerebellum,** and **brain stem** (**Figure 8-3**). The cerebrum consists of right and left hemispheres that can be subdivided into several lobes. The dominant hemisphere contains the language center and is the left side in virtually all right-handed individuals and 85% of left-handed individuals. The cerebrum is separated from the cerebellum by an extension of the dura mater called the **tentorium cerebelli**. The cerebellum is located in the posterior fossa of the cranium, behind the

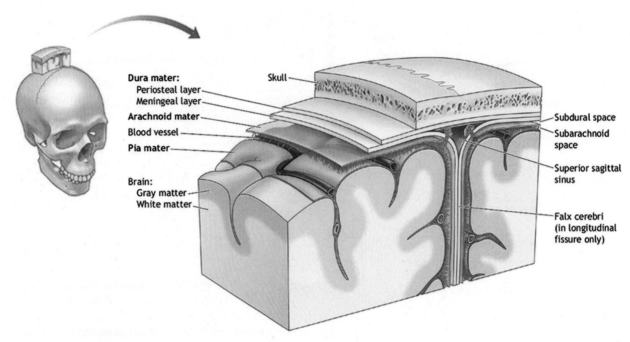

Figure 8-2 Meningeal coverings of the brain.
Courtesy of the American College of Surgeons.

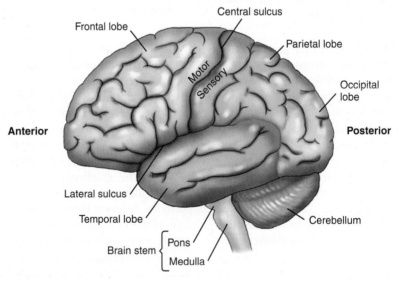

Figure 8-3 Regions of the brain.
© National Association of Emergency Medical Technicians (NAEMT).

brain stem and beneath the cerebrum. The brain stem is inferior to the cerebrum and anterior to the cerebellum. **Table 8-1** lists all of the major regions of the brain and their functions. Much of the **reticular activating system**, the portion of the brain responsible for arousal and alertness, is also found in the brain stem. Blunt trauma can impair the reticular activating system, leading to a transient loss of consciousness.

The brain receives 14% of the cardiac output, which is continuously flowing in and out of the brain at about 700 milliliters (ml) per minute. At any time, the intracranial blood volume is 15% arterial, 40% venous, and 45% within the microcirculation. The brain is surrounded by **cerebrospinal fluid (CSF)**, which is produced in the ventricular system of the brain and also surrounds the spinal cord. CSF helps cushion the brain and is contained in the

Table 8-1 The Brain	
Region	**Function**
Cerebrum	Sensory function, motor function, intelligence, memory
Frontal	Emotions, motor function, and expression of speech on the dominant side
Parietal	Sensory function, spatial orientation
Temporal	Regulation of certain memory functions; speech reception and integration in all right-handed and the majority of left-handed individuals
Occipital	Vision
Cerebellum	Movement
Brain stem	Signal relay between brain and spinal cord
Midbrain	Arousal and alertness via the reticular activating system
Pons	Respiratory apnea centers, conveyance of signals from cerebrum to medulla and cerebellum
Medulla	Cardiopulmonary centers (breathing, heart rate)

subarachnoid space as well. The amount of CSF is small (100 ml) compared to brain parenchyma and cerebral blood flow. The pressure inside the skull is known as **intracranial pressure (ICP)** and is the result of the combined pressure of brain tissue, blood, and CSF against the skull. It is important to note that the volume of CSF is small compared to the volume of brain tissue and blood. Although CSF removal can help reduce ICP, its accumulation is rarely the cause of raised ICP in acute traumatic injury.

There are 12 cranial nerves that originate from the brain and brain stem (**Figure 8-4**). Cranial nerve (CN) III (**oculomotor nerve**) controls pupillary constriction and is important in assessing patients with suspected brain injury. It crosses the surface of the tentorium cerebelli, and any hemorrhage or edema that causes downward herniation of the brain will compress the nerve, impairing its function and leading to pupil dilation.

Physiology

Cerebral Blood Flow

It is critical that the brain's neurons receive a constant flow of blood in order to provide oxygen and glucose. This constant cerebral blood flow is maintained by ensuring (1) an adequate pressure (cerebral perfusion pressure) to force blood through the brain and (2) a regulatory mechanism (autoregulation), which ensures constant blood flow by varying the resistance to blood flow as the perfusion pressure changes.

Cerebral Perfusion Pressure

Cerebral perfusion pressure is the amount of pressure available to push blood through the cerebral circulation and, thus, maintain blood flow and oxygen and glucose delivery to the energy-demanding cells of the brain. Cerebral perfusion pressure relates directly to the patient's mean arterial pressure (MAP) and ICP. The MAP is the average pressure in the arteries during one cardiac cycle and is an indicator of perfusion to vital organs.

Cerebral perfusion pressure is expressed by the following formula:

Cerebral perfusion pressure = Mean arterial pressure − Intracranial pressure

or

CPP = MAP − ICP

Normal MAP ranges from about 85 to 95 mm Hg. In adults, ICP is normally below 15 mm Hg. It is usually 3 to 7 mm Hg in children and 1.5 to 6 mm Hg in infants.[1] Therefore, cerebral perfusion pressure is normally about 70 to 80 mm Hg. Sudden increases or decreases in blood pressure and ICP may affect cerebral perfusion.

Autoregulation of Cerebral Blood Flow

The most important factor for the brain, however, is not cerebral perfusion pressure itself but rather cerebral blood flow. The brain works very hard at keeping its cerebral blood flow constant over a wide range of changing conditions. This process is known as **autoregulation**. Autoregulation is crucial to the brain's normal function.

To understand autoregulation, we need to remember that for any flowing system:

Pressure = Flow × Resistance

In the case of the brain, this translates into:

Cerebral perfusion pressure = Cerebral blood flow × Cerebral vascular resistance

or

CPP = CBF × CVR

Anterior

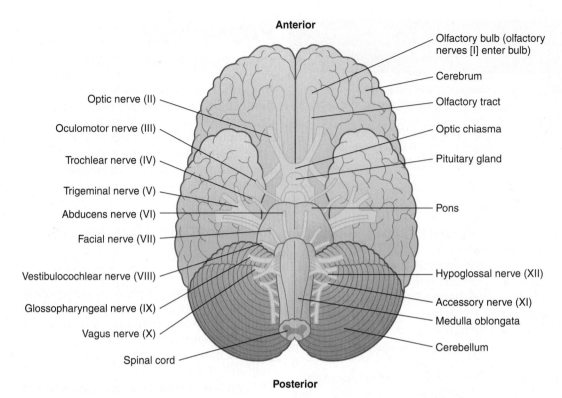

- Optic nerve (II)
- Oculomotor nerve (III)
- Trochlear nerve (IV)
- Trigeminal nerve (V)
- Abducens nerve (VI)
- Facial nerve (VII)
- Vestibulocochlear nerve (VIII)
- Glossopharyngeal nerve (IX)
- Vagus nerve (X)
- Spinal cord

- Olfactory bulb (olfactory nerves [I] enter bulb)
- Cerebrum
- Olfactory tract
- Optic chiasma
- Pituitary gland
- Pons
- Hypoglossal nerve (XII)
- Accessory nerve (XI)
- Medulla oblongata
- Cerebellum

Posterior

Figure 8-4 Inferior surface of the brain showing the origins of the cranial nerves.
© National Association of Emergency Medical Technicians (NAEMT).

Because the brain's principal concern is cerebral blood flow, it is useful to rewrite this equation as:

$$CBF = CPP/CVR$$

If cerebral perfusion pressure decreases, the only way to keep cerebral blood flow constant is by decreasing the cerebral vascular resistance as well. The brain accomplishes autoregulation by adjusting the cerebral vascular resistance (through vasodilation). However, this autoregulatory mechanism requires a certain minimum cerebral perfusion pressure. For example, at a pressure of 0 mm Hg, no amount of vasodilation will cause blood to flow, and there are limits to how much the blood vessels in the head can dilate. Below a cerebral perfusion pressure of about 50 mm Hg, the autoregulatory mechanisms can no longer compensate for the decreased cerebral perfusion pressure, and cerebral blood flow starts to decrease.

Another way to compensate for reduced cerebral blood flow is by extracting more oxygen from the blood that is passing through the brain. The clinical signs and symptoms of ischemia (dizziness and altered mental status) will not be noticed until the diminished perfusion has exceeded the ability of increased oxygen extraction to meet the brain's metabolic needs.[3] As cerebral blood flow begins to fall, cerebral function will decline, and the risk of permanent cerebral injury from ischemia increases.

To make matters worse, injured brains often require higher-than-normal cerebral perfusion pressures to activate autoregulation and keep cerebral blood flow adequate. However, the range of normal flow differs among individuals, and there are no convenient ways to measure cerebral blood flow levels. Therefore, cerebral perfusion pressure is used to estimate the adequacy of cerebral blood flow.

The relationship between cerebral perfusion pressure, ICP, and MAP is important in trauma. Acute intracranial bleeding causes compression to surrounding tissues and an increased ICP. This is termed *mass effect*. As the ICP increases, the amount of pressure needed to push blood through the brain also increases. The MAP will subsequently increase to maintain CPP. If the MAP cannot keep up with the increase in ICP or if treatment to decrease the ICP is not rapidly instituted, the amount of blood flowing through the brain will start to decrease, leading to ischemic brain damage and impaired brain function. Therefore, in the absence of an ICP monitor, the best practice is to maintain a high-normal MAP. The Brain Trauma Foundation recommends maintaining systolic blood pressure greater than 90 mm Hg for neurologically injured patients.[4-8]

Cerebral Venous Drainage

Cerebral venous drainage is an often overlooked but significant contributor of ICP and autoregulation. A network of superficial and deep cerebral veins drains the blood from various regions of the brain into a system of venous sinuses. Ultimately the superior sagittal sinus (from above) and the straight sinus (from the middle and below) join together at the confluence of sinuses (**torcula**) before draining laterally into the left and right transverse sinuses. Cerebral drainage into the transverse sinuses is asymmetric in the majority of patients, with the superior sagittal sinus draining primarily into the right transverse sinus and the straight sinus draining primarily into the left transverse sinus.[9] The left and right transverse sinuses eventually empty into their respective jugular veins, which drain into the superior vena cava. It should be noted that except for subdural hematoma, acute emergencies involving the cerebral veins are exceedingly rare.[9] The vast majority of neurologic vascular conditions arise as a result of arterial compromise.[9]

Venous sinuses are susceptible to dilation and compression. For example, when cerebral blood inflow rises, venous drainage increases as an autoregulatory mechanism. However, there is a point at which the limits of compliance increase and inadequate venous drainage can result in venous and intracranial hypertension. Acute compression, such as depressed skull fractures, expanding intracranial hematomas, and sinus thrombosis, can also impair venous drainage, increasing ICP. Obstruction of the dominant sinus has more effects than obstruction of the nondominant sinus. Extracranial causes, such as jugular venous compression from head flexion or tight cervical collars, can also impair venous drainage by almost 10 mm Hg.[10-12]

Oxygen and Cerebral Blood Flow

The brain is a highly metabolic organ and therefore has high oxygen requirements. Decreased levels of oxygen (hypoxia) cause significant vasodilation in an effort to dramatically increase cerebral blood flow. This response typically does not occur until the arterial oxygen partial pressure (Pao_2) falls below 50 mm Hg. Cerebral blood flow can increase by up to 400% of resting levels.[3]

Carbon Dioxide and Cerebral Blood Flow

The cerebral blood vessels respond to changes in arterial carbon dioxide levels by constricting or dilating. Decreased levels of carbon dioxide (hypocapnia) result in vasoconstriction, while elevated levels (hypercapnia) cause vasodilation. Hyperventilation reduces the arterial carbon dioxide partial pressure ($Paco_2$) by increasing the rate at which carbon dioxide is blown off by the lungs. The resulting hypocapnia changes the acid–base balance in the brain, resulting in vasoconstriction. This cerebral vasoconstriction reduces the intravascular volume of the brain, reducing cerebral blood volume and, therefore, often ICP.[13,14] Hyperventilation has been used to reduce ICP but also adversely impacts cerebral blood flow. In fact, data suggest that hyperventilation more reliably reduces cerebral blood flow than ICP.[15-17]

Under normal circumstances, autoregulation ensures adequate cerebral blood flow by maintaining the correct cerebral vascular resistance for the available cerebral perfusion pressure to ensure continuing adequate cerebral blood flow. However, hyperventilation of a patient bypasses the autoregulation mechanisms of the brain. Thus, hyperventilation-induced cerebral vasoconstriction may reduce cerebral blood volume enough to reduce ICP, but it also increases cerebral vascular resistance, regardless of whether cerebral perfusion pressure is adequate to maintain cerebral blood flow. As a result, hyperventilation can reduce cerebral blood flow, placing the injured brain at greater risk for ischemic injury. A $Paco_2$ of less than 35 mm Hg increases the risk of cerebral ischemia, and a $Paco_2$ greater than the normal range of 35 to 45 mm Hg (hypercapnia) leads to dilation of cerebral arterioles, thus increasing cerebral blood flow while at the same time increasing intravascular volume and potentially increasing ICP. Management of TBI using hyperventilation is discussed later in this chapter.

Pathophysiology

TBI can be divided into two categories: primary and secondary.

Primary Brain Injury

Primary brain injury occurs at the time of the original insult and is any injury that occurs because of the initial trauma. This includes injury to the brain, its coverings, and associated vascular structures. Primary brain injuries include brain contusions, hemorrhages, and damage to nerves and brain vessels. Because neural tissue does not regenerate well and because little possibility exists for repair, there is minimal expectation of recovery of the structure and function lost with primary injury.

Secondary Brain Injury

Secondary brain injury refers to further injury to structures that were originally unharmed by the primary injury. At the time of injury, pathophysiologic processes are initiated, resulting in further injury to the brain for hours to weeks after the initial insult. The primary focus in the prehospital (and hospital) management of TBI is to identify and limit or stop these secondary injury mechanisms. The secondary effects are insidious in nature, and there can often be significant, ongoing damage that is not immediately apparent or appreciated. These effects play a significant role in death and disability after TBIs. By understanding what type of secondary injury is likely to occur as a result of the primary trauma, we can prepare for and intervene to correct or prevent these complications from occurring.

Pathologic mechanisms related to intracranial mass effect, elevated ICP, and mechanical shifting of the brain,

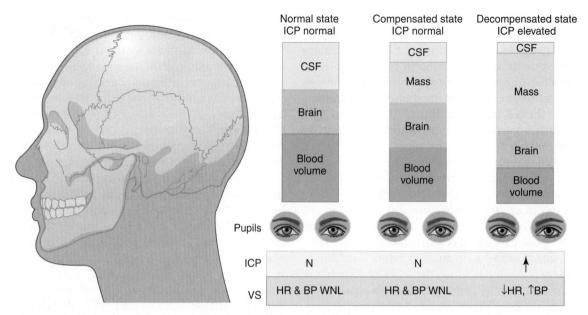

Figure 8-5 Monro-Kellie doctrine: The volume of intracranial contents must remain constant. If the addition of a mass such as a hematoma results in the decrease of an equal volume of CSF and blood, the ICP remains normal. However, when this compensatory mechanism is exhausted, an exponential increase in ICP occurs for minute increases in the volume of the hematoma.

© National Association of Emergency Medical Technicians (NAEMT).

can lead to herniation. These mechanisms cause significant morbidity and mortality if not addressed rapidly, but their management has been revolutionized by computed tomography (CT) scanning and other advanced imaging modalities, ICP monitoring, and immediate surgery. In the prehospital environment, the identification of patients at high risk for herniation from mass effect and their rapid transport to a hospital with the facilities to address these issues are still the key priorities.

Two other important causes of secondary injury are hypoxia and hypotension. Unrecognized and untreated hypoxia and hypotension are as damaging to the injured brain as elevated ICP. In addition, impaired delivery of oxygen or energy substrate (e.g., glucose) to the injured brain has a much more devastating impact than that in the normal brain. Therefore, hypoxia and hypotension should be treated and avoided as much as possible.[7,8,18-20]

Intracranial Causes of Secondary Brain Injury

Mass Effect and Herniation

The secondary injury mechanisms most often recognized are those related to mass effect. These mechanisms are the result of the complex interactions between the brain, CSF, and blood against the skull, described by the **Monro-Kellie doctrine**. This doctrine states that the sum of the volume of brain tissue, blood, and CSF must remain constant with an intact skull. Therefore, an increase in one component

(such as from a hematoma, cerebral swelling, or tumor) must cause a decrease in one or two of the other components or the ICP will increase (**Figure 8-5**).[10]

In response to an expanding mass, the initial compensatory mechanism is to decrease the volume of intracranial CSF. The CSF naturally circulates within and around the brain, brain stem, and spinal cord. However, as the mass expands, CSF will be forced out of the head. Venous drainage will also increase to help reduce intravascular blood volume within the cranial vault. These two mechanisms prevent ICP from rising during the early phase of mass accumulation. As such, the patient can appear asymptomatic. However, as the mass size increases past the threshold of blood and CSF removal, the ICP will begin increasing rapidly. The effect of the mass is to shift the brain across and through fixed structures within the skull, eventually causing the portions of the brain to herniate through or around some of these structures. This causes compression of the brain's most vital centers and jeopardizes their arterial blood supply (**Figure 8-6**). The consequences of this herniation toward and through the foramen magnum are described as the various herniation syndromes (**Figure 8-7** and **Table 8-2**).

Clinical Herniation Syndromes

Clinical features of the herniation syndromes can help identify a patient who is herniating. In uncal herniation, compression of CN III results in a dilated or blown pupil on the same (ipsilateral) side of the herniation. Loss of function of the motor tract will result in weakness on the

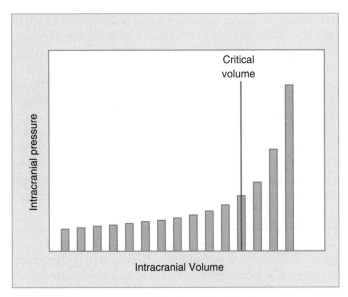

Figure 8-6 This graph demonstrates the relationship between intracranial volume and ICP. As the volume increases, the pressure remains relatively constant as CSF and blood are forced out. Eventually, a point is reached when no additional compensation can occur and ICP rises dramatically.

© National Association of Emergency Medical Technicians (NAEMT).

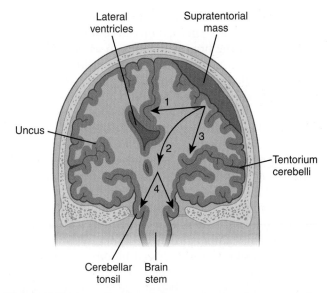

Figure 8-7 The various herniation syndromes that can result from mass effect and increased ICP: (1) cingulate herniation, (2) central herniation, (3) uncal herniation, (4) cerebellotonsillar herniation. These syndromes can occur in combination with each other.

Table 8-2 Description of the Various Herniation Syndromes	
Herniation Type	**Movement**
Uncal (transtentorial)	The medial portion of the temporal lobe (uncus) is pushed toward the tentorium and puts pressure on the brain stem. Progressive herniation will compress CN III, the motor tract, and the reticular activating system on the same side, resulting in a dilated or blown pupil on the same side, motor weakness on the opposite side, and respiratory dysfunction, progressing to coma.
Central (downward herniation)	Parts of the temporal lobes of both cerebral hemispheres are squeezed through a notch in the tentorium (transtentorial). Downward herniation causes tearing of the basilar artery branches, resulting in small hemorrhages. The disrupted brain stem will result in decorticate posturing, respiratory center depression, and death.
Cingulate (subfalcine or transfalcine)	Most common; innermost part of the frontal lobe is scraped under the falx cerebri, which is the dura mater that separates the two hemispheres of the brain. This can cause injury to the medial cerebral hemispheres and the midbrain. It usually occurs in addition to uncal herniation and can present with abnormal posturing and coma.
Cerebellar (upward transtentorial)	The midbrain is pushed upward through the tentorium. This movement can also occur in conjunction with uncal herniation.
Tonsillar (downward cerebellar herniation)	Cerebellar tonsils move downward through the foramen magnum, causing compression of the cerebellum and medulla and upper cervical spinal cord. Injury to the lower medulla results in cardiac and respiratory arrest, a common final event for patients with herniation. This is also referred to as "coning."[21]

© National Association of Emergency Medical Technicians (NAEMT).

opposite (contralateral) side of the body and the Babinski reflex. More extensive herniation can result in destruction of structures in the brain stem known as the *red nucleus* or the **vestibular nuclei**. This can result in **decorticate posturing**, which involves abnormal flexion of the upper extremities and rigidity and extension of the lower extremities. A more ominous finding is **decerebrate posturing**, in which all extremities extend and arching of the spine may occur. Decerebrate posturing occurs with injury and damage to the brain stem (**Figure 8-8**). After herniation, a terminal event may ensue, and the extremities become flaccid and motor activity is absent.[22,23]

As herniation progresses to central and tonsillar herniation, the reticular activating system is affected and results in abnormal ventilatory patterns or apnea, with worsening hypoxia and significantly altered blood carbon dioxide levels. *Cheyne-Stokes ventilations* are a repeating cycle of slow, shallow breaths that become deeper and more rapid and then return to slow, shallow breaths. Brief periods of apnea may occur between cycles. **Central neurogenic hyperventilation** refers to consistently rapid, deep breaths, while ataxic breathing refers to erratic ventilatory efforts that lack any discernible pattern. Spontaneous respiratory function ceases with compression of the brain stem, a common final pathway for herniation (**Figure 8-9**).[21]

As tissue hypoxia develops in the brain, reflexes are activated in an effort to maintain cerebral oxygen delivery. To overcome rising ICP, the autonomic nervous system is activated to increase systemic blood pressure (and MAP) in an effort to maintain a normal cerebral perfusion pressure. Systolic pressures can reach up to 250 mm Hg. However, as the baroreceptors in the carotid arteries and aortic arch sense a greatly increased blood pressure, messages are sent to the brain stem to activate the parasympathetic nervous system. A signal then travels via the 10th cranial nerve, the vagus nerve, to slow the heart rate. **Cushing phenomenon** describes the combination of findings that occur with increased ICP: bradycardia, increased blood pressure associated with a widened pulse pressure, and irregular respirations, such as Cheyne-Stokes breathing.[24]

Ischemia and Herniation

The herniation syndromes describe how increased ICP can result in compression and further brain injury. However, elevated ICP from cerebral swelling can also cause injury to the brain through decreased oxygen delivery and subsequent cerebral ischemia. Based on the cerebral perfusion pressure formula (CPP = MAP – ICP), an increase in ICP will result in a decrease in cerebral perfusion pressure and threatens cerebral perfusion. This is compounded by the ischemic insults sustained from other causes, such as systemic hypotension. These mechanical and ischemic insults bring about an endless cascade, resulting in more cerebral swelling that causes further mechanical and ischemic damage. This process will ultimately lead to herniation and death without intervention. Limiting this secondary

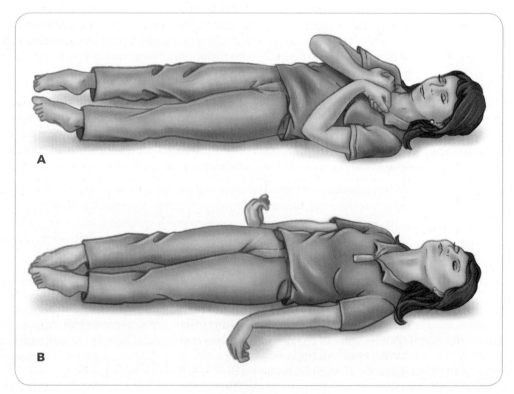

Figure 8-8 A. Decorticate posturing. **B.** Decerebrate posturing.

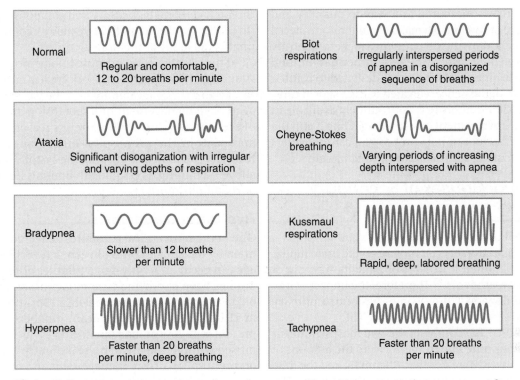

Figure 8-9 This image demonstrates the various types of breathing patterns that may occur after head and brain trauma.

Modified from *Mosby's Guide to Physical Examination*, Seidel HM, Ball JW, Dains JE, et al. Copyright Elsevier (Mosby), 1999.

injury and breaking this cycle of injury are the principal goals of TBI management.

Cerebral Edema

Cerebral edema (brain swelling) often occurs at the site of a primary brain injury. Direct injury to the neuronal cell membranes allows intracellular fluid to collect within damaged neurons, leading to cerebral edema. In addition, injury can activate inflammatory responses that further injure neurons and the cerebral capillaries, leading to fluid collection within the neurons and interstitial spaces, leading to further cerebral edema. As the edema develops, the mechanical and ischemic injury previously described occurs, which aggravates these processes in an endless cycle of increasing edema and injury.

Cerebral edema can occur in association with or as a result of intracranial hematomas, as a result of direct injury to the brain parenchyma in the form of cerebral contusion, or as a result of diffuse brain injury from hypoxia or hypotension.

Intracerebral Hematomas

In trauma, mass effect results from the accumulation of blood in the intracranial space. Intracranial hematomas, such as epidural, subdural, or intracerebral hematomas, are major sources of mass effect. Because mass effect is due to the hematoma size, rapid removal of these hematomas can break the cycle of edema and injury described earlier.

Unfortunately, these hematomas often have associated cerebral edema, and other interventions in addition to removing the hematoma are required to stop the cycle of injury and edema. Specific cerebral hematomas are described later.

Venous Obstruction

Venous obstruction can also be an occult but clinically significant cause of increased ICP. The two main causes of intracranial venous obstruction are external compression and focal internal thrombosis. With external compression, the thin walls of the dural venous sinuses can be focally compressed by depressed skull fractures or expanding masses, preventing venous outflow. The most worrisome injury is the occipital skull fracture over the right transverse sinus. Compression can also result in venous thrombosis, which will further exacerbate venous obstruction.

Focal internal obstructions such as dural sinus thromboses are rare but associated with high mortality. Treatment of both usually requires some type of urgent surgical intervention. Both processes can begin an endless cycle of venous hypertension, further cerebral swelling, and further venous compression, all resulting in intracranial hypertension.

Intracranial Hypertension

The combination of cerebral edema, brain ischemia, venous obstruction, and mass effect result in intracranial hypertension. ICP is measured as a way to quantify and assess the degree of cerebral edema. ICP monitors are placed in the hospital to allow health care providers to quantify the cerebral swelling, assess the risk of herniation, and monitor the effectiveness of therapies designed to combat cerebral edema. In this sense, elevated ICP is a sign of cerebral swelling. ICP monitoring is not routinely available in the prehospital environment, but understanding it and the reasons for its control can help prehospital care providers with decision making for the brain-injured patient.

Extracranial Causes of Secondary Brain Injury

Hypotension

Brain ischemia is extremely common in severe brain injury. Studies have identified it in 90% of patients who die of TBI and in many survivors.[25] Therefore, the impact of low cerebral blood flow on TBI outcomes has been a primary focus for limiting secondary injury after TBI.

In the national TBI database, the two most significant predictors of poor outcome from TBI were the amount of time spent with an ICP greater than 20 mm Hg and the time spent with a systolic blood pressure less than 90 mm Hg. In fact, a single episode of systolic blood pressure less than 90 mm Hg can lead to a poorer outcome.[7] Several studies have confirmed the profound impact of low systolic blood pressure on the outcome after TBI.

Many patients with TBI sustain other injuries, often involving hemorrhage and subsequent hypotension. Fluid resuscitation, as well as rapid definitive treatment of these injuries to maintain systolic blood pressure of at least 90 mm Hg is essential to limit the secondary injury to the brain that can result from failing to meet this goal.

In addition to hemorrhage, a second factor threatens cerebral blood flow after TBI, especially in the most severe injuries. A typical normal cortical cerebral blood flow is 50 ml per 100 grams (g) of brain tissue per minute (or 50 ml/100 g/minute [min]). After severe TBI, this value can drop to 30 ml or even as low as 20 ml/100 g/min in the most severe injuries. The cause of this decline in cerebral blood flow is unclear, but the decline may be due to a loss of autoregulation or a protective mechanism to downregulate the brain in response to injury. Regardless, this decreased cerebral blood flow, compounded with hemorrhagic shock, further increases the ischemic threat to the brain.[7,14,26]

As previously discussed, injury to the brain also impairs the autoregulation mechanisms, and higher cerebral perfusion pressures are required to maintain adequate cerebral blood flow. Severely injured areas of the brain can lose almost all ability to autoregulate. In these areas, the blood vessels become dilated, causing hyperemia and shunting of blood toward the most severely injured brain areas and away from areas that could still be saved by adequate perfusion.[27,28] Last, aggressive hyperventilation can further

threaten cerebral blood flow and compound the ischemic threat by constricting blood vessels to compromised and unaffected areas of the brain.

This combination of physiologic downregulation, shunting, and hemorrhagic shock creates multiple ischemic threats to the salvageable areas of the brain and makes the aggressive management of hypotension an essential part of the management of TBI. For this reason, an aggressive approach in the prehospital environment, with fluid resuscitation aimed at keeping the systolic blood pressure above 90 mm Hg, is essential to limiting secondary injury in the brain-injured patient.

Hypoxia and Hyperoxia

One of the most critical substrates delivered to the injured brain by the circulation is oxygen. Irreversible brain damage can occur after only 4 to 6 minutes of cerebral anoxia. Studies have also demonstrated a profound impact of an oxygen saturation of hemoglobin (Spo_2) less than 90% in TBI patients.[4,7,20] A significant number of TBI patients present with low or inadequate Spo_2, which may be easily missed without the use of pulse oximetry.[19] The emphasis on prehospital airway management and oxygen delivery for brain-injured patients has partly been the result of these studies. Adequate ventilation and blood flow are critical in maintaining adequate oxygen delivery to the brain. One study of patients with severe TBI demonstrated a mortality rate of 26.9% if neither hypoxemia nor hypotension occurred, 28% with hypoxemia alone, and 57.2% if both were noted.[29] Therefore, prehospital care providers must ensure adequate circulation by minimizing blood loss and adequate oxygenation by maintaining a patent airway and adequate ventilation.

It is important to note that too much oxygen delivery, or hyperoxia, has also been associated with worse outcomes. Ventilation with high oxygen levels has been associated with injury to many cell types, including the brain, lung, heart, and eyes.[30] The exact mechanism within the brain is unclear, but the injury may be due to several factors, including free radical toxicity, altered metabolites, and/or cerebral vasoconstriction. One hundred percent oxygen can also cause cerebral vasoconstriction, which may subsequently alter cerebral metabolism. The few available studies evaluating the effects of high levels of Fio_2 and high Pao_2 have demonstrated poor functional outcomes.[31,32] They have been associated with higher mortality rates, lower discharge GCS scores, and longer hospital length of stay compared with patients with normal oxygen levels. None of these studies has investigated the effects of short periods of hyperoxia in the prehospital environment, however. These studies suggest that there is likely an ideal therapeutic window for Pao_2 levels after TBI between 100 mm Hg and 200 mm Hg. While both hyperoxia and hypoxia outside those ranges can be dangerous, the preponderance of the evidence available to date is that, with specific regard to the prehospital environment, hypoxia is more dangerous on even a transient basis.

Anemia

Also, critical to the delivery of oxygen to the brain is the oxygen-carrying capacity of the blood, which is determined by the amount of hemoglobin it contains. A 50% drop in hemoglobin has a much more profound effect on oxygen delivery to the brain than a 50% drop in the partial pressure of oxygen (Pao_2). For this reason, anemia from blood loss can impact the outcome of TBI.

Hypocapnia and Hypercapnia

As discussed earlier in this chapter, both hypocapnia (decreased $Paco_2$) and hypercapnia (increased $Paco_2$) can worsen brain injury. When cerebral blood vessels constrict from significant hypocapnia, cerebral blood flow is compromised, leading to a decrease in oxygen delivery to the brain. Hypercapnia can result from hypoventilation from many causes, including drug or alcohol intoxication and abnormal ventilation patterns seen in patients with increased ICP. Hypercapnia causes cerebral vasodilation, which can further increase ICP.

Hypoglycemia and Hyperglycemia

When cerebral blood flow decreases, there is a decrease in oxygen delivery, as well as the delivery of glucose and other necessary brain metabolites. Glucose is the primary fuel source of the adult brain, and changes in cerebral glucose metabolism are a hallmark response to TBI. Imaging studies have demonstrated a rapid transient increase in glucose uptake shortly after injury, followed by a prolonged period of depressed glucose metabolism. Glucose metabolism depression is greater in severely injured TBI patients, and the duration of this depression increases with age. The location of depressed metabolism is important, as higher metabolic rates in the thalamus, brain stem, and cerebellum have a significant positive correlation with levels of consciousness.[36-39]

Both elevations (hyperglycemia) and decreases (hypoglycemia) in blood glucose can jeopardize ischemic brain tissue. The disastrous impact of significant hypoglycemia on the nervous system, during injury and at other times, is well known. Neurons are unable to store glucose and thus require a continual supply of glucose to carry out cellular metabolism. In the absence of glucose, ischemic neurons can be permanently damaged. However, it is also true that a prolonged serum glucose level greater than 150 milligrams/deciliter (mg/dl), and probably greater than 200 mg/dl, may be harmful to the injured brain. Elevated blood glucose levels have been associated with poorer neurologic outcome and should therefore be avoided.[40,41]

In the prehospital environment, the emphasis should be on avoiding hypoglycemia because the physiologic threat from low glucose is much more immediate than the danger from elevated serum glucose. Blood-glucose measurement should be performed in the field in all patients with altered mentation and, if found to be below normal values, treated with glucose administration. In addition, any induced hyperglycemia is likely to be transient, and the tight glucose control required to manage these patients properly will be established upon admission to the hospital.

Seizures

A patient with acute TBI is at risk for seizures for several reasons. Hypoxia from either airway or breathing problems can induce generalized seizure activity, as can hypoglycemia and electrolyte abnormalities. Ischemic or damaged brain tissue can serve as an irritable focus to produce **grand mal seizures** or **status epilepticus**. Seizures, in turn, can aggravate preexisting hypoxia caused by impairment of respiratory function. Additionally, the massive neuronal activity

---

Box 8-1 Alcohol Use and TBI

Alcohol use is a known risk factor for TBI, particularly subdural hematoma.[33,34] There are multiple factors that contribute to this known increase in risk. Physical shrinkage of the brain (cerebral atrophy) is commonly seen in patients who chronically ingest moderate to heavy volumes of alcohol over long periods. As the volume of the brain decreases, increasing tension is placed on the bridging veins, similar to how the cables on a suspension bridge hold the roadway in place. As this tension increases, it takes less shearing force to cause damage. Heavy alcohol consumption is also known to reduce clotting ability due to interference with the liver's ability to effectively produce clotting factors.[35]

Patients with a history of alcohol abuse or those who are acutely intoxicated may lack the ability to fully articulate the perceived extent of their injuries. This can confound physical assessment findings and make them less reliable—possibly obscuring the manifestations of a serious head injury.

The combined influence of these factors in individuals with a history of alcohol abuse or acute alcohol intoxication should lead to a lower threshold of suspicion for serious TBI in these patients. The forces necessary to cause serious injury in these patients may be significantly lower than those necessary to cause injury in individuals without a known history of alcohol abuse. Even patients who have suffered relatively minor head trauma should be evaluated fully, and transport to the hospital for in-depth medical evaluation should be strongly encouraged.

associated with generalized seizures rapidly depletes oxygen and glucose levels, further worsening cerebral ischemia.

Venous Obstruction

In addition to intracranial venous obstruction, as discussed previously, there are also extracranial causes of venous obstruction that can indirectly raise ICP. The venous tracts drain into the jugular veins, so any compression of the jugular veins can cause an upstream effect of intracranial venous obstruction. Poor head position, such as flexion or flexion with rotation, can cause significant increases in ICP (from a mean ICP of 8.8 to 16.2 mm Hg). This is even higher in children who have larger occiputs and floppier necks.[9,42] Cervical collars can increase the ICP from 4 mm Hg to 14.5 mm Hg.[12] Increased intrathoracic and intra-abdominal pressure can also cause increased jugular venous pressure, affecting cerebral venous outflow. As a result, efforts should be made to keep the head in a neutral position and to avoid tight-fitting cervical collars.

Assessment

A quick survey of the physics of trauma that caused the injury, combined with a rapid primary survey, will help identify potential life-threatening problems in a patient with suspected TBI. It is also critical to continually reassess these patients, perhaps more often than usual, because the pathophysiology of TBI is a dynamic process. Examination findings may fluctuate significantly as the condition of the patient changes over time.

Physics of Trauma

Knowledge of injury mechanisms is critical with all trauma patients, as it can aid in identifying specific injury patterns, especially in TBI. Key data about the physics of trauma will frequently come from observation of the scene or from bystanders. The windshield of the patient's vehicle may have a "spiderweb" pattern, suggesting an impact with the patient's head, or a bloody object may be present that was used as a weapon during an assault. A lateral impact on the side of the head can cause fracture of the temporal bone of the skull with injury to the underlying middle meningeal artery leading to epidural hematoma. High-impact injuries or rapid acceleration–deceleration injuries, such as high-speed motor vehicle collisions, can result in a **coup-contrecoup injury**. This occurs when the head strikes a fixed object, causing a coup injury at the site of impact and a contrecoup injury on the opposite side, where the brain collides with the opposite side of the skull. This important information should be reported to personnel at the receiving facility because it may be essential for proper diagnosis and management of the patient, not only as it relates to possible brain injury but also for other injuries.

Primary Survey

Exsanguinating Hemorrhage

In the primary survey of a trauma patient, life-threatening external hemorrhage must be immediately identified and managed. If exsanguinating external hemorrhage is present, it must be controlled even before assessing the airway (or simultaneously, if adequate assistance is present at the scene). This type of bleeding typically involves arterial bleeding from an extremity but may also occur from the scalp or at the junction of an extremity with the trunk (junctional bleeding) and other sites.

Airway

The patency of the patient's airway should be examined and ensured. In unconscious individuals, the tongue may completely occlude the airway. Noisy ventilations indicate partial obstruction by either the tongue or foreign material. Emesis, hemorrhage, and swelling from facial trauma are common causes of airway compromise in patients with TBI.

Breathing

Adequate oxygen delivery to the injured brain is essential to minimize secondary brain injury. Maintaining SpO_2 above 90% is critical; failure to do so results in poorer outcomes for brain-injured patients. Evaluation of respiratory function must also include an assessment of the rate, depth, and adequacy of breathing. As noted previously, several different breathing patterns can result from severe brain injury. In multisystem trauma patients, thoracic injuries can further impair both oxygenation and ventilation. Cervical spine fractures occur in about 2% to 5% of patients with TBI and may result in spinal cord injuries that significantly interfere with ventilation.

Circulation

Maintaining a systolic blood pressure greater than 90 mm Hg is also critical to preventing secondary brain injury. Therefore, any hemorrhage should be rapidly controlled to prevent and/or minimize hypotension. Uncontrolled bleeding from a scalp injury can be an unrecognized cause of hemorrhagic shock and should therefore be controlled as best as possible with direct pressure or a pressure dressing. If possible, the prehospital care provider should also note and quantify evidence of external bleeding. In the absence of significant external blood loss, a weak, rapid pulse in a victim of blunt trauma suggests life-threatening internal hemorrhage in the pleural spaces, peritoneum, retroperitoneum, or soft tissues surrounding long-bone fractures. In an infant with open fontanelles, sufficient blood loss can occur inside the cranium to produce hypovolemic shock.

Autoregulatory mechanisms to maintain cerebral perfusion pressure in the setting of increased ICP can lead to a recognized series of cardiovascular changes, mainly manifested as increased blood pressure. Attempts to treat hypertension should be avoided, because this will result in decreased cerebral perfusion pressure in the setting of high ICP, causing secondary brain injury. As discussed earlier, the Cushing phenomenon may be seen in severe intracranial hypertension, which is the combination of bradycardia, increased blood pressure associated with a widened pulse pressure, and irregular respirations, such as Cheyne-Stokes breathing.[20] These findings may indicate impending herniation. In a patient with potentially life-threatening injuries, transport should not be delayed to measure blood pressure; it should be performed en route as time permits.

Disability

After the initiation of appropriate measures to treat problems identified during the primary survey, a rapid neurologic examination should be performed. This includes obtaining a baseline GCS score and pupillary assessment. The GCS score is calculated by using the best response noted when evaluating the patient's eyes, verbal response, and motor response status. Each component of the score should be recorded individually, rather than just providing a total, so that specific changes can be noted over time. Of note, the score was updated in 2014 to address variations in techniques and to promote a more consistent use of the GCS score (**Table 8-3**).[43,44] How to determine a patient's GCS score is covered in detail in the Patient Assessment and Management chapter.

The GCS score is important because it can help to classify the severity of TBI and whether a patient is able to protect his or her airway in the setting of a TBI. The lowest total GCS score is 3 and maximum total score is 15. A total GCS score of 13 to 15 likely indicates a mild TBI while a score of 9 to 12 is indicative of moderate TBI. A GCS score of 3 to 8 suggests severe TBI. Standard guidelines recommend intubation for GCS scores equal to or less than 8.[29,45] Many other factors can also affect the GCS score, including the presence of intoxicants or other drugs.

The most critical portion of the GCS score is the motor score. Studies have demonstrated equal sensitivity and specificity between both motor and total GCS scores for neurologic assessment and prognostication. Obtaining the motor score in the prehospital setting is especially important because it is a dynamic score that often deteriorates from the field to the hospital. Admission values are often lower than field values due to field intubation, paralysis, and/or sedation, making the full GCS score impossible to obtain.

Table 8-3 Glasgow Coma Scale			
Subcategory	**1974 Classification**	**2014 Classification**	**Points**
Eye opening	Spontaneous	Spontaneous	4
	To speech (command)	To sound	3
	To pain	To pressure	2
	None	None	1
Verbal response	Orientation	Oriented	5
	Confused conversation	Confused	4
	Inappropriate speech	Words	3
	Incomprehensible speech	Sounds	2
	None	None	1
Motor response	Follows commands	Obey commands	6
	Localizes painful stimuli	Localizing	5
	Withdraws from pain (nonlocalizing)	Normal flexion	4
	Abnormal flexion (decorticate)	Abnormal flexion	3
	Abnormal extension (decerebrate)	Extension	2
	Gives no motor response	None	1

Studies have demonstrated that the field GCS motor score predicts 6-month mortality better than admission motor scores. Given these findings and the simplicity of the motor score, use of the motor score alone has been advocated in the prehospital triage setting.[45,46]

In addition to determining the GCS score, the pupils are examined quickly for symmetry and response to light. In adults, the resting pupil diameter is generally between 3 and 5 mm.[47] A difference of greater than 1 mm in pupil size is considered abnormal. A fixed pupil is defined as a response to bright light of less than 1 mm.[29] The combination of motor GCS score and admission pupillary reactivity has been demonstrated to accurately assess and predict TBI outcomes. Acute pupillary dilation indicates a neurologic emergency and can indicate brain stem ischemia and/or uncal herniation. Uncal herniation from brain edema or mass effect can cause compression of the oculomotor nerve (CN III), causing pupil dilation. Decreased blood flow to the brain stem and brain stem ischemia also cause pupillary dilation. Of note, a portion of the population has **anisocoria**, or unequal pupils, which is either congenital or acquired as the result of ophthalmic trauma. However, it is not always possible in the field to distinguish between pupillary inequality caused by trauma and congenital or preexisting posttraumatic anisocoria. Therefore, pupillary inequality should always be treated as secondary to the acute trauma until the appropriate workup has ruled out cerebral edema or motor or ophthalmic nerve injury.[48]

Expose/Environment

Patients who have sustained a TBI frequently have other injuries, which threaten life and limb as well as the brain. All such injuries must be identified. The entire body should be examined for other potentially life-threatening problems.

Secondary Survey

Once life-threatening injuries have been identified and managed, a thorough secondary survey should be completed if time permits. The patient's head and face should be palpated carefully for wounds, depressions, and **crepitus**. The pupillary size and response should be rechecked at this time. Because of the incidence of associated cervical spine fractures in patients with TBI, as noted previously, the neck should be examined for tenderness and bony deformities.

Any drainage of clear fluid from the nose or ear canals may be CSF. In most cases, however, the CSF will be mixed with blood, making formal recognition of this finding difficult. One method that is often suggested is to place a drop of the suspected blood–CSF mixture onto a gauze pad. When placed on a gauze pad or white cloth, CSF may diffuse out from blood, producing a characteristic yellowish "halo."[49] If time permits, this test may be attempted during transport; however, there are many false positive results, thus limiting its usefulness.

The single most important observation is assessment of the patient's mental status and how it changes over the course of the time you are with the patient. Patients who are initially found with an impaired mental status that improves are much less concerning than those patients whose mental status deteriorates during your management and transport.

In a cooperative patient, a more thorough neurologic examination may also be performed. This will include assessing the cranial nerves, sensation, and motor function in all extremities. Looking for complete or partial deficits as well as asymmetry in function may reveal important clues to a possible neurologic injury. Findings such as **hemiparesis** (weakness) or **hemiplegia** (paralysis), present on only one side of the body, are considered "lateralizing signs" and usually are indicative of TBI.

History

A SAMPLE history (*s*ymptoms, *a*llergies, *m*edications, *p*ast history, *l*ast meal, *e*vents) can be obtained from the patient, family members, or bystanders if time and circumstances allow. Diabetes mellitus, seizure disorders, and drug or alcohol intoxication can mimic TBI. Any evidence of drug use or overdose should be noted. The patient may have a history of prior head injury and may complain of persistent or recurring headache, visual disturbances, nausea and vomiting, or difficulty speaking.[50]

Serial Examinations

It is important to reevaluate the GCS score and determine what changes are occurring over time. The patient who initially presented with a GCS score that is now decreasing is of much greater concern for serious TBI than a patient who has an improving GCS score. A small number of patients with apparently mild brain injury (GCS score 14 or 15) may experience an unexpected deterioration in their mentation. During transport, both the primary survey and assessment of the GCS score should be repeated at frequent intervals. Patients whose GCS score deteriorates by more than two points during transport are at particularly high risk for an ongoing pathologic process.[48,51,52] These patients need rapid transport to an appropriate facility. The receiving facility will use GCS score trends during transport in the patient's early management. Trends in the GCS score or vital signs should be reported to the receiving facility and documented on the patient care report. Responses to management should also be recorded.[53]

Specific Head and Neck Injuries

Head trauma usually refers to injuries that result in changes in brain function, such as altered consciousness, confusion, coma, convulsions, or other neurologic deficits. However, head trauma may also refer to injuries to the bones and soft tissues of the face and head that do not involve the brain.[1]

Scalp Injuries

As noted in the anatomy section, the scalp is composed of multiple layers of tissue and is highly vascular. Injuries can vary from simple small lacerations to complex injuries such as a degloving injury, in which a large area of the scalp is torn back from the skull. Uncontrolled hemorrhage from these injuries can result in hypovolemic shock and even **exsanguination** (**Figure 8-10**). This type of injury often occurs in an unrestrained front-seat occupant of a vehicle whose head impacts the windshield, as well as in workers whose long hair becomes caught in machinery. A serious blow to the head may result in the formation of a scalp hematoma, which may be confused with a depressed skull fracture while palpating the scalp.

Skull Fractures

Skull fractures can result from either blunt or penetrating trauma. Linear fractures are usually from blunt trauma. However, a powerful impact may produce a depressed skull fracture, in which fragments of bone are driven toward or into the underlying brain tissue (**Figure 8-11**). Although simple linear fractures can be diagnosed only with a radiographic study, depressed skull fractures can often be palpated during a careful physical examination. A closed, nondepressed skull fracture by itself is of little clinical significance, but its presence increases the risk of an intracranial hematoma. Closed, depressed skull fractures may require neurosurgical intervention because the decrease in intracranial space by the encroaching fracture results in increased ICP. Open skull fractures can result from a particularly forceful impact or a gunshot wound and serve as an entry site for bacteria, predisposing the

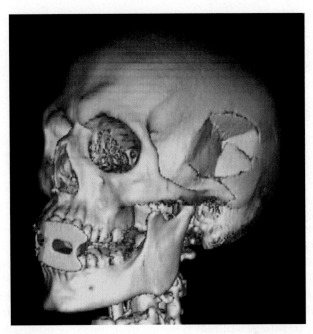

Figure 8-11 A three-dimensional reconstruction of a depressed skull fracture after an assault.
Courtesy of Peter T. Pons, MD, FACEP.

patient to meningitis. If the dura mater is torn, brain tissue or CSF may leak from an open skull fracture. Because of the risk of meningitis, these wounds require immediate neurosurgical evaluation.

Basilar skull fractures are fractures of the base of the skull that most commonly involve temporal bone fractures. These fractures can cause tears in membranes, resulting in leakage of CSF. In approximately 12% to 30% of basilar skull fractures, CSF can leak from the ears through a perforated eardrum (otorrhea) or from the nostrils (rhinorrhea).[54] Periorbital ecchymosis ("raccoon eyes") and Battle's sign, in which ecchymosis is noted over the mastoid area behind the ears, can also occur with basilar skull fractures, although they may take several hours after injury to become apparent. If permitted, examination of the tympanic membrane with an otoscope may reveal blood behind the eardrum, indicating a basilar skull fracture.

Facial Injuries

Injuries to the face range from minor soft-tissue trauma to severe injuries associated with airway compromise or hypovolemic shock. The airway may be compromised by either structural damage or anatomic distortion resulting from the trauma or from fluid or other objects in the airway itself. Structural changes may include deformities of fractured facial bones or hematomas that develop in the tissues. Because the head has a high concentration of blood vessels, injuries to this region frequently result in significant hemorrhage. Blood and blood clots may interfere with the patency of the airway. Facial trauma is often associated

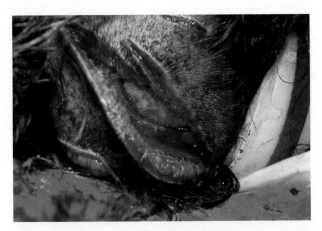

Figure 8-10 Extensive scalp injuries may result in massive external hemorrhage.
Courtesy of Peter T. Pons, MD, FACEP.

with alterations in consciousness and potentially severe trauma to the brain. Trauma to the face may result in fractures or displacement of teeth into the airway lumen. TBIs and swallowed blood from facial injuries may lead to vomiting, which also may lead to airway obstruction.

Trauma to the Eye and Orbit

Injury to the structures of the orbit and eye are common and often result from direct trauma to the face. Although injury of the globe (eyeball) itself is not often encountered, it must be considered whenever trauma to the face and orbit is noted, as proper management of a globe injury increases the salvage rate of the patient's vision.

Eyelid Laceration

In the prehospital setting, laceration of an eyelid must cause consideration of the possibility that the globe itself has been penetrated. Field treatment consists of immediately covering the eye with a protective rigid shield (*not* a pressure patch) that is placed over the bony orbit. The primary consideration is to avoid any pressure on the eye that might do further harm by forcing intraocular contents out through a corneal or scleral laceration.

Corneal Abrasion

A corneal abrasion is disruption of the protective **epithelial** covering of the cornea. This abrasion results in intense pain, tearing, light sensitivity (photophobia), and increased susceptibility to infection until the defect has healed (usually in 2 to 3 days). There is typically a history of **antecedent** trauma or contact lens use. Prehospital management for this disorder is to cover the eye with a patch, shield, or sunglasses to reduce the discomfort caused by light sensitivity.

Subconjunctival Hemorrhage

Subconjunctival hemorrhage over the sclera of the eye results from bleeding between the **conjunctiva** and the **sclera** (**Figure 8-12**). It is easily visible without the use of any diagnostic equipment. This injury is innocuous and resolves over a period of several days to several weeks without treatment. In the presence of antecedent trauma, one should be alert for another, more serious injury. For example, an occult globe rupture should be suspected if hemorrhage results in massive swelling of the conjunctiva, known as (**chemosis**). Prehospital management of this disorder consists solely of transporting the patient to the hospital so that the diagnosis can be confirmed and other associated disorders ruled out.

Hyphema

The term **hyphema** refers to blood in the anterior chamber of the globe between the **iris** and the **cornea**. This condition is usually seen in the setting of acute trauma from a direct blow to the eye. The eye should be examined with the victim sitting upright. If enough blood is present, it collects at the bottom of the anterior chamber and is visible as a layered hyphema (**Figure 8-13**). This blood may not be appreciated if the victim is examined while in a supine position or if the amount of blood is very small. Hyphema patients should have a protective shield placed over the eye and be transported to the hospital in a sitting position (if there is no other contraindication) so that a complete eye examination can be performed.

Open Globe

If there is a history of trauma and penlight inspection of the eye reveals an obvious **open globe** (wound that goes through the cornea or sclera into the interior of the eyeball), the remainder of the physical examination of the eye should be discontinued and a protective shield immediately placed onto the bony orbit over the eye to protect it from further injury. Do *not* apply a pressure patch or instill any topical medication.

There are two primary concerns in the management of this condition. The first is to minimize manipulation of or

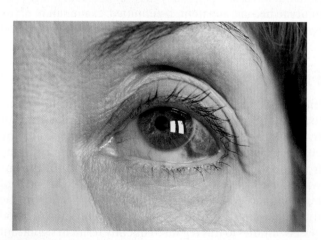

Figure 8-12 Subconjunctival hemorrhage.

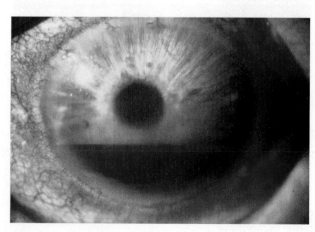

Figure 8-13 Hyphema.

additional trauma to the eye that might raise intraocular pressure and result in expulsion of intraocular contents through the corneal or scleral defect. The second is to prevent the development of **posttraumatic endophthalmitis**, an infection of the interior portion of the eye. This typically has devastating visual results. Expeditious transport to the hospital is warranted for ophthalmologic evaluation and surgical repair.

A penetrating injury to the eye or a ruptured globe may not always be obvious. Clues to occult rupture include the mechanism of injury as well as clinical findings of large subconjunctival hemorrhage with chemosis, dark uveal tissue (the colored iris) present at or protruding through the junction of the cornea and the sclera, a distorted pupil (teardrop shaped), a leak from a lacerated or punctured corneal wound, or a decrease in vision. If an occult globe rupture is suspected, the patient should be treated as described previously for an obvious open globe. The relatively less severe appearance of the injury does not eliminate the threat of endophthalmitis, so rapid transport to the hospital is still warranted.

Nasal Fractures

Fracture of the nasal bones is the most common fracture in the face. Indications that a nasal fracture is present include **ecchymosis**, **edema**, nasal deformity, swelling, and epistaxis (nosebleed). On palpation, bony crepitus may be noted.

High-force midface traumas may cause nasal bone fractures as well as fractures of the cribriform plate (the thin, horizontal bone in the skull through which the olfactory [cranial nerve 1] nerve passes). Any clear rhinorrhea (CSF leak from the nose) occurring after significant force to the midface is significant for possible cribriform plate fracture.

Midface Fractures

Midface fractures can be categorized according to the Le Fort classification, shown in **Figure 8-14**.

- *Le Fort I fracture* involves a horizontal detachment of the maxilla from the nasal floor. Although air passage through the nares (nostrils) may not be affected, the oropharynx may be compromised by a blood clot or edema in the soft palate.
- *Le Fort II fracture*, also known as a pyramidal fracture, includes the right and left maxillae, the medial portion of the orbital floor(s), and the nasal bones. The sinuses are well vascularized, so this fracture may be associated with airway compromise from significant hemorrhage.
- *Le Fort III fracture* involves fracture completely separating the facial bones from the skull (craniofacial disjunction). Because of the forces involved, this injury may be associated with airway compromise, presence of TBI, injuries to the tear ducts, malocclusion (misalignment) of teeth, and CSF leakage from the nares.

Patients with a midface fracture generally have loss of normal facial symmetry. The face may appear flattened, and the patient may be unable to close the jaws or teeth. If conscious, the patient may complain of facial pain and numbness. On palpation, crepitus may be noted over fracture sites.

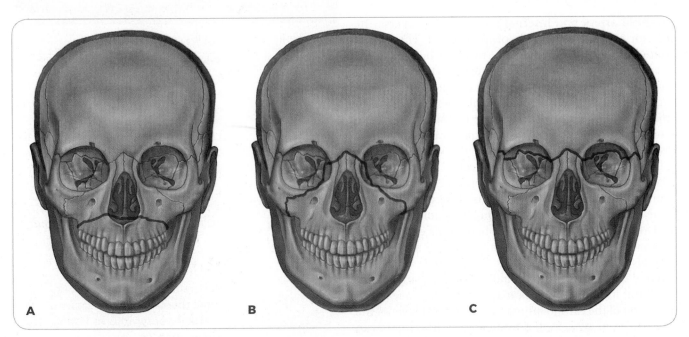

Figure 8-14 Types of Le Fort fractures of the midface. **A.** Le Fort I fracture. **B.** Le Fort II fracture. **C.** Le Fort III fracture.

Mandibular Fractures

Following fractures of the nasal bones, mandibular fractures are the second most common type of facial fracture. Often, the mandible (jawbone) is broken in more than one location. The most common complaint of a patient with a mandibular fracture, in addition to pain, is malocclusion of the teeth where the upper and lower teeth no longer meet in their usual alignment. Visual examination may reveal a step-off or misalignment of the teeth. On palpation, a step-off type of deformity and crepitus may be noted. In a supine patient with a mandibular fracture, the tongue may occlude the airway as the bony support structure of the tongue is no longer intact.

Laryngeal Injuries

Fractures of the larynx typically result from a blunt blow to the anterior neck, such as when a motorcycle or bicycle rider's anterior neck is struck by an object. The patient may complain of a change in voice (usually lower in tone). On inspection, the prehospital care provider may note a neck contusion or loss of the prominence of the thyroid cartilage (Adam's apple). A fracture of the larynx may result in the patient coughing up blood (hemoptysis) or the development of subcutaneous emphysema in the neck, which may be detected on palpation. Endotracheal intubation is generally contraindicated in the presence of a laryngeal fracture because this procedure may dislodge fracture segments. If a patient with a suspected laryngeal fracture has a compromised airway, a surgical cricothyrotomy may be lifesaving.

Injuries to Cervical Vessels

A carotid artery and internal jugular vein traverse the anterior neck on either side of the trachea. The carotid arteries supply blood to the majority of the brain, and the internal jugular veins drain this region. Open injury to one of these vessels can produce profound hemorrhage. An added danger from internal jugular vein injuries is air embolism. If a patient is sitting up or the head is elevated, venous pressure may fall below atmospheric pressure during inspiration, permitting air to enter the venous system. A large air embolus can be fatal because it can interfere with both cardiac function and cerebral perfusion. An additional concern of trauma to the cervical vasculature is the development of an expanding hematoma that may lead to airway compromise as the hematoma expands and impinges on and distorts the normal airway anatomy. It may also cause jugular venous compression, occluding cerebral venous outflow and indirectly increasing ICP.

Blunt injury to the neck may also result in a tear and dissection of the carotid intima (the innermost layer of the carotid artery) away from the outer layers. This injury can lead to occlusion of the carotid artery and a resultant stroke secondary to decreased brain perfusion. Carotid artery intimal flaps or dissections often occur when a restrained occupant in a vehicle collision impacts the shoulder strap located across the neck.

Brain Injuries

Cerebral Concussion

The diagnosis of a "concussion" is made as a result of the presence of symptoms persisting after mild TBI. Most people associate a loss of consciousness with the diagnosis of concussion, but it is not required to make the diagnosis of concussion. The hallmark of concussion is actually posttraumatic amnesia, which is a state of confusion following trauma where the patient is disoriented and unable to recall events that occurred before (retrograde) and after (anterograde) injury.[55] Retrograde amnesia can extend from minutes to days before the head trauma, while anterograde amnesia tends to be shorter. Its duration tends to correlate with the duration of loss of consciousness and the severity of head injury. **Table 8-4** lists a grading system for concussion.

These patients may become agitated because they do not understand or recall what is going on. Other neurologic changes include the following:

- Vacant stare (befuddled facial expression)
- Delayed verbal and motor responses (slow to answer questions or follow instructions)

Table 8-4 Cantu Concussion Grading System	
Severity	**Description**
Grade 1: Mild	No loss of consciousness Posttraumatic amnesia or postconcussion signs or symptoms lasting less than 30 minutes
Grade 2: Moderate	Loss of consciousness lasting less than 1 minute Posttraumatic amnesia or postconcussion signs or symptoms lasting longer than 30 minutes but less than 24 hours
Grade 3: Severe	Loss of consciousness lasting more than 1 minute Posttraumatic amnesia lasting more than 24 hours; postconcussion signs or symptoms lasting longer than 7 days

- Confusion and inability to focus attention (easily distracted and unable to follow through with normal activities)
- Disorientation (walking in the wrong direction; unaware of time, date, and place)
- Slurred or incoherent speech (making disjointed or incomprehensible statements)
- Lack of coordination (stumbling, inability to walk tandem/straight line)
- Emotions inappropriate to the circumstances (distraught, crying for no apparent reason)
- Memory deficits (exhibited by patient repeatedly asking the same question that has already been answered)
- Inability to memorize and recall (e.g., three out of three words or three out of three objects in 5 minutes)[56]

Severe headache, dizziness, nausea, and vomiting frequently accompany a concussion. Patients exhibiting signs of concussion, especially patients with nausea, vomiting, or neurologic findings on secondary survey, should be immediately transported for further evaluation. The formal diagnosis of a concussion will be made in the hospital once the patient has been evaluated and a head CT scan result shows no observable intracranial pathology. Although most of these findings last several hours to a couple days, some patients experience a postconcussive syndrome with headaches, dizziness, and difficulty concentrating for weeks, and even months, after a severe concussion.

It is also important to determine whether the patient has had a recent concussion and, if so, whether the symptoms from that episode have completely resolved. Patients who have sustained a concussion and sustain a second concussion before the symptoms from the first one have fully resolved are at risk for sudden deterioration in neurologic status. This phenomenon, termed **secondary impact syndrome**, has become particularly concerning in athletic events where athletes sustain a concussion and are eager to return to the game before they have fully recovered from the effects of the initial trauma.[55,56,78] In these cases, the brain is already compromised from the first impact, and the second trauma results in the loss of autoregulation, producing sudden and massive edema, which leads to herniation and death. This process can occur in as little as 5 minutes. Controversy exists as to whether this is, in fact, a unique and distinct entity or rather a progressive form of cerebral edema.[78] Regardless, patients (especially athletes) who have sustained a concussion should be carefully evaluated to determine the persistence of symptoms. If the patient has not fully recovered from the initial insult, he or she should avoid

---

Box 8-2 Impact of Head Injuries on Sleep

Disturbance of the sleep–wake cycle is one of the most persistent and commonly seen complications in the patient who has suffered a head injury. TBIs across the entire spectrum of severity, during both the acute and chronic phases, are subject to potential sleep–wake cycle disturbances. The most profound sleep–wake disturbances are seen in patients who have suffered from a severe TBI.[57-59] Around 30% of patients will complain of sleep–wake disturbances within 10 days of the injury. This number increases to over 50% at 6 weeks post injury.[60-62] The most commonly seen sleep–wake disturbances were:

- Insomnia (50%)
- Difficulty staying asleep (50%)
- Waking up earlier than intended (38%)
- Disturbing dreams or nightmares (27%)[63]

Careful and specific questioning while obtaining the patient history can help identify and characterize these disturbances. Ask about excessive daytime sleepiness (seen in 50% to 80% of patients post TBI).[64-67] This is distinct from fatigue, in that patients with fatigue generally get tired during physical and mental activity, whereas excessive daytime sleepiness is typically seen when the patient is sedentary.[68,69] Patients may fall asleep at inappropriate times despite feeling as if they had adequate sleep the night before.[68,69] It is also important to ask about insomnia and the increased need for sleep above what they required prior to the injury. Patients may also see changes to their internal clock (circadian rhythm) and discover that they have an increased desire to sleep during the day and are more alert during the nighttime hours.[70-72]

A variety of treatments for sleep–wake disturbances post TBI are used, including behavioral modifications and pharmacologic therapy.[73,74] For many patients, good sleep hygiene is sufficient treatment until symptoms resolve. When sleep hygiene alone is not effective, a physician specializing in sleep disorders or a neurologist may decide to prescribe medication.

The majority of patients with sleep–wake cycle disturbances after a TBI will have full resolution of symptoms within 6 months following the injury. A minority of patients may require behavioral modifications and medication therapy past 6 months, with their sleep–wake habits never fully recovering. This is rare, however, and typically seen in more severe head injuries.[75-77]

repeat trauma to the head and brain and, in the case of athletes, not be allowed to return to play.

The effects of repetitive concussion on the brain, particularly as it relates to sports injuries, have garnered more attention in recent years. Concussions are frequently seen in contact sports. Most concussions are minor and the majority of athletes will recover within a few days or weeks. However, a small number will sustain permanent damage, resulting in a progressive degenerative brain disease known as **chronic traumatic encephalopathy (CTE)**.[55,79]

CTE is thought to occur primarily in athletes with a history of repetitive brain trauma and is primarily seen with contact sport athletes, such as boxers and football players. The severity of the disorder correlates with the length of time in the sport and the number of traumatic injuries. The symptoms are initially insidious, such as deteriorating attention, concentration, and memory; disorientation and confusion; and occasional dizziness and headaches. Some patients are affected by a prominent mood disturbance, which is usually depression. However, with progressive deterioration, more severe symptoms begin manifesting, including lack of insight, poor judgment, and overt dementia. Other symptoms that occur during the three stages of clinical deterioration are listed in **Table 8-5**. Documented cases of CTE have demonstrated a symptom onset as early as 25 years, with a variable progression from between 2 and 46 years.[56,79]

Intracranial Hematoma

Intracranial hematomas are divided into four general types: epidural, subdural, subarachnoid, and intracerebral. Because the signs and symptoms of each of these have significant overlap, specific diagnosis in the prehospital setting (as well as the ED) is almost impossible, although the prehospital

Table 8-5	Three Stages of Clinical Deterioration in Chronic Traumatic Encephalopathy
Stages	**Description**
1	Affective disturbances and psychotic symptoms
2	Initial symptoms of Parkinson disease, social instability, erratic behavior, memory loss
3	General cognitive dysfunction progressing to dementia, full-blown Parkinson disease, speech and gait abnormalities, ocular abnormalities such as ptosis

Box 8-3 Return to Play

"When can I get back in the game?" is a question posed frequently by athletes after suffering a head injury. Athletes participating at highly competitive levels may be influenced to prematurely return to play, especially when scholarships and future careers in professional sports may hang in the balance. With this being the case, objective criteria have been developed for use in determining an athlete's ability to safely return to athletic activities. This is generally referred to as the graduated "return to play" protocol, or RTP protocol for short.

Prior to beginning the RTP protocol, an athlete should return to full academic activities and be fully off of any medications prescribed as a result of the head injury. If the athlete is symptom-free, does not require medications for the head injury, has regained his or her baseline cognitive performance, and has a completely normal neurologic examination, then it is generally considered safe to begin the RTP protocol. Until these criteria have been met and a health care professional has given permission, it is generally considered *unsafe* for the athlete to return to sports participation.[80,81]

It is recommended that at least 1 to 2 days of complete physical and mental rest be completed prior to beginning the RTP protocol. Each step should take a minimum of 24 hours and if, at any point, the symptoms worsen during the progression, the athlete should return to the previous symptom-free stage. Any time symptoms last longer than 14 days for an adult or 30 days for a child, the athlete should be seen by a physician with specific training in head injury and concussion management.

This protocol is typically managed by an athletic trainer or physician and falls outside the scope of most EMS professionals. It is important for EMS professionals to have some understanding of this protocol, however. When transporting a patient with a suspected head injury, asking about previous head injuries and whether or not those head injuries were fully recovered prior to returning to play are important points to determine during the history and physical examination.[82,83] Finally, consideration should be given when transporting patients with complaints related to a previous head injury, and the RTP protocol information can be used as a source for the development of protocols and procedures for EMS agencies to follow when encountering patients with these types of histories or injuries.

care provider may suspect a particular type of hematoma based on the characteristic clinical presentation. Even so, a definitive diagnosis can be made only after a CT scan is performed at the receiving facility. Because these hematomas occupy space inside the rigid skull, they may produce rapid increases in ICP, especially if they are sizable.

Epidural Hematoma

Epidural hematomas often result from a relatively low-velocity blow to the temporal bone, such as the impact from a punch or baseball. A fracture of this thin bone damages the middle meningeal artery, which results in arterial bleeding that collects between the skull and dura mater (**Figure 8-15**). This high-pressure arterial blood can

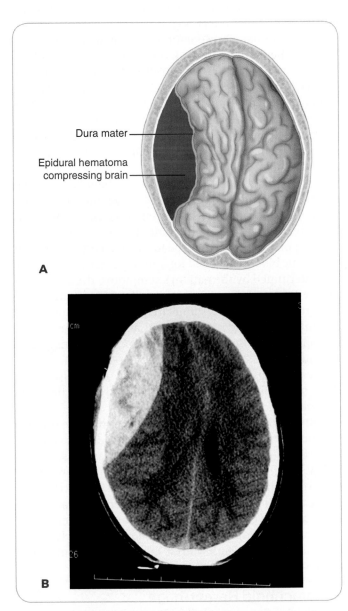

Dura mater

Epidural hematoma
compressing brain

A

B

Figure 8-15 A. Epidural hematoma. **B.** CT scan of epidural hematoma.

Courtesy of Peter T. Pons, MD, FACEP.

start to dissect, or peel, the dura off of the inner table of the skull, creating an epidural space full of blood. Such an epidural hematoma has a characteristic lens shape, as seen on the CT scan, created by the dura holding the hematoma against the inner table of the skull. The principal threat to the brain is from the expanding mass of blood displacing the brain and threatening herniation.

The classic history for an epidural hematoma is a patient experiencing a brief loss of consciousness, then regaining consciousness, and then experiencing a rapid decline in consciousness. During the period of consciousness, the lucid interval, the patient may be oriented, lethargic, or confused or may complain of a headache. However, the majority of patients with epidural hematomas do not experience this "lucid interval," and it may also occur with other types of intracranial hemorrhages, making it nonspecific for epidural hematoma. Nonetheless, a patient who experiences a "lucid interval," followed by a decline in GCS score, is at risk for a progressive intracranial process and needs emergency evaluation.

As a patient's consciousness worsens, the physical examination may reveal a dilated and sluggish or nonreactive pupil, most commonly on the ipsilateral side of the herniation. Because motor nerves cross over to the other side above the spinal cord, hemiparesis or hemiplegia typically occurs on the contralateral side. The mortality rate for an epidural hematoma is about 20%. However, with rapid recognition and hematoma evacuation, the mortality rate can be as low as 2%. This improved rate of outcome is because an epidural hematoma is usually an isolated space-occupying lesion, with little injury to the brain beneath. If the hematoma is quickly recognized and removed, the pathologic mass effect is corrected, and the patient can make an excellent recovery. Rapid removal reduces mortality as well as neurologic morbidity.

Subdural Hematoma

Subdural hematomas account for about 30% of severe brain injuries, with a male-to-female ratio of 3:1.[84] In young adults, 56% of subdural hematomas are due to motor vehicle crashes and 12% are due to falls, while in older adults, 22% are due to motor vehicle crashes and 56% are due to falls.[85]

In addition to being more common than epidural hematomas, subdural hematomas also differ in etiology, location, and prognosis. Unlike the epidural hematoma, which is caused by arterial hemorrhage, a subdural hematoma generally results from a venous bleed. In this case, bridging veins are torn during a violent blow to the head. Blood collects in the subdural space, between the dura mater and the underlying arachnoid membrane (**Figure 8-16**).

Subdural hematomas present in two different ways. In patients who have experienced significant trauma, the disruption of the bridging veins results in relatively rapid accumulation of blood in the subdural space, with rapid

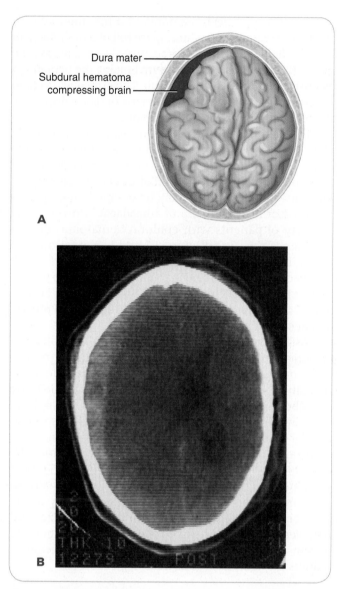

Figure 8-16 A. Subdural hematoma. **B.** CT scan of subdural hematoma.

Courtesy of Peter T. Pons, MD, FACEP.

onset of mass effect. Direct injury to the brain parenchyma beneath the subdural hematoma occurs concomitantly with venous disruption. As a result, the mass effect of subdural hematomas is often caused by both blood accumulation and cerebral edema of the underlying injured brain. Patients presenting with this type of acute mass effect will have an acutely depressed mental status and will need rapid identification of the emergency in the field with emergent transport to an appropriate receiving facility for CT scan, ICP monitoring and management, and possibly surgery.

However, clinically occult subdural hematomas can occur in other patients. In older adult or debilitated patients, such as those with chronic disease, the subdural space is enlarged secondary to brain atrophy. In such patients, blood may accumulate in the subdural space without exerting

mass effect and is therefore asymptomatic. Such subdural hematomas can occur during falls in older adults or during minor trauma. Older patients receiving anticoagulants such as warfarin (Coumadin) are at higher risk. Because these falls are minor, patients often do not present for evaluation and the bleeds are not identified. Many patients in whom chronic subdural hematoma is eventually identified do not even recall the traumatic event that caused the bleed because it seemed so minor.

In some patients with an occult subdural hematoma, the subdural blood liquefies but is retained within the subdural space. Over time, through a mechanism that includes repeated small bleeds into the liquid hematoma, the now-chronic subdural hematoma can expand and slowly start to exert mass effect on the brain. Because the onset of the mass effect is gradual, the patient will not have the dramatic presentation associated with an acute subdural hematoma. Instead, the patient is more likely to present with headache, visual disturbances, personality changes, difficulty speaking (**dysarthria**), and hemiparesis or hemiplegia of a slowly progressive nature. Only when some of these symptoms become pronounced enough to prompt the patient or caregiver to seek help is the chronic subdural hematoma discovered. On CT scan, a chronic subdural hematoma has a distinct appearance compared with the more emergent, acute subdural hematoma. Often the event precipitating transport for evaluation and care is the most recent of the small, repetitive subdural bleeds that create chronic subdural hematomas, and a small amount of acute blood may be found in a larger collection of chronic blood. The need for and the urgency of surgery are determined by the patient's symptoms, the amount of mass effect, and the patient's overall medical condition.

Prehospital care personnel frequently encounter these patients when called to facilities that care for chronically ill populations. Because the symptoms are nonspecific, diagnosing a chronic subdural hematoma in the field is rarely possible, and the symptoms may be confused with those of a stroke, infection, dementia, or even a generalized decline in the patient.

Although many subdural hematomas in these patients will be chronic, patients taking anticoagulants, after an apparently insignificant trauma, may have a subdural hematoma that expands over several hours and progresses to herniation resulting from the patient's inability to clot. These patients can have a benign presentation and then deteriorate several hours after their trauma. Older adults, especially patients receiving anticoagulants who have experienced apparently minor falls, should be managed with a heightened sense of urgency and care.

Subarachnoid Hemorrhage

Subarachnoid hemorrhage (SAH) is bleeding that occurs beneath the arachnoid membrane, which lies under the subdural space covering the brain. Blood in the subarachnoid space cannot enter the subdural space. Many of the brain's blood vessels are located in the subarachnoid space, so injury to these vessels will cause subarachnoid bleeding, a layering of blood beneath the arachnoid membrane on the surface of the brain. This layering of blood is typically thin and rarely causes mass effect.

SAH is usually associated with spontaneous rupture of cerebral aneurysms and causing the sudden onset of the worst headache of the patient's life. In reality, trauma is the most common cause of subarachnoid bleeding. These patients will usually complain of headaches, which may be severe in nature, as well as nausea, vomiting, and dizziness. In addition, the presence of blood in the subarachnoid space may cause meningeal signs such as pain and stiffness of the neck, visual complaints, and photophobia (aversion to bright light). Bleeding from the posterior communicating artery can cause oculomotor nerve abnormalities or loss of movement on the ipsilateral side; the affected eye will look down and outward, and patients will not be able to lift their eyelids. These patients may also develop seizures, although seizure development is more common in cerebral aneurysm rupture or arteriovenous malformations.

Because subarachnoid bleeding rarely causes mass effect, it does not require surgery for decompression. In fact, patients with SAH and a GCS score of 13 or greater generally do extremely well.[86] However, traumatic SAH can be a marker for potentially severe brain injury whose presence increases the risk for other space-occupying lesions, elevated ICP, and intraventricular hemorrhage. They have a 63% to 73% increased risk of a cerebral contusion and a 44% risk of developing subdural hematomas. Patients with greater than 1 centimeter (cm) of blood thickness or blood in the suprasellar or ambient cisterns have a positive predictive value of 72% to 78% for a poor outcome, and traumatic SAH doubles the incidence of death in brain-injured patients.[87,88]

Cerebral Contusions

Damage to the brain itself may produce cerebral contusions. If this damage includes injury to the blood vessels within the brain, there will be bleeding within the brain, known as intracerebral hematomas. Cerebral contusions are relatively common both in patients with severe brain injuries and in those with moderate head injuries. Although they are typically the result of blunt trauma, these injuries may also occur from penetrating trauma, such as a gunshot wound to the brain. In blunt trauma, cerebral contusions may be multiple. Cerebral contusions result from a complex pattern of transmission and reflection of forces within the skull. As a result, contusions often occur in locations remote from the site of impact, often on the opposite side of the brain—the familiar coup-contrecoup injury.

Cerebral contusions often take 12 to 24 hours to appear on CT scans, and these patients may initially have a normal head CT scan. The only clue to its presence may be a depressed GCS score, with many patients showing moderate head injuries (GCS score 9 to 13). As the contusion evolves after injury, it becomes apparent on the head CT scan and can cause increased mass effect and increasing headaches. Of particular concern, cerebral contusions may cause moderate head injuries to deteriorate to severe head injuries in about 10% of patients.[89]

Penetrating Cranial Injury

Penetrating trauma of the brain is one of the most devastating neurologic injuries. The penetrating object will cause direct injury to the brain tissue as it passes into and, in some cases, through the brain parenchyma. The nature of the neurologic injury produced depends on the area of the brain injured. Gunshot wounds are particularly destructive because of the energy associated with the missile (as described in the Physics of Trauma chapter). Not only does a bullet cause direct injury as it passes through tissue, the associated shock wave damages tissue along the cavitation pathway. In particular, gunshot wounds that cross the midline and pass from one side of the brain to the other, thus involving both sides of the brain, are associated with a dismal outcome. In rare instances, such as when the bullet traverses only the frontal lobes, the patient may survive, albeit with significant impairment. The potential for survival is also better if the bullet passes from front to back on one side of the brain. Again, however, the patient will have persistent, significant neurologic deficit.

All penetrating brain injury results in open fracture of the skull. The potential for subsequent infection, if the patient survives, is high. In addition, penetrating injuries of the skull may damage other important organs such as the eyes, ears, and face, leading to impaired function of the involved organs.

Management

Effective management of a patient with TBI begins with orderly interventions focused on treating any life-threatening problems identified in the primary survey. Once these problems are addressed, the patient should be rapidly packaged and transported to the nearest facility capable of caring for TBI.

Exsanguinating Hemorrhage

Hemorrhage control is essential. Direct pressure or pressure dressings should be applied to any external hemorrhage. Complex scalp wounds can produce significant external blood loss. Several gauze pads held in place by an elastic roller bandage create an effective pressure dressing to control bleeding. If this approach fails to control bleeding, the bleeding can often be controlled by applying direct pressure along the wound edges, thereby compressing the scalp vasculature between the skin and soft tissues and the galea. A pressure dressing should not be applied to a

Box 8-4 Refusal of Treatment

Patients who refuse medical treatment and/or transport are encountered frequently by EMS professionals. These encounters become more complicated when EMS professionals believe that it is in the patient's best interest to be transported and assessed by a physician, yet the patient refuses because he or she feels well and has no signs of neurologic impairment or deficit at the time of assessment. Often, TBI patients with severe mechanisms of injury may not experience the full severity of their injury until hours or days later. Consider patients with an epidural bleed, where there is often a lucid interval, during which the patient feels well, before suffering the potentially fatal effects of hemorrhage hours later.

Patients who have suffered a possible head injury should be evaluated fully, with particular attention being paid to their decision-making capacity. In addition, the following signs and symptoms indicate the need for further medical attention, and this should be communicated to the patient:

- Unequal pupils
- Worsening headache
- Nausea and vomiting
- Drowsiness or difficulty wakening
- Slurring of speech
- Confusion or change in behavior
- Loss of consciousness
- Seizures
- Physical fatigue
- Numbness
- Decreased coordination
- Trouble recognizing people or locations

When the EMS provider feels that it is in the best interest of the patient to be transported to the hospital for further assessment, and a patient with full decision-making capacity refuses transport, every attempt should be made to clearly articulate the risks of refusal and benefits of care. This includes very direct warnings about the possibility of death and permanent disability that can result from delayed medical care. Contacting medical direction sooner rather than later in these situations can be helpful, as patients may be more willing to listen to the advice of a physician in some cases. In the event that the patient still refuses transport and further treatment, it should be made clear that he or she can change his or her mind at any time that and EMS will be available to return and evaluate him or her.

When patients do not clearly possess full decision-making capacity, medical direction and law enforcement should be involved to the extent necessary to do what is in the best interest of the patients—transport them to the hospital for further evaluation. Use of the information contained in this section can provide the necessary arguments to medical direction, law enforcement, and for the patient chart to support treatment decisions made in the best interests of the patient.

Protocols, medical direction instructions, and local legal statutes should always be the followed when making treatment decisions. Discussions regarding the proper course of action to take in scenarios similar to those discussed here are best had before the incident takes place and should be routinely incorporated into continuing education and initial employee training. The dictum of "first do no harm" should be foundational in the approach to care for all patients encountered by EMS professionals. Patients with questionable capacity are certainly no exception.

depressed or open skull fracture unless significant hemorrhage is present, because it may aggravate brain injury and lead to an increase in ICP. Direct gentle pressure may also limit the size of extracranial (scalp) hematomas. Gentle handling and immobilization to a long backboard or scoop stretcher in anatomic alignment can minimize interstitial blood loss around fractures.

Hemorrhage from the carotid arteries and internal jugular veins may be massive. In most circumstances, direct pressure will control such external hemorrhage. Injuries to these vessels from penetrating trauma may be associated with internal bleeding, presenting as an expanding hematoma. These hematomas may compromise the airway, and endotracheal intubation may be necessary.

However, attempts to intubate a conscious patient with an expanding neck hematoma but no external bleeding may stimulate a cough, which may be sufficient to disrupt a clot that may have formed at a knife or bullet wound, resulting in massive external hemorrhage.

Airway

Patients with a depressed level of consciousness may be unable to protect their airway, and adequate oxygenation of the injured brain is critical to preventing secondary injury. As noted earlier, facial injuries can be associated with hemorrhage and edema that may compromise the airway. Hematomas in the floor of the mouth or in the soft palate may occlude the airway. The manual and simple airway skills, such as the jaw thrust maneuver, are appropriate initial airway interventions. (See the Airway and Ventilation chapter.) Both oral and nasal airways may become obstructed by edema or blood clots, and intermittent suctioning may be necessary. Definitive airway management of patients with TBI has historically been focused on endotracheal intubation. However, many of the alternative devices such as supraglottic airways can serve to maintain a patent airway in the prehospital setting. Suction equipment should always be readily available. Airway management interventions and TBI will often precipitate episodes of vomiting.

Patients with facial fractures and laryngeal or other neck injuries will typically assume a position that maintains their airway. Attempts to force a patient to lie supine or wear a cervical collar may be met with extreme combativeness if the patient becomes hypoxic as a result of positional airway impairment. In these situations, airway patency takes precedence over spinal immobilization, and patients may be transported in a sitting or semi-sitting position. Cervical collars may also be deferred if thought to compromise the airway, although manual stabilization of the spine should still be provided. Conscious patients can often assist in managing their own airways by suctioning themselves when they feel it is needed. Facial trauma, including those injuries caused by gunshot wounds, is not a contraindication to endotracheal intubation; however, many of these patients will need to be managed using percutaneous transtracheal ventilation or a needle or surgical cricothyroidotomy.

Securing the airway is considered to be the first treatment priority, and prehospital endotracheal intubation is traditionally advocated for patients with a GCS score of 8 or less. However, this prehospital intervention is controversial. An early study reported that victims of TBI who were intubated appeared to do better than those who were not intubated.[90] However, more recent studies have suggested that prehospital endotracheal intubation may be associated with increased mortality.[91-96] A 2015 meta-analysis demonstrated that prehospital intubation by providers with limited experience was associated with a twofold increase in the odds of mortality, while intubation by experienced providers demonstrated no difference in mortality.[97] Several factors likely contribute to the higher mortality rates associated with inexperienced providers, including unrecognized episodes of hypoxia and/or hypotension.[85] Prolonged or failed intubation attempts result in hypoxia, and medications used to facilitate intubation have hemodynamic effects including hypotension. After successful intubation, inappropriate ventilation, including unintentional hyperventilation, can further complicate the course. As a result, poorly performed intubation appears to be more harmful than no intubation at all.

Furthermore, any delays in reaching the hospital and receiving definitive surgical intervention are associated with poorer outcomes. In urban settings, short transport times allow patients to be managed using alternate techniques and delivered fairly urgently to the ED where the airway can be managed in a more controlled setting. Conversely, in systems with longer transport times, intubation may be more beneficial than no intubation at all, even when done by a less experienced prehospital care provider. It is important to note that all studies have demonstrated the importance of provider experience in overall outcomes. Intubations by experienced providers do not increase scene time or total prehospital time and are associated with significantly lower mortality.[97,98] As such, the decision to intubate a patient depends on both the length of transport and prehospital care provider experience.

With these qualifiers in mind, prehospital care providers should consider active airway management for all patients with a severe TBI (GCS score ≤ 8). Such management can be extremely challenging due to patient combativeness, clenched jaw muscles (trismus), vomiting, and the need to maintain in-line cervical spine stabilization. As a result, intubation, if that is the method of airway management chosen, should be performed by the most skilled provider available. It is essential that the patient's SpO_2 be monitored continuously and hypoxia (SpO_2 less than 90%) be avoided. Blind nasotracheal intubation can serve as an alternative technique, but the presence of midface trauma is a relative contraindication due to the possibility of inadvertent cranial and cerebral penetration with the nasotracheal tube in these patients. However, this complication is rare and has been reported only twice in head trauma patients.[99,100]

The use of neuromuscular blocking agents as part of a rapid-sequence intubation (RSI) protocol may facilitate successful intubation.[101] However, the safety and efficacy of RSI in the prehospital setting is undetermined. RSI with the use of lidocaine, fentanyl, and/or esmolol as premedication has not been demonstrated to decrease morbidity or mortality. However, some studies demonstrate that even though RSI improves intubation success, it can contribute to worse outcomes. Consequently, the routine use of paralytics in patients who are spontaneously breathing and maintaining SpO_2 greater than 90% on supplemental oxygen is not recommended.[29]

There is no one ideal airway management technique that is preferred over any other. Instead, manual and simple airway skills should be used as initial interventions, and complex airway interventions should be performed only if the airway cannot be maintained by less invasive means. In many cases, bag-mask ventilation with a nasal or oral airway is sufficient to oxygenate and ventilate the patient. Prolonged attempts at complex airway interventions should be avoided, especially with a short transport time.

Breathing

All patients with suspected TBI should receive supplemental oxygen. All patients should be monitored with continuous pulse oximetry because hypoxia is often difficult to clinically detect otherwise. Oxygen concentration can be titrated by pulse oximetry for a goal SpO_2 of at least 90%, with 94% or higher as optimal. If hypoxia persists despite oxygen therapy, the prehospital care provider should attempt to identify and treat all likely etiologies, including aspiration and tension pneumothoraces. Use of positive end-expiratory pressure (PEEP), if available, may be considered to improve oxygenation. However, levels of PEEP greater than 15 centimeters of water (cm H_2O) may increase ICP.[102,103]

Because both hypocapnia and hypercapnia can aggravate TBI, controlling the ventilator rate is important.[29,104] In the hospital, arterial blood gases (ABGs) are available to directly measure and maintain $PaCO_2$ in a normal range of 35 to 40 mm Hg. End-tidal carbon dioxide ($ETCO_2$) can also be used to estimate serum $PaCO_2$ in hemodynamically stable patients. Because the measured values for $ETCO_2$ and $PaCO_2$ vary widely from patient to patient, each in-hospital patient must have a unique "offset" between $PaCO_2$ and $ETCO_2$ determined by comparison of the $ETCO_2$ value with an ABG to obtain acceptable accuracy from the use of $ETCO_2$. New ABGs are obtained each time the patient's condition changes.

In the prehospital environment, ABGs and $PaCO_2$ are not routinely available to determine the "offset" with $ETCO_2$. In addition, other patient factors, such as changes in pulmonary perfusion, cardiac output, and patient temperature, can cause alterations in $ETCO_2$. These changes cannot be differentiated from changes in $ETCO_2$ that result from actual changes in $PaCO_2$. Furthermore, physiologic changes occur rapidly during resuscitation in the prehospital phase, which prevents $ETCO_2$ from being used with any accuracy. Although $ETCO_2$ is an excellent tool for monitoring ventilation, it is not accurate enough to guide hyperventilation therapy meaningfully in the prehospital setting.[105-115]

Instead, it is simpler to judge the degree of ventilation by counting breaths per minute. Normal ventilatory rates should be used when assisting ventilation in patients with TBI: 10 breaths/minute for adults, 20 breaths/minute for children, and 25 breaths/minute for infants. Excessively fast ventilatory rates and subsequent hypocapnia produce cerebral vasoconstriction, which, in turn, leads to a decrease in cerebral oxygen delivery. Routine prophylactic hyperventilation has been shown to worsen neurologic outcome and should not be used. A subgroup analysis of patients enrolled in the San Diego Paramedic RSI trial showed that both hyperventilation and severe hypoxia in the prehospital setting were associated with an increase in mortality. For adult patients, ventilating with a tidal volume of 350 to 500 ml at a rate of 10 breaths/minute should be sufficient to maintain adequate oxygenation without inducing hypocarbia.[29]

Hyperventilation of a patient in a controlled fashion may be considered in the specific circumstance of signs of herniation. These signs include asymmetric pupils, dilated and nonreactive pupils, extensor posturing or no response on motor examination, or progressive neurologic deterioration defined as a decrease in the GCS score of more than 2 points in a patient whose initial GCS score was 8 or less. In such cases, mild, controlled hyperventilation in the field may be performed during the prehospital phase of care. Mild hyperventilation is defined as an $ETCO_2$ of 30 to 35 mm Hg as measured by capnography or by careful control of the breathing rate (20 breaths/minute for adults, 25 breaths/minute for children, and 30 breaths/minute for infants less than 1 year of age).[29]

Circulation

Both blood loss and hypotension are important causes of secondary brain injury, so efforts should be made to prevent or treat these conditions.

Because hypotension further worsens brain ischemia, standard measures should be employed to combat shock. In patients with TBI, the combination of hypoxia and hypotension is associated with a high mortality rate. If shock is present and major internal hemorrhage is suspected, prompt transport to a trauma center takes priority over other interventions. Hypovolemic and neurogenic shock are aggressively treated by resuscitation with intravenous (IV) fluids such as blood products and isotonic crystalloid solutions. To preserve cerebral perfusion, adequate fluid should be given to maintain a systolic blood pressure of at least 90 mm Hg. For adult TBI patients with normal vital signs and no other suspected injuries, IV fluid at a rate of no more than 125 ml/hour should be administered and adjusted if signs of shock develop.[104] However, transport should not be delayed to establish IV access.

A randomized trial of patients with severe TBI showed that those who received prehospital resuscitation with hypertonic saline had almost identical neurologic functioning 6 months after injury compared to those treated with crystalloid.[104] Because of its increased cost and lack of benefit compared to normal saline or lactated Ringer solution, hypertonic saline is not recommended for routine prehospital volume replacement.

Disability

Assessment of the motor portion of the GCS score and the pupils should be integrated into the primary survey of all trauma patients after circulation is addressed. Use of the GCS score helps evaluate the patient's status and may impact transport and triage decisions.

Prehospital management of TBI patients primarily consists of measures aimed at reversing and preventing factors that cause secondary brain injury. Prolonged or multiple grand mal seizures can be treated with IV administration of a benzodiazepine, such as diazepam, lorazepam, or midazolam. These drugs should be cautiously titrated because hypotension and ventilatory depression may occur.

Because of the significant incidence of cervical spine fractures, patients with suspected TBI as a result of blunt trauma should be placed in spinal immobilization. Some degree of caution must be exercised when applying a cervical collar to a patient with TBI. A tightly fitted cervical collar can impede venous drainage of the head, thereby increasing ICP. *Application of a cervical collar is not mandatory as long as the head and neck are sufficiently immobilized.* Victims of penetrating head wounds generally do not require spine immobilization unless clinical findings clearly demonstrate spinal cord neurologic damage.

Transport

To achieve the best possible outcome, patients with moderate and severe TBI should be transported directly to a trauma center that can perform CT imaging and provide prompt neurosurgical consultation and intervention (including ICP monitoring if indicated). If such a facility is not available, aeromedical transport from the scene to an appropriate trauma center should be considered.[53]

The patient's pulse rate, blood pressure, SpO_2, and GCS score should be reassessed and documented every 5 to 10 minutes during transport. PEEP valves may be used cautiously if persistent hypoxia exists up to levels of 15 cm of H_2O; PEEP greater than 15 cm H_2O may increase ICP. The patient's body heat should be preserved during transport. In general, patients with TBI should be transported in a supine position because of the presence of other injuries.[116] Although elevating the head on the ambulance stretcher or long backboard (reverse Trendelenburg position) may decrease ICP, cerebral perfusion pressure may also be jeopardized, especially if the head is elevated higher than 30 degrees.

The receiving facility should be notified as early as possible so that appropriate preparations can be made before the patient's arrival. The radio report should include information regarding the mechanism of injury, initial GCS score and any changes en route, focal signs (e.g., motor examination asymmetry, unilaterally or bilaterally dilated pupils) and vital signs, other serious injuries, and response to management.[117]

Prolonged Transport

Prolonged transport times may lower the threshold for performing advanced airway management. RSI may be used in this setting, especially if aeromedical transport is considered, because a combative patient in the confines of a helicopter threatens the crew, pilot, and himself or herself. Efforts to control the airway should be performed while cervical spine stabilization is being applied. Oxygen should be administered to maintain an appropriate SpO_2

level. Because of the risk of developing pressure ulcers from lying on a hard backboard, the patient may be placed on a padded long backboard, especially if the anticipated transport time is lengthy. Patients should be attached to continuous pulse oximetry, and serial vital signs, including ventilations, pulse, blood pressure, and GCS score, should be measured. Pupils should be periodically checked for response to light and symmetry.

When there is a delay in transport or a prolonged transport time to an appropriate facility, additional management options can be considered. For patients with an abnormal GCS score, the blood glucose level should be checked. If the patient is hypoglycemic, a 50% dextrose solution can be administered intravenously until the blood glucose is restored to a normal level. Benzodiazepines may be titrated intravenously if recurrent or prolonged seizures occur.

External hemorrhage should be controlled, and crystalloid fluids administered if signs of shock are apparent. Fluids should be titrated to maintain the systolic blood pressure greater than 90 mm Hg in the patient with suspected TBI. Associated injuries should be managed en route to the receiving facility. Fractures should be appropriately splinted to control both internal hemorrhage and pain.

Appropriate management of increased ICP in the prehospital setting is extremely challenging because the ICP is not monitored in the field unless the patient is undergoing interfacility transfer and already has an ICP monitor or ventriculostomy in place. Although a declining GCS score may represent increasing ICP, it may also be the result of worsening cerebral perfusion from hypovolemic shock. Warning signs of possible increased ICP and herniation include the following:

- Decline in GCS score of two points or more
- Development of a sluggish or nonreactive pupil
- Development of hemiplegia or hemiparesis
- Cushing phenomenon

The decision to intervene and manage increased ICP is based on written protocol or made in consultation with medical control at the receiving facility. Possible temporizing management options include sedation, chemical paralysis, the use of osmotically active agents such as mannitol, and controlled hyperventilation (**Figure 8-17**). Small doses of benzodiazepine sedatives should be titrated cautiously because of the potential side effects of hypotension and ventilatory depression. Use of a long-acting neuromuscular blocking agent, such as vecuronium, may be considered if the patient is intubated. If the cervical collar is too tight, it may be loosened slightly or removed, provided that the head and neck are adequately immobilized with other measures.

Osmotherapy with mannitol (0.25 to 1.0 g/kg) can be given intravenously. However, aggressive diuresis may produce hypovolemia, which can worsen cerebral perfusion. Mannitol should be avoided for patients in whom systemic resuscitation has not been achieved—that is,

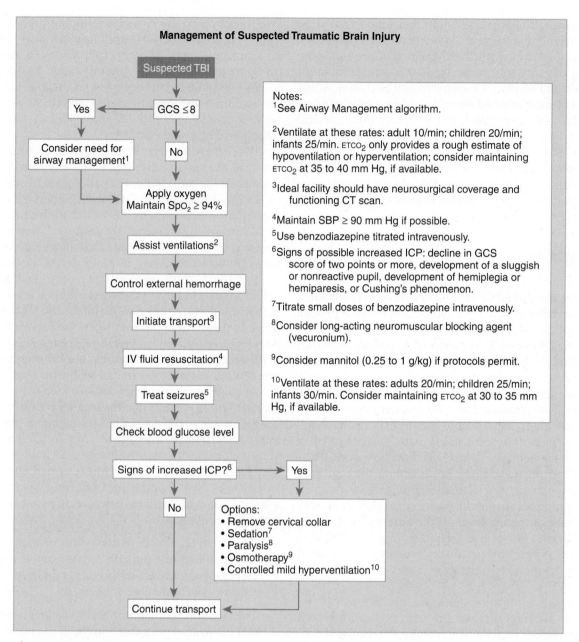

Figure 8-17 Management of suspected TBI.

© National Association of Emergency Medical Technicians (NAEMT).

patients with systolic blood pressure less than 90 mm Hg. If an osmotic agent is used, the patient should be maintained in a euvolemic state. In addition, a Foley catheter should be placed to monitor urine output if transport will be extremely prolonged.

An increased rate of ventilation (controlled, mild therapeutic hyperventilation) aimed at maintaining the ETCO₂ at 30 to 35 mm Hg may be considered for obvious signs of herniation. The following ventilatory rates should be used: 20 breaths/minute for adults, 25 breaths/minute for children, and 30 breaths/minute for infants. As stated previously, *prophylactic hyperventilation has no role in TBI, and therapeutic hyperventilation, if instituted, should be stopped if signs of intracranial hypertension resolve.* Steroids have not been shown to improve the outcome of patients with TBI and should not be administered.[29]

The primary focus for the TBI patient during prolonged transport or in austere environments is the best possible maintenance of cerebral oxygenation and perfusion and the best efforts possible to control cerebral edema.

SUMMARY

- Knowledge of head and brain anatomy is essential to understanding the pathophysiology of traumatic brain injury (TBI).
- Providers must understand the mechanisms by which the brain compensates for reduced cerebral blood flow following trauma.
- Primary brain injury occurs at the time of the original insult and is any injury that occurs because of the initial trauma.
- Secondary brain injury refers to further injury to structures that were unharmed by the primary injury. In the prehospital environment, recognition of pathophysiologic processes representative of secondary injury, including herniation from mass effect, hypoxia, and hypotension, and rapid transport are the key priorities.
- Knowing the mechanism of injury allows providers to anticipate certain injury patterns,

which is crucial in identifying the rapidly escalating conditions associated with brain injury.
- The severity of TBI may not be immediately apparent; therefore, serial neurologic evaluations of the patient, including Glasgow Coma Scale (GCS) scores, particularly the motor score, and pupillary response, are necessary to recognize changes in the patient's condition.
- Prehospital management of the TBI patient involves controlling hemorrhage from other injuries, maintaining a systolic blood pressure of at least 90 mm Hg, and providing oxygen to maintain oxygen saturation of at least 90%.
- Providers should consider active airway management for all patients with a severe TBI (GCS score ≤8). If intubation is chosen, it should be performed by the most skilled prehospital care provider available.

SCENARIO RECAP

On an 85°F (29°C) summer day, you and your partner are dispatched to the finish line of a marathon race for a 30-year-old man who fell 14 ft (4.3 m) off a ladder while attempting to secure the finish line banner. Upon your arrival, the patient is supine and unresponsive. A bystander is holding the patient's head and neck in-line.

You note an irregular breathing rate that increases and then decreases in depth. You also note that there is bloody fluid coming from both ears and both nostrils of the patient. The patient's airway is maintained with an oropharyngeal airway once absence of the gag reflex is noted. Your partner ventilates the patient with a bag-mask device at a rate of 12 breaths/minute. You notice that the patient's right pupil is dilated. The radial pulse is 54 and regular. Oxygen saturation (SpO_2) is 96%. The patient's skin is cool, dry, and pale. His GCS score is calculated to be 7 (E2V1M4).

You rapidly prepare the patient for transport and place him into your ambulance to perform the secondary survey while en route to the hospital. Palpation of the occiput generates a painful moan from the patient. You cover the patient with a warm blanket and measure his blood pressure, which is 184/102 mm Hg. An electrocardiogram reveals sinus bradycardia with infrequent premature ventricular beats noted. The right pupil remains widely dilated.

- What injury is most likely present given the patient's presenting signs?
- What are your management priorities at this point?
- What actions may you need to take to combat increased ICP and maintain cerebral perfusion during a prolonged transport?

SCENARIO SOLUTION

En route to the hospital, the patient begins to show palmar flexion of both hands. With this sign of impending herniation, you increase the ventilation rate to 16 to 20 breaths/minute. The patient remains unconscious. You consider insertion of a complex airway; however, since the Spo$_2$ is at 96% and transport time to the trauma center is only a few minutes, you decide to maintain him with the oral airway and bag-mask device with 100% oxygen.

References

1. Hyder AA, Wunderlich CA, Puvanachandra P, et al. The impact of traumatic brain injuries: a global perspective. *Neuro Rehabilitation*. 2007;22:341-353.

2. Centers for Disease Control and Prevention, National Center for Injury Prevention and Control, Division of Unintentional Injury Prevention. Traumatic brain injury and concussion. https://www.cdc.gov/traumaticbraininjury/index.html. Updated July 6, 2017. Accessed October 23, 2017.

3. Cipolla MJ. *The Cerebral Circulation*. San Rafael, CA: Morgan & Claypool Life Sciences; 2009.

4. Chestnut RM, Marshall LF, Klauber MR, et al. The role of secondary brain injury in determining outcome from severe head injury. *J Trauma*. 1993;34:216.

5. Fearnside MR, Cook RJ, McDougall P, et al. The West-mead Head Injury Project outcome in severe head injury: a comparative analysis of prehospital, clinical, and CT variables. *Br J Neurosurg*. 1993;7:267.

6. Gentleman D. Causes and effects of systemic complications among severely head-injured patients transferred to a neurosurgical unit. *Int Surg*. 1992;77:297.

7. Marmarou A, Anderson RL, Ward JL, et al. Impact of ICP instability and hypotension on outcome in patients with severe head trauma. *J Neurosurg*. 1991;75:S59.

8. Miller JD, Becker DP. Secondary insults to the injured brain. *J R Coll Surg Edinb*. 1982;27:292.

9. Mtui E, Gruener G, Dockery P. *Fitzgerald's Clinical Neuroanatomy and Neuroscience*. 7th ed. Edinburgh: Elsevier Saunders; 2017.

10. Wilson MH. Monro-Kellie 2.0: the dynamic vascular and venous pathophysiological components of intracranial pressure. *J Cereb Blood Flow Metab*. 2016;36(8):1338-1350.

11. Mavrocordatos P, Bissonnette B, Ravussin P. Effects of neck position and head elevation on intracranial pressure in anaesthetized neurosurgical patients: preliminary results. *J Neurosurg Anesthesiol*. 2000;12:10-14.

12. Sundstrøm T, Asbjørnsen H, Habiba S, et al. Prehospital use of cervical collars in trauma patients: a critical review. *J Neurotrauma*. 2014;31:531-540.

13. Obrist WD, Gennarelli TA, Segawa H, et al. Relation of cerebral blood flow to neurological status and outcome in head injured patients. *J Neurosurg*. 1979;51:292.

14. Obrist WD, Langfitt TW, Jaggi JL, et al. Cerebral blood flow and metabolism in comatose patients with acute head injury. *J Neurosurg*. 1984;61:241.

15. Coles JP, Minhas PS, Fryer TD, et al. Effect of hyperventilation on cerebral blood flow in traumatic head injury: clinical relevance and monitoring correlates. *Crit Care Med*. 2002;30(9):1950-1959.

16. Imberti R, Bellinzona G, Langer M. Cerebral tissue PO$_2$ and SjvO$_2$ changes during moderate hyperventilation in patients with severe traumatic brain injury. *J Neurosurg*. 2002;96(1):97-102.

17. Stocchetti N, Maas AI, Chieregato A, van der Plas AA. Hyperventilation in head injury: a review. *Chest*. 2005;127(5):1812-1827.

18. Miller JD, Sweet RC, Narayan RK, et al. Early insults to the injured brain. *JAMA*. 1978;240:439.

19. Silverston P. Pulse oximetry at the roadside: a study of pulse oximetry in immediate care. *BMJ*. 1989;298:711.

20. Stochetti N, Furlan A, Volta F. Hypoxemia and arterial hypotension at the accident scene in head injury. *J Trauma*. 1996;40:764.

21. Plum F. *The Diagnosis of Stupor and Coma*. 3rd ed. New York, NY: Oxford University Press; 1982.

22. Langfitt TW, Weinstein JD, Kassell NF, et al. Transmission of increased intracranial pressure. I. Within the craniospinal axis. *J Neurosurg*. 1964;21:989.

23. Langfitt TW. Increased intracranial pressure. *Clin Neurosurg*. 1969;16:436.

24. Ayling J. Managing head injuries. *Emerg Med Serv*. 2002;31(8):42.

25. Graham DI, Ford I, Adams JH, et al. Ischeaemic brain damage is still common in fatal non-missile head injury. *J Neurol Neurosurg Psychiatry*. 1989;52:346.

26. Obrist WD, Wilkinson WE. Regional cerebral blood flow measurement in humans by xenon-133 clearance. *Cerebrovasc Brain Metab Rev*. 1990;2:283.

27. Darby JM, Yonas H, Marion DW, et al. Local "inverse steal" induced by hyperventilation in head injury. *Neurosurgery*. 1988;23:84.

28. Marion DW, Darby J, Yonas H. Acute regional cerebral blood flow changes caused by severe head injuries. *J Neurosurg*. 1991;74:407.

29. Badjatia N, Carney N, Crocco TJ, et al. Guidelines for prehospital management of traumatic brain injury: 2nd edition. *Prehosp Emerg Care*. 2007;12(1):S1-S52.

30. Bostek CC. Oxygen toxicity: an introduction. *AANA J*. 1989;57(3):231-237.

31. Brenner M, Stein D, Hu P, et al. Association between early hyperoxia and worse outcomes after traumatic brain injury. *Arch Surg*. 2012;147(11):1042-1046.

32. Tolias CM, Reinert M, Seiler R, Gilman C, Scharf A, Bullock MR. Normobaric hyperoxia-induced improvement in cerebral metabolism and reduction in intracranial pressure

in patients with severe head injury: a prospective historical cohort matched study. *J Neurosurg.* 2004;101(3):435-444.

33. Mechtcheriakov S, Brenneis C, Egger K, Koppelstaetter F, Schocke M, Marksteiner J. A widespread distinct pattern of cerebral atrophy in patients with alcohol addiction revealed by voxel-based morphometry. *J Neurol Neurosurg Psychiatry.* 2007;78(6):610-614.

34. Mayer S, Rowland L. Head injury. In: Rowland L, ed. *Merritt's Neurology.* Philadelphia: Lippincott Williams & Wilkins; 2000:401.

35. Dimmitt SB, Rakic V, Puddey IB, et al. The effects of alcohol on coagulation and fibrinolytic factors: a controlled trial. *Blood Coagul Fibrinolysis.* 1998;9(1):39-45.

36. Caron MJ, Hovda DA, Mazziotta JC, et al. The structural and metabolic anatomy of traumatic brain injury in humans: a computerized tomography and positron emission tomography analysis. *J Neurotrauma.* 1993;10(suppl 1):S58.

37. Caron MJ, Mazziotta JC, Hovda DA, et al. Quantification of cerebral glucose metabolism in brain-injured humans utilizing positron emission tomography. *J Cereb Blood Flow Metab.* 1993;13(suppl 1):S379.

38. Caron MJ. PET/SPECT imaging in head injury. In: Narayan RK, Wilberger JE, Povlishock JT, eds. *Neurotrauma.* New York, NY: McGraw-Hill; 1996.

39. Jalloh I, Carpenter KLH, Helmy A, et al. Glucose metabolism following human traumatic brain injury: methods of assessment and pathophysiologic findings. *Metab Brain Dis.* 2015;30:615-632.

40. Lam AM, Winn HR, Cullen BF, et al. Hyperglycemia and neurological outcome in patients with head injury. *J Neurosurg.* 1991;75:545.

41. Young B, Ott L, Dempsey R, et al. Relationship between admission hyperglycemia and neurologic outcome of severely brain-injured patients. *Ann Surg.* 1989;210:466.

42. Brightbill TC, Martin SB, Bracer R. The diagnostic significance of large superior ophthalmic veins in patients with normal and increased intracranial pressure: CT and MR evaluation. *Neuro Ophthal.* 2001;26:93-101.

43. Teasdale G. The Glasgow structured approach to assessment of the Glasgow Coma Scale: what's new with the Glasgow Coma Score. http://www.glasgowcomascale.org/whats-new/. Accessed October 23, 2017.

44. Teasdale G, Allen D, Brennan P, et al. The Glasgow Coma Scale: an update after 40 years. *Nurs Times.* 2014;110:12-16.

45. Majdan M, Steyerberg EW, Nieboer D, et al. Glasgow Coma Scale motor score and pupillary reaction to predict six-month mortality in patients with traumatic brain injury: comparison of field and admission assessment. *J Neurotrauma.* 2015;32(2):101-108.

46. Ross SE, Leipold C, Terregino C, et al. Efficacy of the motor component of the Glasgow Coma Scale in trauma triage. *J Trauma.* 1998;45(1):42-44.

47. Jarvis C, ed. *Physical Examination and Health Assessment.* 6th ed. St. Louis, MO: Elsevier Publishers; 2012:71.

48. Brain Trauma Foundation. Glasgow Coma Score. In: Gabriel EJ, Ghajar J, Jagoda A, et al. *Guidelines for Prehospital Management of Traumatic Brain Injury.* New York, NY: Brain Trauma Foundation; 2000.

49. Dula DJ, Fales W. The "ring sign": is it a reliable indicator for cerebral spinal fluid? *Ann Emerg Med.* 1993;22:718.

50. American College of Surgeons. *Advanced Trauma Life Support.* Chicago, IL: American College of Surgeons; 2012.

51. Servadei F, Nasi MT, Cremonini AM. Importance of a reliable admission Glasgow Coma Scale score for determining the need for evacuation of posttraumatic subdural hematomas: a prospective study of 65 patients. *J Trauma.* 1998; 44:868.

52. Winkler JV, Rosen P, Alfrey EJ. Prehospital use of the Glasgow Coma Scale in severe head injury. *J Emerg Med.* 1984;2:1.

53. Brain Trauma Foundation. Hospital transport decisions. In: Gabriel EJ, Ghajar J, Jagoda A, et al. *Guidelines for Prehospital Management of Traumatic Brain Injury.* New York, NY: Brain Trauma Foundation; 2000.

54. Prosser JD, Vender JR, Solares CA. Traumatic cerebrospinal fluid leaks. *Otolaryngol Clin N Am.* 2011;44:857-873.

55. American Academy of Neurology. The management of concussion in sports (summary statement). *Neurology.* 1997;48:581.

56. Bey T, Ostick B. Secondary impact syndrome. *West JEM.* 2009;10:6-10.

57. Duclos C, Dumont M, Wiseman-Hakes C, et al. Sleep and wake disturbances following traumatic brain injury. *Pathol Biol (Paris).* 2014;62(5):252-261.

58. Orff HJ, Ayalon L, Drummond SP. Traumatic brain injury and sleep disturbance: a review of current research. *J Head Trauma Rehabil.* 2009;24(3):155-165.

59. Sandsmark DK, Elliott JE, Lim MM. Sleep-wake disturbances after traumatic brain injury: synthesis of human and animal studies. *Sleep.* 2017;40(5).

60. Chaput G, Giguère JF, Chauny JM, Denis R, Lavigne G. Relationship among subjective sleep complaints, headaches, and mood alterations following a mild traumatic brain injury. *Sleep Med.* 2009 Aug;10(7):713-716.

61. King NS, Crawford S, Wenden FJ, Moss NE, Wade DT. The Rivermead Post Concussion Symptoms Questionnaire: a measure of symptoms commonly experienced after head injury and its reliability. *J Neurol.* 1995 Sep;242(9):587-592.

62. Haboubi NH, Long J, Koshy M, Ward AB. Short-term sequelae of minor head injury (6 years experience of minor). *Disabil Rehabil.* 2001 Sep 20;23(14):635-638.

63. Mathias JL, Alvaro PK. Prevalence of sleep disturbances, disorders, and problems following traumatic brain injury: a meta-analysis. *Sleep Med.* 2012;13(7):898-905.

64. Collen J, Orr N, Lettieri CJ, Carter K, Holley AB. Sleep disturbances among soldiers with combat-related traumatic brain injury. *Chest.* 2012;142(3):622-630.

65. Masel BE, Scheibel RS, Kimbark T, Kuna ST. Excessive daytime sleepiness in adults with brain injuries. *Arch Phys Med Rehabil.* 2001;82(11):1526-1532.

66. Watson NF, Dikmen S, Machamer J, Doherty M, Temkin N. Hypersomnia following traumatic brain injury. *J Clin Sleep Med.* 2007;3(4):363-368.

67. Young, TB. Epidemiology of daytime sleepiness: definitions, symptomatology, and prevalence. *J Clin Psychiatry.* 2004;65(suppl 16):12-16.

68. Sullivan KA, Edmed SL, Allan AC, Karlsson LJE, Smith SS. Characterizing self-reported sleep disturbance after mild traumatic brain injury. *J Neurotrauma.* 2015;32(7):474-486.

69. American Academy of Sleep Medicine. *International Classification of Sleep Disorders.* 3rd ed. Darien, IL: American Academy of Sleep Medicine; 2014.

70. Williams BR, Lazio SE, Ogilvie RD. Polysomnographic and quantitative EEG analysis of subjects with long-term insomnia complaints associated with mild traumatic brain injury. *Clin Neurophysiol.* 2008;119(2):429-438.

71. Ouellet MC, Morin CM. Efficacy of cognitive-behavioral therapy for insomnia associated with traumatic brain injury: a single-case experimental design. *Arch Phys Med Rehabil.* 2007;88(12):1581-1592.

72. Seda G, Sanchez-Ortuno MM, Welsh CH, Halbower AC, Edinger JD. Comparative meta-analysis of prazosin and imagery rehearsal therapy for nightmare frequency, sleep quality, and posttraumatic stress. *J Clin Sleep Med.* 2015;11(1):11-22.

73. Menn SJ, Yang R, Lankford A. Armodafinil for the treatment of excessive sleepiness associated with mild or moderate closed traumatic brain injury: a 12-week, randomized, double-blind study followed by a 12-month open-label extension. *J Clin Sleep Med.* 2014;10(11):1181-1191.

74. Kaiser PR, Valko PO, Werth E, et al. Modafinil ameliorates excessive daytime sleepiness after traumatic brain injury. *Neurology.* 2010;75(20):1780-1785.

75. Meehan WP III. Medical therapies for concussion. *Clin Sports Med.* 2011;30(1):115-124, ix.

76. Mazwi NL, Fusco H, Zafonte R. Sleep in traumatic brain injury. *Handb Clin Neurol.* 2015;128:553-566.

77. Arciniegas DB, Anderson CA, Topkoff J, McAllister TW. Mild traumatic brain injury: a neuropsychiatric approach to diagnosis, evaluation, and treatment. *Neuropsychiatr Dis Treat.* 2005;1(4):311-327.

78. McCrory P. Does second impact syndrome exist? *Clin J Sport Med.* 2001;11:144-149.

79. McKee AC, Cantu RC, Nowinski CJ, et al. Chronic traumatic encephalopathy in athletes: progressive tauopathy following repetitive head injury. *J Neuropathol Exp Neurol.* 2009;68(7):709-735.

80. Centers for Disease Control. Get a heads up on concussion in sports policies: information for parents, coaches, and school and sports professionals. https://www.cdc.gov/headsup/pdfs/policy/headsuponconcussioninsportspolicies-a.pdf. Accessed March 23, 2018.

81. Centers for Disease Control. Implementing return to play: learning from the experiences of early implementers. https://www.cdc.gov/headsup/pdfs/policy/rtp_implementation-a.pdf. March 23, 2018.

82. McCrory P, Meeuwisse W, Dvořák J, et al. Consensus statement on concussion in sport: the 5th International Conference on Concussion in Sport. Berlin, October 2016. *Br J Sports Med.* 2017;51(11):838-847.

83. Halstead ME, Walter KD, Council on Sports Medicine and Fitness, American Academy of Pediatrics. Clinical report: sport-related concussion in children and adolescents. *Pediatrics.* 2010;126(3):597-615.

84. Meagher RL, Young WF. Subdural hematoma. eMedicine, Medscape. http://emedicine.medscape.com/article/1137207-overview. Updated August 04, 2016. Accessed May 23, 2017.

85. Coughlin RF, Moser RP. Subdural hematoma. In: Domino FJ, ed. *The 5-Minute Clinical Consult 2013.* 21st ed. Philadelphia, PA: Wolters Kluwer Health/Lippincott Williams & Wilkins; 2013:1246-1247.

86. Quigley MR, Chew BG, Swartz CE, Wilberger JE. The clinical significance of isolated traumatic subarachnoid hemorrhage. *J Trauma Acute Care Surg.* 2013;74:581-584.

87. Brain Trauma Foundation. CT scan features. In: Bullock MR, Chesnut RM, Clifton GL, et al. *Management and Prognosis of Severe Traumatic Brain Injury.* 2nd ed. New York, NY: Brain Trauma Foundation; 2000.

88. Kihtir T, Ivatury RR, Simon RJ, et al. Early management of civilian gunshot wounds to the face. *J Trauma.* 1993;35:569.

89. Rimel RW, Giordani B, Barth JT. Moderate head injury: completing the clinical spectrum of brain trauma. *Neurosurgery.* 1982;11:344.

90. Winchell RJ, Hoyt DB. Endotracheal intubation in the field improves survival in patients with severe head injury. *Arch Surg.* 1997;132:592.

91. Davis DP, Hoyt DB, Ochs M, et al. The effect of paramedic rapid sequence intubation on outcome in patients with severe traumatic brain injury. *J Trauma Injury Infect Crit Care.* 2003;54:444.

92. Bochicchio GV, Ilahi O, Joshi M, et al. Endotracheal intubation in the field does not improve outcome in trauma patients who present without an acutely lethal traumatic brain injury. *J Trauma Injury Infect Crit Care.* 2003;54:307.

93. Davis DP, Peay J, Sise MJ, et al. The impact of prehospital endotracheal intubation in moderate to severe traumatic brain injury. *J Trauma.* 2005;58:933.

94. Bulger EM, Copass MK, Sabath DR, et al. The use of neuromuscular blocking agents to facilitate prehospital intubation does not impair outcome after traumatic brain injury. *J Trauma.* 2005;58:718.

95. Wang HE, Peitzman AB, Cassidy LD, et al. Out-of-hospital endotracheal intubation and outcome after traumatic brain injury. *Ann Emerg Med.* 2004;44:439.

96. Chi JH, Knudson MM, Vassar MJ, et al. Prehospital hypoxia affects outcome in patients with traumatic brain injury: a prospective multi-center study. *J Trauma.* 2006;61:1134.

97. Bossers SM, Schwarte LA, Loer SA, et al. Experience in prehospital endotracheal intubation significantly influences mortality of patients with severe traumatic brain injury: a systematic review and meta-analysis. *PLoS One.* 2015;10(10):1-26.

98. Meizoso JP, Valle EJ, Allen CJ, et al. Decreased mortality after prehospital interventions in severely injured trauma patients. *J Trauma Acute Care Surg.* 2015;79:227-231.

99. Marlow TJ, Goltra DD, Schabel SI. Intracranial placement of a nasotracheal tube after facial fracture: a rare complication. *J Emerg Med.* 1997;15:187.

100. Horellou MD, Mathe D, Feiss P. A hazard of nasotracheal intubation. *Anaesthesia.* 1978;22:78.

101. Davis DP, Ochs M, Hoyt DB, et al. Paramedic-administered neuromuscular blockade improves prehospital intubation success in severely head-injured patients. *J Trauma Injury Infect Crit Care.* 2003;55:713.

102. Cooper KR, Boswell PA, Choi SC. Safe use of PEEP in patients with severe brain injury. *J Neurosurg.* 1985;63:552.

103. McGuire G, Crossley D, Richards J, et al. Effects of varying levels of positive end-expiratory pressure on intracranial pressure and cerebral perfusion pressure. *Crit Care Med.* 1997;25:1059.

104. Warner KJ, Cuschieri J, Copass MK, et al. The impact of prehospital ventilation on outcome after severe traumatic brain injury. *J Trauma.* 2007;62:1330.

105. Christensen MA, Bloom J, Sutton KR. Comparing arterial and end-tidal carbon dioxide values in hyperventilated neurosurgical patients. *Am J Crit Care.* 1995;4:116.

106. Grenier B, Dubreuil M. Noninvasive monitoring of carbon dioxide: end-tidal versus transcutaneous carbon dioxide. *Anesth Analg.* 1998;86:675.

107. Grenier B, Verchere E, Mesli A, et al. Capnography monitoring during neurosurgery: reliability in relation to various intra-operative positions. *Anesth Analg.* 1999;88:43.

108. Isert P. Control of carbon dioxide levels during neuroanaesthesia: current practice and an appraisal of our reliance upon capnography. *Anaesth Intensive Care.* 1994;22:435.

109. Kerr ME, Zempsky J, Sereika S, et al. Relationship between arterial carbon dioxide and end-tidal carbon dioxide in mechanically ventilated adults with severe head trauma. *Crit Care Med.* 1996;24:785.

110. Mackersie RC, Karagianes TG. Use of end-tidal carbon dioxide tension for monitoring induced hypocapnia in head-injured patients. *Crit Care Med.* 1990;18:764.

111. Russell GB, Graybeal JM. Reliability of the arterial to end-tidal carbon dioxide gradient in mechanically ventilated patients with multisystem trauma. *J Trauma Injury Infect Crit Care.* 1994;36:317.

112. Sanders AB. Capnometry in emergency medicine. *Ann Emerg Med.* 1989;18:1287-1290.

113. Sharma SK, McGuire GP, Cruise CJE. Stability of the arterial to end-tidal carbon dioxide difference during anaesthesia for prolonged neurosurgical procedures. *Can J Anaesthesiol.* 1995;42:498.

114. Warner KJ, Cuschieri J, Garland B, et al. The utility of early end-tidal capnography in monitoring ventilation status after severe trauma. *J Trauma.* 2009;66:26-31.

115. Davis DP, Dunford JV, Poste JC, et al. The impact of hypoxia and hyperventilation on outcome after paramedic rapid sequence intubation of severely head injured patients. *J Trauma.* 2004;57:1.

116. Feldman Z, Kanter MJ, Robertson CS. Effect of head elevation on intracranial pressure, cerebral perfusion pressure and cerebral blood flow in head-injured patients. *J Neurosurg.* 1992;76:207.

117. Schott JM, Rossor MN. The grasp and other primitive reflexes. *J Neurol Neurosurg Psychiatry.* 2003;74:558-560.

Suggested Reading

American College of Surgeons Committee on Trauma. Head trauma. In: *Advanced Trauma Life Support for Doctors, Student Course Manual.* 10th ed. Chicago, IL: American College of Surgeons; 2017.

Badjatia N, Carney N, Crocco TJ, et al. Guidelines for prehospital management of traumatic brain injury: 2nd edition. *Prehosp Emerg Care.* 2007;12(1):S1-S52.

Post AF, Boro T, Ecklund JM. Injury to the brain. In: Mattox KL, Feliciano DV, Moore EE. *Trauma.* 7th ed. New York, NY: McGraw-Hill; 2013.

Teasdale G, Allen D, Brennan P, et al. The Glasgow Coma Scale: an update after 40 years. *Nurs Times.* 2014;110:12-16.

CHAPTER **9**

Spinal Trauma

Lead Editors:
Steven C. Ludwig, MD
Luke Brown, MD
Ian Bussey
Alyssa Nash, BS

CHAPTER OBJECTIVES   At the completion of this chapter, you will be able to do the following:

- Describe the epidemiology of spinal injuries.
- Compare and contrast the most common mechanisms that produce spinal injury in adults with those in children.
- Recognize patients with the potential for spinal trauma.
- Relate the signs and symptoms of spinal injury and neurogenic shock with their underlying pathophysiology.
- Integrate principles of anatomy and pathophysiology with assessment data and principles of trauma management to formulate a treatment plan for the patient with obvious or potential spinal injury.

- Describe the multifaceted decision-making process required to determine if spinal motion restriction is appropriate for a given patient.
- Discuss factors associated with prehospital findings and interventions that may affect spinal injury morbidity and mortality.
- Understand the principles of selective spinal immobilization and how the application of these principles may change, depending on the patient and the situation.
- Understand the controversy surrounding steroid administration for spinal cord injury, and understand novel treatments currently under investigation.

SCENARIO

You have been dispatched to the scene of a bicyclist who is reported down alongside a roadway. On arrival, the scene is safe, with traffic being controlled by the police. The patient, a young woman, is lying supine on the side of the road away from traffic. A police officer is kneeling beside her and trying to talk to her, but she is not responding.

As you begin your primary survey, you are unable to ascertain the specific cause of the fall. It appears the woman fell from her bike while riding along the roadway, but you do not know whether she was struck by a motor vehicle. The police tell you there were no witnesses. The patient is wearing full cycling gear, including

(continued)

SCENARIO (CONTINUED)

helmet and gloves. She has abrasions on her forehead and an obvious deformity of the right wrist. Her airway is open, and she is breathing regularly. She shows no obvious signs of external blood loss. Her skin appears dry and warm, with normal color. As you are performing your primary survey, she begins to awaken but remains confused as to what happened.

- What pathologic processes explain the patient's presentation?
- What immediate interventions and further assessments are needed?
- What are the management goals for this patient?

INTRODUCTION

Traumatic spine injury (TSI) is potentially life threatening, with severity largely dependent on the region of the spine injured and whether damage includes nearby structures, such as the spinal cord. The injury most often results from high-energy forces but may occur with a lower energy mechanism of injury in vulnerable populations such as older adults. Injury to the skeletal components of the spine may not result in damage to the spinal cord, and, in some cases, the spinal cord, blood vessels, and nerves may be damaged without fracture or dislocation of the vertebrae. Damaged bony structures and supportive ligaments may result in structural instability of the vertebral column, making the spinal cord and other nearby structures susceptible to injury unless spinal motion is appropriately restricted. Severe injuries may irreparably damage the spinal cord and leave the patient with a lifelong neurologic disability. Immediate spinal cord damage occurs as a result of the trauma event, or primary injury. Secondary injury may follow the initial injury and result in worsened neurologic deficit. This secondary injury can be provoked or exacerbated by pathologic motion from an injured spinal column. Failure to suspect, properly assess, and stabilize a patient with a potential spine injury may produce a poor outcome. Prompt recognition and prehospital management of these injuries are important for timely stabilization in the critically injured patient, may guide future diagnostic and management decisions, and will reduce the risk of secondary injury.

Sudden violent forces acting on the body can stress the osseous and ligamentous structures in the spine beyond their normal limits of motion. The following four concepts help clarify the possible effect of energy on the spine when evaluating the potential for injury:

1. The head is similar to a bowling ball perched on top of the neck, and its mass often moves in a different direction from the torso, resulting in strong forces being applied to the neck (cervical spine, spinal cord).

2. Objects in motion tend to stay in motion, and objects at rest tend to stay at rest (Newton's first law).

3. Sudden or violent movement of the upper legs displaces the pelvis, resulting in forceful movement of the lower spine. Because of the weight and inertia of the head and torso, force in an opposite (contra) direction is applied to the upper spine.

4. Lack of neurologic deficit does not rule out bone or ligament injury to the spinal column or conditions that have stressed the spinal cord to the limit of its tolerance.

About 52 people per 1 million of the population in the United States (approximately 11,000 people) will sustain some type of spinal cord injury (SCI) annually, with an estimated 245,000 to 353,000 people living with the ensuing disability. SCI can occur at any age; however, nearly half of all injuries occur between 16 and 30 years of age. This age group is involved in the most violent and high-risk activities. The average age at injury was 42 years in 2010–2016, up from age 29 years in the 1970s; this trend is predictable given the increasing average age of the U.S. population.[1] Males overwhelmingly outnumber females and account for over 80% of SCIs. Common causes are motor vehicle crashes (48%), falls (21%), penetrating injuries (15%), sports injuries (14%), and other injuries (2%).[2] In the older adult population, falls outnumber motor vehicle crashes as the primary cause of SCI.[3]

SCI can have profound effects on physical function, lifestyle, and financial circumstances. In addition, when compared to the general population, those who survive the initial SCI generally have a shorter life expectancy.[3] The spinal cord may be injured at any level, and the two main categories of SCI include complete and incomplete injury. Complete SCI affects both sides of the body and results in total loss of all function, including movement and sensation, below the level of the injury. Incomplete injury describes any SCI without complete loss of neurologic function. Movement, sensation, or both are preserved but may be asymmetric in a patient with an incomplete

SCI. In general, physiologic dysfunction and long-term impairment increase along the spine, with a cervical spine injury being the most devastating. Complete injury at the highest level in the cervical spine is catastrophic and often fatal before emergency personnel arrive on scene. The loss of motor and sensory function after SCI can range from mild weakness to requiring a wheelchair or even a ventilator.

Patients with severe injuries may experience profound changes to daily activity levels and independence. SCI also impacts the financial circumstances of the patient as well as the population in general.[4] A patient with this injury requires both acute and long-term care. The lifetime cost of this care is estimated to be between $1.6 and $4.8 million per patient who sustains a permanent SCI, with cost rising with injury severity and age at time of injury.[3]

Neurologic deficits may result from trauma to a number of different central and peripheral nervous system structures or may be the result of inadequate oxygenation or perfusion to the brain or spinal cord. Patients may have injuries to multiple organ systems in addition to peripheral nerve injuries, which can manifest as a deficit. For example, a multitrauma patient may have sustained a direct blow to the head resulting in direct neurologic injury, a significant vascular injury resulting in shock and inadequate perfusion and thus an anoxic injury to neurologic structures, and an extremity injury that directly injures a peripheral nerve. Recovery from such injuries is variable, and while permanent in some cases, the potential for recovery is possible and must be assumed during the initial care of a patient. While the presentation of these patients may be complex, spinal injury should be a considered in any of the following mechanisms[5,6]:

- Any blunt mechanism that produced a violent impact on the head, neck, torso, or pelvis
- Incidents that produce sudden acceleration, deceleration, or lateral bending forces to the neck or torso
- Any fall from a height, especially in older adults
- Ejection or a fall from any motorized or otherwise powered transportation device
- Any shallow-water diving incident

The practice of prehospital spinal immobilization using the traditional rigid long backboard has evolved significantly since first gaining support in the 1960s. The decision to perform spinal motion restriction is made after careful consideration of the mechanism of injury, comorbidities and unique risk factors, and physical examination of the patient. Understanding the limitations and potential complications of this intervention is equally important in clinical decision making. More recently, the safety and efficacy of immobilization using the rigid long backboard has been challenged by researchers and has resulted in a paradigm shift away from traditional immobilization practices. The

evolution in prehospital management of spine trauma has generated widespread adoption of evidence-based protocols for spinal motion restriction and management of acute SCI that reduce widely recognized complications associated with immobilization using a rigid backboard, while effectively limiting spinal motion in patients with an injured spine. The patient with a suspected spinal injury should be manually stabilized in a neutral in-line position until the need for continued spinal motion restriction has been assessed. The initial management of a patient with suspected spinal trauma must include aggressive resuscitation to ensure uninterrupted perfusion of neurologic tissue and spinal motion restriction to prevent secondary injury and worsened neurologic decline.

Anatomy and Physiology

Vertebral Anatomy

The spine is a complex structure that primarily functions to facilitate movement in all three planes and disperse the forces from loads of the head and trunk to the pelvis, while simultaneously shielding the tenuous neurologic tissue of the spinal cord. The spinal column comprises 33 bones called vertebrae, which are stacked on top of one another. Except for the first (C1) and second (C2) vertebrae at the top of the cervical spine and the fused sacral and coccygeal vertebrae at the lower spine, all of the vertebrae are similar in form, structure, and motion (**Figure 9-1**). The *body* is situated anteriorly and represents the largest part of each vertebra. Each vertebral body bears most of the weight of the vertebral column and torso superior to it. Two curved sides called the **neural arches** are formed by the pedicle and posteriorly by the lamina projecting back from the body. The spinous process is a midline bony protuberance from the posterior aspect of the lamina that serves as an attachment for muscles and ligaments. In the lower five cervical vertebrae, this **spinous process** points directly posterior; in the thoracic and lumbar vertebrae, it points slightly downward in a caudal direction (toward the feet). Each vertebra has a pair of facet joints on the posterior aspect. These joints are covered in cartilage, allowing the vertebrae to articulate with one another.

Arising laterally from the junction of the pedicles and the vertebral bodies are additional bony structures called **transverse processes** that also serve as additional points for attachment of the paraspinal muscles. Several neural and vascular structures, including the root of each spinal nerve, spinal artery, and dorsal root ganglion, pass through an opening called the **intervertebral foramen** (also called neural foramen) present between every pair of vertebrae. The neural arches and the posterior part of each vertebral body form a near-circular shape with an opening in the

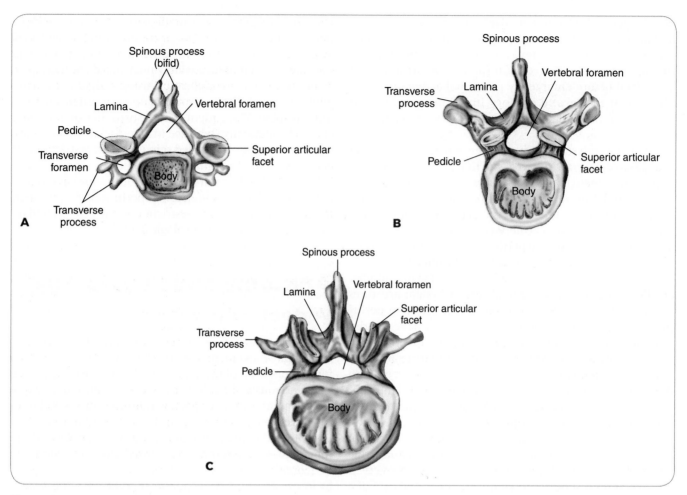

Figure 9-1 The body (anterior portion) of each vertebra becomes larger and stronger in the lower spine because it must support increasing mass as it approaches the pelvis. **A.** Fifth cervical vertebra. **B.** Thoracic vertebra. **C.** Lumbar vertebra.

© National Association of Emergency Medical Technicians (NAEMT).

center called the **vertebral foramen** (spinal canal). The spinal cord, surrounded by the thecal sac that contains cerebrospinal fluid, passes through this space. The spinal cord is protected somewhat from injury by the bony vertebrae surrounding it, but it remains vulnerable to direct penetrating injury through the interlaminar space. Each vertebral foramen lines up with that of the vertebrae above and the vertebrae below to form the hollow spinal canal through which the spinal cord passes. Variability in the size of the foramen can result from pathologic processes (e.g., arthritic change, tumor, and spinal disc herniation), spinal loading, and posture. The risk of damaging the neurovascular structures that pass through these openings may increase if the foramen becomes narrowed.

Vertebral Column

The individual vertebrae are stacked in an **S**-shaped column (**Figure 9-2**). This organization allows extensive multidirectional movement while imparting maximum strength. The spinal column is divided into five individual regions for reference. Beginning at the top of the spinal column and descending downward, these regions are the cervical, thoracic, lumbar, sacral, and coccygeal regions. Vertebrae are identified by the first letter of the region in which they are found and their sequence from the top of that region. The first cervical vertebra is called *C1*, the third thoracic vertebra *T3*, the fifth lumbar vertebra *L5*, and so on throughout the entire spinal column. Each vertebra supports increasing body weight as the vertebrae progress down the spinal column. Appropriately, the vertebrae from C3 to L5 become progressively larger to accommodate the increased weight and workload (see Figure 9-1).

Located at the cranial aspect of the spinal column are the seven *cervical* vertebrae that support the head and form the skeletal component of the neck. The cervical region is flexible to allow for total movement of the head. It is important to note that the vertebral arteries that supply the posterior aspect of the brain run through separate foramina in the cervical vertebra, usually entering at C6. In the case of significant displacement or fracture, this artery can become compromised, resulting in decreased

The thoracic spine is more rigid and allows less movement than the cervical spine. The increased stability provided by the ribs extending between the thoracic vertebrae and sternum is a major reason why injury of the thoracic spine in a healthy adult patient typically requires the significant physical forces of high-energy mechanisms. However, the incidence of thoracic spine injury is higher in the older adult population and in those with factors that reduce the relative strength of the thoracic spine. Below the thoracic vertebrae are the five *lumbar* vertebrae. The lumbar spine is flexible, allowing for movement in several directions. The five *sacral* vertebrae fuse by adulthood to form a single bony structure called the **sacrum**. Similarly, the four *coccygeal* vertebrae fuse and form the *coccyx* (tailbone). The incidence of traumatic vertebral fracture is highest in the thoracic and lumbar spine (75–90%), with most localized to the thoracolumbar junction.[9-11] Conversely, SCI and the overall incidence of TSI (including injuries without fracture) occur most frequently in the cervical region.[7,8]

Each vertebra is separated from the one above and below it by the intervertebral disc (**Figure 9-3**). This disc consists of a fibrous annulus that is filled with a gelatinous interior called the nucleus pulposus. The discs serve as soft cushions that allow the spine to bend in multiple directions. They also act as shock absorbers by attenuating the gravitational and mechanistic axial load of the spine. If damaged, the intervertebral disc may protrude into the spinal canal, compressing the cord or the nerves that come through the intervertebral foramina.

Ligaments and muscles tether the spine from the base of the skull to the pelvis. These ligaments and muscles form a web that sheathes the entire bony part of the spinal column, holding it in normal alignment, providing stability, and allowing for movement. The anterior and posterior longitudinal ligaments connect the vertebral bodies anteriorly and inside the canal. Ligaments between the spinous processes provide support for flexion–extension (forward and backward) movement, and those between

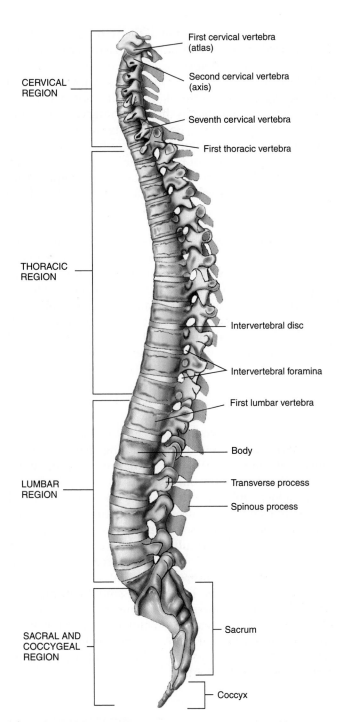

First cervical vertebra (atlas)

Second cervical vertebra (axis)

Seventh cervical vertebra

First thoracic vertebra

CERVICAL REGION

THORACIC REGION

Intervertebral disc

Intervertebral foramina

First lumbar vertebra

Body

Transverse process

Spinous process

LUMBAR REGION

SACRAL AND COCCYGEAL REGION

Sacrum

Coccyx

Figure 9-2 The vertebral column is not a straight rod but a series of blocks that are stacked to allow for several bends or curves. At each of the curves, the spine is more vulnerable to fractures; hence the origin of the phrase "breaking the S in a fall."
© National Association of Emergency Medical Technicians (NAEMT).

perfusion to the brain, and the patient may present with stroke-like symptoms. Compared with lower regions of the spine, the cervical spine has relatively unrestricted mobility and is most commonly injured.[7,8] Next are 12 *thoracic* vertebrae. Each pair of ribs connects posteriorly to one of the thoracic vertebrae at the costovertebral joints.

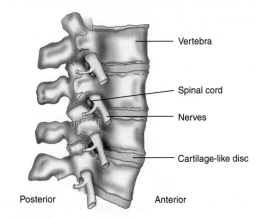

Vertebra

Spinal cord

Nerves

Cartilage-like disc

Posterior

Anterior

Figure 9-3 The cartilage between adjacent vertebral bodies is called the intervertebral disc.
© National Association of Emergency Medical Technicians (NAEMT).

the lamina provide support during lateral flexion (side bending) (**Figure 9-4**). If the soft-tissue structures that stabilize the spine are torn, excessive movement of one vertebra in relation to another can occur. This excessive movement may result in dislocation of the vertebrae and could potentially narrow the space occupied by the spinal cord, called the spinal canal, severely enough to cause SCI. It is important to note that in children, more ligamentous laxity exists. Unlike the adult spine, the increased laxity of the pediatric spine allows enough displacement of the spinal column to damage the cord without radiographic evidence of spinal column injury. This is called SCI without radiographic abnormality (SCIWORA).

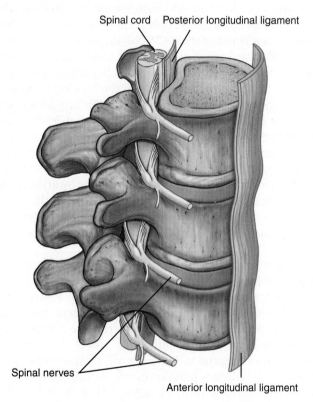

Spinal cord   Posterior longitudinal ligament

Spinal nerves

Anterior longitudinal ligament

Figure 9-4 Anterior and posterior longitudinal ligaments of the vertebral column.
© National Association of Emergency Medical Technicians (NAEMT).

The head balances on top of the spine, and the spine is connected to the pelvis though the sacroiliac joints. The skull perches on the ring-shaped first cervical vertebra (C1), referred to as the **atlas**. Very little bony stability is imparted by the joints of C1 and the skull, and the primary stabilization of this articulation is through strong craniocervical ligaments. The **axis**, C2, has a peg-like structure called the odontoid process (similar to a tooth) that protrudes upward. It is located just behind the anterior arch of the atlas, and it forms a rotational articulation (**Figure 9-5**). The articulation between C1 and C2 imparts 50% of the cervical spine's rotational motion.

The human head weighs between 16 and 22 pounds (lb; 7 to 10 kilograms [kg]), somewhat more than the average weight of a bowling ball. The cervical spine is particularly susceptible to injury due to a number of factors: position of the head atop the thin and flexible neck, normal forces that act upon the head, the small size of the supporting muscles, and the lack of protective bony structures (such as ribs). The cervical spinal canal narrows after the level of C1/C2, and the spinal cord consequently occupies 95% of the available space with minimal clearance between the cord and wall of the canal. Even a minor dislocation at this point can produce compression of the spinal cord. In contrast, the spinal cord occupies only 65% of the spinal canal as it terminates in the upper lumbar region. The posterior neck muscles are strong, permitting up to 60% of the range of flexion and 70% of the range of extension of the head without any stretching of the spinal cord. However, when sudden violent acceleration, deceleration, or lateral force is applied to the body, the momentum surpasses the stabilizing force of the osseous and ligamentous structures of the cervical spine, resulting in cord compromise. An example of this scenario would be a rear-end collision without the headrest properly adjusted.

The sacrum is the base of the spinal column, the platform on which the spinal column rests. The sacrum supports between 70% and 80% of the body's total weight. The sacrum is a part of both the spinal column and the pelvic girdle, and it is joined to the rest of the pelvis by immovable sacroiliac joints.

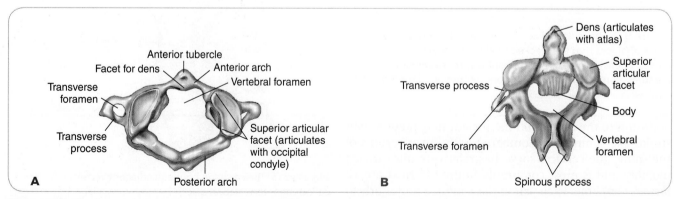

Figure 9-5 The first and second cervical vertebrae are uniquely shaped. **A.** Atlas (C1). **B.** Axis (C2).
© National Association of Emergency Medical Technicians (NAEMT).

Spinal Cord Anatomy

The spinal cord is a collection of neurons that carries outgoing and incoming signals between the brain and the rest of the body. It is continuous with the brain, beginning at the termination of the medulla oblongata, passing through the foramen magnum (the hole at the base of the skull) and respective vertebrae via the spinal canal to the level of the second lumbar (L2) vertebra. Blood is supplied to the spinal cord by the anterior and posterior spinal arteries.

The spinal cord is covered by three membranes, known as meninges: the pia, arachnoid, and dura mater, from innermost to outermost membrane, respectively. This meningeal covering continues to the second sacral vertebrae, where it terminates in a sac-like reservoir. The space between the pia mater and arachnoid mater contains cerebrospinal fluid (CSF), which is produced by the brain and encases the brain and spinal cord. In addition to removal of waste products from the brain, CSF protects against injury during rapid changes in acceleration that cause the brain to be pushed against the skull.

The spinal cord itself consists of gray matter and white matter. The gray matter consists primarily of the neuronal cell bodies. The white matter contains the long myelinated axons that make up the anatomic spinal tracts and serve as the communication pathways for nerve impulses. Spinal tracts are divided into two types: ascending and descending (**Figure 9-6**).

Ascending nerve tracts carry sensory impulses from distal body parts through the spinal cord up to the brain. Ascending nerve tracts can be further divided into those that carry different sensations: pain and temperature; touch and pressure; and sensory impulses of motion, vibration, position, and light touch. The tracts that carry pain and temperature sensation decussate or "cross over" in the spinal cord itself, meaning that the neuronal tract with the information from the right side of the body crosses over to the left side of the spinal cord and then travels up to the brain. In contrast, the nerve tract that carries the sensory

information for position, vibration, and light touch does not cross over in the spinal cord, but more cranially at the level of the medulla. Thus, this sensory information is carried up to the brain on the same side of the spinal cord as the nerve roots.

Descending nerve tracts are responsible for carrying motor impulses from the brain through the spinal cord down to the body, and they control all muscle movement and muscle tone. These descending tracts do not cross over in the spinal cord. Therefore, the motor tract on the right side of the spinal cord controls motor function on the right side of the body. These motor tracts do cross over in the brain stem, however, so the left side of the brain controls motor function on the right side of the body, and vice versa.

As the spinal cord continues to descend, pairs of nerves branch off from the spinal cord at each vertebra and extend to the various parts of the body (**Figure 9-7**). The spinal

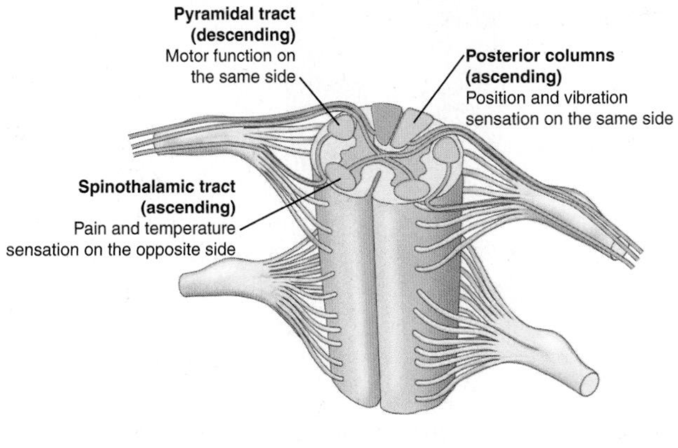

Figure 9-6 Spinal cord tracts.
© National Association of Emergency Medical Technicians (NAEMT).

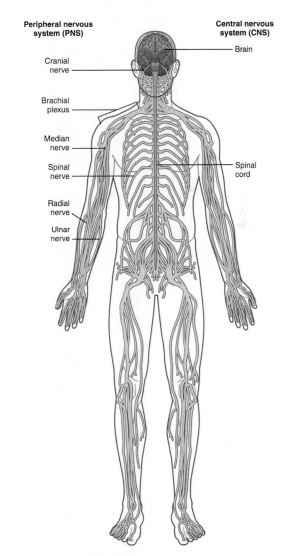

Figure 9-7 Nerves of the central nervous system (CNS) and peripheral nervous system (PNS).
© National Association of Emergency Medical Technicians (NAEMT).

cord has 31 pairs of spinal nerves, named according to the level from which they arise. Each nerve has two roots (one dorsal and one ventral) on each side.

The **dorsal root** carries information for sensory impulses, and the ventral root carries motor impulse information. Neurologic stimuli pass between the brain and each part of the body through the spinal cord and respective pairs of these nerves. As they branch from the spinal cord, these nerves pass through a notch in the inferior lateral side of the vertebra, posterior to the vertebral body, called the intervertebral foramen.

A **dermatome** is the sensory area on the skin surface of the body innervated by a single dorsal root. Collectively,

dermatomes allow the body areas to be mapped out for each spinal level (**Figure 9-8**). Dermatomes help determine the level of an SCI. Three landmarks to keep in mind are the clavicles, which are the C4–C5 dermatome; the nipple level, which is the T4 dermatome; and the umbilicus level, which is the T10 dermatome. Remembering these three levels can help to quickly locate an SCI.

The process of inhalation and exhalation requires both chest excursion and proper changes in the shape of the diaphragm. The intercostal muscles as well as accessory respiratory muscles such as the trapezius also contribute to breathing. The diaphragm is innervated by the left and right phrenic nerves, which originate from the nerves arising

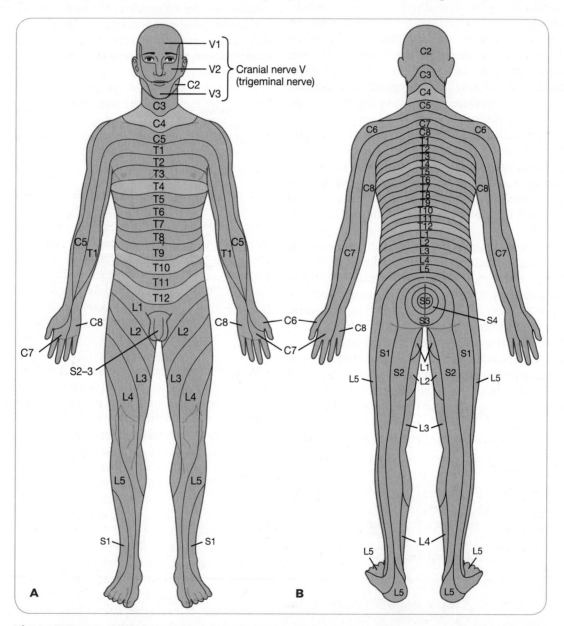

Figure 9-8 Dermatome map showing the relationship between areas of touch sensation on the skin and the spinal nerves that correspond to these areas. Loss of sensation in a specific area may indicate injury to the corresponding spinal nerve or level of injury of the spinal cord. **A.** Frontal view. **B.** Posterior view.

from the spinal cord between levels C3 and C5. If the spinal cord is injured above the level of C3 or the phrenic nerves are cut, a patient will lose the ability to breathe spontaneously. A patient with this injury may asphyxiate before the arrival of providers unless bystanders initiate rescue breathing. Therefore, it is critical to maintain control of the airway in a patient with suspected SCI. Positive-pressure ventilation may need to be continued during transport.

Pathophysiology

The bony spine can normally withstand forces of up to 1,000 foot-pounds (1,360 joules) of energy. High-speed travel and contact sports can routinely exert forces on the spine well in excess of this amount. Even in a low- to moderate-speed vehicle crash, the body of an unrestrained 150-lb (68-kg) person can easily place 3,000 to 4,000 foot-pounds (4,080 to 5,440 joules) of force against the spine if the head is suddenly stopped by the windshield or roof. Similar force can occur when a motorcyclist is thrown over the front of the motorcycle or when a high-speed skier collides with a tree. Compression strength of the vertebral column increases caudally, likely reflecting the differences in vertebral size, shape, and bone mineral density (BMD) at various spine levels.[12-15] The large forces needed to cause TSI often result in associated injuries to visceral, vascular, and pulmonary structures, which further complicate patient management. Cervical injury has the highest risk of associated injury to structures other than the spine (65%), followed by injury to the lumbar (52%) and thoracic (50%) levels. Thoracic spine trauma should raise a particularly high index of suspicion for associated injury to the lung, diaphragm, ribs, and sternum. In addition to the region of spine injured, the risk of associated injury increases with increasing number of spine fractures or injured spine segments.[16]

Skeletal Injuries

Various types of injuries can occur to the spine, including the following[17]:

- Compression fractures, which produce wedge compression or total flattening of the body of the vertebra
- Burst fractures, which can violate the posterior vertebral wall and may produce small fragments of bone that may lie in the spinal canal near the cord
- Subluxation, which is a partial dislocation of a vertebra from its normal alignment in the spinal column
- Discoligamentous injury, which results from overstretching or tearing of the ligaments and muscles, producing instability between the vertebrae with or without bony injury

While simple compression fractures are usually stable injuries, any of these injuries may immediately result in severe compression or (less commonly) transection of the spinal cord resulting in irreversible injury. In some patients, however, damage to the vertebrae or ligaments results in an *unstable* spinal column injury but does not produce an immediate SCI. Should the fragments in an unstable spine shift position, they may then damage the spinal cord secondarily. In addition, patients who have one spine fracture have a 10% to 20% chance of having another, noncontiguous spinal column injury. Therefore, the entire spine should be considered when determining the need for spinal immobilization in a patient with a suspected injury to a particular spine segment.

A lack of neurologic deficit does not rule out a bony fracture or an unstable spine. Although the presence of good motor and sensory responses in the extremities indicates that the spinal cord is currently intact, it does not exclude a damaged vertebra or associated bony, ligamentous, or soft-tissue injury. The majority of patients with spine fractures have no neurologic deficit. A full assessment is required to determine the need for immobilization.

Specific Mechanisms of Injury That Cause Spinal Trauma

Axial loading of the spine can occur in several ways. Most often, this compression of the spine occurs when the head strikes an object and the weight of the still-moving body bears against the stopped head, such as when the head of an unrestrained occupant strikes the windshield or when the head strikes an object in a shallow-water diving incident. Compression and axial loading also occur when a patient sustains a fall from a substantial height and lands in a standing position. This type of injury drives the weight of the head and thorax down against the lumbar spine while the sacral spine remains stationary. About 20% of falls from a height greater than 15 feet (4.6 meters [m]) involve an associated lumbar spine fracture; however, it is important to recognize that certain patient populations, particularly older adults, have a significantly higher rate of spinal fracture after falling from much shorter distances than 15 ft (5 m).[18] During such an extreme energy exchange, the spinal column tends to exaggerate its normal curvature, and fractures and compressions occur at such areas. Many compression or burst fractures that result from axial loading occur at the apices of the lumbar lordosis or thoracic kyphosis.

Excessive flexion (**hyperflexion**), excessive extension (**hyperextension**), and excessive rotation (**hyper-rotation**) can cause osseous or ligamentous damage, resulting in impingement on or stretching of the spinal cord.

Sudden or excessive lateral bending requires much less movement than flexion or extension before tensile or compressive failure of the spinal column occurs, as motion in this direction is limited to begin with. During lateral impact, the torso and the thoracic spine are moved laterally. The head tends to remain in place until it is pulled along by the cervical attachments. The center of gravity of the head is above and anterior to its seat and attachment to the cervical spine; therefore, the head will tend to roll sideways. This movement often results in dislocations and bony fractures.

Distraction (over-elongation of the spine) occurs when one part of the spine is stable and the rest is in longitudinal motion. This pulling apart of the spine can easily cause stretching and tearing of the spinal cord. Distraction-type TSI is a common mechanism in pediatric playground injuries, hangings, and certain types of motor vehicle crashes.

There are many recognized mechanisms of SCI; however, over 90% result from the following four major causes, listed in order of frequency[19]:

- Motor vehicle crashes (42%)
- Falls (27%)
- Acts of violence (15%)
- Sports-related activities, including shallow-water diving (8%)

Major causes of TSI and SCI in pediatric patients vary significantly by age and race. A significant proportion (17.5%) of spinal injuries in patients younger than 2 years result from violent physical abuse, while motor vehicle crashes and falls remained a common cause regardless of patient age.[20-23] Adolescents are more likely to sustain an injury during a sports-related activity than are younger children or adults.[24] Firearm-related injuries are responsible for nearly a quarter of all SCI in black adolescents in the United States.[25]

In practice, determining the exact mode of failure of the spinal column is difficult as the injury mechanism can result in complex force patterns. One must always assume that an injury severe enough to cause fracture or neurologic injury has caused spinal instability until proven otherwise by further clinical and radiographic evaluation.

Spinal Cord Injuries

Primary injury occurs at the time of impact or force application and may cause spinal cord compression, direct SCI (usually from sharp unstable bony fragments or projectiles), and interruption of spinal cord blood flow. Secondary injury occurs after the initial insult and can include swelling, ischemia, or movement of bony fragments.[26]

Cord concussion results from the temporary disruption of spinal cord functions distal to the injury. **Cord contusion** involves bruising or bleeding into the tissues of the spinal cord, which may also result in a temporary (and sometimes permanent) loss of spinal cord functions distal to the injury (spinal "shock"). **Spinal shock** is a neurologic phenomenon that occurs for a variable amount of time after SCI (usually less than 48 hours), resulting in temporary loss of sensory and motor function, muscle flaccidity and

paralysis, and loss of reflexes below the level of the SCI. Cord contusion is often caused by a penetrating type of injury or movement of bony fragments against the spinal cord. The severity of injury resulting from the contusion is related to the amount of bleeding into the spinal cord tissue. Damage to or disruption of the spinal blood supply can result in local cord tissue ischemia.

Cord compression is pressure on the spinal cord caused by swelling of local tissues but also may occur from traumatic disc rupture and bone fragments or development of a compressive hematoma. Cord compression may result in tissue ischemia and in some cases may require surgical decompression to prevent a permanent loss of function; thus prompt transport for imaging and definitive evaluation is important. **Cord laceration** occurs when spinal cord tissue is torn or cut. This type of injury usually results in irreversible neurologic injury.

Spinal cord transection can be categorized as complete or incomplete. In **complete cord transection**, all spinal tracts are interrupted, and all spinal cord functions distal to the site are lost. Because of the additional effects of swelling, determination of the extent of loss of function may not be accurate until 24 hours after the injury. Most complete spinal cord transections result in either paraplegia or quadriplegia, depending on the level of the injury. In **incomplete cord transection**, some tracts and motor/sensory functions remain intact. Prognosis for recovery is greater in these cases than with complete transection.

It is not possible in the prehospital environment to discern whether the resulting neurologic deficit is due to cord contusion, spinal shock, or a more severely damaged spinal cord. Therefore, all suspected SCI patients should be evaluated and managed without consideration of this distinction.

Types of incomplete cord injuries include the following:

- **Anterior cord syndrome** is typically a result of bony fragments or pressure on anterior spinal arteries resulting in infarction or damage to the anterior aspect of the spinal cord (**Figure 9-9**). Symptoms include loss of motor function and pain, temperature, and light touch sensations. However, some light touch, motion, position, and vibration sensations are spared through the intact posterior column.

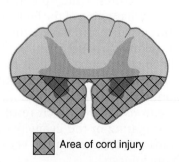

■ Area of cord injury

Figure 9-9 Anterior cord syndrome.
© National Association of Emergency Medical Technicians (NAEMT).

- **Central cord syndrome** usually occurs with hyperextension of the cervical area, especially in patients who may have preexisting stenosis from degenerative or congenital etiologies (**Figure 9-10**). Symptoms include weakness or paresthesias in the upper extremities but less significant loss of strength and sensation in the lower extremities. This syndrome causes varying degrees of bladder dysfunction.
- **Brown-Séquard syndrome** is caused by penetrating injury and involves hemi-transection of the spinal cord, involving only one side of the spinal cord (**Figure 9-11**). Symptoms include complete spinal cord damage and loss of function on the affected side (motor, vibration, motion, and position) with loss of pain and temperature sensation on the side opposite the injury.[27]

While *spinal shock* represents a loss of motor and sensory signal transmission in the spinal cord secondary to injury, this must be discriminated from *neurogenic shock*, a type of distributive shock with pathophysiologic signs caused by loss of sympathetic outflow to the heart and peripheral vessels. Without appropriate sympathetic stimulation, unopposed parasympathetic transmission results in bradycardia and dilation of peripheral arteries and veins. Dilation of arteries results in loss of peripheral systemic vascular resistance, and dilation of veins results in venous pooling. These findings reduce cardiac preload—the venous return to the right side of the heart. In combination with bradycardia, a serious decrease in cardiac output may occur. Recall that the hypovolemic shock patient presents with

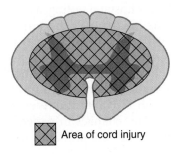

Area of cord injury

Figure 9-10 Central cord syndrome.
© National Association of Emergency Medical Technicians (NAEMT).

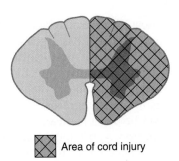

Area of cord injury

Figure 9-11 Brown-Séquard syndrome.
© National Association of Emergency Medical Technicians (NAEMT).

tachycardia in response to hypotension, and the skin is cool and clammy as the peripheral blood vessels constrict to shunt blood volume to vital organs in an attempt to maintain blood pressure. Conversely, the classic finding of the physiology associated with spinal shock is "hypotensive bradycardia" that may require treatment with atropine (or other parasympathetic blocking agent) in addition to other methods of aggressive resuscitation. Other findings related to the unopposed parasympathetic tone include warm, flushed skin and priapism (abnormal, prolonged erection of the penis) as a result of vasodilation. In practice, patients with SCIs and spinal shock often have other injuries that may result in hypovolemic shock in addition to neurogenic shock, making assessment and management more challenging.

Spinal Cord Perfusion

Spinal cord blood flow is determined partially by the spinal cord perfusion pressure (SCPP):

Spinal cord perfusion pressure (SCPP) = Mean arterial pressure (MAP) − Extrinsic pressure

Several factors can affect spinal cord perfusion and oxygenation as well as extrinsic pressure on the cord:

1. *Mean arterial pressure (MAP).* The MAP primarily determines cord perfusion. Adequate resuscitation to a target MAP of 90 mm Hg with both fluid administration and medication is crucial to maintaining SCPP. Systemic hypotension (defined as a systolic blood pressure < 90 mm Hg) at any point acutely following SCI is associated with worsened neurologic outcome.[28]
2. *Spinal venous congestion.* This can be the effect of venous thrombosis or the result of extrinsic compression of the spinal veins resulting in inadequate blood outflow. On a microvascular level, the MAP must be higher in the setting of spinal venous congestion to push blood through the area of venous congestion in order to achieve adequate oxygen exchange.
3. *Hypoxia.* Trauma patients often have pulmonary issues that may result in decreased oxygen exchange in the lungs resulting in low partial pressure of arterial oxygen in the blood. Administering supplemental oxygen and maintaining control over the airway are crucial to maintaining adequate blood flow to the spinal cord.
4. *Medications.* Many common anesthetic agents, including morphine and other opioids, can reduce cardiac output due to negative inotropic effects on cardiac muscle.[29] While pain control in a trauma patient is important, these agents must be used judiciously to allow for adequate cord perfusion and oxygenation.

Initial Resuscitation

Aggressive resuscitation plays a critical role in the prehospital management of SCI-related shock and in reducing neurologic deficit and preventing secondary neurologic damage. The pathogenesis of secondary neurologic injury stems from loss of autoregulation, leading to loss of spinal microcirculation, leading to further ischemic damage. Early, aggressive volume and blood pressure augmentation can improve this microcirculation and decrease the risk of secondary insults to the cord.[30] Additionally, up to 30% of SCI cases are associated with multitrauma and severe hemorrhage. This reflects the 20% mortality rate prior to hospital admission in SCI patients and the emphasis needed on adequate resuscitation efforts in the field.[31]

Ideally, initial resuscitation of the SCI patient should include measures to maintain a target MAP of at least 90 mm Hg for 7 days following the injury.[32,33] This is often accomplished using crystalloids, colloids, or blood products through appropriate venous access to restore as much neurologic blood flow as possible.[31] In the polytrauma SCI patient, it is important that prehospital providers weigh the potential risk and benefit of permissive hypotension. Given the risks of worsening SCI severity with transient low perfusion states, permissive hypotension should generally be avoided whenever SCI is suspected.[34-36] Volume-based resuscitation that includes glucose in the infusion fluids should be avoided for two reasons. First, glucose is metabolized quickly, leaving an excess of free water more likely to support the formation of edema. Second, too much glucose leads to hyperglycemia, which results in increased anaerobic cell metabolism, leading to increased lactate, decreased systemic pH, and a poorer outcome.[31]

It is also important to remember high SCIs (C5 or above) are more likely to require cardiovascular interventions such as vasopressors and pacemakers. Vasomotor sympathetic fibers exit the spinal cord between the levels of the first and fourth thoracic vertebrae and may be transected with higher cervical injuries while parasympathetic fibers travel in the vagus nerve outside of the spinal cord to the chest. This results in unabated parasympathetic flow and the paradox of bradycardia with hypotension.[37] Studies have shown that the average MAP of patients with complete cervical injuries is only 66 mm Hg when they arrived at the intensive care unit, far below the 90–mm Hg target MAP needed to maintain adequate perfusion of the spinal cord. One study revealed that 40% of patients with complete cervical SCI presented with signs of neurogenic shock and immediately required pressor support.[30] While first responders must be vigilant in their resuscitation efforts for all spinal injuries, it must be emphasized in cervical SCI patients to produce the best possible neurologic outcomes for this subset of patients.

Assessment

Spinal injury, as with other conditions, should be assessed in the context of other injuries and conditions present. After ensuring provider and scene safety, the primary survey is the first priority. A rapid scene assessment and history of the event should determine if the possibility of a spinal injury exists, which would require the need for protection of the spinal column with external immobilization. The head is brought into a neutral in-line position, unless contraindicated (see the Manual In-Line Stabilization of the Head discussion later in this chapter). The head is maintained in that position until the assessment reveals no indication for immobilization, or the manual stabilization is replaced with a spinal motion restriction device, such as cervical collar with a backboard, vacuum mattress, or vest-type device. If the mechanism of injury is unclear or the scene assessment cannot be adequately performed or is otherwise unreliable, one must assume the presence of spinal column injury and initiate external immobilization until a more thorough assessment can be performed.

Neurologic Examination

In the field, a rapid neurologic examination is performed to identify obvious deficits potentially related to an SCI. The patient is asked to move the arms, hands, and legs, and any inability to do so is noted. Then the patient is checked for the presence or absence of sensation, beginning at the shoulders and moving down the body to the feet. A complete neurologic examination does not need to be performed in the prehospital setting, as it will not provide additional information that will affect the decisions about needed prehospital care and serves only to expend precious time on scene and delay transport.

The rapid neurologic examination should be repeated after the patient has been immobilized, any time the patient is moved, and upon arrival to the receiving facility. This will help identify any changes in patient condition that may have occurred after the primary survey.

Using Mechanism of Injury to Assess SCI

Traditionally, prehospital care providers were taught that suspicion for a spinal injury is based solely on the mechanism of injury and that spinal immobilization is required for any patient with a suggestive mechanism of injury. Until recently, this generalization has caused a lack of clear clinical guidelines for assessment of SCIs. Mechanism of injury should never be the sole means of determining the need for spinal motion restriction, as it represents only one factor in a multifaceted decision-making process to determine whether spinal motion restriction is appropriate.

Assessment of the neck and spine for spinal immobilization should also include assessment of the motor and sensory function, presence of pain or tenderness, and patient reliability as predictors of SCI. In addition, the patient may not complain of pain in the spinal column because of pain associated with a more distracting painful injury, such as a fractured femur.[37] The definition of what constitutes a distracting injury remains controversial; however, the prehospital provider should take associated injuries into consideration while assessing a patient for potential TSI and potentially lower the threshold for applying spinal motion restriction if a distracting injury may exist.[38-41] Alcohol or drugs that the patient may have ingested as well as traumatic brain injury (TBI) may also blunt the patient's perception of pain and mask serious injury. Spinal motion restriction is likely not indicated in conscious patients with a reliable examination, no neurologic deficit, no neck or back pain, and no significant distracting injury. In patients with any of these factors positive on examination or who are unable to provide a reliable examination, spinal motion restriction should be continued.

Blunt Trauma

Blunt trauma is a common mechanism for TSI and warrants careful evaluation by the prehospital provider. Motor vehicle crashes and falls are responsible for the more than half of all spine fractures related to blunt trauma.[19] Large meta-analyses that included over 500,000 patients have determined the rate of thoracolumbar fracture in all blunt trauma to be about 7%, with over a quarter severe enough to cause SCI.[19] Injuries of the cervical spine result in higher risk of SCI and resulting neurologic impairment compared with the thoracic or lumbar spine.[16] In studies evaluating similarly large numbers of patients, the cervical spine is injured in over 6% of cases of blunt trauma and considerably higher in those who are unconscious or have suffered a head injury.[42,43] Almost half of all cervical injuries from blunt trauma are unstable; thus, a critical opportunity exists for prehospital intervention to prevent secondary injury.[44]

As a general guideline, the presence of spinal injury and a potentially unstable spine should be presumed, manual stabilization of the cervical spine immediately performed, and an assessment of the spine conducted to determine the need for immobilization with the following situations:

- Any blunt mechanism that produced a violent impact on the head, neck, torso, or pelvis (e.g., assault, entrapment in a structural collapse)
- Incidents that produced sudden acceleration, deceleration, or lateral bending forces to the neck or torso (e.g., moderate- or high-speed motor vehicle crashes, pedestrians struck by vehicle, involvement in explosion)
- Any fall, especially in older adults

- Ejection or fall from any motorized or otherwise powered transportation device (e.g., scooters, skateboards, bicycles, motor vehicles, motorcycles, recreational vehicles)
- Any shallow-water incident (e.g., diving, body surfing)

Other situations often associated with spinal damage include the following:

- Head injuries with any alteration in level of consciousness
- Significant helmet damage
- Significant blunt injury to the torso
- Impacted or other deceleration fractures of the legs or hips
- Significant localized injuries to the area of the spinal column

These mechanisms of injury should mandate a thorough and complete examination of the patient to determine whether indications are present that necessitate spinal motion restriction. If no indications are found, manual stabilization of the cervical spine can be discontinued.

Use of proper seat belt restraints has proven to save lives and reduce head, face, and thoracic injuries. However, the use of proper restraints does not completely rule out the possibility of spinal injury. In significant frontal-impact collisions when sudden severe deceleration occurs, the restrained torso stops suddenly as the seat and shoulder belts engage, but the unrestrained head can continue its forward movement. If the force of deceleration is strong enough, the head will move down until the chin strikes the chest wall, frequently rotating across the diagonal strap of the shoulder restraint. Such rapid, forceful hyperflexion and rotation of the neck can result in compression fractures of the cervical vertebrae, "jumped" facets (dislocation of the articular processes), and stretching of the spinal cord. Different mechanisms can also cause spinal trauma in restrained victims of rear or lateral collisions. The amount of damage to the vehicle and the patient's other injuries are the key factors in determining if a patient needs to be immobilized.

Penetrating Trauma

Penetrating injury represents a special consideration regarding the potential for spinal trauma.[45] In general, if a patient did not sustain definite neurologic injury at the moment that the penetrating trauma occurred, there is little concern for subsequent development of an SCI (**Box 9-1**). This is because of the mechanism of injury and the kinematics associated with the force involved. Penetrating objects generally do not produce unstable spinal fractures because penetrating trauma, unlike blunt injury, produces minimal risk of creating unstable ligamentous or bony injury. A penetrating object causes injury along the path of penetration. Gunshot wounds are common causes of cord contusion. While the bullet can transect the cord, causing irreversible injury, the ballistic shock of the bullet passing close to the cord more frequently results in a cord contusion that may recover. Knife injuries rarely result in SCI; however, injury is still possible. In addition to lacerating neurologic structures, knife injuries can cause local tissue swelling, resulting in cord contusion.

Indications for Spinal Motion Restriction

The mechanism of injury can be used as an aid to determine indications for spinal immobilization (**Figure 9-12**). The key point is that a complete physical assessment coupled with good clinical judgment will guide decision making.

In 2018, the American College of Surgeons Committee on Trauma, the National Association of EMS Physicians, and the American College of Emergency Physicians updated recommendations regarding the use of spinal motion restriction. Based on these recommendations and current literature, spinal motion restriction should be considered when a blunt mechanism of injury exists with any of the indications listed in **Box 9-2**.

Several important signs and symptoms are concerning for serious spinal trauma (**Box 9-3**). However, the absence of these signs does not definitively rule out spinal injury.

In an effort to reduce the unnecessary use of spinal motion restriction, particularly with a rigid long backboard, these professional bodies also recommend that immobilization on a backboard is not necessary if the patient meets all of the criteria listed in **Box 9-4**.[47]

Patients with a penetrating injury (e.g., gunshot or stab wound) to the head, neck, or torso and no evidence of spinal injury, such as neurologic signs or symptoms (e.g., numbness, tingling, and loss of motor or sensory function or actual loss of consciousness), should not be immobilized.[47-50] Numerous studies have shown that unstable spinal injuries rarely occur from penetrating trauma to the head, neck, or torso,[51-58] and isolated penetrating injuries by themselves are not indications for spinal motion restriction. Because of the very low risk of an unstable spinal injury and because the other injuries created by the penetrating trauma often require a higher priority in management, patients with penetrating trauma should *not* undergo spinal immobilization. In fact, a retrospective study using the National Trauma Data Bank documented that patients with penetrating trauma who received spinal immobilization in the field had a higher overall mortality rate than those who did not.[59]

Box 9-2 Indications for Spinal Motion Restriction

- *Midline spinal pain and/or tenderness.*[46,47] This includes subjective pain or pain on movement, point tenderness, or guarding of the structures in the midline spinal area.
- *Altered level of consciousness or clinical intoxication* (e.g., TBI, under the influence of alcohol or intoxicating substances)[46,47]
- *Paralysis or focal neurologic signs and/ or symptoms* (e.g., numbness and/or motor weakness).[46,47] This includes bilateral paralysis, partial paralysis, paresis (weakness), numbness, prickling or tingling, and neurogenic spinal shock below the level of the injury. In males, a continuing erection of the penis (priapism) may be an additional indication of SCI.
- *Anatomic deformity of the spine.*[46,47] This includes any deformity of the spine noted on physical examination of the patient.
- *Presence of a distracting injury*[46]
- *Inability to communicate*[47]

Box 9-3 Signs and Symptoms of Spinal Trauma

- Pain in the neck or back
- Pain on movement of the neck or back
- Pain on palpation of the posterior neck or midline of the back
- Deformity of the spinal column
- Guarding or splinting of the muscles of the neck or back
- Paralysis, paresis, numbness, or tingling in the legs or arms at any time after the incident
- Signs and symptoms of neurogenic shock
- Priapism (in male patients)

Box 9-4 Criteria to Determine When Spinal Motion Restriction Is Unnecessary

- Normal level of consciousness (Glasgow Coma Scale score of 15)
- No spine tenderness or anatomic abnormality
- No distracting injury
- No intoxication
- No neurologic findings or complaints

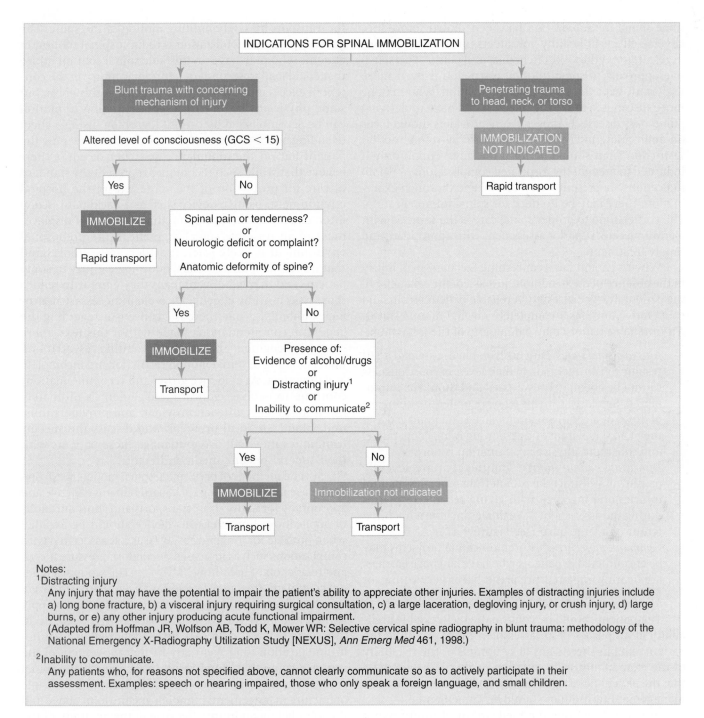

Figure 9-12 Indications for spinal immobilization.

© National Association of Emergency Medical Technicians (NAEMT).

Penetrating injuries by themselves are not indications for spinal immobilization. Unless a secondary mechanism exists or there is evidence of spinal injury, spinal motion restriction should not routinely be performed in patients with penetrating injuries.

The primary focus of prehospital care is to recognize the indications for spinal motion restriction rather than to attempt to clear the spine.[60-67] Because many patients do not have a spinal injury, a selective approach to performing spinal motion restriction is appropriate, especially since spinal immobilization has been shown to produce adverse effects in healthy volunteers, including increases in respiratory effort, skin ischemia, and pain.[68] This selective approach to spinal motion restriction is even more important with the older adult population, who may be more susceptible to skin breakdown and have underlying pulmonary disease. Prehospital care providers should focus on appropriate indications for performing spinal motion restriction[69] but should perform the intervention only if indicated to prevent the associated complications.[46,47] If no indications are present after a careful and thorough examination, there may be no need for spinal immobilization. The cornerstone to proper spinal care is the same as with all trauma care: superior assessment with appropriate and timely treatment.

When a patient has a concerning mechanism of injury in the absence of the conditions just listed, the reliability of the patient must be assessed. A reliable patient is calm and cooperative and has a completely normal mental status. An unreliable patient may exhibit any of the following:

- *Altered mental status.* Patients who have sustained a TBI resulting in an alteration in their levels of consciousness cannot be adequately evaluated and should be immobilized. Similarly, patients who are under the influence of drugs or alcohol are immobilized and managed as if they had spinal injury until they are calm, cooperative, and sober and physical examination is normal.
- *Distracting painful injuries.* Injuries that are severely painful may distract the patient from other, less painful injuries and interfere with giving reliable responses during the assessment.[37] Examples include a fractured femur or a large burn (see Figure 9-12).
- *Communication barriers.* Communication problems may be encountered in patients who have language barriers, are hearing impaired, are preverbal or very young, or for any reason cannot communicate effectively.

The patient should be continually rechecked for reliability at all phases of an assessment. If at any time the patient exhibits these signs or symptoms or the reliability of the examination is in question, it should be assumed that the patient has a spinal injury, and full immobilization management techniques should be implemented.

In many situations the mechanism of injury is not suggestive of neck injury (e.g., falling on an outstretched hand and producing a Colles' fracture [distal radius and ulna fracture]). In these patients, in the presence of a normal examination and proper assessment, spinal immobilization is not indicated.

Management

If TSI is suspected and spinal motion restriction is appropriate, the prehospital provider should prepare the patient for transport by safely limiting motion of the spine. The goal of spinal immobilization is to limit spinal motion in patients who may have an unstable spinal column injury that could lead to secondary neurologic injury in the context of excess motion. It is controversial at this point, but some physicians believe that such limitation to motion can be accomplished by careful logrolling, using a sheet or sliding board to accomplish transfers, and keeping the patient flat on the ambulance stretcher or cot. Others believe that while such techniques represent the standard of care for protection of the spine within the hospital environment, using a device such as a backboard, scoop litter, or vacuum mattress to reduce the risk of displacement of an unstable spinal segment in the prehospital environment is likely safer. Providers must understand that there is risk of secondary neurologic injury in some patients and that whatever means they employ to reduce those risks must be effective to avoid unnecessary neurologic disability. While there is a consensus regarding the general recommendations made within this text, there is acknowledgment that current scientific research and understanding of spinal motion restriction are incomplete and imperfect. As evidence grows and recommendations continue to evolve, clinical management is ultimately the responsibility of each provider, and providers must understand the local protocols and discuss the specific techniques they will use to manage these patients with their supervisors and medical director.

Several methods of performing spinal motion restriction can be used. The rigid long backboard remains effective and appropriate for many short transports and short durations of application; however, this device should be avoided when possible for longer transports, as it is associated with complications such as increased discomfort, pressure ulcers, and restriction of breathing.[46-48,50,70-72] The scoop stretcher or vacuum mattress may be used as an alternative to a rigid long backboard, as these devices are often easier to apply and may be more comfortable (**Box 9-5**). The head, neck, torso, and pelvis should each be immobilized in a neutral in-line position to prevent any further movement of the unstable spine that could result in damage to the spinal cord. Spinal immobilization follows the common principle of fracture management: immobilizing the joint above and the joint below an injury. Because of the anatomy of the spine, this principle of immobilization must be extended beyond just the joint above and below a suspected vertebral injury. The joint above the spine means the head, and the joint below means the pelvis.

The vacuum mattress was invented by Loed and Haederlé in France (**Box 9-6**). Other sources give credit to Erik Runereldt, a Swede, who reportedly got the idea for it in the late 1960s after seeing a package of coffee beans being vacuum packed.

As with most medical tools, there are many different makes of vacuum mattresses; therefore, prehospital care

Box 9-5 The Scoop Stretcher

The scoop stretcher (also known as clamshell stretcher, Robertson orthopedic stretcher, and scoop) was invented in 1943 by Wallace W. Robinson from Portland, Maine, and was patented in 1947.[73] It used just one opening joint at the foot end of the stretcher. The form we know today, with two opening joints, was patented by Ferno in 1970.

The scoop stretcher (Figure 9-13) has traditionally been made out of metal (aluminum or other lightweight metals), but modern plastics are now used more commonly. It is a two-part device, allowing the separated halves to be placed under each side of the patient without excessive manipulation. After fastening the two halves together, the patient can be lifted and transferred to an ambulance stretcher or vacuum mattress.

In its collapsed state, the scoop stretcher is roughly 5 ft, 5 inches (1.6 m) long and 16 inches (0.4 m) wide, but it can be extended to about 6 ft, 6 inches (2.0 m) to suit the size of the patient. The weight of a scoop is roughly the same as a long backboard. The acceptable patient weight limits vary according to the manufacturer's specifications (generally, 350 to 660 lb [160 to 300 kg]). The scoop stretcher can be used as a tool for transporting a patient over a long distance, provided the patient is properly secured with belts. There is some evidence that the scoop stretcher causes less discomfort than the rigid long backboard and may result in less spine movement during application of the device.[74]

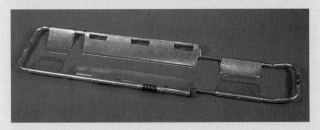

Figure 9-13 Scoop stretcher.
© Jones and Bartlett Publishers. Courtesy of MIEMSS.

Box 9-6 The Vacuum Mattress Splint

The vacuum mattress (Figure 9-14) is a transport and immobilization tool that is used after the patient has been transferred to it with a scoop stretcher. The splint is an airtight polymer bag filled with small polystyrene balls and a valve. When the air inside the vacuum mattress is removed, the atmospheric pressure outside presses the balls together, forming a rigid "bed" for the patient that molds to the patient's body contours.

The vacuum mattress has evolved considerably in the past decade. It is now wider and longer than the original version, and it has an improved valve system to more easily remove the air from within the mattress. Removal of the air from the mattress involves using a vacuum pump (either an electric suction unit or a hand pump).

The mattress shown here has a V shape, enabling prehospital care providers to package the patient more securely. The belts for fixation and carrying are sewn onto the mattress, which makes it easy to use and handle.

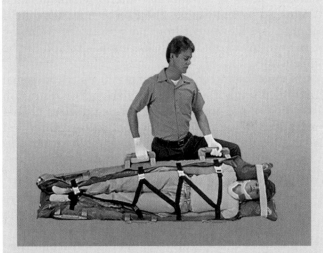

Figure 9-14 Vacuum mattress splint.
Courtesy of Hartwell Medical.

providers must be familiar with their particular device and participate in frequent trainings.

Several studies have demonstrated that the vacuum mattress provides a much higher degree of comfort to the patient when compared to the long rigid backboard.[75-80] Of particular importance, the vacuum mattress is, similar to most backboards, x-ray penetrable, so the patient does not need to be removed from the immobilizing systems while being evaluated in the emergency department.

Moderate anterior flexion or extension of the arms may cause significant movement of the shoulder girdle. Any movement or angulation of the pelvis results in movement of the sacrum and of the vertebrae attached to it. For example, lateral movement of both legs together can result in angulation of the pelvis and lateral bending of the spine.

Fractures of one area of the spine are often associated with fractures of other areas of the spine.[57] Therefore, the traditional teaching has been that the entire weight-bearing spine (cervical, thoracic, lumbar, and sacral) should be considered as one entity, and the entire spine immobilized and supported to achieve proper immobilization if there is suspicion of underlying injury. The supine position is the most stable position to ensure continued support during handling, carrying, and transporting a patient. It also provides the best access for further examination and additional resuscitation and management of a patient. When the patient is supine, the airway, mouth and nose, eyes, chest, and abdomen can be accessed simultaneously.

Patients usually present in one of four general postures: sitting, semi-prone, supine, or standing. If spinal column injury is suspected, the patient's spine needs to be protected and stabilized immediately and continuously from the time the patient is discovered until the patient is mechanically secured. Techniques and equipment, such as manual stabilization, half-spine boards, immobilization vests, scoop stretchers, proper logroll methods, and rapid extrication with full manual stabilization, are interim techniques used to protect a patient's spine. These techniques allow for a patient's safe movement from the position in which he or she was found until full supine immobilization can be implemented.

In some instances, the patient may benefit from spinal precautions rather than complete spinal motion restriction using one of the previously mentioned devices. Spinal precautions can be performed by applying a rigid cervical collar and firmly securing the patient to the stretcher. This is likely more appropriate in the following situations[47]:

- Patients who are ambulatory on the scene
- Patients who have mild to moderate neck pain, are reliable, have no neurologic deficit or complaints, and have no back or other thoracolumbar pain
- Patients for whom a backboard or other spinal restricting device is not otherwise indicated based on the presence of a distracting injury, decreased level of consciousness, or evidence of intoxication

Often, too much focus is placed on particular immobilization devices without an understanding of the principles of immobilization and how to modify these principles to meet individual patient needs. Specific devices and immobilization methods can be safely used only with an understanding of the anatomic principles that are generic to all methods and equipment. Any inflexible, detailed method for using a device will not meet the varying conditions found in the field. Regardless of the specific equipment or method used, the management of any patient with an

unstable spine should follow the general steps described in the next section.

General Method

When the decision is made to immobilize a trauma patient, follow these principles:

1. Move the patient's head into a proper neutral in-line position (unless contraindicated; see next section). Continue manual support and in-line stabilization without interruption.
2. Evaluate the patient by performing the primary survey, and provide any immediately required intervention.
3. Check the patient's motor ability, sensory response, and circulation in all four extremities, if the patient's condition allows.
4. Examine the patient's neck, and measure and apply a properly fitting, effective cervical collar.
5. Depending on the situation and how critical the patient's injuries are, either position a short backboard or vest-type device on the patient or use a rapid extrication maneuver if the patient is in a motor vehicle. Place the patient on a long backboard or other appropriate immobilization device if he or she is lying on the ground.
6. Immobilize the patient's torso to the device so that it cannot move up, down, left, or right.
7. Evaluate and pad behind the adult patient's head or pediatric patient's chest as needed.
8. Immobilize the patient's head to the device, maintaining a neutral in-line position.
9. Once the patient is on the immobilization device (if a short device is used), immobilize the legs so that they cannot move anteriorly or laterally.
10. Secure the patient's arms if indicated.
11. Reevaluate the primary survey, and reassess the patient's motor ability, sensory response, and circulation in all four extremities, if the patient's condition allows.

Manual In-Line Stabilization of the Head

Once it has been determined from the mechanism of injury that an injured spine may exist, the first step is to provide manual in-line stabilization. The patient's head is grasped and carefully moved into a neutral in-line position unless contraindicated (see the following discussion). A proper neutral in-line position is maintained without any significant traction on the head and neck. Only enough pull should be exerted on a sitting or standing patient to cause axial unloading (taking the weight of the head off the axis and the rest of the cervical spine). The head should be constantly maintained in the manually stabilized neutral in-line position until mechanical immobilization of the torso and head is completed or the examination reveals no need for spinal immobilization. In this way, the patient's head and neck are immediately immobilized and remain so if indicated until after examination at the hospital. Moving the head into a neutral in-line position presents less risk than if the patient were carried and transported with the head left in an angulated position. In addition, both immobilization and transport of the patient are much simpler with the patient's head in a neutral position.

Contraindications

Movement of the patient's head into a neutral in-line position is contraindicated in a few cases. If careful movement of the head and neck into a neutral in-line position results in any of the following, the movement must be stopped:

- Resistance to movement
- Neck muscle spasm
- Increased pain
- Commencement or increase of a neurologic deficit, such as numbness, tingling, or loss of motor ability
- Compromise of the airway or ventilation

Neutral in-line movement should not be attempted if a patient's injuries are so severe that the head presents with such misalignment that it no longer appears to extend from the midline of the shoulders. In these situations, the patient's head must be immobilized in the position in which it was initially found. Fortunately, such cases are rare.

Rigid Cervical Collars

Rigid cervical collars alone do not provide complete immobilization; they simply aid in supporting the neck and promote a lack of movement. Stabilization of the body to a spinal motion restriction device or to the ambulance cot must be accomplished in order to effectively limit spinal motion during transfer and transport of patients.

Prehospital methods of spinal motion restriction (using a vest, a short backboard, or a long backboard device) necessarily still allow some movement of the patient and the spine because these devices only fasten to the patient externally, and the skin and muscle tissue move slightly on the skeletal frame even when the patient is extremely well immobilized. Most rescue situations involve some movement of the patient and spine when extricating, carrying, and loading the patient. This type of movement also occurs when an ambulance accelerates and decelerates in normal driving conditions.

An effective cervical collar sits on the chest, posterior thoracic spine and clavicle, and trapezius muscles, where the tissue movement is minimal. It still allows movement at C6, C7, and T1, but it helps limit compression of these vertebrae. The head is secured under the angle of the mandible and at the occiput of the skull. The rigid collar allows the unavoidable loading between the head and the torso to be transferred from the cervical spine to the collar, limiting the cervical compression that could otherwise result.

Even though it does not fully immobilize the spine and head, a cervical collar aids in limiting head movement. The rigid anterior portion of the collar also provides a safe pathway for the lower head strap across the anterior collar as the patient is further immobilized.

The collar must be the correct size for the patient. A collar that is too short will not be effective and will allow significant flexion or compression of the spine from axial loading; a collar that is too large will cause distraction of the spine, hyperextension, or full motion if the chin slips inside of it.[81] Also, a collar must be applied properly. A collar that is too loose will be ineffective in limiting head movement and can accidentally cover the anterior chin, mouth, and nose, obstructing the patient's airway; a collar that is too tight can compress the veins of the neck, causing increased intracranial pressure.

There are many different rigid cervical collars available. The method of determining the correct size and the application of the device should be done according to the manufacturer's recommendations. An ill-fitting, improperly sized cervical collar will not help the patient and may be detrimental if an unstable spinal column is present (**Box 9-7**).

The collar is applied after bringing the patient's head into a neutral in-line position. If the head cannot be returned to a neutral in-line position, use of any collar is difficult and should not be considered. In this case, the improvised use of a blanket or towel roll may assist in stabilization. A collar that does not allow the mandible to move down and the mouth to open without motion of the spine will produce aspiration of gastric contents into the lungs if the patient vomits and, therefore, should not be used. Alternative methods to immobilize a patient when a collar cannot be used may include use of such items as blankets, towels, and tape. In the prehospital setting, the prehospital care provider may need to be creative when presented with these types of patients. Whatever method is used, the basic concepts of immobilization should be followed (**Box 9-8**).

There have been reports of increased intracranial pressure associated with cervical collar use in patients with

---

Box 9-7 Proper Cervical Collar Sizing

An ill-fitting, improperly sized cervical collar will not help the patient and may be detrimental if an unstable spinal column is present.

Box 9-8 Guidelines for Rigid Cervical Collars

Rigid cervical collars:

- Do not adequately immobilize by their use alone
- Must be properly sized for each patient
- Must not inhibit a patient's ability to open the mouth or the prehospital care provider's ability to open the patient's mouth if vomiting occurs
- Should not obstruct or hinder ventilation in any way

TBI. If a patient with suspected TBI shows obvious signs of increasing intracranial pressure, loosening or opening the collar should be considered to provide some relief.[82,83]

Immobilization of Torso to the Board Device

Regardless of the specific device used, the patient must be immobilized so that the torso cannot move up, down, left, or right. The device is secured to the patient's torso so that the head and neck will be supported and immobilized when affixed to it. The patient's torso and pelvis are immobilized to the device so that the thoracic, lumbar, and sacral sections of the spine are supported and cannot move. The torso should be immobilized to the device before the head is secured. In this way, any movement of the device that may occur when fastening the torso straps is prevented from angulating the cervical spine. The head should also be unrestrained from the backboard first upon arrival to the trauma center in order to protect the cervical spine from any torso movement during the initial evaluation.

There are many different methods for immobilizing the device to the torso. Protection against movement in any direction—up, down, left, or right—should be achieved at both the upper torso (shoulders or chest) and the lower torso (pelvis) to avoid compression and lateral movement of the vertebrae of the torso. Immobilization of the upper torso can be achieved with several specific methods; an understanding of the basic anatomic principles common to each method must be applied. Cephalad movement of the upper torso is prohibited by use of a strap on each side, fastened to the board inferior to the upper margin of each shoulder, which then passes over the shoulder and is fastened at a lower point (**Figure 9-15**). Caudad movement of the torso can be prohibited by use of straps that pass snugly around the pelvis and legs (**Figure 9-16**).

In one method, two straps are used to produce an X. A strap goes from each side of the board over the shoulder, then across the upper chest and through the opposite armpit, to fasten to the board on the armpit side. This approach stops any upward, downward, left, or right movement of the upper torso (**Figure 9-17**).

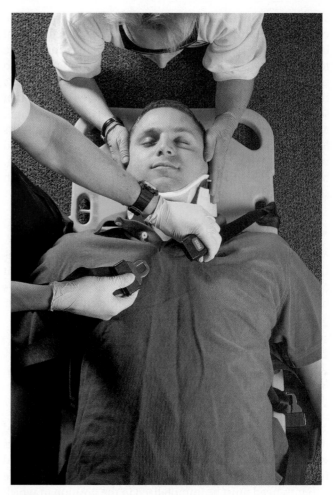

Figure 9-15 Cephalad movement of the upper torso is prohibited by use of an oblique strap on each side.

© Jones & Bartlett Learning. Photographed by Darren Stahlman.

The same immobilization can be achieved by fastening one strap to the board and passing it through one armpit, then across the upper chest and through the opposite armpit, to fasten to the second side of the board. A strap, or cravat, is then added to each side and passed over the shoulder to fasten it to the armpit strap, similar to a pair of suspenders.

Immobilization of the upper torso of a patient with a fractured clavicle is accomplished by placing backpack-type loops around each shoulder through the armpit and fastening the ends of each loop in the same handhold. The straps remain near the lateral edges of the upper torso and do not cross the clavicles. With any of these methods, the straps are over the upper third of the chest and can be fastened tightly without producing the ventilatory compromise typically produced by tight straps placed lower on the thorax.

Immobilization of the lower torso can be achieved by use of a single strap fastened tightly over the pelvis at the iliac crests. If the long backboard will have to be upended or carried on stairs or over a distance, a pair of groin loops will provide stronger immobilization than the single strap across the iliac crests.

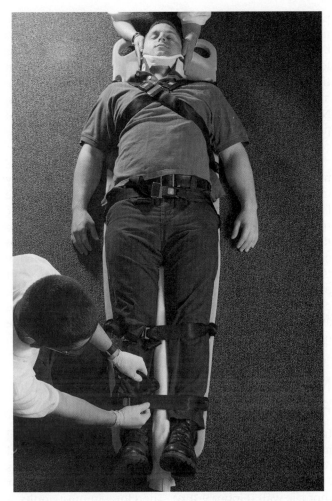

Figure 9-16 Caudad movement of the torso can be prohibited by use of straps that pass snugly around the pelvis and legs.

© Jones & Bartlett Learning. Photographed by Darren Stahlman.

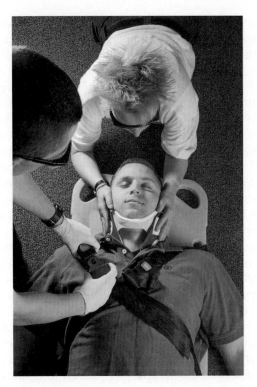

Figure 9-17 Use of two straps to produce an X across the upper chest helps to stop any upward, downward, left, or right movement of the upper torso.

© Jones & Bartlett Learning. Photographed by Darren Stahlman.

Lateral movement or anterior movement away from the rigid device at the midtorso can be prevented by use of an additional strap around the midtorso. Any strap that surrounds the torso between the upper thorax and the iliac crests should be snug but not so tight that it inhibits chest excursion, impairing ventilatory function, or causes a significant increase in intra-abdominal pressure. Regardless of which strapping device or technique is used, the principle is to secure the torso and then the head to the backboard. The particular device and technique chosen depend on the judgment of the prehospital care provider and the given situation.

The Backboard Debate

While the backboard provides motion restriction of the entire spine, it is important to understand a number of facts about the backboard itself. Being placed onto a rigid board is an extremely uncomfortable experience for the patient. An unpadded board will lead to complaints of back discomfort after a relatively short time on the board. In addition, being immobilized onto a rigid backboard leads to a significant amount of pressure being placed on bony prominences in contact with the board. Over time, circulation to these areas can become compromised, leading to skin ischemia, necrosis, and decubitus ulcers. All of these factors should prompt the prehospital care provider to place some padding under the patient and to minimize the amount of time a patient spends on the board.

In addition, some patients, especially bariatric individuals, may experience respiratory compromise from being strapped supine onto a board.

All of these concerns have led to a growing move to decrease or completely cease the use of the backboard or to remove patients from the board once the patient has been placed on the stretcher. While it is clear that too many patients are unnecessarily immobilized based solely on the mechanism of injury, the conceptual framework surrounding the backboard cannot be disregarded. Like any intervention, the application of these management strategies must be carefully considered. In addition, while not the only method to achieve spinal motion restriction due to recognition of potential complications, the backboard is useful in select circumstances such as short transports.

It is certainly possible to maintain spinal alignment and limit motion by simply laying a patient on an ambulance cot in a supine position with a cervical collar in place. This is the technique used to immobilize patients in the hospital even after an unstable cervical or thoracolumbar injury has been formally diagnosed. If thoracolumbar injury cannot be excluded, however, it is not safe to allow such a patient to sit up with the head at all elevated. If head elevation is desired to enhance airway protection, consider moving the stretcher to a reverse Trendelenburg position so that the spine remains in complete vertical alignment throughout. In the hospital, however, while patients can be safely moved by transfers using sheets and multiple personnel, and while they can be safely repositioned by logrolling to avoid pressure sore development, there is typically no need to move them vertically and potentially over uneven terrain as is often the case during operations in the field. There is also no need to transport them by vehicle over bumps and potholes and through traffic. Thus, the needs for spinal column stabilization are not as profound in the hospital as they are in the field.

Furthermore, given that most EMS transport times in the United States are relatively short and that the length of time patients in the hospital need to maintain spinal motion restriction or immobilization is relatively long, the degree of discomfort associated with use of a longboard in the hospital is much greater than in the prehospital environment, and the risk of secondary spinal column displacement and resultant secondary neurologic injury is relatively small. This is the reason that patients should be (and routinely are) removed from backboards or immobilization devices soon after arrival at hospitals or trauma centers.

It is also possible to safely extricate patients from vehicles using temporary devices such as short backboards and sliding boards and to immediately position them onto ambulance cots without ever employing a long backboard. This technique requires increased attention to detail during patient transfers and a high degree of awareness of the need to maintain spinal precautions during all transfers by all personnel involved in such moves. Maintaining this level of control can be difficult, as it is not uncommon in the prehospital environment to employ the help of relatively untrained personnel in executing such transfers. Nonetheless, this technique has the advantage of increased patient comfort and decreased scene time for physiologically unstable patients.

Elimination of the use of long backboards in the prehospital environment has occurred with increasing frequency in the United States and Europe without evidence in the literature to date of an increase in the incidence of catastrophic secondary neurologic injury. While some EMS agencies in the United States are beginning to consider elimination of the use of long backboards, others have chosen to modify their use of backboarding techniques to attempt to limit discomfort rather than expose patients to the potential risk of secondary catastrophic injury. EMS providers should be aware of the changes in their system and remain up-to-date on the latest evidence and protocol changes.

Maintenance of Neutral In-Line Position of the Head

In many patients, when the head is placed in a neutral in-line position, the posterior-most portion of the occipital region at the back of the head is between 0.5 and 3.5 inches (1.3 to 8.9 centimeters [cm]) anterior to the posterior thoracic wall (**Figure 9-18A**). Therefore, in most adults, a space exists between the back of the head and the board device when the head is in a neutral in-line position; thus, suitable padding should be added before securing the patient's head to the board device (**Figure 9-18B**). To

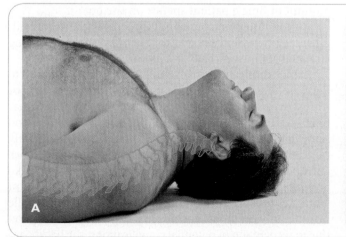
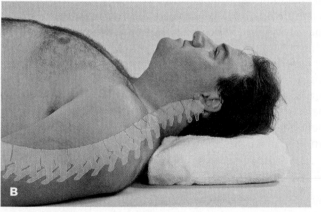

Figure 9-18 **A.** In some patients, allowing the skull to fall back to the level of the backboard can produce severe hyperextension of the spine. **B.** Padding is needed between the back of the head and the backboard in these patients to prevent hyperextension.

be effective, this padding must be made of a material that does not readily compress. Firm, semirigid pads designed for this purpose or folded towels can be used. The amount of padding needed must be individualized for each patient; some individuals require none. If too little padding is inserted or if the padding is of an unsuitable spongy material, the head will be hyperextended when head straps are applied. If too much padding is inserted, the head will be moved into a flexed position. Both hyperextension and flexion of the head can increase spinal cord damage and should be avoided.

The same anatomic relationship between the head and back applies when most people are supine, whether on the ground or on a backboard. When most adults are supine, the head falls back into a hyperextended position. On arrival, the head should be moved into a neutral in-line position and manually maintained in that position, which in many adults will require holding the head up off the ground. Once the patient is placed on the long backboard and the head is about to be fastened to the board, proper padding (as described) should be inserted between the back of the head and the board to maintain the neutral position. These principles should be used with all patients, including athletes with shoulder pads and patients with abnormal curvature of the spine, such as those with severe kyphosis.

In small children, generally those with the body size of a 7-year-old or younger, the size of the head is much larger relative to the rest of the body than it is in adults, and the muscles of the back are less developed.[84] When a small child's head is in a neutral in-line position, the back of the head usually extends 1 to 2 inches (2.5 to 5 cm) beyond the posterior plane of the back. Therefore, if a small child is placed directly on a rigid surface, the head will be moved into a position of flexion (**Figure 9-19A**).

The placement of small children on a standard long backboard results in unwanted flexion of the head and neck. The long backboard needs to be modified either by creating a recess in the board for the occiput to fit into or by inserting padding under the torso to maintain the head in a neutral position (**Figure 9-19B**). The padding placed under the torso should be of the appropriate thickness so that the head lies on the board in a neutral position; too much will result in extension, too little in flexion. The padding under the torso must also be firm and evenly shaped. Use of irregularly shaped or insufficient padding or placing it only under the shoulders can result in movement and misalignment of the spine (**Box 9-9**).

Completing Immobilization

Head

Once the patient's torso has been immobilized to the rigid device selected and appropriate padding inserted behind the head as needed, the head should be secured to the

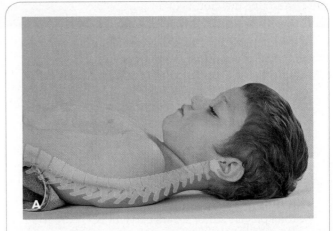
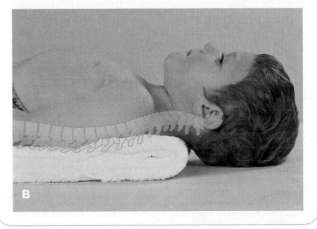

Figure 9-19 A. The larger size of a child's head relative to body size, combined with the reduced development of the posterior thoracic muscles, produces hyperflexion of the head when a child is placed on a backboard. **B.** Padding beneath the shoulders and torso will prevent this hyperflexion.

© National Association of Emergency Medical Technicians (NAEMT).

device. Because of its rounded shape, the head cannot be stabilized on a flat surface with only straps or tape. Use of these alone allows the head to rotate and move laterally. Also, because of the angle of the forehead and the slippery nature of oily and moist skin and hair, a simple strap over the forehead is unreliable and can easily slide off. Although the human head weighs about the same as a bowling ball, it has a significantly different shape. The head is ovoid, longer than it is wide with almost completely flat lateral sides, resembling a bowling ball with about 2 inches (5 cm) cut off to form left and right sides. Adequate external immobilization of the head, regardless of method or device, can be achieved only by placing pads or rolled blankets on these flat sides and securing them with straps or tape. In the case of vest-type devices, this is accomplished with hinged side flaps that are part of the vest.

The side supports, whether they are preshaped foam blocks or rolled blankets, are placed next to both sides of

Box 9-9 Athletic Equipment Removal

While relatively rare, spinal trauma in athletes represents a potentially career-ending and life-altering event. Trauma during sporting activities comprises nearly 15% of all TSIs, 10% of all SCIs, and 2% to 3% of all sports-related hospital admissions in the United States.[85-87] The mechanism in which injury occurs varies based on the activity. Similarly, certain sporting activities carry higher risk of SCI than do others. Athletes in the United States who participate in wrestling, gymnastics, and football sustain a large proportion of cervical SCIs.[87] High school–aged football players suffer severe cervical SCI more than any other age group involved in this sport.[88] Hockey, a sport that also carries a relatively higher risk of spine injury, will likely result in rising sports-related TSI as the popularity of the sport in the United States continues to rise.[87,89] It is important that prehospital providers are aware of the unique challenges faced while treating athletes (e.g., protective equipment such as helmets and face masks) to ensure that they can confidently and appropriately assess and manage these patients when a TSI is suspected. Similarly, EMS systems must collaborate with athletic trainers and recreational sporting programs in their community to ensure that all stakeholders are prepared with the equipment and training necessary for safe, effective prehospital management of an injured athlete.

The assessment and management of sports-related TSI must begin wherever the patient is encountered, with care taken before the patient is transferred from the field to a more controlled environment. Whenever an athlete is exposed to a traumatic mechanism of injury and complains of midline pain or tenderness of the spine, reduced range of motion, and/or neurologic signs or symptoms, manual stabilization of the spine should be performed with careful physical examination. If continued spinal motion restriction is appropriate (see criteria discussed previously in this chapter), providers should carefully prepare the patient for transfer to an appropriate hospital for further evaluation. In addition, any athlete found unconscious after a traumatic mechanism of injury should be treated as if a TSI has occurred until this can be ruled out by further diagnostic testing.[87] While there is limited evidence to better guide this decision, it is currently recommended that whenever there are persistent neurologic complaints, pain, or reduced range of motion in the spine, the athlete should not be permitted to return to play.[90]

While special care for helmeted athletes is needed, the general principles of spinal immobilization taught in Prehospital Trauma Life Support (PHTLS) courses are appropriate and need to be followed. If the patient is not wearing any protective equipment, such as padding, helmet, or face mask, he or she should be treated in the same fashion as any other patient undergoing spinal motion restriction. There have been recent changes in recommendations from professional organizations, such as the National Athletic Trainers' Association (NATA) and National Association of State EMS Officials (NAEMSO), regarding the removal of protective equipment.[89,91] If a helmet with a face mask is still in place when the athlete is encountered, careful removal of the face mask should be completed to ensure adequate access to effectively manage the airway.[87-89] The helmet should be removed only when enough trained personnel are available to assist.[87-89] Ideally, the helmet and shoulder pads should be removed as one unit. However, it is still possible to immobilize a player to a long backboard without causing hyperextension of the cervical spine when the helmet alone is removed. This is accomplished by the appropriate use of padding behind the head to maintain the head in neutral alignment with the rest of the spine if the shoulder pads are not removed.

Prehospital care providers must determine the specific medical needs for an injured athlete and take appropriate steps to meet those needs, which may often include immediate removal of the athletic equipment. While some organizations (e.g., NATA) recommend the removal of protective equipment in the field,[89] the decision remains an area of controversy. Regardless of the decision, the methods of spinal motion restriction should be made with careful consideration of how protective athletic equipment may influence the ability to maintain neutral alignment of the spine, how excessive spinal motion can be prevented during transfer and transport, and whether the equipment will restrict the ability to assess or manage the patient in the prehospital environment. Athletic equipment should be removed by personnel trained and experienced in the removal of sports equipment. If the decision is made not to remove the equipment at the scene, someone knowledgeable in sports equipment removal should accompany the patient to the hospital.

the head. The sidepieces should be at least as wide as the patient's ears, or larger, and be at least as high as the level of the patient's eyes with the patient supine. Two straps or pieces of tape surrounding these headpieces draw the sides together. When it is packaged between the blocks or blankets, the head now has a flat posterior surface that can be fixed to a flat device. The upper forehead strap is placed snugly across the front of the lower forehead (across the supraorbital ridge) to help prevent anterior movement of the head. If tape is used, avoid placing it directly onto the eyebrows. This strap should be pulled tightly enough to indent the blocks or blankets and rest firmly on the forehead.

The device, regardless of type, that holds the head also requires a lower strap to help keep the sidepieces firmly pressed against the lower sides of the head and to anchor the device further and prevent anterior movement of the lower head and neck. The lower strap passes around the sidepieces and across the anterior rigid portion of the cervical collar. This strap should not place too much pressure on the front of the collar, which could produce airway compression or a venous return problem at the neck.

Sandbags are not recommended for use as side supports because of the weight that may be placed on the head and neck when the immobilized patient is turned on his or her side.[92] The use of sandbags secured to the long backboard on the sides of the head and neck represents a dangerous practice. Regardless of how well they are secured, these heavy objects can shift and move. Should the need arise to rotate the patient and board to the side, such as when the patient needs to vomit, the combined weight of the sandbags can produce localized lateral pressure against the head and cervical spine, forcing them to move. Raising or lowering the head of the board when moving and loading the patient or any sudden acceleration or deceleration of the ambulance can also produce shifting of the bags and movement of the head and neck.

The use of chin cups or straps encircling the chin prevents opening of the mouth to vomit, so these devices should not be used.

Whatever method of stabilization is chosen, it is essential that the provider recognize that rigid immobilization of the cervical spine with these devices will impede the ability to manipulate the patient's mouth and gain access to his or her airway in a way that would allow for airway protection in the event of decreasing level of consciousness. It also potentially decreases the ability of the patient to protect his or her airway in the event of vomiting or bleeding in the oropharynx. In addition, restrictive supine positioning that often results from spinal motion restriction has been shown to reduce airway patency in unconscious trauma patients when compared to lateral positioning.[93] This results in an increased risk of airway compromise.

The jaw-thrust maneuver results in less motion at unstable cervical injuries when compared with other airway maneuvers.[94] If airway management is required, it is recommended that the jaw-thrust maneuver be performed while a separate provider maintains neutral stabilization of the cervical spine. It is important to remember that the risk of secondary catastrophic neurologic injury in these patients, even with endotracheal intubation using direct laryngoscopy in the presence of an unstable cervical spine,[95] is small, regardless of the presenting signs, symptoms, and mechanism. It is also important to remember that the risk of airway compromise and aspiration in a patient with a decreased level of consciousness who is vomiting or bleeding into his or her oropharynx is real, substantial, and potentially devastating. Never allow the process of immobilization of the cervical spine to result in compromise of the ability to maintain and secure a patient's airway.

Legs

Significant outward rotation of the legs may result in anterior movement of the pelvis and movement of the lower spine; tying the feet together eliminates this possibility. Placing a rolled blanket or piece of padding between the legs will increase comfort for the patient.

The patient's legs are secured to the immobilization device with two or more straps: one strap proximal to the knees at about midthigh and one strap distal to the knees. The average adult measures 14 to 20 inches (35 to 50 cm) from one side to the other at the hips and only 6 to 9 inches (15 to 23 cm) from one side to the other at the ankles. When the feet are placed together, a V shape is formed from the hips to the ankles. Because the ankles are considerably narrower than the device, a strap placed across the lower legs can prevent anterior movement but will not prevent the legs from moving laterally from one edge of the immobilization device to the other. If the device is angled or rotated, the legs will fall to the lower edge of the device, which can angulate the pelvis and produce movement of the spinal column.

One way to hold the patient's lower legs effectively in place is to encircle them several times with the strap before attaching it to the immobilization device. The legs can be kept in the middle of the device by placing blanket rolls between each leg and the edges of the device before strapping. It is important to ensure that the straps are not so tight that they impair distal circulation.

Arms

For safety, the patient's arms may be secured to the device or across the torso before moving the patient. One way to achieve this is with the arms placed at the sides on the device with the palms in, secured by a strap across the forearms and torso. This strap should be snug but not so tight as to compromise the circulation in the hands.

The patient's arms should not be included in the strap at the iliac crests or in the groin loops. If the straps are tight enough to provide adequate immobilization of the lower torso, they can compromise the circulation in the hands. If the straps are loose, they will not provide adequate immobilization of the torso or arms. Use of an additional strap exclusively to hold the arms allows the strap to be opened for taking a blood pressure measurement or starting an intravenous line once the patient is in the ambulance without compromising the immobilization. If the arm strap is also a torso strap, loosening it to free just an arm has the side effect of loosening the torso immobilization as well.

Rapid Extrication Versus Short Device for the Seated Patient

The decision to use a rapid extrication technique over a short device should be based on the clinical presentation of the patient, the findings during the primary survey, and the situation at the scene. If the patient is found to have critical injuries; has airway, breathing, or circulation issues; or is in shock or impending shock, rapid extrication techniques and rapid transport are appropriate. The benefit in rapidly accessing the patient and treating these conditions outweighs the risk of the extrication procedure for these patients. Fortunately, few patients fall into this category. In most stable patients, a short device can be employed.

Most Common Immobilization Mistakes

The following are the most common immobilization errors:

1. Failing to adequately provide spinal motion restriction such that the torso can move significantly up or down on the board device or the head can still move excessively.
2. Improperly sizing or improperly applying the cervical collar.
3. Immobilizing the patient with the head hyperextended. The most common cause is a lack of appropriate padding behind the head.
4. Immobilizing the head before the torso or readjusting the torso straps after the head has been secured. This causes movement of the device relative to the torso, which results in movement of the head and cervical spine.
5. Inadequately padding. Failure to fill the voids under a patient can allow for inadvertent movement of the spine, resulting in additional injury as well as increased discomfort for the patient.
6. Placing someone in spinal immobilization who does not meet immobilization criteria.
7. Taking excessive time to achieve immobilization in the context of a physiologically unstable or potentially unstable patient.
8. Using overly aggressive immobilization techniques that fail to prioritize maintaining and protecting airway integrity.

Complete spinal motion restriction is generally not a comfortable experience for the patient. As the degree and quality of the immobilization increase, the patient's comfort decreases. Spinal immobilization is a balance between the need to protect and immobilize the spine completely, the need to maintain and protect airway access, the need to expeditiously initiate transport, and the need to make it tolerable for the patient. This is why proper evaluation of the need for spinal immobilization is indicated (**Box 9-10**).

Obese Patients

With the increasing number of obese patients, care of the *bariatric* (overweight, obese) patient is becoming more common. Transport of a 400-lb (182-kg) patient is becoming an all-too-common occurrence, and special bariatric transport cots have been developed for this purpose. However, a review of commercially available long backboards shows that most long backboards measure 16 by 72 inches (40 by 183 cm), with a few measuring 18 inches (46 cm) wide. The weight limit for these long backboards varies from 250 lb (113 kg) to 600 lb (272 kg). When using backboards on bariatric trauma patients, special care is needed to ensure that the safe operating limits are not exceeded. Also, additional personnel must be present to help lift and extricate bariatric patients to avoid causing further injury to the patient or prehospital care providers. This subgroup of trauma patients presents the challenge of balancing safe packaging and moving procedures against the short scene times normally recommended for critically injured trauma patients.

Some obese patients may demonstrate an increased work of breathing to the point of respiratory failure if placed supine on a backboard. This phenomenon occurs secondary to the increased pressure being placed on the diaphragm by the adipose tissue of the abdomen. In these cases, the principles of immobilization should still be followed, but the practice may have to be changed. An obese patient with a potential cervical injury may have his or her cervical spine manually maintained by the prehospital care provider's hands and a cervical collar, while the patient is allowed to remain sitting upright on the stretcher during transport. This approach will provide cervical stabilization without causing increased respiratory distress.

Box 9-10 Criteria for Evaluating Immobilization Skills

Prehospital care providers must practice their immobilization skills in hands-on sessions using mock patients before use with real patients. At least one study has shown that appropriate immobilization was not performed in a significant number of patients with potential spinal injury.[81] When practicing or when evaluating new methods or equipment, the following criteria will serve as good tools for measuring how effective the intervention has been at restricting spinal motion:

1. Initiate manual in-line stabilization immediately, and maintain it until it is replaced mechanically.
2. Check neurologic function distally.
3. Apply an effective, properly sized cervical collar.
4. Secure the torso before the head.
5. Prevent movement of the torso up or down the device.
6. Prevent movement of the upper and lower torso left or right on the immobilization device.
7. Ensure ties crossing the chest do not inhibit chest excursion or result in ventilatory compromise.
8. Effectively immobilize the head so that it cannot move in any direction.
9. Provide padding behind the head, if necessary.
10. Maintain the head in a neutral in-line position.

11. Ensure that nothing inhibits or prevents the mouth from being opened and that sufficient access to the airway is present to effectively allow the provider to maintain and protect airway integrity.
12. Immobilize the legs so that they cannot move anteriorly, rotate, or move from side to side, even if the board and patient are rotated to the side.
13. Maintain the pelvis and legs in a neutral in-line position.
14. Ensure that the arms are appropriately secured to the device or torso.
15. Ensure that any ties or straps do not compromise distal circulation in any limb.
16. Reevaluate the patient if bumped, jostled, or in any way moved in a manner that could compromise an unstable spine while the device was being applied.
17. Complete the procedure within an appropriate time frame.
18. Recheck distal neurologic function.

Many methods and variations can meet these objectives. The selection of a specific method and specific equipment should be based on the situation, the patient's condition, and available resources.

Pregnant Patients

Occasionally a pregnant patient will require spinal immobilization. Depending on the gestational age, placing the patient in a fully supine position may cause compression of the inferior vena cava by the gravid uterus, leading to a decrease in venous blood return to the heart, thus decreasing the mother's blood pressure. In these circumstances, the patient should be secured to the backboard using standard techniques. Once secured, the backboard is tipped on an angle to place the patient in a relative left lateral position (left side down with blanket or padding under the right side of the patient sufficient to support this position). This position will move the uterus off of the vena cava, restoring blood pressure (**Figure 9-20**).

Use of Steroids

Steroids are not currently recommended in the hospital or prehospital management of SCI. Several older studies[96] suggested that high doses of the steroid methylprednisolone improve the neurologic outcome of some patients with acute SCIs resulting from blunt trauma when started within 8 hours of the injury.[97-99] SCIs in children or those

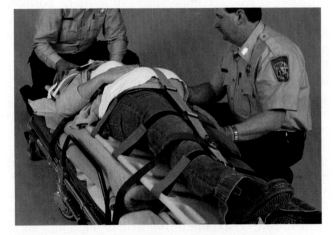

Figure 9-20 Tipping a pregnant female onto her left side helps displace the uterus from the inferior vena cava and improves blood return to the heart, thus restoring blood pressure.
© Jones & Bartlett Learning. Courtesy of MIEMSS.

resulting from penetrating trauma were not studied, and steroids are never indicated for neurologic deficits resulting from stab or gunshot wounds.

Because steroids have known adverse effects, including suppression of adrenal gland and immune functioning and because of concerns regarding the scientific validity of these studies, administration of steroids to patients with SCIs was questioned.[92] In fact, the complications associated with steroid administration may significantly outweigh any benefit, if any, they may confer. Numerous publications no longer recommend steroid use for spinal injury, either in the field or in the hospital.[100-104] In summary, the current medical literature does not support a role for the administration of steroids to the spinal cord–injured patient in the hospital or prehospital setting.[105,106]

Prolonged Transport

As with other injuries, the prolonged transport of patients with suspected or confirmed spine and spinal cord injuries presents special considerations. While backboards may be valuable for transfers over short distances or duration, they should not be used as immobilization devices for periods exceeding 30 minutes. Such efforts should help reduce the risk for the development of pressure ulcers in a patient with SCI. Any areas where there could be pressure on the patient's body, especially over bony prominences, should be sufficiently padded. For transports that will exceed 30 minutes, consideration should be given to using a scoop stretcher to carefully lift a patient, removing the long backboard, and then placing the patient down onto the ambulance cot.

Patients who are immobilized in a supine position are at risk for aspiration should they regurgitate. In the event the patient begins to vomit, the backboard and patient should immediately be tipped onto the side. Suction should be kept near the head of the patient so it is readily accessible should vomiting occur. Insertion of a gastric tube (either nasogastric or orogastric), if allowed, and the judicious use of antiemetic medications may help reduce this risk.

Patients with high SCIs may have involvement of their diaphragm and accessory respiratory muscles (i.e., intercostal muscles), predisposing them to respiratory failure. Impending respiratory failure may be aggravated and hastened by straps placed across the trunk for spinal immobilization that further restrict respiration. Prior to initiating a prolonged transport, providers must double-check that the patient's torso is secured at the shoulder girdle and at the pelvis and that any straps do not limit chest wall excursion.

As described earlier, patients with high SCIs may experience hypotension from loss of sympathetic tone (neurogenic "shock"). Although these patients rarely suffer from widespread hypoperfusion of their tissues, crystalloid boluses are generally sufficient to restore their blood pressure to normal. Vasopressors are rarely, if ever, necessary to treat neurogenic shock. Another hallmark of a high cervical spine injury is bradycardia. If associated with significant hypotension, bradycardia may be treated with intermittent doses of atropine, 0.5 to 1.0 mg administered intravenously.

The presence of tachycardia combined with hypotension should raise suspicion for the presence of hypovolemic (hemorrhagic), rather than neurogenic, shock. Careful assessment may pinpoint the source of hemorrhage, although intra-abdominal sources and pelvic fractures are most likely. Insertion of a urinary catheter will allow urine output to be used as another guide to tissue perfusion. In an adult, a urine output of greater than 30 to 50 milliliters per hour (ml/hour) generally indicates satisfactory end-organ perfusion. The loss of sensation that accompanies an SCI may prevent a conscious patient from perceiving peritonitis or other injuries below the level of the sensory deficit.

Patients with spinal injuries may have significant back pain or pain from associated fractures. Pain may be managed with small doses of intravenous narcotics titrated until pain is relieved. (See the Musculoskeletal Trauma chapter for further details.) Narcotics may exaggerate the hypotension associated with neurogenic shock.

Patients with SCIs lose some ability to regulate body temperature, and this effect is more pronounced with injuries higher in the spinal cord. Thus, these patients are sensitive to the development of hypothermia, especially when they are in a cold environment. Patients should be kept warm (normothermic), but providers must remember that covering them with too many blankets may lead to hyperthermia.

Spine and spinal cord injuries are best managed at facilities that have excellent orthopedic or neurosurgical services and are experienced in the management of these injuries. All level I and II trauma centers should be capable of managing the SCI and any associated injuries. Some facilities that specialize in the management of spine and spinal cord injuries may directly accept a patient who has suffered only an SCI (e.g., a shallow-water diving injury with no evidence of aspiration).

SUMMARY

- The vertebral column is comprised of 24 separate vertebrae plus the sacrum and coccyx stacked on top of one another.
- The major functions of the spinal column are to support the weight of the body and allow movement.
- The spinal cord is enclosed within the vertebral column and is vulnerable to injury from abnormal movement and positioning. When support for the vertebral column has been lost as a result of injury to the vertebrae or to the muscles and ligaments that help hold the spinal column in place, injury to the spinal cord can occur.
- After ensuring provider and scene safety, the primary survey is the first priority. A rapid scene assessment and history of the event should determine if the possibility of a spinal injury exists.
- Mechanism of injury should never be the sole means of determining the need for spinal motion restriction, as it represents only one factor in a multifaceted decision-making process to determine if spinal motion restriction is appropriate. Assessment of the neck and spine for spinal immobilization should also include assessment of motor and sensory function, presence of pain or tenderness, and patient reliability as predictors of SCI.
- Prehospital care providers must be familiar with the devices (e.g., scoop stretchers, vacuum mattresses, rigid cervical collars) and the techniques (e.g., manual in-line stabilization, maintenance of in-line position of the head) used to restrict spinal motion. They must participate in frequent trainings and stay up-to-date on local protocols.
- Special patient populations, including patients who are obese or pregnant, and prolonged transport times may require modifications to standard immobilization practices. The device selected should immobilize the head, chest, and pelvis areas in a neutral in-line position without causing or allowing movement. Dependent on the patient, the severity of the patient's injuries, and the availability of equipment, the technique chosen should be based on the judgment of the prehospital care provider with the guidance of local EMS medical direction. Properly fitting and applying equipment are paramount for the successful immobilization of the trauma patient.

SCENARIO RECAP

You have been dispatched to the scene of a bicyclist who is reported down alongside a roadway. On arrival, the scene is safe, with traffic being controlled by the police. The patient, a young woman, is lying supine on the side of the road away from traffic. A police officer is kneeling beside her and trying to talk to her, but she is not responding.

As you begin your primary survey, you are unable to ascertain the specific cause of the fall. It appears the woman fell from her bike while riding along the roadway, but you do not know whether she was struck by a motor vehicle. The police tell you there were no witnesses. The patient is wearing full cycling gear, including helmet and gloves. She has abrasions on her forehead and an obvious deformity of the right wrist. Her airway is open, and she is breathing regularly. She shows no obvious signs of external blood loss. Her skin appears dry and warm with normal color. As you are performing your primary survey, she begins to awaken but remains confused as to what happened.

- What pathologic processes explain the patient's presentation?
- What immediate interventions and further assessments are needed?
- What are the management goals for this patient?

SCENARIO SOLUTION

The patient's vital signs are as follows: pulse 66 beats/minute, ventilatory rate 14 breaths/minute, and blood pressure 96/70 mm Hg. As you continue your examination, you note that the patient is not moving her arms or legs. The physical findings along with the vital signs are suggestive of neurogenic shock. Interruption of the sympathetic nervous system and unopposed parasympathetic influence on the vascular system below the point of spinal injury result in an increased size of the vascular container and a relative hypovolemia. The patient's response to the spinal cord injury is a low blood pressure and bradycardia.

The first priorities of care are to continue to maintain a patent airway and oxygenation and assist ventilation as necessary to ensure an adequate minute volume while concurrently providing manual stabilization of the cervical spine. You immobilize the patient effectively and efficiently on a spinal motion restriction device and transport her to an appropriate facility 9 minutes away. You manage the hypotension caused by neurogenic shock with two separate 250-ml boluses of intravenous fluids. You splint the fractured arm while en route.

The goals of prehospital management for this patient are to prevent additional spinal cord trauma, maintain tissue perfusion, care for extremity trauma en route, and transport without delay to an appropriate facility for definitive care.

References

1. Ortman JM, Velkoff VA, Hogan H. *An Aging Nation: The Older Population in the United States*. Suitland, MD: US Census Bureau; May 2014:P25-1140.

2. *Spinal Cord Injury: Facts and Figures at a Glance* [SCI data sheet]. Birmingham, AL: National SCI Statistical Center; 2017.

3. Singh A, Tetreault L, Kalsi-Ryan S, Nouri A, Fehlings MG. Global prevalence and incidence of traumatic spinal cord injury. *Clin Epidemiol*. 2014;6:309-331.

4. DeVivo MJ. Causes and costs of spinal cord injury in the United States. *Spinal Cord*. 1997;35:809.

5. Meldon SW, Moettus LN. Thoracolumbar spine fractures: clinical presentation and the effect of altered sensorium and major injury. *J Trauma*. 1995;38:1110.

6. Ross SE, O'Malley KF, DeLong WG, et al. Clinical predictors of unstable cervical spine injury in multiply-injured patients. *Injury*. 1992;23:317.

7. Greenbaum J, Walters N, Levy PD. An evidence-based approach to radiographic assessment of cervical spine injuries in the emergency department. *J Emerg Med*. 2009;36(1):64-71.

8. Stein DM, Knight WA IV. Emergency neurological life support: traumatic spine injury. *Neurocrit Care Soc*. 2017;27:S170-S180.

9. Hu R, Mustard CA, Burns B. Epidemiology of incident spinal fracture in a complete population. *Spine*. 1996;21(4):492-499.

10. Wood KB, Buttermann GR, Phukan R, et al. Operative compared with nonoperative treatment of a thoracolumbar burst fracture without neurological deficit: a prospective randomized study with follow-up at 16 and 22 years. *J Bone Joint Surg Am*. 2015;97:3-9.

11. Wood KB, Buttermann GR, Mehob A, Garvey T, Jhanjee R, Sechriest V. Operative compared with nonoperative treatment of a thoracolumbar burst fracture without neurological deficit: a prospective, randomized study. *J Bone Joint Surg Am*. 2003;85(5):773-781.

12. Adams MA, Dolan P. Spine biomechanics. *J Biomech*. 2005;38(10):1972-1983.

13. Izzo R, Guarnieri G, Guglielmi G, Muto M. Biomechanics of the spine. Part 1: spinal stability. *Eur J Radiol*. 2013;82:118-126.

14. Dreischarf M, Shirazi-Adl A, Arjmand N, Rohlmann A, Schmidt H. Estimation of loads on human lumbar spine: a review of *in vivo* and computational model studies. *J Biomech*. 2016;49:833-845.

15. Oxland TR. Fundamental biomechanics of the spine: what we have learned in the past 25 years and future directions. *J Biomechan*. 2016;49:817-832.

16. Leucht P, Fischer K, Muhr G, Mueller EJ. Epidemiology of traumatic spine fractures. *Injury*. 2009;40:166-172.

17. Lindsey RW, Gugala Z, Pneumaticos SG. Injury to the vertebrae and spinal cord. In: Feliciano DV, Mattox KL, Moore EE, eds. *Trauma*. New York, NY: McGraw Hill; 2008:479-510.

18. Jawa RS, Singer AJ, Rutigliano DN, et al. Spinal fractures in older adult patients admitted after low-level falls: 10-year incidence and outcomes. *J Am Geriatr Soc*. 2017;65(5):909-915.

19. Katsuura Y, Osborn JM, Cason GW. The epidemiology of thoracolumbar trauma: a meta-analysis. *J Orthop*. 2016;13:383-388.

20. Shin JI, Lee NJ, Cho SK. Pediatric cervical spine and spinal cord injury: a national database study. *Spine*. 2016;41(4):283-292.

21. Mohseni S, Talving P, Castelo Branco B, et al. Effect of age on cervical spine injury in pediatric population: a National Trauma Data Bank review. *J Pediatr Surg*. 2011;46:1771-1776.

22. Easter JS, Barkin R, Rosen CL, Ban K. Cervical spine injuries in children, part 1: mechanism of injury, clinical presentation, and imaging. *J Emerg Med*. 2011;41(2):142-150.

23. Patel JC, Tepas JJ III, Mollitt DL, Pieper P. Pediatric cervical spine injuries: defining the disease. *J Pediatr Surg*. 2001;36(2):373-376.

24. Parent S, Mac-Thiong J-M, Roy-Beaudry M, Sosa JF, Labelle H. Spinal cord injury in the pediatric population: a systematic review of the literature. *J Neurotrauma.* 2011;28:1515-1524.

25. Piatt JH Jr. Pediatric spinal injury in the US: epidemiology and disparities. *J Neurosurg Pediatr.* 2015;16:463-471.

26. Tator CH, Fehlings MG. Review of the secondary injury theory of acute spinal cord trauma with special emphasis on vascular mechanisms. *J Neurosurg.* 1991;75:15.

27. Tator CH. Spinal cord syndromes: physiologic and anatomic correlations. In: Menezes AH, Sonntag VKH, eds. *Principles of Spinal Surgery.* New York, NY: McGraw-Hill; 1995.

28. Ahuja CS, Martin AR, Fehlings M. Recent advances in managing a spinal cord injury secondary to trauma. *F1000Res.* 2016;5:ii.

29. Wu C, Fry CH, Henry J. The mode of action of several opioids on cardiac muscle. *Exp Physiol.* 1997;82:261-272.

30. Vale FL, Burns J, Jackson AB, Hadley MN. Combined medical and surgical treatment after acute spinal cord injury: results of a prospective pilot study to assess the merits of aggressive medical resuscitation and blood pressure management. *J Neurosurg.* 1997;87:239-246.

31. Bernhard M, Gries A, Kremer P, Bottiger BW. Spinal cord injury (SCI)—prehospital management. *Resuscitation.* 2005;66:127-139.

32. Section on Disorders of the Spine and Peripheral Nerves of the American Association of Neurologic Surgeons/Congress of Neurologic Surgeons. Blood pressure management after acute spinal cord injury. *Neurosurgery.* 2002;50:S58.

33. Catapano JS, Hawryluk GWJ, Whetstone W, et al. Higher mean arterial pressure values correlate with neurologic improvement in patients with initially complete spinal cord injuries. *World Neurosurg.* 2016;96:72-79.

34. Carrick MM, Leonard J, Slone DS, Mains CW, Bar-Or D. Hypotensive resuscitation among trauma patients. *Biomed Res Int.* 2016;2016:8901938.

35. Catapano JS, Hawryluk GWJ, Whetstone W, et al. Higher mean arterial pressure values correlate with neurologic improvement in patients with initially complete spinal cord injuries. *World Neurosurg.* 2016;96:72-79.

36. Ryken TC, Hurlbert RJ, Hadley MN, et al. The acute cardiopulmonary management of patients with cervical spinal cord injuries. *Neurosurgery.* 2013;72:84-92.

37. Bilello JP, Davis JW, Cunningham MA, et al. Cervical spinal cord injury and the need for cardiovascular intervention. *Arch Surg.* 2003;138:1127.

38. Heffernan DS, Schermer CR, Lu SW. What defines a distracting injury in cervical spine assessment? *J Trauma Inj Infect Crit Care.* 2005;59(6):1396-1399.

39. Cason B, Rostas J, Simmons J, Frotan MA, Brevard SB, Gonzalez RP. Thoracolumbar spine clearance: clinical examination for patients with distracting injuries. *J Trauma Acute Care Surg.* 2015;80(1):125-130.

40. Konstantinidis A, Plurad D, Barmparas G, et al. The presence of nonthoracic distracting injuries does not affect the initial clinical examination of the cervical spine in evaluable blunt trauma patients: a prospective observational study. *J Trauma Inj Infect Crit Care.* 2011;71(3):528-532.

41. Lindborg R, Jambhekar A, Chan V, Laskey D, Rucinski A, Fahoum B. Distracting injury defined: does an isolated hip fracture constitute a distracting injury for clearance of the cervical spine? *Emerg Radiol.* 2018 Feb;25(1):35-39.

42. Young AJ, Wolfe L, Tinkoff G, Duane TM. Assessing incidence and risk factors of cervical spine injury in blunt trauma patients using the National Trauma Data Bank. *Am Surg.* 2015;81:879-883.

43. Hills MW, Deane SA. Head injury and facial injury: is there an increased risk of cervical spine injury. *J Trauma.* 1993; 34(4):549-553.

44. Shekhar H, Kahn S. Cervical spine injuries. *Orthopaed Trauma.* 2016;30(5):390-401.

45. Connell RA, Graham CA, Munro PT. Is spinal immobilization necessary for all patients sustaining isolated penetrating trauma? *Injury.* 2003;34:912.

46. EMS management of patients with potential spine injury. American College of Emergency Physicians website. https://www.acep.org/Clinical—Practice-Management /EMS-Management-of-Patients-with-Potential-Spinal-In jury/#sm.00016r6fxtacmdlozd61o8v0zxwcw. Published 2015. Accessed February 4, 2018.

47. National Association of EMS Physicians and American College of Surgeons Committee on Trauma. EMS spinal precautions and the use of the long backboard, prehospital emergency care. *Prehosp Emerg Care.* 2013;17(3):392-393.

48. Stuke LE, Pons PT, Guy JS, Chapleau WP, Butler FK, McSwain NE. Prehospital spine immobilization for penetrating trauma—review and recommendations from the Prehospital Trauma Life Support Executive Committee. *J Trauma Inj Infect Crit Care.* 2011;71(3):763-770.

49. Haut ER, Kalish BT, Efron DT, et al. Spine immobilization in penetrating trauma: more harm than good? *J Trauma Inj Infect Crit Care.* 2010;68(1):115-121.

50. Abram S, Bulstrode C. Routine spinal immobilization in trauma patients: what are the advantages and disadvantages? *Surgeon.* 2010;8:218-222.

51. Kennedy FR, Gonzales P, Beitler A, et al. Incidence of cervical spine injuries in patients with gunshot wounds to the head. *Southern Med J.* 1994;87:621.

52. Chong CL, Ware DN, Harris JH. Is cervical spine imaging indicated in gunshot wounds to the cranium? *J Trauma.* 1998;44:501.

53. Kaups KL, Davis JW. Patients with gunshot wounds to the head do not require cervical spine immobilization and evaluation. *J Trauma.* 1998;44:865.

54. Lanoix R, Gupta R, Leak L, Pierre J. C-spine injury associated with gunshot wounds to the head: retrospective study and literature review. *J Trauma.* 2000;49:860.

55. Barkana Y, Stein M, Scope A, et al. Prehospital stabilization of the cervical spine for penetrating injuries of the neck: is it necessary? *Injury.* 2003;34:912.

56. Cornwell EE, Chang, DC, Boner JP, et al. Thoracolumbar immobilization for trauma patients with torso gunshot wounds—is it necessary? *Arch Surg.* 2001;136:324.

57. American College of Surgeons Committee on Trauma. *Advanced Trauma Life Support for Doctors.* 9th ed. Chicago, IL: American College of Surgeons; 2012.

58. Stuke LE, Pons PT, Guy JS, Chapleau WP, Butler FK, McSwain NE. Prehospital spine immobilization for penetrating trauma—review and recommendations from the Prehospital Trauma Life Support Executive Committee. *J Trauma.* 2011;71:763.

59. Haut ER, Kalish BT, Efron DT, et al. Spine immobilization in penetrating trauma: more harm than good? *J Trauma.* 2010;68:115-121.

60. Ullrich A, Hendey GW, Geiderman J, et al. Distracting painful injuries associated with cervical spinal injuries in blunt trauma. *Acad Emerg Med*. 2001;8:25.

61. Domeier RM, Evans RW, Swor RA, et al. Prospective validation of out-of-hospital spinal clearance criteria: a preliminary report. *Acad Emerg Med*. 1997;4:643.

62. Domeier RM, Swor RA, Evans RW, et al. Multicenter prospective validation of prehospital clinical spinal clearance criteria. *J Trauma*. 2002;53:744.

63. Hankins DG, Rivera-Rivera EJ, Ornato JP, et al. Spinal immobilization in the field: clinical clearance criteria and implementation. *Prehosp Emerg Care*. 2001;5:88.

64. Stroh G, Braude D. Can an out-of-hospital cervical spine clearance protocol identify all patients with injuries? An argument for selective immobilization. *Ann Emerg Med*. 2001;37:609.

65. Dunn TM, Dalton A, Dorfman T, et al. Are emergency medical technician-basics able to use a selective immobilization of the cervical spine protocol? A preliminary report. *Prehosp Emerg Care*. 2004;8:207.

66. Domeier RM, Frederiksen SM, Welch K. Prospective performance assessment of an out-of-hospital protocol for selective spine immobilization using clinical spine clearance criteria. *Ann Emerg Med*. 2005;46:123.

67. Domeier RM, National Association of EMS Physicians Standards and Practice Committee. Indications for prehospital spinal immobilization. *Prehosp Emerg Care*. 1997;3:251.

68. Kwan I, Bunn F. Effects of prehospital spinal immobilization: a systematic review of randomized trials on healthy subjects. *Prehosp Disast Med*. 2005;20:47.

69. National Association of EMS Physicians and American College of Surgeons Committee on Trauma. Position Statement: EMS spinal precautions and the use of the long backboard. *Prehosp Emerg Care*. 2013;17:392-393.

70. Akkuş Ş, Çorbacıoğlu Ş, Çevik Y, Akinci E, Uzunosmanoğlu H. Effects of spinal immobilization at 20° on respiratory functions. *Am J Emerg Med*. 2016;34:1959-1962.

71. Ham WHW, Shoonhoven L, Schuurmans MJ, Leenen LPH. Pressure ulcer development in trauma patients with suspected spinal injury; the influence of risk factors present in the emergency department. *Int Emerg Nurs*. 2017;30:13-19.

72. Ham WHW, Shoonhoven L, Schuurmans MJ, Leenen LPH. Pressure ulcers, indentation marks and pain from cervical spine immobilization with extrication collars and headblocks: an observational study. *Injury*. 2016;47:1924-1931.

73. Robinson WW, inventor. Scoop stretcher. US patent 2417378. December 28, 1943.

74. Krell JM, McCoy MS, Sparto PJ, Fisher GL, Stoy WA, Hostler DP. Comparison of the Ferno Scoop Stretcher with the long backboard for spinal immobilization. *Prehosp Emerg Care*. 2006;10(1):46-51.

75. Lovell ME, Evans JH. A comparison of the spinal board and the vacuum stretcher, spinal stability and interface pressure. *Injury*. 1994;25(3):179-180.

76. Chan D, Goldberg RM, Mason J, Chan L. Backboard versus mattress splint immobilization: a comparison of symptoms generated. *J Emerg Med*. 1996;14(3):293-298.

77. Johnson DR, Hauswald M, Stockhoff C. Comparison of a vacuum splint device to a rigid backboard for spinal immobilization. *Am J Emerg Med*. 1996;14(4):369-372.

78. Hamilton RS, Pons PT. The efficacy and comfort of full-body vacuum splints for cervical-spine immobilization. *J Emerg Med*. 1996;14(5):553-559.

79. Cross DA, Baskerville J. Comparison of perceived pain with different immobilization techniques. *Prehosp Emerg Care*. 2001;5(3):270-274.

80. Luscombe MD, Williams JL. Comparison of a long spinal board and vacuum mattress for spinal immobilisation. *Emerg Med J*. 2003;20(5):476-478.

81. Ben-Galim P, Dreiangel N, Mattox KL, Reitman CA, Kalantar SB, Hipp JA. Extrication collars can result in abnormal separation between vertebrae in the presence of a dissociative injury. *J Trauma*. 2010;69(2):447-450.

82. Ho AMH, Fung KY, Joynt GM, Karmakar KM, Peng Z. Rigid cervical collar and intracranial pressure of patients with severe head injury. *J Trauma*. 2002;53:1185-1188.

83. Mobbs RJ, Stoodley MA, Fuller JF. Effect of cervical hard collar on intracranial pressure after head injury. *Anz J Surg*. 2002;72:389-391.

84. DeBoer SL, Seaver M. Big head, little body syndrome: what EMS providers need to know. *Emerg Med Serv*. 2004;33:47.

85. Nalliah RP, Anderson IM, Lee MK, Rampa S, Allareddy V, Allareddy V. Epidemiology of hospital-based emergency department visits due to sports injuries. *Pediatr Emerg Care*. 2014;30(8):511-515.

86. UAB Spinal Cord Injury Model System Information Network. The UAB-SCIMS information network. University of Alabama School of Medicine website. www.spinalcord.uab.edu. Accessed February 4, 2018.

87. Puvanesurajah V, Qureshi R, Cancienne JM, Hassanzadeh H. Traumatic sports-related cervical spine injuries. *Trauma Spine Inj*. 2017;30(2):50-56.

88. Banerjee R, Palumbo MA, Fadale PD. Catastrophic cervical spine injuries in the collision sport athlete, part 1: epidemiology, functional anatomy, and diagnosis. *Am J Sports Med*. 2004;32(4):1077-1087.

89. Appropriate care of the spine injured athlete: updated from 1998 document. National Athletic Trainers' Association website. https://www.nata.org/sites/default/files/Executive-Summary-Spine-Injury-updated.pdf. Updated August 5, 2015. Accessed February 4, 2018.

90. Schroeder GD, Vaccaro AR. Cervical spine injuries in the athlete. *J Am Acad Orthop Surg*. 2016;24(9):e122-e133.

91. Response to the National Athletic Trainers Association: appropriate care of the spine injured athlete; inter-association consensus statement. National Association of State EMS Officials website. https://www.nasemso.org/Councils/Medical Directors/documents/NASEMSO-Response-to-NATA-Care-of-Spine-Injured-Athlete.pdf. Published October 27, 2015. Accessed March 4, 2018.

92. Nesathurai S. Steroids and spinal cord injury: revisiting the NASCIS 2 and NASCIS 3 trials. *J Trauma*. 1998;45:1088.

93. Hyldmo PK, Vist GE, Feyling AC, et al. Is the supine position associated with loss of airway patency in unconscious

trauma patients? A systematic review and meta-analysis. *Scan J Trauma Resusc Emerg Med*. 2013;23:50.

94. Prasarn ML, Horodyski EB, Scott NE, Konopka G, Conrad B, Rechtine GR. Motion generated in the unstable upper cervical spine during head tilt–chin lift and jaw thrust maneuvers. *Spine J*. 2014;14:609-614.

95. Hindman BJ, From RP, Fontes RB, et al. Intubation biomechanics: laryngoscope force and cervical spine motion during intubation in cadavers—cadavers vs. patients, the effect of repeated intubations, and the effect of type II odontoid fracture on C1-C2 motion. *Anesthesiology*. 2015;123(5):1042-1058.

96. Hall ED, Springer JE. Neuroprotection and acute spinal cord injury: a reappraisal. *NeuroRx*. 2004;1(1):80-100.

97. Bracken MB, Shepard MJ, Collins WF, et al. A randomized, controlled trial of methylprednisolone or naloxone in the treatment of acute spinal-cord injury. Results of the Second National Acute Spinal Cord Injury Study. *N Engl J Med*. 1997;322(20):1405-1411.

98. Bracken MB, Shepard MJ, Collins WF, et al. Methylprednisolone or naloxone treatment after acute spinal cord injury: 1-year follow-up data. Results of the Second National Acute Spinal Cord Injury Study. *J Neurosurg*. 1992;76(1):23-31.

99. Otani K, Abe H, Kadoya S, et al. Beneficial effect of methyl-prednisolone sodium succinate in the treatment of acute spinal cord injury. *Sekitsui Sekizui J*. 1996;7:633-647.

100. Bledsoe BE, Wesley AK, Salomone JP. High-dose steroids for acute spinal cord injury in emergency medical services. *Prehosp Emerg Care*. 2004;8:313.

101. American College of Surgeons Committee on Trauma. Spine and spinal cord trauma. In: *Advanced Trauma Life Support for Doctors*. Chicago, IL: American College of Surgeons; 2008.

102. Short DJ, El Masry WS, Jones PW. High dose methylprednisolone in the management of acute spinal cord injury—a systematic review from the clinical perspective. *Spinal Cord*. 2000;38:273.

103. Coleman WP, Benzel D, Cahill DW, et al. A critical appraisal of the reporting of the National Acute Spinal Cord Injury Studies (II and III) of methylprednisolone in acute spinal cord injury. *J Spinal Disord*. 2000;13:185.

104. Hurlbert RJ. The role of steroids in acute spinal cord injury: an evidence-based analysis. *Spine*. 2001;26:S39.

105. Bracken MB. Steroids for acute spinal cord injury (review). *Cochrane Database Syst Rev*. 2012.

106. Evaniew N, Noonan VK, Fallah N, et al. Methylprednisolone for the treatment of patients with acute spinal cord injuries: a propensity score-matched cohort study from a Canadian multi-center spinal cord injury registry. *J Neurotrauma*. 2015;32(21):1674-1683.

Suggested Reading

American College of Surgeons Committee on Trauma. *Advanced Trauma Life Support for Doctors, Student Course Manual*. 9th ed. Chicago, IL: American College of Surgeons; 2012.

Pennardt AM, Zehner WJ. Paramedic documentation of indicators for cervical spine injury. *Prehosp Disaster Med*. 1994;9:40.

White CC, Domeier RM, Millin MG; Standards and Clinical Practice Committee, National Association of EMS Physicians. EMS spinal precautions and the use of long backboard—resource document to the position statement of the National Association of EMS Physicians and the American College of Surgeons Committee on Trauma. *Prehosp Emerg Care*. 2014;18(2):306-314.

SPECIFIC SKILLS

Spine Management

These skills are meant to demonstrate the principles of spinal immobilization. The specific preference as to the particular device used will be determined by each agency, jurisdictional medical oversight, and local protocols.

Cervical Collar Sizing and Application

Principle: To select and apply an appropriate-sized cervical collar to assist in providing neutral alignment and stabilization of the patient's head and neck.

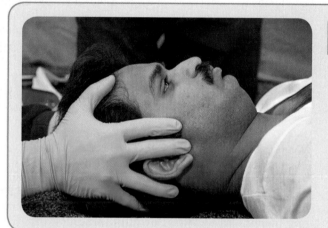

1 The first prehospital care provider provides manual neutral in-line stabilization of the patient's head and neck.

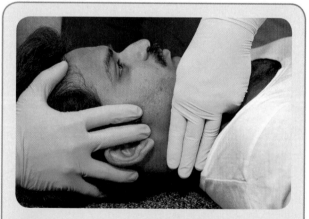

2 The second prehospital care provider uses his or her fingers to measure the patient's neck between the patient's lower jaw and shoulder.

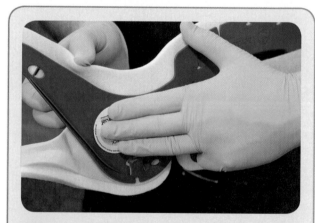

3 The second prehospital care provider uses this measurement to select a properly sized collar or adjust an adjustable collar to the correct size.

Spine Management (*continued*)

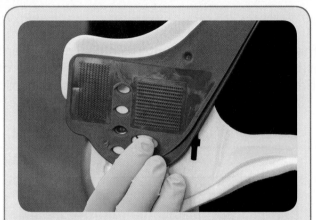

4 If an adjustable collar is utilized, make sure the collar is locked into the proper size.

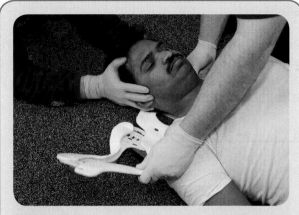

5 The second prehospital care provider applies the properly sized collar, while the first prehospital care provider continues to maintain the neutral in-line head and neck stabilization.

6 After applying and securing the cervical collar, manual in-line stabilization of the head and neck is maintained until the patient is secured to an immobilization device.

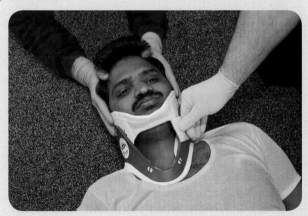

(*continued*)

Logroll

Principle: To turn a patient while maintaining manual stabilization with minimal movement of the spine. The logroll is indicated for (1) positioning a patient onto a long backboard or other device to facilitate movement of the patient and (2) turning a patient with suspected spinal trauma to examine the back.

A. *Supine Patient*

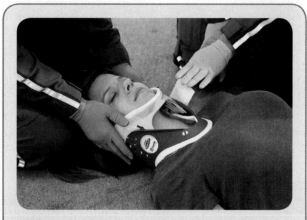

1 While one prehospital care provider maintains neutral in-line stabilization at the patient's head, a second prehospital care provider applies a properly sized cervical collar.

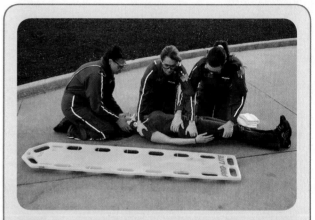

2 While one prehospital care provider maintains neutral in-line stabilization, a second prehospital care provider kneels at the patient's midthorax, and a third prehospital care provider kneels at the level of the patient's knees. The patient's arms are straightened and placed palms-in next to the torso while the patient's legs are brought into neutral alignment. The patient is grasped at the shoulder and hips in such a fashion as to maintain a neutral in-line position of the lower extremities. The patient is "logrolled" slightly onto his or her side.

Spine Management *(continued)*

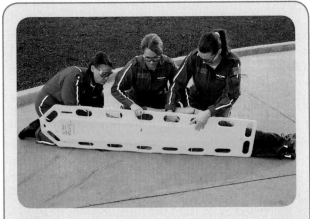

3 The long backboard is placed with the foot end of the board positioned between the patient's knees and ankles (the head of the long backboard will extend beyond the patient's head). The long backboard is held against the patient's back, the patient is logrolled back onto the long backboard, and the board is lowered to the ground with the patient.

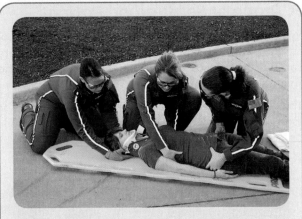

4 Once on the ground, the patient is grasped firmly by the shoulders, the pelvis, and the lower extremities.

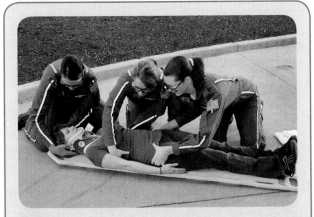

5 The patient is moved upward and laterally onto the long backboard. Neutral in-line stabilization is maintained without pulling on the patient's head and neck.

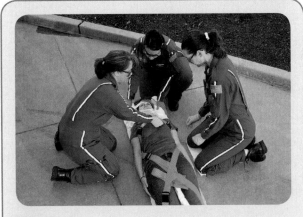

6 The patient is positioned onto the long backboard with the head at the top of the board and the body centered and secured to the device.

(continued)

Spine Management (continued)

B. Prone or Semi-prone Patient

When a patient presents in a prone or semi-prone position, a stabilization method similar to that used for the supine patient can be used. The method incorporates the same initial alignment of the patient's limbs, the same positioning and hand placement of the prehospital care providers, and the same responsibilities for maintaining alignment.

The patient's arms are positioned in anticipation of the full rotation that will occur. When using the semi-prone logroll method, a cervical collar can be safely applied only after the patient is in an in-line position and supine on the long backboard, not before.

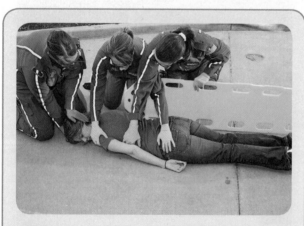

1 Whenever possible, the patient should be rolled away from the direction in which the patient's face initially points. One prehospital care provider establishes in-line manual stabilization of the patient's head and neck. Another prehospital care provider kneels at the patient's thorax and grasps the patient's opposite shoulder and wrist and pelvis area. A third prehospital care provider kneels at the patient's knees and grasps the patient's wrist and pelvis area and lower extremities.

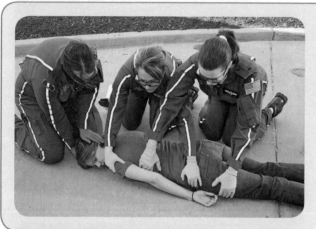

2 The long backboard is placed on the lateral edge and brought into position between the patient and the prehospital care providers.

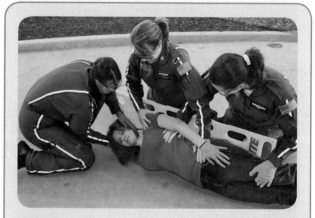

3 The board is placed with the foot of the board between the patient's knees and ankles, and the patient is logrolled onto his or her side. The patient's head rotates less than the torso, so by the time the patient is on his or her side (perpendicular to the ground), the head and torso have come into proper alignment.

Spine Management (continued)

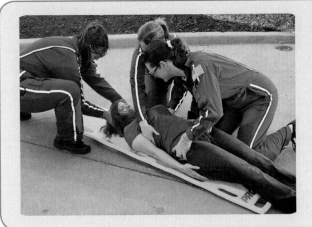

4 Once the patient is supine on the long back-board, the patient is moved upward and toward the center of the board. The prehospital care providers should take care not to pull the patient but to maintain neutral in-line stabilization. Once the patient is positioned properly on the long backboard, a properly sized cervical collar can be applied, and the patient can be secured to the backboard.

© National Association of Emergency Medical Technicians (NAEMT).

Sitting Immobilization (Vest-Type Extrication Device)

Principle: To immobilize a trauma patient without critical injuries before moving the patient from a sitting position.

This type of immobilization is used when spinal stabilization is indicated for a sitting trauma patient without life-threatening conditions. Several brands of vest-type extrication devices are available. Each model is slightly different in design, but any model can serve as a general example. The Kendrick Extrication Device (KED) is used in this demonstration. The details (but not the general sequence) are modified when using a different model or brand of extrication device. Also, during this demonstration, the windshield of the vehicle has been removed for clarification purposes.

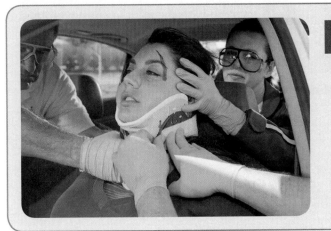

1 Manual in-line stabilization is initiated and a properly sized cervical collar applied.

(continued)

Spine Management (continued)

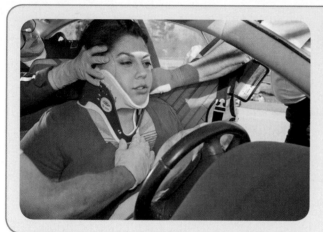

2 The patient is maintained in an upright position slightly forward to provide an adequate amount of space between the patient's back and the vehicle seat for placement of the vest-type device. *Note:* Before placing the vest-type device behind the patient, the two long straps (groin straps) are unfastened and placed behind the vest device.

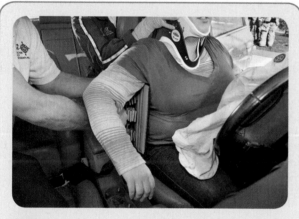

3 After placing the vest device behind the patient, the side flaps are placed around the patient and moved until the side flaps are touching the patient's armpits.

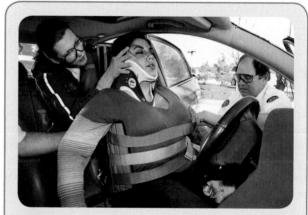

4 The torso straps are positioned and fastened, starting with the middle chest strap and followed by the lower chest strap. Each strap is tightened after attachment. Use of the upper chest strap at this time is optional. If the upper chest strap is used, the prehospital care provider should ensure that it is not so tight that it impedes the patient's ventilations. The upper chest strap should be tightened just before moving the patient.

Spine Management *(continued)*

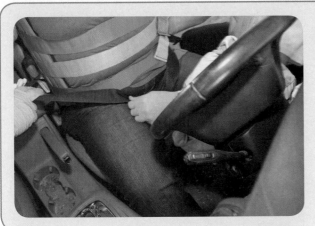

5 Each groin strap is positioned and fastened. Using a back-and-forth motion, each strap is worked under the patient's thigh and buttock until it is in a straight line in the intergluteal fold from front to back. Each groin strap is placed under the patient's leg and attached to the vest on the same side as the strap's origin. Once in place, each groin strap is tightened. The patient's genitalia should not be placed under the straps but to the side of each strap.

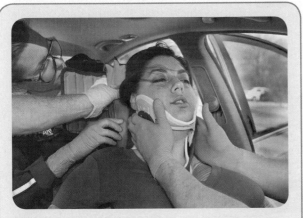

6 Padding is placed between the patient's head and the vest to maintain neutral alignment.

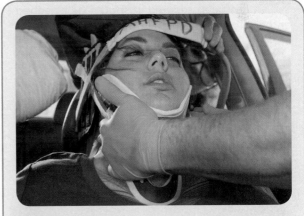

7 The patient's head is secured to the head flaps of the vest device. The prehospital care provider should be careful not to seat the patient's mandible or obstruct the airway. *Note:* The torso straps should be evaluated and readjusted as needed.

(continued)

Spine Management (continued)

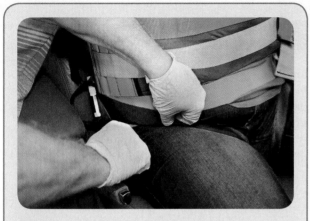

8 All straps should be rechecked before moving the patient. If the upper chest strap has not been secured, it should be attached and tightened.

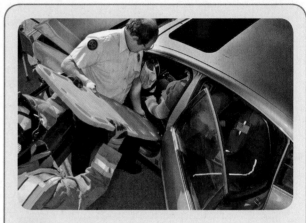

9 If possible, the ambulance cot with a long backboard should be brought to the opening of the vehicle door. The long backboard is placed under the patient's buttocks so that one end is securely supported on the vehicle seat and the other end on the ambulance cot. If the ambulance cot is not available or the terrain will not allow the placement of the cot, other prehospital care providers can hold the long backboard while the patient is rotated and lifted out of the vehicle.

10 While rotating the patient, the patient's lower extremities must be elevated onto the seat. If the vehicle has a center console, the patient's legs should be moved over the console one at a time.

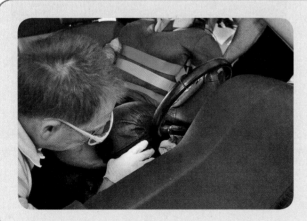

Spine Management (*continued*)

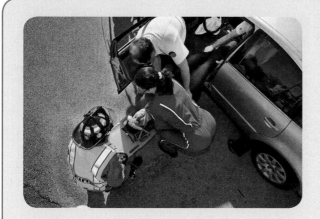

11 Once the patient is rotated with his or her back to the center of the long backboard, the patient is lowered onto the board while keeping the legs elevated. After placing the patient on the long backboard, the two groin straps are released, and the patient's legs are lowered. The patient is positioned by moving him or her up on the board with the vest device in place. The prehospital care provider should consider releasing the upper chest strap at this time.

Once the patient is positioned on the long backboard, the vest device is left secured in place to continue to immobilize the patient's head, neck, and torso. The patient and vest device are secured to the long backboard. The patient's lower extremities are immobilized to the board, and the long backboard is secured to the ambulance cot.

Rapid Extrication

Principle: To manually stabilize a patient with critical injuries before and during movement from a sitting position.

A. *Three or More Prehospital Care Providers*

Sitting patients with life-threatening conditions and indications for spinal immobilization (see Figure 9-12) can be rapidly extricated. Immobilization to an interim device before moving the patient provides more stable immobilization than when using only the manual (rapid extrication) method. However, it requires an additional 4 to 8 minutes to complete. The prehospital care provider will use the vest or short backboard methods when (1) the scene and patient's condition are stable and time is not a primary concern, or (2) a special rescue situation involving substantial lifting or technical rescue hoisting exists and significant movement or carrying of the patient will be needed before it is practical to complete the supine immobilization to a long backboard.

Rapid extrication is indicated in the following situations:

- When the patient has life-threatening conditions identified during the primary survey that cannot be corrected where the patient is found
- When the scene is unsafe and clear danger to the prehospital care provider and patient exists, necessitating rapid removal to a safe location
- When the patient needs to be moved quickly to access other, more seriously injured patients

Note: Rapid extrication is selected only when life-threatening conditions are present and not on the basis of personal preference.

(*continued*)

Spine Management (continued)

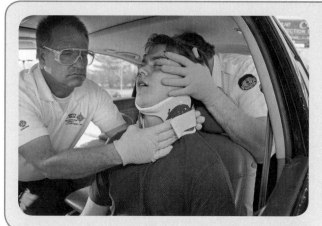

1 Once the decision is made to extricate a patient rapidly, manual in-line stabilization of the patient's head and neck in a neutral position is initiated. This is best accomplished from behind the patient. If a prehospital care provider is unable to get behind the patient, manual stabilization can be accomplished from the side. Whether from behind the patient or the side, the patient's head and neck are brought into a neutral alignment, a rapid assessment of the patient is performed, and a properly sized cervical collar is applied.

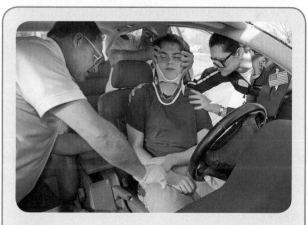

2 While manual stabilization is maintained, the patient's upper torso and lower torso and legs are controlled. The patient is rotated in a series of short, controlled movements.

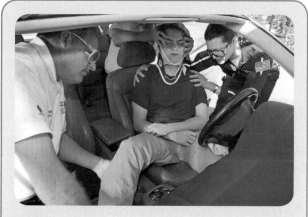

3 If the vehicle has a center console, the patient's legs should be moved one at a time over the console.

Spine Management *(continued)*

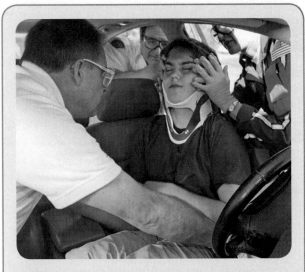

4 The prehospital care provider continues to rotate the patient in short, controlled movements until control of manual stabilization can no longer be maintained from behind and inside the vehicle. A second prehospital care provider assumes manual stabilization from the first prehospital care provider while standing outside of the vehicle.

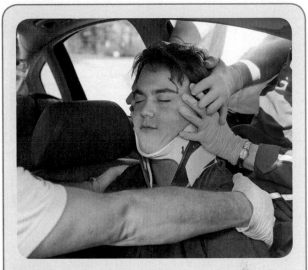

5 The first prehospital care provider can now move outside the vehicle and reassume manual stabilization from the second prehospital care provider.

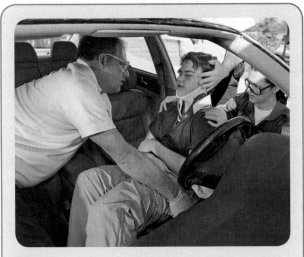

6 The rotation of the patient is continued until the patient can be lowered out of the vehicle door opening and onto the long backboard.

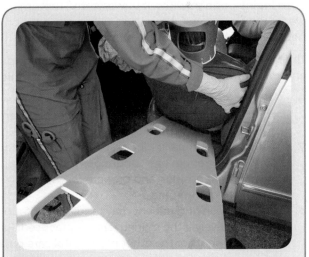

7 The long backboard is placed with the foot end of the board on the vehicle seat and the head end on the ambulance cot. If the cot cannot be placed next to the vehicle, other prehospital care providers can hold the long backboard while the patient is lowered onto it.

(continued)

Spine Management *(continued)*

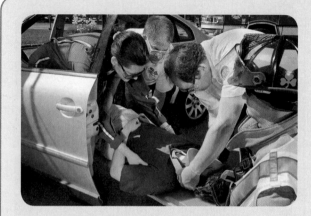

8 Once the patient's torso is down on the board, the weight of the patient's chest is controlled while the patient's pelvis and lower legs are controlled. The patient is moved upward onto the long backboard. The prehospital care provider who is maintaining manual stabilization must be careful not to pull the patient and should continue to support the patient's head and neck.

After the patient is positioned onto the long backboard, the prehospital care providers can secure the patient to the board and the board to the ambulance cot. The patient's upper torso is secured first, then the lower torso and pelvis area, then the head. The patient's legs are secured last. If the scene is unsafe, the patient should be moved to a safe area before being secured to the board or cot.

Note: This procedure represents only one example of rapid extrication. Because few field situations are ideal, prehospital care providers may need to modify the steps for extrication for the particular patient and situation. The principle of rapid extrication should remain the same regardless of the situation: Maintain manual stabilization throughout the extrication process without interruption, and maintain the entire spine in an in-line position without unwarranted movement. Any positioning of the prehospital care providers that works can be successful. However, numerous position changes and hand position takeovers should be avoided because they invite a lapse in manual stabilization.

The rapid extrication technique can effectively provide manual in-line stabilization of the patient's head, neck, and torso throughout a patient's removal from a vehicle. The following are three key points of rapid extrication:

1. One prehospital care provider maintains stabilization of the patient's head and neck at all times, another rotates and stabilizes the patient's upper torso, and a third moves and controls the patient's lower torso, pelvis, and lower extremities.
2. Maintaining manual in-line stabilization of the patient's head and neck is impossible if attempting to move the patient in one continuous motion. The prehospital care providers need to limit each movement, stopping to reposition and prepare for the next move. Undue haste will cause delay and may result in movement of the spine.
3. Each situation and patient may require adaptation of the principles of rapid extrication. This can only work effectively if the maneuvers are practiced. Each prehospital care provider needs to know the actions and movements of the other prehospital care providers.

B. Two Prehospital Care Providers

In some situations, an adequate number of prehospital care providers may not be available to extricate a critical patient rapidly. In these situations, a two-provider technique is useful.

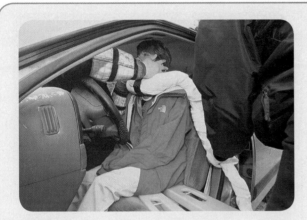

1 One prehospital care provider initiates and maintains manual in-line stabilization of the patient's head and neck. A second prehospital care provider places a properly sized cervical collar on the patient and places a prerolled blanket around the patient. The center of the blanket roll is placed at the patient's midline on the rigid cervical collar. The ends of the blanket roll are wrapped around the cervical collar and placed under the patient's arms.

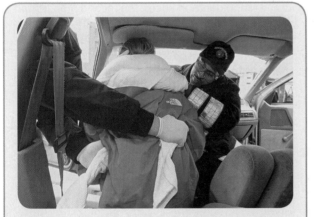

2 The patient is turned using the ends of the blanket roll and until the patient's back is centered on the door opening.

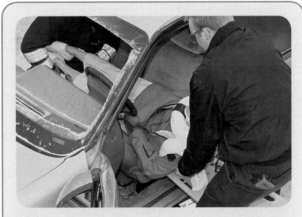

3 The first prehospital care provider takes control of the blanket ends, moving them under the patient's shoulders, and moves the patient by the blanket, while the second prehospital care provider moves and controls the patient's lower torso, pelvis, and legs.

(continued)

Spine Management (continued)

Child Immobilization Device

Principle: To provide spinal immobilization to a child with a suspected spinal injury.

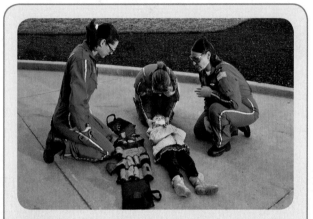

1 The first prehospital care provider kneels above the patient's head and provides manual in-line stabilization of the patient's head and neck. The second prehospital care provider sizes and applies a cervical collar while the first prehospital care provider maintains neutral in-line stabilization. The second prehospital care provider straightens the patient's arms and legs, if needed.

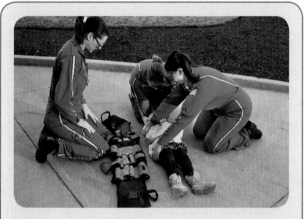

2 The second prehospital care provider now kneels at the patient's side between the shoulders and knees. The second prehospital care provider grasps the patient at the shoulder and hips in such a fashion as to maintain a neutral in-line position of the lower extremities. On command from the first prehospital care provider, the patient is logrolled slightly onto his or her side.

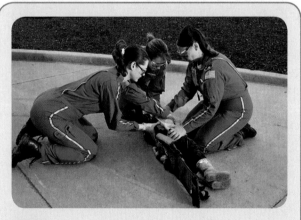

3 A third prehospital care provider positions the immobilization device behind the patient and holds it in place.

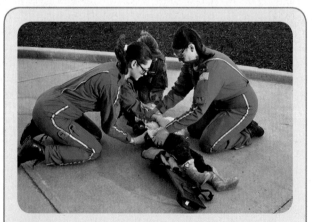

4 The device is held against the patient's back, the patient is logrolled onto the device, and the device is lowered to the ground with the patient.

Spine Management (continued)

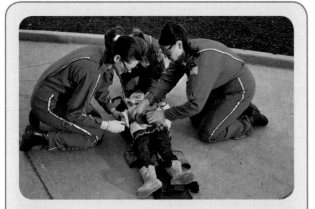

5 The patient is now secured to the immobilization device by the second and third prehospital care provider while the first prehospital care provider maintains head and neck stabilization.

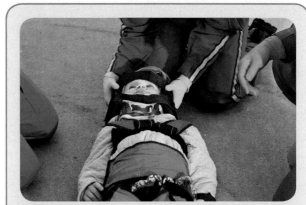

6 After securing the patient's torso and lower extremities to the immobilization device, the patient's head is secured to the immobilization device.

© National Association of Emergency Medical Technicians (NAEMT).

Helmet Removal

Principle: To remove a safety helmet while minimizing the risk of additional injury.

Patients who are wearing full-face helmets must have the helmet removed early in the assessment process. This provides immediate access for the prehospital care provider to assess and manage a patient's airway and ventilatory status. Helmet removal ensures that hidden bleeding is not occurring into the posterior helmet and allows the prehospital care provider to move the head (from the flexed position caused by large helmets) into neutral alignment. It also permits complete assessment of the head and neck in the secondary survey and facilitates spinal immobilization when indicated (see Figure 9-12). The prehospital care provider explains to the patient what will occur. If the patient verbalizes that the prehospital care provider should not remove the helmet, the prehospital care provider will explain that properly trained personnel can remove it by protecting the patient's spine. Two prehospital care providers are required for this maneuver.

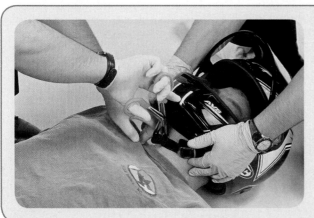

1 One prehospital care provider takes a position above the patient's head. With palms pressed on the sides of the helmet and fingertips curled over the lower margin, the first prehospital care provider stabilizes the helmet, head, and neck in as close to a neutral in-line position as the helmet allows. A second prehospital care provider kneels at the side of the patient, opens or removes the face shield if needed, removes eyeglasses if present, and unfastens or cuts the chin strap.

(continued)

Spine Management *(continued)*

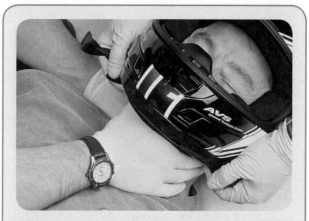

2   The patient's mandible is grasped between the thumb and the first two fingers at the angle of the mandible. The other hand is placed under the patient's neck on the occiput of the skull to take control of manual stabilization. The prehospital care provider's forearms should be resting on the floor or ground or on his or her own thighs for additional support.

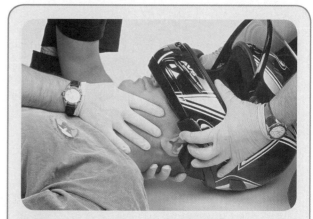

3   The first prehospital care provider pulls the sides of the helmet slightly apart, away from the patient's head, and rotates the helmet with up-and-down rocking motions while pulling it off of the patient's head. Movement of the helmet is slow and deliberate. The prehospital care provider takes care as the helmet clears the patient's nose.

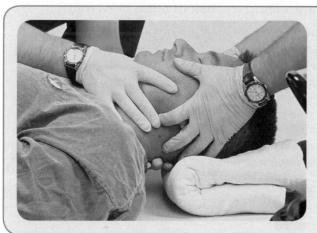

4   Once the helmet is removed, padding should be placed behind the patient's head to maintain a neutral in-line position. Manual stabilization is maintained, and a properly sized cervical collar is placed on the patient.

Note: Two key elements are involved in helmet removal, as follows:

1. While one prehospital care provider maintains manual stabilization of the patient's head and neck, the other prehospital care provider moves. At no time should both prehospital care providers be moving their hands.
2. The prehospital care provider rotates the helmet in different directions, first to clear the patient's nose and then to clear the back of the patient's head.

Spine Management *(continued)*

Vacuum Mattress Application

It is important to take proper care when using a vacuum mattress. Any sharp object on the ground or in the patient's clothes may pierce the mattress, rendering it useless.

The steps involved in applying a vacuum splint may vary from the following steps, depending upon the particular vacuum mattress available. Prehospital care providers should become familiar with the steps specific to the particular device used in their agency.

The prehospital care provider places the vacuum mattress on the lowered stretcher, partially deflated. The valve of the vacuum mattress should be at the head. The plastic balls inside the vacuum mattress should be evenly spread out to form a relatively flat surface.

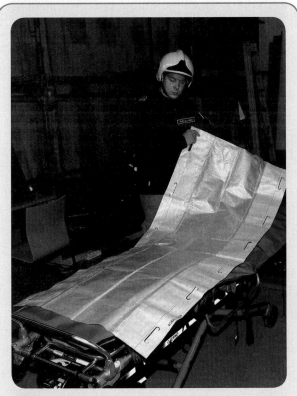

1 A prehospital care provider places a vacuum mattress on a lowered stretcher. The mattress should be deflated partially with the valve of the mattress at the head. The plastic balls inside the mattress should be spread out evenly to form a relatively flat surface. A prehospital care provider then places a sheet on the vacuum mattress.

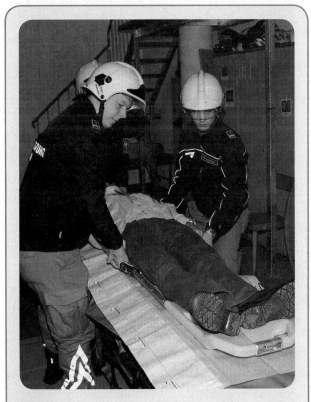

2 A scoop stretcher is used to transfer the patient onto the vacuum mattress.

(continued)

Spine Management (continued)

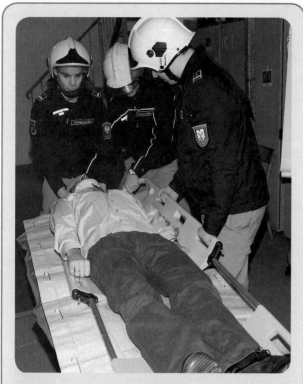

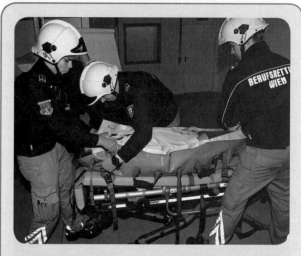

4 The vacuum mattress is molded to the body contours of the patient while one prehospital care provider maintains manual in-line stabilization of the patient's head. Once the mattress is molded to the patient, the valve of the vacuum mattress is opened and suction is applied to deflate the mattress.

3 The scoop stretcher is removed carefully from beneath the patient.

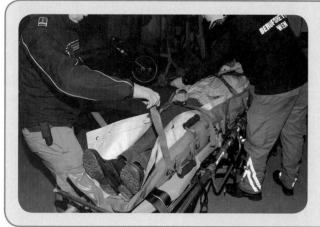

5 Then the valve is closed and the patient secured with belts. A sheet or blanket should be placed over the patient.

CHAPTER 10

© Ralf Hiemisch/Getty Images.

Thoracic Trauma

Lead Editor:
Mark Gestring, MD, FACS

CHAPTER OBJECTIVES   At the completion of this chapter, you will be able to do the following:

- Discuss the normal anatomy and physiology of the thoracic organs.
- Explain the alterations in anatomy and physiology that result from thoracic injury.
- Discuss the relationships among the kinematics of trauma, thoracic anatomy and physiology, and various assessment findings, leading to an index of suspicion for various injuries.
- Differentiate between patients in need of rapid stabilization and transport and patients in whom further on-scene assessment and management are warranted or appropriate.
- Relate the signs, symptoms, pathophysiology, and management of the following specific thoracic injuries:

- Rib fractures
- Flail chest
- Pulmonary contusion
- Pneumothorax (simple, open, and closed)
- Tension pneumothorax
- Hemothorax
- Blunt cardiac injury
- Cardiac tamponade
- Commotio cordis
- Traumatic aortic disruption
- Tracheobronchial disruption
- Traumatic asphyxia
- Diaphragmatic rupture

SCENARIO

You and your partner are dispatched to an industrial construction area for a worker who was struck by a piece of metal. Upon arrival, you are met at the gate by the site safety officer, who leads you to an interior work area. En route to the work area, the safety officer states the patient was helping to install metal studs. When he turned to grab another stud, he ran into the end of a stud his partner had just trimmed, cutting through his shirt and puncturing his chest.

In the work area, you find an approximately 35-year-old man sitting upright on a pile of lumber, leaning forward and holding a rag to the right side of his chest. You ask the patient what happened, and he tries to tell you but has to stop after every five to six words to catch his breath. As you move the rag, you notice an open laceration approximately 2 inches (5 centimeters [cm]) long with a small amount of blood-tinged, "bubbling"

(continued)

fluid. The patient is diaphoretic and has a rapid radial pulse. Decreased breath sounds are noted on the right side with auscultation. No other abnormal physical findings are noted.

- Is this patient in respiratory distress?
- Does he have life-threatening injuries?
- What interventions should you undertake in the field?
- What modality should be used to transport this patient?
- How would a different location (e.g., rural) impact your management and plans during prolonged transport?
- What other injuries do you suspect?

INTRODUCTION

As with other forms of injury, thoracic trauma can result from blunt or penetrating mechanisms. Blunt force applied to the thoracic cage in motor vehicle crashes, high falls, beatings, or crush injuries can cause disruption of the normal anatomy and physiology of the thoracic organs. Similarly, penetrating wounds from firearms, knives, or impalement on objects such as rebar can injure the thorax. Definitive management of most thoracic injuries does not require *thoracotomy* (opening the chest cavity operatively). In fact, only 15% to 20% of all chest injuries require thoracotomy. The remaining 85% are well managed with relatively simple interventions, such as supplemental oxygen, ventilatory support, analgesia, and tube *thoracostomy* (chest tube placement) when necessary.[1-3]

Nevertheless, thoracic injuries can be deadly. The thoracic organs are intimately involved in the maintenance of oxygenation, ventilation, perfusion, and oxygen delivery. Injury to the chest, especially if not promptly recognized and appropriately managed, can lead to significant morbidity. *Hypoxia* (insufficient oxygen in the blood), **hypercarbia** (excessive carbon dioxide in the blood), *acidosis* (excessive acid in the blood), and *shock* (insufficient oxygen reaching the body's organs and tissues) can result from inadequate management of chest injury in the short term and thereby contribute to late complications, such as multisystem organ failure, which accounts for the 25% of trauma deaths that result from thoracic injury.[1-3]

Anatomy

The chest is basically a hollow cylinder formed by its bony and muscular structures. There are 12 paired ribs. The upper 10 pairs attach to the spinal column in the back and either the sternum or the rib above in the front. The lower two pairs of ribs attach only in back to the spine. In the front they are free and thus referred to as "floating ribs." This bony cage provides a great deal of protection to the internal organs of the chest cavity and, thanks to the lower ribs, even shields the organs of the upper abdomen (most notably the spleen and liver). This framework of ribs is reinforced with muscle. The **intercostal muscles** lie between and connect the ribs to one another.

A number of muscle groups move the upper extremity and are part of the chest wall, including the major and minor *pectoral muscles*, anterior and posterior *serratus muscles*, and *latissimus dorsi muscles*, along with the various muscles of the back (**Figure 10-1**). All this "padding" means it takes a considerable amount of force to injure the internal organs.

Also found in the thorax are muscles involved in the process of breathing (ventilation), including the intercostal muscles; the *diaphragm*, which is a dome-shaped muscle attached around the lower aspect of the chest; and muscles in the neck that attach to upper ribs. An artery, vein, and nerve course along the lower edge of each rib and provide blood and stimulation to the intercostal muscles.

Lining the cavity formed by these structures is a thin membrane called the **parietal pleura**. A matching thin membrane covers the two lungs within the chest cavity, called the **visceral pleura**. There is normally no space between these two membranes. In fact, a small amount of fluid between the two membranes holds them together, much as a thin layer of water will hold two sheets of glass together. This pleural fluid creates a surface tension, which opposes the elastic nature of the lungs, preventing their otherwise natural tendency to collapse.

The lungs occupy the right and left sides of the chest cavity (**Figure 10-2**). Between them and enveloped by them is a space called the **mediastinum**, which contains the trachea, the main bronchi, the heart, the major arteries and veins to and from the heart, and the esophagus.

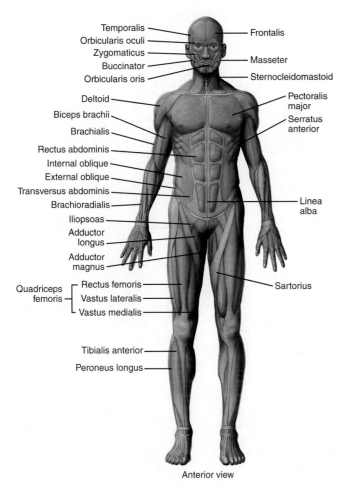

Figure 10-1 The muscular system.

Background image © Carol and Mike Werner/Science Source.

Physiology

The two components of chest physiology that are most likely to be impacted by injury are *breathing* and *circulation*.[1-3] Both processes need to be working properly and in conjunction with one another for oxygen to reach the body's organs, tissues, and ultimately cells and to expel carbon dioxide. To best understand what happens to patients when their chests are injured and how to manage their injuries, it is important to understand the physiology of these two processes.

Ventilation

The lay terms *breathing* and *respiration* actually refer to the physiologic process of ventilation. *Ventilation* is the mechanical act of drawing air through the mouth and nose into the trachea and bronchi and then into the lungs, where it arrives in small air sacs known as *alveoli*. **Respiration** is ventilation plus the delivery of oxygen to the cells. The process of drawing air in is called **inhalation**. Oxygen in the inhaled air is transported across the lining membrane of the alveoli, into adjacent small blood vessels known as **capillaries**, where it attaches to hemoglobin in the red blood cells for transport to the rest of the body. This process is known as **oxygenation**. Simultaneously, carbon dioxide, which is dissolved in the blood, diffuses out into the air within the alveoli for expulsion when that air is blown out again in the process of exhalation (**Figure 10-3**). **Cellular respiration** is the use of oxygen by the cells to produce energy. (See the Shock: Pathophysiology of Life and Death chapter and the Airway and Ventilation chapter.)

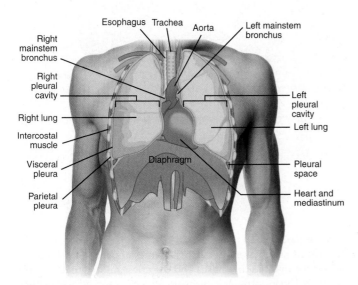

Figure 10-2 The thoracic cavity, including the ribs, intercostal muscles, diaphragm, mediastinum, lungs, heart, great vessels, bronchi, trachea, and esophagus.

© MariyaL/Shutterstock.

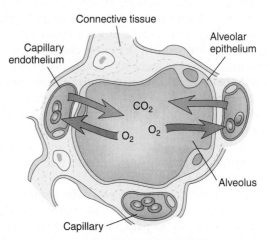

Figure 10-3 The capillaries and alveoli lie in close proximity; therefore, oxygen (O_2) can easily diffuse through the capillary, alveolar walls, capillary walls, and red blood cells. Carbon dioxide (CO_2) can diffuse in the opposite direction.

© National Association of Emergency Medical Technicians (NAEMT).

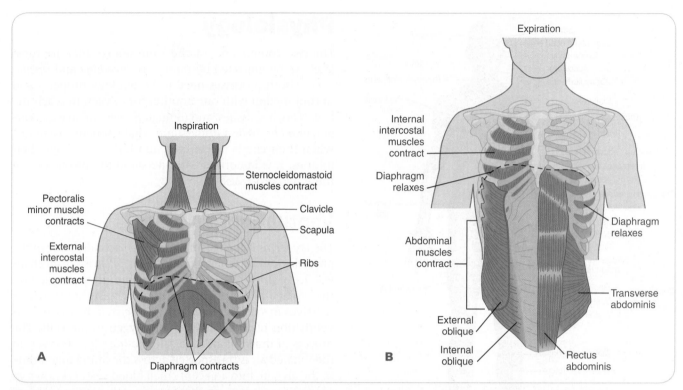

Figure 10-4 **A.** During inspiration, the diaphragm contracts and flattens. Accessory muscles of inspiration—such as the external intercostal, pectoralis minor, and sternocleidomastoid muscles—lift the ribs and sternum, which increases the diameter and volume of the thoracic cavity. **B.** In expiration during quiet breathing, the elasticity of the thoracic cavity causes the diaphragm and ribs to assume their resting positions, which decreases the volume of the thoracic cavity. In expiration during labored breathing, muscles of expiration—such as the internal intercostal and abdominal muscles—contract, causing the volume of the thoracic cavity to decrease more rapidly.

© National Association of Emergency Medical Technicians (NAEMT).

Inhalation is brought about by contraction of the muscles of respiration (primarily the intercostal muscles and the diaphragm), which results in a lifting and separating of the ribs and downward motion of the diaphragm. This action increases the size of the thoracic cavity and creates a negative pressure within the chest compared with the air pressure outside the body. As a result, air flows into the lungs (**Figure 10-4** and **Figure 10-5**). *Expiration* is achieved by relaxing the intercostal muscles and diaphragm, resulting in the return of the ribs and diaphragm to their resting positions. This return causes the pressure within the chest to exceed the pressure outside the body, and air from the lungs is emptied through the bronchi, trachea, mouth, and nose to the outside.

Ventilation is under the control of the respiratory center of the brain stem. The brain stem controls ventilation through monitoring of the partial pressure of arterial carbon dioxide ($Paco_2$) and partial pressure of arterial oxygen (Pao_2) by specialized cells known as **chemoreceptors**. Chemoreceptors are located in the brain stem and in the aorta and carotid arteries. If the chemoreceptors detect increased $Paco_2$, they stimulate the respiratory center to increase

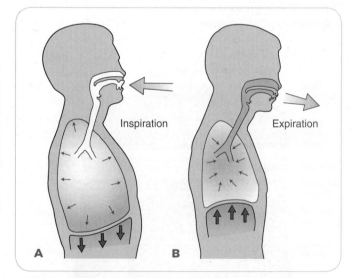

Figure 10-5 When the chest cavity expands during inspiration, the intrathoracic pressure decreases and air goes in the lungs. When the diaphragm relaxes and the chest returns to its resting position, the intrathoracic pressure increases and air is expelled. When the diaphragm is relaxed and the glottis is open, the pressure inside and outside the lungs is equal. **A.** Inspiration. **B.** Expiration.

© National Association of Emergency Medical Technicians (NAEMT).

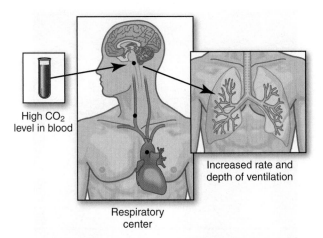

Figure 10-6 An increased level of carbon dioxide is detected by nerve cells sensitive to this change, stimulating the lung to increase both depth and rate of ventilation.
© National Association of Emergency Medical Technicians (NAEMT).

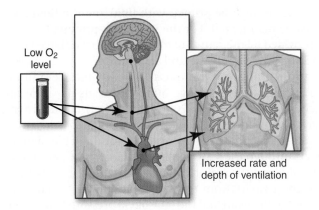

Figure 10-7 Receptors located in the aorta and carotid arteries are sensitive to the blood's oxygen level and will stimulate the lungs to increase air movement into and out of the alveolar sacs.
© National Association of Emergency Medical Technicians (NAEMT).

the depth and frequency of breaths, eliminating more carbon dioxide and returning $Paco_2$ to normal (**Figure 10-6**). This process is very efficient and can increase the volume of air moved in and out of the lungs per minute by a factor of 10. Mechanoreceptors, found in the airways, lungs, and chest wall, measure the degree of stretch in these structures and provide feedback to the brain stem about lung volume.

In certain lung diseases, such as emphysema, or chronic obstructive pulmonary disease (COPD), the lungs are not able to eliminate carbon dioxide as effectively. This results in a chronic elevation of the carbon dioxide level in the blood. The chemoreceptors become insensitive to changes in $Paco_2$. As a result, the chemoreceptors in the aorta and carotid arteries stimulate breathing when the Pao_2 falls. Similar to when the brain stem chemoreceptors detect an increase in $Paco_2$ and stimulate increased respirations to lower the carbon dioxide level, the oxygen chemoreceptors send feedback to the respiratory center that stimulate the respiratory muscles to be more active, increasing the ventilatory rate and depth to raise the Pao_2 to more normal values (**Figure 10-7**). This mechanism is often referred to as "hypoxic drive," as it is related to falling levels of oxygen in the blood.

The concept of the hypoxic drive has led to recommendations to limit the amount of oxygen given to trauma patients with preexisting COPD for fear of suppressing their impetus to breathe. Trauma patients who are hypoxic should never be deprived of supplemental oxygen in the prehospital setting.[4] The true existence of the hypoxic drive remains controversial. If it truly exists, it will not manifest itself in the acute setting.

Box 10-1 defines several terms that are important in discussing and understanding the physiology of ventilation.[5]

Box 10-1 Pulmonary Volumes and Relationships

- *Dead space.* Amount of air brought into the lungs that does not have the opportunity to exchange oxygen and carbon dioxide with the blood in the alveolar capillaries (e.g., air in trachea and bronchi).
- **Minute ventilation** ($\dot{V}$). Total volume of air moved into and out of the lungs in 1 minute.
- **Tidal volume** (*VT*). Amount of air that is inhaled and then exhaled during a normal breath (0.4 to 0.5 liters).
- **Total lung capacity** (*TLC*). Total volume the lungs contain when maximally inflated. This volume declines with age from 6 liters in young adults to approximately 4 liters in elderly persons.
- **Work of breathing**. Physical work or effort performed in moving the chest wall and diaphragm to breathe. This work increases with rapid breathing, increasing minute ventilation, and when the lungs are abnormally stiff.

Circulation

The other major physiologic process that may be affected following thoracic injury is circulation. The following discussion sets the stage for the pathophysiology of chest injury. The Shock: Pathophysiology of Life and Death chapter covers this topic more extensively.

The heart, which lies in the center of the chest within the mediastinum, functions as a biologic pump. For a pump to work, it must be primed with fluid and the fluid level must be maintained. For the heart, this priming function is provided by the return of blood through two large veins, the **superior vena cava** and the **inferior vena cava**. The heart then normally contracts 70 to 80 times per minute on average (normal range 60 to 100 beats per minute), ejecting approximately 70 milliliters (ml) of blood with each beat out to the body through the aorta.

Processes that interfere with the return of blood to the heart through the superior and inferior venae cavae (e.g., loss of blood through hemorrhage, increased pressure in the chest cavity from tension pneumothorax) cause the output of the heart and thus the blood pressure to decrease. Similarly, processes that injure the heart itself (e.g., blunt cardiac injury) may make the heart a less efficient pump, causing the same physiologic abnormalities. Just as chemoreceptors recognize changes in carbon dioxide or oxygen levels, **baroreceptors** located in the arch of the aorta and the carotid sinuses of the carotid arteries recognize changes in blood pressure and direct the heart to change the rate and forcefulness of its beating to return the blood pressure to normal.

Pathophysiology

As mentioned earlier, both blunt and penetrating mechanisms may disrupt the physiologic processes just described. There are common elements in the disturbances created by these mechanisms.

Penetrating Injury

In penetrating injuries, objects of varying sizes and types traverse the chest wall, enter the thoracic cavity, and possibly injure the organs within the thorax. Normally, no space exists between the pleural membranes. However, when a penetrating wound creates a communication between the chest cavity and the outside world, air can enter into the pleural space through the wound during inspiration when the pressure inside the chest is lower than the pressure outside the chest. Air may be further encouraged to enter a wound if the resistance to airflow through the wound is less than that through the airways. Air in the pleural space (**pneumothorax**) disrupts the adherence between the pleural membranes created by the thin film of pleural fluid. Together, these processes allow the lung to collapse, preventing effective ventilation. Penetrating wounds result in an open pneumothorax only when the size of the chest wall defect is large enough that the surrounding tissues do not close the wound at least partially during inspiration and/or expiration.

Wounds of the lung caused by a penetrating object allow air to escape from the lung into the pleural space and result in collapse of the lung. In either case, the patient becomes short of breath. To make up for the lost ventilation

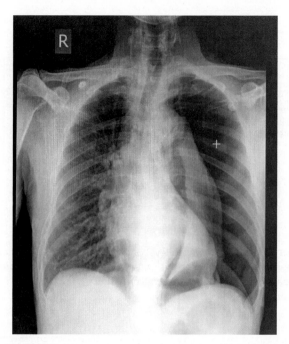

Figure 10-8 An x-ray showing a left tension pneumothorax.
© Noppadon Seesuwan/Shutterstock.

capacity, the respiratory center will stimulate more rapid breathing, increasing the work of breathing. The patient may be able to tolerate the increased workload for a time, but if not recognized and treated, the patient is at risk for ventilatory failure, which will be manifested by increasing respiratory distress as the carbon dioxide levels in the blood rise and the oxygen levels fall.

If there is continued entry of air into the chest cavity without any exit, pressure will begin to build within the pleural space, leading to **tension pneumothorax** (**Figure 10-8**). This condition further impedes the patient's ability to properly ventilate. It will begin to impact circulation negatively as venous return to the heart is reduced by the increasing intrathoracic pressure, and shock may ensue. In extreme cases with displacement of the *mediastinal structures* (organs and vessels located in the middle of the chest between the two lungs) into the opposite side of the chest, venous return is highly compromised, leading to decreased blood pressure and jugular venous distension, and the classic, but late, finding of **tracheal shift** away from the midline toward the uninvolved side of the chest may be detected.

Lacerated tissues and torn blood vessels bleed. Penetrating wounds to the chest may result in bleeding into the pleural space (**hemothorax**) from the chest wall muscles, the intercostal vessels, and the lungs (**Figure 10-9**). Penetrating wounds to the major vessels in the chest result in catastrophic bleeding. Each pleural space can accommodate approximately 3,000 ml of fluid. Thoracic bleeding into the pleural space may not be readily apparent externally, but it may be of sufficient magnitude to create a shock state. The presence of large volumes of blood in the pleural space

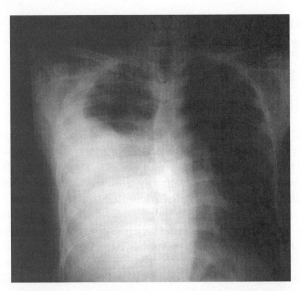

Figure 10-9 An x-ray showing a right hemothorax.
© Medicshots/Alamy Stock Photo.

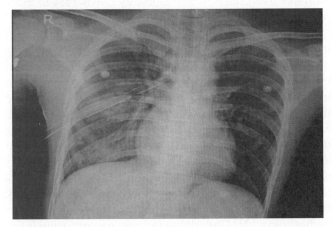

Figure 10-10 An x-ray showing a right pulmonary contusion.
© Richman Photo/Shutterstock.

will impede the patient's ability to breathe; the blood in the pleural space prevents expansion of the lung on that side. It is not uncommon for an injury to the lung to result in both a hemothorax and a pneumothorax, termed a *hemopneumothorax*. A hemopneumothorax results in collapse of the lung and impaired ventilation from both the air in the pleural space and the accumulation of blood in the thoracic cavity.

Wounds of the lung may also result in bleeding into the lung tissue itself. This blood floods the alveoli, preventing them from filling with air. Alveoli filled with blood cannot participate in gas exchange. The more alveoli that are flooded, the more the patient's ventilation and oxygenation may be compromised.

Blunt Force Injury

Blunt force applied to the chest wall is transmitted through the chest wall to the thoracic organs, especially the lungs.

This wave of energy can tear lung tissue, which may result in bleeding into the alveoli. In this setting, the injury is called a **pulmonary contusion** (**Figure 10-10**). A pulmonary contusion is essentially a bruise of the lung. It can be made worse by fluid resuscitation. The impact on oxygenation and ventilation is the same as with penetrating injury.

If the force applied to the lung tissue also tears the visceral pleura, air may escape from the lung into the pleural space, creating a pneumothorax and the potential for a tension pneumothorax, as previously described. Blunt force trauma to the chest can also break ribs, which can then lacerate the lung, resulting in pneumothorax as well as hemothorax (both caused by bleeding from the broken ribs and from the torn lung and intercostal muscles). Blunt force injury typically associated with sudden deceleration incidents may cause shearing or rupture of the major blood vessels in the chest, particularly the aorta, leading to catastrophic hemorrhage. Finally, in some cases, blunt force can disrupt the chest wall, leading to instability of the chest wall and compromise of the changes in intrathoracic pressure, leading to impaired ventilation.

Assessment

As in all aspects of medical care, assessment involves taking a history and performing a physical examination. In trauma situations, we speak of a **SAMPLE history**, in which the patient's symptoms, age and allergies, medications, past history, time of the last meal, and events surrounding the injury are elucidated (see the Patient Assessment and Management chapter).[6]

Besides the overall mechanism that resulted in injury, patients are asked about any symptoms they may be experiencing if they are conscious and able to communicate. Victims of chest trauma will likely be experiencing chest pain, which may be sharp, stabbing, or constricting. Frequently, the pain is worse with respiratory efforts or movement. The patient may report a sense of being short of breath or being unable to take in an adequate breath. The patient may feel apprehensive or light-headed if shock is developing. It is important to remember that the absence of symptoms does not equal to the absence of injury.

The next step in assessment is the performance of a physical examination. There are four components to the physical examination: observation, palpation, percussion, and auscultation. The assessment should also include a determination of vital signs. Placement of a pulse oximeter to assess arterial oxygen saturation is a useful adjunct in the assessment of the injured patient.[6,7]

- *Observation.* The patient is observed for pallor of the skin and sweating, which may indicate the presence of shock. The patient may also appear apprehensive. The presence of **cyanosis** (bluish discoloration of skin, especially around the mouth and lips) may be evident in advanced hypoxia. The frequency of respirations and whether the patient appears to be having trouble breathing (gasping, contractions of the accessory muscles of respiration in the neck, nasal flaring) should be noted. Is the trachea in the midline, or deviated to one side or the other? Are the jugular veins distended? The chest is examined for contusions, abrasions, lacerations, and whether the chest wall expands symmetrically with breathing. Does any portion of the chest wall move paradoxically with respiration? (That is, instead of moving out during inspiration, does it collapse inward, and vice versa during exhalation?) If any wounds are identified, they are carefully examined to see if they are bubbling air as the patient breathes in and out.

- *Auscultation.* The entire chest is evaluated. Decreased breath sounds on one side compared to the other may indicate pneumothorax or hemothorax on the examined side. Pulmonary contusions may result in abnormal breath sounds (crackles). Although often difficult to discern in the field, muffled heart sounds from blood collecting around the heart and murmurs from valvular damage may also be noted on auscultation of the heart.
- *Palpation.* By gently pressing the chest wall with hands and fingers, assessment for the presence of tenderness, crepitus (either bony or **subcutaneous emphysema**), and bony instability of the chest wall is performed.
- *Percussion.* This examination technique is difficult to perform in the field because the environment is often noisy, making evaluation of the percussion note difficult. In addition, there is little additional information to be obtained from percussion that will change the prehospital management.
- *Pulse oximetry.* The level of oxygen bound to hemoglobin should be assessed and monitored to detect changes in the patient's condition and responses to therapy. The oxygen saturation should be maintained at 94% or greater.
- *Waveform capnography.* Whether by sidestream assessment with a nasal probe, by mask, or by in-line assessment in an intubated patient, capnography (end-tidal carbon dioxide) is used to assess the level of carbon dioxide in expired air and is monitored to detect changes in the patient's condition and responses to therapy. In-line sampling measures the end-tidal carbon dioxide directly at the point of sampling, whereas sidestream assessment takes a sample of expired air and performs the carbon dioxide determination at the monitor location, which is remote from the sampling site.

Repeat determinations of the ventilatory rate during patient reassessment may be the most important assessment tool in recognizing that a patient is deteriorating. As patients become hypoxic and compromised, an early clue to this change is a gradual increase in the ventilatory rate.

Assessment and Management of Specific Injuries

Rib Fractures

Rib fractures are commonly encountered by prehospital care providers and are present in approximately 10% of all trauma patients.[8] Several factors have been shown to contribute to the morbidity and mortality of patients with multiple rib fractures, including total number of ribs fractured, the presence of bilateral fractures, and increased age (65 years or older).[9] The elderly are especially susceptible to rib fractures, likely due to loss of cortical bone mass (osteoporosis), which allows the ribs to fracture after sustaining less kinetic force. Regardless of age, mortality increases as more ribs are fractured. The mortality rate for a single rib fracture is 5.8%, increasing to 10% in those with five fractured ribs. The mortality rate is 34% in those with eight rib fractures.[10,11]

Despite the ribs being fairly well protected by overlying musculature, rib fractures are a common occurrence in thoracic trauma. The upper ribs are broad, thick, and particularly well protected by the shoulder girdle and muscles.[1-3] Because it requires great energy to fracture the upper ribs, patients with upper rib fractures are at risk for harboring other significant injuries, such as traumatic disruption of the aorta. Rib fractures occur most often in ribs 4 to 8 laterally, where they are thin and have less overlying musculature. The broken ends of the ribs may tear muscle, lung, and blood vessels, with the possibility of an associated pulmonary contusion, pneumothorax, or hemothorax.[1,3,12] Underlying pulmonary contusion is the most commonly associated injury seen with multiple rib fractures. Compression of the lung may rupture the alveoli and lead to pneumothorax, as discussed previously. Fracture of the lower ribs[12-14] may be associated with injuries of the spleen and liver and may indicate the potential for other intra-abdominal injuries. These injuries may present with signs of blood loss or shock.[1,3,12]

Assessment

Patients with simple rib fractures will most often complain of chest pain with breathing or movement and difficulty breathing. They may have labored respirations. Careful palpation of the chest wall will usually reveal point tenderness directly over the site of the rib fracture, and crepitus may be felt as the broken ends of the rib grind against each other. The prehospital care provider assesses vital signs, paying particular attention to the ventilatory rate and depth of breathing. Pulse oximetry also should be performed, as well as capnography if available.[1,15,16]

Management

Pain relief is a primary goal in the initial management of patients with rib fractures. This may involve reassurance and positioning of the patient's arms using a sling and swath. It is important to reassure and continuously reassess the patient, keeping in mind the potential for deterioration in ventilation and the development of shock. Establishing intravenous (IV) access should be considered, depending on the patient's condition and anticipated transport time. Administration of IV analgesics may be appropriate in some situations for advanced units with appropriate protocols and medical control and in situations where the pain from the rib fractures is impeding the patient's ability to breathe effectively. The patient is encouraged to take deep breaths and cough to prevent the collapse of the alveoli (**atelectasis**) and the potential for pneumonia and other complications. Rigid immobilization of the rib cage with tape or straps should be avoided because these interventions predispose to the development of atelectasis and pneumonia.[1,3] Administering supplemental oxygen and assisting ventilations may be necessary to ensure adequate oxygenation.

Flail Chest

Flail chest occurs when two or more adjacent ribs are fractured in more than one place along their length. The result is a segment of chest wall that is no longer in continuity with the remainder of the chest. When the respiratory muscles contract to raise the ribs up and out and lower the diaphragm, the flail segment paradoxically moves inward in response to the negative pressure being created within the thoracic cavity (**Figure 10-11**). Similarly, when these muscles relax, the segment may move outward as pressure inside the chest increases. This paradoxical motion of the flail segment makes ventilation less efficient. The degree of inefficiency is directly related to the size of the flail segment.

The significant force necessary to produce such a lesion is generally transmitted to the underlying lung, resulting in a pulmonary contusion. The patient thus may have two mechanisms to compromise ventilation and gas exchange, the flail segment and the underlying pulmonary contusion (which is the bigger problem when it comes to compromising ventilation). As described earlier, the pulmonary contusion does not allow for gas exchange in the contused portion of the lung because of alveolar flooding with blood.

Assessment

As with a simple rib fracture, assessment of flail chest will reveal a patient in pain. The pain is typically more severe,

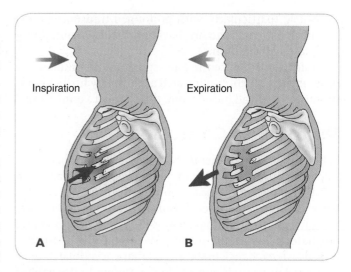

Figure 10-11 Paradoxical motion. **A.** If stability of the chest wall has been lost by ribs fractured in two or more places, as intrathoracic pressure decreases during inspiration, the external air pressure forces the chest wall inward. **B.** When intrathoracic pressure increases during expiration, the chest wall is forced outward.

© National Association of Emergency Medical Technicians (NAEMT).

however, and the patient usually appears to be in distress. The ventilatory rate is elevated, and the patient does not take deep breaths because of the pain. Hypoxia may be present, as demonstrated by pulse oximetry or cyanosis. Paradoxical motion may or may not be evident or easily recognized. Initially, the intercostal muscles will be in spasm and tend to stabilize the flail segment. As these muscles fatigue over time, the paradoxical motion becomes increasingly evident. The patient will have tenderness and potentially bony crepitus over the injured segment. The instability of the segment may also be appreciated on palpation.

Management

Management of flail chest is directed toward pain relief, ventilatory support, and monitoring for deterioration. The ventilatory rate may be the most important parameter to follow and carefully measure. Patients who are developing underlying pulmonary contusion and respiratory compromise will demonstrate an increase in their ventilatory rate over time. Pulse oximetry, if available, is also useful to detect hypoxia.[7] Oxygen should be administered to ensure an oxygen saturation of at least 94%.

IV access may be obtained, except in cases of extremely short transport times. Narcotic analgesics may be carefully titrated to provide pain relief.

Support of ventilation with bag-mask device assistance, continuous positive airway pressure (CPAP), or endotracheal intubation and positive-pressure ventilation may be necessary (particularly with prolonged transport times) for those patients who are having difficulty maintaining adequate oxygenation.[15]

Efforts to stabilize the flail segment with sandbags or other means are contraindicated as they may further compromise chest wall motion and, thus, impair ventilations.[1]

Pulmonary Contusion

When lung tissue is lacerated or torn by blunt or penetrating mechanisms, bleeding into the alveolar air spaces can result in *pulmonary contusion*. As the alveoli fill with blood, gas exchange is impaired because air cannot enter these alveoli from the terminal airways. In addition, blood and edematous fluid in the tissue between the alveoli further impede gas exchange in the alveoli that are ventilated. Pulmonary contusion is almost always present in the patient with a flail segment and is a common—and potentially lethal—complication of thoracic injury.[3,12] Deterioration to the point of respiratory failure may occur over the first 24 hours after injury.

Assessment

Assessment findings of the patient are variable depending on the severity of the contusion (percentage of involved lung). Early assessment typically reveals no respiratory compromise. As the contusion progresses, the ventilatory rate will increase and rales may be heard on auscultation. In fact, a rising ventilatory rate is often the earliest clue that a patient is deteriorating from a pulmonary contusion. A high index of suspicion is necessary, particularly in the presence of a flail segment.

Management

Management is directed toward support of ventilation. The prehospital care provider should repeatedly reassess the ventilatory rate and any signs of respiratory distress. Continuous pulse oximetry and capnography, if available, should be utilized. Supplemental oxygen should be provided to all patients with suspected pulmonary contusion with a goal of maintaining oxygen saturation in the normal range (≥ 94%). CPAP can be used to improve oxygenation in patients in whom supplemental oxygen alone proves to be inadequate for maintaining acceptable oxygen saturation levels.[17] Support of ventilation with a bag-mask device or endotracheal intubation may be necessary.[16]

In the absence of hypotension (systolic blood pressure less than 90 millimeters of mercury [mm Hg]), aggressive IV fluid administration may further increase edema and compromise ventilation and oxygenation. Instead, IV fluids should be administered judiciously and only as necessary to maintain blood pressure greater than 80 mm Hg. Pulmonary contusion is another example in which fluid resuscitation may worsen outcome and therefore must be balanced with the patient's need to maintain a blood pressure of at least 80 mm Hg. (See the Shock: Pathophysiology of Life and Death chapter.)

Pneumothorax

Pneumothorax is present in up to 20% of severe chest injuries.[10] The three types of pneumothoraces represent increasing levels of severity: simple, open, and tension.

Simple pneumothorax is the presence of air within the pleural space. As the amount of air in the pleural space increases, the lung on that side collapses (**Figure 10-12**). **Open pneumothorax** ("sucking chest wound") involves a pneumothorax associated with a defect in the chest wall that allows air to enter and exit the pleural space from the outside with ventilatory effort. *Tension pneumothorax* occurs when air continues to enter and is trapped in the pleural space with gradual increase in intrathoracic pressure. This leads to a shift of the mediastinum and results in decreased venous blood return to the heart and compromised circulatory function.

Simple Pneumothorax

Assessment

Assessment in simple pneumothorax is likely to demonstrate findings similar to those in patients with a rib fracture. The patient frequently complains of pleuritic chest pain (pain while breathing) and shortness of breath that may vary from mild to severe and may exhibit varying symptoms and signs of respiratory dysfunction. The classic findings are decreased breath sounds on the side of injury. Any patient with respiratory distress and diminished breath sounds should be assumed to have a pneumothorax.

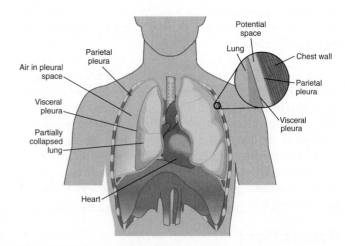

Figure 10-12 Air in the pleural space forces the lung in, decreasing the amount that can be ventilated and, therefore, decreasing oxygenation of the blood leaving the lung.

© National Association of Emergency Medical Technicians (NAEMT).

Management

The prehospital care provider administers supplemental oxygen, obtains IV access, and prepares to treat shock if it develops. Monitoring of pulse oximetry and waveform capnography, if available, is essential to expectant management of the patient in order to detect early signs of respiratory deterioration.[10-14,18,19] If spinal immobilization is not necessary, the patient may be more comfortable in a semi-recumbent position. Rapid transport is essential.[14,16,18] If the prehospital care provider is functioning at the basic level and transport time will be prolonged, rendezvous with an advanced life support (ALS) unit should be considered.

A key point in management is the recognition that a simple pneumothorax may quickly evolve into a tension pneumothorax. The patient needs to be continuously monitored for the development of tension pneumothorax so that timely intervention can occur before there is a serious compromise of circulation.

Open Pneumothorax

Open pneumothorax, as with simple pneumothorax, involves air entering the pleural space, causing the lung to collapse. A defect in the chest wall that results in a communication between the outside air and the pleural space is the hallmark of an open pneumothorax. Mechanisms leading to open pneumothorax include gunshot wounds, shotgun blasts, stabbings, impalements, and (rarely) blunt trauma. When the patient attempts to inhale, air crosses the open wound and enters the pleural space because of the negative pressure created in the thoracic cavity as the muscles of respiration contract. In larger wounds, there may be free flow of air in and out of the pleural space with the different phases of respiration (**Figure 10-13**). Audible

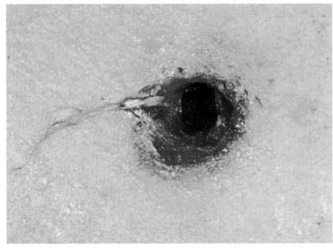

Figure 10-13 A gunshot or stab wound to the chest produces a hole in the chest wall through which air can flow both into and out of the pleural cavity.

Courtesy Norman McSwain, MD, FACS, NREMT-P.

noise is often created as air travels into and out of the hole in the chest wall; thus, this wound has been referred to as a "sucking chest wound."

Because airflow follows the path of least resistance, this abnormal airflow through the chest wall may occur preferentially to the normal flow through the upper airway and trachea into the lung, especially if the open defect is similar or larger in size than the glottic opening to the lower airway. Resistance to the flow of air through a wound decreases as the defect size increases. Effective ventilation is then inhibited both by the collapse of the lung on the injured side and with the preferential flow of air into the pleural space through the wound rather than via the trachea into the alveoli of the lung. Though the patient is breathing, oxygen is prevented from entering the circulatory system.

Assessment

Assessment of the patient with open pneumothorax generally reveals obvious respiratory distress. The patient will typically be anxious and tachypneic (breathing rapidly). The pulse rate will be elevated and potentially thready. Examination of the chest wall will reveal the wound, which may make audible sucking sounds during inspiration, with bubbling during expiration.

Management

Initial management of an open pneumothorax involves sealing the defect in the chest wall and administering supplemental oxygen. Airflow through the wound into the pleural cavity is prevented by applying an occlusive dressing; using a commercial product such as the Halo, Asherman, or Bolin chest seals; or using improvised methods, such as application of aluminum foil or plastic wrap (unlike plain gauze, these materials do not allow airflow through them). Petroleum gauze is a viable option if a commercial device is not available.

A patient with an open pneumothorax virtually always has an injury to the underlying lung, allowing for two sources of air leak, the first being the hole in the chest wall and the second being the hole in the lung. Even if an injury to the chest wall is sealed with an occlusive dressing, air leakage into the pleural space can continue from the injured lung, setting the stage for the development of a tension pneumothorax (**Figure 10-14**).

The traditional teaching has been that for an open pneumothorax, the occlusive dressing is secured on three sides.[1] This prevents airflow into the chest cavity during inspiration while allowing air to escape through the loose side of the dressing during exhalation and, hopefully, preventing the development of a tension pneumothorax (**Figure 10-15**). In contrast, taping the occlusive dressing on all four sides has been advocated as preferable to taping only on three sides; however, no definitive answer to this issue has been determined.

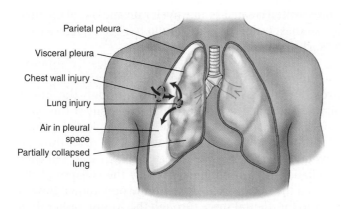

Parietal pleura
Visceral pleura
Chest wall injury
Lung injury
Air in pleural space
Partially collapsed lung

Figure 10-14 Because of the proximity of the chest wall to the lung, it would be extremely difficult for the chest wall to be injured by penetrating trauma and the lung not to be injured. Stopping the hole in the chest wall does not necessarily decrease air leakage into the pleural space; leakage can also come from the lung.

© National Association of Emergency Medical Technicians (NAEMT).

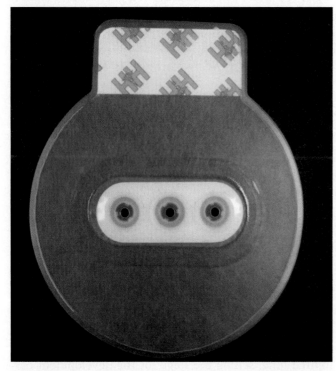

Figure 10-15 Vented chest seals have been shown in animal studies to prevent the development of tension pneumothorax after sealing of an open chest wound.

Courtesy of H & H Medical Corporation.

A study in animals compared the physiologic response of an open pneumothorax that has been completely sealed with a commercial unvented occlusive dressing to the response in those cases sealed with a vented dressing.[20] This study showed that both seals improved the respiratory

physiology associated with an open pneumothorax; however, the vented seal prevented the development of tension pneumothorax, which the unvented seal did not. This finding has led the military's Committee on Tactical Combat Casualty Care to recommend that, if available, a vented chest seal is preferred over an unvented chest seal.[21] An unvented chest seal is an acceptable alternative if the vented type is not available; however, the patient must be carefully observed for the subsequent development of a tension pneumothorax.

In view of the research, Prehospital Trauma Life Support (PHTLS) now recommends the following approach to the management of an open pneumothorax:

- Place a vented chest seal over the open chest wound.
- If a vented seal is not available, place a plastic or foil square over the wound and tape on three sides.
- If none of these are available, an unvented chest seal or a material such as petroleum gauze that prevents ingress and egress of air may be used; however, this approach may allow the development of tension pneumothorax, so the patient must be observed carefully for signs of deterioration.
- If the patient develops tachycardia, tachypnea, or other indications of respiratory distress, remove the dressing for a few seconds, and assist ventilations as necessary.
- If respiratory distress continues, assume the development of a tension pneumothorax, and perform a needle thoracostomy using a large-bore (10- to 16-gauge) needle that is 3.5 inches (8 cm) in length in the second intercostal space at the midclavicular line or in the fifth intercostal space along the anterior axillary line.

If these measures fail to support the patient adequately, endotracheal intubation and positive-pressure ventilation may be necessary.[15] If positive pressure is utilized and a dressing has been applied to seal the open wound, the prehospital care provider needs to monitor the patient carefully for the development of tension pneumothorax. If signs of increasing respiratory distress develop, the dressing over the wound should be vented or removed to allow for decompression of any accumulating tension. If this is ineffective, needle decompression should be considered.[22]

In cases in which positive-pressure ventilation is being performed, the wound does not need to be sealed, although a sterile dressing is still valuable from the standpoint of limiting further wound contamination. The positive-pressure ventilation effectively manages the pathophysiology usually associated with the open pneumothorax by ventilating the lung directly.

Tension Pneumothorax

Tension pneumothorax is a life-threatening emergency. As air continues to enter the pleural space without any exit or release, intrathoracic pressure builds up. As intrathoracic

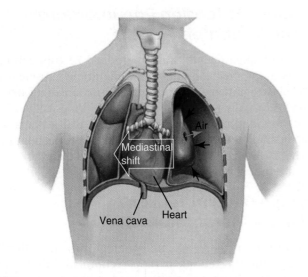

Figure 10-16 Tension pneumothorax. If the amount of air trapped in the pleural space continues to increase, not only is the lung on the affected side collapsed, but the mediastinum is shifted to the opposite side. The lung on the opposite side is then compressed and intrathoracic pressure increases, which kinks the vena cava and decreases blood return to the heart.

© National Association of Emergency Medical Technicians (NAEMT).

pressure rises, ventilatory compromise increases and venous return to the heart decreases. The decreasing cardiac output coupled with worsening gas exchange results in profound shock (**Figure 10-16**). The increasing pressure on the injured side of the chest may eventually push the structures in the mediastinum toward the other side of the chest. This distortion of anatomy may further impede venous return to the heart through the kinking of the inferior vena cava as it passes through the diaphragm. Additionally, inflation of the lung on the uninjured side is increasingly restricted, and further respiratory compromise results.

Any patient with a thoracic injury is at risk for developing tension pneumothorax. Patients at particular risk are those who likely have a pneumothorax (e.g., patient with signs of rib fracture), those who have a known pneumothorax (e.g., patient with a penetrating wound to the chest), and those with chest injury who are undergoing positive-pressure ventilation. Such patients must be continuously monitored for signs of increasing respiratory distress associated with circulatory impairment and rapidly transported to an appropriate facility.

Assessment

The findings during assessment depend on how much pressure has accumulated in the pleural space (**Box 10-2**). Initially, patients will exhibit apprehension and discomfort. They will generally complain of chest pain and difficulty breathing. As the tension pneumothorax worsens, they

---

Box 10-2 Signs of Tension Pneumothorax

Although the following signs are frequently discussed with a tension pneumothorax, many may not be present or are difficult to identify in the field.

Observation

- *Cyanosis* may be difficult to see in the field. Poor lighting, variation in skin color, and dirt and blood associated with trauma often render this sign unreliable.
- *Distended neck veins* are described as a classic sign of tension pneumothorax. However, since a patient with a tension pneumothorax may also have lost a considerable amount of blood, distended neck veins may not be prominent.

Palpation

- *Subcutaneous emphysema* is a common finding. As the pressure builds up within the chest cavity, air will begin to dissect through the tissues of the chest wall. Because tension pneumothorax involves significantly elevated intrathoracic pressure, the subcutaneous emphysema can often be palpated across the entire chest wall and neck and sometimes can involve the abdominal wall and face as well.
- *Tracheal deviation* is usually a late sign. Even when it is present, it can be difficult to diagnose by physical examination. In the neck, the trachea is bound to the cervical spine by fascial and other supporting structures; thus, the deviation of the trachea is more of an intrathoracic phenomenon, although deviation may be palpated in the jugular notch if it is severe. Tracheal deviation is not often noted in the prehospital environment.

Auscultation

- *Decreased breath sounds on the injured side*. The most helpful part of the physical examination is checking for decreased breath sounds on the side of the injury. However, to use this sign, the prehospital care provider must be able to distinguish between normal and decreased sounds. Such differentiation requires a great deal of practice. Listening to breath sounds during every patient contact will help.

---

will exhibit increasing agitation, tachypnea, and respiratory distress. In severe cases, cyanosis and apnea may occur.

The classic findings are tracheal deviation away from the side of injury, diminished breath sounds on the side of injury, and a tympanitic percussion note. It is difficult to detect diminished breath sounds in the field environment. Constant practice with auscultation of all patients will hone the prehospital care provider's skill and make detection of this important finding more likely. Detection of a tympanitic percussion note in the field is basically impossible, but the finding is mentioned for the sake of completeness. Transport and treatment should never be delayed for purposes of performing percussion of the chest.

Other physical findings that may be evident are jugular venous distension, chest wall crepitus, and cyanosis. Tachycardia and tachypnea become increasingly prominent as the intrathoracic pressure builds and the pulse pressure narrows, culminating in hypotension and uncompensated shock.

Management

The priority in management involves decompressing the tension pneumothorax.[15] Decompression should be performed when the following three findings are present:

1. Worsening respiratory distress or difficulty ventilating with a bag-mask device
2. Unilateral decreased or absent breath sounds
3. Decompensated shock (systolic blood pressure less than 90 mm Hg with a narrowed pulse pressure)[15-19,22]

Depending on the clinical setting and the training level of the prehospital care provider, several options (discussed next) for pleural decompression exist. If decompression is not an option (i.e., only basic life support [BLS] is available and no occlusive dressing to remove), rapid transport to an appropriate facility while administering high-concentration oxygen (fraction of inspired oxygen [F_{IO_2}] ≥ 85%) is imperative. Positive-pressure ventilatory assistance should be used only if the patient is hypoxic and fails to respond to supplemental oxygen, as this situation may rapidly worsen the tension pneumothorax. Assisting ventilations may result in air accumulating more rapidly in the pleural space. If ALS intercept is an option, it should be accomplished, but only if the intercept will be faster than delivery to an appropriate facility.

Removal of an Occlusive Dressing

In the patient with an open pneumothorax, if an occluding dressing has been applied, it should be briefly opened or removed. This should allow the tension pneumothorax to decompress through the wound with a rush of air. This procedure may need to be repeated periodically during transport if symptoms of tension pneumothorax recur. If removing the dressing for several seconds is ineffective or if there is no open wound, an ALS provider may proceed with a needle thoracostomy.

Suspected Tension Pneumothorax in the Intubated Patient

In an intubated patient, a malpositioned ET tube can be mistaken for a tension pneumothorax. If the ET tube has slipped farther down from the trachea into one of the main bronchi (usually the right), the opposite lung will not be ventilated and breath sounds and chest wall expansion may be markedly diminished. In these cases, the position of the ET tube should be assessed and confirmed prior to any attempt at chest decompression.

Needle Decompression (Needle Thoracostomy)

Insertion of a needle (angiocatheter) into the pleural space on the affected side permits accumulated air, under pressure, to escape. Successful decompression converts a tension pneumothorax into an open pneumothorax and reverses the hemodynamic compromise associated with decreased venous return caused by the shift of mediastinal contents away from the collapsed lung.[23] This, along with the immediate improvement in ability to oxygenate and ventilate, can be lifesaving.

Needle decompression has historically been performed through the second intercostal space in the midclavicular line on the affected side of the chest. Recent evidence, however, supports using the fifth intercostal space along the anterior axillary line (lateral approach) as the preferred location for needle decompression (**Figure 10-17**).[24]

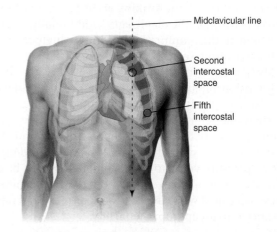

Midclavicular line

Second intercostal space

Fifth intercostal space

Figure 10-17 Needle decompression of the thoracic cavity for treatment of suspected tension pneumothorax. The procedure is performed using a large-bore (10- to 16-gauge) IV needle that is at least 8 cm (3.5 inches) in length. The needle can be placed at the fifth intercostal space along the anterior axillary line.

© MariyaL/Shutterstock.

Each location has advantages and disadvantages. Decompression in the midclavicular line has the advantage of ease of access for the prehospital care provider, but chest wall thickness at this location can result in the inability of the catheter to reach the thoracic cavity or kinking of the catheter during patient movement. In addition, there is a small risk of inducing major hemorrhage from inadvertent placement of the catheter into the subclavian vessels (superiorly) or internal mammary artery, heart, or pulmonary vessels (medially).[25,26] For these reasons, the lateral approach is now preferred as the first-line technique for tension pneumothorax decompression in the prehospital environment.

Advantages of the midaxillary placement of the catheter include its relative safety and efficacy. The chest wall is thinner in this location across all body mass index (BMI) quartiles in both males and females. In addition, higher success rates have been reported using this location,[27,28] and evidence suggests that catheters placed at the fifth intercostal space at the anterior axillary line are more stable during transport and less likely to become dislodged,[29] although kinking may be an issue.[30]

Regardless of the location chosen, decompression should be performed with a large-bore (10- to 16-gauge) IV needle that is at least 8 cm (3.5 inches) in length. The needle and catheter should be advanced until a rush of air is encountered, but not beyond that point. The lung on the affected side is collapsed and shifted toward the contralateral side; therefore, it is unlikely to be injured during the procedure. Once the decompression is achieved, the needle is removed and the catheter is taped to the chest to prevent dislodgment. Careful monitoring of the patient following the procedure is mandatory. One study noted a 26% mechanical failure rate due to kinking, obstruction, or dislodgment of the angiocatheter, with 43% of decompression attempts ultimately failing to relieve the tension pneumothorax.[31]

This procedure, when successfully performed, converts the tension pneumothorax into a negligible open pneumothorax. The relief to respiratory effort far outweighs the negative effect of the open pneumothorax. Because the diameter of the decompression catheter is significantly smaller than the patient's airway, it is unlikely that any air movement through the catheter will significantly compromise ventilatory effort. Thus, creation of a one-way valve (Heimlich valve) is probably unnecessary from a clinical standpoint. Using a manufactured valve is costly, and fashioning a valve from a glove is time consuming. Continued provision of supplemental oxygen, as well as ventilatory support as needed, is appropriate.

As a general rule, bilateral tension pneumothorax is exceedingly rare in patients who are not intubated and ventilated with positive pressure. The first step in reassessing the patient is to confirm the location of the ET tube, ensure that it has no kinks or bends causing compression of the tube, and ensure that the tube has not inadvertently moved down into a main bronchus. Extreme caution should be exercised with bilateral needle decompression in patients who are not being ventilated with positive-pressure ventilation. If the prehospital care provider's assessment is in error, the creation of bilateral pneumothoraces can cause severe respiratory distress.

The patient should be rapidly transported to an appropriate facility. IV access should be obtained en route unless transport time is particularly short. The patient must be closely observed for deterioration. Repeat decompression and endotracheal intubation may become necessary.

Tube Thoracostomy (Chest Tube Insertion)

In general, insertion of a chest tube (tube thoracostomy) is not performed in the prehospital setting because of concerns of time, procedural complications, infection, and training issues. Needle decompression can be accomplished in a fraction of the time required to perform a tube thoracostomy because fewer steps are necessary and less equipment is used. Published complication rates with tube thoracostomy range from 2.8% to 21%[32,33] and include damage to the heart or lungs and malposition in the subcutaneous tissues of the chest wall or in the peritoneal cavity. This procedure requires a sterile field, which is challenging to create in the field. A break in sterile technique, such as contamination of the chest tube or instruments, may result in the development of an empyema (collection of pus in the pleural space), requiring surgical intervention and drainage. Significant training is required to develop this skill, and ongoing practice is required to maintain skill proficiency.

Patients being transported with a chest tube in place are still at risk for the development of a tension pneumothorax, particularly if they are undergoing positive-pressure ventilatory assistance. If signs of a tension pneumothorax begin to manifest, first ensure that there are no kinks in the chest tube or connecting tubing. Next, ensure that the connecting tubing is correctly connected to a water seal and drainage device. Even with no identified problems, the patient with signs of an increasing tension pneumothorax may require needle decompression. Do not delay just because there is already a chest tube in place (**Box 10-3**).

Hemothorax

Hemothorax occurs when blood enters the pleural space. Because this space can accommodate a large volume of blood (2,500 to 3,000 ml), hemothorax can represent a source of significant blood loss. In fact, the loss of circulating blood volume from bleeding into the pleural space represents a greater physiologic insult to the patient with chest injury than the collapse of the lung that the

Box 10-3 Troubleshooting Tube Thoracostomy

Three Basic Components of Chest Tube Drainage Systems

1. *Seal.* Allows air to escape pleural space but not return. The seal is generally a water seal that bubbles as air escapes the pleural space and rises with inspiratory negative pressure.
2. *Collecting system.* Collects and measures output. Observe for changes in volume of output and nature.
3. *Suction.* Provides negative pressure to assist drainage and expansion. Ensure that suction is appropriately attached and functioning. Review the basic operation of any drainage system with the patient's health care team prior to transfer of the patient (Figure 10-18).

Changes in Respiratory Status in Patients With Chest Tubes

- *Assess vital signs, including pulse oximetry.* If the chest tube is not working properly, the patient may become tachycardic, tachypneic, and hypoxic. If tension pneumothorax is developing, subcutaneous emphysema, increasing respiratory distress, narrowing pulse pressure, and hypotension may result.
- *Assess lung sounds.* The lung sounds may become diminished in the involved side if the chest is no longer functioning and instead is allowing air to reaccumulate within the chest.
- *Assess ventilatory effort.* Ventilatory effort will increase when the chest tube is not functioning.
- *Assess circulation.* If the chest tube is not working properly and is allowing air to accumulate within the chest, the patient may become tachycardic. If tension pneumothorax is developing, narrowing pulse pressure and hypotension may result.
- *Assess level of consciousness.* If hypoxia or signs of shock develop, the patient may become agitated and anxious. As these complications progress, the patient's level of consciousness will decrease.

Troubleshooting Steps

- Assess the dressing and tube site to ensure that the chest tube has not been dislodged during transfers.

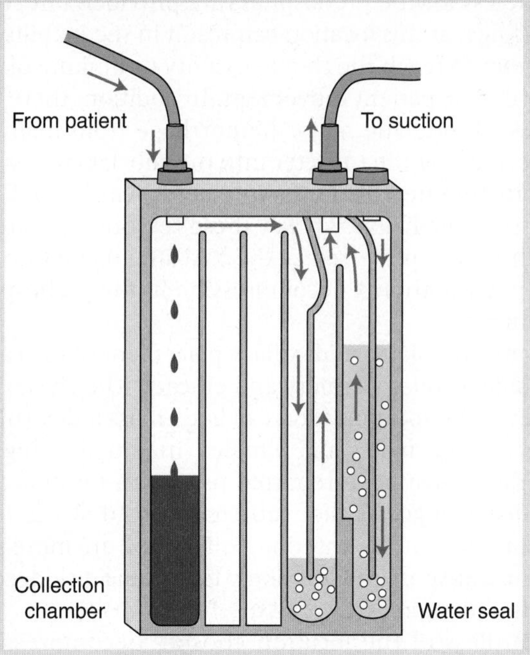

Figure 10-18 A chest drainage system provides negative pressure to assist drainage and expansion of the patient's chest.

© National Association of Emergency Medical Technicians (NAEMT).

- Check that the chest tubing is tightly connected and unobstructed, with no kinks or clamps.
- Check that the chest seal is intact and functioning. Is there any bubbling and/or variation with ventilations?
- Assess whether the chest tube is fogging and/or drainage is continuing.
- Ensure that the suction is functioning. Is there continuous bubbling or a negative pressure indicator throughout the ventilation cycle?
- If the patient's ventilatory status continues to deteriorate, assess closely for signs of developing tension pneumothorax. If indicated, disconnect the chest tube from the drainage system, which should allow release of tension if the chest tube is properly placed and unobstructed. If this step does not relieve the condition, consider needle decompression, and contact online medical control.

hemothorax produces (**Figure 10-19**). It is rare that enough blood accumulates to create a "tension hemothorax." The mechanisms resulting in hemothorax are the same as those causing the various types of pneumothoraces. The bleeding may come from the chest wall musculature, intercostal vessels, lung parenchyma, pulmonary vessels, or great vessels of the chest.

Assessment

Assessment reveals a patient in some distress, depending on the amount of blood lost into the chest and the resultant compression of the lung on the involved side. Chest pain and shortness of breath are again prominent features, generally with signs of significant shock. The prehospital care

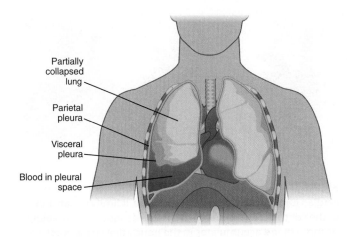

Figure 10-19 Hemothorax. The blood loss associated with hemorrhage into the thoracic cavity (leading to hypovolemia) is a much more severe problem than the amount of lung compressed by this blood.

© National Association of Emergency Medical Technicians (NAEMT).

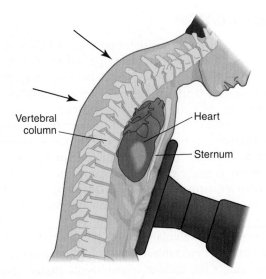

Figure 10-20 The heart can be compressed between the sternum (as the sternum stops against the steering column or dashboard) and the posterior thoracic wall (as the wall continues its forward motion). This compression can contuse the myocardium.

© National Association of Emergency Medical Technicians (NAEMT).

provider monitors the patient for signs of shock: tachycardia, tachypnea, confusion, pallor, and hypotension. Breath sounds on the side of the injury are diminished or absent, but the percussion note is dull (compared to tympanitic for a pneumothorax). Pneumothorax may be present in conjunction with hemothorax, increasing the likelihood for cardiorespiratory compromise. Because of loss of circulating blood volume, distended neck veins often are not present.

Management

Management includes constant observation to detect physiologic deterioration while providing appropriate support. High-concentration oxygen should be administered and ventilation supported if necessary with a bag-mask device or endotracheal intubation, if available and indicated. Hemodynamic status is closely monitored. IV access should be obtained and appropriate fluid therapy provided with a goal of maintaining adequate perfusion without large volumes indiscriminately administered. Rapid transport to an appropriate facility that is capable of immediate blood transfusion and surgical intervention completes the management algorithm for hemothorax. Needle decompression of the chest for hemothorax is not effective and not indicated.

Blunt Cardiac Injury

Cardiac injury most often results from application of force to the anterior chest, especially in a deceleration event such as a motor vehicle crash with violent frontal impact.[1,2,34] The heart is then compressed between the sternum anteriorly and the spinal column posteriorly (**Figure 10-20**). This compression of the heart causes an abrupt increase in the pressure within the ventricles to several times normal,

which results in cardiac contusion, sometimes valvular injury, and (rarely) cardiac rupture, as follows:

- *Cardiac contusion*. The most common result of cardiac compression is cardiac contusion. The heart muscle is bruised, with varying amounts of injury to the myocardial cells. This injury most often results in abnormal heart rhythms, such as sinus tachycardia.[34] Of greater concern, but less common, are premature ventricular contractions or nonperfusing rhythms such as ventricular tachycardia and ventricular fibrillation. If the septal region of the heart is injured, the electrocardiogram (ECG) may demonstrate intraventricular conduction abnormalities, such as right bundle branch block. If a sufficient volume of myocardium is injured, the contractility of the heart may be impaired, and cardiac output falls, resulting in cardiogenic shock. Unlike the other forms of shock usually encountered in the trauma setting, this shock does not improve with fluid administration and may actually worsen.
- *Valvular rupture*. Rupture of the supporting structures of the heart valves or the valves themselves typically renders the valves incompetent. The patient will present in varying degrees of shock with symptoms and signs of congestive heart failure (CHF), such as *tachypnea*, rales, and new-onset heart murmur.
- *Blunt cardiac rupture*. A rare event, blunt cardiac rupture occurs in less than 1% of patients with blunt chest trauma.[34-36] Most of these patients will die at the scene from *exsanguination* into the chest or fatal cardiac tamponade. The surviving patients will typically present with cardiac tamponade.

Assessment

Assessment of the patient with the potential for blunt cardiac injury reveals a mechanism that imparted a frontal impact to the center of the patient's chest. A bent steering column accompanied by bruising over the sternum implies such a mechanism. As with other chest injuries, the patient is likely to complain of chest pain and/or shortness of breath. If a dysrhythmia is present, the patient may complain of palpitations. Physical findings of concern are bruising over the sternum, crepitus over the sternum, and sternal instability. With a floating sternum (**flail sternum**), the ribs on either side of the sternum are broken, allowing it to move paradoxically with respirations, similar to flail chest, as described earlier. If valvular disruption has occurred, a harsh murmur may be detectable over the precordium along with signs of acute CHF, such as hypotension, jugular venous distension, and abnormal breath sounds. ECG monitoring may demonstrate tachycardia, premature ventricular contractions, other rhythm disturbances, or ST-segment elevation.

Management

The key management strategy is correct assessment that blunt cardiac injury may have occurred and transmission of that concern along with the clinical findings to the receiving hospital. In the meantime, high-concentration oxygen is administered and IV access established for judicious fluid therapy. The patient should be placed on a cardiac monitor to detect dysrhythmias and ST-segment elevations, if present. If dysrhythmias are present and ALS providers are present, standard antidysrhythmic pharmacotherapy should be instituted. There are no data to support prophylactic antidysrhythmic therapy in blunt cardiac injury. As always, ventilatory support measures should be implemented as indicated.

Cardiac Tamponade

Cardiac tamponade occurs when a wound of the heart allows fluid (usually blood) to acutely accumulate between the pericardial sac and the heart.[1,34] The pericardial sac is comprised of a fibrous, inelastic tissue. Normally, there is a small amount of fluid in the pericardial sac, similar to the pleural space, as described earlier. Because the pericardium is inelastic, pressure begins to rise rapidly within the pericardial sac as fluid accumulates within it acutely. This rising pericardial pressure impedes venous return to the heart. This, in turn, leads to diminished cardiac output and blood pressure. With each contraction of the heart, additional blood may enter the pericardial sac, further impeding the heart's ability to fill in preparation for the next contraction (**Figure 10-21**). This condition can become profound enough to precipitate **pulseless electrical activity**, a life-threatening injury requiring coordinated response by prehospital care providers in all phases of care to achieve

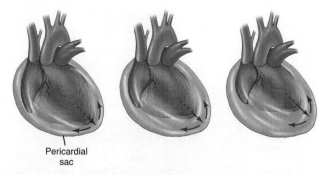

Peicardial
sac

Figure 10-21 Cardiac tamponade. As blood courses from the cardiac lumen into the pericardial space, it limits expansion of the ventricle. Therefore, the ventricle cannot fill completely. As more blood accumulates in the pericardial space, less ventricular space is available to accumulate blood, and cardiac output is reduced.
© National Association of Emergency Medical Technicians (NAEMT).

an optimal outcome. The normal adult pericardium may be able to accommodate as much as 300 ml of fluid before pulselessness occurs, but as little as 50 ml is usually enough to impede cardiac return and, thus, cardiac output.[1]

Most often, cardiac tamponade is caused by a stab wound to the heart. This mechanism of injury may result in penetration into one of the cardiac chambers or just a laceration of the myocardium. The right ventricle is the most anterior chamber in the heart and is therefore the most commonly injured chamber in penetrating trauma. Regardless of the anatomic location of injury, bleeding into the pericardial sac occurs. The rising pressure within the pericardium results in the cardiac tamponade physiology. At the same time, the increased pressure within the pericardium may temporarily impede further bleeding from the cardiac wound, allowing the patient to survive long enough to reach definitive medical care. In the case of gunshot wounds to the heart, the damage to the heart and pericardium is usually so severe that the pericardium cannot contain the hemorrhage, resulting in rapid exsanguination into the chest cavity. The same is true in the case of impalements. Blunt rupture of a cardiac chamber can result in cardiac tamponade but more often causes exsanguinating hemorrhage.

Cardiac tamponade should be kept in mind as a possibility when evaluating any patient with a thoracic penetration. This index of suspicion should be raised to the level of "present until proven otherwise" when the penetrating injury is within a rectangle (the cardiac box) formed by drawing a horizontal line along the clavicles, vertical lines from the nipples to the costal margins, and a second horizontal line connecting the points of intersection between the vertical lines and the costal margin (**Figure 10-22**). The presence of such a wound should be communicated to the receiving institution as soon as it is recognized to allow for appropriate preparation to manage the patient.

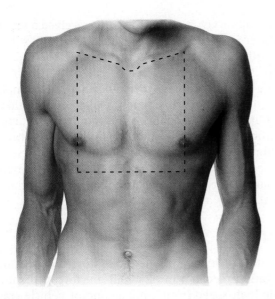

Figure 10-22 The index of suspicion for penetrating cardiac injury should be high if the penetrating wound occurs within the "cardiac box."

© MariyaL/Shutterstock.

Box 10-4 Paradoxical Pulse

The **paradoxical pulse**, also known as pulsus paradoxus, is actually an accentuation of the normal, slight drop in systolic blood pressure (SBP) that occurs during inspiration. As the lungs expand, there is preferential filling and ejection of blood from the right side of the heart at the expense of the left side. Thus, peripheral blood pressure falls. This decrease in SBP is usually less than 10 to 15 mm Hg. A greater decrease in SBP constitutes the so-called paradoxical pulse.

Assessment

Assessment involves quickly recognizing the presence of at-risk wounds, as previously described, in combination with an appreciation for the physical findings of pericardial tamponade. Beck's triad is a constellation of findings indicative of cardiac tamponade: (1) distant or muffled heart sounds (the fluid around the heart makes it difficult to hear the sounds of the valves closing), (2) jugular venous distension (caused by the increasing pressure in the pericardial sac backing blood up into the neck veins), and (3) low blood pressure. Another physical finding described in cardiac tamponade is paradoxical pulse (**Box 10-4**).

Detection of some of these signs is difficult in the field, especially muffled heart tones and paradoxical pulse. Additionally, the components of Beck's triad are present in only 22% to 77% of cases of tamponade.[37,38] Thus, the prehospital care provider needs to maintain a high index of suspicion, based on the location of the wounds and hypotension, and implement therapy accordingly.

Management

Management requires rapid monitored transport to a facility that can perform immediate surgical repair.[14,17,39-43] The prehospital care provider first needs to recognize that cardiac tamponade likely exists and to inform the receiving facility so that preparations can be made for emergent surgical intervention. Oxygen in high concentration should be administered. IV access should be obtained and judicious fluid therapy initiated, because this can augment central venous pressure and thus improve cardiac filling for a time. The prehospital care provider should strongly consider endotracheal intubation and positive-pressure ventilation if the patient is hypotensive.[19,41,42]

Definitive therapy requires release of the tamponade and repair of the cardiac injury. A patient with a suspected cardiac tamponade should be transported directly to a facility capable of immediate surgical intervention, if available. Draining some of the pericardial fluid by **pericardiocentesis** (insertion of a needle into the pericardial space) is often an effective temporizing maneuver (**Figure 10-23**). Risks of

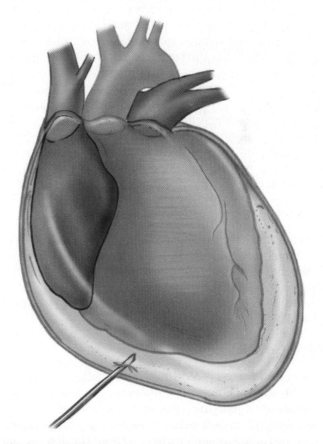

Figure 10-23 Draining some of the pericardial fluid by pericardiocentesis is often an effective temporizing maneuver for cardiac tamponade.

© Jones & Bartlett Learning.

pericardiocentesis include injury to the heart and coronary arteries, resulting in increased tamponade and injury to the lung, great vessels, and liver. In very rare cases, resuscitative thoracotomy (opening the chest to control bleeding and repair internal wounds) has been performed in the field by physicians in systems in which they respond to field emergencies.[44,45]

Commotio Cordis

The term **commotio cordis** refers to the clinical situation in which an apparently innocuous blow to the anterior chest results in sudden cardiac arrest.[46,47] A 2003 study reported 128 cases of commotio cordis in the United States, predominantly in children and adolescents (mean age about 13 years).[48] Most experts theorize that commotio cordis results from a relatively minor, nonpenetrating blow to the precordium (area over the heart), occurring at an electrically vulnerable portion of the cardiac cycle, whereas some believe that coronary artery vasospasm may play a role in its development. Regardless of the mechanism, the terminal result is a cardiac dysrhythmia resulting in ventricular fibrillation and sudden cardiac arrest.

This condition most frequently occurs during amateur sporting events in which the victim is struck in the midanterior chest by a projectile or object, such as a baseball (most common), ice hockey puck, lacrosse ball, or softball. However, commotio cordis has also been reported after bodily impacts (e.g., karate blows), a low-velocity motor vehicle crash, and the collision of two outfielders trying to catch a baseball. After the impact, victims have been known to walk a step or two and then suddenly drop to the ground in cardiac arrest. Typically, no injury is noted to the ribs, sternum, or heart at autopsy. Most victims have no known history of heart disease. It is possible that the condition may be prevented through the use of equipment such as safety baseballs.[49]

Assessment

Patients who have sustained commotio cordis are found in cardiopulmonary arrest. In some victims, a minor bruise is noted over the sternum. Ventricular fibrillation is the most common rhythm, although complete heart block and left bundle branch block with ST-segment elevations have also been seen.

Management

Once cardiac arrest is confirmed, cardiopulmonary resuscitation (CPR) is initiated. Commotio cordis is managed in a manner similar to cardiac arrests resulting from myocardial infarction rather than those resulting from trauma and blood loss. The cardiac rhythm should be determined as expeditiously as possible, with rapid defibrillation administered if ventricular fibrillation is identified. Prognosis is poor, with the chance of survival at 15% or less.[47]

Virtually all survivors of this condition received both rapid, bystander-initiated CPR and immediate defibrillation, often with an automated external defibrillator. Precordial thumps have not been shown to consistently terminate ventricular fibrillation; however, they may be attempted if a defibrillator is not immediately available. The initiation of CPR and electrical defibrillation should not be delayed to perform a precordial thump.[50] If immediate attempts at defibrillation are unsuccessful, the airway is secured and IV access initiated. Epinephrine and antidysrhythmic pharmacologic agents may be administered as outlined in medical cardiac arrest protocols.

Traumatic Aortic Disruption

Traumatic aortic disruption results from a deceleration/acceleration mechanism of significant force.[51] Examples include high-speed frontal-impact motor vehicle crashes and high falls in which the patient lands flat.

The aorta arises from the upper portion of the heart in the mediastinum. The heart, ascending aorta, and aortic arch are relatively mobile within the chest cavity. As the arch of the aorta transitions to the descending aorta, it is "wrapped" with an investing layer of tissue and becomes adherent to the vertebral column. Thus, the descending aorta is relatively immobile. When there is a sudden deceleration of the body, such as occurs in a high-speed frontal impact, the heart and the aortic arch continue to move forward relative to the fixed (immobile) descending aorta. This contrast in velocity produces shear forces in the aortic wall at the junction between these two segments of the aorta.[42] Thus, the typical location for a traumatic aortic injury is just distal to the takeoff of the left subclavian artery. This shear force can disrupt the wall of the aorta in varying degrees (**Figure 10-24**). When the tear extends through the full thickness of the aortic wall, the patient rapidly exsanguinates into the pleural cavity. However, if the tear is only partially through the wall, leaving the outer layer (adventitia) intact, the patient may survive for a variable length of time, making rapid identification and treatment essential for a successful outcome.[51]

Assessment

Assessment of aortic disruption hinges on index of suspicion. A high index should be maintained in situations involving high-energy deceleration/acceleration mechanisms. For such a devastating injury, there may be little external evidence of chest injury. The prehospital care provider needs to assess the adequacy of the airway and breathing and should carefully auscultate and palpate the chest. Careful examination may demonstrate that the pulse quality may be different between the two upper extremities (pulse stronger in the right arm than the left) or between the upper (brachial artery) and lower extremities (femoral artery). Blood pressures, if measured, may be higher in the upper

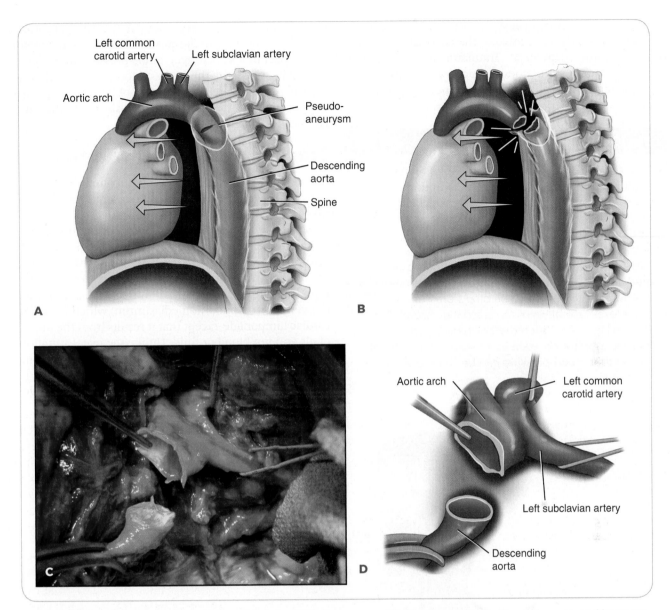

Figure 10-24 **A.** The descending aorta is a fixed structure that moves with the thoracic spine. The arch, aorta, and heart are freely movable. Acceleration of the torso in a lateral-impact collision or rapid deceleration of the torso in a frontal-impact collision produces a different rate of motion between the arch-heart complex and the descending aorta. This motion may result in a tear of the inner lining of the aorta that is contained within the outermost layer, producing a pseudoaneurysm. **B.** Tears at the junction of the arch and descending aorta may also result in a complete rupture, leading to immediate exsanguination in the chest. **C.** and **D.** Operative photograph and drawing of a traumatic aortic tear.

A, B, and D: © National Association of Emergency Medical Technicians (NAEMT); C: Courtesy Norman McSwain, MD, FACS, NREMT-P.

extremities than in the lower extremities, comprising the signs of a pseudo-coarctation (narrowing) of the aorta.

Definitive diagnosis of aortic disruption requires radiographic imaging in the hospital. Plain chest radiographs may demonstrate a variety of signs suggesting the injury is present. The most reliable of these is widening of the mediastinum. The injury can be definitively demonstrated with **aortography**, computed tomography (CT) of the chest, and **transesophageal echocardiography**.[51]

Management

Management of traumatic aortic disruption in the field is supportive. A high index of suspicion for its presence is maintained when the appropriate mechanism exists. High-concentration supplemental oxygen is administered and IV access is obtained, except in cases of extremely short transport times. Communication with the receiving facility about the mechanism and suspicion for aortic disruption should occur at the earliest opportunity. Strict blood pressure control is imperative to the successful outcome of these injuries (**Box 10-5**). Traumatic aortic disruption represents another situation in which balanced resuscitation is clinically useful. Fluid resuscitation that results in normal or elevated blood pressure may result in rupture of the remaining tissue of the aorta and rapid exsanguination. If transport times are longer, blood pressure management should be guided by the highest blood pressure obtained, typically in the right arm. Control of both blood pressure and contractile force may be accomplished with the administration of beta blockers.[52]

Box 10-5 Blood Pressure Maintenance

Caution: When performing interhospital transfer of patients with suspected aortic disruption, it is important not to raise the patient's blood pressure aggressively because this may lead to exsanguinating hemorrhage (see the Shock: Pathophysiology of Life and Death chapter). Many of these patients may be given infusions of medications, such as beta blockers (e.g., esmolol, metoprolol), to maintain the blood pressure at a lower level, typically a mean arterial pressure of 70 mm Hg or less. Such therapy typically requires invasive monitoring, such as insertion of an arterial line, so that blood pressure can be monitored much more carefully.

Tracheobronchial Disruption

Tracheobronchial disruption is an uncommon, but potentially highly lethal, condition.[52] All lacerations of the lung involve disruption of airways to some degree; however, in these cases, the intrathoracic portion of the trachea itself or one of the main or secondary bronchi is disrupted. This disruption results in high flow of air through the injury into the mediastinum or pleural space (**Figure 10-25**). Pressure rapidly accumulates, resulting in tension pneumothorax or even tension pneumomediastinum, which is similar to cardiac tamponade except that it results from the presence of air and not blood or fluid. Unlike the usual situation in tension pneumothorax, needle thoracostomy may result in the continuous flow of air through the catheter and may fail to relieve the tension. This is caused by the ongoing

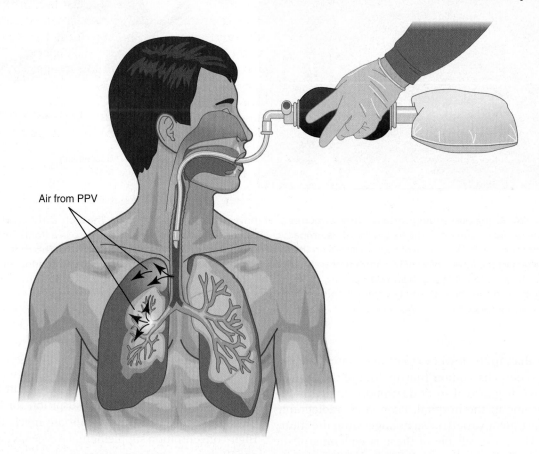

Air from PPV

Figure 10-25 Tracheal or bronchial rupture. Positive-pressure ventilation can directly force large amounts of air through the trachea or bronchus, rapidly producing a tension pneumothorax.

high flow of air across these major airways into the pleural space. Respiratory function may be significantly impaired because of preferential airflow across the lesion as well as the pressure. Positive-pressure ventilation efforts may worsen the tension. Penetrating trauma is more likely to cause this injury than blunt trauma. However, blunt injury of high energy may also cause tracheobronchial disruption.[53]

Assessment

Assessment of the patient with tracheobronchial disruption demonstrates an individual in obvious distress. The patient may be pale and diaphoretic and will demonstrate signs of respiratory distress, such as use of accessory muscles of respiration, grunting, and nasal flaring. Extensive subcutaneous emphysema, especially in the upper chest and neck, may be identified (**Figure 10-26**). Although traditionally taught as important findings, jugular venous distension may be obscured by subcutaneous emphysema, and deviation of the trachea may only be noted upon palpation of the trachea in the jugular notch. Ventilatory rate will be elevated, and oxygen saturation may be diminished. The patient may or may not be hypotensive and may cough up blood (hemoptysis). The hemorrhage associated with penetrating trauma may not be present in the blunt cases, but hemothorax is a possibility in both penetrating and blunt trauma.

Management

Successful management of tracheobronchial disruption requires administration of supplemental oxygen and judicious use of ventilatory assistance. If assisted ventilation makes the patient more uncomfortable, only oxygen is administered and the patient is transported as quickly as possible to an appropriate facility. Continuous monitoring for signs of progression toward a tension pneumothorax is imperative, and rapid needle decompression should be attempted if these signs present. Complex advanced airway management, such as selective main bronchus intubation, is difficult to accomplish in the field and has the potential for worsening a major bronchial injury.

Traumatic Asphyxia

Traumatic asphyxia is so named because the victims physically resemble strangulation patients. They exhibit the same bluish discoloration of the face and neck (and in the case of traumatic asphyxia, upper chest) as patients who have been strangled. Unlike strangled patients, however, traumatic asphyxia patients do not suffer from true asphyxia (cessation of air and gas exchange). The similarity in appearance to strangulation patients results from the impaired venous return from the head and neck that is present in both groups of patients.

The mechanism for traumatic asphyxia is an abrupt, significant increase in thoracic pressure resulting from a crush to the torso (e.g., car falling off a jack onto the patient's chest). This pressure results in blood being forced back out of the heart and into the veins in a retrograde direction. Because the veins of the arms and lower extremities contain valves, backward flow into the extremities is limited. However, the veins of the neck and head lack such valves, and blood is preferentially forced into these areas. Subcutaneous venules and small capillaries rupture and blood leaks out, resulting in the purplish discoloration of the skin. Rupture of small vessels in the brain and retina may result in brain and eye dysfunction. Traumatic asphyxia is reported to be a marker for blunt cardiac rupture.[54]

Assessment

The hallmark of traumatic asphyxia is plethora, a bodily condition characterized by an excess of blood and turgescence (i.e., swelling and distension of blood vessels), with a reddish coloration of the skin. This appearance is most prominent above the level of the crush (**Figure 10-27**).

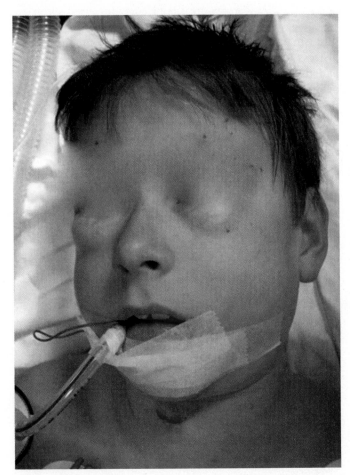

Figure 10-26 Patient with trauma to the anterior neck causing a tracheal disruption and subcutaneous emphysema of the face (eyelids) and neck.

Photograph provided courtesy of J. C. Pitteloud, MD, Switzerland.

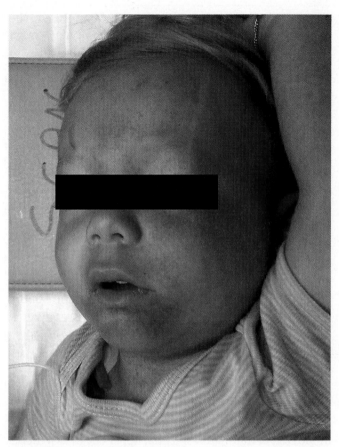

Figure 10-27 Child with traumatic asphyxia. Note the purple discoloration, particularly on the chin, and the multiple petechiae on the face and forehead.

Photograph provided courtesy of J.C. Pitteloud M.D., Switzerland.

The skin below the level of injury is normal. Because of the force applied to the chest necessary to cause this injury, many of the injuries already discussed in this chapter may be present, as well as injuries to the spine and spinal cord.

Management

Management is supportive. High-concentration oxygen is administered, IV access obtained, and judicious ventilatory support provided, if indicated. The reddish-purple discoloration typically fades within 1 to 2 weeks in survivors.

Diaphragmatic Rupture

Small lacerations of the diaphragm may occur in penetrating injuries to the thoracoabdominal region.[1] Because the diaphragm rises and falls with respiration, any penetration that is below the level of the nipples anteriorly or the level of the scapular tip posteriorly is at risk for having traversed the diaphragm. Generally, these lesions do not present any acute problems on their own, but they usually require surgical repair because of the risk in the future for herniation

and strangulation of abdominal contents through the defect. Significant injuries to thoracic or abdominal organs may accompany these otherwise apparently innocuous injuries.

Blunt diaphragmatic rupture results from the application of sufficient force to the abdomen to increase abdominal pressure acutely, abruptly, and sufficiently to disrupt the diaphragm. Unlike the small tears that usually accompany penetrating injury, the tears resulting from blunt mechanisms are frequently large and allow acute herniation of the abdominal viscera into the chest cavity[1] (**Figure 10-28**). Respiratory distress results from the pressure of the herniated organs on the lungs, preventing effective ventilation, as well as from contusion of the lungs. This impairment of ventilation may be life threatening. In addition to the ventilatory dysfunction, rib fractures, hemothorax, and pneumothorax may occur. Injury of intra-abdominal organs may also accompany the injury to the diaphragm, including injuries to the liver, spleen, stomach, or intestines, as these organs are forced through the tear in the diaphragm into the pleural cavity. These patients are frequently in acute distress and require rapid intervention to recover.

Assessment

Assessment frequently reveals a patient in acute respiratory distress who appears anxious, tachypneic, and pale. The patient may have contusions of the chest wall, bony crepitus, or subcutaneous emphysema. Breath sounds on the affected side may be diminished, or bowel sounds may be auscultated over the chest. The abdomen may be scaphoid if enough of the abdominal contents have herniated into the chest.

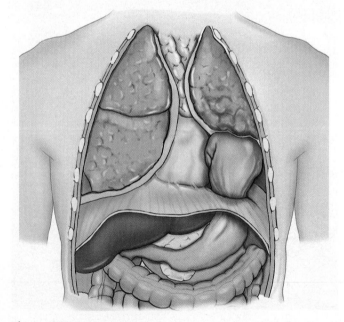

Figure 10-28 Diaphragmatic rupture may cause the bowel or other structures to herniate through the tear, causing partial compression of the lung and respiratory distress.

© National Association of Emergency Medical Technicians (NAEMT).

Management

Prompt recognition that diaphragmatic rupture may be present is necessary. Supplemental oxygen in high concentration should be administered and ventilation supported as necessary. The patient should be rapidly transported to an appropriate facility.

Prolonged Transport

Priorities for managing patients with known or suspected thoracic injuries during prolonged transport remain fundamental, including managing the airway, supporting ventilation and oxygenation, controlling hemorrhage, and providing appropriate volume resuscitation. When faced with a prolonged transport, prehospital care providers may have a lower threshold for securing the airway with endotracheal intubation. Indications for performing endotracheal intubation include increasing respiratory distress or impending respiratory failure (after exclusion or treatment of a tension pneumothorax), a flail chest, open pneumothorax, or multiple rib fractures. Oxygen should be provided to maintain oxygen saturation at 94% or greater.

Ventilations should be assisted as necessary. Pulmonary contusions worsen over time, and the use of CPAP, positive end-expiratory pressure (PEEP) with a transport ventilator, or PEEP valves with bag-mask device may facilitate oxygenation. Any patient with significant thoracic trauma may have or develop a tension pneumothorax, and ongoing assessment should look for the hallmark signs. In the presence of decreased or absent breath sounds, worsening respiratory distress, difficulty squeezing the bag-mask device, increasing peak inspiratory pressures in patients on a ventilator, and hypotension, pleural decompression should be performed. A tube thoracostomy (insertion of a chest tube) may be performed by authorized personnel, typically air medical flight crews, if the patient requires needle decompression or is found to have an open pneumothorax. IV access should be secured and IV fluids administered judiciously.

Patients with suspected intrathoracic, intra-abdominal, or retroperitoneal hemorrhage should be maintained with systolic blood pressure in the range of 80 to 90 mm Hg. Overaggressive volume resuscitation may significantly worsen pulmonary contusions, as well as lead to recurrent internal hemorrhage (see the Shock: Pathophysiology of Life and Death chapter).

Patients with severe pain from multiple rib fractures may benefit from small doses of narcotics titrated intravenously. If narcotic administration results in hypotension and respiratory failure, volume resuscitation and ventilatory support should be provided.

Patients with cardiac dysrhythmias associated with blunt cardiac injury may benefit from the use of antidysrhythmic medications. Any interventions performed should be carefully documented on the patient care report, and the receiving facility must be made aware of the procedures.

SUMMARY

- Thoracic injuries are particularly significant because of the potential for compromise of respiratory and circulatory function and because thoracic injuries are frequently associated with multisystem trauma.
- When responding to penetrating injuries to the chest, prehospital care providers should be prepared to manage a hemothorax or a pneumothorax, or both, which is termed a *hemopneumothorax*.
- When responding to blunt force trauma to the chest, injuries that prehospital care providers should be on the lookout for include pulmonary contusion, tears of the visceral pleura, broken ribs, shearing or rupture of the major blood vessels in the chest, and disruption of the chest wall. Associated conditions include hemothorax, pneumothorax, and catastrophic hemorrhage. Pulse oximetry and sidestream or in-line waveform capnography are useful adjuncts for assessing ventilatory status and responses to therapy.
- Patients with chest injury need to be managed aggressively and transported quickly to definitive care.
- Prehospital care providers must be prepared to recognize and manage the three types of pneumothoraces:
  - Simple pneumothorax is the presence of air within the pleural space.
  - Open pneumothorax ("sucking chest wound") involves a defect in the chest wall that allows air to enter and exit the pleural space from the outside with ventilatory effort.
  - Tension pneumothorax occurs when air continues to enter and is trapped in the pleural space with gradual increase in intrathoracic pressure. Signs of tension pneumothorax should be carefully sought because treatment in the

(continued)

SUMMARY (CONTINUED)

field with needle decompression may correct this possible, and rapidly fatal problem.

- Because of the high risk of multisystem trauma in patients with blunt thoracic injury, spinal immobilization should be employed when transporting these patients.
- Electrocardiographic monitoring may suggest blunt cardiac injury.
- Particular attention should be paid to the administration of supplemental high-concentration

oxygen and the need for ventilatory support in any patient suspected of having chest trauma.

- Intravenous access should be obtained en route to the medical facility and fluid therapy administered with appropriate goals in mind.
- Although many thoracic injuries can be managed without surgical intervention, the patient with a chest injury must still be evaluated and managed at an appropriate medical facility.

SCENARIO RECAP

You and your partner are dispatched to an industrial construction area for a worker who was struck by a piece of metal. Upon arrival, you are met at the gate by the site safety officer, who leads you to an interior work area. En route to the work area, the safety officer states the patient was helping to install metal studs. When he turned to grab another stud, he ran into the end of a stud his partner had just trimmed, cutting through his shirt and puncturing his chest.

In the work area, you find an approximately 35-year-old man sitting upright on a pile of lumber, leaning forward and holding a rag to the right side of his chest. You ask the patient what happened, and he tries to tell you but has to stop after every five to six words to catch his breath. As you move the rag, you notice an open laceration approximately 2 inches (5 cm) long with a small amount of blood-tinged, "bubbling" fluid. The patient is diaphoretic and has a rapid radial pulse. Decreased breath sounds are noted on the right side with auscultation. No other abnormal physical findings are noted.

- Is this patient in respiratory distress?
- Does he have life-threatening injuries?
- What interventions should you undertake in the field?
- What modality should be used to transport this patient?
- How would a different location (e.g., rural) impact your management and plans during prolonged transport?
- What other injuries do you suspect?

SCENARIO SOLUTION

The scene report, patient complaints, and physical examination lead you to suspect that this patient may have serious and potentially life-threatening injuries. He is awake and speaking coherently, indicating that he has a stable airway. He is experiencing severe respiratory distress. The location of the wound, bubbling fluid, and decreased breath sounds indicate an open pneumothorax.

You move quickly to apply an occlusive dressing, provide the patient with supplemental oxygen, and consider ventilatory assistance with a bag-mask device as necessary. The first priorities in this scenario are to recognize the seriousness of the injuries, stabilize the patient, and initiate transfer to an appropriate facility. Given this patient's respiratory distress and findings, he is at significant risk for complications. Transport to the closest trauma center is appropriate. IV access should be obtained en route.

There is risk for respiratory deterioration, and the patient's ventilatory status needs to be monitored closely. Signs of progressing circulatory compromise and respiratory distress would prompt you to first remove the occlusive dressing and, if there is no improvement, to perform needle decompression. If transport time will be extended, air transport should be considered.

References

1. American College of Surgeons Committee on Trauma. Thoracic trauma. In: *Advanced Trauma Life Support for Doctors, Student Course Manual*. 9th ed. Chicago, IL: American College of Surgeons; 2012.

2. Wall MJ, Huh J, Mattox KL. Thoracotomy. In: Mattox KL, Feliciano DV, Moore EE, eds. *Trauma*. 5th ed. New York, NY: McGraw-Hill; 2004.

3. Livingston DH, Hauser CJ. Trauma to the chest wall and lung. In: Mattox KL, Feliciano DV, Moore EE, eds. *Trauma*. 5th ed. New York, NY: McGraw-Hill; 2004.

4. Howes DS, Bellazzini MA. Chronic obstructive pulmonary disease. Wolfson AB, Hendey GW, Ling LJ, et al., eds. *Harwood-Nuss' Clinical Practice of Emergency Medicine*. 5th ed. Philadelphia, PA: Wolters Kluwer/Lippincott Williams & Wilkins; 2010.

5. Wilson RF. Pulmonary physiology. In: Wilson RF. *Critical Care Manual: Applied Physiology and Principles of Therapy*. 2nd ed. Philadelphia, PA: Davis; 1992.

6. American College of Surgeons Committee on Trauma. Initial assessment. In: *Advanced Trauma Life Support for Doctors*. 9th ed. Chicago, IL: American College of Surgeons; 2012.

7. Silverston P. Pulse oximetry at the roadside: a study of pulse oximetry in immediate care. *BMJ*. 1989;298:711.

8. Ziegler DW, Agarwal NN. The morbidity and mortality of rib fractures. *J Trauma Acute Care Surg*. 1994;37(6):975-979.

9. Pressley CM, Fry WR, Philip AS, et al. Predicting outcome of patients with chest wall injury. *Am J Surg*. 2012;204(6):900-904.

10. Flagel BT, Luchette FA, Reed RL, et al. Half-a-dozen ribs: the breakpoint for mortality. *Surgery*. 2005;138:717-725.

11. Jones KM, Reed RL, Luchette FA. The ribs or not the ribs: which influences mortality? *Am J Surg*. 2011;202(5);598-604.

12. Richardson JD, Adams L, Flint LM. Selective management of flail chest and pulmonary contusion. *Ann Surg*. 1982;196:481.

13. Di Bartolomeo S, Sanson G, Nardi G, et al. A population-based study on pneumothorax in severely traumatized patients. *J Trauma*. 2001;51(4):677.

14. Regel G, Stalp M, Lehmann U, et al. Prehospital care: importance of early intervention outcome. *Acta Anaesthesiol Scand Suppl*. 1997;110:71.

15. Barone JE, Pizzi WF, Nealon TF, et al. Indications for intubation in blunt chest trauma. *J Trauma*. 1986;26:334.

16. Mattox KL. Prehospital care of the patient with an injured chest. *Surg Clin North Am*. 1989;69(1):21.

17. Simon B, Ebert J, Bokhari F, et al. Management of pulmonary contusion and flail chest: an Eastern Association for the Surgery of Trauma practice management guideline. *J Trauma Acute Care Surg*. 2012 Nov;73(5 suppl 4):S351-S361.

18. Cooper C, Militello P. The multi-injured patient: the Maryland Shock Trauma Protocol approach. *Semin Thorac Cardiovasc Surg*. 1992;4(3):163.

19. Barton ED, Epperson M, Hoyt DB, et al. Prehospital needle aspiration and tube thoracostomy in trauma victims: a six-year experience with aeromedical crews. *J Emerg Med*. 1995;13:155.

20. Kheirabadi BS, Terrazas IB, Koller A, et al. Vented vs. unvented chest seals for treatment of pneumothorax (PTx) and prevention of tension PTx in a swine model. *J Trauma Acute Care Surg*. 2013;75:150-156.

21. Butler FK, Dubose JJ, Otten EJ, et al. Management of open pneumothorax in tactical combat casualty care: TCCC guidelines change 13-02. *J Special Ops Med*. 2013;13(3):81-86.

22. Eckstein M, Suyehara DL. Needle thoracostomy in the pre-hospital setting. *Prehosp Emerg Care*. 1998;2:132.

23. Holcomb JB, McManus JG, Kerr ST, Pusateri AE. Needle versus tube thoracostomy in a swine model of traumatic tension hemopneumothorax. *Prehosp Emerg Care*. 2009;13(1):18-27.

24. American College of Surgeons. *Advanced Trauma Life Support for Doctors*. 10th ed. Chicago, IL: American College of Surgeons; 2018.

25. Netto FA, Shulman H, Rizoli SB, et al. Are needle decompressions for tension pneumothoraces being performed appropriately for appropriate indications? *Am J Em Med*. 2008;26;597-602.

26. Riwoe D, Poncia H. Subclavian artery laceration: a serious complication of needle decompression. *Em Med Aust*. 2011;23:651-653.

27. Inaba K, Branco BC Exkstein M, et al. Optimal positioning for emergent needle thoracostomy: a cadaver-based study. *J Trauma*. 2011;71:1099-1103.

28. Inaba K, Karamanos E, Skiada D, et al. Cadaveric comparison of the optimal site for needle decompression of tension pneumothorax by prehospital care providers. *J Trauma*. 2015;79(6):1044-1048.

29. Leatherman ML, Held JM, Fluke LM, et al. Relative device stability of anterior versus axillary needle decompression for tension pneumothorax during casualty movement: preliminary analysis of a human cadaver model. *J Trauma*. 2017;83(1):S136-S141.

30. Beckett A, Savage E, Pannell D, et al. Needle decompression for tension pneumothorax in tactical combat casualty care: do catheters placed in the midaxillary line kink more often than those in the midclavicular line? *J Trauma*. 2011;71:S408-S412.

31. Martin M, Satterly S, Inaba K, Blair K. Does needle thoracostomy provide adequate and effective decompression of tension pneumothorax? *J Trauma*. 2012;73(6):1410-1415.

32. Davis DP, Pettit K, Rum CD, et al. The safety and efficacy of prehospital needle and tube thoracostomy by aeromedical personnel. *Prehosp Emerg Care*. 2005;9:191.

33. Etoch SW, Bar-Natan MF, Miller FB, et al. Tube thoracostomy: factors related to complications. *Arch Surg*. 1995;130:521.

34. Newman PG, Feliciano DV. Blunt cardiac injury. *New Horizons*. 1999;7(1):26.

35. Ivatury RR. The injured heart. In: Mattox KL, Feliciano DV, Moore EE, eds. *Trauma*. 5th ed. New York, NY: McGraw-Hill; 2004:555.

36. Symbas NP, Bongiorno PF, Symbas PN. Blunt cardiac rupture: the utility of emergency department ultrasound. *Ann Thorac Surg*. 1999;67(5):1274.

37. Demetriades D. Cardiac wounds. *Ann Surg*. 1986;203(3):315-317.

38. Jacob S, Sebastian JC, Cherian PK, et al. Pericardial effusion impending tamponade: a look beyond Beck's triad. *Am J Em Med*. 2009;27:216-219.

39. Ivatury RR, Nallathambi MN, Roberge RJ, et al. Penetrating thoracic injuries: in-field stabilization versus prompt transport. *J Trauma*. 1987;27:1066.

40. Bleetman A, Kasem H, Crawford R. Review of emergency thoracotomy for chest injuries in patients attending a UK accident and emergency department. *Injury*. 1996;27(2):129.

41. Durham LA III, Richardson RJ, Wall MJ Jr, et al. Emergency center thoracotomy: impact of prehospital resuscitation. *J Trauma*. 1992;32(6):775.

42. Honigman B, Rohweder K, Moore EE, et al. Prehospital advanced trauma life support for penetrating cardiac wounds. *Ann Emerg Med*. 1990;19(2):145.

43. Lerer LB, Knottenbelt JD. Preventable mortality following sharp penetrating chest trauma. *J Trauma*. 1994;37(1):9.

44. Wall MJ Jr, Pepe PE, Mattox KL. Successful roadside resuscitative thoracotomy: case report and literature review. *J Trauma*. 1994;36(1):131.

45. Coats TJ, Keogh S, Clark H, et al. Prehospital resuscitative thoracotomy for cardiac arrest after penetrating trauma: rationale and case series. *J Trauma*. 2001;50(4):670.

46. Zangwill SD, Strasburger JF. Commotio cordis. *Pediatr Clin North Am*. 2004;51(5):1347-1354.

47. Perron AD, Brady WJ, Erling BF. Commodio cordis: an underappreciated cause of sudden cardiac death in young patients: assessment and management in the ED. *Am J Emerg Med*. 2001;19(5):406-409.

48. Maron BJ, Gohman TE, Kyle SB, Estes NAM III, Link MS. Clinical profile and spectrum of commotio cordis. *JAMA*. 2002;287:1142–1146.

49. Madias C, Maron BJ, Weinstock J, et al. Commotio cordis—sudden cardiac death with chest wall impact. *J Cardiovasc Electrophysiol*. 2007;18(1):115-122.

50. 2010 American Heart Association Guidelines for Cardiopulmonary Resuscitation and Emergency Cardiovascular Care Science. *Circulation*. 2010;122:S745-S746.

51. Mattox KL, Wall MJ, Lemaire SA. Injury to the thoracic great vessels. In: Mattox KL, Feliciano DV, Moore EE, eds. *Trauma*. 5th ed. New York, NY: McGraw-Hill; 2004.

52. Fabian TC, Roger T. Sherman Lecture: advances in the management of blunt thoracic aortic injury: Parmley to the present. *Am Surg*. 2009;75(4):273-278.

53. Riley RD, Miller PR, Meredith JW. Injury to the esophagus, trachea, and bronchus. In: Mattox KL, Feliciano DV, Moore EE, eds. *Trauma*. 5th ed. New York, NY: McGraw-Hill; 2004.

54. Rogers FB, Leavitt BJ. Upper torso cyanosis: a marker for blunt cardiac rupture. *Am J Emerg Med*. 1997;15(3):275.

Suggested Reading

Bowley DM, Boffard KD. Penetrating trauma of the trunk. *Unfallchirurg*. 2001;104(11):1032.

Brathwaite CE, Rodriguez A, Turney SZ, et al. Blunt traumatic cardiac rupture: a 5-year experience. *Ann Surg*. 1990;212(6):701.

Helm M, Schuster R, Hauke J. Tight control of prehospital ventilation by capnography in major trauma victims. *Br J Anaesth*. 2003;90(3):327.

Lateef F. Commotio cordis: an underappreciated cause of sudden death in athletes. *Sports Med*. 2000;30:301.

Papadopoulos IN, Bukis D, Karalas E, et al. Preventable prehospital trauma deaths in a Hellenic urban health region: an audit of prehospital trauma care. *J Trauma*. 1996;41(5):864.

Rozycki GS, Feliciano DV, Oschner MG, et al. The role of ultrasound in patients with possible penetrating cardiac wounds: a prospective multicenter study. *J Trauma*. 1999;46:542.

Ruchholtz S, Waydhas C, Ose C, et al. Prehospital intubation in severe thoracic trauma without respiratory insufficiency: a matched-pair analysis based on the Trauma Registry of the German Trauma Society. *J Trauma*. 2002;52(5):879.

Streng M, Tikka S, Leppaniemi A. Assessing the severity of truncal gunshot wounds: a nation-wide analysis from Finland. *Ann Chir Gynaecol*. 2001;90(4):246.

SPECIFIC SKILLS

Thoracic Trauma Skills

Needle Decompression

Principle: To decrease intrathoracic pressure from a tension pneumothorax affecting the patient's breathing, ventilation, and circulation.

In patients with increasing intrathoracic pressure from a developing tension pneumothorax, the side of the thoracic cavity that has the increased pressure should be decompressed. If this pressure is not relieved, it will progressively limit the patient's ventilatory capacity and compromise venous return, producing inadequate cardiac output and death.

In patients in whom an open pneumothorax has been treated by the use of an occlusive dressing and a tension pneumothorax develops, decompression can usually be achieved through the wound, which provides an existing opening into the thorax. Opening the occlusive dressing over the wound for a few seconds should initiate a rush of air out of the wound as increased pressure in the thorax is relieved.

Once this pressure has been released, the wound is resealed with the occlusive dressing to allow for proper alveolar ventilation and to stop air from "sucking" into the wound. The patient should be monitored carefully, and, if any signs of tension recur, the dressing should be "burped" again to release the intrathoracic pressure.

Decompression in a closed tension pneumothorax is achieved by providing an opening—a thoracostomy—in the affected side of the chest. Different methods for performing a thoracostomy exist. Because needle thoracostomy is the most rapid method and does not require special equipment, it is the preferred method for use in the field.

Needle decompression carries minimal risk and can greatly benefit the patient by improving oxygenation and circulation. Needle decompression should be performed only when the following three criteria are met:

1. Evidence of worsening respiratory distress or difficulty with a bag-mask device
2. Decreased or absent breath sounds
3. Decompensated shock (systolic blood pressure less than 90 mm Hg)

Necessary equipment for needle chest decompression includes a needle, a syringe, ½-inch adhesive tape, and alcohol swabs. The needle used should be a large-bore, over-the-needle IV catheter between 10 and 14 gauge, at least 3.5 inches (8 cm) in length. A 16-gauge catheter can be used if a larger bore is not available.

One prehospital care provider attaches the needle to the syringe while a second prehospital care provider auscultates the patient's chest to confirm which side has the tension pneumothorax, which is indicated by absent or diminished breath sounds.

(continued)

Thoracic Trauma Skills (continued)

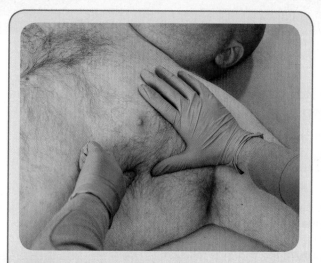

1 After confirmation of a tension pneumothorax, the anatomic landmarks are located on the affected side (second intercostal space along the midclavicular line *or* fifth intercostal space along the anterior axillary line).

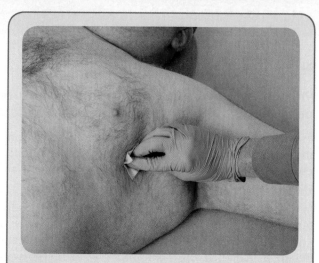

2 The site is swabbed with an antiseptic wipe.

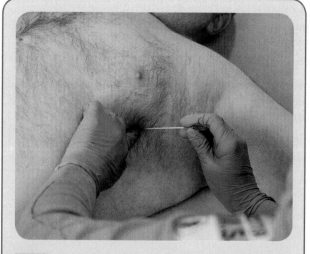

3 The skin over the site is stretched between the fingers of the nondominant hand. The needle and syringe are positioned over the top of the rib.

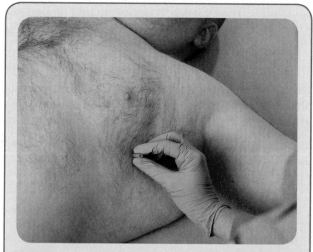

4 Once the needle enters into the thoracic cavity, air will escape into the syringe, and the needle should not be advanced further.

Thoracic Trauma Skills (*continued*)

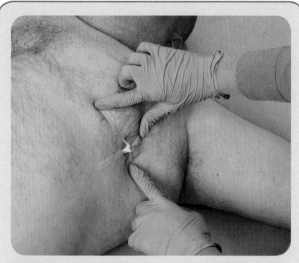

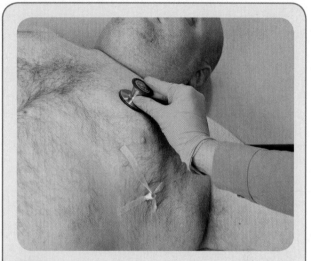

5 The catheter should be left in place and the needle removed, with care not to kink the catheter. As the needle is removed, a rush of air from the hub of the catheter should be heard. If no air escapes, the catheter should be left in place to indicate that needle decompression of the chest was attempted.

6 After the needle is removed, the catheter is taped in place with adhesive tape. After securing the catheter, the chest is auscultated to check for increased breath sounds. The patient is monitored and transported to an appropriate facility. The prehospital care provider need not waste time applying a one-way valve. Needle decompression may need to be repeated if the catheter becomes occluded with a blood clot and tension pneumothorax reoccurs.

CHAPTER **11**

Abdominal Trauma

Lead Editors:
Thomas Scalea, MD
Ronald Tesoriero, MD, FACS
Jason Weinberger, DO

CHAPTER OBJECTIVES
At the completion of this chapter, you will be able to do the following:

- Analyze scene assessment data and mechanism of injury to determine the level of suspicion for abdominal or pelvic trauma.
- Understand the anatomy of the abdomen and pelvis to aid in the recognition and triage of patients with abdominal injury.
- Anticipate the pathophysiologic effects of a blunt or penetrating injury to the abdomen.
- Recognize the physical examination findings indicative of intra-abdominal injury.
- Correlate external signs of abdominal injury to the potential for specific abdominal organ injuries.

- Identify the indications for rapid intervention and transport in the context of abdominal or pelvic trauma.
- Understand appropriate field management decisions for patients with suspected abdominal trauma, including those with impaled objects, evisceration, and external genital trauma.
- Correlate the anatomic and physiologic changes associated with pregnancy to the pathophysiology and management of trauma.
- Discuss the effects of maternal trauma on the fetus and the priorities of management.

SCENARIO

You are called to a construction site for a male patient in his mid-20s who fell 3 hours earlier and is now complaining of increasing abdominal pain. He states that he tripped on a piece of wood at the site and fell, striking his left lower chest and abdomen on some stacked wood. The patient notes moderate pain over his lower left rib cage when he takes deep breaths and complains of mild difficulty breathing. His coworkers wanted to call for assistance when he fell, but he said the symptoms weren't so bad and told them to hold off. He states that the discomfort has been increasing in intensity and that he is now feeling light-headed and weak.

You find the patient sitting on the ground in visible discomfort. He is holding the left side of his lower chest and upper abdomen. He has a patent airway, a respiratory rate of 28 breaths/minute, a heart rate of 124 beats/minute, and a blood pressure of 94/58 millimeters of mercury (mm Hg). The patient's skin is pale and diaphoretic. You lay him down, and on physical examination, he has tenderness on palpation of the left lower ribs without obvious bony crepitus. His abdomen is nondistended and soft to palpation, but he has tenderness and voluntary guarding in the left upper quadrant. No external ecchymosis or subcutaneous emphysema is present.

- What are the patient's possible injuries?
- What are the priorities in the care of this patient?
- Are signs of peritonitis present?

INTRODUCTION

Unrecognized abdominal injury is one of the major causes of preventable death in the trauma patient. Because of the limitations of prehospital assessment, patients with suspected abdominal injuries are best managed by prompt transport to the closest appropriate facility.

Early death from severe abdominal trauma typically results from massive blood loss caused by either penetrating or blunt injuries. Any patient with unexplained shock after sustaining a traumatic injury to the trunk of the body should be assumed to have an intra-abdominal hemorrhage until proven otherwise. The absence of local signs and symptoms does not rule out the possibility of abdominal trauma; signs and symptoms often take time to develop and are especially difficult to identify in the patient whose level of consciousness is altered by alcohol, drugs, or traumatic brain injury (TBI). Complications and death may occur from liver, spleen, colon, small intestine, stomach, or pancreatic injuries that were not initially detected. Consideration of the kinematics can raise the index of suspicion and alert the prehospital care provider to possible abdominal trauma and intra-abdominal hemorrhage. It is not necessary to be concerned with pinpointing the exact extent of abdominal trauma but rather to recognize the likelihood of injury, treat the clinical findings, and triage to the appropriate facility.

Anatomy

The abdomen contains the major organs of the digestive, endocrine, and urogenital systems and major vessels of the circulatory system. The abdominal cavity is located below the diaphragm; its boundaries include the anterior abdominal wall, the pelvic bones, the vertebral column, and the muscles of the abdomen and flanks. The abdominal cavity is divided into two regions based upon the relationship to the *peritoneum*, which covers many of the organs of the abdomen. The **peritoneal cavity** (the "true" abdominal cavity) contains the spleen, liver, gallbladder, stomach, portions of the large intestine (transverse and sigmoid colon), most of the small intestines (primarily the jejunum and ileum), and female reproductive organs (uterus and ovaries) (**Figure 11-1**). The **retroperitoneal space** is the area in the abdominal cavity that is located behind the peritoneum and contains the kidneys, ureters, inferior vena cava, abdominal aorta, pancreas, much of the duodenum, ascending and descending colon, and rectum (**Figure 11-2**).

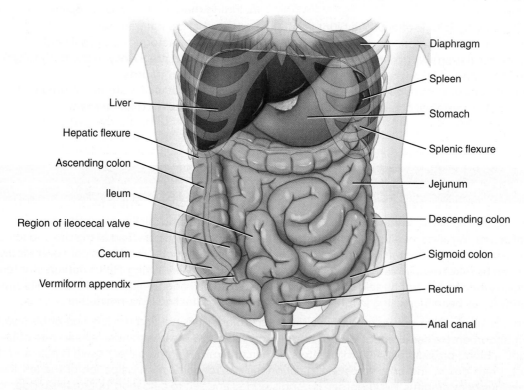

Figure 11-1 The organs inside the peritoneal cavity (shown above) frequently produce peritonitis when injured. Organs in the peritoneal cavity include solid organs (spleen and liver), hollow organs of the gastrointestinal tract (stomach, small intestine, and colon), and reproductive organs.

© National Association of Emergency Medical Technicians (NAEMT).

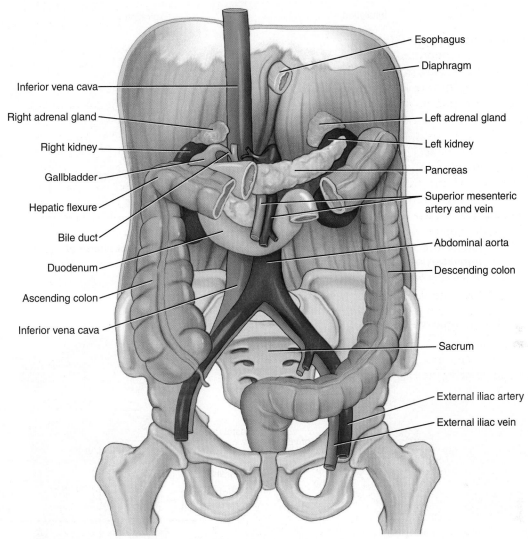

Inferior vena cava

Right adrenal gland

Right kidney

Gallbladder

Hepatic flexure

Bile duct

Duodenum

Ascending colon

Inferior vena cava

Esophagus

Diaphragm

Left adrenal gland

Left kidney

Pancreas

Superior mesenteric artery and vein

Abdominal aorta

Descending colon

Sacrum

External iliac artery

External iliac vein

Figure 11-2 The abdomen is divided into two spaces: peritoneal cavity and retroperitoneal space. The retroperitoneal space shown here includes the portion of the abdomen behind the peritoneum. Because the retroperitoneal organs are not within the peritoneal cavity, injury to these structures generally does not produce peritonitis; however, injury to the large blood vessels and solid organs may produce rapid and massive hemorrhage.

© National Association of Emergency Medical Technicians (NAEMT).

The urinary bladder and male reproductive organs (penis, testes, and prostate) lie inferior to the peritoneal cavity.

A portion of the abdomen lies in the lower thorax. This is because the dome shape of the diaphragm allows the upper abdominal organs to rise up into the lower chest. This superior portion of the abdomen, sometimes referred to as the thoracoabdomen, is protected in front and along the flanks by the ribs and in back by the vertebral column. The thoracoabdomen contains the liver, gallbladder, spleen, and parts of the stomach anteriorly and the lower lobes of the lungs posteriorly, separated by the diaphragm. Because of their location, the same forces that fracture ribs may injure the underlying lungs, liver, or spleen.

The relationship of these abdominal organs to the lower portion of the thoracic cavity changes with the respiratory cycle. At peak expiration, the dome of the relaxed diaphragm

rises to the level of the fourth intercostal space (nipple level in the male), providing greater protection to abdominal organs from the rib cage. Conversely, at peak inspiration, the dome of the contracted diaphragm lies at the level of the sixth intercostal space; the inflated lungs almost fill the thorax and largely push these abdominal organs out from under the rib cage. Thus, the organs injured by penetrating trauma to the thoracoabdomen may differ depending on which phase of respiration the patient was in when injured (**Figure 11-3**).

The most inferior portion of the abdomen is protected on all sides by the pelvis. This area contains the rectum, a portion of the small intestine (especially when the patient is upright), the urinary bladder, and, in the female, the reproductive organs. Retroperitoneal hemorrhage associated with a fractured pelvis is a major concern in this portion of the abdominal cavity.

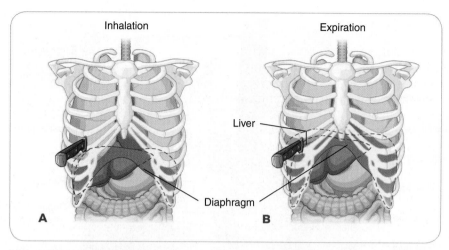

Figure 11-3 Relationship of abdominal organs to the thorax in different phases of respiration in a patient with a stab wound. **A.** Inhalation. **B.** Exhalation.
© National Association of Emergency Medical Technicians (NAEMT).

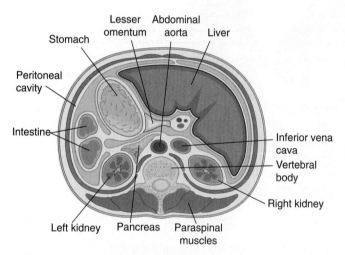

Figure 11-4 This transverse section of the abdominal cavity provides an appreciation of the organ's positions in the anteroposterior direction and the relatively limited protection, particularly anteriorly and laterally.
© National Association of Emergency Medical Technicians (NAEMT).

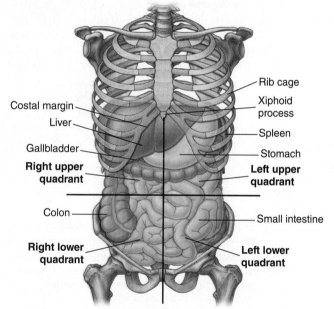

Figure 11-5 As with any part of the body, the better the description of pain, tenderness, guarding, and other signs, the more accurate the diagnosis. The most common system of identification divides the abdomen into four quadrants: left upper, right upper, left lower, and right lower.
© National Association of Emergency Medical Technicians (NAEMT).

The abdomen between the rib cage and the pelvis is protected only by the abdominal muscles and other soft tissues anteriorly and laterally. Posteriorly, the lumbar vertebrae and the thick, strong *paraspinal* muscles located along the length of the spine provide more protection (**Figure 11-4**).

For purposes of patient assessment, the surface of the abdomen is divided into four quadrants. These quadrants are formed by drawing two lines: one in the middle from the tip of the xiphoid to the symphysis pubis and one perpendicular to this midline at the level of the umbilicus (**Figure 11-5**). Knowledge of anatomic landmarks is important because of the high correlation of organ location to pain response. The

right upper quadrant includes the liver and gallbladder, the left upper quadrant contains the spleen and stomach, and the right lower quadrant and left lower quadrant contain primarily the intestines, the distal ureters, and, in women, the ovaries. A portion of the intestinal tract exists in all four quadrants. The urinary bladder and the uterus in women are midline between the lower quadrants.

Pathophysiology

Dividing the abdominal organs into hollow, solid, and vascular (blood vessel) groups helps explain manifestations of injury to these structures. When injured, solid organs (liver, spleen) and blood vessels (aorta, vena cava) bleed, whereas hollow organs (intestine, gallbladder, urinary bladder) primarily spill their contents into the peritoneal cavity or retroperitoneal space (they too bleed but often not as briskly as do solid organs). Loss of blood into the abdominal cavity, regardless of its source, can contribute to or can be the primary cause of the development of hemorrhagic shock. The release of acids, digestive enzymes, and/or bacteria from the gastrointestinal tract into the peritoneal cavity results in **peritonitis** (inflammation of the peritoneum, or the lining of the abdominal cavity) and **sepsis** (systemic infection) if not recognized and promptly treated by surgical intervention. Because urine and bile are generally sterile (do not contain bacteria) and do not contain digestive enzymes, perforation of the gallbladder or urinary bladder does not produce peritonitis as quickly as material spilled from the intestine. Similarly, because it lacks acids, digestive enzymes, and bacteria, blood in the peritoneal cavity does not cause peritonitis for a number of hours. Bleeding from intestinal injury is typically minor, unless the larger blood vessels in the *mesentery* (the folds of peritoneal tissue that attach the bowel to the posterior wall of the abdominal cavity) are damaged.

Injuries to the abdomen can be caused by either penetrating or blunt trauma. Penetrating trauma, such as a gunshot or stab wound, is more readily visible than blunt trauma. Multiple organs may be damaged as a result of penetrating trauma, more commonly with gunshot wounds versus stab wounds given the high energy associated with the "missile"-type injury and the relatively low energy and limited length of most objects used to stab a patient. A mental visualization of the potential trajectory of the penetrating object, such as a bullet or the path of a knife blade, can help identify possible injured internal organs.

The diaphragm extends superiorly to the fourth intercostal space anteriorly, the sixth intercostal space laterally, and the eighth intercostal space posteriorly during maximum expiration (see Figure 11-3). Patients who sustain a penetrating injury to the thorax below these anatomic locations may also have sustained an abdominal injury. Penetrating wounds of the flanks and buttocks may involve organs in the abdominal cavity as well. These penetrating injuries may cause bleeding from a major vessel or solid organ and perforation of a segment of the intestine, the most frequently injured organ in penetrating trauma.

Blunt trauma injuries are often more challenging to recognize than those caused by penetrating trauma. These injuries to abdominal organs result from either compression or shear forces. In **compression injuries**, the organs of the abdomen are crushed between solid objects, such as between the steering wheel and spinal column. **Shear forces** create rupture of the solid organs or rupture of blood

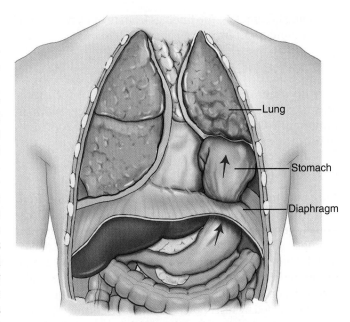

Figure 11-6 With increased pressure inside the abdomen, the diaphragm can rupture, allowing intra-abdominal organs such as the stomach or small intestine to herniate into the chest.
© National Association of Emergency Medical Technicians (NAEMT).

vessels in the cavity because of the tearing forces exerted against their supporting ligaments. The liver and spleen can shear and bleed easily, and blood loss can occur at a rapid rate. Increased intra-abdominal pressure produced by compression can rupture the diaphragm, causing the abdominal organs to move upward into the pleural cavity (**Figure 11-6**). (See the Kinematics of Trauma chapter and the Thoracic Trauma chapter.) The intra-abdominal contents forced into the chest cavity can compromise lung expansion and affect both respiratory and cardiac function. Although rupture of each half of the diaphragm is now believed to occur equally, rupture of the left *hemidiaphragm* (half of the diaphragm) is diagnosed more often, as the underlying liver on the right side often prevents herniation of abdominal contents into the right chest and makes the diagnosis of a right-side diaphragm injury more difficult.

Pelvic fractures may be associated with the loss of large volumes of blood caused by damage to the many smaller blood vessels adjacent to the pelvis. Other injuries associated with pelvic fractures include damage to the urinary bladder and the rectum, as well as injuries to the urethra in the male and the vagina in the female.

Assessment

The assessment of abdominal injury can be difficult, especially with the limited diagnostic capabilities available in the prehospital setting. A high index of suspicion for abdominal injury should develop from a variety of sources of information, including kinematics, the findings from the physical examination, and input from the patient or bystanders.

Kinematics

As with other types of trauma, knowledge of the mechanism of injury, whether blunt or penetrating, plays an important role in shaping the prehospital care provider's index of suspicion for abdominal trauma.

Penetrating Trauma

Most penetrating trauma in the civilian setting results from stab wounds and gunshot wounds from handguns. Occasionally, impalement with or onto an object occurs when, for example, someone falls onto a projecting piece of wood or metal. These low to moderate kinetic energy forces lacerate or cut abdominal organs along the pathway of the knife, projectile, or penetrating object. High-velocity injuries, such as those created by high-powered rifles and assault weapons, tend to create more serious injuries because of the larger temporary cavities created as the projectile moves through the peritoneal cavity. Projectiles may strike bones (ribs, spine, or pelvis), resulting in fragments that may perforate internal organs. Stab wounds are less likely to penetrate the peritoneal cavity than projectiles fired from a handgun, rifle, or shotgun.

When the peritoneum is penetrated, stab wounds are most likely to injure the liver (40%), small bowel (30%), diaphragm (20%), and colon (15%), whereas gunshot wounds most commonly damage the small bowel (50%), colon (40%), liver (30%), and abdominal vessels (25%).[1] Because of the thicker musculature of the back, penetrating trauma to the back is less likely to result in injuries of intraperitoneal structures than wounds to the anterior abdominal wall. Overall, only about 15% of patients with stab wounds to the abdomen will require surgical intervention, whereas about 85% of patients with gunshot wounds will need surgery for definitive management of their abdominal injuries. Tangential gunshot wounds may pass through subcutaneous tissues but never enter the peritoneal cavity. Explosive devices may also propel fragments that penetrate the peritoneum and injure internal organs.

Blunt Trauma

Numerous mechanisms lead to the compression and shear forces that may damage abdominal organs. A patient may experience considerable deceleration or compression forces when involved in motor vehicle and motorcycle crashes, when struck or run over by a vehicle, or after falling from a significant height. Although abdominal organs are most often injured in events associated with significant kinetic injury, such as those with rapid deceleration or severe compression, abdominal injuries may result from more innocuous-appearing mechanisms, such as assaults, falls down a flight of stairs, and sporting activities (e.g., being tackled in football). Any protective devices or gear used by the patient should be noted, including seat belts, air bags, or sports padding.

Compression of a solid organ may result in splitting of its structure (e.g., hepatic laceration), whereas similar forces applied to a hollow structure, such as a loop of bowel or the bladder, may cause the structure to burst open ("rupture"), spilling its contents into the abdomen. Shearing forces may result in tears of structures at sites of tethering to other structures, such as where the more mobile small bowel joins the ascending colon, which is fixed in the retroperitoneum. The organs most commonly injured following blunt trauma to the abdomen include the spleen, liver, and small bowel. Not all injuries to solid organs require surgical intervention (**Box 11-1**). Many of these types of solid organ injuries are just observed carefully in the hospital, as they often stop bleeding on their own.

Box 11-1 Nonoperative Management of Solid Organ Injuries

Suspected injuries of the spleen, liver, or kidney no longer mandate surgical exploration in the modern trauma center. Experience has shown that many of these injuries stop bleeding prior to the development of shock and then heal without surgical repair. Research has shown that even significant solid organ injuries may be safely observed, provided the patient is not experiencing hypovolemic shock or peritonitis. Patients are admitted to the hospital for close monitoring of their vital signs, blood count, and abdominal exam, initially in the intensive care unit. The advantage of this approach is that it prevents the patient from undergoing a potentially unnecessary operation. Because the spleen performs an important role in fighting infections, removal of the spleen (splenectomy) predisposes patients (especially children) to certain bacterial infections.

Successful nonoperative management of these injuries was first reported for splenic injuries in children, but this approach is now often applied to adult patients, as well as to patients suffering injuries to the liver and kidney. Following blunt trauma, data indicate that about 84% of splenic injuries can be managed in this manner, with reported success rates over 90% at high-volume trauma centers.[2] Similarly, many liver injuries are managed nonoperatively, with a success rate of over 90%.[3] Nonoperative management often includes angiographic embolization of bleeding, not simply observation.

The risk of failure of this technique (rebleeding, with the development of shock requiring surgical intervention) is greatest in the first 10 days following injury. Prehospital care providers should be aware of this approach, as they may respond to patients who are experiencing rebleeding after discharge from the hospital.

History

History may be obtained from the patient, family, or bystanders, and it should be documented on the patient care report and relayed to the receiving facility. Obtaining a photograph of the scene and sharing this with emergency department personnel may be valuable in communicating the mechanism of injury clearly. In addition to the components of the SAMPLE history (**s**ymptoms, **a**llergies and **a**ge, **m**edications, **p**ast medical/surgical history, **l**ast meal, **e**vents preceding injury), questions should be tailored to the mechanism of injury and the presence of comorbid conditions that can potentially increase mortality or morbidity. For example, in the case of a motor vehicle crash, questions may be asked to determine the following:

- Type of collision, position of patient in the vehicle, or ejection from the vehicle
- Estimated vehicle speed at time of crash
- Extent of vehicle damage, including intrusion into the passenger compartment, steering wheel deformity, windshield damage, and requirement for prolonged extrication
- Use of safety devices, including seat belts, deployment of air bags, and presence of child safety seats

In the case of penetrating injury, questions may be asked to determine the following:

- Type of weapon (handgun or rifle, caliber, length of knife)
- Number of times the patient was shot or stabbed
- Distance from which the patient was shot
- Amount of blood at the scene (although accurate estimation is often difficult)
- Previous history of penetrating injury (may have retained ballistic fragments)

Physical Examination

Primary Survey

Most severe abdominal injuries present as abnormalities identified in the primary survey, primarily in the evaluation of breathing and circulation. Unless there are associated injuries, patients with abdominal trauma generally present with a patent airway. The alterations found in the breathing, circulation, and disability assessments generally correspond to the degree of shock present. Patients with early, compensated shock may have a mild increase in their respiratory rate, whereas those with severe hemorrhagic shock demonstrate marked tachypnea. Rupture of a hemidiaphragm often compromises respiratory function when abdominal contents herniate into the chest on the affected side, and bowel sounds may be heard over the thorax when breath sounds are auscultated. Similarly, shock from intra-abdominal hemorrhage may range from mild tachycardia, with few other findings, to severe tachycardia, marked hypotension, and pale, cool, clammy skin.

The most reliable indicator of intra-abdominal bleeding is the presence of hypovolemic shock from an unexplained source. When assessing disability, the prehospital care provider may note only subtle signs, such as mild anxiety or agitation, in the patient with compensated shock from abdominal trauma, whereas patients with life-threatening hemorrhage may have serious depression in their mental status. When abnormalities are found in the assessment of these systems and while preparing for immediate transport, the abdomen should be exposed and examined for evidence of trauma, such as bruising or penetrating wounds.

Secondary Assessment

During the secondary assessment, the abdomen is examined in greater detail. This examination primarily involves inspection and palpation of the abdomen and should be approached systematically.

Inspection

The abdomen is examined for soft-tissue injuries and distension. Intra-abdominal injury may be suspected when soft-tissue trauma is noted over the abdomen, flanks, or back. Such injuries may include contusions, abrasions, stab or gunshot wounds, obvious bleeding, and unusual findings such as evisceration, impaled objects, or tire marks. The "seat belt sign" (ecchymosis or abrasion across the abdomen resulting from compression of the abdominal wall against the shoulder harness or lap belt) indicates that significant force was applied to the abdomen as a result of sudden deceleration (**Figure 11-7**) and increases the likelihood of intra-abdominal injury eightfold.[4] The incidence of intra-abdominal injuries in pediatric patients with seat belt signs is greater than the incidence in adults. The injuries associated with restraints are typically to the bowel and its supporting mesentery, as they are compressed and crushed between the seat belt and anterior abdominal wall and the spinal column posteriorly, and often present

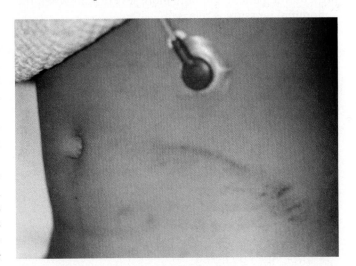

Figure 11-7 An abdominal "seat belt sign" resulting from the patient decelerating against a lap belt.

Courtesy of Peter T. Pons, MD, FACEP.

in a delayed fashion. *Grey-Turner's sign* (ecchymosis involving the flanks) and *Cullen's sign* (ecchymosis around the umbilicus) indicate retroperitoneal bleeding; however, these signs are often delayed and may not be seen in the first few hours after injury.

The contour of the abdomen should be noted, assessing if it is flat or distended. Distension of the abdomen may indicate significant internal hemorrhage; however, the adult peritoneal cavity can hold up to 1.5 liters of fluid before showing any obvious signs of distension. Abdominal distension may also be the result of a stomach filled with air, as can occur during artificial ventilation with a bag-mask device. Although these signs may indicate intra-abdominal injury, some patients with substantial internal injury may lack these findings.

Palpation

Palpation of the abdomen is undertaken to identify areas of tenderness. Ideally, palpation is begun in an area in which the patient does not complain of pain. Then, each of the abdominal quadrants is palpated. While palpating a tender area, the prehospital care provider may note that the patient "tenses up" the abdominal muscles in that area. This reaction, called **voluntary guarding**, protects the patient from the pain resulting from palpation. **Involuntary guarding** represents rigidity or spasm of the abdominal wall muscles in response to peritonitis. **Box 11-2** lists physical findings consistent with the presence of peritonitis. Unlike voluntary guarding, involuntary guarding remains when the patient is distracted (e.g., with conversation) or the abdomen is surreptitiously palpated (e.g., with pressure on the stethoscope while appearing to auscultate bowel sounds). Although the presence of **rebound tenderness** has long been considered an important finding indicating peritonitis, many surgeons now believe that this maneuver—pressing deeply on the abdomen and then quickly releasing the pressure—causes excessive pain. If rebound tenderness is present, the patient will note more severe pain when the abdominal pressure is released.

Deep or aggressive palpation of an obviously injured abdomen should be avoided because, in addition to the pain it causes, palpation may theoretically aggravate bleeding or other injury. Great care during palpation should also be exercised if there is an impaled object in the abdomen. In fact, there is little additional useful information to be gained by palpating the abdomen in a patient with an impaled object.

Box 11-2 Findings From the Physical Examination That Support a Diagnosis of Peritonitis

- Significant abdominal tenderness on palpation or with coughing (either localized or generalized)
- Involuntary guarding
- Percussion tenderness
- Diminished or absent bowel sounds

Although tenderness is an important indicator of intra-abdominal injury, several factors may confound the assessment of tenderness. Patients with altered mental status, such as those with a TBI or those under the influence of drugs or alcohol, may have an *unreliable* examination; that is, the patient may not report tenderness or respond to palpation even when significant internal injuries are present. Pediatric and geriatric patients are more likely to have unreliable abdominal examinations because of impaired pain responses. Conversely, patients with lower rib fractures or a pelvic fracture may have an *equivocal* (ambiguous) examination, with tenderness resulting from either the fractures or associated internal injuries. If the patient has distracting pain from injuries, such as extremity or spinal fractures, abdominal pain may not be elicited on palpation.

Palpation of the pelvis in the prehospital setting provides little information that will alter the management of the patient. If time is taken to perform this examination, it is performed only once, because any clot that has formed at the site of an unstable fracture may be disrupted, thus exacerbating hemorrhage. During this examination, the pelvis is palpated gently to assess for instability and tenderness. This evaluation involves two steps:

1. Pressing inward on the iliac crests
2. Pressing posteriorly on the pubic symphysis

If instability or pain is noted during any step of the examination, no further palpation of the pelvis should take place.

Auscultation

Hemorrhage and spillage of intestinal contents in the peritoneal cavity may result in an *ileus*, a condition in which the peristalsis of the bowel ceases. This results in a "quiet" abdomen, as bowel sounds are diminished or absent. Auscultation of bowel sounds is generally not a helpful prehospital assessment tool. Time should not be wasted trying to determine their presence or absence because this diagnostic sign will not alter the prehospital management of the patient. If bowel sounds are heard over the thorax during auscultation of breath sounds, however, the presence of a diaphragmatic rupture may be considered.

Percussion

Although percussion of the abdomen may reveal tympanic or dull sounds, this information does not alter prehospital management of the trauma patient and only expends valuable time; therefore it is not recommended as a prehospital assessment tool. Significant tenderness on percussion or pain when the patient is asked to cough represents a key finding of peritonitis. Peritoneal signs are summarized in Box 11-2.

Special Examinations and Key Indicators

Surgical evaluation and, in many cases, intervention remain key needs for most patients who have sustained abdominal injuries; time should not be wasted in attempts to determine the exact details of injury. In many patients, identification of specific organ injury will not be revealed until the abdomen is further evaluated by computed tomography (CT) scanning or surgical exploration.

In the emergency department, ultrasound has become the primary bedside modality used to assess a trauma patient for intra-abdominal hemorrhage.[1,5-8] The focused assessment with sonography for trauma (FAST) examination involves three views of the peritoneal cavity and a fourth view of the pericardium to assess for the presence of fluid, presumably blood, around the heart (**Figure 11-8** and **Box 11-3**). Because fluid does not reflect the ultrasound waves back to the device, fluid appears anechoic (sonographically

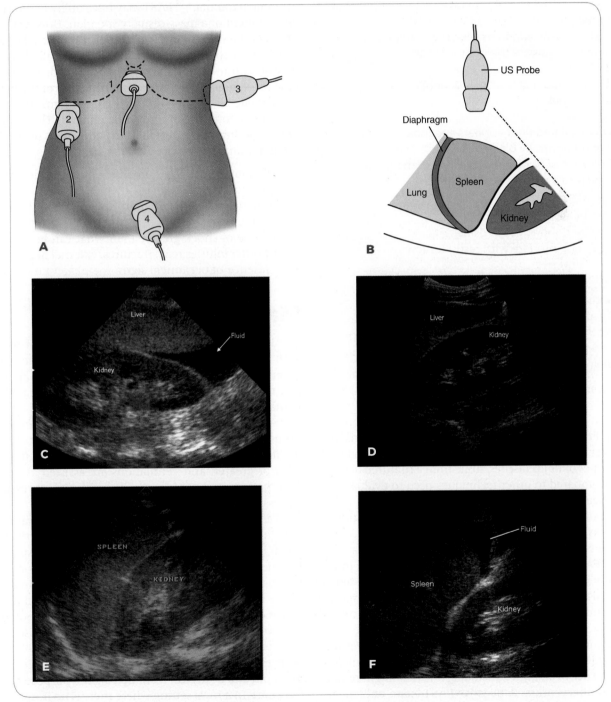

Figure 11-8 Focused assessment with sonography for trauma (FAST). **A.** Four views constituting the FAST examination. **B.** Normal splenorenal view identifying organs. **C.** Normal view of the right upper quadrant. **D.** Abnormal view of the right upper quadrant demonstrating the presence of fluid (blood). **E.** Normal view of the left upper quadrant. **F.** Abnormal view of the left upper quadrant demonstrating the presence of fluid (blood).

Box 11-3 FAST Examination*

The FAST examination has value in the trauma patient because most significant intra-abdominal injuries are associated with hemorrhage into the peritoneal cavity. Although ultrasound cannot differentiate the type of fluid present, any fluid in the trauma patient is presumed to be blood.

Technique
- Four acoustic windows (views) are imaged, three of which evaluate the peritoneal cavity:
  1. Pericardial
  2. Perihepatic (Morrison's pouch)
  3. Perisplenic
  4. Pelvic
- Accumulated fluid appears anechoic (sonographically black).
- Presence of fluid in one or more of the areas indicates a positive scan.

Advantages
- Can be rapidly performed
- Can be done at the bedside
- Does not interfere with resuscitation
- Is noninvasive
- Is less costly than CT

Disadvantages
- Results are compromised in patients who are obese, who have subcutaneous air, or who have had previous abdominal surgery.
- Skill at imaging is operator dependent.

*FAST has been studied in several prehospital systems.[9-12]

---

black). Presence of fluid in one or more areas is worrisome; however, ultrasonography cannot differentiate blood from other types of fluids (ascites, urine from a ruptured bladder, etc.). Compared to other techniques used to evaluate the peritoneal cavity, FAST can be rapidly performed at the patient's bedside, does not interfere with resuscitation, is noninvasive, does not involve radiation exposure, and is much less costly than CT scanning. The primary disadvantage of FAST is that it does not definitively diagnose injury but only indicates the presence of fluid that may be blood. Other disadvantages of the FAST exam are that imaging is dependent on the operator's skill and experience and its utility is compromised in patients who are obese, have subcutaneous air, or have had previous surgery. Perhaps most important, a negative FAST exam does not rule out the presence of an injury, including one that might require surgical intervention. A negative FAST exam only means that, at the moment when the exam was performed, fluid was not visualized in the abdomen. This result could be because no injury exists or because not enough blood had accumulated in the abdomen to be seen (which is a real

possibility given a rapid response by emergency medical services [EMS] to the trauma incident scene).

Because of ease of use and improved ultrasound technology, some ground and air EMS systems and military teams have explored the use of FAST in the prehospital setting. The FAST exam has been shown to be feasible in the field, but no published data have demonstrated that use of this technology results in improved outcomes for patients with abdominal trauma.[9-15] FAST may have utility in the austere environment or a mass-casualty situation. However, use of FAST is not recommended by Prehospital Trauma Life Support (PHTLS) for routine prehospital care, especially because it may delay transport to the receiving facility or may provide false reassurance about the actual condition of the patient.

Despite all of these different components, the assessment of abdominal injury can be difficult. The following are key indicators for establishing the index of suspicion for abdominal injury:

- Obvious signs of trauma (e.g., soft-tissue injuries, gunshot wounds)
- Presence of hypovolemic shock without another obvious cause
- Degree of shock greater than what can be explained by other injuries (e.g., fractures, external hemorrhage)
- Presence of peritoneal signs

Management

The key aspects of prehospital management of patients with abdominal trauma are to recognize the presence of potential injury and initiate rapid transport, as appropriate, to the closest appropriate facility that is capable of managing the patient.

Abnormalities in vital functions identified in the primary survey are supported during transport. Supplemental oxygen is administered to maintain saturation at 94% or greater, and ventilations are assisted as needed. External hemorrhage is controlled with direct pressure or a pressure dressing.

Patients with abdominal trauma often require transfusion and surgical intervention to control internal hemorrhage and repair injuries; therefore, patients should be transported to facilities that have immediate surgical capability, such as a trauma center, if available. Findings particularly indicative of the need for prompt surgical intervention include evidence of abdominal trauma associated with hypotension or peritoneal signs, and the presence of an evisceration or impaled object. Taking a patient with intra-abdominal injuries to a facility that does not have an available operating room and a surgical team defeats the purpose of rapid transport. In a rural setting where there is no hospital with general surgeons on staff, consideration should be given to direct transfer to a trauma center, either by ground or air, as early surgical intervention is the key to survival of the unstable patient with abdominal trauma. Case reports describe prehospital use of resuscitative endovascular balloon occlusion of the aorta (REBOA) by highly trained teams to control hemorrhage in torso trauma in order to allow time for transfer to definitive care[16] (**Figure 11-9**). Given the requirement for specialized training, the unclear benefit to outcomes, and potential for significant complications, this intervention is not currently available for prehospital care and is not recommended by PHTLS.

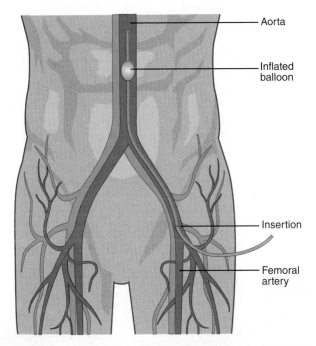

Figure 11-9 Resuscitative endovascular balloon occlusion of the aorta (REBOA) for uncontrolled hemorrhage in the torso.
© National Association of Emergency Medical Technicians (NAEMT).

Labels: Aorta, Inflated balloon, Insertion, Femoral artery

If the patient has sustained blunt trauma that also could have produced spinal or pelvic injury, stabilization is performed as appropriate. For proper instructions on spinal immobilization, see the Spinal Trauma chapter. In hemodynamically unstable blunt trauma patients with suspected pelvic injury, prehospital providers are advised to stabilize, or "close," the pelvis by securing it with a sheet or applying a commercial pelvic binder (**Figure 11-10**). Securing the pelvis in this fashion reduces pelvic volume and stabilizes fracture fragments, thus helping to reduce the risk of major hemorrhage during transport to definitive care.

During transport, intravenous (IV) access is obtained. The decision to administer crystalloid fluid replacement en route depends on the patient's clinical presentation. Abdominal trauma represents one of the key situations in which balanced resuscitation is indicated. Aggressive administration of IV fluid may elevate the patient's blood pressure to levels that will disrupt any clot that has formed and result in recurrence of bleeding that had ceased because of blood clotting and hypotension. (Further discussion of IV fluid administration is provided in the Shock: Pathophysiology of Life and Death chapter.) Although prehospital teams equipped with blood products and strict protocols to guide transfusion in hypotensive trauma patients have been established in some areas, the long-term outcomes of this strategy are uncertain.[17] Whether crystalloid or blood products are available, prehospital care providers must achieve a delicate balance: maintain a blood pressure that provides perfusion to vital organs without restoring blood pressure to elevated or even normal ranges, which may reinitiate bleeding sites in the abdomen or pelvis. In the absence of TBI, the target systolic blood pressure is 80 to 90 mm Hg (mean arterial pressure of 60 to 65 mm Hg). For patients with suspected

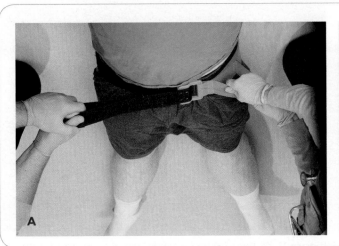
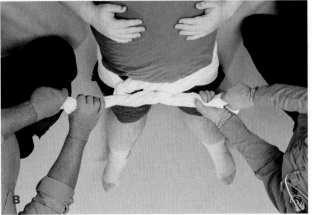

Figure 11-10 Examples of prehospital pelvic stabilization techniques. **A.** Commercially available pelvic binder. **B.** Sheet used for binding.
© Jones & Bartlett Learning. Photographer by Darren Stahlman.

intra-abdominal bleeding and a TBI, the systolic blood pressure is maintained at a minimum of 90 mm Hg.

Tranexamic acid (TXA) is a clot-stabilizing medication that has been used for years to control bleeding and has started to make its way into the prehospital environment. TXA works by binding to plasminogen and preventing it from becoming plasmin, thereby preventing the breakdown of fibrin in a clot. Ongoing studies will assist in determining the appropriate prehospital role for TXA. Shock: Pathophysiology of Life and Death discusses TXA in greater detail.

Special Considerations

Impaled Objects

Because removal of an impaled object may cause additional trauma and because the object may be actively controlling (*tamponade effect*) the bleeding, removal of an impaled object from the abdomen in the prehospital environment is contraindicated (**Figure 11-11**). The prehospital care provider should neither move nor remove an object impaled in a patient's abdomen. In the hospital, these objects are not removed until their shape and location have been identified by radiographic evaluation and until blood replacement and a surgical team are present and ready. Often these objects are removed in the operating room.

A prehospital care provider may stabilize the impaled object, either manually or mechanically, to prevent any further movement in the field and during transport. In some circumstances the impaled object may need to be cut in order to free the patient and permit transport to the trauma center. If bleeding occurs around it, direct pressure should be applied around the object to the wound with the palm

of the hand. Psychological support of the patient is important, especially if the impaled object is visible to the patient.

The abdomen should not be palpated or percussed in these patients because these actions may produce additional organ injury from the distal end of the object. Further examination is unnecessary because the presence of impaled objects indicates the need for management by a surgeon.

Evisceration

In an abdominal **evisceration**, a section of intestine or other abdominal organ is displaced through an open wound and protrudes outside the abdominal cavity (**Figure 11-12**). The tissue most often visualized is the fatty **omentum** that lies over the intestines. Attempts should not be made to replace the protruding tissue into the abdominal cavity. The **viscera** should be left on the surface of the abdomen or protruding as found.

Treatment efforts should focus on protecting the protruding segment of intestine or other organ from further damage. Most of the abdominal contents require a moist environment. If the intestine or some of the other abdominal

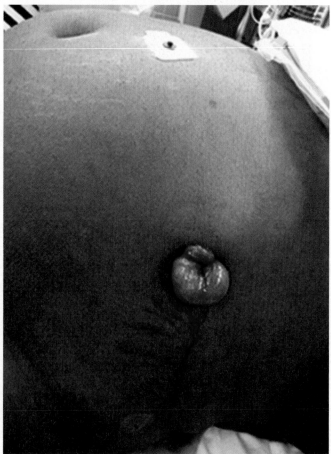

Figure 11-12 Bowel eviscerated through a wound in the abdominal wall.

Courtesy of Lance Stuke, MD, MPH.

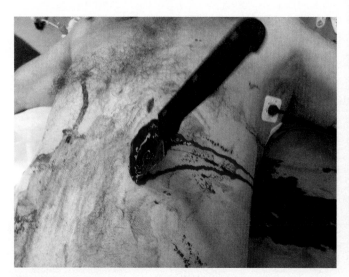

Figure 11-11 Removal of an impaled object from the abdomen is contraindicated in the prehospital environment.

Courtesy of Lance Stuke, MD, MPH.

organs become dry, cell death will occur. Therefore, the eviscerated abdominal contents should be covered with a clean or sterile dressing that has been moistened with saline (normal saline IV fluid can be used). These dressings should be periodically remoistened with saline to prevent them from drying out. Wet dressings may be covered with a large, dry or occlusive dressing to keep the patient warm.

Psychological support is extremely important for patients with an abdominal evisceration, and care should be taken to keep the patient calm. Any action that increases pressure within the abdomen, such as crying, screaming, or coughing, can force more of the organs outward. These patients should be expeditiously transported to a trauma center.

Trauma in the Obstetric Patient

Anatomic and Physiologic Changes

Pregnancy causes both anatomic and physiologic changes to the body's systems. These changes can affect the patterns of injuries seen and make the assessment of an injured pregnant patient especially challenging. The prehospital care provider is dealing with two or more patients and must be aware of the changes that have occurred to the woman's anatomy and physiology throughout the pregnancy.

A human pregnancy typically lasts about 40 weeks from conception to birth, and this gestational period is divided into three sections, or trimesters. The first trimester ends at about the 12th week of gestation, and the second trimester is slightly longer than the other two, ending at about week 28.

Following conception and implantation of the fetus, the uterus continues to enlarge through the 38th week of pregnancy. Until about the 12th week, the growing uterus remains protected by the bony pelvis. By the 20th week of gestation, the top of the uterus (fundus) is at the umbilicus,

and the fundus approaches the xiphoid process by the 38th week. This anatomic change makes the uterus and its contents more susceptible to both blunt and penetrating injury (**Figure 11-13**). Injury to the uterus can include rupture, penetration, *abruptio placentae* (when a portion of the placenta is pulled away from the uterine wall), and premature rupture of the membranes (**Figure 11-14**). The placenta and gravid uterus are highly vascular; injuries to these structures can result in profound hemorrhage. Because the hemorrhage can be concealed inside the uterus or peritoneal cavity, it may not be externally visible.

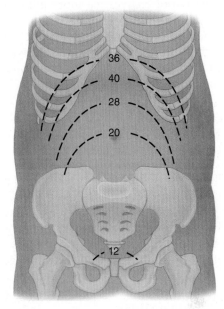

Figure 11-13 Fundal height. As pregnancy progresses, the uterus becomes more susceptible to injury.
© National Association of Emergency Medical Technicians (NAEMT).

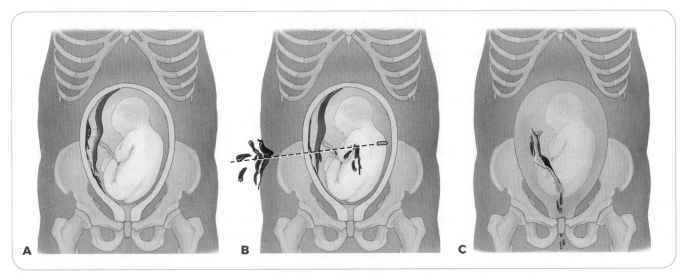

Figure 11-14 Diagram of uterine trauma. **A.** Abruptio placentae. **B.** Gunshot to the uterus. **C.** Ruptured uterus.
© National Association of Emergency Medical Technicians (NAEMT).

Although a marked protuberance of the abdomen is obvious in late pregnancy, the rest of the abdominal organs remain essentially unchanged, with the exception of the uterus. Intestine that is displaced superiorly is shielded by the uterus in the last two trimesters of pregnancy. The increased size and weight of the uterus alter the patient's center of gravity and increase the risk of falls. Because of its prominence, the gravid abdomen is often injured in a fall.

In addition to these anatomic changes, physiologic changes occur during pregnancy. The woman's heart rate normally increases throughout pregnancy by 15 to 20 beats/minute above normal by the third trimester. This makes the interpretation of tachycardia more difficult. Systolic and diastolic blood pressures normally drop 5 to 15 mm Hg during the second trimester but often return to normal at term. By the 10th week of pregnancy, the woman's cardiac output increases by 1 to 1.5 liters/minute. By term, the woman's blood volume has increased by about 50%. *Because of these increases in cardiac output and blood volume, the pregnant patient may lose 30% to 35% of her blood volume before signs and symptoms of hypovolemia become apparent.*[18] Hypovolemic shock may induce premature labor in patients in the third trimester. Oxytocin, which is released along with antidiuretic hormone in response to loss of circulating blood volume, stimulates uterine contractions.

Some women may have significant hypotension when supine. This supine hypotension of pregnancy typically occurs in the third trimester and is caused by the compression of the inferior vena cava by the enlarged uterus. This dramatically decreases venous return to the heart, and because there is less filling, cardiac output and blood pressure fall[18] (**Figure 11-15**).

The following maneuvers may be used to relieve supine hypotension (**Figure 11-16**):

1. The woman may be placed on her left side (left lateral decubitus position), or if spinal immobilization is indicated, 4 to 6 inches (10 to 15 centimeters [cm]) of padding should be placed under the right side of the long backboard.
2. If the patient cannot be rotated, her right leg should be elevated to displace the uterus to the left.
3. The uterus may be manually displaced toward the patient's left side.

These three maneuvers reduce compression on the vena cava, increasing venous return to the heart and improving cardiac output.

During the third trimester, the diaphragm is elevated and may be associated with mild dyspnea, especially when the patient is supine. Peristalsis (propulsive, muscular movements of intestines) is slower during pregnancy, so

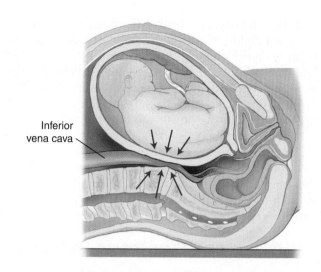

Figure 11-15 Full-term uterus compressing the vena cava.
© National Association of Emergency Medical Technicians (NAEMT).

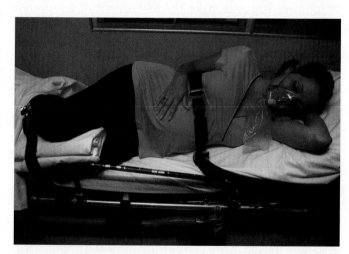

Figure 11-16 Tipping a pregnant female onto her left side helps displace the uterus from the inferior vena cava and improves blood return to the heart, thus restoring blood pressure.
© Jones & Bartlett Learning. Courtesy of MIEMSS.

food may remain in the stomach many hours after eating. Therefore, the pregnant patient is at greater risk for vomiting and subsequent aspiration.

Toxemia of pregnancy (also known as eclampsia) is a late complication of pregnancy. Whereas *pre-eclampsia* is characterized by edema and hypertension, **eclampsia** is characterized by mental status changes and seizures, thus mimicking TBI. A careful neurologic assessment and asking about potential complications of pregnancy and other medical conditions such as known diabetes, hypertension, or seizure history are important.

Assessment

Pregnancy typically does not alter the woman's airway, but significant respiratory distress may occur when a patient in her third trimester is placed supine on a long backboard. The decrease in peristalsis of the gastrointestinal tract makes vomiting and aspiration more likely. Airway patency and pulmonary function are assessed, including auscultation of breath sounds and monitoring of pulse oximetry.

As with hemoperitoneum from other sources, intra-abdominal bleeding associated with uterine injury may not produce peritonitis for hours. More likely, blood loss from an injury may be masked by the pregnant female's increased cardiac output and blood volume. Therefore, a high index of suspicion and assessment for subtle changes (e.g., skin color) may provide important clues.

In general, the condition of the fetus will depend on the condition of the woman; however, the fetus may be in jeopardy while the woman's condition and vital signs appear hemodynamically normal. This occurs because the body shunts blood away from the uterus (and fetus) to the vital organs. Neurologic changes should be noted and documented, although the exact etiology may not be identifiable in the prehospital setting.

As with the nonpregnant patient, auscultation of bowel sounds is generally not helpful in the prehospital setting. Similarly, spending valuable minutes searching for fetal heart tones at the scene is not useful; their presence or absence will not alter prehospital management. The external genitalia should be checked for evidence of vaginal bleeding, and the patient should be asked about the presence of contractions and fetal movement. Contractions may indicate that premature labor has begun, whereas a decrease in fetal movement may be an ominous sign of profound fetal distress.

Palpation of the abdomen may reveal tenderness. A firm, hard, tender uterus is suggestive of abruptio placentae, which is associated with visible vaginal bleeding in approximately 70% of cases.[18]

Management

With an injured pregnant patient, the survival of the fetus is best ensured by focusing on the woman's condition. In essence, for the fetus to survive, usually the woman needs to survive. Priority is given to ensuring an adequate patent airway and supporting respiratory function. Sufficient oxygen should be administered to maintain a pulse oximetry reading of 95% or higher. Ventilations may need to be assisted, especially in the later stages of pregnancy. It is wise to anticipate vomiting and have suction nearby.

The goals of shock management are essentially the same as for any patient and include judicious IV fluid administration, especially if evidence of decompensated shock is present. Any evidence of vaginal bleeding or a rigid, board-like abdomen with external bleeding in the last trimester of pregnancy may indicate abruptio placentae or a ruptured uterus. These conditions threaten not only the life of the fetus but also that of the woman because exsanguination can occur rapidly. No good data exist to define the best target blood pressure for an injured pregnant patient. However, restoration of normal systolic and mean blood pressures will most likely result in better fetal perfusion, despite the risk of promoting additional internal hemorrhage in the woman.

Transport of the pregnant trauma patient should not be delayed. Every pregnant trauma patient—even those who appear to have only minor injuries—should be rapidly transported to the closest appropriate facility. An ideal facility is a trauma center that has both surgical and obstetric capabilities immediately available. Adequate resuscitation of the woman is the key to survival of the woman and fetus.

Genitourinary Injuries

Injuries to the kidneys, ureters, and bladder are most often present with *hematuria* (blood in the urine). This sign will generally not be noted unless the patient has a urinary catheter inserted. Because the kidneys receive a significant portion of cardiac output, blunt or penetrating injuries to these organs may result in life-threatening retroperitoneal hemorrhage.

Pelvic fractures may be associated with lacerations of the urinary bladder and the walls of the vagina or the rectum. Open pelvic fractures, such as those with deep groin or perineal lacerations, may result in severe external hemorrhage.

Trauma to the external genitalia may occur from multiple mechanisms, although injuries resulting from ejection from a motorcycle or motor vehicle, an industrial accident, straddle-type mechanisms, gunshot wounds, or sexual assault predominate. Because of the numerous nerve endings in these organs, these injuries are associated with significant pain and psychological concern. These organs contain numerous blood vessels, and copious amounts of blood may be seen. In general, this type of bleeding can be controlled with direct pressure or a pressure dressing. Dressings should not be inserted into the vagina or the urethra to control bleeding, particularly in pregnant women. If direct pressure is not required to control hemorrhage, these injuries should be covered with moist, clean, saline-soaked gauze. Any amputated parts should be managed as described in the Musculoskeletal Trauma chapter. Further evaluation of all genital injuries should occur at the hospital.

SUMMARY

- Intra-abdominal injuries are often life threatening because of internal hemorrhage and spillage of gastrointestinal contents into the peritoneal cavity.
- The extent of internal injuries is not identifiable in the prehospital setting; therefore mechanism of injury in combination with signs of abdominal trauma should increase the prehospital care provider's index of suspicion.
- Management of the patient with abdominal trauma includes oxygenation, hemorrhage control, and rapid packaging for transport. Spinal immobilization precautions should be taken in blunt trauma patients with torso injury and the pelvis further stabilized with a binder if hemodynamically unstable.

- Balanced resuscitation with crystalloid solutions permits perfusion of vital organs while potentially minimizing the risk of aggravating internal hemorrhage.
- Because emergent surgical intervention may be lifesaving, a patient with abdominal trauma should be transported to a trauma center with immediate surgical capability.
- The anatomic and physiologic changes of pregnancy have implications for the pattern of injury, presentation of signs and symptoms of trauma, and management of the pregnant trauma patient.
- Management of potential fetal compromise caused by trauma is accomplished through effective resuscitation of the woman.

SCENARIO RECAP

You are called to a construction site for a male patient in his mid-20s who fell 3 hours earlier and is now complaining of increasing abdominal pain. He states that he tripped on a piece of wood at the site and fell, striking his left lower chest and abdomen on some stacked wood. The patient notes moderate pain over his lower left rib cage when he takes deep breaths and complains of mild difficulty breathing. His coworkers wanted to call for assistance when he fell, but he said the symptoms weren't so bad and told them to hold off. He states that the discomfort has been increasing in intensity and that he is now feeling light-headed and weak.

You find the patient sitting on the ground in visible discomfort. He is holding the left side of his lower chest and upper abdomen. He has a patent airway, a respiratory rate of 28 breaths/minute, a heart rate of 124 beats/minute, and a blood pressure of 94/58 mm Hg. The patient's skin is pale and diaphoretic. You lay him down, and on physical examination, he has tenderness on palpation of the left lower ribs without obvious bony crepitus. His abdomen is nondistended and soft to palpation, but he has tenderness and voluntary guarding in the left upper quadrant. No external ecchymosis or subcutaneous emphysema is present.

- What are the patient's possible injuries?
- What are the priorities in the care of this patient?
- Are signs of peritonitis present?

SCENARIO SOLUTION

The patient is tender over his left lower ribs and left upper quadrant. These findings can represent injuries to the thorax, intra-abdominal organs, or both. His vital signs are consistent with compensated hypovolemic shock, and a hemothorax or intra-abdominal bleeding must be considered. More likely, the tenderness over the lower ribs may indicate fractured ribs with an associated laceration of the spleen, resulting in intraperitoneal hemorrhage.

Oxygen is administered, and the patient is packaged for transport. En route to the trauma center, intravenous access is obtained; however, given the patient's blood pressure, crystalloid fluid is administered judiciously, as aggressive fluid infusion may raise his blood pressure and lead to increased bleeding.

References

1. American College of Surgeons (ACS) Committee on Trauma. Abdominal trauma. In: *Advanced Trauma Life Support for Doctors, Student Course Manual*. 8th ed. Chicago, IL: ACS; 2008:111-126.

2. Banerjee A, Duane TM, Wilson SP, et al. Trauma center variation in splenic artery embolization and spleen salvage: a multicenter analysis. *J Trauma Acute Care Surg*. 2013;75(1):69-75.

3. Boese CK, Hackl M, Müller LP, et al. Nonoperative management of blunt hepatic trauma: a systematic review. *J Trauma Acute Care Surg*. 2015;79(4):654-660.

4. Velmahos GC, Tatevossian R, Demetriades D. The "seat belt mark" sign: a call for increased vigilance among physicians treating victims of motor vehicle accidents. *Am Surg*. 1999;65(2):181.

5. Rozycki GS, Ochsner MG, Schmidt JA, et al. A prospective study of surgeon-performed ultrasound as the primary adjuvant modality for injured patient assessment. *J Trauma Injury Infect Crit Care*. 1995;39(3):492.

6. Rozycki GS, Ochsner MG, Feliciano DV, et al. Early detection of hemoperitoneum by ultrasound examination of the right upper quadrant: a multicenter study. *J Trauma Injury Infect Crit Care*. 1998;45(5):878.

7. Rozycki GS, Ballard RB, Feliciano DV, et al. Surgeon-performed ultrasound for the assessment of truncal injuries: lessons learned from 1540 patients. *Ann Surg*. 1998;228(4):557.

8. Polk JD, Fallon WF Jr. The use of focused assessment with sonography for trauma (FAST) by a prehospital air medical team in the trauma arrest patient. *Prehosp Emerg Care*. 2000;4(1):82.

9. Melanson SW, McCarthy J, Stromski CJ, et al. Aeromedical trauma sonography by flight crews with a miniature ultrasound unit. *Prehosp Emerg Care*. 2001;5(4):399.

10. Walcher F, Kortum S, Kirschning T, et al. Optimized management of polytraumatized patients by prehospital ultrasound. *Unfall-chirurg*. 2002;105(11):986.

11. Strode CA, Rubal BJ, Gerhardt RT, et al. Wireless and satellite transmission of prehospital focused abdominal sonography for trauma. *Prehosp Emerg Care*. 2003;7(3):375.

12. Heegaard WG, Ho J, Hildebrandt DA. The prehospital ultrasound study: results of the first six months (abstract). *Prehosp Emerg Care*. 2009;13(1):139.

13. Heegard WG, Hildebrandt D, Spear D, et al. Prehospital ultrasound by paramedics: results of field trial. *Acad Em Med*. 2010;17(6):624-630.

14. Jorgensen H, Jensen CH, Dirks J. Does prehospital ultrasound improve treatment of the trauma patient? A systematic review. *Eur J Emerg Med*. 2010;17(5):249-253.

15. Rooney KP, Lahham S, Lahham S, et al. Pre-hospital assessment with ultrasound in emergencies: implementation in the field. *World J Emerg Med*. 2016;7(2):117-123.

16. Sadek S, Lockey DJ, Lendrum RA, Perkins Z, Price J, Davies GE. Resuscitative endovascular balloon occlusion of the aorta (REBOA) in the pre-hospital setting: an additional resuscitation option for uncontrolled catastrophic haemorrhage. *Resuscitation*. 2016;107:135-138.

17. Smith IM, James RH, Dretzke J, Midwinter MJ. Prehospital blood product resuscitation for trauma: a systematic review. *Shock*. 2016;46(1):3-16.

18. American College of Surgeons (ACS) Committee on Trauma. Trauma in pregnancy and intimate partner violence. In: *Advanced Trauma Life Support for Doctors, Student Course Manual*. 9th ed. Chicago, IL: ACS; 2012:288-297.

Suggested Reading

Berry MJ, McMurray RG, Katz VL. Pulmonary and ventilatory responses to pregnancy, immersion and exercise. *J Appl Physiol*. 1989;66(2):857.

Coburn M. Genitourinary trauma. In: Moore EE, Feliciano DV, Mattox KL, eds. *Trauma*. 7th ed. New York, NY: McGraw-Hill; 2012:669.

Knudson MM, Yeh D. Trauma in pregnancy. In: Moore EE, Feliciano DV, Mattox KL, eds. *Trauma*. 7th ed. New York, NY: McGraw-Hill; 2012:709.

Raja AS, Zabbo CP. Trauma in pregnancy. *Emerg Med Clin North Am*. 2012;30:937-948.

Melville SC, Melville DE. Abdominal trauma. In: Stone C, Humphries RL, eds. *Current Diagnosis and Treatment Emergency Medicine*. 7th ed. New York, NY: McGraw-Hill; 2011.

CHAPTER 12

Musculoskeletal Trauma

Lead Editors:
Robert O'Toole, MD
David Potter, MD

CHAPTER OBJECTIVES

At the completion of this chapter, you will be able to do the following:

- List the three categories used to classify patients with extremity injuries, and relate this classification to priority of care.
- Describe the primary and secondary surveys as related to extremity trauma.
- Discuss the significance of hemorrhage in both open and closed fractures of the long bones and pelvis.
- List the five major pathophysiologic problems associated with extremity injuries that may require management in the prehospital setting.

- Explain the management of extremity trauma as an isolated injury and in the presence of multisystem trauma.
- Given a scenario involving an extremity injury, select an appropriate splint and splinting method.
- Describe the special considerations involved in femur fracture management.
- Discuss the management of amputations.

SCENARIO

It is a beautiful Saturday afternoon in June. You have been dispatched to a local motorcycle racetrack for a rider who has been injured. Upon arrival, you are escorted by track officials to an area on the track just in front of the grandstand where the track's medical crew (two-person, emergency medical responders, nontransport) is attending to a single patient lying supine on the track.

One of the emergency medical responders tells you that the patient was a rider in a 350-cc class race with 14 other motorcycles and that three of them collided in front of the grandstand. The other two riders were not injured, but the patient was unable to stand or move without significant pain in his right leg and pelvis. There was no loss of consciousness and no complaints other than leg pain. The medical crew has maintained the patient in a supine position with manual stabilization of the right lower extremity.

As you assess the patient, you find that he is a 19-year-old man, conscious and alert without past medical or trauma history. The patient's initial vital signs are as follows: Blood pressure is 104/68 millimeters of mercury (mm Hg), pulse is 112 beats/minute, respirations are 24 breaths/minute, and skin is pale and diaphoretic. The patient

(continued)

SCENARIO (CONTINUED)

states that he collided with another rider when he came out of a corner and that the collision caused him to lose balance and slide across the track. He states his right leg was run over by at least one other bike. Visual inspection of his right leg reveals shortening of the leg and no open wounds when compared to the left side, tenderness, and bruising of the mid-anterior thigh area.

· What does the mechanism of injury from this event tell you about the potential injuries for this patient?
· What type of injury do you suspect, and what would your management priorities be?

INTRODUCTION

Musculoskeletal injury, although common in trauma patients, rarely poses an immediate life-threatening condition. Skeletal trauma can be life threatening, however, when it produces significant blood loss (hemorrhage), either externally or from internal bleeding into the extremity or into the pelvis.

When caring for a critical trauma patient, the prehospital care provider has three primary considerations with regard to extremity injuries:

1. Maintain assessment priorities. Do not be distracted by dramatic, non-life-threatening musculoskeletal injuries (**Figure 12-1**).
2. Recognize potentially life-threatening musculoskeletal injuries.
3. Recognize the mechanism of injury and the force that created the musculoskeletal injuries and the potential for other life-threatening injuries caused by that energy transfer.

If a life-threatening or potentially life-threatening condition is discovered during the primary survey, the secondary survey should not be started. Any problems found during the primary survey should be corrected before moving to the secondary survey (see later discussion). This may mean delaying the secondary survey until the patient is en route to the hospital or even, in some cases, waiting until arrival at the emergency department (ED).

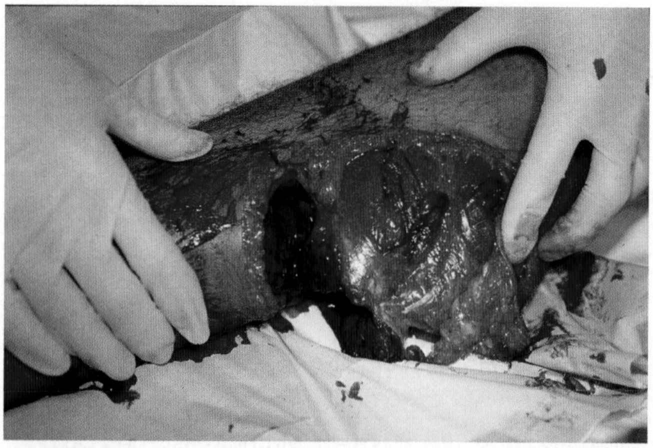

Critical trauma patients may be secured to and transported on long backboards to facilitate moving the patient and to allow for resuscitation and treatment of both critical and noncritical injuries. Use of a long backboard allows for immobilization of the entire patient and all of his or her injuries, when appropriate, on a single platform that makes it possible to move the victim without disturbing the splinting. Details of long backboard/backboard immobilization are discussed in the Spinal Trauma chapter. The prehospital provider must consider the risk of delayed transport time versus the benefit of splinting extremities that have musculoskeletal pain without obvious deformity or crepitus. In general, any deformity in the extremities should be straightened, or otherwise generally realigned, and then immobilized for transport. The prehospital provider is unlikely to impart any more force or injury than what was sustained during the time of the trauma, and there are substantial downsides to leaving a limb in a severely deformed position for a prolonged time.

Figure 12-1 Some extremity injuries, although dramatic in appearance, are not life threatening.

Courtesy of Peter T. Pons, MD, FACEP.

Anatomy and Physiology

Understanding the gross anatomy and physiology of the human body is an important piece of the prehospital care provider's fund of knowledge. Although this textbook does not discuss all of the anatomy and physiology of the musculoskeletal system, it reviews some of the basics.

The mature human body has approximately 206 bones (**Figure 12-2**). The skeleton is divided into two primary divisions: the axial skeleton and the **appendicular skeleton**. The axial skeleton comprises the bones of the central part of the body, including the skull, spine, sternum, and ribs. The appendicular skeleton is made up of the bones of the upper and lower extremities, shoulder girdle, and pelvis (excluding the sacrum).

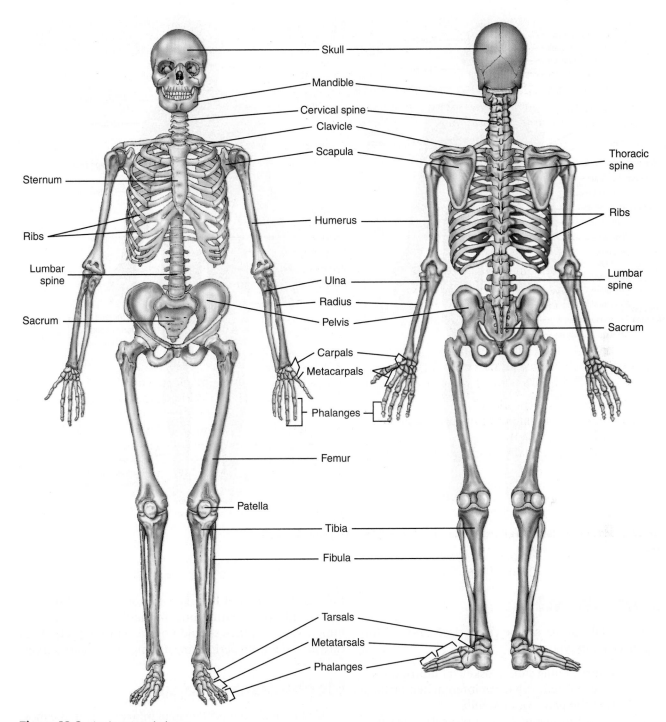

Figure 12-2 The human skeleton.
© National Association of Emergency Medical Technicians (NAEMT).

The human body has almost 650 individual muscles, which are categorized by their function. The muscles that are specific to this chapter are the voluntary, or skeletal, muscles. These muscles are categorized as *skeletal* because they move the skeletal system. Muscles in this category voluntarily move the structures of the body (**Figure 12-3**).

Other important structures discussed in this chapter are tendons and ligaments. A **tendon** is a band of tough, inelastic, fibrous tissue that connects a muscle to bone. It is the white part at the end of a muscle that directly attaches a muscle to the bone that it will move. A **ligament** is a band of tough, fibrous tissue connecting bone to bone; its function is to hold joints together.

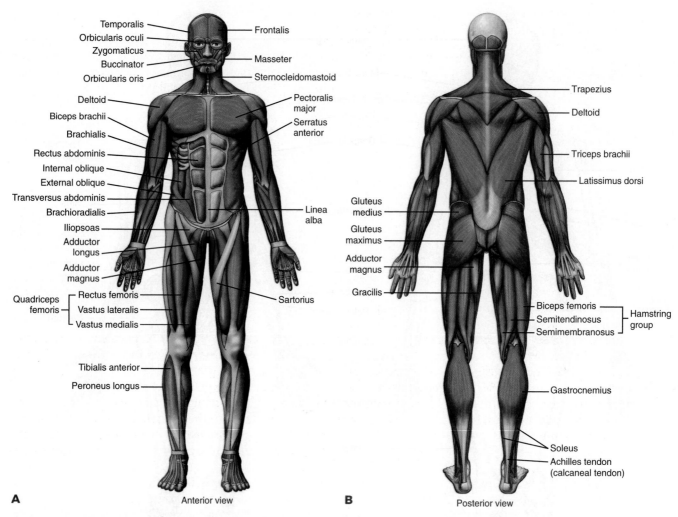

Figure 12-3 Major muscles of the human body. **A.** Anterior view. **B.** Posterior view.
© National Association of Emergency Medical Technicians (NAEMT).

Assessment

Musculoskeletal trauma can be categorized into the following three main types:

1. Life-threatening musculoskeletal injuries, such as external hemorrhage or internal hemorrhage within the pelvis or extremity
2. Non-life-threatening musculoskeletal trauma associated with multisystem life-threatening trauma (life-threatening injuries plus limb fractures)
3. Isolated non-life-threatening musculoskeletal trauma (isolated limb fractures)

The purpose of the primary survey is to identify and treat life-threatening conditions. The presence of a non-life-threatening musculoskeletal injury can be an indicator of force involved with the injury and should alert the prehospital provider to assess for possible multisystem trauma. Care should be taken to not become distracted by non-life-threatening but dramatic musculoskeletal injury. These injuries should not prevent the prehospital care provider from performing a complete primary survey.

Mechanism of Injury

Understanding the mechanism of injury is one of the most important functions of the assessment and management of a trauma patient. Rapidly determining the mechanism of injury and its associated energy (e.g., falling from standing vs. being thrown from a motorcycle at high speed) will help the prehospital care provider to suspect and recognize the most critical injuries or conditions. The best source for determining the mechanism of injury is directly from the patient. If the patient is unresponsive, details of the injury can be obtained from witnesses. If none of these options is available, collect observations at the scene and the pattern of injuries found on physical examination, and present this information directly to the receiving facility. This information should also be documented on the patient care report (PCR).

Based on the mechanism of injury, the prehospital care provider may develop a high index of suspicion for the injuries that a patient might have sustained. This consideration and knowledge of various injury patterns may bring to mind additional injuries for which the patient should be assessed. Consider the following examples:

- If a patient jumps out of a window feetfirst, the primary injury suspicion would be fractures of the lower extremity, pelvis, and spine. Secondary injuries to consider would be abdominal injuries due to possible shearing mechanisms.
- If a patient is involved in a motorcycle collision with a telephone pole and hits his or her head on the pole, primary injuries will include head, cervical spine, and thoracic injury. A secondary injury might include a femur fracture from "striking" the femur on the handlebars of the motorcycle.
- If a passenger in a motor vehicle crash sustains a side-impact collision, consideration to musculoskeletal trauma would include upper and lower extremity fractures and pelvis injury. Associated injury patterns to consider include head injury, rib or lung injury, and abdominal injury.

Primary and Secondary Surveys

Primary Survey

The first steps of any patient assessment are to ensure scene safety and evaluate the situation. Once the scene is as safe as possible, the patient can be assessed. The primary survey is based on components necessary for sustaining life: airway, breathing, and circulation.

Although angulated fractures or partial amputations may draw the prehospital care provider's attention because of their visual impact, life-threatening conditions must take priority. Exsanguinating hemorrhage, airway, breathing, circulation, disability, and expose/environment (XABCDE) remain the most important parts of the primary survey. For a patient with life-threatening conditions identified in the primary survey, management of musculoskeletal trauma should be delayed until those problems are corrected. Exsanguinating external hemorrhage (X) is often due to musculoskeletal causes and should be addressed first in the primary survey, typically with direct pressure followed by immediate proximal tourniquet application. If the patient has life-threatening injuries, the prehospital care provider will next assess and address airway, breathing, and circulation. If the patient has no life-threatening injuries, the provider can proceed to the secondary survey.

Secondary Survey

With the exception of assessing and addressing exsanguinating extremity hemorrhage, which occurs during the primary survey, assessment of the extremities occurs during the secondary survey. To facilitate the physical examination, the prehospital care provider considers removing any clothing that was not removed during the primary survey, as allowed by the environment. If the mechanism of injury is not obvious, every effort should be made to safely expose the pelvis and both upper and lower extremities including the hands and feet. Additionally, the patient or bystanders can be questioned about how the injuries occurred. The patient should also be queried about the presence of pain in the extremities. Most patients with significant musculoskeletal injuries have pain, unless a spinal cord injury is present.

Assessment of the extremities includes evaluating any pain, weakness, or abnormal sensations in the extremities. Specific attention is paid to the following:

- *Injury to the bones and joints.* This evaluation is accomplished by inspecting for deformities that may represent fractures or dislocations (**Table 12-1**) and palpating the extremity for tenderness and crepitus. The lack of these physical findings does not exclude the possibility of fracture or other musculoskeletal injury. Crepitus is the grinding feeling that bones make when the fractured ends rub against one another. Crepitus can be elicited by palpating the site of injury and by movement of the extremity. Crepitus sounds like a "snap, crackle, and pop" or the popping of plastic "bubble wrap" used for packing. This feeling of bones grating against one another during the assessment of a patient can produce further injury; therefore, once the crepitus is noted, no additional or repetitive steps should be taken to produce it. Crepitus is a distinct feeling that is not easily forgotten, and immediate immobilization is indicated once it has been identified.
- *Soft-tissue injuries.* The prehospital care provider visually inspects for swelling, lacerations, abrasions, hematomas, skin color, and wounds. Consider the possibility that a wound close to an apparent fracture is an open fracture. Firmness and tenseness of the soft tissues along with pain that appears out of proportion to the general findings may indicate the presence of a **compartment syndrome**. Compartment syndrome is a limb-threatening injury and should be communicated to the hospital provider (management of compartment syndrome is discussed later in this chapter).
- *Perfusion.* Perfusion should be evaluated by identifying the most distal palpable pulse (radial or ulnar in the upper extremity and dorsalis pedis or posterior tibial in the lower extremity) and noting capillary refilling time in the fingers or toes. Absence of distal pulses in

Table 12-1 Common Joint Dislocation Deformities

Joint	Direction	Deformity
Shoulder	Anterior	Squared off rotated
	Posterior	Locked in internal rotation
Elbow	Posterior	Olecranon prominent posteriorly
Hip	Anterior	Extended, abducted, externally rotated
	Posterior	Flexed, adducted, internally rotated
Knee	Anteroposterior	Loss of normal contour, extended*
Ankle	Lateral is most common	Externally rotated, prominent medial malleolus
Subtalar joint	Lateral is most common	Laterally displaced os calcis (calcaneus)

*May spontaneously reduce prior to evaluation

Source: American College of Surgeons Committee on Trauma: *Advanced Trauma Life Support*, ed 10, page 155, Chicago, 2018, ACS.

Table 12-2 Peripheral Nerve Assessment of Upper Extremities

Nerve	Motor	Sensation	Anticipated Injury Location
Ulnar	Index and little finger abduction	Little finger	Elbow injury
Median distal	Thenar contraction with opposition	Distal tip of index finger	Wrist fracture or dislocation
Median, anterior interosseous	Index tip flexion	None	Supracondylar fracture of humerus (children)
Musculocutaneous	Elbow flexion	Radial forearm	Anterior shoulder dislocation
Radial	Thumb, finger metacarpophalangeal extension	First dorsal web space	Distal humeral shaft, anterior shoulder dislocation
Axillary	Deltoid	Lateral shoulder	Anterior shoulder dislocation, proximal humerus fracture

Source: American College of Surgeons Committee on Trauma, *Advanced Trauma Life Support*, ed 10, page 161, Chicago, 2018, ACS.

the extremities can indicate disruption of an artery, compression of the vessel by a hematoma or bone fragment, or a compartment syndrome. Large or expanding hematomas may indicate the presence of an injury to a large vessel.

- *Neurologic function.* The prehospital care provider's neurologic assessment should include both motor and sensory function in both upper and lower extremities. For most situations in the prehospital setting, evaluating gross neurologic functioning is sufficient. **Table 12-2** shows large nerve motor and sensory distributions with the most common associated location of injury. Lack of injury at the anticipated site in the presence of nerve dysfunction should prompt providers to ask more questions and the need of further examination.

- *Motor function.* Motor function can be assessed by first asking the patient if any weakness is noted. Motor function in the upper extremity is evaluated by having

Table 12-3 Peripheral Nerve Assessment of Lower Extremities

Nerve	Motor	Sensation	Injury
Femoral	Knee extension	Anterior knee	Pubic rami fractures
Obturator	Hip adduction	Medial thigh	Obturator ring fractures
Posterior tibial	Toe flexion	Sole of foot	Knee dislocation
Superficial peroneal	Ankle eversion	Lateral dorsum of foot	Fibular neck fracture, knee dislocation
Deep peroneal	Ankle/toe dorsiflexion	Dorsal first to second web space	Fibular neck fracture, compartment syndrome
Sciatic nerve	Ankle dorsiflexion or plantar flexion	Foot	Posterior hip dislocation
Superior gluteal	Hip abduction	Upper buttocks	Acetabular fracture
Inferior gluteal	Gluteus maximus hip extension	Lower buttocks	Acetabular fracture

Source: American College of Surgeons Committee on Trauma, *Advanced Trauma Life Support*, ed 10, page 161, Chicago, 2018, ACS.

the patient open and close a fist and by testing the patient's grip strength (the patient squeezes the prehospital care provider's fingers), while lower extremity motor function is tested by having the patient wiggle his or her toes and push-pull against the examiner's hands with his or her feet. A patient's ability to clinch gluteal muscles and squeeze the buttock cheeks does not eliminate the need for a rectal examination during a full neurologic examination once the patient reaches the hospital.

- *Sensory function.* Sensory function is evaluated by asking about the presence of any deficits or changes in sensations. Sensory function should be tested at the most distal aspect of each extremity. Table 12-2 and **Table 12-3** provide information on performing more detailed evaluations of motor and sensory function of the extremities.

Repeat evaluation of extremity perfusion and neurologic functioning should be performed after any splinting procedure.

Associated Injuries

While performing the secondary survey, clues based on the mechanism of injury may help uncover particular commonly associated injury patterns. Such injury patterns can prompt the prehospital care provider to assess for occult injuries associated with specific fractures. **Table 12-4** provides some examples of associated injuries.

Specific Musculoskeletal Injuries

Injuries to the extremities result in two primary problems that require management in the prehospital setting: hemorrhage and pulselessness.

Hemorrhage

Bleeding can be dramatic or subtle. Regardless of the wound's appearance, it is the amount of blood lost and the rate of its loss that determines whether the patient will be able to compensate for the loss of blood volume or whether he or she will descend into shock. A good rule to remember is, "No bleeding is minor; every red blood cell counts." Even a small trickle of blood can add up to substantial blood loss if it is ignored for a long enough period.

External Hemorrhage

External arterial bleeding should be identified during the primary survey, as it can be life threatening. Generally, this type of bleeding is easily recognized, but assessment can be difficult when blood is hidden underneath a patient or in heavy or dark clothing. Obvious hemorrhage requires immediate attention and should be assessed and controlled while or even before the patient's airway and breathing are being managed.

Table 12-4 Injuries Associated With Musculoskeletal Injuries

Injury	Missed/Associated Injury
■ Clavicular fracture ■ Scapular fracture ■ Fracture and/or dislocation of shoulder	■ Major thoracic injury, especially pulmonary contusion and rib fractures ■ Scapulothoracic dissociation
Fracture/dislocation of elbow	■ Brachial artery injury ■ Median, ulnar, and radial nerve injury
Femur fracture	■ Femoral neck fracture ■ Ligamentous knee injury ■ Posterior hip dislocation
Posterior knee dislocation	■ Femoral fracture ■ Posterior hip dislocation
■ Knee dislocation ■ Displaced tibial plateau	■ Popliteal artery and nerve injuries
Calcaneal fracture	■ Spine injury or fracture ■ Fracture-dislocation of talus and calcaneus ■ Tibial plateau fracture
Open fracture	70% incidence of associated nonskeletal injury

Source: American College of Surgeons Committee on Trauma, *Advanced Trauma Life Support*, ed 10, page 164, Chicago, 2018, ACS.

Estimation of external blood loss can be extremely difficult. Although less experienced individuals tend to overestimate the amount of external hemorrhage, underestimation is also possible, as overt signs of external blood loss are not always apparent. One study suggested that prehospital estimates of blood loss were inaccurate and not clinically beneficial.[1] The reasons for these inaccurate blood loss estimates are many and include that the patient may have been moved from the site of injury or that lost blood may have been absorbed by clothing or soil or washed away in water or by rain.

Internal Hemorrhage

Internal hemorrhage is common with musculoskeletal trauma, and it is often missed. It may result from damage to major blood vessels (many of which are located in close proximity to the long bones of the body), from disrupted muscle, and from fractured bones. Continued swelling of an extremity or a cold, pale, pulseless extremity could indicate internal hemorrhage from major arteries or veins. Significant internal blood loss can be associated with fractures (**Table 12-5**). The thigh and pelvis can hold enough volume to make the blood loss life threatening.

Both the potential internal and the external blood loss associated with extremity trauma must be considered when evaluating the patient. This will help the prehospital care

provider anticipate the potential for the development of shock, prepare for the possibility of systemic deterioration, and intervene appropriately to minimize its occurrence.

Table 12-5 Approximate Internal Blood Loss Associated With Fractures

Bone Fractured	Internal Blood Loss (milliliters [ml]) per Fracture*
Rib	125
Radius or ulna	250–500
Humerus	500–750
Tibia or fibula	500–1,000
Femur	1,000–2,000
Pelvis	1,000–massive

*(Average total blood volume in an adult = 5,000 to 6,000 ml)

Note: This table describes common amounts of blood loss from an isolated bone fracture. Injury to underlying organs and tissues can significantly increase these numbers. For example, a rib fracture that also lacerates an intercostal artery or damages the spleen could lead to major hemorrhage in the chest or abdomen, respectively.

Management

The initial management of external hemorrhage involves the application of direct pressure to the wound. Elevation of an extremity has not been shown to slow hemorrhage, and in musculoskeletal trauma, it may aggravate injuries that are present. (See discussion in the Shock: Pathophysiology of Life and Death chapter.) If hemorrhage is not immediately and completely controlled with direct pressure or a pressure dressing, a tourniquet should be applied. (Follow the principles described in the Shock: Pathophysiology of Life and Death chapter.) A second tourniquet should be applied next to the first if hemorrhage control is not achieved with placement of the first tourniquet. A recommended topical hemostatic agent can be considered for hemorrhage that is not amenable to use of a tourniquet, such as in the groin or axilla. Such agents may also be considered for prolonged transport situations.

Tourniquet use is the standard of care in the prehospital management of exsanguinating extremity injuries. See the Shock: Pathophysiology of Life and Death chapter for an in-depth discussion of prehospital tourniquet use.

After controlling bleeding in patients with life-threatening hemorrhage from an extremity, prehospital care providers can repeat the primary survey and focus on airway, breathing, and circulation resuscitation and rapid transport to the facility that can best treat the patient's condition. During transport, administration of oxygen and initiation of intravenous (IV) fluid resuscitation for patients with shock can begin, keeping in mind that when internal hemorrhage is suspected, the target systolic blood pressure is 80 to 90 mm Hg (mean blood pressure is 60 to 65 mm Hg) and 90 to 100 mm Hg for patients with suspected traumatic brain injury. For patients with minor bleeding and no signs of shock or other life-threatening problems, bleeding can be controlled with direct pressure, and the secondary survey should be performed.

Pulseless Extremity

During your assessment of the patient, when trying to locate and identify distal pulses on each of the extremities, one thing to consider is that the fracture deformity may be the cause of decreased limb perfusion. In general, once the primary survey has been completed (ABCs), if there is a deformed limb that is noted to be without a pulse, attempt to realign the limb to the general appearance of an uninjured extremity. At that point, recheck pulses to see if the realignment helped restore blood flow. It is important to note that the purpose of this realignment is not to reduce an open fracture, restore function, or definitively treat the injury. The purpose is simply to provide a direct path for blood flow and remove any kink or compression of the vessels that may be caused by the deformity.

If pulses are restored or capillary refilling is appropriate, this is the position in which the extremity should be splinted. This information should be communicated to the receiving hospital facility.

The same mechanism of action that creates compartment syndrome can also cause distal occlusion from bleeding and associated swelling within isolated compartments proximally in the extremities. Assessing for compartment syndrome (discussed later in this chapter) should be considered in evaluation of a pulseless extremity. Remember, a pulseless extremity is a limb-threatening injury, and transport time to a hospital with immediate surgical capabilities is crucial.

Pelvic Fracture

Severe pelvic fractures present a number of challenging problems for prehospital care providers (**Figure 12-4**). The first is identification of a patient who is hemodynamically unstable from a pelvis fracture. In the field, consideration of the mechanism of injury, amount of energy imparted on the body during the injury, and the lower extremity deformity are additional ways to assess for pelvic injury. Potentially, an accurate assessment can mean the difference between life and death. Few injuries in orthopaedics are truly life threatening, but pelvic ring disruptions can be.

The greatest immediate concern in pelvic fracture is internal hemorrhage, which can be very difficult to manage. Pelvic fractures can range from minor, relatively insignificant fractures to life-threatening injuries associated with massive internal and external hemorrhage (**Box 12-1**). Fractures of the **pelvic ring** are associated with overall mortality rates

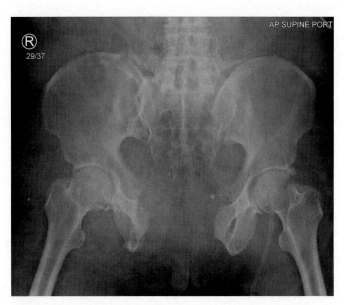

Figure 12-4 Fracture of the pelvis. The arrows show multiple fractures involving the pubic rami and the acetabulum.
Courtesy of Andrew Pollak, MD.

Box 12-1 Pelvic Binders

At least three pelvic binders are commercially available: Pelvic Binder (Pelvic Binder, Inc.), Sam Sling (Sam Products), and Trauma Pelvic Orthotic Device (TPOD; BioCybernetics International).

Rationale

Some pelvic ring fractures are associated with an increase in the pelvic volume, permitting large amounts of intra-abdominal hemorrhage. Because the volume is increased, there is less tissue surrounding the pelvis to **tamponade** bleeding. Patients with hemodynamic instability often undergo surgical application of pelvic external fixation to help reduce the volume and assist with hemodynamic stability. This measure should be an afterthought to field application of a binder.

Binder Use

The concern for causing further injury during the application of a potential lifesaving pelvic binder should not prevent the application of a binder. The energy imparted on the body at the time of the initial trauma is far greater than that caused by a logroll or positioning while applying the binder. The literature has shown no detrimental effect to applying a binder early, even after full radiographic evaluation suggested it was not warranted. Not applying one, however, in the context of major pelvic ring disruption with increased intrapelvic volume, could result in fatal exsanguination.

ranging from 9% to 20%. Furthermore, the presence of a pelvic ring fracture in blunt trauma is an independent risk factor for death and doubles the chance of death.[2] Patients with pelvic fractures frequently have associated injuries, including traumatic brain injuries, long-bone fractures, thoracic injuries, urethral disruption in men, splenic trauma, and liver and kidney trauma.

To assess the pelvis, rocking or gentle manual pressure anterior to posterior and from the sides may identify crepitus or instability. Palpation over the mons pubis region may demonstrate a large gap between the left and right hemipelvis, indicating significant pelvic ring disruption. Once identified by physical exam, further examination to assess pelvic stability is contraindicated, as it could lead to worsening hemorrhage or clot disruption.

Open fractures of the pelvis may lacerate the rectum or vagina, and an obvious source of external blood loss may not be readily apparent. It is not the role of the prehospital care provider to identify and classify pelvic fracture patterns or to determine whether there is a hidden laceration making it an open fracture. The primary goal is to identify life-threatening pelvic fractures and provide appropriate treatment.

Some pelvic ring fractures are associated with an increase in pelvic volume due to the fracture pattern and degree of displacement, thus allowing large volumes of intrapelvic hemorrhage to occur that can be life threatening. Closed reduction of the pelvis by application of a binder requires simple, but specific, placement to ensure it does what it is supposed to do. A binder is designed for hemodynamic stabilization by limiting intrapelvic volume and therefore decreasing blood loss associated with pelvis fractures; it is not designed for fracture stabilization.

The binder should be centered over the greater trochanters, not the pelvic brim. Commonly, binders are placed too superiorly, which can compress the abdomen and, in extreme cases, make it difficult to ventilate. Confirming the proper location allows for the transfer of compression from the binder to the pelvis regardless of body habitus. The result of proper placement is a reduction of pelvic volume, stabilization of the pelvis, and, ideally, a decrease in ongoing bleeding.

Femur Fracture

Femur fractures, like pelvis injuries, can be life threatening due to the large amount of associated hemorrhage into each thigh. An adult can lose 1,000 to 2,000 ml of blood into each thigh and thus develop hemodynamic instability and shock. In the absence of life-threatening conditions, a traction splint should be applied to stabilize suspected midshaft femoral fractures. The application of traction, both manually and by use of a mechanical device, can help decrease internal bleeding as well as decrease the patient's pain.

Splinting the femur represents a unique splinting situation because of the musculature of the thigh. The powerful thigh muscles often make reduction, realignment, and immobilization with splinting or traction difficult.

Contraindications to the use of a traction splint include the following:

- Avulsion or amputation of the ipsilateral ankle and foot
- Suspected fractures adjacent to the knee (A traction splint may be used as a rigid splint in this situation, but traction should not be applied.)

Instability (Fractures and Dislocations)

Tears of the supporting structures of a joint, fracture of a bone, and major muscle or tendon injury contribute to the instability of an injured extremity.

Fractures

If a bone is fractured, immobilizing it may decrease pain. The energy imparted at the time of injury to cause a fracture causes more damage and injury than anything a prehospital provider can do by realigning an extremity and immobilizing it with a splint or traction.

In general, fractures are classified as either closed or open. In a **closed fracture**, the skin is not open to bone, whereas in an **open fracture**, the integrity of the skin has been interrupted and bone is functionally or even potentially grossly exposed (**Figure 12-5A**). Orthopaedic surgeons may classify fractures by their patterns, but knowledge of the fracture pattern does not alter field management, whereas knowledge of the associated skin integrity might.

Closed Fractures

Closed fractures are fractures in which the bone has been broken but the patient has no associated loss of skin integrity (i.e., the skin is not broken in the region of the fracture) (**Figure 12-5B**). Signs of a closed fracture include pain, tenderness, deformity, hematomas, swelling, and crepitus. In some patients, however, pain and tenderness may be the only findings. Pulses, skin color, and motor and sensory function should be assessed distal to the suspected fracture site. It is not always true that an extremity is not fractured because the patient can voluntarily move it or, in the case of a lower extremity, even walk on it; adrenalin from a traumatic event may motivate patients to endure pain they would not tolerate normally. Additionally, some patients have a remarkably high pain tolerance.

Open Fractures

Open fractures usually occur when a sharp bone end penetrates the skin from the inside out or, less commonly, when the trauma or an object lacerates the skin and muscle at a fracture site (from the outside in) (**Figure 12-5C**). When a fracture is open to the outside environment, the ends of the fractured bone become contaminated with bacteria from the overlying skin or from the environment. This contamination can lead to the serious complication of a bone infection (*osteomyelitis*), which can interfere with healing of the fracture. Although the skin wound associated with an open fracture often is not associated with significant hemorrhage, persistent bleeding may come from the canal of the bone or from the decompression of a hematoma deep inside the tissue.

Any open wound near a possible fracture needs to be considered an open fracture and treated as such. Generally, a protruding bone or bone end should not be intentionally replaced; however, the bones occasionally return to a near-normal position when realigned for splinting or immobilization.

Open fractures may not always be easy to identify in a trauma patient. Although bone protruding from a wound is obvious, soft-tissue injuries in proximity to a fracture/deformity may have resulted from a bone end that broke through the surface of the skin only to recede back into the tissue.

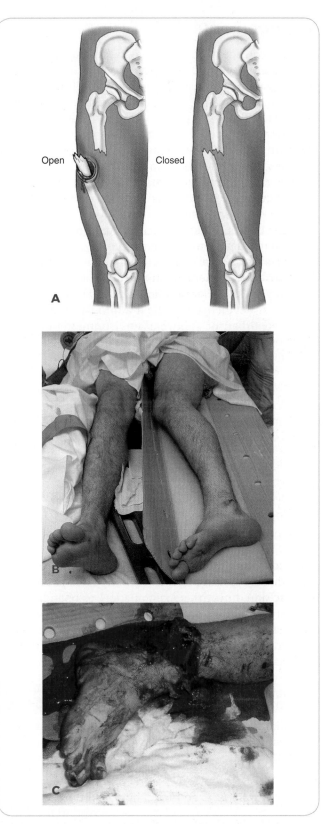

Figure 12-5 A. Open versus closed fracture. **B.** Closed fracture of the femur. Note the internal rotation and shortening of the left leg. **C.** Open fracture of the tibia.

A: © National Association of Emergency Medical Technicians (NAEMT); **B:** Courtesy Norman McSwain, MD, FACS, NREMT-P; **C:** Courtesy of Peter T. Pons, MD FACEP.

Management

The first consideration in managing fractures is to control hemorrhage and treat for shock. Direct pressure and pressure dressings will control virtually all external hemorrhage encountered in the field. Open wounds or exposed bone ends should be covered with a sterile dressing moistened with sterile normal saline or water. Consider realigning the deformed extremity at time of splinting for pain control, ease of splinting, fracture stabilization, and possibly, to improve perfusion by restoration of gross limb alignment. If the bone ends of an open fracture retract into the wound during reduction or splinting, this information must be documented on the PCR and reported to ED personnel. Some recent literature supports the administration of weight-based antibiotics, and some data show that earlier delivery of antibiotics may reduce infection rates. Antibiotic administration is controversial. There is no evidence that field administration of antibiotics in urban or suburban environments decreases infection rates.

Prior to splinting, an injured extremity should generally be returned to its normal anatomic position, including the use of gentle traction if necessary to realign an extremity to its normal length as best as possible and within reasonable clinical judgment. A "reduced fracture," one that is returned to normal anatomic alignment, is easier to splint. Second, restoring alignment may alleviate compression of arteries or nerves and result in improved perfusion and neurologic functioning. Realigning fractures also decreases hemorrhage and assists with pain control.

If the fracture is open and bone is exposed, the bone end should be gently rinsed with sterile water or normal saline (as time allows) to remove obvious contamination prior to an attempt to restore normal anatomic position. It is not of major concern if the bone ends retract back into the skin during this manipulation, as open fractures require irrigation and **debridement** in the operating room regardless. However, the fact that the bone was exposed prior to reduction is key information that should be passed on during the patient report at the receiving facility. No more than two attempts should be made to restore an extremity to normal position, and, if unsuccessful, the extremity should be splinted "as is."

The primary objective of splinting is to prevent movement of the fractured body part. Doing so will help decrease the patient's pain and stabilize the fragments. To immobilize any long bone in an extremity effectively, the entire limb should be immobilized. To do this, the injured site should be supported manually while the joint and bone above (proximal to) and the joint and bone below (distal to) the injury site are immobilized. Numerous types of splints are available, and most can be used with both open and closed fractures (**Box 12-2**). With virtually all splinting techniques, further inspection of the extremity is limited, and therefore a thorough assessment should be performed before splinting.

Four additional points are important to remember when applying any type of splint:

1. Pad splints to prevent movement of the extremity inside the splint, to help increase the patient's comfort, and to prevent pressure sores.
2. Remove jewelry and watches so that these objects will not inhibit circulation as additional swelling occurs. Lubrication with soap, lotion, or a water-soluble jelly may facilitate removal of tight rings.
3. Assess neurovascular functions distal to the injury site before and after applying any splint and periodically thereafter. A pulseless extremity indicates either a vascular injury or a compartment syndrome, and rapid transport to an appropriate facility becomes even more of a priority.
4. After splinting, consider elevating the extremity, if possible, to decrease edema and throbbing. Ice or cold packs can also be used to decrease pain and swelling and may be placed on the splinted extremity near the suspected fracture site.

Box 12-2 Types of Splints

Various splints and splinting materials are available (**Figure 12-6**), including the following:

- *Rigid splints* cannot be changed in shape. They require that the body part be positioned to fit the splint's shape. Examples of rigid splints include board splints (wood, plastic, or metal) and the long backboard. Rigid splints are best used for long-bone injuries.
- *Formable splints* can be molded into various shapes and combinations to accommodate the shape of the injured extremity. Examples of formable splints include vacuum splints, air splints, pillows, blankets, cardboard splints, wire-ladder splints, and foam-covered moldable metal splints. Formable splints are best used for ankle, wrist, and long-bone injuries.
- *Traction splints* are designed to maintain mechanical in-line traction to help realign fractures. Traction splints are most often used to stabilize femur shaft fractures.

Box 12-2 Types of Splints (*continued*)

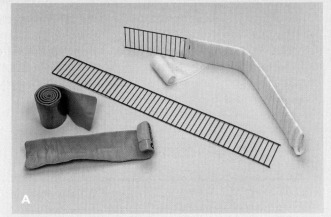
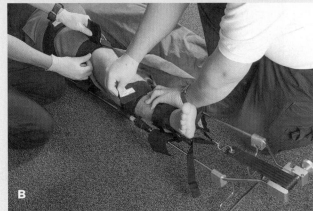
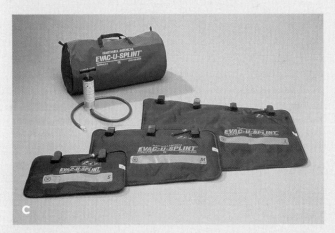
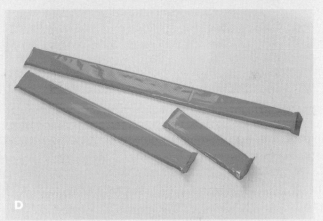

Figure 12-6 A. Formable splint. **B.** Traction splint. **C.** Vacuum splint. **D.** Board splint.

A, D: © National Association of Emergency Medical Technicians (NAEMT); B: © Jones & Bartlett Learning. Photographed by Darren Stahlman. C: Courtesy of Hartwell Medical.

Dislocations

Joints are held together by ligaments. The bones that make up a joint are attached to their muscles by tendons. Movement of an extremity is accomplished by the contraction (shortening) of muscles. This reduction of muscle length pulls the tendons that are attached to a bone and moves the extremity at a joint. A dislocation is a separation of two bones at the joint, resulting from significant disruption to the ligaments that normally provide supporting structure and stability at a joint (**Figure 12-7** and **Figure 12-8**). A dislocation, similar to a fracture, produces an area of instability that the prehospital care provider needs to secure. Dislocations can produce great pain. A dislocation can be difficult to distinguish clinically from a fracture without an x-ray and may be associated with fractures as well (fracture-dislocation). Deformity of a joint provides a clue to the type and direction of dislocation.

The proper description to provide to the hospital provider should be based on the more distal segment when

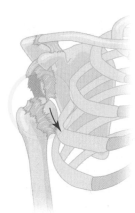

Figure 12-7 A dislocation is a separation of a bone from a joint; the picture depicts a typical anterior shoulder dislocation.

describing the dislocation. For example, a knee dislocation is based on the direction the tibia travels in relation to the femur. A posterior knee dislocation means the tibia is posterior to the femur.

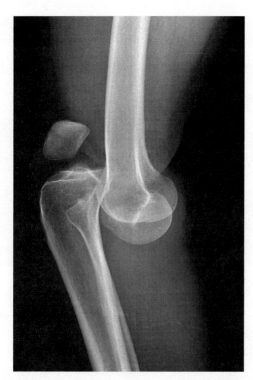

Figure 12-8 Right anterior knee dislocation with overriding tibia on the femur. Note the tibia (distal segment) has traveled anterior to the femur (proximal segment).

© Steven Needell/Science Source.

Individuals who have had prior dislocations have ligaments that are more lax than normal and may be prone to more frequent dislocations unless the problem is corrected surgically. Unlike those sustaining a dislocation for the first time, these patients are often familiar with their injury and can help in assessment and stabilization. Chronic or frequent dislocators do not necessarily need a field reduction attempted. Taking them to the hospital with dislocated joints when they are unable to self-reduce them is often less dangerous and better tolerated from a pain and discomfort standpoint than it is for patients with first-time dislocations.

Management

As a general rule, suspected dislocations should be splinted in the position found. Gentle manipulation of the joint can be done to try to return blood flow when the pulse is absent or weak. Realignment may improve the vascular status of the patient's limb. When faced with a brief transport time to the hospital, however, the better decision is to initiate transport rather than attempt manipulation. This manipulation will cause the patient great pain, so the patient should be prepared before moving the extremity. A splint should be used to immobilize most dislocations, while a sling is used for shoulder injuries. Documentation of how the injury was sustained and found and of the presence of pulses, movement, sensation, and color before and after splinting is important. During transport, ice or cold packs can be used to decrease pain and swelling. Analgesia can be provided as necessary to reduce pain.

Attempted reduction of a dislocation should be undertaken only when permitted by written protocols or online medical control and when the prehospital care provider has been properly trained in the appropriate techniques. All attempts at reduction of a dislocation should be properly documented and communicated to the hospital provider.

Special Considerations

Critical Multisystem Trauma Patient

Adherence to the primary survey priorities in patients with multisystem trauma that includes injured extremities does not imply that extremity injuries should be ignored or that injured extremities should not be protected from further harm. Rather, it means that *life takes precedence over limb* when faced with a critically injured trauma patient with extremity injuries that are not life threatening. The focus should be on maintaining vital functions through resuscitation, and only limited measures should be taken to address the extremity injuries, regardless of how dramatic the injuries appear. By properly immobilizing a patient to a long backboard, all extremities and the entire skeleton are essentially splinted in an anatomic position and the patient is easily moved. A secondary survey can be omitted if the life-threatening problems identified in the primary survey require ongoing interventions and if transport time is short. If a secondary survey is deferred, the prehospital care provider can simply document the findings that precluded performing the secondary survey.

Compartment Syndrome

Compartment syndrome refers to a limb-threatening condition in which the blood supply to an extremity is compromised by increased pressure within that limb. The muscles of extremities are enveloped by dense connective tissue called **fascia**. This fascia forms numerous compartments in the extremities in which the muscles are contained. Muscle fascia has minimal stretch, and anything that increases the pressure inside the compartments may result in a compartment syndrome.

The two most common causes of compartment syndrome are hemorrhage within a compartment from a fracture or vascular injury and third-space edema that forms when ischemic muscle tissue is reperfused after a period of diminished or absent blood flow. However, a splint or cast that is applied too tightly may produce a compartment syndrome by external compression. As the pressure in the compartment increases beyond that of capillary pressure, blood flow is impaired through the capillaries. The tissue served by these vessels then becomes ischemic. The pressure may continue to build to the point that even arterial flow and nerve function are compromised by compression.

The two early signs of a developing compartment syndrome are (1) *pain* that is above the baseline pain appropriate to the trauma and that does not respond to pain-relieving measures and (2) altered sensation (abnormal sensations or reduced/absent sensation) of the involved extremity. Pain is often described as out of proportion to the injury. This pain may be dramatically increased on passive movement of a finger or toe in that extremity. Nerves are extremely sensitive to their blood supply, and any compromised blood flow will manifest as paresthesia. The fact that these symptoms are normally associated with a fracture underscores the need for baseline circulatory, motor, and sensory examinations and repeated serial examinations so that the prehospital care provider can identify changes.

The other three "classic" signs of compartment syndrome—pulselessness, pallor, and paralysis—are late findings and indicate a clear compartment syndrome and a limb in jeopardy of muscle death (necrosis). Compartments may be extremely tense and firm to palpation, although it is difficult to judge the compartment pressures by physical examination alone.

Management

In the hospital, compartment pressures can be measured by hospital providers in extremities where compartment syndrome is suspected. Compartment syndrome must be definitively managed with emergent surgical intervention (*fasciotomy*), which involves an incision through the skin and fascia into the affected compartments to decompress the affected muscle tissue.

Only basic maneuvers can be attempted in the field. Any tightly applied splint or dressings should be removed and distal perfusion reassessed. Splinting the extremity provides stability. Elevation of the extremity is not recommended. Keeping the extremity level with the heart is ideal. Additionally, the ankle should be dorsiflexed when splinted to reduce anterior compartment pressure on the lower leg. Because compartment syndrome may develop during a long-distance transfer, serial examinations are essential for early identification of this problem.

Mangled Extremity

A "mangled extremity" refers to a complex injury resulting from high-energy transfer in which significant injury occurs to two or more of the following: (1) skin and muscle, (2) tendons, (3) bone, (4) blood vessels, and (5) nerves (**Figure 12-9**). Common mechanisms producing mangled extremities include motorcycle crash, ejection from a motor vehicle, and a pedestrian being struck by an automobile. When encountered, patients may be in shock from either external blood loss or hemorrhage from associated

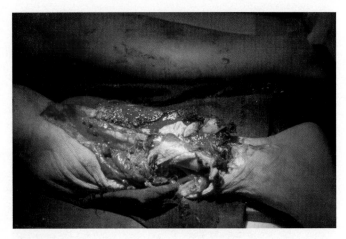

Figure 12-9 Mangled extremity resulting from crushing injury between two vehicles. The patient has fractures and extensive soft-tissue injury.
Courtesy of Peter T. Pons, MD, FACEP.

injuries, which are common because of the high-energy mechanism. Most mangled extremities involve severe open fractures, and amputation is frequently necessary. Limb salvage is possible in some patients, typically involving multiple surgical procedures, and substantial long-term disability is common.

Management

Even with a mangled extremity, the focus is still on the primary survey to rule out or address life-threatening conditions. Hemorrhage control, including the use of a tourniquet, may be required. The mangled extremity should be splinted, if the patient's condition allows. These patients are probably best cared for at high-volume level I trauma centers.

Amputations

When tissue has been totally separated from an extremity, the tissue is completely without nutrition and oxygenation. This type of injury is termed an *amputation*. An amputation is the loss of part or all of a limb. All amputations may be accompanied by significant bleeding, but it is more common with partial amputations. When vessels are completely transected, they retract and constrict, and blood clots may form, decreasing or stopping hemorrhage; however, when a vessel is only partially transected, the two ends cannot retract, and blood continues to pour out of the hole.

Amputations are often evident on the scene (**Figure 12-10**). This type of injury receives great attention from bystanders, and the patient may or may not know that the extremity is missing. Psychologically, the prehospital care provider needs to deal with this injury cautiously (**Box 12-3**).

The missing extremity should be located for possible reattachment. This is especially true for the upper extremity and thumb. Lower extremity amputations are generally not reattached in the setting of traumatic amputations because

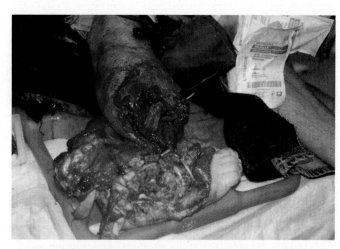

Figure 12-10 Complete amputation of the right leg after it became entangled in machinery.

Courtesy of Peter T. Pons, MD, FACEP.

Box 12-3 Phantom Pain

In some circumstances, the patient may complain of pain distal to the amputation. This "phantom pain" is the sensation that pain exists in a missing extremity. The reason for phantom pain is not understood completely, but the brain may not realize that the extremity is not present. This sensation usually is not present at the time of the injury.

---

lower extremity prostheses are effective and the success of replantation in the lower extremity is poor.

The primary survey should be performed before looking for a missing extremity, unless adequate numbers of emergency response personnel are present to assist. The appearance of an amputation may be horrifying, but if the patient does not have a patent airway or is not breathing, the loss of the limb is secondary to the life-threatening priorities.

Amputations can be very painful. Pain management should be employed as necessary once life-threatening problems have been excluded in the primary survey (**Figure 12-11**).

Management

Principles of managing an amputated part include the following:

1. Clean the amputated part by gentle rinsing with lactated Ringer (LR) solution.
2. Wrap the part in sterile gauze moistened with LR solution and place it in a plastic bag or container.
3. After labeling the bag or container, place it in an outer container filled with crushed ice.

4. Do not freeze the part by placing it directly on the ice or by adding another coolant such as dry ice.
5. Transport the part along with the patient to the closest appropriate facility.[3]

The longer the amputated portion is without oxygen, the less likely that it can be replaced successfully. Cooling the amputated body part, without freezing it, will reduce the metabolic rate and prolong this critical time. However, replantation is not a guarantee of successful attachment or ultimate function. Because lower extremity prostheses, particularly in the case of amputations below the knee, often allow the patient to resume a near-normal life, lower extremities are rarely considered for replantation. Furthermore, only cleanly separated amputations in otherwise healthy, younger individuals are usually considered for replantation. Smokers are less likely to have successful replantation because the nicotine in tobacco is a potent vasoconstrictor and may compromise blood flow to the replanted segment. Patients who are candidates for replantation of fingers (particularly the thumb) or a hand/forearm should be transported to a level I trauma center with specific replantation capabilities because level II and III facilities often lack replantation capability. Ultimately, it will be up to the surgical team to determine whether a replantation is possible.

Transport of a patient should not be delayed to locate a missing amputated part. If the amputated part is not readily found, law enforcement officials or other emergency responders should remain at the scene to search for it. When the amputated part is transported in a separate vehicle from the patient, the prehospital care provider must ensure that the transporters of the amputated part understand clearly where the patient is being transported and how to handle the part once it is located. The receiving facility should be notified as soon as the part is located, and transport of the part should be initiated as soon as possible.

Field Amputation

In general, many extremities that appear hopelessly entrapped can be released with additional extrication expertise. If the patient has an extremity entangled in a machine, an often-overlooked expert is the maintenance person who repairs the machine. This person usually has the technical knowledge to expeditiously disassemble and remove parts from a machine, allowing extrication. On rare occasions, however, a patient may have an entrapped extremity for which a field amputation may be the only reasonable option. A regional trauma system should consider development of an appropriately equipped field amputation team (**Box 12-4**). While rarely used, such a team has been shown to save lives.[4] Although formal field amputation is not considered part of the scope of practice of prehospital care providers in the United States, some entrapped extremities may be connected by only a small strand of tissue. The decision to

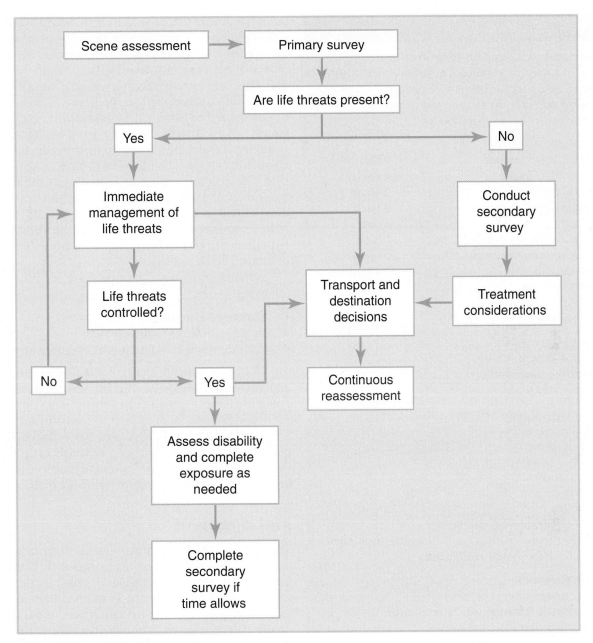

Figure 12-11 Primary survey algorithm.
© National Association of Emergency Medical Technicians (NAEMT).

cut this tissue or wait for a physician to arrive at the scene must be made in consultation with medical oversight. If a substantial amputation is necessary, it should ideally be performed by a trained physician because of the anatomic knowledge and technical expertise required. Significant sedation may need to be administered for the procedure, including general anesthesia and intubation.

Crush Syndrome

An extremity that is crushed during a traumatic injury can cause a reaction called rhabdomyolysis. This condition is associated with death of the muscle in the affected extremity

and release of **myoglobin**. Clinically, it is characterized by renal failure, end-organ injury, and potentially, death. The timing of the impact from this myoglobin is after the crushing force is removed from the extremity.

Traumatic injury to the muscle causes release of both myoglobin and potassium. Once the patient has been extricated, the affected limb suddenly becomes reperfused with new blood; at the same time, the old blood with elevated levels of myoglobin and potassium is washed out of the injured area and into the rest of the body. Elevated potassium can result in life-threatening cardiac dysrhythmias, and free myoglobin will produce tea- or cola-colored urine and will eventually result in renal failure.

Crush syndrome was first described in World War I in German soldiers rescued from collapsed trenches, then again in World War II in patients rescued from collapsed buildings during the London Blitz. In World War II, crush syndrome had a mortality rate in excess of 90%. During the Korean War, mortality was 84%, but after the advent of hemodialysis, mortality decreased to 53%. In the Vietnam War, the mortality rate was approximately the same, at 50%.

The importance of crush syndrome, however, should not be limited to historical or military interest. Approximately 3% to 20% of the survivors of earthquakes have sustained a crush injury, and approximately 40% of survivors from collapsed buildings will have crush injuries.[5,6] In 1978, an earthquake near Beijing, China, injured more than 350,000 persons, with 242,769 deaths. More than 48,000 of these people died from crush syndrome. More commonly, mechanisms of crush syndrome include entrapment from a trench collapse, construction collapse, or motor vehicle collision.

Patients with crush syndrome are identified by the following:

- Prolonged entrapment
- Traumatic injury to muscle mass
- Compromised circulation to the injured area

Of note, traumatic rhabdomyolysis can also occur in patients, often the elderly, who fall, perhaps fracture a hip, and are unable to get up or in patients who fall in a bathroom and become wedged next to the bathtub and toilet. They are found hours or days later, having lain in the same position, often on a hard surface. The weight of their body on the muscles for a prolonged period of time leads to muscle breakdown and the findings of traumatic rhabdomyolysis.

Management

The key in improving outcomes in crush syndrome is early and aggressive fluid resuscitation. It is important for the prehospital care provider to remember that toxins are accumulating within the entrapped limb during the extrication process. Once the entrapped limb is freed, the accumulated toxins wash into the central circulation, similar to a bolus of poison. Therefore, success will depend on minimizing the toxic effects of accumulated myoglobin and potassium before release of the limb. Resuscitation needs to occur before extrication.[7] A delay in fluid resuscitation will result in renal failure in 50% of the patients, and a delay of 12 hours or more produces renal failure in almost 100% of the patients. Some authors have advocated that final extrication be delayed until the patient has been adequately resuscitated.[8] A poorly resuscitated patient may go into cardiac arrest during extrication because of the sudden release of metabolic acid and potassium into the bloodstream when the compression on the extremity is released.[9]

Fluid resuscitation should proceed with normal saline at a rate of up to 1,500 ml per hour to ensure adequate renal output of 150 to 200 ml per hour. LR solution is avoided until urine output is adequate because of the presence of potassium in the IV fluid. The addition of 50 milliequivalents (mEq) of sodium bicarbonate and 10 grams of mannitol to each liter of fluid used during the extrication period may help decrease the incidence of renal failure. Once the patient has been extricated, the normal saline fluids can be slowed to 500 ml per hour, alternating with 5% dextrose in water (D_5W), with one ampule of sodium bicarbonate per liter.[10]

Once the blood pressure is stabilized and volume status restored, attention is turned toward prophylaxis against **hyperkalemia** and the toxic effects of serum myoglobin. Hyperkalemia in the field can be recognized by the development of peaked T waves on the cardiac monitor. Treatment of the increased potassium follows standard protocols for hyperkalemia, including IV sodium bicarbonate administration, inhaled beta-agonists (albuterol), administration of dextrose and insulin (if available), and, if life-threatening cardiac dysrhythmias occur, IV calcium chloride. Alkalinization of the urine will provide some degree of protection to the kidneys; however, the key is to maintain increased urine output (typically in the range of 50 to 100 ml/hr).

Sprains

A **sprain** is an injury in which ligaments are stretched or torn. Sprains are caused by a sudden twisting of the joint beyond its normal range of motion. They are characterized by significant pain, swelling, and possible hematoma. Externally, sprains may resemble a fracture or dislocation. Definitive differentiation between a sprain and a fracture is accomplished only through a radiographic study. In the prehospital setting, it is reasonable to splint a suspected sprain in case it turns out to be a fracture or dislocation. An ice or cold pack may help relieve pain. Use of narcotic pain medication is generally not necessary or desirable and should be reserved for cases with significant pain that is unresponsive to splinting, elevation, and ice.

Management

The general management for suspected sprain includes the following steps:

1. Identify and treat any and all life-threatening injuries found in the primary survey.
2. Stop any external bleeding, and treat the patient for shock.
3. Evaluate for distal neurovascular function.
4. Support the area of injury.
5. Immobilize the injured extremity.
6. Apply ice or cold packs to control pain and swelling.
7. Reevaluate the injured extremity after immobilization for changes in distal neurovascular function.

Prolonged Transport

Patients with extremity trauma often have coexisting injuries. Ongoing internal blood loss may be from abdominal or thoracic injuries, and during a prolonged transport, the primary survey will need to be reassessed frequently to ensure that all life-threatening conditions are identified and no new ones have emerged. Vital signs should be obtained at regular intervals. Intravenous crystalloid solutions should be administered at a rate to maintain adequate perfusion, unless significant internal hemorrhage is suspected in the pelvis, abdomen, or thorax. In settings where compartment syndrome is suspected, pulses are diminished, or active hemorrhage has occurred, frequent checks are necessary.

During long transports, the prehospital care provider needs to focus greater attention on extremity perfusion. In limbs with compromised vascular supply, the provider can attempt to restore normal anatomic positioning to optimize the chance for improved blood flow. Similarly, in the face of prolonged transport times, consideration should be given to reduction of dislocations with impaired distal circulation prior to initiation of transport. Distal perfusion, including pulses, color, and temperature, as well as motor and sensory function, should be examined in a serial manner. Compartments should be monitored for the development of potential compartment syndrome. These examinations, including any changes that develop, should be carefully recorded and communicated to the provider at the receiving facility.

Measures to ensure patient comfort should be taken. Splinting devices should be comfortable and well padded. The limbs should be assessed for any pressure points inside the splint where pressure could contribute to the creation of an ulcer, especially in an extremity with compromised perfusion. Parenteral narcotic analgesia should be given at regular intervals if necessary, with careful monitoring of ventilatory rate, blood pressure, pulse oximetry, and capnography.

Contaminated wounds should be flushed with normal saline irrigation so that gross particulate matter (e.g., soil, grass) is removed. Antibiotics may be administered for open fractures if there is a prolonged transport or a delay to receiving care from a hospital provider. Guidelines exist for antibiotic type, and gram-positive coverage is typical (cephalosporin, e.g., Ancef), with many authors advocating addition of gram-negative coverage for more severe and contaminated injuries (aminoglycosides). Penicillin is added for farm injuries. If a body part has been amputated, it should also be periodically assessed so that it remains cool but does not freeze or become macerated (softened) by soaking in water.

SUMMARY

- In patients with multisystem trauma, attention is directed toward the primary survey first and the identification and management of all life-threatening injuries, including internal or external hemorrhage in the extremities.
- Prehospital care providers must be careful not to be distracted from addressing life-threatening conditions by the gross, dramatic appearance of any noncritical injuries or by the patient's request for their management.
- Once the patient has been fully assessed and found to have only isolated injuries without

systemic implication, then noncritical injuries should be addressed.
- Musculoskeletal injuries should be immobilized for stability and to provide comfort and some relief from pain.
  - Rapidly determining the mechanism of injury and energy transferred will help the prehospital care provider suspect and recognize the most critical injuries or conditions.
  - The first consideration in managing fractures is to control hemorrhage and treat for shock.
  - As a general rule, suspected dislocations should be splinted in the position found.

SCENARIO RECAP

It is a beautiful Saturday afternoon in June. You have been dispatched to a local motorcycle racetrack for a rider who has been injured. Upon arrival, you are escorted by track officials to an area on the track just in front of the grandstand where the track's medical crew (two-person, emergency medical responders, nontransport) is attending to a single patient lying supine on the track.

One of the emergency medical responders tells you that the patient was a rider in a 350-cc class race with 14 other motorcycles and that three of them collided in front of the grandstand. The other two riders were not injured, but the patient was unable to stand or move without significant pain in his right leg and pelvis. There was no loss of consciousness and no complaints other than leg pain. The medical crew has maintained the patient in a supine position with manual stabilization of the right lower extremity.

As you assess the patient, you find that he is a 19-year-old man, conscious and alert without past medical or trauma history. The patient's initial vital signs are as follows: Blood pressure is 104/68 mm Hg, pulse is 112 beats/minute, respirations are 24 breaths/minute, and skin is pale and diaphoretic. The patient states that he collided with another rider when he came out of a corner and that the collision caused him to lose balance and slide across the track. He states his right leg was run over by at least one other bike. Visual inspection of his right leg reveals shortening of the leg and no open wounds when compared to the left side, with tenderness, and bruising of the mid-anterior thigh area.

- What does the mechanism of injury of this event tell you about the potential injuries for this patient?
- What type of injury do you suspect, and what would your management priorities be?

SCENARIO SOLUTION

After completing the primary survey and ensuring that this was an isolated musculoskeletal injury, with your partner's help, you were able to apply a traction splint to the midshaft femur fracture of the right leg. After securing your patient to a long backboard, you were able to move the patient to the ambulance for transport to the hospital. Once in the ambulance, oxygen via mask was administered, and an IV was established. The patient stated that after the splint was applied, his pain improved significantly and that he did not need any analgesic at the moment. The patient's vital signs remained unchanged throughout the transport.

References

1. Williams B, Boyle M. Estimation of external blood loss by paramedics: is there any point? *Prehosp Disaster Med.* 2007;22(6):502-506.
2. Shulman JE, O'Toole RV, Castillo RC, et al. Pelvic ring fractures are an independent risk factor for death after blunt trauma. *J Trauma.* 2010;68:930-934.
3. Seyfer AE, American College of Surgeons Committee on Trauma. *Guidelines for Management of Amputated Parts.* Chicago, IL: American College of Surgeons; 1996.
4. Sharp CF, Mangram AJ, Lorenzo M, Dunn EL. A major metropolitan "field amputation" team: a call to arms . . . and legs. *J Trauma.* 2009;67(6):1158-1161.
5. Pepe E, Mosesso VN, Falk JL. Prehospital fluid resuscitation of the patient with major trauma. *Prehosp Emerg Care.* 2002;6:81.
6. Better OS. Management of shock and acute renal failure in casualties suffering from crush syndrome. *Ren Fail.* 1997;19:647.
7. Michaelson M, Taitelman U, Bshouty Z, et al. Crush syndrome: experience from the Lebanon war, 1982. *Isr J Med Sci.* 1984;20:305.
8. Pretto EA, Angus D, Abrams J, et al. An analysis of pre-hospital mortality in an earthquake. *Prehosp Disaster Med.* 1994;9:107.
9. Collins AJ, Burzstein S. Renal failure in disasters. *Crit Care Clin.* 1991;7:421.
10. Sever MS, Vanholder R, Lameire N. Management of crush-related injuries after disasters. *N Engl J Med.* 2006;354:1052.

Suggested Reading

American College of Surgeons Committee on Trauma. Musculoskeletal trauma. In: ACS Committee on Trauma. *Advanced Trauma Life Support.* 9th ed. Chicago, IL: American College of Surgeons; 2012:206-229.

Ashkenazi I, Isakovich B, Kluger Y, et al. Prehospital management of earthquake casualties buried under rubble. *Prehosp Disast Med.* 2005;20:122.

Coppola PT, Coppola M. Emergency department evaluation and treatment of pelvic fractures. *Emerg Med Clin North Am.* 2003;18(1):1.

SPECIFIC SKILLS

Traction Splint for Femur Fractures

Principle: To immobilize femur fractures to minimize ongoing internal thigh hemorrhage.

This type of immobilization is used for fractures of the shaft of the femur. The application of traction and immobilization helps to reduce muscle spasm and pain while at the same time decreasing the potential for the fractured ends of the bone to produce additional damage and increased bleeding. Traction splints should be applied only if the patient's condition is stable and time permits. Traction splints should not be used if there are associated fractures or injuries to the knee or tibia. The Hare traction splint is shown for illustrative purposes. Other traction splints, such as the Sager traction splint, may be used in accordance with local protocol and policy.

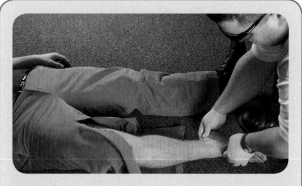

1 The prehospital care provider exposes the leg and assesses the patient's neurovascular status both before and after any manipulation. The provider explains to the patient what is going to happen and then performs the action.

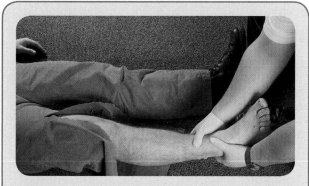

2 If the fractured extremity has marked deformity, the second prehospital care provider grasps the ankle and foot and applies gentle traction to straighten out the fracture and restore the patient's leg to length.

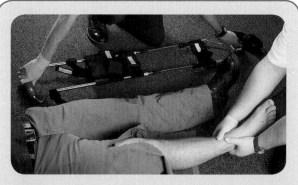

3 The splint is measured against the uninjured leg and adjusted to the appropriate length (approximately 8 to 10 inches [20 to 25 cm] beyond the heel of the leg).

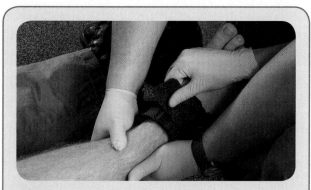

4 The ankle strap is applied to the injured leg. The strap may be used to maintain traction as necessary.

Traction Splint for Femur Fractures (*continued*)

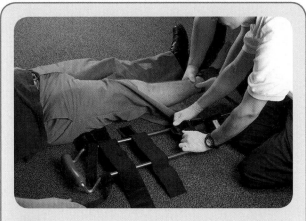

5 All Velcro securing straps are opened.

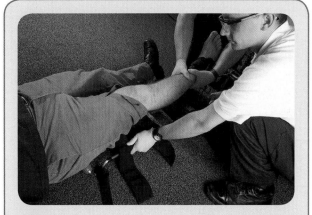

6 The patient's leg is elevated, and the proximal end of the traction splint is seated against the ischial tuberosity of the pelvis.

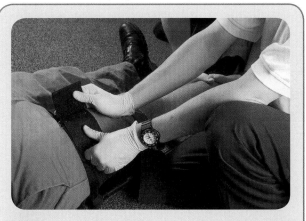

7 The prehospital care provider applies the proximal (pubic) strap around the proximal thigh to secure it in place.

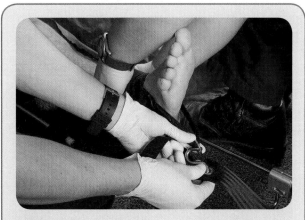

8 The ankle strap is attached to the traction hitch at the distal end of the splint.

(*continued*)

Traction Splint for Femur Fractures *(continued)*

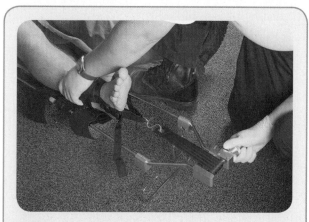

9 While maintaining manual traction, the prehospital care provider slowly turns the traction hitch mechanism to take over the traction function. Once the patient's leg has been restored to the same length as the uninjured leg, the provider stops turning the traction hitch mechanism.

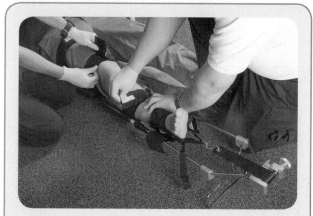

10 The prehospital care provider applies all remaining Velcro straps to secure the leg to the traction splint.

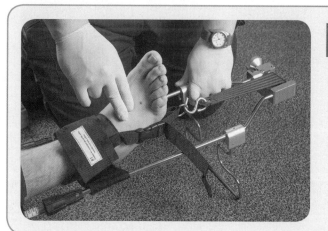

11 The prehospital care provider reassesses the patient's neurovascular status.

Burn Injuries

Lead Editors:
Brian H. Williams, MD, FACS
Spogmai Komak, MD

CHAPTER OBJECTIVES

At the completion of this chapter, you will be able to do the following:

- Describe the etiology, pathophysiology, and systemic effects of burn injury.
- Describe the underlying fluid shift in burn injury.
- Define various depths of burns.
- Describe the zones of burn injuries.
- Explain how ice can deepen the depth of burns.
- Estimate burn size using the rule of nines.
- Calculate fluid resuscitation using the Parkland formula.
- Calculate fluid resuscitation using the Rule of Ten.
- Describe the additional fluid needs in pediatric patients with burns.

- Describe the unique aspects of pediatric burns and child abuse.
- Describe appropriate burn dressings for prehospital care.
- Explain the unique concerns of electrical injuries.
- Describe the special considerations in radiation and chemical burns.
- Relate the management concerns in patients with circumferential burns.
- Describe the three elements of smoke inhalation.
- Discuss the criteria for the transfer of patients to burn centers.

SCENARIO

You are called to a residential structure fire. When your unit arrives, you witness a two-story house that is fully involved with fire and has thick black smoke pouring out of the roof and windows. You are directed to a victim who is being cared for by emergency medical responders (EMRs). They tell you that the patient reentered the burning building in an attempt to rescue his dog, and he was carried out unconscious by fire fighters.

Your patient is a man who appears to be in his thirties. The majority of his clothes have been burned off. He has obvious burns to his face, and his hair has been singed. He is unconscious; he is breathing spontaneously, but with snoring respirations. The EMRs have placed the patient on high-flow oxygen with a nonrebreathing mask. On physical examination, his airway is patent with manual assistance (jaw thrust); he ventilates easily. The sleeves of his shirt have been burned off. His arms have circumferential burns, but his radial pulse is easily palpable. His heart rate is 118 beats/minute, blood pressure is 148/94 millimeters of mercury (mm Hg), ventilatory

(continued)

INTRODUCTION

Acute thermal injury continues to be a significant medical problem, claiming an estimated 180,000 lives worldwide annually.[1] An estimated 11 million people worldwide were treated for burn injuries in 2004 alone.[1] Over 95% of fatal fire-related burns occur in low- and middle-income countries, with children and the elderly being the most vulnerable population with the highest mortality.[2] Major burn injury is a subset of acute trauma. It is unique in that it is almost always associated with significant disfigurement and deformity, in addition to repeated episodes of sepsis, wound infection, and multiorgan involvement seen in other forms of traumatic injury.

Etiology of Burn Injury

The majority of burns are a result of thermal injury due to flame (55%), followed by scald (40%) injury. Fire is the most common cause of burn in adults, while scald burns from hot liquids are the most common burns to children and older adults. House fires are related to approximately 4% of burn admissions but have a 12% fatality rate (in patients hospitalized from house fires); this rate is much higher than the 3% fatality rate of patients with burns from other causes and is presumably associated with inhalation injury.[3] The impact of low incomes on fire and burn fatalities is tied to older buildings that were not built to meet current fire safety codes, crowded living conditions, and the absence of smoke detectors.

The elderly and young are the most susceptible populations to burn injury. Scald burns are the most common burns seen in the pediatric population age 1 to 5 years. Child abuse accounts for a large proportion of immersion scald burns.[4] Intentional burn injuries can be distinguished from accidental burns based on the pattern and site of the burn. Nonaccidental burns often have clear-cut edges as found in a stocking or glove distribution, where a child's foot or hand has been held in scalding water. Accidental burns, such as those caused by a child spilling hot liquid, most often occur on the head, trunk, and palmar surface of the hands and feet. Other causes of burn injury include cold temperature, electricity, chemical agents, and radiation injury.

Pathophysiology of Burn Injury

Skin is a relatively poor conductor of heat; as such, it provides an extensive barrier to heat injury. Heat transfer within the skin is influenced by thermal conductivity of the heated material, the area through which heat is transferred, and the temperature gradient within the material. The methods of heat transfer include conduction, convection, and radiation. The simplest method of heat transfer is conduction, which occurs when a solid object comes in direct contact with skin, while convection is the mechanism of energy transfer between the skin and a heated liquid or gas.

Acute transfer of heat to skin results in burn injury with immediate dysregulation of the barrier function of skin, impairing the most basic of functions, including temperature regulation, protection against infection, and maintenance of fluid homeostasis. Burn injury causes alteration in systemic circulation due to loss of vascular wall integrity, with resultant loss of protein into the interstitium. Fluid translocation into the interstitial space increases due to increased capillary permeability, and an imbalance in hydrostatic and oncotic forces causing rapid fluid shifts from the intravascular compartment. With large burn injuries, the dramatic loss of fluids, electrolytes, and protein results in loss of effective circulating plasma volume, massive edema formation, decreased end-organ perfusion, and depressed cardiovascular function.

Fluid Shifts in Burn Injury

Burn injury is characterized by the disruption of the integumentary system with resultant changes both directly at the site of injury and at a systemic level. Direct thermal injury causes changes in microvascular circulation manifested by local hyperemia, edema, and resultant capillary leakage. Edema formation follows as a result of mediators directly influencing vascular permeability. Such mediators include histamine and bradykinin, which are thought to drive the early phase of edema formation (12 to 24 hours) post burn. This edema formation can be profound, leading to shock.

Microvascular injury disrupts the capillary barriers separating the intravascular and interstitial compartments.

This results in dramatic depletion of plasma volume, with a marked increase in extracellular fluid that manifests clinically as profound burn wound edema and systemic hypovolemia. The aim of fluid resuscitation in burn injury is to restore intravascular volume and support the patient through the initial 24 hours of severe post-burn hypovolemia.

Massive fluid shifts occur in burn injury because of the disruption between the intravascular and extravascular compartment, with intracellular and interstitial volumes increasing at the expense of plasma volume.[5] This is the critical concept underlying the burn shock and burn injury fluid shifts and informs the modern basis for early targeted resuscitation.

Several different resuscitation formulas may be used, with variability in the composition of resuscitation fluid. The consensus is to give the least amount of fluid necessary to maintain adequate end-organ perfusion and that the replacement of extracellular salt lost in the burned tissue is essential.[6-8]

Systemic Effects of Burn Injury

Burn injury results in a dramatic hypermetabolic response driven by multifold increases in circulating catecholamines after injury. Burns exceeding 30% of the total body surface area (TBSA) are characterized by massive release of cytokines and inflammatory mediators into the systemic circulation.

Early cardiovascular response to burn injury is a reduction in cardiac output accompanied by an elevation in peripheral vascular resistance. This response is seen immediately after burn injury, secondary to the intravascular volume depletion from movement of fluid into the interstitium. After initiation of fluid resuscitation and replacement of plasma volume, cardiac output increases, surpassing normal cardiac output due to a hyperdynamic state, driven by an attenuated hypermetabolic response.

Release of catecholamines, vasopressin, and angiotensin causes peripheral and splanchnic bed vasoconstriction, which can affect end-organ function. Glomerular filtration rate and renal blood flow are decreased initially secondary to a decrease in intravascular volume. Additionally, there is decreased mesenteric blood flow, decreased bowel mucosal integrity, and integumentary capillary leakage after burn injury. This leads to gastrointestinal (GI) dysfunction and translocation of bacteria into the portal circulation.

Pulmonary function is also altered in burn injury, as it is in other forms of traumatic injury. There is an increase in respiratory rate and tidal volume after resuscitation, resulting in increased minute ventilation. Circulating cytokines cause an increase in pulmonary vascular resistance, which results in deceased pulmonary capillary hydrostatic pressure and may contribute to pulmonary dysfunction during the initial resuscitation phase of injury.

Anatomy of the Skin

The skin is the largest organ in the human body. It serves multiple complex functions, including protection from the external environment, regulation of fluids, thermoregulation, sensation, and metabolic adaptation (**Figure 13-1**). The skin covers about 1.5 to 2.0 square meters in the average adult. It is made up of two layers: the **epidermis** and the **dermis**. The outer epidermis is about 0.05 millimeters (mm) thick in areas such as the eyelids and can be as thick as 1 mm on the sole of the foot. The epidermis is derived from ectoderm and is capable of regenerative healing. The epidermis is connected to the dermis via the basement membrane zone, which contains epidermal projection (rete ridges) that interdigitate with dermal projections (papillae).

The dermis layer of skin is derived from mesoderm and is divided into the papillary dermis and the reticular dermis. The papillary dermis is extremely bioactive and is the reason that superficial partial-thickness burns generally heal faster than deeper partial-thickness burns (as the papillary component is lost in deeper burns).

The deeper dermis is on average 10 times thicker than the epidermis. The subcutaneous layer, or *hypodermis*, is made up of adipose (fat) and connective tissue that helps keep the outer layers of the skin attached to the underlying structures. The subcutaneous layer also contains some of the larger blood vessels and nerves.

The skin of males is thicker than the skin of females, and the skin of children and older adults is thinner than that of the average adult. These facts explain why one individual can sustain burns of varying depths from exposure to a singular burning agent, why a child might experience a deep burn while an adult with the same exposure has only a superficial injury, or why an elderly person will sustain a deeper burn than a younger adult.

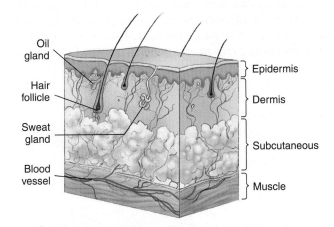

Figure 13-1 Normal skin. The skin in composed of two layers: epidermis and dermis. The subcutaneous layer and associated muscle are located below the skin. Some layers contain structures such as glands, hair follicles, blood vessels, and nerves. All of these structures are interrelated in the maintenance, loss, and gain of body temperature.

© National Association of Emergency Medical Technicians (NAEMT).

Burn Characteristics

Burn injury is caused by applied heat with resultant damage to the skin, subcutaneous tissue, fat, muscle, and even bone. Changes at the cellular level following acute thermal injury cause denaturation of proteins and loss of plasma membrane integrity. Temperature and duration of contact are important determinants in the depth of burn injury.

Acute thermal injury causes tissue necrosis at the center of injury with progressively less damage at the periphery. The depth of heat injury depends on the degree of heat exposure and depth of heat penetration.

Injury to the skin can occur in two phases: immediate and delayed. Immediate injury is from acute thermal exposure resulting in immediate loss of plasma membrane integrity and protein denaturation. Delayed injury results from inadequate resuscitation, desiccation, edema, and wound infection. Skin is capable of tolerating temperatures of 104°F (40°C) for brief periods. However, once temperatures exceed this point, there is a *logarithmic* increase in the magnitude of tissue destruction.[9]

A full-thickness burn has three zones of tissue injury that essentially form concentric circles (**Figure 13-2**).[10] The central zone is known as the **zone of coagulation**, and this is the region of greatest tissue destruction. The tissue in this zone is *necrotic* (dead) and is not capable of tissue repair.

Adjacent to the zone of necrosis is a region of lesser injury. This zone, referred to as the **zone of stasis**, is characterized by the presence of both viable and nonviable cells. This zone often has tenuous blood flow immediately after injury with associated capillary vasoconstriction and ischemia. Timely and appropriate burn care, including systemic fluid resuscitation and avoidance of vasoconstriction, is critical in prevention of necrosis in this zone of injury. Local wound care, including nondesiccating dressings, topical antimicrobials, and frequent monitoring of the wound for infection, can further ensure that damaged cells do not progress to tissue necrosis. Failure to resuscitate the patient appropriately results in death of the cells in the injured tissue and in tissue necrosis.

A common error that results in damage to the zone of stasis is the application of ice by a bystander or prehospital care provider. Ice applied to the skin in an effort to stop the burning process can cause vasoconstriction, preventing reestablishment of blood flow that is critically needed for the injured tissue. It is argued that when ice is applied to a burn the patient will experience some reduction in pain; however, the *analgesia* (pain relief) will be at the expense of additional tissue destruction. For these reasons, ice should be withheld, any ongoing burning should be arrested with the use of ambient or room-temperature water, and analgesia should be provided with oral or parenteral (all other routes) medications.

The outermost zone of injury is known as the **zone of hyperemia**. This zone has minimal cellular injury and is characterized by increased blood flow secondary to an inflammatory reaction initiated by the burn injury. The zone of hyperemia is characterized by viable cells and usually recovers unless complicated by hypoperfusion or wound infection.

Burn Depth

Estimation of burn depth can be deceptively difficult for even the most experienced prehospital care provider. Often, a burn that appears to be **partial thickness** will prove to be **full thickness**. The surface of a burn may appear to be partial thickness at first glance, but later, after **debridement** in the hospital, the superficial epidermis separates, revealing a white, full-thickness burn **eschar** underneath. Often it is best to simply tell patients that the injury is either superficial or deep and that further evaluation is required to determine ultimate burn depth. Furthermore, the prehospital care provider should never attempt to estimate burn depth until attempts have been made to initially debride the wound in the hospital.

Superficial Burns

Superficial burns involve only the epidermis and are characterized as red and painful (**Figure 13-3**). These burns extend into the papillary dermis and characteristically form blisters. These wounds blanch with pressure, and blood flow to this area is increased compared to adjacent normal skin. Superficial dermal wounds usually heal within 2 to 3 weeks without scar formation. These wounds do not require surgical excision and grafting. Burns of this depth are not included when calculating the percentage of TBSA that is burned or used for fluid administration.

Partial-Thickness Burns

Partial-thickness burns, once referred to as *second-degree burns*, are those that involve the epidermis and varying portions of the underlying dermis (**Figure 13-4**). They can be

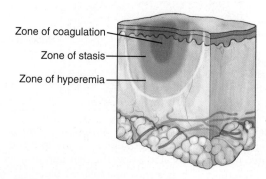

Zone of coagulation

Zone of stasis

Zone of hyperemia

Figure 13-2 Three zones of burn injury.

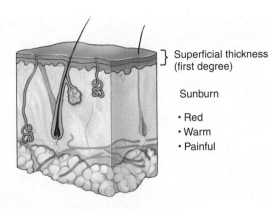

Figure 13-3 Superficial burn.
© National Association of Emergency Medical Technicians (NAEMT).

Superficial thickness
(first degree)

Sunburn

- Red
- Warm
- Painful

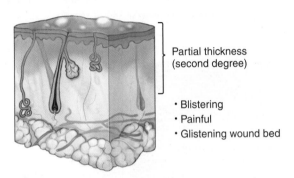

Figure 13-4 Partial-thickness burn.
© National Association of Emergency Medical Technicians (NAEMT).

Partial thickness
(second degree)

- Blistering
- Painful
- Glistening wound bed

further classified as either *superficial* or *deep*. Partial-thickness burns will appear as blisters (**Box 13-1**) or as **denuded** burned areas with a glistening or wet-appearing base. Superficial dermal burns extend into the papillary dermis. These wounds blanch with pressure, and the blood flow to the dermis is increased over that of normal skin due to vasodilation. These wounds are painful. Because remnants of the dermis survive, these burns can often heal but generally take approximately 3 weeks to do so. A deep partial-thickness burn involves destruction of most of the dermal layer, with few viable epidermal cells. Blisters do not generally form because the nonviable tissue is thick and adheres to underlying viable dermis (eschar). Blood flow is compromised, and it is often difficult to distinguish between a deep partial-thickness and full-thickness burn wound; however, the presence of sensation to touch indicates that the burn is a deep partial-thickness injury. Deep partial-thickness wounds that do not heal by 3 weeks should be excised and grafted.

In partial-thickness burns, the zone of necrosis involves the entire epidermis and varying depths of the superficial dermis. If not well cared for, the zone of stasis in these injuries can progress to necrosis, making these burns larger and perhaps converting the wound to a full-thickness burn. A superficial partial-thickness burn will heal with vigilant wound care. Deep partial-thickness burns often require

Box 13-1 Blisters

Much discussion has been generated about blisters, including whether or not to open and debride them and how to approach the blister associated with partial-thickness burns. A blister occurs when the epidermis separates from the underlying dermis and fluid that is leaking from nearby vessels fills the space between the layers. The presence of *osmotically active* proteins in the blister fluid draws additional fluid into the blister space, causing the blister to continue to enlarge. As the blister enlarges, it creates pressure on the injured tissue of the wound bed, which increases the patient's pain.

Many think that the skin of the blister acts as a dressing and prevents contamination of the wound. However, the skin of the blister is not normal and, therefore, cannot serve as a protective barrier. Additionally, maintaining the blister intact prevents application of topical antibiotics directly on the injury. For these reasons, most burn specialists open and debride blisters after arrival of the patient to the hospital.[11]

In the prehospital setting, blisters are generally best left alone during the relatively short transport time—in most cases, to the hospital where the burn injury can be managed in a cleaner environment. Blisters that have already ruptured should be covered with a clean, dry dressing.

surgery in order to minimize scarring and prevent functional deformities of high-function areas such as the hands.

Full-Thickness Burns

A full-thickness burn results in complete destruction of the epidermis and dermis, leaving no residual epidermal cells to repopulate the wound. Full-thickness burns may have several appearances (**Figure 13-5**). Most often these wounds will appear as thick, dry, white, leathery burns, regardless of the patient's race or skin color (**Figure 13-6**). This thick, leathery damaged skin is referred to as *eschar*. In severe cases, the skin will have a charred appearance with visible *thrombosis* (clotting) of blood vessels (**Figure 13-7**).

There is a common misconception that full-thickness burns are pain free, owing to the fact that the injury destroys the nerve endings in the burned tissue. Patients with these burns have varying degrees of pain. Full-thickness burns are typically surrounded by areas of partial- and superficial-thickness burns. The nerves in these areas are intact and continue to transmit pain sensation. Burns of this depth can be disabling and life threatening. Prompt surgical excision and intensive rehabilitation at a specialized center are required.

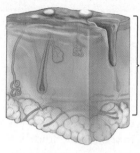

Full thickness
(third degree)
• Leathery
• White to charred
• Dead tissue
• Victims will have pain from burned
  areas adjacent to the full-thickness burn.

Figure 13-5 Full-thickness burn.

© National Association of Emergency Medical Technicians (NAEMT).

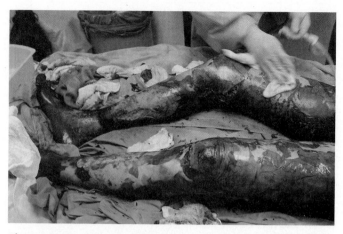

Figure 13-7 Example of deep, full-thickness burn with charring of the skin and visible thrombosis of blood vessels.

Courtesy of Dr. Jeffrey Guy.

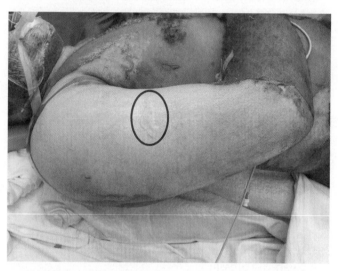

Figure 13-6 This patient has suffered from partial-thickness burns and a full-thickness burn, characterized as white and leathery in appearance.

Courtesy of Dr. Jeffrey Guy.

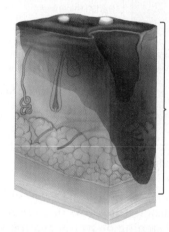

Fourth degree
(full thickness with
deep tissue damage)

Figure 13-8 Fourth-degree burn.

© National Association of Emergency Medical Technicians (NAEMT).

Subdermal Burns

Subdermal burns (previously referred to as fourth-degree burns) are those that not only burn all layers of the skin but also burn underlying fat, muscles, bone, or internal organs (**Figure 13-8** and **Figure 13-9**). These burns are, in fact, full-thickness burns with deep tissue damage. These burns can be extremely debilitating and disfiguring as a result of the damage done to the skin and underlying tissues and structures. Significant debridement of dead and **devitalized** tissue may result in extensive soft-tissue defects.

Burn Assessment

Primary Survey and Resuscitation

The goal of the primary survey is to systematically evaluate and treat life-threatening disorders in order of importance to preserve life. The XABCDE (exsanguinating hemorrhage, airway, breathing, circulation, disability, and expose/environment) method of trauma care applies to the management of the burn patient, although burn patients provide unique challenges in every step of the resuscitation.

Major burns are often a highly morbid injury. However, aside from burn-related compromise of the airway or breathing, burns by themselves are not typically an immediately life-threatening injury. The overall appearance of the burns can be dramatic and even grotesque. The sophisticated prehospital care provider will be mindful that the patient may also have suffered from a mechanical trauma and have less apparent internal injuries that pose a more immediate life threat.

Control of Severe External Bleeding

Burn patients are trauma patients, and they may have sustained injuries other than the thermal injuries. Burns are obvious and sometimes intimidating injuries, but it is

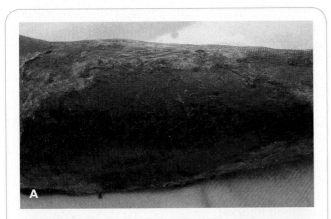

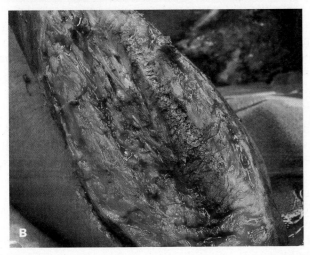

Figure 13-9 Subdermal burns are full-thickness burns with deep tissue damage. **A.** Skin. **B.** Subcutaneous fat, muscle, and bone.

Courtesy of Dr. Jeffrey Guy.

vital to assess for other less obvious internal injuries that may be more immediately life threatening than the burns. For example, in attempts to escape being burned, patients may leap from the windows of buildings, elements of the burning structure may collapse and fall on the patient, or the patient may be trapped in the burning wreckage of a motor vehicle crash. In all of these cases, the patient may have sustained both burns and associated trauma. The immediate life threat is hemorrhage from the traumatic injury and not the burn.

Airway

Burn injury is a subset of acute traumatic injury, and as in all trauma patients, attention to airway is paramount. Thermal injury from acute exposure to flame can cause edema of the airway above the level of the vocal cords and can occlude the airway. Therefore, careful initial, as well as continuous, evaluation is required. Prehospital care providers who are likely to experience prolonged

transport times need to be particularly vigilant about airway assessment. Airway management in the burn patient is more challenging when there is a concern for smoke injury or when the initial thermal injury is from fire in an enclosed space. More than 30% of thermally injured patients admitted to burn centers in the United States have a concomitant smoke inhalation injury.[12] Direct thermal insult to the upper airways results in edema formation leading to progressive swelling of mucosa, which can increase resistance to the inflow of air during inhalation. Initially, 100% humidified oxygen should be given to all patients when no signs of obvious respiratory distress are present. The patient should be thoroughly inspected, paying particular attention to the presence of chest rise and circumferential torso burns, which may restrict adequate chest rise and ventilation.

Endotracheal intubation is necessary for patients in acute respiratory distress, those with increasing work of breathing, and those who have sustained burns to the face or neck, which may result in edema and airway obstruction. It is imperative to pay particular attention to the cervical spine, especially in patients who have sustained burn injury from an explosion or deceleration accident.

If the patient is intubated, special precautions must be taken when securing the endotracheal (ET) tube to prevent inadvertent dislodgment or extubation. Following facial burns, the skin of the face will often peel or weep fluid, rendering adhesive tapes unsuitable for securing the ET tube. The ET tube can be secured using two umbilical tapes (**Figure 13-10A**) or pieces of intravenous (IV) tubing wrapped around the head. One piece should be draped over the ear and the second under the ear (**Figure 13-10B**). Commercially available cloth and Velcro devices are also suitable.

Breathing

As with any trauma patient, breathing can be adversely affected by such problems as fractured ribs, pneumothoraces, and other closed or open chest wounds. In the event of a circumferential chest wall burn, the chest wall compliance progressively decreases to such an extent that it inhibits the patient's ability to inhale. Prompt escharotomies of the chest wall should be performed in this case. An **escharotomy** is a surgical procedure that involves making an incision through the hardened burn eschar, allowing the burn and chest to expand and move with the patient's respiratory movements.

Circulation

The process of evaluating and managing circulation includes the measurement of blood pressure, evaluation of circumferential burns (see the Circumferential Burns section in this chapter), and establishment of IV catheters. Accurate measurement of blood pressure becomes difficult or impossible with burns to the extremities, and if a

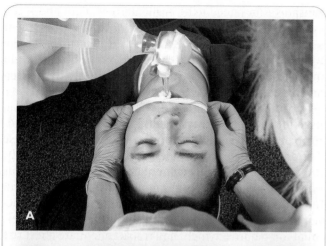

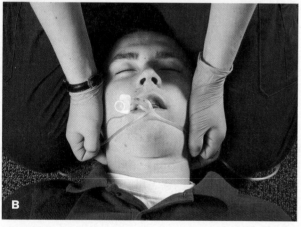

Figure 13-10 Prehospital care providers can use umbilical tape or IV tubing to secure an ET tube if the patient has burns to the face. **A.** Umbilical tape. **B.** IV tubing.

© Jones & Bartlett Learning. Photographed by Darren Stahlman.

blood pressure can be obtained, it may not correctly reflect systemic arterial blood pressure because of full-thickness burns and edema of the extremities. Even if the patient has adequate arterial blood pressure, distal limb perfusion may be critically reduced because of circumferential injuries. Burned extremities should be elevated during transport to reduce the degree of swelling in the affected limb.

Establishment of two large-bore IV catheters capable of the rapid flow rate needed for large-volume resuscitation is a requirement for burns that involve more than 20% of the total body surface area. Ideally, the IV catheters should not be placed through or adjacent to burned tissue; however, placement through the burn is appropriate if no alternative sites are available. When the catheter is placed in or near a burn, special measures must be taken to ensure that the catheter is not inadvertently dislodged. Adhesive tapes and dressings typically used to secure IV catheters will be ineffective when applied on or adjacent

to burned tissue. Alternative means to secure the lines include wrapping the site with Kerlix or Coban rolls. In some patients, the prehospital care provider may not be able to obtain venous access. Intraosseous (IO) access is a reliable alternative method to administer IV fluids as well as narcotics.

Disability

A source of life-threatening neurologic disability that is unique to burn victims is the effect of inhaled toxins such as carbon monoxide and hydrogen cyanide gas. These toxins can produce asphyxiation (see the section on Smoke Inhalation Injuries).

Evaluate the patient for neurologic and motor deficits as one would do for any other trauma patient. Identify and splint fractures of long bones after applying a clean sheet or dressing if the extremity is burned. Perform spinal immobilization if you suspect a potential spinal injury.

Expose/Environment

The next priority is to expose the patient completely. All jewelry should be promptly removed because the gradually developing swelling of burned areas will cause jewelry to act as a constricting band and compromise distal circulation. In the event of mechanical trauma, all of the patient's clothes are removed in order to identify injuries that might be concealed by the clothing. In a burn victim, removal of the clothing can potentially have a therapeutic benefit. Clothing and jewelry can retain residual heat, which may continue to injure the patient. Following chemical burns, the clothing may be soaked with the agent that burned the patient. In the case of chemical burns, improper handling of the victim's clothing that has been saturated with a potentially hazardous material can result in injury to both the patient and the prehospital care provider.

Controlling the environmental temperature is critical when caring for patients with large burns. Patients with large surface area burns are unable to retain their own body heat and are extremely susceptible to hypothermia. The burn leads to vasodilation in the skin, which, in turn, allows for increased heat loss. In addition, as open burn wounds weep and leak fluid, evaporation further exacerbates the patient's body heat loss. Make every effort to preserve the patient's body temperature. Apply several layers of blankets. Keep the passenger compartment of the transporting ambulance or aircraft warm, regardless of the time of year. As a general rule, if the prehospital care providers are comfortable, then ambient temperature is not warm enough for the patient.

Secondary Survey

After completing the primary survey, the next objective is completion of the secondary survey. The secondary survey of a patient with a burn injury is no different from that of any other trauma patient. The prehospital care provider should conduct a complete head-to-toe evaluation. The appearance of the burns can be dramatic; however, these wounds typically are not immediately life threatening. A thorough and systematic evaluation needs to be performed the same as would be done for any other trauma patient. IV access should be attempted, but there should not be a delay in transporting the patient to an emergency facility due to an inability to establish access. If the transport time to the nearest facility is less than 60 minutes, then transport should not be delayed for access. If IV access is established, then lactated Ringer solution should be infused at a rate of 500 milliliters per hour (ml/hr) in an adult and 250 ml/hr in a child over the age of 5 years.

Burn Size Estimation (Assessment)

A careful evaluation of burn wounds is conducted once the primary and secondary surveys are complete. The wounds are cleansed and assessed. Estimation of burn size is necessary to resuscitate the patient appropriately and prevent the complications associated with hypovolemic shock from burn injury. Burn size determination is also used as a tool for stratifying injury severity and triage. The most widely applied method is the rule of nines, which applies the principle that major regions of the body in adults are considered to be 9% of the total body surface area (**Figure 13-11**). The perineum, or genital area, represents 1%.

Burns can be assessed using the rule of palms (**Figure 13-12**). The use of the patient's palm has been a widely accepted and long-standing practice for estimating the size of smaller burns. However, there has not been uniform acceptance of what defines a palm and how large it is.[13] The average area of the palm alone (not including the extended fingers) is 0.5% TBSA in males and 0.4% in females. Including the palmar aspect of all five extended digits along with the palm increases the area to 0.8% total body surface area (TBSA) for males and 0.7% TBSA for females.[13] Aside from gender differences of palm size, the size of the palm also

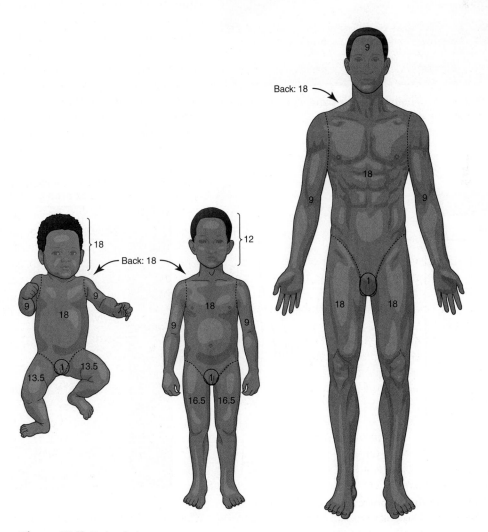

Figure 13-11 Rule of nines.

varies with body weight of the patient. As the patient's body mass index (BMI) increases, the total skin surface area of the body increases, and the TBSA percentage of the palm decreases.[14] Therefore, in most cases, the palm plus the fingers of the patient can be considered to be approximately 1% of the patient's TBSA.

Estimation of burn size in children is different from that for adults due to the relative increase of TBSA in the head. Additionally, the proportion of TBSA of children's heads and lower extremities differs with, age. The *Lund-Browder chart* is a diagram that takes into account age-related changes in children. Using these charts, a prehospital care

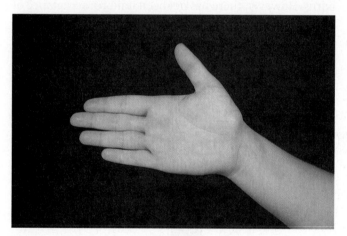

Figure 13-12 The rule of palms uses the patient's palm plus the fingers to estimate the size of smaller burns.

© Jones & Bartlett Learning. Photographed by Kimberly Potvin.

provider maps the burn and then determines burn size based on an accompanying reference table (**Figure 13-13**). This method requires drawing a map of the burns and then converting the map to a calculated burned surface area. The complexity of this method makes it difficult to use in a prehospital situation.

Dressings

Before transport, the wounds should be dressed. The goal of the dressings is to prevent ongoing contamination and airflow over the wounds, which will help with pain control.

Dressings in the form of a dry sterile sheet or towel are sufficient before transporting the patient. Several layers of blankets are then placed over the sterile burn sheets to help the patient maintain body heat. Topical antibiotic ointments and creams should not be applied until the patient has been evaluated by the burn center.

Transport

Patients who have multiple injuries in addition to their burns should first be transported to a trauma center, where immediate life-threatening injuries can be identified and surgically treated, if necessary. Once stabilized at a trauma center, the patient with burns can be transported to a burn center for definitive burn care and rehabilitation. The American Burn Association and the American College of Surgeons have identified criteria for transport or transfer of burn patients to a burn center, as outlined in **Box 13-2**.

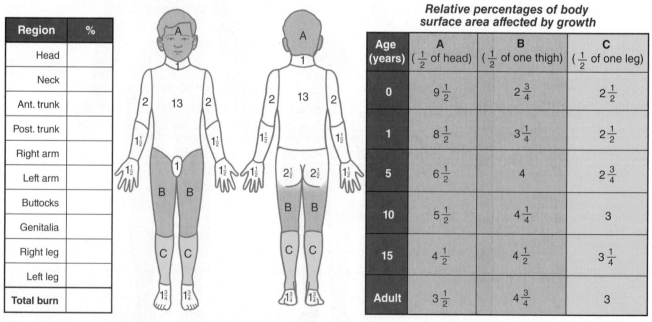

Figure 13-13 Lund-Browder chart.

Modified from Lund, C. C., and Browder, N. C. *Surg. Gynecol. Obstet.* 1944; 79:352-358.

Region	%
Head	
Neck	
Ant. trunk	
Post. trunk	
Right arm	
Left arm	
Buttocks	
Genitalia	
Right leg	
Left leg	
Total burn	

Relative percentages of body surface area affected by growth

Age (years)	A ($\frac{1}{2}$ of head)	B ($\frac{1}{2}$ of one thigh)	C ($\frac{1}{2}$ of one leg)
0	$9\frac{1}{2}$	$2\frac{3}{4}$	$2\frac{1}{2}$
1	$8\frac{1}{2}$	$3\frac{1}{4}$	$2\frac{1}{2}$
5	$6\frac{1}{2}$	4	$2\frac{3}{4}$
10	$5\frac{1}{2}$	$4\frac{1}{4}$	3
15	$4\frac{1}{2}$	$4\frac{1}{2}$	$3\frac{1}{4}$
Adult	$3\frac{1}{2}$	$4\frac{3}{4}$	3

Patients with extensive burns should receive care at centers that have special expertise and resources. Initial transport or early transfer to a burn unit results in a lower mortality rate and fewer complications. A burn unit may treat adults, children, or both.

The Committee on Trauma of the American College of Surgeons recommends referral to a burn unit for patients with burn injuries who meet the following criteria:

1. Inhalation injury
2. Partial-thickness burns over greater than 10% of TBSA
3. Full-thickness (third-degree) burns in any age group
4. Burns that involve the face, hands, feet, genitalia, perineum, or major joints
5. Electrical burns, including lightning injury
6. Chemical burns
7. Burn injury in patients with preexisting medical disorders that could complicate management, prolong recovery, or affect mortality
8. Any patients with burns and concomitant trauma (e.g., fractures) in which the burn injury poses the greatest risk of morbidity or mortality; if trauma poses the greater immediate risk, the patient may be initially stabilized in a trauma center before transfer to a burn unit
9. Children with burns in hospitals without qualified personnel or equipment for the care of children
10. Burn injury in patients who will require special social, emotional, or long-term rehabilitative intervention

Data from the American College of Surgeons (ACS) Committee on Trauma: *Resources for Optimal Care of the Injured Patient: 1999.* Chicago: ACS; 1998.

In geographic areas with no easy access to a burn center, local medical direction will determine the preferred destination for such cases.

Management

Initial Burn Care

The initial step in the care of a burn patient is to stop the burning process. The most effective and appropriate method of terminating the burning is irrigation with copious volumes of room-temperature water. The application of ice will stop the burning and provide analgesia, but it also will increase the extent of tissue damage in the zone of stasis (**Box 13-3**). Remove all clothing and jewelry; these items maintain residual heat and will continue to burn the patient. In addition, jewelry may constrict digits or extremities as the tissues begin to swell.

To effectively dress a recent burn, sterile, nonadherent dressings are applied, and the area is covered with a clean, dry sheet. If a sheet is not readily available, substitute a sterile surgical gown, drapes, towels, or Mylar rescue blanket. The dressing will prevent ongoing environmental contamination while helping to prevent the patient from experiencing pain from air flowing over the exposed nerve endings (**Box 13-4**).

Prehospital care providers have often been unsatisfied and frustrated with the simple application of sterile sheets to a burn. However, topical ointments and conventional topical antibiotics should not be applied because they prevent a direct inspection of the burn. Such topical ointments and antibiotics are removed on admission to the burn center to allow direct visualization of the burn and determination of burn severity. Also, some topical medications may complicate the application of tissue-engineered products used to aid wound healing.

High-concentration antimicrobial-coated dressings have become the mainstay of wound care in burn centers (**Figure 13-14**). These dressings are coated with a form of silver, which is time-released over several days when applied to an open burn wound. The released silver provides rapid antimicrobial coverage of the common organisms contaminating and infecting wounds. Recently, these dressings have been adapted from burn center use to prehospital applications. These large antimicrobial sheets can be rapidly applied to the burn and can eradicate any contaminating organisms. This method of wound care allows prehospital care providers to apply a non-pharmaceutical device that greatly reduces burn wound contamination within 30 minutes of application.[19-21] An advantage of these dressings in wilderness and military applications is their compact size and light weight. An entire adult can be covered with antibiotic dressings that can be stored in a container the size of a manila envelope with minimal weight.

Fluid Resuscitation

Burn injury results in direct disruption of cellular integrity and ongoing release of inflammatory mediators, causing vascular permeability and an increase in microvascular hydrostatic pressure. This drives the large efflux of fluid from the intravascular space into the interstitium. The underlying goal of early initial fluid resuscitation is to replace the intravascular volume and support the patient through the hypovolemia in the first 24 to 48 hours.

Box 13-3 Burn Cooling

A potentially controversial topic is the practice of burn cooling. Several investigators have evaluated the effect of various cooling methods on the microscopic appearance of the burned tissue, as well as the impact on wound healing. In one study, the researchers concluded that burn cooling had a beneficial effect on the experimental burn wound.[15] Burns treated with cooling had less cellular damage than those that were not cooled.

Investigators have been able to directly measure the impact of cooling on the temperature of the burned dermis, the microscopic structure of the tissue, and wound healing. A study evaluated the outcomes of various cooling methods. These investigators compared burns cooled with tap water (59°F [15°C]) to application of a commercially available gel. Each of these methods was applied immediately after the burns as well as after a 30-minute delay. Immediate tap water cooling was almost twice as effective in reducing the temperature within the burned tissue. In this trial, wounds that were cooled had better microscopic appearance and wound healing at 3 weeks after injury.[16]

Overaggressive cooling with ice is harmful and will increase the injury to the tissue already damaged by the burn. This finding was demonstrated in an animal model; cooling the burn immediately by the application of ice was more harmful than application of tap water or no treatment at all.[17] The application of ice water at a temperature of 34–46°F (1–8°C) resulted in more tissue destruction than was seen in burns that received no cooling treatment at all. In contrast, cooling with tap water at a temperature of 54–64°F (12–18°C) showed less tissue necrosis and a faster rate of healing than was observed in wounds not cooled.[18]

An important consideration is that the research on cooling was performed on experimental animals, and the burns were very limited in size. Ten percent TBSA was the largest burn size evaluated.

In summary, not all methods of burn cooling are equivalent. In the prehospital setting, cooling can be performed to stop the acute burning process; however, it should not extend beyond this as cooling that is too aggressive will lead to tissue damage. Additionally, ongoing cooling (beyond that which stops the acute burning process) will contribute to hypothermia in patients with large burns. Another potential hazard of cooling a burn is that in the patient with both burns and mechanical trauma, systemic hypothermia has predictable and detrimental effects on the ability of blood to form a clot.

Box 13-4 Prevent Airflow Over Patient's Burn

Most adults have experienced the pain associated with a dental cavity. The pain is intensified when air is inhaled over the exposed nerve. With a partial-thickness burn, thousands of nerves are exposed, and the air currents in the environment produce pain in the patient when they come into contact with the exposed nerves of the wound. By keeping burns covered, the patient will experience less pain.

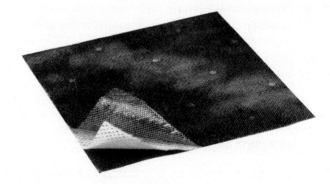

Figure 13-14 Acticoat dressing.
Courtesy of Smith & Nephew.

The resuscitation of a patient with a burn injury is aimed not only at the restoration of the loss of intravascular volume but also at the replacement of anticipated intravascular losses at a rate that mimics those losses as they occur (**Box 13-5**). In trauma patients, the prehospital care provider is replacing the volume that the patient has already lost from hemorrhage from an open fracture or bleeding viscera. In contrast, when treating the patient with a burn injury, the objective is to calculate and replace the fluids that the patient has already lost as well as replace the volume that the prehospital care provider anticipates the patient will lose over the first 24 hours after the burn injury. Early aggressive fluid resuscitation is aimed at preventing progression of patients to burn shock.

Adult Patient

The use of IV fluids, especially lactated Ringer solution, is the best way to initially manage a burn patient. The amount of fluids administered in the first 24 hours after injury is typically 2 to 4 ml/kilogram (kg)/% TBSA burned (using only the total of the partial- and full-thickness burn). Current recommendations are to initiate fluid resuscitation at 2 ml/kg/% TBSA burned. There are several formulas that guide fluid resuscitation in the burn patient. The most notable is the *Parkland formula*, which delivers 4 ml × body weight in kg × percentage of area burned. Half of this fluid needs to be administered within the first 8 hours of injury and the remaining half of the volume from hours 8 to 24.

Note, the first half of the fluid is administered within 8 hours from the time the patient was injured, not from the time the prehospital care provider started to resuscitate the patient. This detail is especially important in wilderness or military settings, in which there may be an initial delay in treatment. For example, if the patient presents for emergency care 3 hours after the injury with no or little fluid administration, the first half of the calculated total needs to be administered over the next 5 hours. Thus, the patient will have received the target volume by hour 8 after the injury.

Lactated Ringer solution is preferred to 0.9% normal saline for burn resuscitation. Burn patients typically require large volumes of IV fluids. Patients who receive large amounts of normal saline in the course of burn resuscitation will often develop a condition known as **hyperchloremic**

acidosis because of the large amounts of chloride in the normal saline solution.

Calculation of Fluid Resuscitation Measures

For example, consider a 176-pound (lb; 80-kg) man who has sustained third-degree burns to 30% of his TBSA and who is managed on scene shortly after the injury. The fluid resuscitation volume would be calculated as follows:

$$24\text{-hour fluid total} = 4\ ml/kg \times \text{weight in kg} \times \%\ \text{TBSA burned}$$
$$= 4\ ml/kg \times 80\ kg \times 30\%\ \text{TBSA burned}$$
$$= 9{,}600\ ml$$

Note that in this formula, the units of kilograms and percent cancel out so that only ml is left, thus making the calculation 4 ml × 80 × 30 = 9,600 ml.

Once the 24-hour total is calculated, divide that number by 2:

$$\text{Amount of fluid to be given from time of}$$
$$\text{injury to hour 8} = 9{,}600\ ml/2 = 4{,}800\ ml$$

To determine the hourly rate for the first 8 hours, divide this total by 8:

$$\text{Fluid rate for the first 8 hours} = 4{,}800$$
$$ml/8\ \text{hours} = 600\ ml/hour$$

The fluid requirement for the next period (hours 8 to 24) is calculated as follows:

$$\text{Amount of fluid to be given from hours 8 to 24}$$
$$= 9{,}600\ ml/2 = 4{,}800\ ml$$

To determine the hourly rate for the final 16 hours, divide this total by 16:

$$\text{Fluid rate for final 16 hours} =$$
$$4{,}800\ ml/16\ \text{hours} = 300\ ml/hour$$

The Rule of Ten for Burn Resuscitation

In an effort to simplify the process of calculating fluid requirements for burn patients in the prehospital setting, researchers from the U.S. Army Institute of Surgical Research developed the Rule of Ten to help guide initial fluid resuscitation.[22] The percentage of body surface area burned is calculated and rounded to the nearest 10. For example, a burn of 37% would be rounded to 40%. The percentage is then multiplied by 10 to get the number of ml per hour of crystalloid. Thus, in the previous example, the calculation would be 40 × 10 = 400 ml per hour. This formula is used for adults weighing 88 to 154 lb (40 to 70 kg). If the patient exceeds this weight range, for each 10 kg in body weight over 70 kg, an additional 100 ml per hour is given.

If the Rule of Ten is compared to the Parkland formula, it will immediately become apparent that the fluid volumes calculated differ to a small extent. Regardless of which method is used to calculate fluid requirements, the calculated volume is an estimate of the fluid needs, and the actual volume given to the patient must be adjusted based on the clinical response of the patient.

Pediatric Patient

Resuscitation in burned children is often initiated following a smaller TBSA burned (10% to 20%) compared to adults.[23,24] Pediatric patients require relatively larger volumes of IV fluids than adults with similar-sized burns (reported in some cases to range from 5.8 to 6.2 ml/kg/% TBSA burned).[23-25] Fluid losses are proportionally greater in children due to their small body weight to body surface ratio.[26] Additionally, children have less metabolic glycogen reserves in their livers to maintain adequate blood glucose during the periods of burn resuscitation. For these reasons, children should receive 5% dextrose-containing IV fluids (D_5LR) at a standard maintenance rate in addition to burn resuscitation fluids.

Smoke Inhalation: Fluid Management Considerations

The patient with both thermal burns and smoke inhalation requires significantly more fluid than the burn patient without smoke inhalation.[27] Resuscitation in this group has been reported to require significantly more fluid compared to similar burns without inhalation injury.[27,28]

Analgesia

Burns are extremely painful and, as such, require appropriate attention to pain relief beginning in the prehospital setting. Narcotic analgesics such as fentanyl (1 microgram [mcg] per kg body weight) or morphine (0.1 milligram [mg] per kg body weight) in adequate dosages will be required to control pain.

Special Considerations

Electrical Burns

Electrical injuries are devastating injuries, with underlying tissue destruction and necrosis that is not often apparent from the associated skin injury. The severity of electrical injury is determined by voltage, current, path of current flow, duration of contact, and resistance at the point of contact.

Electrical injury is the result of electric current, either alternating current (AC) or direct current (DC). Electrical injuries can be low voltage (< 1,000 volts [V]) or high voltage (> 1,000 V). Electric current generally follows the path of least resistance (through nerves and blood vessels), although high-voltage current may take a direct path between the point of entrance and the ground. Current is concentrated at its entrance point and then diverges

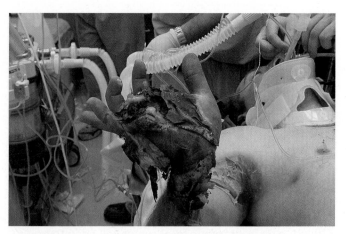

Figure 13-15 Patient after electrical injury from high-tension wires.
Courtesy of Dr. Jeffrey Guy.

and reconverges before exiting, causing the most severe tissue damage to occur at sites of contact (**Figure 13-15**). High-voltage electrical wounds are often charred, deep burns that leave a black metallic coating on the skin. Severity of damage to tissue is greatest around the contact sites, with damage to vital organs occurring in relation to the path of current.

In the treatment of electrical burns, prehospital care providers must keep in mind that the fluid resuscitation requirements usually cannot be estimated using skin surface measurements, as the damage to underlying tissues is often underestimated. Underlying devitalized tissue is often extensive and involves muscular tissue damage. Often, fascia surrounding the affected muscle limits limb swelling, with resultant rising pressures in the affected compartment. This can create a compartment syndrome within the affected limb.

Continued ischemia secondary to the initial electrical injury and ongoing increasing compartment pressures can result in irreversible muscle damage after 6 to 8 hours. Muscle necrosis within the compartment results in further release of cytokine mediators, increasing vascular permeability and extravasation of fluid into the injury site. Release of hemoglobin from necrotic muscle is circulated through the kidney. Release of myoglobin results in obstruction of the renal collecting tubules, leading to acute renal failure.

Electrical and crush injuries share many similarities. In both injuries, there is massive destruction of large muscle groups with resultant release of both potassium and myoglobin. (See the Musculoskeletal Trauma chapter.) The release of muscle potassium causes a significant increase in the serum level, which can result in cardiac dysrhythmias. Elevated potassium levels can make administration of the depolarizing muscle relaxant succinylcholine prohibitively dangerous.[29] If chemical paralysis of the patient is required, such as for rapid-sequence intubation, nondepolarizing agents such as vecuronium or rocuronium may be used.

Myoglobin is a molecule found in the muscle that assists the muscle tissue in the transportation of oxygen. When released into the bloodstream in considerable amounts, the myoglobin is toxic to the kidneys and can cause kidney failure. This condition, **myoglobinuria**, is evidenced by tea- or cola-colored urine (**Figure 13-16**).

Prehospital care providers are commonly called on to provide interhospital transfers of patients after electrical injuries. Patients with electrical burns should ideally be transported with a urinary catheter in place. Patients with myoglobinuria require aggressive fluid administration to maintain a urine output of greater than 100 ml/hour in adults or 1 ml/kg/hour in children to avoid acute kidney injury. Sodium bicarbonate is administered in some cases to make the myoglobin more soluble in urine and reduce the likelihood of renal injury; however, its actual benefit in preventing acute kidney injury remains a topic of debate.

The electrical burn patient may have associated mechanical injuries as well. Approximately 15% of patients with electrical injuries also have traumatic injuries. This rate is twice that seen in patients burned by other mechanisms.[30] Tympanic membranes may rupture, resulting in hearing difficulties. Intense and sustained muscle contraction (*tetany*) can result in shoulder dislocations and compression fractures of multiple levels of the spine as well as long bones, and for this reason, spinal immobilization or spinal motion restriction should be considered for patients with electrical injury. Long-bone fractures should be splinted when detected or suspected. Intracranial bleeds and cardiac dysrhythmias may also occur.

Electrical flash burns are the result of superheated air. Nevertheless, because of the catastrophic and occult nature of conduction injuries, it is imperative that providers maintain a high index of suspicion for the presence of a transmission type of injury.

Circumferential Burns

Circumferential burns of the trunk or limbs are capable of producing a life- or limb-threatening condition as a result of the thick, inelastic eschar that is formed. Circumferential burns of the chest can constrict the chest wall to such a degree that the patient suffocates from the inability to inhale. Circumferential burns of the extremities create a tourniquet-like effect that can render an arm or leg pulseless. Therefore, all circumferential burns should be handled as emergencies and patients transported to a burn center or to the local trauma center, if a burn center is not available. As discussed previously, escharotomies are surgical incisions made through the burn eschar to allow expansion of the deeper tissues and decompression of previously compressed and often occluded vascular structures (**Figure 13-17**).

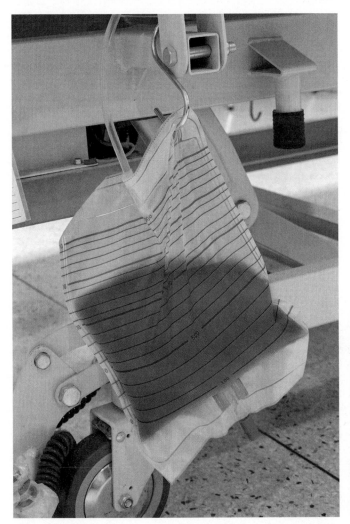

Figure 13-16 Urine of patient after electrical injury from high-tension wires. The patient has myoglobinuria after extensive muscle destruction.

© Suphatthra olovedog/Shutterstock.

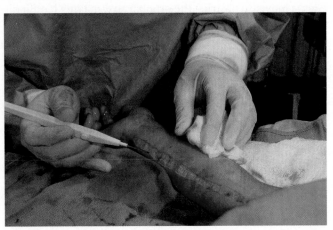

Figure 13-17 Escharotomies are performed to release the constricting effect of circumferential burns.

Courtesy of Dr. Jeffrey Guy.

> **Box 13-6** Conditions Suggesting Smoke Inhalation
>
> - Burn in a confined space
> - Confusion or agitation
> - Burns to face or chest
> - Singeing of eyebrows or nasal hair
> - Soot in the sputum
> - Hoarseness, loss of voice, or stridor

> **Box 13-7** Symptoms of Carbon Monoxide Poisoning
>
> - Mild
>   - Headache
>   - Fatigue
>   - Nausea
> - Moderate
>   - Severe headache
>   - Vomiting
>   - Confusion
>   - Drowsiness/sleepiness
>   - Increased heart rate and ventilatory rate
> - Severe
>   - Seizures
>   - Coma
>   - Cardiorespiratory arrest
>   - Death

Smoke Inhalation Injuries

The leading cause of death in fires is not thermal injury; it is the inhalation of toxic smoke. Any patient with a history of exposure to smoke in an enclosed space should be considered to be at risk of having an inhalation injury. Victims with burns to the face or soot in the sputum are at risk for a smoke-inhalation injury; however, the absence of these signs does not exclude the diagnosis of a toxic inhalation (**Box 13-6**). Maintaining a high index of suspicion is vitally important because signs and symptoms may not manifest for days after the exposure.

Inhalation injury is caused by steam, hot air, gases, or toxic fumes. Inhalation injury can result in upper airway injury, lower airway injury, pulmonary parenchymal injury, and systemic toxicity. Depending on the setting of the fire, a wide variety of materials and chemicals may be part of the combustion process; many of these compounds may act together to increase injury and morbidity. The extent of injury is affected by the ignition source, temperature, concentration, and solubility of gases generated.

Edema formation in the oropharynx, bronchial areas, and lung parenchyma accounts for many of the effects of smoke inhalation injury. Ongoing edema contributes to the microvascular disruption, inhibiting gas exchange. The edema may also obstruct the oropharynx, making it difficult for the patient to breathe and also making intubation of the patient perilous.

Toxic Gas Inhalational Injury

Two gaseous products that are clinically important are *carbon monoxide* and *hydrogen cyanide*. Both molecules are classified as asphyxiants and, thus, cause cell death by cellular hypoxia. Patients with asphyxia from smoke containing one or both of these compounds will have inadequate delivery of oxygen to tissues despite an adequate blood pressure or pulse oximeter reading.

Carbon Monoxide

Carbon monoxide is an odorless, colorless gas that is produced by incomplete combustion of products such as wood, paper, and cotton. Carbon monoxide binds to hemoglobin with much greater affinity than oxygen does. This competitive binding to hemoglobin reduces delivery of oxygen to tissues, leading to severe hypoxia, especially in tissues with high oxygen extraction (i.e., the brain and heart). The symptoms of carbon monoxide inhalation depend on the duration or severity of exposure and the resultant serum levels. Symptoms can range from mild headache to confusion, unconsciousness, convulsions, and death (**Box 13-7**). Traditional teaching is that patients poisoned with carbon monoxide develop "classic" cherry-red skin coloration. Unfortunately, this is often a late sign and should not be relied on when considering the diagnosis. Diagnosis should be based on direct measurements of carboxyhemoglobin in arterial or venous blood. The inability to differentiate oxyhemoglobin from carboxyhemoglobin limits the use of pulse oximetry.

Portable pulse carbon monoxide monitors that noninvasively measure the amount of carbon monoxide in the bloodstream are available for use in the prehospital setting (**Figure 13-18**). These monitors look and operate like pulse oximeters. Patients will generally complain of mild symptoms with levels of 10% to 20% carboxyhemoglobin. As the level of carbon monoxide in the blood increases, symptoms progressively get worse. As levels exceed 50% to 60%, seizures, coma, and death result.

Pulse oximeters cannot be used to guide recognition or treatment of carbon monoxide poisoning. Pulse oximetry will give a falsely normal or elevated reading because the detection of oxyhemoglobin depends on the colorimetric analysis performed by the oximeter, and that analysis is limited by the similar color of carboxyhemoglobin.

Treatment of carbon monoxide toxicity is removal of the patient from the source and administration of oxygen.

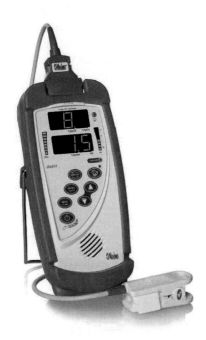

Figure 13-18 Masimo prehospital carbon monoxide monitor, Rad-57.

Courtesy of Masimo Corporation.

When breathing room air (21% oxygen), the body will eliminate half the carbon monoxide in 250 minutes.[31] When the patient is placed on 100% oxygen, the half-life of the carbon monoxide–hemoglobin complex is reduced to 40 to 60 minutes.[32]

The use of hyperbaric oxygen therapy is controversial but may be considered if carbon monoxide elimination is not achieved as expected with the use of normobaric (100% oxygen). Hyperbaric treatment is delivered in a hyperbaric chamber with a typical regimen consisting of several sessions at 2 to 3 atmospheres. Limited studies have shown an improvement in neurologic complications from carbon monoxide poisoning with the use of hyperbaric treatment.[33] A review of seven randomized trials compared hyperbaric oxygen treatment to 100% oxygen therapy. It found mixed results regarding improvement of neurologic sequelae.[34] The role of hyperbaric treatment in inhalation injury at the present time remains controversial and should only be considered on a patient-specific basis if treatment with normobaric oxygen is not achieving adequate clearance of oxygen and if there is significant underlying neurologic compromise as a result of carbon monoxide exposure.

Hydrogen Cyanide

Cyanide gas is produced from the burning of plastics or polyurethane. Cyanide poisons the cellular processes of energy production, preventing the body's cells from using oxygen. Hydrogen cyanide inhibits cellular oxygenation with resultant tissue anoxia, which is caused by reversible inhibition of cytochrome c oxidase. The patient can die from asphyxia despite having adequate amounts of oxygen available in the blood. Symptoms of cyanide toxicity include altered level of consciousness, dizziness, headache, and tachycardia or tachypnea. Patients with carbon monoxide toxicity from a structure fire should also be considered to be at risk for cyanide poisoning.

The treatment of cyanide poisoning is rapid administration of an antidote. The preferred antidote for cyanide poisoning is a medication that directly binds to the cyanide molecule, rendering it harmless. *Hydroxocobalamin* (Cyanokit) detoxifies the cyanide by directly binding to it and forming cyanocobalamin (vitamin B_{12}), which is nontoxic. Hydroxocobalamin is available for prehospital use in Europe and the United States. A second chelating agent that has been used in Europe for cyanide poisoning is *dicobalt edetate*; however, if this medication is administered in the absence of cyanide poisoning, cobalt toxicity is a risk.

The "Lilly kit" or "Pasadena kit" has been the traditional cyanide antidote kit used in the United States and may still be utilized in some settings. This method of treating cyanide poisoning was developed in the 1930s and found to be effective in detoxifying animals poisoned with 21 times the lethal dose of cyanide.[35] The goal of this antidote therapy is to induce the formation of a second poison (methemoglobin) in the patient's blood. This therapeutically induced poison binds with the cyanide and allows the body to slowly detoxify and excrete the cyanide.

The Lilly kit contains three medications. The first medication to be administered for victims of cyanide poisoning is a nitrate, either amyl nitrate or sodium nitrate, both of which are provided in the kit. Amyl nitrate comes in an ampule that is broken open, releasing fumes that the patient inhales; sodium nitrate, which is given IV, is the preferred method of administration, as it is a more efficient delivery modality and avoids exposure of health care providers to amyl nitrate fumes. The nitrate medications change some of the patient's hemoglobin into a form called methemoglobin, which attracts the cyanide away from the site of toxic action in the mitochondria of the cell. Once the cyanide binds with the methemoglobin, the mitochondria can once again begin to produce energy for the cell. Unfortunately, methemoglobin is toxic because it does not carry oxygen to cells as well as hemoglobin does. This decrease in oxygen delivery can exacerbate the tissue hypoxia associated with increased carbon monoxide levels that the victim may also have as a result of smoke inhalation.[36,37]

The third medication in the kit is sodium thiosulfate, which is given IV after the nitrate. The thiosulfate and cyanide from the methemoglobin are metabolized to thiocyanate, which is safely excreted in the patient's urine.

Because of the toxicity of methemoglobin and the time needed to administer the full Lilly kit, hydroxocobalamin has become the preferred antidote for the treatment of cyanide poisoning.

Toxin-Induced Lung Injury

In simplified terms, smoke is the product of incomplete combustion—that is, chemical dust. The chemicals in the smoke react with the lining of the trachea and lungs and damage the cells lining the airways and lungs.[38-40] Compounds such as ammonia, hydrogen chloride, and sulfur dioxide form corrosive acids and alkalis when they are inhaled and react with water.[41] These poisons cause necrosis of the cells lining the trachea and bronchioles. Normally, these cells have tiny hair-like structures called *cilia*. On these cilia is a blanket of mucus that captures and transports normally inhaled debris to the oropharynx, where the debris is swallowed into the GI tract. Several days after an inhalation injury, these cells die. The debris from these necrotic cells and the debris these cells typically capture accumulate instead of being removed. The result is an increase in secretions, plugging of the airways with mucus and cellular debris, and an increased rate of life-threatening pneumonia.

Prehospital Management

The initial and most important element of caring for a patient with smoke exposure is determining the need for orotracheal intubation. Continuous reevaluation of airway patency is required in order to recognize developing signs of airway obstruction. Change in the character of the voice, difficulty handling secretions, or drooling are signs of impending airway occlusion. Whenever patency of the patient's airway is in doubt, the prehospital care provider can proceed with securing the airway using orotracheal intubation.[42,43] In some cases, rapid-sequence intubation may be necessary, if allowed, to manage the airway. In the event of long transport times, rendezvous with an agency capable of providing definitive airway management should be considered.

Patients with smoke inhalation should be transported to burn centers even in the absence of cutaneous burns. Burn centers treat a greater volume of patients with smoke inhalation and offer unique modes of mechanical ventilation and occasionally hyperbaric oxygen therapy.

Cold Temperature Injury

Cold injuries are the result of either direct tissue freezing (frostbite) or chronic exposure to cold temperatures slightly above freezing. Frostbite is a more severe form of cold injury and is caused by direct ice crystal formation at the cellular level, with cellular dehydration and microvascular occlusion. In addition to direct cellular damage, frostbite causes progressive tissue ischemia, accounting for a more delayed loss of tissue.

Direct exposure to cold temperature causes the formation of extracellular and intracellular ice crystals, which causes a transmembrane osmotic shift that drives water from within the cell, causing intracellular dehydration. The dehydration affects intracellular electrolytes and causes changes in intracellular protein and lipid conformation. In addition to direct cellular effects, severe cold temperature affects the microvascular pathophysiology. Frostbite causes a transient vasoconstriction of both arterioles and venules, with occlusion and resumption of blood flow. This process is thought to be associated with production of mediators of tissue injury such as reactive oxygen species.

Severe injury leads to a progressive edema and loss of range of motion, with progression to tissue necrosis, gangrene, and eventual full-thickness tissue loss with ongoing freezing. Initial treatment of frostbite injury is rapid rewarming of the affected tissues. Gradual, spontaneous rewarming is inadequate, particularly for deeper injuries. Rapid rewarming should be achieved by immersing the tissue in a large water bath of 104–108°F (40–42°C). The water should be warm but not hot to the normal hand. Adequate analgesia is important, as the rewarming process can often be painful. After rewarming, the affected skin should be cleaned, dried, and elevated to minimize edema. Care should be taken to avoid pressure ulceration.

Child Abuse

Burn injuries are the third most common injury causing death in children.[4] Approximately 20% of all child abuse is the result of intentional burning. The majority of the children intentionally burned are 1 to 2 years of age.[44] Many jurisdictions require health care providers to report cases of suspected child abuse.

The most common form of burn seen in child abuse is forcible immersion. These injuries typically occur when an adult places a child in hot water, often as a punishment related to toilet training.[45] Immersion scalds are often deep because of the prolonged skin exposure (although water temperature may not be as high as in other forms of burns). Factors that determine the severity of injury include age of the patient, temperature of the water, and duration of exposure. The child may sustain deep partial- or full-thickness burns of the hands or feet in a glove-like or stocking-like pattern. Such findings are especially suspicious when the burns are symmetric and lack splash patterns (**Figure 13-19** and **Figure 13-20**).[46] In cases of intentional scalding, the child will tightly flex the arms and legs into a defensive posture because of fear or pain. The resultant burn pattern will spare the flexion creases of the popliteal fossa (knees), the antecubital fossa (elbows), and the groin. Sharp lines of demarcation will also be seen between burned and unburned tissue, essentially indicating a dip (**Figure 13-21**).[47,48]

In accidental scald injuries, the burns will have variable burn depth, irregular margins, and smaller burns remote from the large burns, indicating splash.[49]

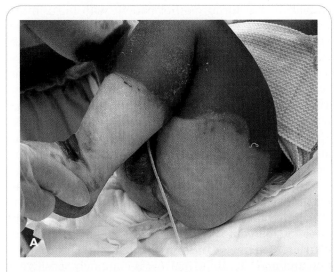

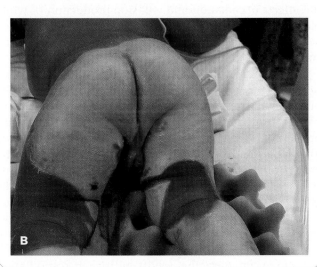

Figure 13-19 The straight lines of the burn pattern and absence of splash marks indicate that this burn is the result of abuse. **A.** Side view. **B.** Posterior view.

Courtesy of Dr. Jeffrey Guy.

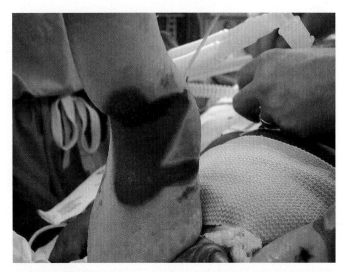

Figure 13-20 The sparing of the areas of flexion and the sharp lines of demarcation between burned and unburned skin indicate that this child was in a tightly flexed, defensive position before injury. Such a posture indicates that the scald is not accidental.

Courtesy of Dr. Jeffrey Guy.

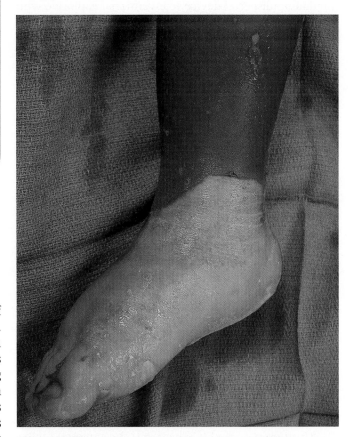

Figure 13-21 The stocking-type scald of the child's foot indicates intentional immersion burn injury consistent with child abuse.

Courtesy of Dr. Jeffrey Guy.

Contact Burns

Contact burns are the second most common mechanism of burn injury in children, whether accidental or intentional. All body surfaces have some degree of curvature. When an accidental contact burn occurs, the burning agent makes contact with the curved body surface area. The burning instrument is deflected off the curved surface, or the victim withdraws from the hot object. The resultant injury has an irregular burn edge and depth. When a child receives an intentional contact burn, the inflicting implement is pressed onto the child's skin. The resultant injury has sharp lines of demarcation between burned and unburned tissue and uniform depth.[48] Common objects involved in contact burns include curling irons, steam irons, radiators, and hot pots and pans.

Radiation Burns

The severity of burns produced from various forms of radiation is a product of the amount of energy absorbed by the target tissue. The various forms of radiation include electromagnetic radiation, x-rays, gamma rays, and particulate radiation. The different forms of radiation are able to transfer varying degrees of energy to tissue. Additionally, some forms of radiation (e.g., electromagnetic) can pass through tissue or an individual, resulting in no damage. In contrast, other forms of radiation (e.g., neutron exposure) are absorbed by the target tissue and result in significant injury. It is the absorption of the radiation that results in damage to the absorbing tissue. The absorption capacity of the radiation is more damaging than the actual dose of radiation. Equivalent doses of different forms of radiation will have dramatically different effects on an individual.

The typical exposure to radiation occurs in the setting of an industrial or occupational incident. However, with the increasing threat of global terrorism, the detonation of a radiation dispersal device (conventional explosive with radioactive material added) or a small, improvised nuclear device is a possibility. (See the Explosions and Weapons of Mass Destruction chapter for more detail.)

The detonation of a nuclear weapon in a metropolitan area, on the other hand, would injure and kill many people by three mechanisms: thermal burns from the initial firestorm, supersonic destructive blast causing blunt and penetrating trauma, and production of radiation. Mortality from a combination of thermal and radiation burns is greater than that from either thermal or radiation burns alone of equal magnitude. The combination of thermal and radiation burns has a synergistic effect on mortality.[50]

Radioactive materials are a type of hazardous material, and many of the initial priorities are the same as for any patient exposed to a hazardous material. The initial priorities are to utilize appropriate personal protective equipment, remove the patient from the source of contamination, remove contaminated clothing, and irrigate the patient with water. Remember that any removed clothing should be considered contaminated and should be handled with caution. Irrigation is performed carefully to remove any radioactive debris or particles from contaminated areas without spreading the injury to uncontaminated body surfaces. Irrigation should continue until contamination has been minimized to a steady state, as determined by a full-body survey with a Geiger counter.[51]

The exception to this approach is the patient who has sustained major trauma in addition to radiation injury. In these cases, clothing should be removed immediately, the traumatic injury dealt with, and the patient stabilized. Patients with burns should undergo fluid resuscitation similar to that for any other patient with burn injury. Irradiated patients may experience vomiting and diarrhea, which will necessitate an increase in resuscitation fluids.

The physiologic consequences of whole-body irradiation are termed **acute radiation syndrome** (ARS). The initial symptoms of ARS typically appear within hours of exposure. The cells of the body that are most sensitive to the effects of radiation are those that typically undergo rapid division. These rapidly dividing cells are found in the skin, GI tract, and bone marrow; therefore, these tissues manifest the first signs of ARS. Within a few hours after significant radiation exposure, the patient will experience nausea, vomiting, and cramping abdominal pain. Aggressive fluid management is required to prevent the development of renal failure. Over the following days, the patient may develop bloody diarrhea, ischemia of the bowel, and overwhelming infection and may die. Bone marrow is extremely sensitive to the effects of radiation and will stop production of white blood cells needed to fight infections and platelets needed to make blood clots. The resultant infections and bleeding complications are often fatal.

After a nuclear event, IV supplies, infusion pumps, and receiving medical facilities may be in short supply. If the prehospital care provider is unable to provide the patient with IV resuscitation, the patient can be resuscitated with oral fluids. A cooperative patient should be encouraged to drink a balanced salt solution to maintain a large urine output; alternatively, fluids can be delivered by nasogastric or nasoenteric tubes. Oral balanced salt solutions include Moyer's solution (4 grams [g] sodium chloride [0.5 teaspoon of salt] and 1.5 g sodium bicarbonate [0.5 teaspoon baking soda] in 1 liter of water) and World Health Organization oral rehydration solution (WHO ORS). Animal research has shown encouraging results with such resuscitation strategies in patients with burns as large as 40% TBSA. Administration of balanced salt solution to the GI tract at a rate of 20 ml/kg provided resuscitation equivalent to standard IV fluid resuscitation.[52]

Chemical Burns

All prehospital care providers need to be familiar with the basics of treating chemical injuries. Prehospital care providers in urban settings may be called to a chemical incident at an industrial setting, whereas a rural prehospital care provider may be summoned to an incident involving agents used in agriculture. Tons of hazardous materials are transported through urban and rural settings daily by both highways and rail systems. Military prehospital care providers may treat casualties of chemical burns caused by weapons or incendiary devices, chemicals used to fuel or maintain equipment, or chemical spills after damage to civilian installations.

Injuries from chemicals are often the result of prolonged exposure to the offending agent, in contrast to thermal injuries, which usually involve a very brief exposure duration. The severity of chemical injury is determined by four factors: nature of the chemical, concentration of the chemical, duration of contact, and mechanism of action of the chemical.

Chemical agents are classified as acid, base, organic, or inorganic. **Acids** are chemicals with a pH between 7 (neutral) and 0 (strong acid). **Bases** are agents with a pH between 7 and 14 (strong base) (**Figure 13-22**). Acids damage tissue by a process called **coagulative necrosis**; the damaged tissue coagulates and transforms into a barrier that prevents deeper penetration of the acid. In contrast, alkali burns destroy the tissue by **liquefaction necrosis**; the base liquefies the tissue, allowing the chemical to penetrate more deeply and cause increasingly deeper tissue damage. Alkali agents dissolve proteins of tissue and form alkaline proteins, which are soluble and allow further reaction deeper into affected tissues. Organic solutions will dissolve the liquid membranes of cell walls and cause disruption of cellular architecture, and cause damage predominantly through this mechanism. Inorganic solutions, in contrast, remain on the exterior of the cell.

Prehospital Management

The greatest priority in the care of a patient exposed to chemical agents is personal and scene safety. As in any emergency, the prehospital care provider should always be protected first. If there is any possibility of exposure to a chemical hazard, ensure scene safety and determine if any special garment or breathing apparatus is required or if any specially trained personnel or equipment are necessary. Avoid contamination of equipment and emergency vehicles; a contaminated vehicle creates an exposure risk to all others in its path. Attempt to obtain identification of the chemical agent as soon as possible.

Remove all clothing from the patient, as it may be contaminated with the chemical agent in either liquid or powder form. The contaminated clothing needs to be discarded with care. If any particulate substance is on the skin, it should be brushed away. Next, wash (*lavage*) the patient with copious amounts of water. Lavage will dilute the concentration of the injurious agent and wash away any remaining reagent. The key to lavage is to use large amounts of water. A common error is to rinse 1 or 2 liters of water across the patient and then stop the lavage process once the water starts to pool and accumulate on the floor. When lavaged with only small amounts of fluid, the offending agent is spread across the patient's body surface area and not flushed away.[53,54]

Failure to provide adequate runoff and drainage of lavage fluid may cause injury to previously unexposed and uninjured areas of the patient's body as the contaminated lavage accumulates beneath the patient. One simple way of promoting runoff in a prehospital setting is to place the patient on a backboard and then tilt it with cribbing or other means to elevate the head. At the lower end of the board, tuck a large plastic garbage bag to capture the contaminated runoff.

Neutralizing agents for chemical burns are typically avoided. In the neutralizing process the neutralizing agents often give off heat in an exothermic reaction. Therefore,

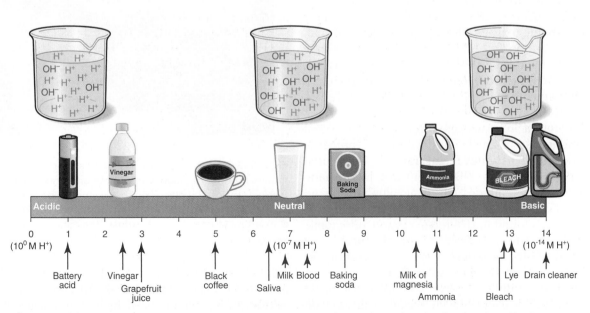

Figure 13-22 Chemical agents are classified as acid, neutral, or base, depending on the amount of hydrogen or hydroxide ions. Many household items are acids or bases and require care in handling.

a well-meaning prehospital care provider may create a thermal burn in addition to the chemical burn. Most commercially available decontamination solutions are made for the purpose of decontaminating equipment, not people.

Chemical Burns to the Eye

Injuries to the eye caused by exposure to alkali may be encountered. A small exposure to the eye can result in a vision-threatening injury. The eyes should be immediately irrigated with large amounts of irrigation fluid. If possible, ocular decontamination with continuous irrigation using a Morgan lens is performed (**Figure 13-23**). If a Morgan lens is not available, continuous irrigation may be accomplished manually with handheld IV tubing or, if both eyes are involved, a nasal cannula placed on the bridge of the nose and attached to IV tubing and an IV bag. Application of an ophthalmic local anesthetic such as proparacaine will simplify the patient's care for the prehospital care provider.

Specific Chemical Exposures

Cement is an alkali that may be retained on the clothing or in the footwear of individuals. The powdered cement reacts with the victim's sweat in a reaction that both gives off heat and excessively dries, or *desiccates,* the skin.[55] This exposure typically presents with a burn injury hours or the day after contact with the cement. The initial treatment includes brushing the cement powder away followed by copious irrigation.

Fuels such as gasoline and kerosene can cause contact burns after prolonged exposure. These organic hydrocarbons can dissolve cell membranes, resulting in skin necrosis.[56] Decontamination of the patient covered with fuel is accomplished by irrigation with large volumes of water. Gasoline contact exposure can lead to full-thickness tissue injury. An exposure of sufficient duration or severity may result in systemic toxicity. Severe cardiovascular, renal, pulmonary, neurologic, and hepatic complications may follow absorption through the topical wounds. In cases of suspected systemic toxicity, prompt surgical debridement may be warranted if there is concern for ongoing absorption of toxins from the wound.

Hydrofluoric acid is a dangerous substance widely used in domestic, industrial, and military settings. It is primarily found in the manufacturing of refrigerants but is also used when making herbicides, pharmaceuticals, high-octane gasoline, aluminum, plastics, electrical components, and fluorescent lightbulbs. In addition, it is used to etch glass and metal and is found in rust removers and automobile wheel cleaners. The real danger of this chemical is the fluoride ion, which produces profound alterations of electrolytes, especially calcium and magnesium.[57] The fluoride ion chelates positively charged ions like calcium and magnesium, causing an efflux of intracellular calcium with resultant cell death. The fluoride ion remains active until it is completely neutralized and can effectively penetrate to

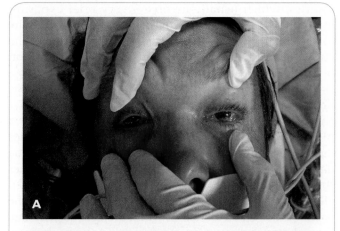

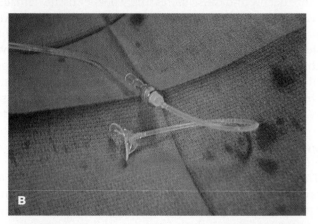

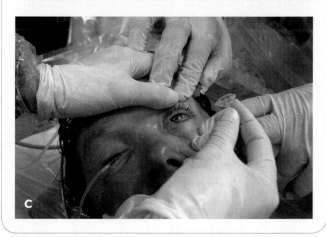

Figure 13-23 Eyes that have sustained a chemical injury require prompt irrigation with copious amounts of saline. A Morgan lens can be placed on the eye to provide appropriate ocular irrigation. **A.** Chemical burn to the eyes. **B.** Morgan lens. **C.** Inserting Morgan lenses to irrigate the patient's eyes.
Courtesy of Dr. Jeffrey Guy.

bone. Even small amounts of hydrofluoric acid can lead to profound, and potentially lethal, *hypocalcemia* (low serum calcium level). Left untreated, hydrofluoric acid will liquefy tissues and leach calcium from the patient's bones. Initial treatment for hydrofluoric acid exposure is irrigation with water, followed by application of calcium gluconate gel at an emergency department. Patients with hydrofluoric acid burns should be promptly transferred to a burn center for additional treatment.

Injuries from phosphorus are often seen in military settings. **White phosphorus** (WP) is a powerful incendiary agent used in the production of munitions. It burns violently when exposed to air, producing brilliant flames and dense smoke. It will continue to burn until all of the agent has been consumed or is deprived of oxygen. When in contact with skin, WP will produce deep chemical and thermal burns.

The initial treatment is to deprive the WP of access to oxygen. All clothing needs to be rapidly removed because it may contain some retained phosphorus particles that could ignite the clothing. Keep the affected areas immersed in water or saline-soaked dressings, and remoisten the dressings during transport. If the dressings dry out, any retained WP will reignite and could ignite the dressings and burn the patient.

Hypochlorite solutions are often used to produce household bleaches and industrial cleaners. These solutions are strong alkalis; the commonly available solutions are 4% to 6% and are not usually lethal unless large areas of the body are exposed to the chemical. **Sulfur** and **nitrogen mustards** are compounds that are classified as **vesicants** or **blister agents**. These agents have been used as chemical weapons and are recognized as a threat in chemical terrorism. These chemicals will burn and blister skin on exposure. They are irritants to the skin and cause irritation to the lungs and the eyes. After exposure, patients will complain of a burning sensation in the throat and eyes. The skin involvement develops several hours later as redness and is followed by blistering in the exposed or contaminated areas. After intense exposure, victims will develop full-thickness necrosis and respiratory failure.[58-60] The principal treatment in the field is decontamination to prevent inadvertent cross-contamination.

In caring for victims of vesicant exposure, prehospital care providers must wear appropriate gloves, garments, and breathing equipment. The Scene Management chapter covers this topic in detail. The patients must be decontaminated and irrigated with water or saline. Other agents used to decontaminate victims, used by specially trained personnel, include dilute hypochlorite solution and Fuller's earth powder, which is available commercially and functions as an absorbent agent. Additional specialized treatment is required when the patient arrives at a burn center.

Tear gas and similar chemicals are known as **riot control agents**. A riot control agent will rapidly and briefly disable those exposed to it by causing irritation to the skin, mucous membranes, lungs, and eyes. The extent of the injury is determined by the magnitude of exposure to the agent. The duration of the irritation typically lasts 30 to 60 minutes. Treatment consists of removing those exposed to the riot control agent from the source of the exposure, removing contaminated clothing, and irrigating the patients' skin and eyes.

SUMMARY

- All burns are serious, regardless of their size.
- Potentially life-threatening burns include large thermal burns, electrical injuries, and chemical burns.
- Unlike in mechanical trauma (e.g., penetrating, blunt), the body has little to no adaptive mechanisms to survive a burn injury.
- Burn injuries are not isolated to the skin; these are systemic injuries of unparalleled magnitude. Patients with major burn injury will experience dysfunction of the cardiovascular, pulmonary, gastrointestinal, renal, and immune systems.
- Failure to provide appropriate fluid resuscitation will lead to refractory shock, multiorgan dysfunction, and even deepening of the burns. The role of the prehospital care provider is, therefore, crucial in optimizing survival after a burn injury.

- Although complicated and dangerous, burns are rarely rapidly fatal. A patient with severe smoke inhalation and large thermal burns may take several hours or days to die. Patients with burns also are likely to have other mechanical trauma.
- Dramatic burns may direct the prehospital care provider's attention away from other, potentially life-threatening injuries. Performing primary and secondary surveys will reduce the likelihood of missing these injuries (e.g., pneumothorax, pericardial tamponade, splenic rupture).
- Constant vigilance is required to avoid becoming a victim. Often the injuring agent still poses a risk for injuring the prehospital care providers.
- Even small burns in areas of high function (hands, face, joints, perineum) may result in long-term impairment from scar formation.

(continued)

SUMMARY (CONTINUED)

- Familiarity with burn center transport criteria will help to ensure that all patients can achieve maximum functional recovery after burn injury.
- The leading cause of death in patients with burns is complications from smoke inhalation: asphyxiation, thermal injury, and delayed toxic-induced lung injury. Patients often do not develop symptoms of respiratory failure for 48 hours or longer. Even without burns to the skin, victims of smoke inhalation should be transported to burn centers.
- Victims of burn injury from hazardous materials, such as chemicals or radioactive agents, should undergo decontamination to avoid inadvertent spread of the material to prehospital and health care providers.

SCENARIO RECAP

You are called to a residential structure fire. When your unit arrives, you witness a two-story house that is fully involved with fire and has thick black smoke pouring out of the roof and windows. You are directed to a victim who is being cared for by EMRs. They tell you that the patient reentered the burning building in an attempt to rescue his dog, and he was carried out unconscious by fire fighters.

Your patient is a man who appears to be in his thirties. The majority of his clothes have been burned off. He has obvious burns to his face, and his hair has been singed. He is unconscious; he is breathing spontaneously, but with snoring respirations. The EMRs have placed the patient on high-flow oxygen with a nonrebreathing mask. On physical examination, his airway is patent with manual assistance (jaw thrust); he ventilates easily. The sleeves of his shirt have been burned off. His arms have circumferential burns, but his radial pulse is easily palpable. His heart rate is 118 beats/minute, blood pressure is 148/94 mm Hg, ventilatory rate is 22 breaths/minute, and oxygen saturation (SpO_2), taken by pulse oximeter, is 92%. On physical examination, you determine that the patient is burned on his entire head and has blistering of the anterior chest and abdomen, along with full-thickness burns of his entire right and left arm and hand.

- What is the extent of burns for this patient?
- What are the initial steps for managing this patient?
- How does the prehospital care provider recognize an inhalation injury?

SCENARIO SOLUTION

The patient has sustained critical injuries. Given that the patient was found collapsed in a burned building with burns to the face and labored respirations, you must be concerned that the patient has inhaled a large amount of smoke.

Evaluate and reevaluate for airway edema and an inhalation injury. Airway patency needs to be a concern; however, the patient currently is managing his own airway. Keeping in mind that often the best person to manage an airway is the patient, you need to balance the time required to transport the patient with the difficulties of airway management in a patient with an edematous airway. If transport will be prolonged or delayed, secure the airway by endotracheal intubation. The patient clearly needs 100% oxygen given the exposure to smoke and concerns about asphyxiants. If you elect to intubate this patient, be careful to secure the ET tube. Anchor the tube securely. A portable carbon monoxide monitor placed on the patient reports a carboxyhemoglobin level of 16%, which is already being treated since the patient is on 100% oxygen. You consult the local protocol regarding management of smoke inhalation with potential cyanide poisoning.

Both upper extremities have deep, full-thickness burns. You are not able to identify any veins to establish an IV line. Neither leg is burned, nor is there evidence of any fractures. An IO line is started in the left tibia, and an infusion of lactated Ringer solution is started.

The patient is burned on the entire head, both upper extremities, and the anterior trunk. Each limb is approximately 9% of TBSA, the anterior trunk is 18%, and the head is approximately 9%. Therefore, the estimated TBSA burned is approximately 45%. The patient weighs approximately 175 pounds, or 80 kg. Estimate the patient's fluid needs using the Parkland formula, as follows:

45% TBSA burned × 80 kg × 4 ml/kg/TBSA burned = 14,400 ml to be administered in first 24 hours

Half this fluid total is administered in the first 8 hours after injury. Therefore, the hourly rate for the first 8 hours is:

14,400 ml/2 = 7,200 ml to be administered in first 8 hours

Calculate the hourly fluid rate:

7,200 ml/8 = 900 ml per hour for hours 0 to 8

References

1. Media centre: burns. World Health Organization website. http://www.who.int/mediacentre/factsheets/fs365/en/. Updated August 2017. Accessed October 11, 2017.

2. Violence and injury prevention: burns. World Health Organization website. http://www.who.int/violence_injury_prevention/other_injury/burns/en/. Accessed October 11, 2017.

3. Vyrosek SB, Annest JL, Ryan GW. Surveillance for fatal and non-fatal injuries—United States, 2001. *MMWR Surveill Summ*. 2004;53(7):1-57.

4. Hoyert DL, Kochanek KD, Murphy SL. Deaths: Final data for 1997. *National Vital Statistics Reports*. 1999;47(19):1-105.

5. Neely AN, Nathan P, Highsmith RF. Plasma proteolytic activity following burns. *J Trauma*. 1988;28:362-267.

6. Shires GT. Proceedings of the Second NIH Workshop on Burn Management. *J Trauma*. 1979;19(11 suppl):862-863.

7. Schwartz, SL. Consensus summary on fluid resuscitation. *J Trauma*. 1979;19(11 suppl):876-877.

8. Moyer CA, Margrave HW, Monafo, WW. Burn shock and extravascular sodium deficiency: treatment with Ringer's solution with lactate. *Arch Surg*. 1965;90:799-811.

9. Mortiz AR, Henrique FC Jr. Studies of thermal injury: the relative importance of time and surface temperature in the causation of cutaneous burn injury. *Am J Pathol*. 1947;23:695.

10. Robinson MC, Del Becarro EJ. Increasing dermal perfusion after burning by decreasing thromboxane production. *J Trauma*. 1980;20:722.

11. Heggers JP, Ko F, Robson MC, et al. Evaluation of burn blister fluid. *Plast Reconstr Surg*. 1980;65:798.

12. Pruitt BA Jr, Goodwin CW, Mason AD Jr. Epidemiological, demographic and outcome characteristics of burn injury.

In: Herndon DN, ed. *Total Burn Care*. London, UK: WB Saunders; 2002:16-32.

13. Rossiter ND, Chapman P, Haywood IA. How big is a hand? *Burns*. 1996;22(3):230-231.

14. Berry MG, Evison D, Roberts AH. The influence of body mass index on burn surface area estimated from the area of the hand. *Burns*. 2001;27(6):591-594.

15. de Camara DL, Robinson MC. Ultrastructure aspects of cooled thermal injury. *J Trauma*. 1981;21:911-919.

16. Jandera V, Hudson DA, de Wet PM, Innes PM, Rode H. Cooling the burn wound: evaluation of different modalities. *Burns*. 2000;26:265-270.

17. Sawada Y, Urushidate S, Yotsuyanagi T, Ishita K. Is prolonged and excessive cooling of a scalded wound effective? *Burns*. 1977;23(1):55-58.

18. Venter TH, Karpelowsky JS, Rode H. Cooling of the burn wound: the ideal temperature of the coolant. *Burns*. 2007;33:917-922.

19. Dunn K, Edwards-Jones VT. The role of Acticoat with nanocrystal-line silver in the management of burns. *Burns*. 2004;30(suppl):S1.

20. Wright JB, Lam K, Burrell RE. Wound management in an era of increasing bacterial antibiotic resistance: a role for topical silver treatments. *Am J Infect Control*. 1998;26:572.

21. Yin HQ, Langford R, Burrell RE. Comparative evaluation of the antimicrobial activity of Acticoat antimicrobial dressing. *J Burn Care Rehabil*. 1999;20:195.

22. Chung KK, Salinas J, Renz EM, et al. Simple derivation of the initial fluid rate for the resuscitation of severely burned adult combat casualties: in silico validation of the rule of 10. *J Trauma*. 2010;69:S49-S54.

23. Merrell SW, Saffle JR, Sullivan JJ, Navar PD, Kravitz M, Warden GD. Fluid resuscitation in thermally injured children. *Am J Surg*. 1986;152:664-669.

24. Graves TA, Cioffi WG, McManus WF, Mason AD Jr, Pruitt BA Jr. Fluid resuscitation of infants and children with massive thermal injury. *J Trauma*. 1988;28:1656-1659.

25. Carvajal HF. Fluid therapy for the acutely burned child. *Compr Ther*. 1977;3:17-24.

26. Herndon DN. *Total Burn Care*. 2nd ed. New York, New York: Saunders; 2002.

27. Navar PD, Saffle JR, Warden GD. Effect of inhalation injury on fluid resuscitation requirements after thermal injury. *Am J Surg*. 1985;150:716.

28. Lalonde C, Picard L, Youn YK, Demling RH. Increased early postburn fluid requirement and oxygen demands are predictive of the degree of airway injury by smoke inhalation. *J Trauma*. 1995;38(2):175-184.

29. Anectine: warnings. RxList website. http://www.rxlist .com/anectine-drug/warnings-precautions.htm. Reviewed January 31, 2011. Accessed September 1, 2013.

30. Layton TR, McMurty JM, McClain EJ, Kraus DR, Reimer BL. Multiple spine fractures from electrical injuries. *J Burn Care Rehabil*. 1984;5:373-375.

31. Forbes WH, Sargent F, Roughton FJW. The rate of carbon monoxide uptake by normal men. *Am J Physiol*. 1945;143:594.

32. Mellins RB, Park S. Respiratory complications of smoke inhalation in victims of fires. *J Pediatr*. 1975;87:1.

33. Weaver LK, Hopkins RO, Chan KJ, et al. Hyperbaric oxygen for acute carbon monoxide poisoning. *N Engl J Med*. 2002;347(14):1057-1067.

34. Juurlink DN, Buckley NA, Stanbrook MB, Isbister GK, Bennett M, McGuigan MA. Hyperbaric oxygen for carbon monoxide poisoning. *Cochrane Database Syst Rev*. 2005;(1):CD002041.

35. Chen KK, Rose CL, Clowes GH. Comparative values of several antidotes in cyanide poisoning. *Am J Med Sci*. 1934;188:767.

36. Feldstein M, Klendshoj NJ. The determination of cyanide in biological fluids by microdiffusion analysis. *J Lab Clin Med*. 1954;44:166.

37. Vogel SN, Sultan TR. Cyanide poisoning. *Clin Toxicol*. 1981;18:367.

38. Herndon DN, Traber DL, Niehaus GD, et al. The pathophysiology of smoke inhalation in a sheep model. *J Trauma*. 1984;24:1044.

39. Till GO, Johnson KJ, Kunkel R, et al. Intravascular activation of complement and acute lung injury. *J Clin Invest*. 1982;69:1126.

40. Thommasen HV, Martin BA, Wiggs BR, et al. Effect of pulmonary blood flow on leukocyte uptake and release by dog lung. *J Appl Physiol Respir Environ Exerc Physiol*. 1984;56:966.

41. Trunkey DD. Inhalation injury. *Surg Clin North Am*. 1978;58:1133.

42. Haponik E, Summer W. Respiratory complications in the burned patient: diagnosis and management of inhalation injury. *J Crit Care*. 1987;2:121.

43. Cahalane M, Demling R. Early respiratory abnormalities from smoke inhalation. *JAMA*. 1984;251:771.

44. Hight DW, Bakalar HR, Lloyd JR. Inflicted burns in children: recognition and treatment. *JAMA*. 1979;242:517.

45. Burn injuries in child abuse. U.S. Department of Justice, Office of Justice Programs, Office of Juvenile Justice and Delinquency Prevention website. https://www.ncjrs.gov /pdffiles/91190-6.pdf. Published May 1997. Reprinted June 2001. Accessed December 17, 2013.

46. Chadwick DL. The diagnosis of inflicted injury in infants and young children. *Pediatr Ann*. 1992;21:477.

47. Adronicus M, Oates RK, Peat J, et al. Nonaccidental burns in children. *Burns*. 1998;24:552.

48. Purdue GF, Hunt JL, Prescott PR. Child abuse by burning: an index of suspicion. *J Trauma*. 1988;28:221.

49. Lenoski EF, Hunter KA. Specific patterns of inflicted burn injuries. *J Trauma*. 1977;17:842.

50. Brooks JW, Evans EI, Ham WT, Reid JD. The influence of external body radiation on mortality from thermal burns. *Ann Surg*. 1953;136:533.

51. American Burn Association. Radiation injury. In: *Advanced Burn Life Support Course*. Chicago, IL: American Burn Association; 1999:66.

52. Michell MW, Oliveira HM, Vaid SU, et al. Enteral resuscitation of burn shock using intestinal infusion of World Health Organization oral rehydration solution (WHO ORS): a potential treatment for mass casualty care. *J Burn Care Rehabil*. 2004;25:S48.

53. Bromberg BF, Song IC, Walden RH. Hydrotherapy of chemical burns. *Plast Reconstr Surg*. 1965;35:85.

54. Leonard LG, Scheulen JJ, Munster AM. Chemical burns: effect of prompt first aid. *J Trauma*. 1982;22:420.

55. Alam M, Moynagh M, Orr DS, Lawlor C. Cement burns—the Dublin national burns experience. *J Burns Wounds*. 2007;7:33-38.

56. Mozingo DW, Smith AD, McManus WF, et al. Chemical burns. *J Trauma*. 1998;28:64.

57. Mistry D, Wainwright D. Hydrofluoric acid burns. *Am Fam Physician*. 1992;45:1748.

58. Willems JL. Clinical management of mustard gas casualties. *Ann Med Milit Belg*. 1989;3S:1.

59. Papirmeister B, Feister AJ, Robinson SI, et al. The sulfur mustard injury: description of lesions and resulting incapacitation. In: Papirmeister B, Feister A, Robinson S, Ford R, eds. *Medical Defense Against Mustard Gas*. Boca Raton, FL: CRC Press; 1990:13.

60. Sidell FR, Takafuji ET, Franz DR. *Medical Aspects of Chemical and Biological Warfare*. Washington, DC: Office of the Surgeon General; 1997.

CHAPTER **14**

Pediatric Trauma

Lead Editors
Ann Dietrich, MD, FAAP, FACEP
David Tuggle, MD
Jessica Naiditch, MD
Katherine Remick, MD, FAAP, FACEP, FAEMS

CHAPTER OBJECTIVES

At the completion of this chapter, you will be able to do the following:

- Identify the anatomic and physiologic differences in children that account for unique pediatric injury patterns.
- Demonstrate an understanding of the special importance of managing the airway and restoring adequate tissue oxygenation in pediatric patients.
- Identify the quantitative vital signs for pediatric patients.
- Demonstrate an understanding of management techniques for the various injuries found in pediatric patients.
- Describe the signs of pediatric trauma suggestive of nonaccidental trauma.

SCENARIO

You are called to the scene of a motor vehicle crash on a heavily traveled highway. Two vehicles were involved in a frontal offset collision. One of the vehicle's occupants is a child who was improperly restrained in a child booster seat. No weather-related factors are involved on this spring afternoon.

On arrival at the scene, you see that the police have secured and blocked traffic from the area around the crash. As your partner and the other arriving crew are assessing the other patients, you approach the child. You see a young boy, approximately 2 years of age, sitting in the booster seat, which is slightly turned at an angle; there is blood on the back of the headrest of the seat in front of him. Despite numerous abrasions and minor bleeding from the head, face, and neck, the child appears very calm.

Your primary and secondary surveys reveal a 2-year-old boy who weakly repeats "ma-ma, ma-ma." His pulse rate is 180 beats/minute, with the radial pulses weaker than the brachial; his blood pressure (BP) is 50 millimeters of mercury (mm Hg) by palpation. His ventilatory rate is 18 breaths/minute, slightly irregular, but without abnormal sounds. As you continue to assess him, you note that he has stopped saying "ma-ma" and seems to just stare into space. You also note that his pupils are slightly dilated, and his skin is pale and sweaty. A woman who identifies herself as the family's nanny tells you that the mother is en route and that you should wait for her.

- What are the management priorities for this patient?
- What are the most likely injuries in this child?
- Where is the most appropriate destination for this child?

INTRODUCTION

Annual data reporting from the Centers for Disease Control and Prevention (CDC) continues to show that injury is the most common cause of death for children in the United States.[1] In 2014, more than 7.5 million unintentional pediatric injuries occurred.[1,2] Tragically, as many as 80% of these deaths due to injury may have been avoidable, either by effective injury-prevention strategies or by ensuring proper care in the acute injury phase.[3]

As with all aspects of pediatric care, proper assessment and management of an injured child require a thorough understanding of not only the unique characteristics of childhood growth and development (including immature anatomy and developing physiology) but also their unique mechanisms of injury.

The adage holds true that "children are not just little adults." Children have distinct, reproducible patterns of injury, different physiologic responses, and special treatment needs, based on their physical and psychosocial development at the time of injury.

This chapter begins by describing the special characteristics of the pediatric trauma patient, then reviews optimal trauma management and its rationale. Although the unique characteristics of pediatric injury are important for the prehospital care provider to understand, the fundamental basic and advanced life support treatment approach using the primary and secondary surveys is the same for every patient, regardless of age or size.

The Child as Trauma Patient

Demographics of Pediatric Trauma

The unique needs and characteristics of pediatric patients require special attention when assessing the acutely injured child. The relative incidence of blunt (vs. penetrating) trauma is highest in the pediatric population, with penetrating trauma accounting for only 7.8% of injuries.[4] While penetrating trauma often results in injury to one body system, blunt trauma mechanisms have a greater propensity for multisystem injury.

Falls, pedestrians struck by automobiles, and occupant injury as a result of motor vehicle crashes are the most common causes of pediatric injury in the United States, with falls alone accounting for more than 2.5 million injuries per year.[2] Worldwide, the World Health Organization estimates that approximately 950,000 children die from trauma and tens of millions are hospitalized with nonfatal injuries.[5] As in the United States, traffic-related accidents are the most common cause of death, with burns, homicide, and falls the next most common.

For a variety of reasons, which will be discussed throughout this chapter, multisystem involvement is the rule rather than the exception in major pediatric trauma. Although minimal external evidence of injury may be present, potentially life-threatening internal injury may still exist and must be evaluated at an appropriate trauma center.

The Physics of Trauma and the Pediatric Trauma

A child's size produces a smaller target to which forces from fenders, bumpers, and falls are applied. Minimal cushioning from body fat, increased elasticity of connective tissues, and proximity of the viscera to the surface of the body limit children's ability to dissipate these forces in the same manner as in the adult; therefore, energy is more readily transmitted to underlying organs. Additionally, the skeleton of a child is incompletely calcified, contains multiple active growth centers, and is more resilient than that of an adult. As a result, there may be significant internal injuries without obvious evidence of external trauma.

Common Patterns of Injury

The unique anatomic and physiologic characteristics of children, combined with the age-specific common mechanisms of injury, produce distinct, but predictable, patterns of injury (**Table 14-1**). Improper seat belt usage or front seat placement in the vehicle with resulting air bag impact can lead to significant injury (**Box 14-1**). Trauma is frequently a time-critical illness, and familiarity with these patterns will assist the prehospital care provider in optimizing management decisions for the injured child in an expeditious manner. For example, blunt pediatric trauma involving closed head injury results in apnea, hypoventilation, and hypoxia much more commonly than hypovolemia and hypotension. Therefore, clinical care guidelines for pediatric trauma patients should include greater emphasis on focused management of the airway and breathing.

Thermal Homeostasis

The ratio between a child's body surface area and body mass is highest at birth and diminishes throughout infancy and childhood. Consequently, more surface area exists through which heat can be quickly lost, not only providing additional stress to the child but also altering the child's physiologic responses to metabolic derangements and shock. Profound hypothermia can result in severe *coagulopathy* and potentially irreversible cardiovascular collapse. In addition, many of the clinical signs of hypothermia are similar to those of impending decompensated shock, thereby potentially muddying the prehospital care provider's clinical assessment.

Table 14-1 Common Patterns of Injury Associated With Pediatric Trauma

Type of Trauma	Patterns of Injury
Motor vehicle crash (child is passenger)	Unrestrained: Multisystem trauma (including chest and abdomen), head and neck injuries, scalp and facial lacerations
	Restrained: Chest and abdomen injuries, lower spine fractures
Motor vehicle crash (child is pedestrian)	Low speed: Lower extremity fractures
	High speed: Multisystem trauma (including chest and abdomen), head and neck injuries, lower extremity fractures
Fall from a height	Low: Upper extremity fractures
	Medium: Head and neck injuries, upper and lower extremity fractures
	High: Multisystem trauma (including chest and abdomen), head and neck injuries, upper and lower extremity fractures
Fall from bicycle	Without helmet: Head and neck lacerations, scalp and facial lacerations, upper extremity fractures
	With helmet: Upper extremity fractures
	Striking handlebar: Internal abdominal injuries

Source: Modified from American College of Surgeons Committee on Trauma. Pediatric trauma. *ACS Committee on Trauma: Advanced Trauma Life Support for Doctors, Student Course Manual.* 10th ed. Chicago, IL: American College of Surgeons; 2018.

Box 14-1 Pediatric Injuries Associated With Seat Belts and Air Bags

Despite laws in all 50 states requiring the use of car safety seats or child restraint devices for young children, evidence suggests that child restraints are often installed improperly.[6] Furthermore, if a child is the front-seat occupant in a vehicle with a passenger-side air bag, the child is just as likely to sustain serious injury whether appropriately restrained or not.[7] A child exposed to a passenger-side air bag is twice as likely to sustain significant injury as a front-seat passenger without an air bag.[8]

Children with lap belt or inappropriate seat belt placement are at increased risk for bowel injury in motor vehicle crashes. These types of seat belt injuries can also cause pancreatic, aortic, and lumbar spine injuries, putting these children at risk for serious multisystem trauma. It is reasonable to assume that any child who was restrained by a lap belt and is found with abdominal wall bruising after a motor vehicle crash has an intra-abdominal injury until proven otherwise.

Approximately 1% of all motor vehicle crashes involving children result in exposure of the child to a deployed passenger air bag. Up to 14% of children who were involved in a motor vehicle collision with first-generation air bag deployment suffered serious injury.[9] With improvements in air bag technology, the risk of injury during deployment, while still significant, has decreased recently to 10%.[10,11] These injuries may include minor upper torso and facial burns and lacerations or major chest, neck, face, and upper extremity injury.[9]

Psychosocial Issues

The psychological ramifications for an injured child can present a major challenge. Particularly with a very young child, regressive psychological behavior may result when stress, pain, or other perceived threats impair the child's ability to process frightening events. Unfamiliar individuals in strange surroundings can limit a child's ability to fully cooperate with history taking, physical examination, and treatment. An understanding of these characteristics and a willingness to soothe and comfort an injured child are frequently the most effective means of achieving good rapport and obtaining a comprehensive assessment of the child's physiologic state.

The child's parents or caregivers also frequently require special attention and may be considered "parent patients."

The treatment of all patients begins with effective communication, but communication becomes even more important when dealing with these parent patients. It may consist of simple words of compassion or great lengths of patience, but you cannot be an effective prehospital care provider for the pediatric patient if you are ignorant of the needs of the parents or caregivers. Parents may require information about their child's injuries and planned treatment or reassurance about their child's condition. If ignored, parents might become angry or aggressive and present significant obstacles to effective care. However, when you include them in the process, often they can act as functional members of their child's emergency care team. Furthermore, parental engagement signals to the child that you are endorsed as a "safe" person, increasing the likelihood of the child's cooperation. Providers must remember that whenever a child is sick or injured, the caregivers are also affected and should be considered patients as well.

Recovery and Rehabilitation

Unique to the pediatric trauma patient is the effect that even minor injury may have on subsequent growth and development. Unlike an anatomically mature adult, a child must not only recover from the injury but also continue normal growth. The effect of injury on this process, especially in terms of permanent disability, growth deformity, or subsequent abnormal development, cannot be overestimated. Children sustaining even minor traumatic brain injury (TBI) may have prolonged disability in cerebral function, psychological adjustment, or other regulated organ systems. These disabilities can have a substantial effect on siblings and parents, resulting in a high incidence of family dysfunction, including divorce.

The effects of inadequate or suboptimal care in the acute injury phase may have far-reaching consequences, not only on the child's immediate survival but also, perhaps more important, on the long-term quality of the child's life. Therefore, it is extremely important to maintain a high index of suspicion for injury and to use clinical "common sense" when caring and making transport decisions for the acutely injured child.

Pathophysiology

The final outcome for the injured child may be determined by the quality of care rendered in the first moments following an injury. During this critical period, a coordinated, systematic primary survey is the best strategy to avoid unnecessary morbidity and prevent overlooking a potentially fatal injury. As in the adult patient, the three most common causes of immediate death in the child are hypoxia, massive hemorrhage, and overwhelming central nervous system (CNS) trauma. These three common causes of immediate death are detailed in this section. Expedient triage, stabilizing emergency medical treatment, and transport to the most appropriate center for treatment can optimize the potential for a meaningful recovery.

Hypoxia

Confirming that a child has an open and functioning airway does not preclude the need for supplemental oxygen and assisted ventilation, especially when CNS injury, hypoventilation, or hypoperfusion is present. Well-appearing injured children can rapidly deteriorate from mild tachypnea to a state of total exhaustion and apnea. Once an airway is established, the rate and depth of ventilation should be carefully evaluated to confirm adequate ventilation. If ventilation is inadequate, merely providing an excessive concentration of oxygen will not prevent ongoing or worsening hypoxia.

The effects of even *transient* (brief) hypoxia on the traumatically injured brain deserve special attention. A child may have significant alteration in level of consciousness (LOC) yet retain an excellent potential for a complete functional recovery if cerebral hypoxia is avoided.

Pediatric patients who require aggressive airway management should be preoxygenated before attempting to place an advanced airway device. This simple maneuver may not only begin the reversal of existing hypoxia but also provide sufficient reserves to improve the margin of safety when placement of an advanced airway is performed. A period of hypoxia during multiple or prolonged attempts at placing an advanced airway may be more detrimental to the child than simply ventilating the child with a bag-mask device and transporting rapidly.[12-14] Attempting advanced airway management is unnecessary and potentially harmful if the child is adequately ventilated and oxygenated using good basic life support skills, such as bag-mask ventilation.

Hemorrhage

Most pediatric injuries do not cause immediate exsanguination. However, children who sustain injuries that result in major blood loss frequently die within moments of the injury or shortly after arrival at a receiving facility. These fatalities frequently result from multiple injured internal organs, with at least one significant injury causing acute blood loss. This bleeding may be minor, such as a simple laceration or contusion, or may be a life-threatening hemorrhage, such as a ruptured spleen, lacerated liver, or avulsed kidney.

As in adults, the injured child compensates for hemorrhage by increasing systemic vascular resistance; however, this is at the expense of peripheral perfusion. Children are physiologically more adept at this response because pediatric vasoconstriction is not limited by preexisting peripheral vascular disease. Using blood pressure measurements alone is an inadequate strategy to identify the early signs of shock. Tachycardia, although it may be the result of fear or pain, should be considered to be secondary to hemorrhage or hypovolemia until proven otherwise. A narrowing pulse pressure and increasing tachycardia may be the first subtle signs of impending shock.

Furthermore, the prehospital care provider must pay close attention to signs of ineffective organ perfusion as evidenced by alterations in respiratory efforts, decreased LOC, and diminished skin perfusion (decreased temperature, poor color, and prolonged capillary refilling time). Unlike in the adult, these early signs of hemorrhage in the child may be subtle and difficult to identify, leading to a delayed recognition of shock. If the provider misses these early signs, a child may lose enough circulating blood volume that compensatory mechanisms fail. When this happens, cardiac output plummets, organ perfusion decreases, and the child can rapidly decompensate, often leading to irreversible, fatal hypotension and shock. Therefore, every child who sustains blunt trauma should be carefully monitored to detect these subtle signs that might signal that there is ongoing hemorrhage, long before frank vital sign abnormalities.

A major reason for the rapid transition to decompensated shock is the loss of red blood cells (RBCs) and their corresponding oxygen-carrying capacity. Restoration of lost intravascular volume with crystalloid solutions will provide a transient increase in blood pressure, but circulating volume will dissipate quickly as the fluid shifts across capillary membranes. It is generally thought that when replacing the intravascular volume with isotonic crystalloid solutions, a 3:1 ratio of crystalloid to the suspected blood loss is needed to compensate for this fluid shift. As blood is lost and intravascular volume is replaced with crystalloids, the remaining RBCs are diluted in the bloodstream, reducing the blood's ability to carry oxygen to the tissues. Therefore, it should be assumed that any child who requires more than one 20-milliliter-per-kilogram (ml/kg) bolus of crystalloid solution may be rapidly deteriorating and not only needs intravascular volume resuscitation with crystalloid solution but will likely also require a transfusion of RBCs so that oxygen-delivery capacity is restored in parallel to the intravascular volume.

However, once vascular access has been secured, there is a tendency to inadvertently over-resuscitate an injured child who is not in frank shock. In the child with moderate bleeding, no evidence of end-organ hypoperfusion, and normal vital signs, fluid resuscitation should be limited to no more than one or two normal saline boluses of 20 ml/kg. The intravascular component of one bolus represents approximately 25% of a child's blood volume. Therefore, if more than two boluses are required, the prehospital care provider must take care to reassess the child for sources of previously undetected ongoing bleeding.

In the child with TBI, fluid resuscitation should be given to prevent hypotension, a known and preventable contributor to secondary head injury.[15,16] The cerebral perfusion pressure is the difference between the intracranial pressure (the pressure inside the skull) and the mean arterial pressure (the pressure driving blood into the skull). TBI can cause an increase in intracranial pressure, therefore even though blood may be adequately oxygenated, if the systemic blood pressure is low, oxygenated blood may not perfuse the brain; thus, hypoxic brain injury can still occur. Although over-resuscitation should be avoided to prevent an **iatrogenic** cerebral edema, hypotension must be prevented or quickly treated with fluid resuscitation, as a single episode of hypotension can increase mortality by as much as 150%.[17] Careful assessments of the child's vital signs and frequent reevaluation after therapeutic interventions should guide ongoing management decisions.

Isotonic crystalloid solutions should be the fluid of choice for resuscitation of the child with TBI, because hypotonic crystalloid solutions (e.g., dextrose in water) are known to increase cerebral edema. Furthermore, although hypertonic crystalloid solutions (e.g., hypertonic saline) may be useful for treatment of cerebral edema in the pediatric intensive care unit where there is extensive monitoring, evidence to date has not demonstrated improved outcomes of pediatric trauma patients when administered in the field. In the setting of impending herniation (evidence of blown pupil or markedly decreased Glasgow coma score) and in the context of prolonged transport, hypertonic saline might be considered in the out of hospital environment.

Central Nervous System Injury

The pathophysiologic changes after CNS trauma begin within minutes. Early and adequate resuscitation is the key to increased survival of children with CNS trauma. Although some CNS injuries are overwhelmingly fatal, many children with the appearance of a devastating neurologic injury go on to a complete and functional recovery after deliberate, coordinated efforts to prevent secondary injury. These recoveries are achieved through the prevention of subsequent episodes of hypoperfusion, hypoventilation, hyperventilation, and ischemia. Adequate ventilation and oxygenation (while avoiding hyperventilation) are as critical in the management of TBIs as the avoidance of hypotension.[16]

For given degrees of CNS injury severity, children have lower mortality and a higher potential for survival than adults. However, the addition of injuries outside the brain lessens the child's chances of a favorable outcome, illustrating the potentially negative effect of shock from associated injuries.

Children with TBI frequently present with an alteration in consciousness, possibly sustaining a period of unconsciousness not witnessed during the initial evaluation. A history of loss of consciousness is one of the most important prognostic indicators of potential CNS injury and should be recorded for every case. In the event that the injury was not witnessed, amnesia to the event is commonly used as a surrogate for a loss of consciousness. Furthermore, complete documentation of baseline neurologic status is important, including the following:

1. Glasgow Coma Scale score (modified for pediatrics)
2. Pupillary reaction
3. Response to sensory stimulation
4. Motor function

These are essential steps in the initial pediatric trauma assessment for neurologic injury. The absence of an adequate baseline assessment makes ongoing follow-up and evaluation of interventions extremely difficult.

Attention to detail in history taking is especially important in pediatric patients with possible cervical spine injury. A child's skeleton is incompletely calcified with multiple active growth centers, often preventing radiographic diagnosis of injury from a mechanism causing a stretching, contusion, or blunt injury to the spinal cord. This condition is called spinal cord injury without radiographic abnormality, or SCIWORA. A transient neurologic deficit that resolves prior to facility arrival may be the only indicator of a significant spinal cord injury. Despite quick symptom resolution, children with SCIWORA can develop spinal cord edema up to 4 days after the initial injury, with devastating neurologic disabilities if left untreated.

Assessment

Primary Survey

The small and variable sizes of pediatric patients (**Table 14-2**), the diminished caliber and size of the blood vessels and circulating volume, and the unique anatomic characteristics of the airway frequently make the standard procedures used in basic life support extremely challenging and technically difficult. Effective pediatric trauma resuscitation mandates the availability of appropriately sized airways, laryngoscope blades, endotracheal (ET) tubes, nasogastric tubes, blood pressure cuffs, oxygen masks, bag-mask devices, and associated equipment. Attempting to place an overly large intravenous (IV) catheter or an inappropriately sized airway can do more harm than good, not only because of the potential physical damage to the patient but also because it may delay transport to the appropriate facility. Color-coded, length-based resuscitation guides (discussed later in the chapter) provide practical medication and equipment references.[18]

Emergency assessment of children of all ages begins with an initial impression. In children, providers should use a rapid approach to quickly determine criticality of a child (i.e. sick or not sick) based on an understanding of their developmental stage and the visual and auditory appearance of the child. Using the **pediatric assessment triangle (PAT)** at the point of first contact with the patient helps to establish a level of severity, determine urgency for treatment, and identify the general category of the physiologic problem. Serial use of the PAT provides a way to track response to therapy and determine the timing of subsequent interventions (**Figure 14-1**).[4,19,20]

The three components of the PAT are appearance, work of breathing, and circulation to the skin. The first step is to use the TICLS mnemonic to assess the child's overall general appearance:

- *Tone.* Moves spontaneously, resists examination, sits or stands (age appropriate)
- *Interactiveness.* Appears alert and engaged with clinician or caregiver, interacts with people and environment, reaches for toys/objects (e.g., penlight)
- *Consolability.* Has differential response to caregiver versus examiner
- *Look/gaze.* Makes eye contact with clinician, tracks visually
- *Speech/cry.* Has strong cry or uses age-appropriate speech

The second step is to assess the work of breathing. This step involves listening for abnormal airway sounds and looking for abnormal positioning, retractions, and flaring.

Table 14-2 Height and Weight Range for Pediatric Patients			
		Range of Mean Norms	
Group	**Age**	**Average Height (cm [inches])**	**Average Weight (kg [lb])**
Neonate	0 to 1 month	51 to 63 (20 to 25)	4 to 5 (8 to 11)
Infant	1 month to 1 year	56 to 80 (22 to 31)	4 to 11 (8 to 24)
Toddler	1 to 2 years	77 to 91 (30 to 36)	11 to 14 (24 to 31)
Preschooler	3 to 5 years	91 to 122 (36 to 48)	14 to 25 (31 to 55)
School-age child	6 to 12 years	122 to 165 (48 to 65)	25 to 63 (55 to 139)
Adolescent	12 to 15 years	165 to 182 (65 to 72)	62 to 80 (137 to 176)

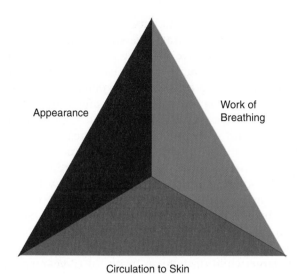

Figure 14-1 Pediatric Assessment Triangle (PAT).

Used with permission of the American Academy of Pediatrics, Pediatric Education for Prehospital Professionals, © American Academy of Pediatrics, 2000.

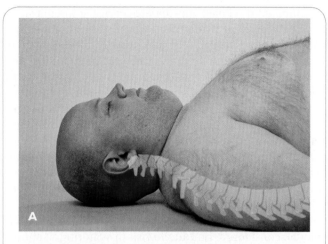

Third, providers must assess the circulation to the skin by looking for pallor, mottling, or cyanosis. Combining these three PAT components forms a general impression. The general impression is the clinician's overall evaluation of the child's physiologic state—sick or not sick.

Stabilization Priorities

The survival rate from immediate exsanguinating injury is low in the pediatric population. Fortunately, the incidence of this type of injury is also low. The initial priority is to identify any exsanguinating external hemorrhage and control the bleeding by direct manual pressure. Once exsanguinating hemorrhage has been addressed or if not present, the provider should manage the pediatric airway.

Airway

As in the injured adult, the immediate priority and focus in the acutely injured child are on airway management. However, there are several anatomic differences that complicate the care of the injured child. Children have a relatively large occiput and tongue and have an anteriorly positioned airway. Additionally, the smaller the child, the greater the size discrepancy between the cranium and the midface. Therefore, the relatively large occiput forces passive flexion of the cervical spine (**Figure 14-2**). These factors predispose children to a higher risk of anatomic airway obstruction than adults. In the absence of trauma, the pediatric patient's airway is best protected by a slightly superior–anterior position of the midface, known as the **sniffing position** (**Figure 14-3**). In the presence of trauma, however, the **neutral position** best protects the cervical spine by keeping it immobilized to prevent the flexion at the fifth and sixth cervical vertebrae (C5 to C6) and the extension at C1 to C2 that occurs with the sniffing

Figure 14-2 Compared to an adult. **A,** a child has a larger occiput and less shoulder musculature. When placed on a flat surface, these factors result in flexion of the neck **B**.

© Jones & Bartlett Learning. Photographed by Darren Stahlman; © National Association of Emergency Medical Technicians (NAEMT).

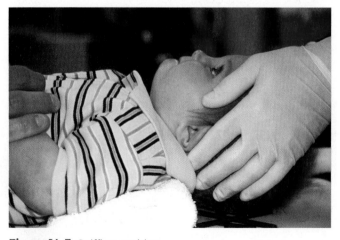

Figure 14-3 Sniffing position.

© American Academy of Orthopaedic Surgeons.

position. In this position, a jaw-thrust maneuver can be used to facilitate airway opening if needed.

Manual stabilization of the cervical spine is performed during airway management and maintained until the child is immobilized with an appropriate cervical immobilization device, whether it is commercially purchased or a simple solution such as towel rolls. Additionally, placing a pad or blanket of 2 to 3 centimeters (cm; about 1 inch) in thickness under an infant's torso can lessen the acute flexion of the neck and help keep the airway patent. Bag-mask ventilation with high-flow (at least 15 liters/minute) 100% oxygen probably represents the best choice when the injured child requires assisted ventilation.[12] Use a properly fitted oxygen mask and the "squeeze-release-release" timing technique. Watch for rise and fall of the chest, and if end-tidal CO_2 ($ETCO_2$) monitoring is available, maintain levels between 35 and 40 mm Hg.

If the child is unconscious, an oropharyngeal airway may be considered, but due to risk of vomiting, it should not be used in the child with an intact gag reflex. This is also true of the laryngeal mask and King LT airways, both of which are supraglottic airways; when sized appropriately, these devices can be considered for airway management in pediatric trauma patients who cannot be ventilated by a simple bag-mask device. In very young children, especially those weighing less than 20 kg, these devices can cause iatrogenic upper airway obstruction by causing the relatively larger pediatric epiglottis to fold into the airway.

In comparison to that of the adult, the child's larynx is smaller in size and is slightly more anterior and *cephalad* (forward and toward the head), making it more difficult to visualize the vocal cords during intubation attempts (**Figure 14-4**). Endotracheal intubation, despite being the most reliable means of ventilation in the child with airway compromise, should be reserved for those situations in which bag-mask ventilation is ineffective. Nasotracheal intubation is not recommended in children. This technique requires a spontaneously breathing patient, involves blind passage around the relatively acute posterior nasopharyngeal angle, and can cause more severe bleeding in children.

Additionally, in the patient with a basilar skull fracture, it can inadvertently penetrate the cranial vault.

If unable to receive effective bag-mask ventilation, a child with craniofacial injuries causing upper airway obstruction may be considered for percutaneous transtracheal jet ventilation with a large angiocatheter. This should be performed only by those skilled in the procedure, as the thin and malleable pediatric trachea can be easily damaged, resulting in permanent iatrogenic airway loss. This procedure is only a temporary measure to improve oxygenation and does not provide adequate ventilation. Increasing hypercarbia dictates that a more definitive airway be established as soon as safely possible. Surgical cricothyroidotomy is usually not indicated in the care of the pediatric trauma patient, though it may be considered in the larger child (usually at the age of 12 years).[21]

Breathing

As in all trauma patients, a significantly traumatized child typically needs an oxygen concentration of 85% to 100% (fraction of inspired oxygen [FIO_2] of 0.85 to 1.0). This concentration is maintained by the use of supplemental oxygen and an appropriately sized clear plastic pediatric mask. When hypoxia occurs in the small child, the body compensates by increasing the ventilatory rate (tachypnea) and by a strenuous increase in ventilatory effort, including increased thoracic excursion efforts and the use of accessory muscles in the neck and abdomen. This increased metabolic demand can produce severe fatigue and result in ventilatory failure, as an increasing percentage of the patient's cardiac output becomes devoted to maintaining this respiratory effort. Ventilatory distress can rapidly progress from a compensated ventilatory effort to ventilatory failure, then respiratory arrest, and ultimately a hypoxic cardiac arrest. Central (rather than peripheral) cyanosis

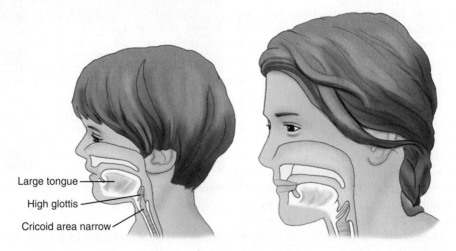

Large tongue
High glottis
Cricoid area narrow

Figure 14-4 Comparison of the adult and child airways.

is a fairly late and often inconsistent sign of respiratory failure. Prehospital care providers should not depend on this finding to identify impending respiratory failure.

Evaluation of the child's ventilatory status with early recognition of the signs of distress and the provision of ventilatory assistance are key elements in the management of the pediatric trauma patient. The normal ventilatory rate of infants and children younger than age 4 years is typically two to three times that of adults (**Table 14-3**).

Tachypnea with signs of increased effort or difficulty may be the first manifestations of respiratory distress and shock. As distress increases, additional signs and symptoms include shallow breathing or minimal chest movement. Breath sounds may be weak or infrequent, and air exchange at the nose or mouth may be reduced or minimal. Ventilatory effort becomes more labored and may include the following:

- Head bobbing with each breath
- Gasping or grunting
- Flared nostrils
- Stridor or snoring respirations
- Suprasternal, supraclavicular, subcostal, or intercostal retractions
- Use of accessory muscles, such as neck and abdominal wall muscles
- Distension of the abdomen when the chest falls (seesaw effect between the chest and abdomen)

The effectiveness of a child's ventilation should be evaluated using the following indicators:

- Rate and depth (minute volume) and effort indicate adequacy of ventilation.
- Pink skin may indicate adequate ventilation.

- Dusky, gray, cyanotic, or mottled skin indicates insufficient oxygenation and perfusion.
- Anxiety, restlessness, and combativeness can be early signs of hypoxia.
- Lethargy, depressed LOC, and unconsciousness are probably advanced signs of hypoxia.
- Breath sounds indicate the depth of exchange.
- Wheezing, rales, or rhonchi may indicate inefficient oxygenation.
- Declining pulse oximetry and/or declining capnography indicate respiratory failure.

A rapid evaluation of ventilation includes assessment of the patient's ventilatory rate (particularly tachypnea), ventilatory effort (degree of labor, nostril flaring, accessory muscle use, retraction, and seesaw movement), auscultation (air exchange, bilateral symmetry, and pathologic sounds), skin color, and mental status.

In the child who initially presents with tachypnea and increased ventilatory effort, normalization of the ventilatory rate and apparent lessening of the respiratory effort should not be immediately interpreted as a sign of improvement as it may indicate exhaustion or impending respiratory failure. As with any change in the patient's clinical status, frequent reassessment is necessary to determine if this is an improvement or deterioration in physiologic status.

Combining a general impression of the child's status, use of the PAT, and an assessment of the child's work of breathing, the prehospital care provider can quickly identify children in need of respiratory support. Children with a good appearance according to the PAT and increased work of breathing are in respiratory distress and require attention to airway positioning (with spinal stabilization), supplemental oxygen, and careful frequent

Table 14-3 Ventilatory Rates for Pediatric Patients			
Group	Age	Ventilatory Rate (breaths/minute)	Ventilatory Rate That Indicates Possible Need for Ventilatory Assistance With Bag-Mask Device (breaths/minute)
Neonate	0 to 1 month	30 to 60	< 30 or > 60
Infant	1 month to 1 year	30 to 53	< 30 or > 53
Toddler	1 to 2 years	22 to 37	< 22 or > 37
Preschooler	3 to 5 years	20 to 28	< 20 or > 28
School-age child	6 to 12 years	18 to 25	< 18 or > 25
Adolescent	12 to 15 years	12 to 20	< 12 or > 20

Source: Data from American Heart Association (AHA). Vital signs in children. *AHA: Pediatric Advanced Life Support.* Dallas, TX: AHA; 2015.

reassessments. Children who have a poor appearance and increased work of breathing are in respiratory failure and should be considered candidates for ventilatory support. Because the main problem is one of inspired volume rather than concentration of oxygen, assisted ventilation is best given by use of a bag-mask device, supplemented with an oxygen reservoir attached to high-concentration oxygen (Fio_2 of 0.85 to 1.0). Because a child's airway is so small, it is prone to obstruction from increased secretions, blood, body fluids, and foreign materials; therefore, early and periodic suctioning may be necessary. In infants, who are obligate nose breathers, the nostrils should be suctioned.

When obtaining a mask seal in infants, caution should be exercised to avoid compressing the soft tissues underneath the chin because doing so pushes the tongue against the soft palate and increases the risk of occluding the airway. Pressure on the uncalcified, soft trachea should also be avoided. One or two hands can be used to obtain a mask seal, depending on the size and age of the child.

Use of the correct-sized bag-mask device is essential for obtaining a proper mask seal, providing the proper tidal volume, and ensuring that the risks of hyperinflation and barotrauma are minimized. Ensure appropriate depth of ventilation by bagging only until chest rise is seen. Adequacy of ventilation can also be assessed by monitoring ETCO$_2$ with a goal level between 35 and 40 mm Hg. Ventilating a child too forcefully or with a tidal volume that is too great can lead to gastric distension. In turn, gastric distension can result in regurgitation, aspiration, or prevention of adequate ventilation by limiting diaphragmatic excursion. Aggressive ventilation can lead to a tension pneumothorax that can result in both severe respiratory distress and sudden cardiovascular collapse, as the mediastinum is more mobile in children. This mobility protects children from traumatic aortic injuries but increases the susceptibility to tension pneumothorax. The more mobile mediastinum compresses easily, allowing for earlier respiratory compromise and cardiovascular collapse than occurs in an adult.

Changes in a child's ventilatory status can be subtle, but ventilatory effort can rapidly deteriorate until ventilation is inadequate and hypoxia ensues. The patient's breathing should be evaluated as part of the primary survey and carefully and periodically reassessed to ensure its continued adequacy. Pulse oximetry should also be monitored, and efforts should be made to keep oxygen saturation (Spo_2) at greater than 94% (at sea level).

Whenever a child is manually ventilated, it is important to carefully control the rate at which ventilations are being administered. It is relatively easy to inadvertently hyperventilate the patient, which will decrease the carbon dioxide level in the blood and cause cerebral vasoconstriction. This can lead to poorer outcomes in patients with TBI. Furthermore, excessive ventilation pressures can lead to gastric insufflation. The distended stomach can subsequently push up into the more pliable pediatric thorax and limit tidal volume capacity. Ensure chest rise when delivering tidal volumes while bagging to avoid underventilation and hypoxia.

Circulation

After stopping any exsanguinating hemorrhage, ensure adequate airway patency and breathing, then proceed to a circulatory assessment. The child's heart rate should be assessed and identified as tachycardic (heart beating too quickly), normal, or bradycardic (heart beating too slowly). If the child is bradycardic, go back and reassess the airway. For normal or fast heart rates, look for signs of hypoperfusion (pallor, mottling, poor capillary refilling time).

A child with hemorrhagic injury can maintain adequate circulating volume by increasing peripheral vascular resistance to maintain mean arterial pressure. Clinical evidence of this compensatory mechanism includes prolonged capillary refilling time, peripheral pallor or mottling, cool peripheral skin temperature, and decreased intensity of the peripheral pulses. In the child, signs of significant hypotension develop with the loss of approximately 30% of the circulating volume. Hypotension is a late sign of hypovolemia. Because of their increased physiologic reserve, children with hemorrhagic injury frequently present with only slightly abnormal vital signs. Initial tachycardia may be from psychological stress, pain, or fear, but in the traumatized child it should always be assumed to be secondary to hypovolemia. If the child is tachycardic but has a normal blood pressure, the child may be in compensated shock. Look for signs of hypoperfusion, and complete frequent reassessments. If increased peripheral vascular resistance is not sufficient to compensate for loss of circulating volume, then the blood pressure will fall. The concept of evolving shock must be of paramount concern in the initial management of an injured child and is a major indication for transport to an appropriate trauma facility for expeditious evaluation and treatment.

A child who is tachycardic with hypotension is experiencing a critical life-threatening emergency (decompensated shock). Stop all external bleeding! If the bleeding is from an extremity injury, tourniquet placement may be lifesaving.[22,23] Fluid resuscitation should be initiated as soon as possible, but transport to a trauma center should not be delayed. Intravenous access and fluids may be initiated en route.

As in the assessment of the airway, a single measurement of heart rate or blood pressure does not equate with physiologic stability. Serial measurements and changing trends of vital signs and perfusion status are critical in gauging a child's evolving hemodynamic state in the acute injury phase. Close monitoring of vital signs is absolutely essential to recognizing the signs of impending shock, enabling the appropriate interventions to be performed to prevent clinical deterioration. **Table 14-4** and **Table 14-5** provide the normal ranges for pulse rate and blood pressure by

Table 14-4 Pulse Rate for Pediatric Patients

Group	Age	Awake Rate (beats/minute)	Asleep Rate (beats/minute)	Pulse Rate That Indicates a Possible Serious Problem* (beats/minute)
Neonate	0 to 1 month	120 to 205	100 to 160	< 100 or > 160
Infant	1 month to 1 year	100 to 180	90 to 160	< 80 or > 150
Toddler	1 to 2 years	98 to 140	80 to 120	< 60 or > 140
Preschooler	3 to 5 years	80 to 120	65 to 100	< 60 or > 130
School-age child	6 to 12 years	75 to 118	60 to 90	< 50 or > 120
Adolescent	12 to 15 years	60 to 100	50 to 90	< 45 or > 100

*Bradycardia or tachycardia.

Source: Data from American Heart Association (AHA). Vital signs in children. *AHA: Pediatric Advanced Life Support.* Dallas, TX: AHA; 2015.

Table 14-5 Blood Pressure for Pediatric Patients

Group	Age	Expected BP Range (mm Hg)*	Lower Limit of Systolic BP (mm Hg)
Neonate	0 to 1 month	Systolic: 67 to 84 Diastolic: 35 to 53 Mean arterial pressure: 45 to 60	> 60
Infant	1 month to 1 year	Systolic: 72 to 104 Diastolic: 37 to 56 Mean arterial pressure: 50 to 62	> 70
Toddler	1 to 2 years	Systolic: 86 to 106 Diastolic: 42 to 63 Mean arterial pressure: 49 to 62	> 70
Preschooler	3 to 5 years	Systolic: 89 to 112 Diastolic: 46 to 72 Mean arterial pressure: 58 to 69	> 75
School-age child	6 to 12 years	Systolic: 97 to 120 Diastolic: 57 to 80 Mean arterial pressure: 66 to 79	> 80
Adolescent	12 to 15 years	Systolic: 110 to 131 Diastolic: 64 to 83 Mean arterial pressure: 73 to 84	> 90

Source: Pediatric data from American Heart Association (AHA). Vital signs in children. *AHA: Pediatric Advanced Life Support.* Dallas, TX: AHA; 2015.

Box 14-2 Pediatric Vital Signs and Quantitative Norms

The term *pediatric*, or child, includes a vast range of physical development, emotional maturity, and body sizes. The approach to the patient and the implications of many injuries vary greatly between an infant and an adolescent.

In most anatomic and therapeutic dosage considerations, a child's weight (or specific height or length) serves as a more accurate indicator than exact chronologic age.[18] Table 14-2 lists the average height and weight for healthy children of varying ages.

The acceptable ranges of vital signs also vary for the different ages within the pediatric population. Adult norms cannot be used as guidelines in smaller children. An adult ventilatory rate of 30 breaths/minute is tachypneic, and an adult heart rate of 120 to 140 beats/minute is tachycardic. Both are considered alarmingly high in an adult and are significant pathologic findings. However, the same findings in an infant may be within the normal ranges.

Normal ranges of vital signs for different age groups may not be consistent across all pediatric references. In an injured child without a previous history of normal vital signs, borderline vital signs may be viewed as pathologic, even though the signs may be

physiologically acceptable in that specific child. The guidelines in Tables 14-4, 14-5, and 14-6 can aid in evaluating vital signs in pediatric patients. These tables present statistically common ranges into which most children in these age groups will fall.

Several commercially available items serve as rapid reference guides for pediatric vital signs and equipment size. These include the length-based resuscitation tape and several slide-rule-type plastic scales. The following guideline formulas can also be used to estimate the expected finding for ages 1 to 10 years:

Weight (kg) = 8 + (2 × Child's age [years])

Lowest acceptable systolic BP (mm Hg) = 70 + (2 × Child's age [years])

Total vascular blood volume (ml) = 80 ml × Child's weight (kg)

Quantitative vital signs in children, although important, are only one piece of information used in making an assessment. A child with a normal set of vital signs can rapidly deteriorate into either critical ventilatory difficulty or decompensated shock. Vital signs should be considered along with mechanism of injury and other clinical findings.

---

pediatric age group. **Box 14-2** presents further discussion of pediatric vital signs and quantitative norms.

Disability

After assessment of exsanguinating hemorrhage, airway, breathing, and circulation, the primary survey must include an assessment of neurologic status. Although the AVPU scale (**A**lert, responds to **V**erbal stimulus, responds to **P**ainful stimulus, **U**nresponsive) is a simple, rapid assessment tool for the child's neurologic status, it is less informative than the Glasgow Coma Scale (GCS). The GCS should be combined with a careful examination of the pupils to determine whether they are equal, round, and reactive to light. As in adults, the GCS provides a more thorough assessment of neurologic status and should be calculated for each pediatric trauma patient. The scoring for the verbal section for children younger than 4 years of age must be modified because of developing communication skills in this age group, and the child's behavior should be observed carefully (**Table 14-6**).

Recent literature suggests that the score of the motor component of the GCS may be as helpful as calculating the total GCS.[24,25] For further discussion of the importance of the motor component, see the Patient Assessment and Management chapter.

Table 14-6 Pediatric Verbal Score

Verbal Response	Verbal Score
Appropriate words or social smile; fixes and follows	5
Crying but consolable	4
Persistently irritable	3
Restless, agitated	2
No response	1

The GCS score should be repeated frequently and used to document progression or improvement of neurologic status during the postinjury period (refer to the Patient Assessment and Management chapter for a review of the GCS). A more thorough assessment of motor and sensory function should be performed in the secondary survey, if time permits.

Expose/Environment

Children should be examined for other potentially life-threatening injuries; however, while exposure is critical and necessary to identify injuries, a child may be frightened at attempts to remove his or her clothes. Explain as you expose each area, and have a parent present whenever possible. In addition, because of children's high body surface area, they are more prone to developing hypothermia. Once the examination to identify other injuries is complete, the pediatric patient should be covered to preserve body heat and prevent further heat loss.

Secondary Survey

The secondary survey of the pediatric patient should follow the primary survey only after life-threatening conditions have been identified and managed. The head and neck should be examined for obvious deformities, contusions, abrasions, punctures, burns, tenderness, lacerations, or swellings. The thorax should be reexamined. Potential pulmonary contusions may become evident after volume resuscitation, manifested by respiratory distress or abnormal lung sounds. Trauma patients are infrequently *nil per os* (NPO [fasting]) at the time of their injuries, so insertion of a nasogastric or orogastric tube may be indicated, if local protocols allow. This protocol is especially important for children who are **obtunded** or who have posttraumatic seizure activity.

Examination of the abdomen should focus on distension, tenderness, discoloration, ecchymosis, and presence of a mass. Careful palpation of the iliac crests may suggest an unstable pelvic fracture and increase the suspicion for possible retroperitoneal or urogenital injury as well as increased risk for hidden blood loss. An unstable pelvis should be noted, but repeated examinations of the pelvis should not be performed, as this may result in further injury and increased blood loss. The pediatric patient should be appropriately immobilized on a long backboard and prepared for transfer to a pediatric trauma facility.

Each extremity should be inspected and palpated to rule out tenderness, deformity, diminished vascular supply, and neurologic deficit. A child's incompletely calcified skeleton, with its multiple growth centers, increases the possibility of epiphyseal (growth plate) disruption. Accordingly, any area of edema, pain, tenderness, or diminished range of motion should be treated as if it were fractured until evaluated by radiographic examination. In children, as in adults, a missed orthopedic injury in an extremity may have little effect on mortality but may lead to long-term deformity and disability.

Management

The keys to pediatric patient survival from a traumatic injury are rapid cardiopulmonary assessment, age-appropriate aggressive management, and transport to a facility capable of managing pediatric trauma. A color-coded, length-based resuscitation tape was devised to serve as a guide that allows for rapid identification of a patient's height with a correlated estimation of weight, the size of equipment

to be used, and appropriate dosages of potential resuscitative drugs. In addition, most prehospital systems have a guideline for selecting appropriate destination facilities for pediatric trauma patients. Be sure to review the protocol prior to arrival at the scene for expedited decisions in critical children.

Control of Severe External Hemorrhage

In the primary assessment of a trauma patient, external hemorrhage must be identified and controlled. If gross exsanguinating external hemorrhage is present, this bleeding must be controlled even before addressing the airway. Control of hemorrhage may be accomplished through direct pressure. This is accomplished by placing 4 × 4 gauze pads directly on the bleeding site and holding pressure. Pressure must be held during the entire transport. Tourniquet placement may be necessary for extremity bleeding when direct pressure does not adequately control the hemorrhage. Control of exsanguinating hemorrhage is imperative. If the patient is having ongoing hemorrhage, perfusion will not improve and the patient will progress to hemorrhagic shock.

Airway

Ventilation, oxygenation, and perfusion are as essential to an injured child as to an adult. Thus, the primary goal of the initial resuscitation of an injured child is restoration of adequate tissue oxygenation as quickly as possible. The first priority of assessment and resuscitation after establishing scene safety and addressing any exsanguinating external hemorrhage is the establishment of a patent airway.

A patent airway should be ensured and maintained with suctioning, manual maneuvers, and airway adjuncts. As in the adult, initial management in the pediatric patient includes in-line cervical spine stabilization. Unless a specialized pediatric spine board that has a depression at the head is used, adequate padding (2 to 3 cm [about 1 inch]) should be placed under the torso of the small child so that the cervical spine is maintained in a straight line rather than forced into slight flexion because of the disproportionately large occiput (**Figure 14-5**). When adjusting and maintaining airway positioning, compressing the soft tissues of the neck and trachea should be avoided.

Once manual control of the airway is achieved, an oropharyngeal airway can be placed if no gag reflex is present. The device should be inserted carefully and gently, parallel to the course of the tongue rather than turned 90 or 180 degrees in the posterior oropharynx as in the adult. Use of a tongue blade to depress the tongue can be helpful in pediatric patients.

Endotracheal intubation under direct visualization of the trachea may be indicated for long transports (**Box 14-3**). However, this procedure should be initiated only by experienced personnel and when adequate oxygenation cannot

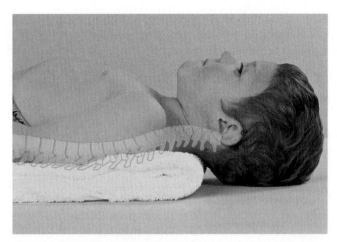

Figure 14-5 Provide adequate padding under the child's torso, or use a spine board with a cutout for the child's occiput.
© National Association of Emergency Medical Technicians (NAEMT).

be maintained by a bag-mask device. Importantly, there are no data to show improved survival or neurologic outcome in pediatric trauma patients intubated early in the field versus those who underwent bag-mask ventilation. In fact, there is some evidence suggesting worse outcomes.[17] A more recent study in a rural setting found that multiple prehospital intubation attempts were associated with significant complications (**Box 14-4**).[26,27]

Although several different supraglottic airway devices have been proven to be effective rescue airway devices for adult trauma victims,[35,36] in some cases, their large size and the lack of smaller sizes make them inadequate as rescue devices for smaller children (under 4 feet [122 cm] in height). The laryngeal mask airway and the smaller sizes of the King LT airways provide an alternate airway device choice in older children (> 8 years of age, when the airway is more similar to that of adults) and are reasonable alternatives to endotracheal intubation in certain situations.[37]

For pediatric patients, the risks may outweigh the benefits of endotracheal intubation and must be carefully considered before attempting the procedure, especially in the pediatric patient in whom bag-mask ventilation is providing adequate ventilation and oxygenation. Consideration of the risks associated with endotracheal intubation is increasingly important as additional nonvisualized advanced airway devices become available and are added into the prehospital care provider's practice.

Breathing

The pediatric patient's minute volume and ventilatory effort should be evaluated carefully. Because of the potential for rapid deterioration from mild hypoxia to ventilatory arrest, ventilation should be assisted if dyspnea and increased ventilatory effort are observed. A properly sized bag-mask device with a reservoir and high-flow oxygen to provide an oxygen concentration of between 85% and 100% (Fio_2 of 0.85 to 1.0) should be used. Continuous pulse oximetry

---

Box 14-3 Pediatric Endotracheal Intubation

Endotracheal intubation of a pediatric patient should include careful attention to cervical spine immobilization. One prehospital care provider should maintain the pediatric patient's spine in a neutral position while another provider intubates.

The narrowest portion of the pediatric airway is the cricoid ring, creating a "physiologic cuff." Although uncuffed ET tubes were previously used in pediatric patients due to this difference, newer recommendations endorse the use of cuffed tubes in all ages. The cuffed tube allows prehospital care providers to inflate the cuff fully, partially, or not at all, depending on the strength of the seal and the child's oxygenation and ventilation. To prevent iatrogenic tracheal injury, cuff pressures should not exceed 25 centimeters of water (cm H_2O). The appropriate size for a cuffed ET tube can be estimated by using the diameter of the child's fifth finger or the external nares or by using the following formula:

Age ÷ 4 + 3.5

Although routine cricoid pressure is no longer recommended, a slight amount of cricoid pressure may be tried to bring the anterior structures of the child's larynx into better view. However, pediatric tracheal rings are relatively soft and pliable, and overzealous cricoid pressure may completely occlude the airway.

A common error that occurs during the intubation of pediatric patients under emergency circumstances is aggressive advancement of the ET tube, resulting in its placement into the right main bronchus. The ET tube should never be advanced more than three times the ET tube size (in centimeters). For example, a 3.0-cm ET tube should rest at a depth no greater than 9 cm.

The chest and epigastrium should always be auscultated after the ET tube is placed and $ETCO_2$ capnometry used whenever available. ET tube placement should be frequently reassessed, especially after any movement of the patient. In addition to confirming ET tube placement, auscultation may rule out the possibility of other pulmonary injury. The pediatric patient with a compromised airway and a pulmonary injury who has been successfully intubated may be in greater jeopardy for the development of a tension pneumothorax as a result of positive-pressure ventilation.

Box 14-4 Prehospital Pediatric Intubation: The Great Debate

It might seem intuitive that providing an ET tube as early as possible in the management of the pediatric patient with TBI would be of benefit. A retrospective review showed improved survival in adult patients with TBI who were intubated prior to arrival at the receiving hospital.[28] Subsequent studies evaluated rapid-sequence intubation (RSI), demonstrating its improved efficiency and success rate in intubation of adults and children.[29,30] However, many retrospective and prospective case-control studies found that prehospital intubation compared with bag-mask ventilation did not improve survival or neurologic outcome and might have been detrimental.[13,31,32] A prospective randomized trial in children comparing endotracheal intubation to bag-mask ventilation in an urban area with short transport times demonstrated no difference in survival or neurologic outcome between the two groups and an increased incidence of complications in the intubated group.[12,33]

Prolonged periods of hypoxia are often associated with the intubation process, as well as periods of overaggressive ventilation following intubation in patients being transported to the trauma center.[14]

Data supporting prehospital pediatric endotracheal intubation are limited and ambiguous. In the spontaneously breathing child, endotracheal intubation with or without pharmacologic assistance is not recommended. Emergency medical services programs that perform pediatric prehospital intubation should include at least the following[34]:

1. Close medical direction and supervision
2. Training and continuing education, including hands-on operating room experience
3. Resources for patient monitoring, drug storage, and ET tube placement confirmation
4. Standardized RSI protocols
5. Availability of an alternate airway such as a laryngeal mask airway or King LT airway
6. Intensive continuing quality assurance/quality control and performance review program

---

serves as an adjunct for ongoing assessment of airway and breathing. The Spo_2 should be kept at greater than 94% (at sea level).

In any intubated pediatric patient, ET tube placement should be confirmed using multiple methods, including directly visualizing the ET tube passing through the vocal folds, listening for the presence of equal bilateral breath sounds, and listening for the absence of sounds over the epigastrium when ventilated. Continuous $ETCO_2$ monitoring should be used to document continuing appropriate ET tube placement and to avoid extremes of hypercarbia and hypocarbia, both of which can be just as detrimental to recovery from a closed head injury as hypoxia. $ETCO_2$ should be targeted at 30 to 40 mm Hg.[14]

Tension Pneumothorax

Children are more susceptible than adults to acute cardiovascular collapse from a tension pneumothorax. Most children with tension pneumothoraces will present with acute cardiac decompensation secondary to decreased venous return before any detectable changes in oxygenation and ventilation have occurred. Any child who acutely decompensates, especially after initiation of positive-pressure ventilation by bag-mask device or advanced airway placement, should be emergently assessed for tension pneumothorax.

Jugular venous distension may be difficult to determine because an extrication collar has been applied or because of the presence of hypovolemia from hemorrhage. Tracheal shift is a late sign of tension pneumothorax and may only be determined by palpating the trachea in the jugular notch. In these pediatric patients, unilateral absent breath sounds, in association with cardiovascular compromise, represent an indication for emergency needle decompression. In the intubated pediatric patient, diminished sounds on the left may indicate a right main bronchus intubation, but when associated with acute cardiac decompensation, these sounds may represent tension pneumothorax. Careful reassessment of the patient's airway and respiratory status is needed to distinguish these subtle differences in the presentation.

Needle decompression of a tension pneumothorax in a pediatric patient should be performed in the second intercostal space at the midclavicular line. This approach is in contrast to a recent change in the adult recommendations for decompression at the midaxillary line at the fifth intercostal space.[38,39] For more on needle decompression, see the Thoracic Trauma chapter. Needle decompression is often more immediately effective in the child because the mediastinum rapidly shifts back to its normal position and venous return is quickly restored. Caution should be taken to watch closely for dislodgment after the angiocatheter is placed.

Circulation

Once the pediatric patient's external hemorrhage is controlled, perfusion should be evaluated. Controlling external hemorrhage involves applying direct manual pressure on the bleeding point, the use of advanced hemostatic dressings, and the use of tourniquets in cases of significant or problematic extremity hemorrhage. Managing external hemorrhage is not just a matter of covering the bleeding site with layer after layer of absorbent dressing. If the initial dressing becomes saturated in blood, it is better to add an additional dressing rather than to replace it, as the removal may dislodge any clot that has begun to form, while at the same time considering additional interventions to stop the ongoing hemorrhage such as wound packing or tourniquet application.

The pediatric vascular system is usually able to maintain a normal blood pressure until severe collapse occurs, at which point it is often unresponsive to resuscitation. Fluid resuscitation should be started whenever signs of compensated hypovolemic shock are present and must be started immediately in pediatric patients who present with decompensated shock. Normal saline solution in 20-ml/kg boluses should be used.

For pediatric trauma patients who display any signs of hemorrhagic shock or hypovolemia, key factors to survival are appropriate volume resuscitation and rapid initiation of transport to a suitable facility. Transport should never be delayed to obtain vascular access or administer IV fluid.

Vascular Access

Fluid replacement in a pediatric patient with severe hypotension or signs of shock must deliver adequate fluid volume to the right atrium to avoid further reduction in cardiac preload. The most appropriate initial sites for IV access are the *antecubital fossa* (anterior aspect of the forearm at the elbow) and the saphenous vein at the ankle. Access through the external jugular vein is another possibility, but airway management takes priority in such a small space and spinal immobilization makes the neck poorly accessible.

In the unstable or potentially unstable pediatric patient, attempts at peripheral access should be limited to two in 90 seconds. If peripheral access is unsuccessful, IO access should be established (**Box 14-5**).

Placement of a subclavian or internal jugular catheter in a pediatric patient should be performed only under the most controlled circumstances within the hospital; this should not be attempted in the prehospital environment.

The determination of which pediatric patients should have intravascular access depends on the severity of injury, the experience of the involved prehospital care providers, and transport times, among other factors. If uncertainty exists regarding which pediatric patients need intravascular access or if fluid replacement is needed during transport, online medical direction should be obtained.

Fluid Therapy

Isotonic crystalloid solution is the initial resuscitation fluid of choice for a hypovolemic pediatric patient. Fluid choices,

---

Box 14-5 Pediatric Intraosseous Infusion

Intraosseous (IO) infusion can provide an excellent alternative site for resuscitative volume replacement in injured children of all ages. This is an effective route for infusion of medications, blood, or high-volume fluid administration.

The most accessible site for IO infusion is the anterior tibia just inferior and medial to the tibial tuberosity. After preparing the skin antiseptically and securing the leg adequately, a site is chosen on the anterior medial portion of the tibia, 1 to 2 cm (0.4 to 0.8 inches) below and medial to the tibial tuberosity. Specially manufactured IO infusion needles are optimal for the procedure, but spinal or bone marrow needles may also be used. Spinal needles that are 18 to 20 gauge work well because they have a trocar to prevent the needle from being obstructed as it passes through the bony cortex into the marrow. Any 14- to 20-gauge needle can be used in an emergency.

A variety of commercially available devices are available that ease the difficulty of placing an IO needle, using various mechanical devices. For example, one device uses a high-speed drill to insert a specially designed IO needle, and another uses a spring-loaded mechanism. The needle is placed at a 90-degree angle to the bone and advanced firmly through the cortex into the marrow.

Evidence that the needle is adequately within the marrow includes the following:

1. A soft "pop" is heard and no resistance is felt after the needle has passed through the cortex.
2. Bone marrow aspirates into the needle.
3. Fluid flows freely into the marrow without evidence of subcutaneous infiltration.
4. The needle is secure and does not appear loose or wobbly.

IO infusion should be considered during initial resuscitation if percutaneous venous cannulation (venous IV insertion) has been unsuccessful. Because the flow rate is limited by the bone marrow cavity, the administration of fluids and medications should normally be done under pressure, and the IO route alone will seldom be sufficient after initial resuscitation.

Proper location of the insertion site is extremely important in the pediatric patient. Failure to properly identify landmarks could lead to misplacement of the IO device and damage of the epiphyseal plate (growth center) of the bone, which, in turn, can result in growth problems of the bone and unequal extremity lengths.

when available, should take into account acidity which may worsen coagulopathy and electrolyte concentrations in the setting of massive tissue injury (i.e. potassium). The time that a crystalloid fluid remains in the intravascular space is relatively short, which is why a 3:1 ratio of crystalloid fluid to blood lost has been recommended. This is discussed in further the Shock: Pathophysiology of Life and Death chapter.

An initial fluid bolus for a pediatric patient is 20 ml/kg, which is approximately 25% of the normal circulating blood volume of the child. The 20-ml/kg bolus of crystalloid can be repeated once. If a pediatric patient requires further fluid resuscitation after the second 20-ml/kg bolus, the patient should receive a transfusion of blood and plasma. The crystalloid bolus may temporarily restore cardiovascular stability as it transiently fills and then leaks from the circulatory system. However, until circulating RBCs are replaced and oxygen transport is restored, hypoxic injury can continue.

Pain Management

As with adults, pain management should be considered for children in the prehospital setting. Small doses of a narcotic analgesia that are appropriately titrated will not compromise the neurologic or abdominal examination. Both morphine and fentanyl are acceptable choices, but they should be administered only according to written prehospital care guidelines or with orders from online medical control. Because of the side effects of hypotension and hypoventilation, all pediatric patients receiving IV narcotics should be monitored with pulse oximetry and serial vital signs. In general, benzodiazepines should not be administered in combination with narcotics because of their synergistic effects on respiratory depression or even respiratory arrest.

Transport

Because timely arrival at the most appropriate facility may be the key element in the pediatric patient's survival, triage is an important consideration in the management of a pediatric patient.

The tragedy of preventable pediatric traumatic death has been documented in multiple studies reported over the past three decades. It is estimated that the majority of pediatric trauma deaths can be classified as preventable or potentially preventable. These statistics have been one of the primary motivations for the development of regionalized pediatric trauma centers, where continuous, coordinated, high-quality, sophisticated care can be provided. Early identification of any physiologic abnormality (heart rate, ventilatory rate, or BP) should increase suspicion for multisystem injury and the need for a pediatric trauma center.

Many urban areas have both pediatric trauma centers and adult trauma centers. Ideally, the pediatric multisystem trauma patient will benefit from the initial resuscitation capability and definitive care available at a pediatric trauma center because of its specialization in treating traumatized children. It may be appropriate to bypass an adult trauma center in favor of transport to a pediatric-capable trauma center. For many communities, however, the nearest specialized pediatric trauma center may be hours away. In these cases, the seriously traumatized child should be transported to the nearest adult trauma center because early resuscitation and evaluation before transport to a pediatric facility may improve the pediatric patient's chances of survival.[40-42]

In areas where no specialized pediatric trauma center is nearby, personnel working in adult trauma centers should be experienced in the resuscitation and treatment of both adult and pediatric trauma patients. In areas where neither facility is close, the seriously injured child should be transported to the nearest appropriate hospital capable of caring for trauma victims, according to local prehospital triage guidelines.

Aeromedical transport may be considered in rural areas to expedite transport. There is little evidence that aeromedical transport provides any benefit in urban areas in which ground transport to a pediatric trauma center is almost as quick.[43] It is becoming increasingly evident that using aeromedical transport exposes both the patient and the crew to a significant amount of risk.[44-46] These concerns must be carefully weighed when deciding whether to utilize this resource.

Review of more than 15,000 records in the National Pediatric Trauma Registry (NPTR) indicates that 25% of the pediatric patients were injured severely enough to require triage to a designated pediatric trauma center. Many EMS and trauma systems use other pediatric triage criteria, which may be dictated by state, regional, or local guidelines. All prehospital care providers need to be familiar with the triage protocols in place within their own systems.

Specific Injuries
Traumatic Brain Injury

TBI is a leading cause of morbidity and mortality in the pediatric population.[47] Although many of the most severe injuries are treatable only by prevention, initial resuscitative measures may minimize secondary brain injury and, consequently, the severity of the pediatric patient's injury. Adequate ventilation, oxygenation, and perfusion are needed to prevent secondary morbidity. While the recovery of pediatric patients sustaining severe TBI is typically considered to be better than in adults, growing evidence indicates that a wide variety of impairments persist, including functional, cognitive, and behavioral abnormalities.

The results of the initial neurologic assessment are useful for prognosis. Even with a normal initial neurologic evaluation, however, any child who sustains a significant head injury may be susceptible to cerebral edema, hypoperfusion, and secondary insults (**Box 14-6**). Furthermore, victims of nonaccidental trauma may have little external evidence of trauma, yet may have sustained considerable intracranial injury. A baseline GCS score should be assessed and frequently repeated during transport. Supplemental oxygen should be administered, and if possible, pulse oximetry should be monitored.

As with hypoxia, hypovolemia may dramatically worsen the original TBI. External hemorrhage must be controlled and the child's fractured extremities immobilized to limit internal blood loss associated with these injuries. An attempt should be made to keep these pediatric patients in a *euvolemic* (normal volume) state with IV volume resuscitation. On rare occasions, infants younger than about 6 months of age may become hypovolemic as a result of intracranial bleeding because they have open cranial sutures and fontanelles. An infant with an open fontanelle may better tolerate an expanding intracranial hematoma and thus not become symptomatic until rapid expansion occurs. An infant with a bulging fontanelle should be considered to have a more severe TBI.

For children with a GCS score of eight or less, adequate oxygenation and ventilation should be the goal at all times, not the placement of an ET tube. Prolonged attempts at securing an endotracheal airway may increase periods of hypoxia and delay transport to an appropriate facility. The best airway for a pediatric patient is the one that is both safest and most effective. Ventilation with a bag-mask device while being prepared to suction emesis, should it occur, is often the best airway for the child with TBI.[12-14]

A pediatric patient with signs and symptoms of intracranial hypertension or increased intracranial pressure, such as a sluggishly reactive or nonreactive pupil, systemic hypertension, bradycardia, and abnormal breathing patterns, may benefit from temporary mild hyperventilation to lower intracranial pressure. However, this effect of hyperventilation is transient and also decreases overall oxygen delivery to the CNS, actually causing additional secondary brain injury.[51] It is strongly recommended that this strategy not be used unless the child is exhibiting signs of active herniation or *lateralizing* signs (distal neurologic abnormalities such as weakness on one side from injury to an area of the brain). $ETCO_2$ monitoring should guide management in the intubated pediatric patient, with the target range about 35 mm Hg. Hyperventilation to an $ETCO_2$ of less than 25 mm Hg has been associated with worse neurologic outcome.[14] If capnography is not available, a ventilation rate of 25 breaths/minute for children and 30 breaths/minute for infants should be used.[52]

During prolonged transports, small doses of mannitol (0.5 to 1 g/kg body weight), or hypertonic saline, may benefit

---

Box 14-6 Pediatric Concussion

The issue of concussion, or mild traumatic brain injury, in pediatric patients, particularly those engaged in sports activities, has become a topic of great importance.[48,49] In 2012, approximately 329,290 children were treated in the emergency department (ED) in the United States for sport and recreation-related diagnosis of concussion or TBI, with the rate of ED visits for these injuries more than doubling from 2001 to 2012.[47] In the past, when a pediatric athlete sustained a concussion, the child was kept out of the game for a short time and was allowed to return to play as soon as he or she felt able to play again. It has been recognized that repeated blows to the head and brain lead to long-term difficulties with cognition, behavior, and function.[50] It is now recommended that any pediatric athlete who has sustained a concussion be removed from play and not be permitted to participate for the duration of the event and until cleared for participation by a qualified physician.

The recognition of concussion is of key importance. Where it was once thought that concussion involved a brief loss of consciousness with a return to normal function, it is now understood that loss of consciousness is not necessary to make the diagnosis. Concussion may involve a variety of symptoms and complaints, including headache, nausea, balance problems, feeling dazed or stunned, confusion, and asking questions slowly or repetitively. It is recommended that medical personnel present at a sporting event have a formal method for assessing pediatric athletes for concussion using a standard sideline assessment tool as well as a neurologic examination.

Full recovery from a concussion may take a week or longer—in some cases, months. Until the pediatric athlete has fully recovered from the concussion and is asymptomatic, the child should not be allowed to return to play. Once the pediatric athlete is asymptomatic, he or she may be returned to activity and play in a graded, structured format with repeat evaluations to assess for relapse of symptoms. Return of symptoms indicates incomplete recovery, and the pediatric athlete should refrain from participation in sports until improvement has occurred. Direction of return to play should be provided by a qualified physician. No child should return to play after a concussion without a thorough evaluation.

pediatric patients with evidence of intracranial hypertension, if local protocols permit. However, the use of mannitol in the setting of insufficient volume resuscitation may result in hypovolemia and worsening shock. Mannitol should not be given in the field without discussing this option with online medical control, unless permitted by standing orders or protocol, in which case the risks and benefits should be carefully weighed. Regardless, use of hypertonic saline or mannitol in the prehospital setting should be reserved for cases of impending herniation. Brief seizures may occur soon after a TBI and, aside from ensuring patient safety, oxygenation, and ventilation, often do not require specific treatment by prehospital care providers. However, recurrent seizure activity is worrisome and may require IV boluses of a benzodiazepine, such as midazolam (0.1 mg/kg/dose). All benzodiazepines should be used with extreme caution in these patients because of the potential side effects of ventilatory depression and hypotension, as well as their ability to cloud the neurologic examination.

Spinal Trauma

The indication for spinal immobilization in a pediatric patient is based on the mechanism of injury and physical findings; the presence of other injuries that suggest violent or sudden movement of the head, neck, or torso; or the presence of specific signs of spine injury, such as deformity, pain, or a neurologic deficit. As with adult patients, the correct prehospital management of a suspected spine injury is in-line manual stabilization followed by the use of a properly fitting cervical collar and immobilization of the pediatric patient to an appropriate device so that the head, neck, torso, pelvis, and legs are maintained in a neutral in-line position. Pediatric patients with a neurologic deficit that quickly resolves may have SCIWORA. Spinal immobilization should be maintained in these patients even if their symptoms resolve prior to hospital arrival. This should be achieved without impairing the child's ventilation or ability to open the mouth or disrupting any other resuscitative efforts.

The threshold for performing spinal immobilization is lower in young children because of their inability to communicate or otherwise participate in their own assessment. No studies have validated the safety of clinically clearing a child's spine in the field. The same immaturity previously discussed also contributes to children's fear and lack of cooperation with immobilization. A child who strongly fights attempts at immobilization may be at increased risk of worsening any existing spinal injuries. It may be valid to decide not to restrain such a pediatric patient if the child can be persuaded to lie quietly without restraints. However, any decision to stop immobilization attempts in the interest of patient safety must be supported by careful and thorough documented reasoning as well as serial assessment of neurologic status during and immediately after transport. Ideally, this decision would be made in concert with online medical control.

When most small children are placed on a rigid surface, the relatively larger size of the child's occiput will result in passive neck flexion. Sufficient padding (2 to 3 cm [about 1 inch]) should be placed under the pediatric patient's torso to elevate it and allow the head to be in a neutral position. The padding should be continuous and flat from the shoulders to the pelvis and extend to the lateral margins of the torso to ensure that the thoracic, lumbar, and sacral spine are on a flat, stable platform without the possibility of anterior–posterior movement. Padding should also be placed between the lateral sides of the pediatric patient and the edges of the board to ensure that no lateral movement occurs when the board is moved or if the pediatric patient and board need to be rotated to the side to avoid aspiration during vomiting episodes.

Various new pediatric immobilization devices are available. The prehospital care provider needs to regularly practice and be familiar with any specialized equipment used in the provider's system as well as the required adjustments necessary when immobilizing a child using adult-sized equipment. If a vest-type device is used on a pediatric patient, adequate immobilization while at the same time preventing respiratory compromise must be ensured. In the past, it was recommended that infants or young children be immobilized in a car safety seat if that is where they were found.[53,54] The National Highway Traffic Safety Administration now recommends that the pediatric patient be immobilized and transported in an appropriately sized pediatric immobilization device instead of the car seat. Keeping the injured child in an upright position in the car seat increases the axial load placed on the spine by the patient's head; therefore, standard immobilization techniques are preferred to the car seat.[55] A child who is not immobilized should not be transported on a caregiver's lap but should be appropriately restrained in a car seat for transport.

Thoracic Injuries

The extremely resilient rib cage of a child often results in less injury to the bony structure of the thorax, but there is still risk for pulmonary injury, such as pulmonary contusion, pneumothorax, or hemothorax. Although rib fractures are rare in childhood, they are associated with a high risk of intrathoracic injury when present. Crepitus may be appreciated on examination and may be a sign of pneumothorax. The risk of mortality increases with the number of ribs fractured. A high index of suspicion is the key to identifying these injuries. Every pediatric patient who sustains trauma to the chest and torso should be carefully monitored for signs of respiratory distress and shock. Abrasions or contusions over the pediatric patient's torso after blunt force trauma may be the only clues to the prehospital care provider that the child has suffered thoracic trauma.

Additionally, when transporting a pediatric patient who has sustained a high-impact blunt thoracic injury, the child's cardiac rhythm should be monitored en route to a medical facility. In all cases, the key items in managing thoracic trauma involve careful attention to ventilation, oxygenation, and timely transport to an appropriate facility.

Abdominal Injuries

The presence of blunt trauma to the abdomen, an unstable pelvis, posttraumatic abdominal distension, rigidity or tenderness, or otherwise unexplained shock can be associated with possible intra-abdominal hemorrhage. A "seat belt sign" (or mark) or a handlebar mark across the abdomen of a pediatric patient is often an indicator of serious internal injuries (**Figure 14-6**).

The key prehospital elements in management of abdominal injuries include fluid resuscitation, supplemental high-concentration oxygen, and rapid transport to an appropriate facility with continued careful monitoring en route. There are really no definitive interventions that prehospital care providers can offer to pediatric patients with intra-abdominal injuries, and, as such, there should be every effort to transport pediatric patients rapidly to the closest, most appropriate facility.

Extremity Trauma

Compared with the adult skeleton, the child's skeleton is actively growing and consists of a large proportion of cartilaginous tissue and metabolically active growth plates. The ligamentous structures that hold the skeleton together are frequently stronger and better able to withstand mechanical

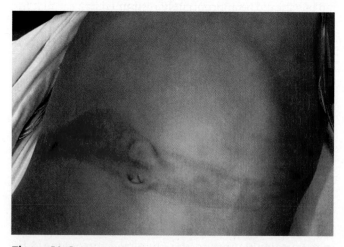

Figure 14-6 "Seat belt sign" in a 6-year-old patient who was found to have a ruptured spleen. Seat belt signs are often associated with serious intra-abdominal injuries.

Courtesy Dr. Jeffrey Guy.

disruption than the bones to which they are attached. As a result, children with skeletal trauma frequently sustain major traumatic forces before developing long-bone fractures, dislocations, or deformities. Incomplete ("greenstick") fractures are common and may be indicated only by bony tenderness and pain on use of the affected extremity.

Primary joint disruption from injury other than penetrating injury is uncommon compared with disruption of the *diaphyseal* (shaft) or *epiphyseal* (end) segments of bone. Fractures that involve the growth plate are unique in that they must be carefully identified and managed in the acute injury phase to not only ensure adequate healing but also prevent subsequent displacement or deformity as the child continues to develop. The association of neurovascular injuries with orthopedic injuries in children should always be considered, and the distal vascular and neurologic examination should be carefully evaluated. Often, the presence of a potentially debilitating injury can be determined only by radiologic study or, when the slightest suggestion of a decrease in distal perfusion exists, by *arteriography* (x-ray study of a blood vessel that has been injected with radio-opaque contrast material).

The apparent gross deformity sometimes associated with extremity injury should not distract focus from potentially life-threatening injuries. Uncontrolled hemorrhage represents the most life-threatening consequence of extremity trauma. In multisystem pediatric and adult trauma patients alike, the initiation of transport to an appropriate facility without delay after completion of the primary survey, resuscitation, and rapid packaging remains paramount in reducing mortality. If basic splinting can be provided en route without detracting from the child's resuscitation, it will help to minimize bleeding and pain from long-bone fractures, but attention to life-threatening injuries should always remain the primary focus.

Burn Injuries

Following motor vehicle crashes and drowning, burns rate third as a cause of pediatric trauma deaths.[1] Caring for an injured child always poses significant physical and emotional challenges to the prehospital care provider, and these difficulties are amplified when caring for the pediatric patient with burns. The child with burns may have an *edematous (swollen) airway*, IV access may be complicated by burns of the extremity, and the pediatric patient may be hysterical from pain.

The primary survey should be followed as in other causes of pediatric trauma, but every step of the primary survey may be more complicated than in a child without thermal injuries. Most deaths related to structure fires are not directly related to soft-tissue burns but are secondary to smoke inhalation. When children are trapped in a structure fire, they often hide from the fire under beds or in closets. These children frequently die, and their recovered bodies often have no burns; they die from carbon monoxide or hydrogen cyanide toxicity and hypoxia.

Thermally induced edema of the airway is always a concern in patients with burns, but especially in pediatric patients. The smaller diameter of the pediatric trachea means that 1 mm of edema will produce a greater magnitude of airway obstruction than in an adult with a larger diameter airway. A pediatric patient with an edematous airway may be sitting forward and drooling or complaining of hoarseness or voice changes. These symptoms should prompt rapid preparations for and initiation of transport to the hospital. While en route, supplemental oxygen is administered and preparations made for airway intervention should the symptoms progress or the child develop respiratory or cardiac arrest.

If an ET tube is placed, it needs to be protected against inadvertent dislodgment or removal. If the pediatric patient accidentally becomes extubated, the prehospital care provider may not be able to intubate the child again due to progressive edema, and the results could be disastrous. Securing an ET tube in a pediatric patient who has peeling facial skin and moist wounds is difficult. Securing the ET tube to the face with adhesive tape should not be attempted in a child with facial burns. The ET tube should be secured with two pieces of umbilical tape, with one piece draped above the ear and the second piece placed below the ear. An effective alternative to umbilical tape is IV tubing. If these supplies are not available but extra hands are, designate a provider to be solely responsible for holding the airway in place.

Fluid Resuscitation

Rapid establishment of intravascular access is vital to prevent the development of shock. Delayed fluid resuscitation in pediatric patients has been associated with significantly worse clinical outcomes and an increased mortality rate, especially in burned infants.[56-58]

After securing an airway and providing adequate ventilation and oxygenation, it is critical that venous access be obtained quickly. Children have a relatively small intravascular volume, and a delay in fluid resuscitation may lead to the rapid development of hypovolemic shock. To provide the large volumes of IV fluids required in critical burns, such pediatric patients usually require two peripheral IV catheters to achieve the required IV flow rates. The insertion of a single large-bore IV catheter is often challenging, so two IV catheters is all the more so. Burns on the extremities may make it difficult to impossible to establish enough access for an appropriate fluid resuscitation.

In children with burns, as in adult patients with burns, fluid needs are calculated from the time of the injury, so a delay of even 30 minutes to the beginning of fluid resuscitation can result in hypovolemic shock. Excessive fluids can result in respiratory complications as well as excessive edema, which can complicate burn care.

The amount of fluids typically given to a patient with burns is calculated based on the estimated percentage of total body surface area (TBSA) burned using the "rule of nines," a rapid and imprecise method of estimating resuscitative fluid needs based on adult battlefield burn casualties. The premise of this method of burn size estimation is that major regions of the adult body (e.g., head, arm, anterior torso) each comprise 9% of the total body surface area. Children's anatomic regions are proportionally different from those in adults; children have larger heads and smaller limbs. There is a tendency to overestimate TBSA of burn in children. Remember that superficial burns (intact erythematous skin) is not included in the TBSA estimation. Estimation of pediatric burn size should use diagrams that are age specific, such as the Lund-Browder chart, and not the rule of nines. Using this chart, each leg can be estimated at 13.5%, arms are 9%, the chest and back are both 18% each, and the head is 18%. If charts and diagrams are not available, the "rule of palms" may be used. Using this method, the size of the pediatric patient's palm plus fingers represents approximately 1% of the body surface area. This is useful when estimating burn area for scattered areas that do not involve an entire body part. (See the Burn Injuries chapter for further discussion of these burn estimation methods.)

Based on the percentage of body surface area burned, the volume of IV fluids needed for resuscitation is determined (see the Burn Injuries chapter). Two important pediatric considerations merit mention. First, small children have a limited reserve of glycogen. Glycogen is essentially glucose molecules strung together, and it is used for carbohydrate storage. Stored glycogen is mobilized in times of stress. If these limited glycogen stores become depleted, the child may rapidly develop hypoglycemia. Second, children have a large volume-to-surface area ratio; the general shape of an adult is a cylinder, whereas children resemble a sphere (**Figure 14-7**). The clinical implication is that a child will require more IV fluids. For the initial prehospital resuscitation, glucose should be checked on any child with an altered mental status. If the child is tachycardic with poor perfusion, a 20-ml/kg fluid bolus should be administered. Total fluids administered should be reported to the hospital upon arrival.

Once peripheral IV access has been obtained, provisions must be made to ensure that the IV line is not inadvertently removed or dislodged. The usual techniques used to secure IV lines are often ineffective when a line is placed in or adjacent to a burn because adhesive tape and dressings may not adhere to burned tissue. If possible, the IV line is secured with a Kerlix dressing, though circumferential dressings must be frequently monitored as edema develops, to prevent the dressing from becoming a constricting band.

When peripheral venous access cannot be obtained, IO catheters should be used for the unstable and/or unconscious pediatric patient. Although previously advocated

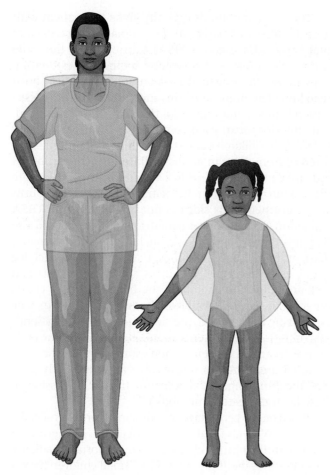

Figure 14-7 Children have a large volume-to-surface area ratio; the general shape of an adult is a cylinder, whereas children resemble a sphere.

© Jones & Bartlett Learning.

only for pediatric patients younger than 3 years of age, IO infusions are now used in older children as well as adults.

Abuse

Between 10% and 20% of all pediatric burn presentations are intentional burns.[59] Up to 50% of these children may experience recurrent abuse, and 30% of this group eventually die from abuse.[59,60] An increased awareness of this problem among prehospital care providers can improve detection of this cause of pediatric trauma. Careful documentation of the situation surrounding the injury, as well as of the injury patterns themselves, can aid officials in the prosecution of the offenders.[61]

The two most common mechanisms by which these children receive burns are scalds and contact burns. Scalds are the most common source of nonaccidental burns. Scalding injuries typically are inflicted on children of toilet-training age. The usual scenario is that the child soils himself or herself and is subsequently immersed in a tub of scalding water. These scald burns are characterized by a pattern of sharp demarcation between burned and unburned tissue

and sparing of flexion creases, as the child will frequently draw his or her legs up to avoid the scalding water (see the Burn Injuries chapter).

Contact burns are the second most common mechanism of abuse burns. Common items used to inflict contact burns are curling irons, clothing irons, and cigarettes. Cigarette burns appear as round wounds measuring slightly over 1 cm (0.4 inches) in diameter (typically 1.3 cm [0.5 inches]). To conceal these injuries, the abuser may place the burns in areas usually covered by clothing, above the hairline in the scalp, or even in the axillae.

All the surfaces of the human body have some degree of curvature; a hot item that accidentally falls onto the body surface will have an initial point of contact and will then deflect from the point of contact. The resultant burns will have irregular borders and uneven depths. In contrast, when a hot item is deliberately used to burn someone, the item is pressed onto the region of the body. The burn will have a pattern with a sharp, regular outline and uniform burn depth (see the Burn Injuries chapter).

A high index of suspicion for abuse is important, and all cases of suspected abuse should be reported. Make meticulous observations of the surroundings, such as the position of various pieces of furniture, presence of curling irons, and depth of bath water. Record the names of the individuals present at the scene. Any pediatric patient suspected of being abused by burns, regardless of the size of the burns, needs to be cared for at a center experienced in pediatric burn care.

Child abuse and neglect are further discussed later in this chapter.

Motor Vehicle Injury Prevention

The American Academy of Pediatrics (AAP) has defined optimal restraint for children in motor vehicles (**Table 14-7**). The AAP recommends that children should always ride in the rear seat and face the rear of the seat until 2 years of age. Children who have outgrown the rear-facing weight or height limit for their convertible seat should use a forward-facing seat with a harness for as long as possible, based on the highest weight and height allowed by the car safety seat manufacturer. They then graduate into a belt-positioning booster seat until they are 8 to 12 years old. At that time, the standard three-point (seat belt–shoulder harness combination) adult restraint can be used. The lap belt alone should never be used. All children should remain in the back seat until they are 13 years of age.

Suboptimal restraint is defined as the lack of use of a child safety seat or booster seat for anyone younger than 8 years of age and lack of a three-point restraint for a child older than 8 years (see Box 14-1).[62] In a review study, when these guidelines were observed, the risk of abdominal injury in children who were appropriately restrained was

Table 14-7 Types of Car Seats		
Age Group	**Type of Seat**	**General Guidelines**
Infants and toddlers	■ Rear-facing only ■ Rear-facing convertible	All infants and toddlers should ride in a **rear-facing seat** until they are at least **2 years of age** or reach the highest weight or height allowed by their car seat manufacturer.
Toddlers and preschoolers	■ Convertible ■ Forward-facing with harness	Children who have outgrown the rear-facing weight or height limit for their convertible seat should use a **forward-facing seat** with a harness for as long as possible, up to the highest weight or height allowed by their car safety seat manufacturer.
School-aged children	■ Booster seats	All children whose weight or height exceeds the forward-facing limit for their car safety seat should use a **belt-positioning booster seat** until the vehicle seat belt fits properly, typically when they have reached 4 feet 9 inches in height and are 8 through 12 years of age. All children younger than 13 should ride in the back seat.
Older children	■ Seat belts	When children are old enough and large enough for the vehicle seat belt to fit them correctly, they should always use **lap and shoulder seat belts** for the best protection. All children younger than 13 years should ride in the back seat.

Source: American Academy of Pediatrics (AAP). Car seats: information for families. https://www.healthychildren.org/English /safety-prevention/on-the-go/Pages/Car-Safety-Seats-Information-for-Families.aspx. Updated March 6, 2018. Accessed April 2, 2018.

3.5 times less than in the suboptimally restrained pediatric population.[63] The protective benefit of the rear-seat position is such that risk of death is decreased by at least 30%, even if restrained with a lap belt only in the rear seat versus three-point restraint in the front seat.[64] For more information on injury prevention, see the Injury Prevention chapter.

Child Abuse and Neglect

Child abuse (maltreatment or nonaccidental trauma) is a significant cause of childhood injury. As mentioned previously, almost 20% of all burns in pediatric patients involve either child abuse or child neglect.[61] Prehospital care providers must always consider the possibility of child abuse when circumstances warrant.

Prehospital care providers should suspect abuse or neglect if they note any of the following scenarios:

- Discrepancy between the history and the degree of physical injury or frequent changes in the reported history.
- Inappropriate response from the family.
- Prolonged interval between time of injury and call for medical care.
- History of the injury inconsistent with the developmental level of the child. For example, a history indicating that a neonate rolled off a bed would be suspect because neonates are developmentally unable to roll over.

Certain types of injuries also suggest abuse, such as the following (**Figure 14-8**):

- Multiple bruises in varying stages of resolution (excluding the palms, forearms, tibial areas, and the forehead in ambulatory children, who are frequently injured in normal falls). Accidental bruises usually occur over bony prominences.
- Bizarre injuries such as bites, cigarette burns, rope marks, or any pattern injury.
- Sharply demarcated burns or scald injuries in unusual areas (see the Burn Injuries chapter).

In many jurisdictions, prehospital care providers are legally mandated reporters if they identify potential child abuse. Generally, providers who act in good faith and in the best interests of the child are protected from legal action. Reporting procedures vary, so providers should be familiar with the appropriate agencies that handle child abuse cases in their location.

Prolonged Transport

Occasionally a situation arises as a result of patient location, triage decisions, or environmental considerations in which transport will be prolonged or delayed and prehospital personnel need to manage the ongoing resuscitation of a pediatric patient. Even though this may be suboptimal

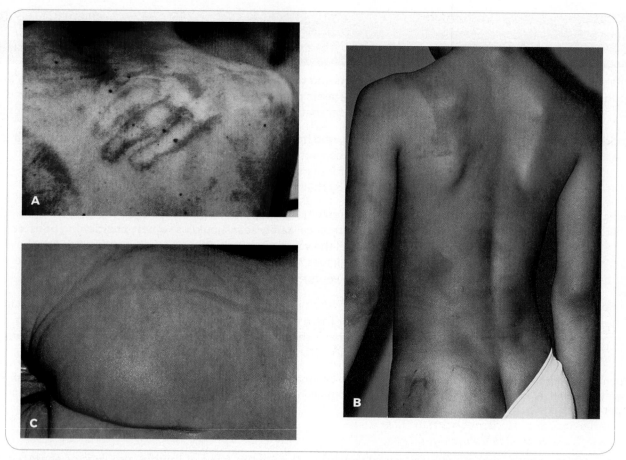

Figure 14-8 Indicators of possible nonaccidental trauma. **A.** Bruises that resemble hand prints. **B.** Bruises that are in multiple stages of healing. **C.** Mongolian blue spots, shown here on the trunk and buttocks of a newborn Asian infant, can be easily confused with bruising.

A: Courtesy of Moose Jaw Police Service. **B:** Courtesy of Ronald Dieckmann, MD. **C:** © Dr. P. Marazzi/Science Source.

because of the lack of field resources (e.g., blood) and the inability to perform diagnostic and therapeutic interventions, by applying the principles discussed in this chapter in an organized fashion, the child can be safely managed until arrival at a trauma center. If radio or cell phone contact with the receiving facility is possible, constant communication and feedback are crucial for both prehospital and hospital-based members of the trauma team.

Management consists of continued serial evaluation of the components of the primary survey. The pediatric patient should be securely stabilized on a backboard with spinal precautions. The board should be padded as well as possible to prevent pressure sores. If the airway is tenuous and the crew is well trained in pediatric airway management, including endotracheal intubation, then airway management should be performed. Otherwise, conscientious bag-mask ventilation is an acceptable management strategy, assuming it provides adequate oxygenation and ventilation.

Pulse oximetry should be monitored and preferably ETCO$_2$ as well, especially in the pediatric patient with a head injury. If signs of shock exist, 20-ml/kg boluses of lactated

Ringer or normal saline solution are administered until the child improves or is transferred to definitive care.

The GCS score should be calculated early and followed serially. Assessment for other injuries should continue, and all efforts to keep the pediatric patient normothermic should be standard practice. Fractures should be splinted and stabilized with serial neurovascular assessments. This cycle of continued reassessment of the primary survey should be repeated until the child can be safely transported or transferred to definitive care.

Any change or decompensation in the pediatric patient's condition requires immediate reassessment of the primary survey. For example, if Spo$_2$ begins to decline, is the ET tube still secure and in the airway? If so, has the child developed a tension pneumothorax? Is the ET tube now in the right main bronchus? If the pediatric patient has received what was thought to be sufficient fluid and is still in shock, is there now cardiac tamponade, severe cardiac contusion, or perhaps an occult source of bleeding, such as intra-abdominal injury or missed scalp laceration? Has the GCS score changed? Are there now lateralizing signs suggesting progressive head injury and requiring more aggressive treatments? Is the circulation and neurologic function of the extremities still intact? Is the child normothermic? If radio contact is available, continued advice and guidance should be sought throughout the resuscitation and transport.

By paying attention to the basics and continually reassessing your pediatric patient, adequate resuscitation can be performed until the pediatric patient can be transferred to definitive care.

SUMMARY

- The primary survey and management of the pediatric patient in the prehospital setting require application of standard trauma life support principles modified to account for the unique characteristics of pediatric patients.
- Traumatic brain injury is the leading cause of death from trauma, as well as the most common injury for which pediatric patients require airway management.
- Children should not be thought of as "little adults." They present unique anatomic and developmental considerations, and both they and their caregivers may require psychological support.
- The pediatric assessment triangle (PAT) helps providers to form a general impression—sick or not sick. The three components of the PAT are appearance, work of breathing, and circulation to the skin.
- Children have the ability to compensate for volume loss longer than adults, but when they decompensate, they deteriorate suddenly and severely.
- Significant underlying organ and vascular injury can occur with few or no obvious signs of external injury.
- Pediatric patients with the following signs are unstable and should be transported without delay to an appropriate facility, ideally a pediatric trauma center:
  - Respiratory compromise
  - Signs of shock or circulatory instability
  - Any alteration to mental status
  - Significant blunt trauma to the head, thorax, or abdomen
  - Any evidence of multiple fractures or significant fractures (ribs or pelvis)
  - Any concern for nonaccidental trauma
- Always consider the possibility of abuse or nonaccidental trauma when the history of the injury does not match the presentation of the patient.

SCENARIO RECAP

You are called to the scene of a motor vehicle crash on a heavily traveled highway. Two vehicles were involved in a frontal offset collision. One of the vehicle's occupants is a child who was improperly restrained in a child booster seat. No weather-related factors are involved on this spring afternoon.

On arrival at the scene, you see that the police have secured and blocked traffic from the area around the crash. As your partner and the other arriving crew are assessing the other patients, you approach the child. You see a young boy, approximately 2 years of age, sitting in the booster seat, which is slightly turned at an angle; there is blood on the back of the headrest of the seat in front of him. Despite numerous abrasions and minor bleeding from the head, face, and neck, the child appears very calm.

Your primary and secondary surveys reveal a 2-year-old boy who weakly repeats "ma-ma, ma-ma." His pulse rate is 180 beats/minute, with the radial pulses weaker than the carotid; his blood pressure is 50 mm Hg by palpation. His ventilatory rate is 18 breaths/minute, slightly irregular, but without abnormal sounds. As you continue to assess him, you note that he has stopped saying "ma-ma" and seems to just stare into space. You also note that his pupils are slightly dilated, and his skin is pale and sweaty. A woman who identifies herself as the family's nanny tells you that the mother is en route and that you should wait for her.

- What are the management priorities for this patient?
- What are the most likely injuries in this child?
- Where is the most appropriate destination for this child?

SCENARIO SOLUTION

You correctly identify this child as a victim of multisystem trauma who is critically injured. His ventilatory rate is low. The first priority is manual cervical spine control and supplemental oxygen with bag-valve mask. You are also acutely aware of the tachycardia and weak peripheral pulses. You quickly search for any obvious signs of bleeding and note there are no obvious sources. You correctly assume the patient is in hypovolemic shock, probably the result of an unrecognized intra-abdominal injury. This child has major multisystem trauma and requires aggressive care to give him a chance to survive.

Because of the nature of the child's injuries, you consult with online medical control, who agrees that helicopter transport to the closest pediatric trauma center is more appropriate than ground transport to a nearby community hospital that has no pediatric critical care, neurosurgical, or orthopedic resources. Brief efforts at peripheral venous access are successful. You begin a crystalloid bolus of 20 ml/kg. The child's mother arrives just as you are transferring care to the helicopter crew.

References

1. National Center for Injury Prevention and Control, Centers for Disease Control and Prevention. 10 leading causes of death reports, 1981–2015. Web-Based Injury Statistics Query and Reporting System (WISQARS). https://webappa.cdc.gov/sasweb/ncipc/leadcause.html. Updated February 19, 2017. Accessed October 17, 2017.

2. National Center for Injury Prevention and Control, Centers for Disease Control and Prevention. Nonfatal injury data. Web-Based Injury Statistics Query and Reporting System (WISQARS). https://www.cdc.gov/injury/wisqars/nonfatal.html. Updated April 20, 2017. Accessed October 17, 2017.

3. Gaines BA, Ford HR. Abdominal and pelvic trauma in children. *Crit Care Med.* 2002;30(suppl 11):S416.

4. American College of Surgeons. National Trauma Data Bank 2013: Pediatric Report. American College of Surgeons; 2013. https://www.facs.org/~/media/files/quality%20programs/trauma/ntdb/ntdb%20pediatric%20annual%20report%202013.ashx. Accessed March 12, 2018.

5. Peden M, Oyegbite K, Ozanne-Smith J, et al., eds. *World Report on Child Injury Prevention.* Geneva, Switzerland: World Health Organization; 2008.

6. Bachman SL, Salzman GA, Burke RV, Arbogast H, Ruiz P, Upperman JS. Observed child restraint misuse in a large, urban community: results from three years of inspection events. *J Safety Res.* 2016 Feb;56:17-22.

7. Grisoni ER, Pillai SB, Volsko TA, et al. Pediatric airbag injuries: the Ohio experience. *J Pediatr Surg.* 2000;35(2):160.

8. Durbin DR, Kallan M, Elliott M, et al. Risk of injury to restrained children from passenger air bags. *Traffic Injury Prev.* 2003;4(1):58.

9. Durbin DR, Kallan M, Elliott M, et al. Risk of injury to restrained children from passenger air bags. *Annu Proc Assoc Adv Auto Med.* 2002;46:15.

10. Ferguson SA, Schneider LW. An overview of frontal air bag performance with changes in frontal crash-test requirements: findings of the Blue Ribbon Panel for the evaluation of advanced technology air bags. *Traffic Inj Prev.* 2008;9(5):421-431.

11. Arbogast KB, Kallan MJ. The exposure of children to deploying side air bags: an initial field assessment. *Annu Proc Assoc Adv Automot Med.* 2007;51:245-259.

12. Gausche M, Lewis RJ, Stratton SJ, et al. Effect of out-of-hospital pediatric endotracheal intubation on survival and neurological outcome: a controlled clinical trial. *JAMA.* 2000;283(6):783.

13. Davis DP, Hoyt DB, Ochs M, et al. The effect of paramedic rapid sequence intubation on outcome in patients with severe traumatic brain injury. *J Trauma Injury Infec Crit Care.* 2003;54(3):444.

14. Davis DP, Dunford JV, Poste JC, et al. The impact of hypoxia and hyperventilation on outcome after paramedic rapid sequence intubation of severely head-injured patients. *J Trauma Injury Infect Crit Care.* 2004;57(1):1.

15. York J, Arrillaga A, Graham R, Miller R. Fluid resuscitation of patients with multiple injuries and severe closed-head injury: experience with an aggressive fluid resuscitation strategy. *J Trauma Injury Infect Crit Care.* 2000;48(3):376.

16. Manley G, Knudson MM, Morabito D, et al. Hypotension, hypoxia, and head injury: frequency, duration, and consequences. *Arch Surg.* 2001;136(10):1118.

17. Chesnut RM, Marshall LF, Klauber MR, et al. The role of secondary brain injury in determining outcome from severe head injury. *J Trauma.* 1993;34(2):216-222.

18. Luten R. Error and time delay in pediatric trauma resuscitation: addressing the problem with color-coded resuscitation aids. *Surg Clin North Am.* 2002;82(2):303.

19. Fernández A, Ares MI, Garcia S, Martinez-Indart L, Mintegi S, Benito J. The validity of the pediatric assessment triangle as the first step in the triage process in a pediatric emergency department. *Pediatr Emerg Care.* 2017 Apr;33(4):234-238.

20. Gausche-Hill M, Eckstein M, Horeczko T, et al. Paramedics accurately apply the pediatric assessment triangle to drive management. *Prehosp Emerg Care.* 2014;18(4):520-530.

21. American College of Surgeons Committee on Trauma. Pediatric trauma. In: *ACS Committee on Trauma: Advanced Trauma Life Support for Doctors, Student Course Manual.* 8th ed. Chicago, IL: American College of Surgeons; 2008:225-245.

22. Sokol KK, Black GE, Azarow KS, Long W, Martin MJ, Eckert MJ. Prehospital interventions in severely injured pediatric patients: rethinking the ABCs. *J Trauma Acute Care Surg.* 2015;79(6):983-989.

23. Kragh JF Jr, Cooper A, Aden JK, et al. Survey of trauma registry data on tourniquet use in pediatric war casualties. *Pediatr Emerg Care.* 2012 Dec;28(12):1361-1365.

24. Chou R, Totten AM, Pappas M, et al., eds. *Glasgow Coma Scale for Field Triage of Trauma: A Systematic Review* [Report No.: 16(17)-EHC041-EF]. Rockville, MD: Agency for Healthcare Research and Quality; 2017.

25. Van de Voorde P, Sabbe M, Rizopoulos D, et al.; PENTA study group. Assessing the level of consciousness in children: a plea for the Glasgow Coma Motor subscore. *Resuscitation.* 2008;76(2):175-179.

26. National Vital Statistics System, Centers for Disease Control and Prevention. Deaths: final data for 1997. *Morb Mortal Wkly Rep.* 1999;47(19):1.

27. Ehrlich PF, Seidman PS, Atallah D, et al. Endotracheal intubation in rural pediatric trauma patients. *J Pediatr Surg.* 2004;39:1376.

28. Winchell RJ, Hoyt DB. Endotracheal intubation in the field improves survival in patients with severe head injury. *Arch Surg.* 1997;132(6):592.

29. Davis DP, Ochs M, Hoyt DB, et al. Paramedic-administered neuromuscular blockade improves prehospital intubation success in severely head-injured patients. *J Trauma Injury Infect Crit Care.* 2003;55(4):713.

30. Pearson S. Comparison of intubation attempts and completion times before and after the initiation of a rapid sequence intubation protocol in an air medical transport program. *Air Med J.* 2003;22(6):28.

31. Stockinger ZT, McSwain NE Jr. Prehospital endotracheal intubation for trauma does not improve survival over bag-valve-mask ventilation. *J Trauma Injury Infect Crit Care.* 2004;56(3):531.

32. Murray JA, Demetriades D, Berne TV, et al. Prehospital intubation in patients with severe head injury. *J Trauma Injury Infect Crit Care.* 2000;49(6):1065.

33. Hansen ML, Lin A, Eriksson C, et al.; CARES surveillance group. A comparison of pediatric airway management techniques during out-of-hospital cardiac arrest using the CARES database. *Resuscitation.* 2017;120:51-56.

34. Davis BD, Fowler R, Kupas DF, Roppolo LP. Role of rapid sequence induction for intubation in the prehospital setting: helpful or harmful? *Curr Opin Crit Care.* 2002;8(6):571.

35. Heins M. The "battered child" revisited. *JAMA.* 1984;251:3295.

36. Davis DP, Valentine C, Ochs M, et al. The Combitube as a salvage airway device for paramedic rapid sequence intubation. *Ann Emerg Med.* 2003;42(5):697.

37. Martin SE, Ochsner MG, Jarman RH, et al. Use of the laryngeal mask airway in air transport when intubation fails. *J Trauma Injury Infect Crit Care.* 1999;47(2):352.

38. Inaba K, Karamanos E, Skiada D, et al. Cadaveric comparison of the optimal site for needle decompression of tension pneumothorax by prehospital care providers. *J Trauma.* 2015;79(6):1044-1048.

39. Leatherman ML, Held JM, Fluke LM, et al. Relative device stability of anterior versus axillary needle decompression for tension pneumothorax during casualty movement: preliminary analysis of a human cadaver model. *J Trauma.* 2017;83(1):S136-S141.

40. McCarthy A, Curtis K, Holland AJ. Paediatric trauma systems and their impact on the health outcomes of severely injured children: an integrative review. *Injury.* 2016;47(3):574-585.

41. Lerner EB, Drendel AL, Cushman JT, et al. Ability of the physiologic criteria of the field triage guidelines to identify children who need the resources of a trauma center. *Prehosp Emerg Care.* 2017;21(2):180-184.

42. Larson JT, Dietrich AM, Abdessalam SF, Werman HA. Effective use of the air ambulance for pediatric trauma. *J Trauma Injury Infect Crit Care.* 2004;56(1):89.

43. Eckstein M, Jantos T, Kelly N, Cardillo A. Helicopter transport of pediatric trauma patients in an urban emergency medical services system: a critical analysis. *J Trauma Injury Infect Crit Care.* 2002;53(2):340.

44. Englum BR, Rialon KL, Kim J, et al. Current use and outcomes of helicopter transport in pediatric trauma: a review of 18,291 transports. *J Pediatr Surg.* 2017;52(1):140-144.

45. Polites SF, Zielinski MD, Fahy AS, et al. Mortality following helicopter versus ground transport of injured children. *Injury.* 2017;48(5):1000-1005.

46. Brown JB, Leeper CM, Sperry JL, et al. Helicopters and injured kids: improved survival with scene air medical transport in the pediatric trauma population. *J Trauma Acute Care Surg.* 2016;80(5):702-710.

47. Faul M, Xu L, Wald M, Coronado V. Traumatic brain injury in the United States: emergency department visits, hospitalizations and deaths 2002–2006. Atlanta, GA: Centers for Disease Control and Prevention; 2010. https://www.cdc.gov/traumaticbraininjury/pdf/blue_book.pdf. Accessed March 12, 2018.

48. Halstead ME, Walter KD, Council on Sports Medicine and Fitness. Clinical report—sport-related concussion in children and adolescents. *Pediatrics.* 2010;126:597.

49. McCrory P, Meeuwisse W, Aubry M, et al. Consensus statement on concussion in sport: the 4th International Conference on Concussion in Sport held in Zurich, November 2012. *J Sci Med Sport.* 2013;16(3):178-189.

50. Centers for Disease Control and Prevention (CDC). Sports-related recurrent brain injuries—United States. *Morb Mortal Wkly Rep.* 1997 Mar 14;46(10):224-227.

51. Carmona Suazo JA, Maas AI, van den Brink WA, et al. CO_2 reactivity and brain oxygen pressure monitoring in severe head injury. *Crit Care Med.* 2000;28(9):3268.

52. Adelson PD, Bratton SL, Carney NA, et al. Guidelines for the acute medical management of severe traumatic brain injury in infants, children, and adolescents. Chapter 4. Resuscitation of blood pressure and oxygenation and prehospital brain-specific therapies for the severe pediatric traumatic brain injury patient. *Pediatr Crit Care Med.* 2003;4(suppl 3):S12.

53. De Lorenzo RA. A review of spinal immobilization techniques. *J Emerg Med.* 1996;14(5):603.

54. Valadie LL. Child safety seats and the emergency responder. *Emerg Med Serv.* 2004;33(7):68.

55. U.S. Department of Transportation, National Highway Traffic Safety Administration. Working group best-practice recommendations for the safe transportation of children in emergency ground ambulances. DOT HS 811 677. September 2012.

56. Williams FN, Herndon DN, Hawkins HK, et al. The leading causes of death after burn injury in a single pediatric burn center. *Crit Care*. 2009;13(6):183.

57. Hollén L, Coy K, Day A, Young A. Resuscitation using less fluid has no negative impact on hydration status in children with moderate sized scalds: a prospective single-centre UK study. *Burns*. 2017;43(7):1499-1505.

58. Müller Dittrich MH, Brunow de Carvalho W, Lopes Lavado E. Evaluation of the "early" use of albumin in children with extensive burns: a randomized controlled trial. *Pediatr Crit Care Med*. 2016;17(6):e280-e286.

59. Peck MD, Priolo-Kapel D. Child abuse by burning: a review of the literature and an algorithm for medical investigations. *J Trauma*. 2002;53(5):1013-1022.

60. Hettiaratchy S, Dziewulski P. ABC of burns: pathophysiology and types of burns. *BMJ*. 2004;328(7453):1427-1429.

61. Hight DW, Bakalar HR, Lloyd JR. Inflicted burns in children: recognition and treatment. *JAMA*. 1979;242:517.

62. American Academy of Pediatrics Committee on Injury and Poison Prevention. Selecting and using the most appropriate car safety seats for growing children: guidelines for counseling parents. *Pediatrics*. 2002;109(3):550.

63. Nance ML, Lutz N, Arbogast KB, et al. Optimal restraint reduces the risk of abdominal injury in children involved in motor vehicle crashes. *Ann Surg*. 2004;239(1):127.

64. Braver ER, Whitfield R, Ferguson SA. Seating positions and children's risk of dying in motor vehicle crashes. *Injury Prev*. 1998;4(3):181.

Suggested Reading

EMSC Partnership for Children/National Association of EMS Physicians model pediatric protocols: 2003 revision [no authors listed]. *Prehosp Emerg Care*. 2004;8(4):343.

CHAPTER 15

Geriatric Trauma

Lead Editors:
Manish Shah, MD, MPH
Michael Lohmeier, MD
Michael Mancera, MD, FAEMS

CHAPTER OBJECTIVES

At the completion of this chapter, you will be able to do the following:

- Discuss the epidemiology of trauma in the older adult population.
- Describe the anatomic and physiologic effects of aging as a factor in causes of geriatric trauma and as a factor in the pathophysiology of trauma.
- Explain the interaction of preexisting medical problems with traumatic injuries in geriatric patients and how these interactions produce differences in the pathophysiology and manifestations of trauma.
- Discuss the physiologic effects of specific common classes of medications on the pathophysiology and manifestations of geriatric trauma.

- Compare and contrast the assessment techniques and considerations used in the older adult population with those used in younger populations.
- Demonstrate modifications in spinal immobilization techniques for safe and effective spinal immobilization of the older adult patient with the highest degree of comfort possible.
- Compare and contrast the management of the older adult trauma patient with that of the younger trauma patient.
- Assess the scene and older patient for signs and symptoms of abuse and neglect.

SCENARIO

Your unit is dispatched to the home of a 78-year-old woman who has fallen down a flight of stairs. Her daughter states that they had spoken on the telephone just 15 minutes earlier and that she was coming to her mother's house to take her to do some shopping. When she got to the house, she found her mother on the floor and called for an ambulance.

Upon initial contact, you find the patient lying at the bottom of a flight of stairs. You note that the patient is an older woman whose appearance matches her reported age. While maintaining in-line stabilization of the spine, you note that the patient is unresponsive to your commands. She has a visible laceration of the forehead and an obvious deformity of the left wrist. She is wearing a Medic Alert bracelet that indicates that she has diabetes.

- Did the fall cause the change in mental status, or was there an antecedent event?
- How do the patient's age, medical history, and medications interact with the injuries received to make the pathophysiology and manifestations different from those in younger patients?
- Should advanced age alone be used as an additional criterion for transport to a trauma center?

INTRODUCTION

The older adult population represents the fastest growing age group in the United States. Over 49 million Americans (15% of the U.S. population) are 65 years of age or older, and this number is expected to double by 2050, with the population of those over the age of 80 expected to triple in that same time frame.[1,2] Similarly, the worldwide number of those older than 60 years of age was just over 900 million in 2015 (12% of the world population) and will increase to just over 2 billion by 2050 (22% of the world population).[3]

Injuries in older adults present unique challenges in prehospital (and hospital) care management. Some of the earliest data that examine the effect of age on outcome are from the Major Trauma Outcome Study by the American College of Surgeons Committee on Trauma.[4] Outcome data from patients aged 65 years and older were compared to those of younger patients. Mortality increased in ages 45 to 55 years and doubled by age 75 years. This age-adjusted risk of death occurred across the spectrum of injury severity. Studies have continued to demonstrate an increased mortality rate for geriatric trauma patients, as compared with younger patients.[5] Despite the increased mortality and morbidity, older adults are historically less likely to receive medical care at a trauma center than younger patients with similar injuries.[6]

With an ever-growing population of older adults, an increasing number of geriatric patients suffer traumatic injuries. Trauma is the fourth leading cause of death in persons aged 55 to 64 years and is the ninth leading cause of death in those aged 65 years and older.[7] Trauma-related deaths in this age group account for 25% of all trauma deaths nationwide.[8] By 2050, an estimated 40% of all trauma patients will be older adults.[9] Specific mechanisms and patterns of injury are also unique to the older adult population.[10] Although motor vehicle crashes are the overall leading cause of trauma deaths, falls are the predominant mechanism of death in patients greater than 75 years of age.

This chapter aims to highlight the unique needs and increased level of risk among older adult trauma patients (**Box 15-1**). Specifically, the aging process and the effects of coexisting medical problems on an older patient's response to trauma and trauma management must be understood. The special considerations outlined in this chapter should be included in the assessment and management of any trauma patient who is 65 years of age or older, physically appears older, or is middle-aged with any medical problems typically associated with the older adult population. Early recognition of traumatic injuries and rapid treatment are paramount for the care of the older trauma patient.

Anatomy and Physiology of Aging

The aging process causes changes in physical structure, body composition, and organ function, which can create unique problems during prehospital care. The aging process influences mortality and morbidity rates.

Aging, or **senescence**, is a natural biologic process that begins during the years of early adulthood. By this time, organ systems have achieved maturation, and a turning point in physiologic growth has been reached. The body gradually loses its ability to maintain **homeostasis** (the state of relative constancy of the body's internal environment), and viability declines over a period of years until death occurs.

The process of aging occurs at the cellular level and is reflected in both anatomic structure and physiologic function. The period of "old age" is generally characterized by frailty, slower cognitive processes, impairment of psychological functions, diminished energy, the appearance of chronic and degenerative diseases, and a decline in sensory acuity. Functional abilities are reduced, and the well-known external signs and symptoms of older age appear, such as skin wrinkling, changes in hair color and quantity, osteoarthritis, and slowness in reaction time and reflexes (**Figure 15-1**). It

Box 15-1 The Value of Older Adults

As is emphasized in the Geriatric Education for Emergency Medical Services program, it is an honor to be involved in the life of an older person in any way. Helping to preserve every trauma patient's life and quality of life is a unique privilege held by prehospital care providers.

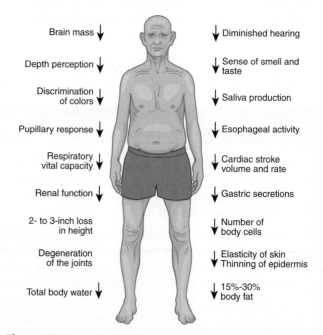

Figure 15-1 Changes caused by aging.

© National Association of Emergency Medical Technicians (NAEMT).

is important to note, however, that quality of life does not necessarily decrease with the aging process.

Influence of Chronic Medical Problems

Although some individuals can reach an advanced age without any serious medical problems, an older person is statistically more likely to have one or more significant medical conditions (**Table 15-1**). Historically, older adults consume health care resources, including the emergency department (ED), at a higher rate than other age groups in the United States.[11,12] Older adult patients also use emergency medical services (EMS) at a higher proportion than younger patients, as older age has been found to be an independent risk factor for EMS transport to the ED.[13]

As a person ages, additional medical problems can occur, often with cumulative negative consequences. The total influence on the body usually is greater than the sum of each individual effect. As each condition progresses and reduces the quality of the body's vital functions, the ability to withstand even modest anatomic or physiologic insults is greatly diminished.

Regardless of whether the patient is pediatric, middle-aged, or geriatric, the priorities, intervention needs, and life-threatening conditions that usually result from serious trauma are the same. However, because of these preexisting physical conditions, older adult patients often die from less severe injuries and die sooner than younger patients. Data show that preexisting conditions impact the mortality of an older trauma patient, and the more conditions a trauma patient has, the higher his or her mortality rate (**Table 15-2**). Several conditions have been shown to increase mortality because they interfere with the physiologic ability to respond to trauma (**Table 15-3**).[14]

Ears, Nose, and Throat

Tooth decay, gum disease, and dental trauma result in the need for various prostheses. The brittle nature of capped

Table 15-1 Percentage of Patients With Preexisting Disease (PED)

Age (years)	PED (%)
13–39	3.5
40–64	11.6
65–74	29.4
75–84	34.7
85+	37.3

Table 15-2 Number of Preexisting Diseases (PEDs) and Patient Outcome After Trauma

Number of PEDs	Survived	Died	Mortality Rate (%)
0	6,341	211	3.2
1	868	56	6.1
2	197	36	15.5
3 or more	67	22	24.7

Table 15-3 Prevalence of Preexisting Diseases (PEDs) and Associated Mortality Rates After Trauma

PED	Number of Patients	PED Present (%)	Total (%)	Mortality Rate (%)
Hypertension	597	47.9	7.7	10.2
Pulmonary disease	286	23	3.7	8.4
Cardiac disease	223	17.9	2.9	18.4
Diabetes	198	15.9	2.5	12.1
Obesity	167	13.4	2.1	4.8
Malignancy	80	6.4	1	20
Neurologic disorder	45	3.6	0.6	13.3
Renal disease	40	3.2	0.5	37.5
Hepatic disease	41	3.3	0.5	12.2

teeth, dentures, and fixed or removable bridges poses a special problem; these foreign bodies can be easily broken and aspirated and can subsequently obstruct the airway.

Changes in the contours of the face result from resorption of the mandible, in part because of the absence of teeth (**edentulism**). This resorption causes a characteristic look of an infolding and shrinking mouth and can adversely affect the ability to create a seal with a bag-mask device or to sufficiently visualize the airway during endotracheal intubation.

The nasopharyngeal tissues become increasingly fragile with age. In addition to the risk this change poses during the initial trauma, interventions such as nasopharyngeal airway insertion may induce profuse bleeding if not performed with care.

Respiratory System

Ventilatory function declines in the older person partly from decreased chest wall elasticity and partly from stiffening of the airway. The increased stiffness in the chest wall is associated with a reduction in expansion of the chest wall and decreased flexibility of cartilaginous connections of the ribs. As a result, the chest cage is less pliable. With declines in the efficiency of the respiratory system, the older person requires more effort to breathe and greater exertion to carry out daily activities.

The alveolar surface area in the lungs decreases with age. A 70-year-old person, for example, would have a 16% reduction in alveolar surface area. Any alteration of the already-reduced alveolar surface further decreases oxygen uptake. Additionally, as the body ages, its ability to saturate hemoglobin with oxygen decreases, leading to lower baseline oxygen saturation and less oxygen reserve available.[15] Because of impaired mechanical ventilation and diminished surface for gas exchange, the older trauma patient is less capable of compensating for physiologic losses associated with trauma.

Changes in the airway and lungs of older adults may not always be related to senescence alone. Cumulative chronic exposure to environmental toxins over the course of their lives may be caused by occupational hazards or tobacco smoke. This can lead to chronic obstructive pulmonary disease (COPD). Impaired cough and gag reflexes, along with poor cough strength and diminished esophageal sphincter tone, result in an increased risk of **aspiration pneumonitis**. A reduction in the number of **cilia** (hairlike projections of

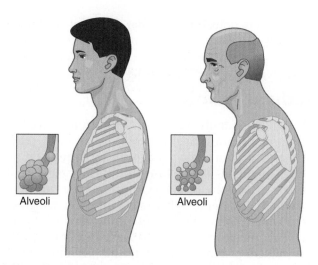

Figure 15-2 Spinal curvature can lead to an anteroposterior hump, which can cause ventilatory difficulties. Reduction in the alveolar surface area can also reduce the amount of oxygen that is exchanged in the lungs.
© National Association of Emergency Medical Technicians (NAEMT).

the cells in the respiratory tract that propel foreign particles and mucus from the bronchi) predisposes the older person to problems caused by inhaled particulate matter.

Another factor that affects the respiratory system is a physical change in the spinal curvature. Curvature changes, primarily increasing **kyphosis**, accompanied by an anteroposterior hump often lead to impaired biomechanics and additional ventilatory compromise (**Figure 15-2**).

Changes that affect the diaphragm can also contribute to ventilatory problems. Stiffening of the rib cage can cause more reliance on the activity of the diaphragm to achieve negative inspiration pressure. This increased reliance on the diaphragm makes an older person especially sensitive to changes in intra-abdominal pressure. Thus, a supine position or a full stomach from a large meal can provoke ventilatory insufficiency.

Injuries to the chest wall may compound these underlying respiratory changes in older patients. In fact, older trauma patients with rib fractures have a significantly increased mortality and risk of complications such as pneumonia, compared with younger patients.[16] The combination of underlying lung disease and physiologic changes of aging may predispose older patients to respiratory compromise after trauma.

Cardiovascular System

In 2015, heart disease was the leading cause of death in people 65 years and older in the United States.[7] In fact, heart disease accounted for so many deaths in this age group that it was the leading cause of death for all age groups combined, despite not being the leading cause of death in any other age group.[7]

Age-related decreases in arterial elasticity lead to increased peripheral vascular resistance. The myocardium and blood vessels rely on their elastic, contractile, and *distensible* (stretchable) properties to function properly. With aging, all of these decline, and the cardiovascular system becomes less efficient at moving fluids around the body.

Atherosclerosis is a narrowing of the blood vessels, a condition in which the inner layer of the arterial wall thickens as fatty deposits build up within the artery. These deposits, called plaques, decrease the inner diameter of the vessel, increasing resistance and making it more difficult to move blood forward. This same luminal narrowing occurs in the coronary vessels. Almost 50% of the U.S. population has coronary artery stenosis by age 65 years.[5]

One result of this narrowing is **hypertension**, a condition that commonly affects adults in the United States. Calcification of the arterial wall reduces compliance and the ability to respond to endocrine and central nervous system stimuli. The decrease in circulation can adversely affect any of the vital organs and is a common cause of heart disease. This is significant because the baseline blood pressure of the older trauma patient may be higher than in younger patients. A common pitfall in the assessment and management of geriatric trauma patients is failure to recognize a "normal"-appearing blood pressure as a sign of shock.

With age, the heart itself shows an increase in fibrous tissue and size (**myocardial hypertrophy**). Atrophy of the cells of the conduction system results in the increased incidence of cardiac dysrhythmias. The normal reflexes in the heart that respond to hypotension diminish with age, reducing the ability of older patients to increase their heart rate and stroke volume to compensate for a low blood pressure. Patients with pacemakers and patients on beta blocker medications have a decreased ability to adjust heart rate and cardiac output to meet the increased demands for oxygen consumption accompanying the stress of trauma.

In the older trauma patient, this reduced circulation contributes to cellular hypoxia. Cellular hypoxia may result in cardiac dysrhythmia, acute heart failure, and even sudden death. The body's ability to compensate for blood loss or other causes of shock is significantly lowered in the older person because of a diminished *inotropic* (cardiac contraction) response to **catecholamines**. In addition, total circulating blood volume decreases, creating less physiologic reserve for blood loss from trauma. Diastolic dysfunction makes the patient more dependent on atrial filling to augment cardiac output, which is diminished in hypovolemic states.

The reduced circulation and circulatory-defense responses, coupled with increasing cardiac failure, produce a significant problem in managing shock in the older trauma patient. Fluid resuscitation needs to be carefully monitored because of the reduced compliance of the cardiovascular system. Care must be taken when treating hypotension and shock to avoid causing volume overload with aggressive fluid resuscitation.[17]

Nervous System

As individuals age, brain weight and the number of neurons (nerve cells) decrease. The weight of the brain reaches its peak (3 pounds [1.4 kg]) at approximately 20 years of age. By 80 years of age, the brain has lost about 10% of its weight, with progressive cerebral atrophy.[18] Additionally, the dural bridging veins become more stretched and thus susceptible to tearing. This results in a lower frequency of epidural hemorrhage and a higher frequency of subdural hemorrhage. The body compensates for the loss of size with increased cerebrospinal fluid. Although this additional space around the brain can protect it from contusion, it also allows for more brain movement in response to acceleration/deceleration injuries. The increased space in the cranial vault also allows significant volumes of blood to accumulate around the brain in the older patient, with minimal or no symptoms.

The speed with which nerve impulses are conducted along certain nerves also decreases. These decreases result in only small effects on behavior and thinking. Reflexes are slower, but not to a significant degree. Compensatory functions can be impaired, particularly in patients with diseases such as Parkinson disease, resulting in an increased incidence of falls. The peripheral nervous system is also affected by the slowing of nerve impulses, resulting in tremors and an unsteady gait.

General information and vocabulary abilities increase or are maintained, whereas skills requiring mental and muscular activity (psychomotor ability) may decline. The intellectual functions that involve verbal comprehension, arithmetic ability, fluency of ideas, experiential evaluation, and general knowledge tend to increase after 60 years of age in those who continue learning activities. Exceptions are those who develop dementia and related disorders such as Alzheimer disease.

Dementia is a general term for a decrease in cognitive capabilities that causes an interference with daily life. Alzheimer disease is the most common form of dementia. Most commonly, memory, attention, communication skills, and judgment may be impaired; however, symptoms may vary. Dementia affects 1 in 10 people age 65 years and older in the United States. It is the fifth leading cause of death for older adults and a major cause of disability.[19] Cognitive effects from dementia are usually gradual in onset. **Delirium** differs from dementia; however, as delirium causes an abrupt change in mental status secondary to an acute medical condition such as infection, and it is generally reversible once the underlying acute process is corrected.

Older adults also have significant mental health burdens. Depression is common in the older population. While depression, dementia, and organic brain disease may be considerations, it is critical that traumatic head injury, hypoxia, and shock take priority when assessing an older trauma patient. (See the Head Trauma chapter.)

Sensory Changes

Vision and Hearing

Overall, men tend to be more likely to have hearing difficulties, whereas both genders have a similar incidence of sight-related impairment.

Poor vision is challenging at any age, but it may be even more problematic for the older person. This may have detrimental effects on reading prescription labels and safe driving abilities. In addition, they have progressive decreases in visual acuity, ability to differentiate colors, and night vision. The cells of the lens of the eye are incapable of restoration to their original molecular structure. Eventually, the lens loses its capability to increase in thickness and curvature. The result is almost universal farsightedness (*presbyopia*) in persons over 40 years of age, requiring glasses for reading.

Because of changes to the various structures of the eye, older persons have more difficulty seeing in dimly lit environments. With age, the lens of the eye begins to become cloudy and impenetrable to light. This gradual process results in a **cataract**, or a milky lens that blocks and distorts light that enters the eye and blurs vision. Over half of people over age 80 are affected by cataracts.[20] This deterioration of vision increases the risk of a motor vehicle crash, particularly when driving at night.

A gradual decline in hearing (*presbycusis*) is also characteristic of aging. **Presbycusis** is usually caused by loss of conduction of sound into the inner ear; the use of hearing aids can compensate for this loss to some degree. This hearing loss is most pronounced when the person attempts to discriminate complex sounds, such as when many people are speaking at once, or with loud, ambient noise present, such as the wailing of sirens.

Pain Perception

Because of the aging process and the presence of diseases such as diabetes, older adults may not perceive pain normally, placing them at increased risk of injury from excesses in heat and cold exposure. Many older adults have conditions such as arthritis that result in chronic pain. Living with

---

Box 15-3 Impact of Sensory Changes With Age

Vision and hearing changes may be so subtle and may occur over such a long period of time that the patient may not realize that changes have occurred. Preventive check-ups with primary care physicians should include screenings to evaluate the older patient for any subtle sensory changes.

---

daily pain can cause an increased tolerance to pain, which may result in a patient's failure to identify areas of injury. When evaluating patients, especially those who usually have pain at baseline, prehospital care providers should locate areas in which the pain has increased or in which the painful area has enlarged. It is also important to note the pain characteristics or exacerbating factors since the trauma occurred.

Renal System

Changes common with aging include reduced levels of filtration by the kidneys and a reduced excretory capacity. These changes should be considered when administering medications normally cleared by the kidneys. Chronic renal insufficiency typically affects older people and contributes to a reduction in a patient's overall health status and ability to withstand trauma. For example, renal dysfunction may be one cause of chronic anemia, which would lower a patient's **physiologic reserve**.

Musculoskeletal System

Bone loses mineral as it ages. The loss of bone (**osteoporosis**) is unequal among the genders. During young adulthood, bone mass is greater in women than in men. However, bone loss is more rapid in women and accelerates after menopause. With this higher incidence of osteoporosis, older women have a greater probability of fractures, particularly of the neck of the femur (hip). Causes of osteoporosis include decreased estrogen levels, increased periods of inactivity, and inadequate intake and inefficient use of calcium.

Osteoporosis contributes significantly to hip fractures and spontaneous compression fractures of the vertebral bodies. The incidence approaches 1% per year for men and 2% for women over age 85 years.[21]

Older persons are sometimes shorter than they were in young adulthood due to a decrease in height of the vertebral discs. As the discs flatten, a loss of approximately 2 inches (5 cm) in height occurs between 20 and 70 years of age. Kyphosis (curvature of the spine) in the thoracic region can also contribute to height loss and is often caused by osteoporosis (**Figure 15-3**). As the bones become more porous and fragile, erosion occurs anteriorly, and compression fractures of the vertebrae may develop. As the thoracic spine becomes more curved, the head and shoulders appear to be pushed forward. If COPD, particularly emphysema, is present, the kyphosis may be more pronounced because of the increased development of the accessory muscles of breathing.

Arthritis is also common in older adults. **Osteoarthritis (OA)** is a degenerative condition that affects joints, leading to damage of the cartilage in joints that normally provide smooth surfaces for joint movement. **Rheumatoid arthritis (RA)**

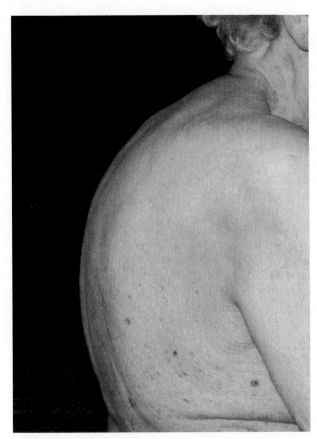

Figure 15-3 Kyphosis, typically caused by osteoporosis.
© Dr. P. Marazzi/Science Source.

is an inflammatory disorder caused by an autoimmune response, which can lead to joint swelling and deformity. These chronic conditions can cause decreased mobility and chronic pain. These limitations need to be considered during assessment and transport of older patients.

Absolute levels of growth hormones decrease with aging, in conjunction with a decline in responsiveness to anabolic hormones. The combined effect is a reduction in muscle mass of older adults. Muscle loss is measured microscopically by both absolute number of muscle cells and reduction in cell size.

Deficits that relate to the musculoskeletal system (e.g., inability to flex the hip or knee adequately with changes in terrain) predispose the older adult to falls. Muscle fatigue can cause many problems that affect movement, especially falls. Changes in the body's normal posture are common, and changes in the spine make the curvature become more acute with aging. Some degree of osteoporosis is universal with aging. Because of this progressive bone resorption, the bones become less pliant, more brittle, and more easily broken. The decrease in bone strength, coupled with reduced muscle strength caused by less active exercise, can result in multiple fractures with only mild

or moderate force. The most common sites of long-bone fracture in older persons include the proximal femur, hip, humerus, and wrist. The increased incidence of falls as a mechanism of injury results in Colles' fractures of the distal radius, as the dorsiflexed hand is outstretched in an effort to break the fall.

The entire vertebral column changes with age, primarily because of the effects of osteoporosis, **osteophytosis** (bone spurs), and calcification of the supporting ligaments. This calcification results in decreased range of motion and narrowing of the spinal canal. The narrowed canal and progressive osteophytic disease put these patients at high risk for spinal cord injury with even minor trauma. The narrowing of the spinal canal is called **spinal stenosis**, and it increases the likelihood of cord compression without any actual break in the bony cervical spine. The thoracic and lumbar spine degenerate progressively as well, and the combined forces of osteoporosis and posture changes lead to increased falls. Even ground-level falls can cause fracture in older patients.[22]

Skin

Significant changes in the skin and connective tissues are associated with aging, and they result in difficulties with response to trauma as well as direct wound healing. Cell numbers decrease, tissue strength is lost, and the skin has impaired functional status. As the skin ages, sweat and sebaceous glands are lost. Loss of sweat glands reduces the body's ability to regulate temperature. Loss of sebaceous glands, which produce oil, makes the skin dry and flaky. Production of melanin, the pigment that gives color to skin and hair, declines, causing an aging pallor. The skin thins and appears translucent, primarily because of changes in underlying connective tissue, and therefore is more prone to sustaining damage from relatively minor trauma. The thinning and drying of the skin also reduce its resistance to minor injury and microorganisms, resulting in an increased infection rate from open wounds. As elasticity is lost, the skin stretches and falls into wrinkles and folds, especially in areas of heavy use, such as those overlying the facial muscles of expression. Thinning of the skin also results in the potential for significant tissue loss and injury in response to relatively low-energy transfers.

Loss of fatty tissue can predispose the older adult to hypothermia. The loss of dermal thickness with advanced age and an associated loss in vascularity are also responsible for impaired thermoregulatory dysfunction. However, hypothermia should also suggest the possibility of occult sepsis, hypothyroidism, or phenothiazine overdose in the older population. This loss of fatty tissue also leads to less padding over bony prominences, such as the head, shoulders, spine, buttocks, hips, and heels. Prolonged immobilization without additional padding can result in tissue necrosis and ulceration as well as increased pain and discomfort during treatment and transport. Therefore, complications from skin breakdown must be considered during the transport and immobilization of older patients.

Nutrition and the Immune System

With aging, a reduction in lean body mass and decreases in metabolic rate cause a reduction in caloric needs. However, because of inefficient utilization, protein needs may actually increase. These competing changes often result in preexisting malnutrition in the older trauma patient. The financial status of retired individuals may also affect their choices of and access to quality nutrition.

The ability of the immune system to function decreases as it ages. Grossly, organs associated with the immune response (thymus, liver, and spleen) all decrease in size. A decrease in cell-mediated and humoral responses to infection also results. Coupled with any preexisting nutritional problems common in the older adult population, there is an increased susceptibility to infection. *Sepsis* is a common cause of late death after severe or even insignificant trauma in the older patient.

Assessment

Prehospital assessment of the older patient is based on the same method used for all trauma patients. Although the methodology is unchanged, the process may be altered in older patients. As with all trauma patients, however, the mechanism of injury should be considered. This section discusses some special considerations in assessing an older trauma patient as these patients are at a high risk for injury.

Physics of Trauma

Falls

Falls are the leading cause of traumatic death and disability in older adults. Approximately one-third of community-dwelling people over 65 years of age fall each year, increasing to 50% by 80 years of age.[23] Although men and women fall with equal frequency, women are more than twice as likely to sustain a serious injury because of more pronounced osteoporosis. Falls, even those that occur from a standing position, can result in serious injury and life-threatening trauma, with up to 25% of those falling suffering a significant injury.[23]

The cause of falls is multifactorial. They result from changes in posture and gait. Declining visual acuity from cataracts, glaucoma, and loss of night vision contributes to the loss of visual cues used to navigate safely. Diseases of the central and peripheral nervous systems and the vascular instability of cardiovascular disease further precipitate falls.

Compounding these preexisting conditions that predispose older adults to fall are the medications used, such as benzodiazepines and beta blockers. Finally, environmental factors are also important contributors to falls. Physical barriers in the environment, such as slippery floors, throw rugs, stairs, poorly fitting shoes, and poor lighting create additional hazards.

Long-bone fractures account for the majority of injuries, with fractures of the hip resulting in the greatest mortality and morbidity rates. The mortality rate from hip fractures is 20% at 1 year after the injury and rises to 33% at 2 years. Mortality is due to multiple causes but is postulated to be related to the effects of decreased mobility. Prehospital care providers must have a high level of suspicion for serious injury given the increased incidence of falls, rate of injury, and severity of complications from falls among older patients. Preventive programs like the Centers for Disease Control and Prevention's Stopping Elderly Accidents, Deaths & Injuries (STEADI) can be effective in decreasing the incidence of these injuries. In addition, many EMS agencies do home visits to help achieve fall prevention.[24]

Vehicular Trauma

From 1999 to 2015, the number of older adult drivers has increased by 50%.[25] Unfortunately, as age increases, so too does the risk of being injured in a vehicle crash (**Box 15-4**). When comparing fatalities per mile driven, an increase in fatality rates is seen in drivers starting at ages 70 to 74 years, with the highest rates being among drivers 85 years and older.[25]

These high fatality rates have been attributed to certain physiologic changes. In particular, subtle changes in memory and judgment together with impaired visual and auditory acuity can result in delayed reaction time. Alcohol is rarely involved, unlike motor vehicle crashes in younger persons. Only 5% of fatally injured older persons are intoxicated, compared with 25% for all other age categories.[25]

Older pedestrians represent nearly one-fifth of all pedestrian fatalities.[26] Because of slower walking speeds, the time allowed by traffic signals may be too short for an older person to traverse the crosswalk safely.

Assault and Domestic Abuse

Abuse is defined as willful infliction of injury, unreasonable confinement, intimidation, or cruel punishment resulting in physical or psychological harm or pain, or the withholding

---

Box 15-4　Older Drivers

The National Highway Traffic Safety Administration (NHTSA) has produced a program called Physician's Guide to Assessing and Counseling Older Drivers. This program is available online at the NHTSA website.

of services that would prevent these conditions. Older adults are highly vulnerable to this crime. Unfortunately, only a small fraction of abuse cases are recognized and reported.[27] (See the later discussion on Elder Maltreatment.)

Burns

Fatalities in older patients occur from burns of smaller size and less severity compared with other age groups. Decreased pain perception and thin skin may result in more severe tissue injury. The presence of preexisting medical conditions, such as cardiovascular disease and diabetes, also results in more complications related to burn injuries. Vascular collapse and infection are the most common causes of death from burns in older patients.

The fatality rate for home fires involving older adults has increased disproportionately compared to other age populations.[28] This may be due to a delayed recognition of a house fire and a decreased ability to escape from a structure fire.

Home oxygen–related fires and burn injury also present a unique risk for older adults, given the higher rate of underlying comorbidities such as COPD. These injuries can result in significant morbidity from facial and airway burn injuries.

Traumatic Brain Injury

The incidence of traumatic brain injury (TBI) among older patients is high, leading to an estimated 12,000 deaths in the United States.[29] There is an increased mortality rate from TBI for older patients compared to younger patients and also an increased need for long-term care facilities and rehabilitation care following injury.

Because of brain atrophy, a fairly large subdural hemorrhage can exist with minimal clinical findings. The combination of head trauma and hypovolemic shock yields a greater fatality rate. Preexisting medical conditions or their treatment may be a cause of altered mentation in older patients. When in doubt as to whether confusion represents an acute or a chronic process, the injured patient should be assumed to have sustained a traumatic brain injury and preferentially transported to a trauma center for evaluation when possible.

Primary Survey

Exsanguinating Hemorrhage

Trauma patients must be assessed for correctable causes of life-threatening hemorrhage. External sites of severe bleeding should be recognized early.

Airway

After establishing scene safety and controlling any exsanguinating hemorrhage, evaluation of the older patient proceeds with assessment of the airway. Changes in mentation may be secondary to hypoxia from partial airway occlusion or obstruction. The oral cavity should be examined for foreign objects, such as dentures or teeth that have become fractured or dislodged.

Breathing

As in any other adult, older patients who breathe at a rate of less than 10 or greater than 30 breaths/minute will not have an adequate minute volume and will require appropriate airway support. In most adults, a ventilatory rate between 12 and 20 breaths/minute is normal and confirms that an adequate minute volume is present. However, in an older patient, reduced tidal volume capacity and pulmonary function may result in an inadequate minute volume, even at rates of 12 to 20 breaths/minute. Because of these changes, breath sounds should be immediately assessed even if the ventilatory rate is normal. Keep in mind, these sounds may be harder to hear because of smaller tidal volumes.

An older patient's vital capacity is often diminished by as much as 50%. Kyphotic changes of the spine (anteroposterior) result in a ventilation–perfusion mismatch at rest. Hypoxia is much more likely to be a consequence of shock than in younger patients. Older patients also have decreased chest excursion. Lower tidal volumes and lower minute volumes are typical. Reductions in capillary oxygen and carbon dioxide exchange are significant. Hypoxemia tends to be progressive.

Circulation

Some findings can only be interpreted properly by knowing the individual patient's pre-event, or baseline, status. Expected ranges of vital signs and other findings usually accepted as normal are not "normal" in every individual, and deviation is much more common in the older patient. Although the typical ranges are broad enough to include most individual adult differences, an individual of any age may vary beyond these norms; therefore, such variation in older patients should be expected.

Medication may contribute to these changes. For example, in the average adult, a systolic blood pressure of 120 millimeters of mercury (mm Hg) is considered normal and generally unimpressive. However, in the chronically hypertensive patient who normally has a systolic blood pressure of 150 mm Hg or higher, a pressure of 120 mm Hg would be a concern, suggestive of occult bleeding (or some other mechanism causing hypotension) of such a degree that decompensation has occurred. Likewise, heart rate is a poor indicator of trauma in older patients because of the effects of medications such as beta blockers and the heart's dampened response to circulating catecholamines (epinephrine). Quantitative information or objective signs should not be used in isolation from other findings.

Failing to recognize that such a change occurred or that it is a serious pathologic finding can lead to a poor outcome for the patient.

Delayed capillary refilling time is common in older patients because of less efficient circulation from peripheral arterial disease and may be a less reliable indicator of acute circulatory changes. Mildly reduced motor, sensory, and circulatory function in the extremities may represent a normal finding in older patients.

Disability

All findings should be viewed collectively to maintain an increased level of suspicion for neurologic injury in the older patient. The older patient's orientation to time and place should be assessed by careful and complete questioning. Wide differences in mentation, memory, and orientation (to the past and present) can exist in older persons. Unless someone on the scene can describe the baseline mental status of the older patient, it should be assumed that any deficits present are indicative of an acute neurologic injury, hypoxia, hypotension, or a combination of the three. Establishing the baseline mental status for the older patient is crucial and may involve obtaining information from the patient, family members, and/or caretakers.

Expose/Environment

Older persons are more susceptible to ambient environmental changes. They have a reduced ability to respond to environmental temperature changes with impairments of both heat production and heat dissipation. Thermoregulation may be related to an imbalance of electrolytes, lower basal metabolic rate, decreased ability to shiver, arteriosclerosis, and the effects of drugs or alcohol. Hyperthermia may result from cerebrovascular accidents (strokes) or medications such as diuretics, antihistamines, and antiparkinsonian drugs. Hypothermia is often associated with decreased metabolism, reduced body fat, less efficient peripheral vasoconstriction, and poor nutrition.

Secondary Survey

The secondary survey of the older trauma patient is performed in the same manner as for younger patients and only after urgent life-threatening conditions have been addressed. However, many factors can complicate the assessment of a geriatric patient, and prehospital care providers should consider how changes of aging may impact presentation when assessing older patients.

Communication Challenges

Many factors come into play when communicating with geriatric patients, from the normal biologic effects of the aging process, to generational expectations of the provider–patient relationship. Understanding how best to communicate with individuals in this age group will help the prehospital care provider deliver prompt, efficient care.

- *Additional patience may be needed because of the older patient's hearing or visual impairments.* Empathy and compassion are essential. A patient's intelligence should not be underestimated merely because communication may be difficult or absent.
- *A significant other or caregiver may need to be involved.* With the patient's permission, involving the caregiver or spouse may be necessary to gather valuable information if the patient is unable to reliably provide a detailed history. Remember to still involve the patient in any discussions as appropriate. Some older patients may be reluctant to give information without the assistance of a relative or support person. Others may not want any others present, and this should be recognized.
- *Be mindful of how impaired hearing, sight, comprehension, and mobility impact your history and physical examination.* Noise, distractions, and interruptions may impact your interaction with the patient. For example, the patient might be unable to hear or understand verbal instructions during an assessment and examination, making it difficult to truly assess acute deficits.
- *Be respectful and avoid language that may be interpreted as condescending.* The patient should be addressed by his or her last name, unless otherwise instructed by the patient. Words that may be considered condescending or dismissive should be avoided, such as "honey" or "dear." It may take the patient a few additional seconds to process questions, especially during the stress of an emergency. Ask the patient one question at a time, and wait for the patient to respond before asking another question.

Physiologic Changes

The prehospital care provider must be prepared for the physiologic distinctions that are often encountered in the geriatric age group.

- *Changes in physiology lead to altered pathophysiology compared to younger patients.* Typical findings of serious illness such as fever, pain, or tenderness may take longer to develop in the older patient and can confuse the presenting signs and symptoms. In addition, many medications can adversely affect the physiologic response to illness and injury. Often a prehospital care provider will have to depend on the patient's history alone.
- *Altered comprehension or neurologic disorders are a significant problem for many older patients.* These impairments can range from delirium to dementia such as Alzheimer disease. Not only may these patients have difficulty in expressing themselves, they also may have difficulty with receiving information or helping in the assessment. They may be restless and sometimes combative.

- *Older patients may not be properly nourished or hydrated.* Shake the patient's hand to feel for grip strength, skin turgor, and body temperature. Look at the patient's state of nourishment. Does the patient appear to be well, thin, or emaciated? Older patients have a decreased thirst response, a drop in the amount of body fat (15% to 30%) as well as total body water.

- *Older patients have a decrease in skeletal muscle weight, widening and weakening of bones, degeneration of joints, and osteoporosis.* They have an increased probability of fractures with comparatively minor injuries and a higher risk of fractures to the vertebrae, hips, and ribs. The ease of rising or sitting should be observed, as it provides clues about muscle strength.

- *Older patients have degeneration of heart muscle cells and fewer pacemaker cells.* Older persons are prone to dysrhythmia as a result of a loss of elasticity of the heart and major arteries. Widespread use of beta blockers, calcium channel blockers, and diuretics further complicates this problem. Often after injury, older patients present with low cardiac output with hypoxia despite the absence of lung injury. Heart rate, stroke volume, and cardiac reserve all decrease, resulting in increased morbidity and mortality after trauma. Consider baseline vital signs when assessing for signs of early decompensation. A blood pressure that would be "normal" for a healthy person may represent significant hypotension for the older patient with comorbid conditions.

Environmental Factors

The environment in which the patient is found can tell you a lot about his or her well-being. Chronic underlying illness may be exacerbated by environmental factors and poor living conditions. Weather-related illness should also be considered in the older patient. Heat- and cold-related death rates increase with age, particularly for those older than 75 years of age.[30]

- *Look for behavioral problems or manifestations that do not fit the scene.* Look at the patient's physical appearance and grooming. Are the attire and grooming appropriate for where and how the patient was found? Does the patient appear capable of accomplishing normal activities of daily living? Is the living space clean and well kept? Is there a potential for elder abuse or neglect? Is the appropriate temperature control and clothing in the living environment consistent with the regional climate?

Detailed History

Medications

Knowledge of a patient's medications can provide key information in determining prehospital care. Preexisting disease in the older trauma patient is a significant finding. The following classes of drugs are of particular interest because of their frequent use by older persons and their potential to impact the physical examination and management of the trauma patient:

- Beta blockers (e.g., propranolol, metoprolol) may account for a patient's absolute or relative bradycardia. In this situation, an increasing tachycardia as a sign of developing shock may not occur. The drug's inhibition of the body's normal sympathetic compensatory mechanisms can mask the true level of the patient's circulatory deterioration. Such patients can rapidly decompensate, seemingly without warning.

- Calcium channel blockers (e.g., diltiazem) may prevent peripheral vasoconstriction and accelerate hypovolemic shock.

- Nonsteroidal anti-inflammatory agents (e.g., ibuprofen) may contribute to platelet dysfunction and increase bleeding.

- Anticoagulants and antiplatelet agents (e.g., clopidogrel, aspirin, warfarin) may increase bleeding and blood loss. Data suggest that use of warfarin increases the risk of adverse outcomes in isolated head injury. Any bleeding from trauma will be more brisk and difficult to control when a patient is taking an anticoagulant. More important, internal bleeding can progress rapidly, leading to shock and death.

- Hypoglycemic agents (e.g., insulin, metformin, rosiglitazone) may be causally related to the events that caused injury, affect mentation, and make blood glucose stabilization difficult if their use is unrecognized.

- Over-the-counter medications, including herbal preparations and supplements, are frequently used. Their inclusion in the list of medications is often omitted by patients, who often do not consider over-the-counter supplements as "medicine." Thus, they should be specifically questioned about their use. These preparations may be unregulated and have unpredictable effects and medication interactions. Complications of these agents include bleeding (garlic) and myocardial infarction (ephedrine/ma huang).

Assessing the older trauma patient's medication list can prove challenging when the patient has impaired awareness or an extensive list of medications with difficult names. In some communities, EMS agencies have promoted programs such as the File of Life Project (www.folife.org). These programs advocate for standardizing the location of detailed medical history to intuitive locations such as the refrigerator door. The patient completes a medical history form that is then placed into a magnetic holder that is applied to the refrigerator, alerting prehospital care providers to the File of Life (**Figure 15-4**). Additionally, many electronic medical records systems used by hospitals and physicians include the most recent medication lists in their discharge instructions, providing another location to find such information.

FILE OF LIFE

KEEP INFORMATION UP TO DATE !!
Review At Least Every Six Months !
MEDICAL DATA REVIEWED AS OF ___ MO. ___ YR.

Name: _____ Sex: M F

Address: _____

Doctor: _____ Phone #: _____

Doctor: _____ Phone #: _____

EMERGENCY CONTACTS

Name: _____ Phone #: _____

Address: _____

Name: _____ Phone #: _____

Address: _____

KEEP INFORMATION UP TO DATE !!
Review At Least Every Six Months !
MEDICAL DATA REVIEWED AS OF ___ MO. ___ YR.

Name: _____ Sex: M F

Address: _____

Doctor: _____ Phone #: _____

Preferred Hospital: _____

EMERGENCY CONTACTS

Name: _____ Phone #: _____

Address: _____

Name: _____ Phone #: _____

Address: _____

MEDICAL DATA

Use pencil for ease in making changes.

Special Conditions/Remarks: _____

Medication	Dosage	Frequency

Pharmacy: _____ Phone: _____

Date of Birth: _____

Blood Type: _____ Religion: _____

Health Care Proxy on file at: _____

Living Will on file at: _____

® FILE OF LIFE   SEE BACK OF CARD FOR ADDITIONAL INFORMATION

Use Pencil for ease in making changes

Recent Surgery: _____ Date: _____

_____

Do you have an EMS-NO CPR Directive or a DNR form ?
YES ☐   NO ☐   Where is it located ?

MEDICAL CONDITIONS

Check all that exist

☐ No known medical conditions   ☐ Hemodialysis
☐ Abnormal EKG   ☐ Hemolytic Anemia
☐ Adrenal Insufficiency   ☐ Hepatitis-Type [   ]
☐ Angina   ☐ Hypertension
☐ Asthma   ☐ Hypoglycemia
☐ Bleeding Disorder   ☐ Laryngectomy
☐ Cancer   ☐ Leukemia
☐ Cardiac Dysrhythmia   ☐ Lymphomas
☐ Cataracts   ☐ Memory Impaired
☐ Clotting Disorder   ☐ Myasthenia Gravis
☐ Coronary Bypass Graft   ☐ Pacemaker
☐ Dementia ☐ Alzheimer's ☐   ☐ Renal Failure
☐ Diabetes/Insulin Dependent   ☐ Seizure Disorder
☐ Eye Surgery   ☐ Sickle Cell Anemia
☐ Glaucoma   ☐ Stroke
☐ Hearing Impaired   ☐ Tuberculosis
☐ Heart Valve Prosthesis   ☐ Vision Impaired
☐ Other:

ALLERGIES

☐ Aspirin   ☐ Insect Stings   ☐ Penicillin
☐ Barbiturate   ☐ Latex   ☐ Sulfa
☐ Codeine   ☐ Lidocaine   ☐ Tetracycline
☐ Demerol   ☐ Morphine   ☐ X-Rays Dyes
☐ Horse Serum   ☐ Novocaine   ☐ No Known Allergies
☐ Environmental:
☐ Other:

MEDICAL INSURANCE

Med Ins Co: _____

Policy #: _____

Other Med Ins Co: _____

Policy #: _____

Medicaid #: _____ Medicare #: _____

Figure 15-4 File of Life.

Courtesy of the File of Life Foundation.

Older patients also have a higher rate of **polypharmacy**, a term used to describe the administration of more than five medications. In fact, nearly half of older patients fit the definition of polypharmacy.[31] This can be a significant cause of morbidity in these patients. One in six hospital admissions for older adults was due an adverse medication event.[32] In an effort to address polypharmacy and its complications, the American Geriatrics Society has established the Beers criteria for identifying potentially inappropriate medication use among older patients.[33] Prehospital care providers should recognize the impact of home medications, especially among older patients with traumatic injuries.

Because older patients often are taking numerous medications, the possibility of medication interactions or inadvertent overdose must be considered as a possible cause of the patient's trauma, altered mental status, or changes in vital signs.

Medical Conditions as a Precursor to Traumatic Injury

A number of medical conditions may predispose individuals to traumatic events, especially those that result in an alteration in the level of consciousness or neurologic deficit. Common examples include seizure disorders, hypoglycemia due to improper insulin dosing, syncope from antihypertensive medication, cardiac dysrhythmia from an acute coronary syndrome, and cerebrovascular accidents. Because the incidence of chronic medical conditions increases with age, geriatric patients are more likely to suffer trauma as a consequence of a medical problem when compared to younger victims. The astute prehospital care provider should note clues from the primary and secondary surveys that may point to a medical problem that precipitated the traumatic event, such as the following:

- Bystander reports that a victim appeared unconscious prior to a crash
- A Medic Alert bracelet that indicates an underlying condition such as diabetes
- An irregular heartbeat or cardiac dysrhythmia seen during electrocardiogram monitoring

The prehospital care provider may be the only source of this information, all of which is highly pertinent to the receiving facility.

Management

Exsanguinating Hemorrhage

Severe external bleeding may lead to exsanguination. This life-threatening bleeding needs to be recognized and addressed rapidly. Direct pressure should be applied to any area of hemorrhage. If severe bleeding involves an extremity site, a tourniquet should be applied to control hemorrhage if direct pressure is unsuccessful.

Airway

The presence of dentures, common among older adults, may affect airway management. Ordinarily, dentures should be left in place to maintain a better seal around the mouth with a mask. However, partial dentures may become dislodged during an emergency and may completely or partially block the airway; these should be removed.

Fragile nasopharyngeal mucosal tissues and the possible use of anticoagulants put the older trauma patient at increased risk of bleeding from placement of a nasopharyngeal airway. This hemorrhage may further compromise the patient's airway and result in aspiration.

Arthritis may affect the temporomandibular joints and cervical spine. The decreased flexibility of these areas may make endotracheal intubation more difficult.

The objective of airway management is primarily to ensure a patent airway for the delivery of adequate tissue oxygenation. Early mechanical ventilation by either bag-mask device or advanced airway interventions should be considered in older trauma patients because of their greatly limited physiologic reserve.

Breathing

In all trauma patients, supplemental oxygen should be administered as soon as possible. Oxygen saturation should generally be kept at greater than or equal to 94%. The older population has a high prevalence of COPD. Even if a patient has severe COPD, it is unlikely that high-flow oxygen administration will be detrimental to the respiratory drive during routine urban or suburban transports. However, if the prehospital care provider notes *somnolence* (a state of drowsiness) or a slowing respiratory rate, ventilations can be assisted with a bag-mask device with consideration for advanced airway management.

Older persons experience increased stiffness of the chest wall. In addition, reduced chest wall muscle power and decreased flexibility of the cartilage make the chest cage less flexible. These and other changes are responsible for reductions in lung volumes. The older patient may need ventilatory support by assisted ventilations with a bag-mask device earlier than younger trauma patients. The mechanical force applied to the resuscitation bag may need to be increased to overcome the increased chest wall resistance. However, as indicated by lower lung volumes at baseline, large tidal volumes are often not needed when providing assisted bag ventilations as this may lead to unintended consequences such as pneumothorax.

Capnography, a measure of end-tidal carbon dioxide ($ETCO_2$), may be another tool used to help assess respiratory status. Capnography measurements for severely injured older trauma patients should be correlated with all other clinical information available.

Circulation

Older persons may have poor cardiovascular reserve. Reduced circulating blood volume, possible chronic anemia, and preexisting myocardial and coronary disease leave the patient with little tolerance for even modest amounts of blood loss.

Because of the laxity of skin or use of anticoagulant agents, geriatric patients are prone to the development of larger hematomas and potentially more significant internal hemorrhage. Early control of hemorrhage through direct pressure on open wounds, stabilization or immobilization of fractures, and rapid transport to a trauma center are essential. Fluid resuscitation should be guided by the index of suspicion for serious bleeding based on the mechanism of injury and an overall appearance of shock. At the same time, overadministration of IV fluids is to be avoided, as the older patient often poorly tolerates an excessive fluid load. Urine output is a poor measure of perfusion in older persons, especially in the prehospital setting.

Immobilization

Protection of the cervical, thoracic, and lumbar spine in trauma patients who have sustained multisystem blunt injury is the standard of care. For patients with normal mentation and no distracting injuries, such spinal immobilization is not necessary in the absence of specific evidence of spinal injury. In the older population, these standards must apply not only in trauma situations but also during acute medical problems in which attempts to maintain airway patency are a priority. Degenerative arthritis of the cervical spine may subject the older patient to spinal cord injury from positioning and manipulating the neck to manage the airway, even without injury to the bony spine. EMS providers must know their local protocols, in addition to understanding the potential value of immobilizing the spine.

A cervical collar applied to an older patient with severe kyphosis should not compress the airway or carotid arteries. Less traditional means of immobilization, such as a rolled towel and head block, may be preferable if standard collars are inappropriate for the specific patient.

Padding may need to be placed under the patient's head and between the shoulders when immobilizing the kyphotic supine older patient (**Figure 15-5**). In systems that have access to one, the vacuum mattress can mold to the patient's anatomy to reduce pressure points and to provide appropriate support and greater comfort. Because of the thin skin and lack of *adipose tissue* (fat) in the frail, older patient, these patients are more likely to develop pressure (*decubitus*) ulcers from lying on their back.

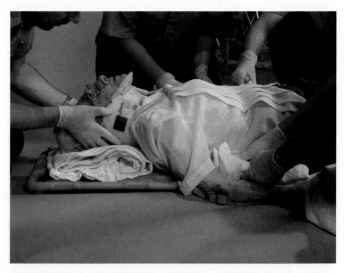

Figure 15-5 Immobilization of a kyphotic patient.
© Jones & Bartlett Learning.

Additional padding may be necessary when the patient is immobilized on a long backboard. It is always a good idea to check for pressure points when the patient is resting on the board and pad appropriately. When applying the straps to secure the patient, the older patient may not be able to straighten his or her legs fully because of decreased range of motion of the hips and knees. This may require the placement of padding under the legs for comfort and security of the patient during transport.[34]

Temperature Control

The older patient should be monitored closely for hypothermia and hyperthermia during treatment and transport. Although it is appropriate to expose the patient to facilitate a thorough examination, older persons are especially prone to heat loss. Once the physical examination is complete, the patient should be covered with a blanket or other available covering to preserve body heat.

The effects of various medications, such as those used to treat Parkinson disease, depression, psychosis, and nausea, may make a patient more prone to overheating. Cooling measures should be considered if the patient cannot be moved quickly to a controlled environment. (See the Environmental Trauma I: Heat and Cold chapter for a detailed discussion of management of hyperthermia.)

Prolonged extrication in the extremes of heat and cold may place the older patient at risk and should be rapidly addressed. External methods of heating or cooling the older trauma patient should be balanced by the possibility of direct thermal injury to the site of application with the patient's attenuated skin structure. Therefore, a sheet or some of the patient's clothing should be placed between the heat or cooling source and the patient's skin.

Legal Considerations

Several legal considerations can become issues when providing care to the older trauma patient. In most of the United States, spouses, siblings, children, spouses of children, and parents have no legal standing in making medical decisions for an adult. Persons with power of attorney or court-appointed conservators may have authority over an individual's financial affairs, but they do not necessarily have control over that individual's personal medical decisions. Court-appointed custodians or guardians may or may not have the power to make medical decisions, depending on the local laws and the specific charge of their appointment. Such powers are considered to exist only when a guardianship of person or a durable power of attorney for health care is specified and clear documentation of such third-party powers is present.

While providing care on a trauma scene, it may be difficult to make such a fine legal distinction. Because the ambulance was summoned and a "call for help" was made, the concept of "implied consent" to care for the patient applies in cases of patients who are unconscious or have reduced mental capacity. If relatives object to the actions of the prehospital care providers or attempt to interfere with care of the patient, law enforcement should be summoned to the scene to assist in dealing with the relatives. In addition, the providers can contact their medical direction and have their online supervising physician speak directly with the relatives. Documentation within the patient's medical record should clearly reflect the decisions made by the providers on scene.

Reporting Elder Abuse

As of 2017, in all states except New York, health care workers, including prehospital care providers, are legally bound to report cases of suspected elder maltreatment to the authorities. Should further clarification be necessary or anyone attempt to interfere with the prehospital care, law enforcement should be called to the scene (if not already present) and the problem presented to the police officer in charge. The law generally provides a protocol for a law enforcement officer to make a timely decision at the scene, with clarification to occur later at the hospital when time allows. Such events should be documented carefully and completely as a part of the EMS medical record.

Elder Maltreatment

Elder abuse is defined as any action by an older person's relative, associated daily household contact (housekeeper, roommate), professional caregiver, or anyone relied upon for daily necessities who takes advantage of the victim's property or emotional state.

Reports and complaints of abuse, neglect, sexual assault, and other related problems among older adults are increasing. The exact extent of elder abuse is not known for the following reasons:

1. Elder abuse has been largely hidden from society.
2. Abuse and neglect of older persons have varying definitions.
3. Elders are reluctant to report the problem to law enforcement agencies or social welfare personnel. A typical victim of elder abuse may be a parent who feels ashamed or guilty because he or she raised the abuser. The abused may also feel traumatized by the situation or fear continued reprisal by the abuser.
4. Some jurisdictions lack formal reporting mechanisms. Some areas do not even have a statutory provision requiring the reporting of elder abuse.

The physical and emotional signs of abuse are often overlooked or perhaps are not accurately identified. Older women are less likely to report incidents of sexual assault to law enforcement agencies. Sensory deficits, dementia, and other causes of mental status change (e.g., medications) may make it difficult or impossible for the victim to accurately report the maltreatment.

Profile of the Abused

Studies have shown an increased association for abuse among patients with the following characteristics[35]:

- Age > 80 years
- Female gender
- Presence of more than three medical conditions
- African American race
- Limited social network
- Annual income > $15,000
- Difficulty with climbing stairs
- Cognitive impairment (Mini-Mental Status Examination score < 23)
- Depression

Profile of the Abuser

The abuser is frequently the spouse of the patient or the middle-aged child or in-law of the patient who is caring for dependent children and dependent parents. Most of these abusers are inadequately trained in the care required and have little relief time from the constant demands of their family. The usual profile of the abuser also includes a history of prior legal troubles as well as unemployment.[36]

Abuse is not restricted to the home. Other environments such as nursing, convalescent, and continuing care centers are sites where the older adults may sustain physical, emotional, or pharmacologic harm. Care providers in these environments may consider older persons to represent management problems or categorize them as obstinate or undesirable patients.

Categories of Maltreatment

Abuse can be categorized in the following ways:

1. *Physical abuse* includes assault, neglect, malnutrition, poor maintenance of the living environment, and poor personal care. The signs of physical abuse or neglect may be obvious, such as the imprint left by an item (e.g., fireplace poker), or may be subtle (e.g., malnutrition). The signs of elder abuse are similar to those of child abuse (**Figure 15-6**). (See the Pediatric Trauma chapter.)

2. *Psychological abuse* can take the forms of neglect, verbal abuse, infantilizing, or deprivation of sensory stimulation.

3. *Financial abuse* can include theft of valuables or embezzlement.

4. *Sexual assault and/or abuse.*

5. *Self-abuse.*

Important Points

Many abused patients are terrorized into making false statements for fear of retribution or because they wish to protect the individual. In the case of elder abuse by family members, fear of removal from the home environment can cause the older patient to lie about the origin of the abuse. In other cases of elder abuse, sensory deprivation or dementia may impair adequate explanation. The prehospital care provider should identify abuse and uncover

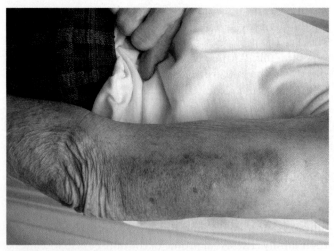

Figure 15-6 Bruises in varying stages of healing are highly suggestive of physical abuse. For example, if a 70-year-old man were brought from his caregiver's home to the ED with bruises such as the ones depicted here, prehospital care providers would need to consider the possibility of abuse.

© Photofusion/Universal Images Group/Getty Images.

Box 15-5 Reporting Elder Abuse and Neglect

In most states, EMS personnel are legally mandated reporters of suspected elder (or adult) abuse, neglect, and exploitation. Mandated reporters must report directly to the social services agency responsible for investigating adult abuse rather than relying on intermediaries such as hospital personnel. If the individual is in immediate danger or has been sexually assaulted, law enforcement must be notified as well. In the event of a death that appears to be the result of abuse or neglect, mandatory reporters must notify the office of the medical examiner or coroner and law enforcement.

Mandatory reporters are liable for failing to report suspected abuse, neglect, and exploitation. They are protected against civil and criminal liability associated with reporting and may be able to keep their identities confidential. Reporting individuals are allowed to share medical information that is pertinent to the case, even though this information would be protected under the Health Insurance Portability and Accountability Act (HIPAA) in normal circumstances. Laws governing the mandatory reporting of elder abuse are enacted at the state level. All prehospital care providers must be aware of the laws in the state in which they work.

---

any pathology reported by the patient. Any history of maltreatment or findings consistent with it should be documented on the patient care report.

Further trauma to a patient may be reduced by identifying and reporting an abusive situation. A high index of suspicion for abuse can allow for referral to protective services from social services and public safety agencies (**Box 15-5**).

Disposition

One of the greatest challenges with prehospital care of the injured patient is defining which patients are most likely to benefit from specialized trauma care and advanced treatment options available at a trauma center. For many of the reasons mentioned previously, traditional triage criteria may be less reliable in the older patient because of physiologic changes or effects of medications. A recommendation from the *Geriatric Trauma Practice Management Guideline* of the Eastern Association for the Surgery of Trauma is that prehospital care providers treating trauma patients of advanced age should consider transport to a trauma center.[37] The Centers for Disease Control and Prevention's *Guidelines for Field Triage of Injured Patients* also recommends that trauma patients over the age of 55 years be considered for transport to a trauma facility.[38]

Because of the differences between injured older and younger patients, and the differences in outcomes, much work is being done to determine if unique criteria are needed to identify older adults who need to be transported to a trauma center. While some studies have shown that using geriatric-specific triage criteria increased the number of older adults meeting criteria for transport to a trauma center, others have failed to demonstrate any increase.[39,40]

Prolonged Transport

The majority of care for the older trauma patient follows the general guidelines for prehospital care of any injured patient. However, several special circumstances exist in prolonged transport scenarios. For example, geriatric patients with less significant anatomic injuries should be triaged directly to trauma centers.

Treatment of shock in the prehospital environment over an extended period requires careful reassessment of vital signs during transport. After control of hemorrhage with local measures, fluid resuscitation should be titrated to physiologic response to optimize resuscitation of intravascular volume status while avoiding potential volume overload in a patient with impaired cardiac function.

Immobilization on a long backboard places the geriatric patient at increased risk for pressure-related skin breakdown over extended transports. Weakened skin structure and impaired vascular supply may lead to earlier complications than in younger trauma patients. Prior to a long transport, consideration should be given to logrolling a patient onto an appropriately padded long backboard or ambulance cot to protect the patient's skin. Agencies in remote regions should consider purchasing a specially designed, low-pressure backboard or vacuum mattress that immobilizes the patient while limiting the potential for skin breakdown.

Environmental control is essential in geriatric patients with a lengthy transport. Limiting body exposure and controlling the ambient temperature of the vehicle are important to limit hypothermia and prevent its complications.

Finally, transport of the geriatric trauma patient from remote regions may be a valid use of aeromedical transport. Transport via helicopter may limit the duration of environmental exposure, reduce the duration of shock, and ensure earlier access to trauma center care, including early surgery and blood transfusion.

Prevention

Given the emergence of mobile integrated health care and community paramedicine programs, prehospital providers may have an increased role in trauma prevention efforts. Many current community paramedicine programs have a specific focus on patients with chronic medical conditions, many of whom are older patients. These programs may represent a unique opportunity to identify safety hazards, such as fall risks, for older patients and allow for education and/or interventions to help prevent injury. EMS systems and providers should consider these types of programs to improve the health of their communities.

SUMMARY

- The older adult population is growing rapidly.
- Although general guidelines for care of the injured patient remain the same, several specific approaches are unique to care of the injured geriatric patient.
- Anatomic and physiologic changes associated with aging, chronic disease, and medications can make certain types of trauma more likely, complicate traumatic injuries, and cause a decreased ability to compensate for shock. Older patients have less physiologic reserve and tolerate physical insult poorly.
- Knowledge of the older trauma patient's medical history and medications is an essential component of care.
- Many factors in geriatric trauma patients can mask early signs of deterioration, increasing the possibility of sudden, rapid decompensation without apparent warning.
- With an older trauma patient, more serious injury may have occurred than indicated by the initial presentation.
- Prehospital care providers should recognize the signs of elder abuse and report any suspicions to the proper authority.
- A lower threshold for direct triage of these patients to trauma centers is important.

SCENARIO RECAP

Your unit is dispatched to the home of a 78-year-old woman who has fallen down a flight of stairs. Her daughter states that they had spoken on the telephone just 15 minutes earlier and that she was coming to her mother's house to take her to do some shopping. When she got to the house, she found her mother on the floor and called for an ambulance.

Upon initial contact, you find the patient lying at the bottom of a flight of stairs. You note that the patient is an older woman whose appearance matches her reported age. While maintaining in-line stabilization of the spine, you note that the patient is unresponsive to your commands. She has a visible laceration of the forehead and an obvious deformity of the left wrist. She is wearing a Medic Alert bracelet that indicates that she has diabetes.

- Did the fall cause the change in mental status, or was there an antecedent event?
- How do the patient's age, medical history, and medications interact with the injuries received to make the pathophysiology and manifestations different from those in younger patients?
- Should advanced age alone be used as an additional criterion for transport to a trauma center?

SCENARIO SOLUTION

When dealing with trauma in the older patient, it cannot always be determined immediately if the trauma was the primary event or was secondary to a medical event, such as a stroke, myocardial infarction, or syncopal episode. Prehospital providers should look for signs of a preceding medical event that may have led to a traumatic injury.

Your primary survey reveals that this patient is maintaining a patent airway and is breathing at a rate of 16 breaths/minute. There is no major external hemorrhage, and the bleeding from the forehead laceration is easily controlled with pressure. The patient's heart rate is 84 beats/minute, and blood pressure is 154/82 mm Hg. You manually control the head and spine and immobilize the patient to a long backboard using appropriate padding underneath the patient. Because the patient is known to have diabetes, you check her blood sugar to see if there is a correctable cause for her altered mentation. Given her age, the apparent head trauma, and the magnitude of the fall, you transport her emergently to the closest trauma center.

References

1. U.S. Census Bureau. State and county quick facts. https://www.census.gov/quickfacts/fact/table/US#viewtop. Accessed February 21, 2018.

2. Mather M, Jacobsen L, Pollard K, Population Reference Bureau. Aging in the United States. *Popul Bull*. 2015;70(2). http://www.prb.org/pdf16/aging-us-population-bulletin.pdf. Accessed February 21, 2018.

3. United Nations, Department of Economic and Social Affairs, Population Division. *World Population Prospects: The 2015 Revision; Key Findings and Advance Tables*. New York, NY: United Nations; 2015.

4. Champion H, Copes WS, Sacco WJ, et al. The Major Trauma Outcome Study: establishing national norms for trauma care. *J Trauma*. 1990;30(11):1356.

5. Hashmi A, Ibrahim-Zada I, Rhee P, et al. Predictors of mortality in geriatric trauma patients: a systematic review and meta-analysis. *J Trauma Acute Care Surg*. 2014;76(3):894-901.

6. Lane P, Sorondo B, Kelly JJ. Geriatric trauma patients: are they receiving trauma center care? *Ann Emerg Med*. 2003;10(3):244-250.

7. Centers for Disease Control and Prevention, National Center for Injury Prevention and Control, Web-Based Injury

Statistics Query and Reporting System (WISQARS). Ten leading causes of death by age group, United States—2010. https://www.cdc.gov/injury/wisqars/LeadingCauses.html. Updated May 2, 2017. Accessed February 21, 2018.

8. American College of Surgeons Committee on Trauma. *Advanced Trauma Life Support for Doctors, Student Course Manual*. 9th ed. Chicago, IL: American College of Surgeons; 2012:272-284.

9. Caterino J, Brown N, Hamilton M, et al. Effect of geriatric-specific trauma triage criteria on outcomes in injured older adults: a statewide retrospective cohort study. *J Am Geriatr Soc*. 2016;64(10):1944-1951.

10. Jacobs D. Special considerations in geriatric injury. *Curr Opin Crit Care*. 2003;9(6):535.

11. U.S. Department of Health and Human Services, Centers for Disease Control and Prevention, National Center for Health Services. Hospitalizations for patients aged 85 and over in the United States, 2000-2010. 2015. https://www.cdc.gov /nchs/data/databriefs/db182.pdf. Accessed February 21, 2018.

12. Roberts D, McKay M, Shaffer A. Increasing rates of emergency department visits for elderly patients in the United States, 1993 to 2003. *Ann Emerg Med*. 2008;51(6): 769-774.

13. Jones C, Wasserman E, Li T, et al. The effect of older age on EMS use for transportation to an emergency department. *Prehosp Disaster Med*. 2017;13:1-8.

14. Milzman DP, Boulanger BR, Rodriguez A, et al. Pre-existing disease in trauma patients: a predictor of fate independent of age and injury severity score. *J Trauma*. 1992;32:236.

15. Smith T. Respiratory system: aging, adversity, and anesthesia. In: McCleskey CH, ed. *Geriatric Anesthesiology*. Baltimore, MD: Williams & Wilkins; 1997.

16. Bergeon E, Lavoie A, Clas D, et al. Elderly trauma patients with rib fractures are at greater risk of death and pneumonia. *J Trauma*. 2003;54(3):478-485.

17. Deiner S, Silverstein JH, Abrams K. Management of trauma in the geriatric patient. *Curr Opin Anaesthesiol*. 2004;17(2):165.

18. Carey J. *Brain Facts: A Primer on the Brain and Nervous System*. Washington, DC: Society for Neuroscience; 2002.

19. Alzheimer's Association. 2017 Alzheimer's disease facts and figures. *Alzheimer's Dement*. 2017;13:325-373.

20. U.S. Department of Health and Human Services, National Institutes of Health, National Eye Institute. Facts about cataracts. https://nei.nih.gov/health/cataract/cataract_facts. Reviewed September 2015. Accessed February 21, 2018.

21. EPOS Group. Incidence of vertebral fracture in Europe: results from the European Prospective Osteoporosis Study (EPOS). *J Bone Miner Res*. 2002;17:716-724.

22. Blackmore C. Cervical spine injury in patients 65 years old and older: epidemiologic analysis regarding the effects of age and injury mechanism on distribution, type, and stability of injuries. *AJR Am J Roentgenol*. 2002;178:573.

23. Tinetti M. Preventing falls in elderly persons. *N Engl J Med*. 2003;348:42.

24. Centers for Disease Control and Prevention. STEADI: Stopping Elderly Accidents, Deaths & Injuries. https://www.cdc .gov/steadi/index.html. Accessed May 4, 2018.

25. Centers for Disease Control and Prevention, National Center for Injury Prevention and Control, Division of Unintentional Injury Prevention. Older adult drivers. https://www.cdc .gov/motorvehiclesafety/older_adult_drivers/index.html. Updated April 7, 2017. Accessed February 21, 2018.

26. National Highway Traffic Safety Administration. Traffic safety facts: 2015 data: pedestrians. https://crashstats.nhtsa .dot.gov/Api/Public/ViewPublication/812375. Published February 2017. Accessed October 25, 2017.

27. National Center for Elder Abuse. Elder abuse and its impact: what you must know. 2013. https://ncea.acl.gov/resources /docs/EA-Impact-What-You-Must-Know-2013.pdf. Accessed February 21, 2018.

28. National Fire Protection Association. Characteristics of home fire victims. 2014. https://www.nfpa.org/News-and-Research /Fire-statistics-and-reports/Fire-statistics/Demographics -and-victim-patterns/Characteristics-of-home-fire-victims. Accessed February 20, 2018.

29. Richmond R, Aldaghlas TA, Burke C, et al. Age: is it all in the head? Factors influencing mortality in elderly patients with head injuries. *J Trauma*. 2011;71(1):E8-E11.

30. Berko J, Ingram D, Saha S, et al. Deaths attributed to heat, cold, and other weather events in the United States, 2006–2010. *Natl Health Stat Rep*. 2014;76.

31. Maher R, Hanlon J, Hajjar E. Clinical consequences of polypharmacy in elderly. *Expert Opin Drug Saf*. 2014;13(1):57-65.

32. Pretorius R, Gataric G, Swedlund S, et al. Reducing the risk of adverse drug reactions in older adults. *Am Fam Physician*. 2013;87(5):331-336.

33. American Geriatrics Society. 2015 Updated Beers criteria for potentially inappropriate medication use in older adults. *J Am Geriatr Soc*. 2015;63(11):2227-2246.

34. National Association of Emergency Medical Technicians, American Geriatrics Society, Snyder, Dr. *Geriatric Education for Emergency Medical Services*. 2nd ed. Burlington, MA: Jones & Bartlett Learning; 2015.

35. Dong X, Simon M. Vulnerability risk index profile for elder abuse in community-dwelling population. *J Am Geriatr Soc*. 2014;62(1):10-15.

36. Amstadter A, Cisler J, McCauley J, et al. Do incident and perpetrator characteristics of elder mistreatment differ by gender of the victim? Results from the National Elder Mistreatment Study. *J Elder Abuse Negl*. 2011;23(1):43-57.

37. Eastern Association for the Surgery of Trauma. *Geriatric Trauma Practice Management Guideline (Update)*. http://www .east.org/content/documents/gpmg-manuscript_2010_final .pdf. Published 2010. Accessed October 25, 2017.

38. Sasser SM, Hunt RC, Faul M. Guidelines for field triage of injured patients: recommendations of the National Expert Panel on Field Triage 2011. *MMWR*. 2012;61(1):1-20.

39. Ichwan N, Darbha S, Shah M, et al. Geriatric-specific triage criteria are more sensitive than standard adult criteria in identifying need for trauma center care in injured older adults. *Ann Emerg Med*. 2015;65(1):92-100.

40. Phillips S, Rond P, Kelly S, et al. The failure of triage criteria to identify geriatric patients with trauma: results from the Florida Trauma Triage Study. *J Trauma*. 1996;40(2):278-283.

Suggested Reading

American College of Surgeons Committee on Trauma. Geriatric trauma. In: *Advanced Trauma Life Support, Student Course Manual.* 9th ed. Chicago, IL: American College of Surgeons; 2012:272-284.

National Association of Emergency Medical Technicians, American Geriatrics Society, Snyder, Dr. *Geriatric Education for Emergency Medical Services.* 2nd ed. Burlington, MA: Jones & Bartlett Learning; 2015.

Reske-Nielsen C, Medzon R. Geriatric trauma. *Emer Med Clin North Am.* 2016;34(3):483-500.

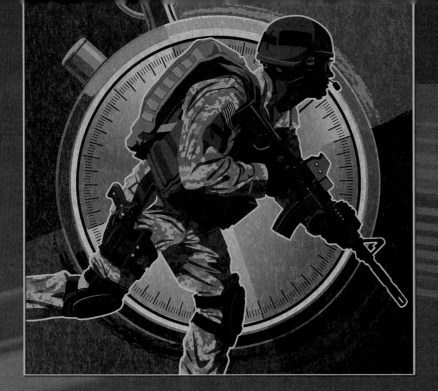

DIVISION **4**

Prevention

CHAPTER **16**　Injury Prevention

Injury Prevention

Lead Editors:
Heidi Abraham, MD, EMT-B, EMT-T, FAEMS
Thomas Colvin, NREMT-P

CHAPTER OBJECTIVES

At the completion of this chapter, you will be able to do the following:

- Describe the concept of energy as a cause of injury.
- Build a Haddon Matrix for a type of injury of interest.
- Relate the importance of accurate, attentive scene observations and documentation of data by prehospital care providers to the success of injury prevention initiatives.
- Assist in the development, implementation, and evaluation of injury prevention programs in your community or emergency medical services (EMS) organization.
- Describe the prevalence of intimate partner violence and what clues EMS should watch for.

- Describe and advocate for the role of EMS in injury prevention, to include:
  - Individual
  - Family
  - Community
  - Professional
  - Organizational
  - Coalitions of organizations
- Identify strategies that prehospital care providers can implement that will reduce the risk of injury.

SCENARIO

You and your partner are on the scene of a motor vehicle collision and are working to rapidly extricate a patient who is overweight from the driver's seat of his vehicle. He was unrestrained in the vehicle during the collision. You and your partner are both wearing approved safety vests over your work gear because you are near the roadway. Law enforcement is on the scene to provide traffic control, and the ambulance is parked to maximize your protection from oncoming vehicles. The patient is properly secured onto your motorized stretcher, which is being used due to the patient's weight. The motorized stretcher allows you and your partner to lift the patient safely into the ambulance without putting excess strain on your bodies.

Once inside the ambulance, you secure yourself in the rear-facing chair and continue care of the patient while your partner operates the siren and the strobe-flashing lights of the ambulance to attract other drivers' attention. She maneuvers safely into her lane and drives to the hospital. The ambulance arrives safely at the hospital, and you transfer the patient to the care of the emergency department staff.

(continued)

SCENARIO (CONTINUED)

While completing paperwork after the call, you consider the overall national injury and death statistics for prehospital care providers. You realize that thanks to the careful attention to all aspects of injury prevention that you and your partner demonstrated, the call was concluded safely for everyone involved.

- Is accident prevention a realistic approach in preventing injury and death in motor vehicle collisions and other causes of traumatic injury?
- Is there evidence that compliance with seat belt and safety seat laws has an impact in preventing injury and death?
- As prehospital care providers, what can we do to prevent deaths and injuries from motor vehicle collisions?

INTRODUCTION

A major impetus in the development of modern emergency medical services (EMS) systems was the publication of the 1966 white paper by the National Academy of Sciences/National Research Council (NAS/NRC), *Accidental Death and Disability: The Neglected Disease of Modern Society*. The paper spotlighted shortcomings in injury management in the United States and helped launch a formal system of on-scene care and rapid transport for patients injured as a result of "accidents." This educational initiative was instrumental in the creation of a more efficient system to deliver prehospital care to sick and injured patients.[1]

The incidence of death and disability from injury in the United States has fallen since the publication of the white paper.[2] Despite this progress, however, injury remains a major public health problem. Nearly 200,000 Americans die from injuries annually, and millions more are adversely affected to some degree.[3,4] Injuries remain a leading cause of death for all age groups.[5,6] For some age groups, particularly children, teenagers, and young adults, injury is the leading cause of death.[7]

Injury is a global problem as well. Over five million people worldwide die from injuries annually.[5] Globally, a person dies from an injury every 6 seconds.[5]

The desire to care for patients stricken by injury draws many into the field of EMS. The Prehospital Trauma Life Support (PHTLS) course teaches prehospital care providers to be efficient and effective in injury management. The need for well-trained providers to care for injured patients will always exist. However, the most efficient and effective method to combat injury is to prevent it from happening in the first place. Health care providers at all levels play an active role in injury prevention to achieve the best results for not only the community at large but also for themselves.

In 1966, the authors of the NAS/NRC white paper recognized the importance of injury prevention when they wrote:

The long-term solution to the injury problem is prevention. . . . Prevention of accidents involves training in the home, in the school, and at work, augmented by frequent pleas for safety in the news media; first aid courses and public meetings; and inspection and surveillance by regulatory agencies.[1]

Prevention of some diseases, such as rabies or measles, has been so effective that the occurrence of a single case makes front-page news. Public health officials recognize that prevention results in the greatest benefit toward the amelioration of disease. Curricula for prehospital care providers have long included formal instruction in scene safety and personal protective equipment as a means of self-injury prevention for the emergency medical technician (EMT). To spur EMS systems to take a more active role in community prevention strategies, the *EMS Agenda for the Future*, developed by and for the EMS community, lists prevention as one of 14 attributes to develop further in order to "improve community health and result in more appropriate use of acute health resources."[8] To this end, the National EMS Education Standards include community injury prevention.

EMS systems are transforming themselves from a solely reactionary discipline to a broader, more effective discipline that includes additional aspects, such as community paramedicine, and places more emphasis on prevention. This chapter introduces key concepts of injury prevention to the prehospital care provider.

Concepts of Injury

Definition of Injury

A discussion of injury prevention should begin with a definition of the term **injury**. Injury is now commonly defined as a harmful event that arises from the release of specific forms of physical energy or barriers to the normal flow of energy.[9] The wide variability of the causes of injury initially represented a major hurdle in its study and prevention. For example, what does a fractured hip caused by an elderly person's fall have in common with a self-inflicted gunshot wound to the head of a young adult? Furthermore, how does one compare a femur fracture from a fall in an older woman to a femur fracture in a young man who crashed his motorcycle? All possible causes of injury—from vehicle crash, to stabbing, to suicide, to drowning—have one factor in common: the transfer of energy to the victim.

Forms of Energy

Energy exists in five physical forms: mechanical, chemical, thermal, radiation, or electrical.

- **Mechanical energy** is the energy that an object contains when it is in motion. For example, mechanical energy, the most common cause of injury, is transferred from a vehicle when an unrestrained driver collides with the windshield during a vehicle crash.
- **Chemical energy** is the energy that results from the interaction of a chemical with exposed human tissue. For instance, chemical energy results in a burn from exposure to an acid or base.
- **Thermal energy** is the energy associated with increased temperature and heat. For example, thermal energy causes injury when a cook sprays lighter fluid on actively burning charcoal in an outdoor grill, which then flashes in his face.
- **Radiation energy** is any electromagnetic wave that travels in rays (such as x-rays) and has no physical mass. Radiation energy produces sunburn in the teenager searching for a golden tan for the summer.
- **Electrical energy** results from the movement of electrons between two points. It is associated with direct injury as well as thermal injury and, for example, damages the skin, nerves, and blood vessels of a prehospital care provider who fails to perform a proper scene assessment before touching a vehicle that hit a utility pole.

Any form of physical energy in sufficient quantity can cause tissue damage. The body can tolerate energy transfer within certain limits; however, an injury results if this threshold is exceeded.

Energy Out of Control

People harness and use all five forms of energy in many productive endeavors every day. In these situations, energy is under control and is not allowed to affect the body adversely. A person's ability to maintain control of energy depends on two factors: task performance and task demand.[10] As long as a person's ability to perform a task exceeds the demands of a task, energy is released in a controlled, usable manner.

In the following three situations, however, demand may exceed performance, leading to an uncontrolled release of energy:

1. *When the difficulty of the task suddenly exceeds the individual's performance ability.* For example, a prehospital care provider may operate an ambulance safely during normal driving conditions but loses control when the vehicle hits a sheet of black ice. The sudden increase in the demands of the task exceeds the provider's performance capabilities and leads to a crash.

2. *When the individual's performance level falls below the demands of the task.* A person who falls asleep at the wheel of a vehicle while driving down a country road experiences a sudden drop in performance with no change in task demand, leading to a crash.

3. *When both factors change simultaneously.* Talking on a cellular phone while driving may reduce a driver's concentration on the road. If an animal darts in front of the vehicle, task demand suddenly rises. Under normal circumstances, the driver may be able to handle the increased demands of the task. A drop in concentration at the very moment when additional skill is required may lead to a crash.

Thus, injury may result when there is a release of energy in an uncontrolled manner in proximity to victims.

Injury as a Disease

The disease process has been studied for years. It is now understood that three factors must be present and interact simultaneously for an illness to occur: (1) an agent that causes the illness, (2) a host in which the agent can reside, and (3) a suitable environment in which the agent and host can come together. Once public health professionals recognized this "epidemiological triad," they discovered how to combat disease (**Figure 16-1**). Eradication of certain infectious diseases has been possible by vaccinating the host, destroying the agent with antibiotics, reducing environmental transmission through improved sanitation, or a combination of all three.

Only since the late 1940s has significant exploration of the **injury process** occurred. Pioneers in the study of injury

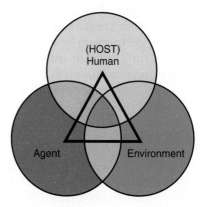

Figure 16-1 Epidemiological triad.
© National Association of Emergency Medical Technicians (NAEMT).

demonstrated that despite the obviously different results, illness and injury are remarkably similar. Both require the presence of the three elements of the epidemiological triad, and therefore, both are treated as a disease:

1. For an injury to occur, a host (i.e., the human) must exist. As with illness, susceptibility of the host does not remain constant from individual to individual; it varies as a result of internal and external factors. *Internal* factors include intelligence, gender, and reaction time. *External* factors include intoxication and social beliefs. Susceptibility also varies over time within the same person.

2. As described previously, the agent of injury is *energy*. Velocity, shape, material, and time of exposure to the object that releases the energy all play a role in whether the host's tolerance level is overwhelmed.

3. The host and agent must come together in an environment that allows the two to interact. Typically, the environment is divided into physical and social components. *Physical* environmental factors can be seen and touched. *Social* environmental factors include attitudes, beliefs, and judgments. For example, teenagers are more likely to participate in risk-taking behavior (the physical component) because they have a greater sense of invincibility (the social component) than other age groups.

The characteristics of the host, agent, and environment change with time and circumstance. Public health professionals Tom Christoffel and Susan Scavo Gallagher describe this dynamic as follows:

> To illustrate, think of the components of the Epidemiological Triad as constantly turning wheels. Inside each wheel are pie-shaped sections, one for each possible circumstantial variable—good and bad. The three wheels turn at different rates, so different characteristics interact (meet) at different times and in different combinations. Some combinations predict that no injury will occur; some predict disaster.[11]

In the case of injury, the host might be a curious, mobile 2-year-old child; the agent of injury might be a swimming pool filled with water with a beach ball floating just beyond the edge; the environment might be a pool gate left open while the babysitter runs inside to answer the telephone. With the host, agent, and environment all coming together at the same time, an unintentional injury—in this case, drowning—can occur.

Haddon Matrix

Dr. William J. Haddon, Jr., is considered the father of the science of injury prevention. Working within the concept of the epidemiological triad, in the mid-1960s, he recognized

that an injury can be broken down into the following three temporal phases:

1. *Pre-event:* Before the injury
2. *Event:* The point when harmful energy is released
3. *Postevent:* The aftermath of the injury (see also the PHTLS: Past, Present, and Future chapter)

By examining the three factors of the epidemiological triad during each temporal phase, Haddon created a nine-cell "phase-factor" matrix (**Table 16-1**). This grid has become known as the **Haddon Matrix**. It provides a means to depict graphically the events or actions that increase or decrease the odds that an injury will occur. It can also be used to identify prevention strategies. The Haddon Matrix demonstrates that *multiple* factors can lead to an injury, and therefore, multiple opportunities exist to prevent or reduce its severity. The matrix played a major role in dispelling the myth that injury is the result of a single cause, bad luck, or fate.

Table 2-1 depicts a Haddon Matrix for an ambulance crash. The components in each cell of the matrix are different, depending on the injury being examined. The *pre-event phase* includes factors that can contribute to the likelihood of a crash; however, energy is still under control. This phase may last from a few seconds to several years. The event phase depicts the factors that influence the severity of the injury. During this time, uncontrolled energy is released, and injury occurs if energy transfer exceeds the body's tolerance. The *event phase* is typically very brief; it may last only a fraction of a second and rarely lasts more than a few minutes. Factors in the *postevent phase* affect the outcome once an injury has occurred. Depending on the type of event, it may last from a few seconds to the remaining life span of the host. (See also the PHTLS: Past, Present, and Future chapter.)

As mentioned previously, a key purpose of the Haddon Matrix is to recognize injury risks so that injury can be avoided. Public health programs have adopted the terminology of primary, secondary, and tertiary prevention.

- *Primary prevention* is aimed at avoiding the injury before it occurs. This type of prevention activity involves education programs to help minimize risk-taking behaviors and the use of protective equipment such as helmets, child safety seats, and vehicle restraint systems.
- *Secondary prevention* refers to those actions taken to prevent the progression of an acute injury once it has occurred—for example, avoiding the occurrence of hypoxia or hypotension after a traumatic brain injury or correcting it as rapidly as possible if it already is present.
- *Tertiary prevention* is directed at minimizing death and the long-term disability following an injury (or disease). Active and aggressive rehabilitation programs fall into this category.

Table 16-1 Haddon Matrix for an Ambulance Crash

| | Epidemiological Triad | | |
Time Phases	Host Factors	Agent Factors	Environment Factors
Pre-event	Driver's visual acuity Experience and judgment Amount of time in the ambulance per shift Level of fatigue Proper nutrition Stress level Adherence to company and community driving laws Quality of driver education courses	Maintenance of brakes, tires, etc. Defective equipment Ambulance's high center of gravity Speed Ease of control	Visibility hazards Road curvature and gradient Surface coefficient of friction Narrow road shoulder Traffic signals Speed limits
Event	Safety belt use Physical conditioning Injury threshold Ejection	Speed capability Ambulance size Automatic restraints Hardness and sharpness of contact surfaces Hardness and sharpness of loose items (e.g., clipboards, flashlights) Steering column Practice of safe driving habits: speed, use of lights/siren, passing, intersections, backing Practice of good partner habits en route: watching road, clearing intersections Safe parking	Lack of guardrails Median barriers Distance between roadway and immovable objects Speed limits Other traffic Attitudes about safety belt use Maintaining an escape route Making no assumptions about an environment being safe (e.g., "nice part of town," high-income home) Weather
Postevent	Age Physical condition Type or extent of injury	Fuel system integrity Entrapment	Emergency communication capability Distance to and quality of responding EMS Training of EMS personnel Availability of extrication equipment Trauma care system of the community Rehabilitation programs in the community

Swiss Cheese Model

British psychologist James Reason proposed another way of thinking about how accidents occur.[12] He likened the process to Swiss cheese. In every situation, a hazard exists that has the potential to cause injury or allow an error to occur. There are usually a series of safeguards or barriers to prevent this from happening. He suggested that each of these barriers or safeguards is like a piece of Swiss cheese. The holes in the cheese are flaws or failures that increase the potential for a hazard or error to cause injury. These flaws may be the result of deficiencies in the organization or administration or may occur following oversight of the system (latent conditions), or they may occur as a result of acts of omission or commission (active failures). Reason argued that every hazard has a trajectory, that a series of failures generally must occur in order for there to be subsequent harm, and that the trajectory must be such that it intersects with holes or failures that have aligned to allow all of the safeguards to fail and injury to occur (**Figure 16-2**).[12]

Classification of Injury

A common method to subclassify injuries is based on intent. Injury may result from either intentional or unintentional causes. Although this is a logical way to view injuries, it underscores the difficulty of injury prevention efforts.

Intentional injury is typically associated with an act of interpersonal or self-directed violence. Problems such as homicide, suicide, assault, sexual assault, domestic violence, child abuse, and war fall into this category.

In the past, **unintentional injuries** were called accidents. The authors of the NAS/NRC white paper appropriately referred to accidental death and disability; this was the vocabulary of the time.[1] Because we now believe that specific factors must come together for an injury to occur, health care providers now realize that the term *accidental* may not accurately portray the degree of preventability associated with unintentional injury resulting from events such as vehicle crashes, drownings, falls, and electrocutions. EMS systems have embraced this concept by using the term *motor vehicle collisions* or *crashes* (often abbreviated

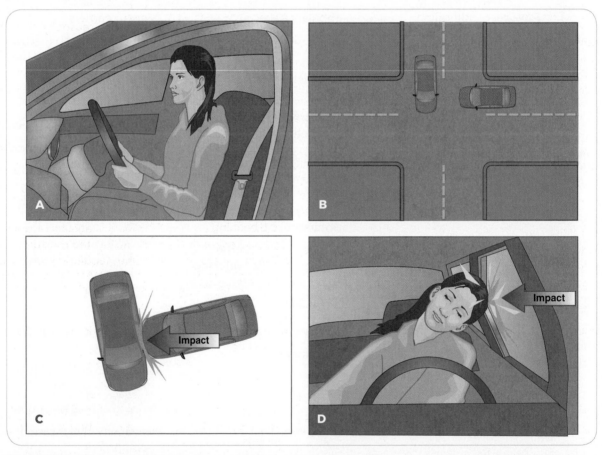

Figure 16-2 The Swiss Cheese model states that in every situation, a hazard exists that has the potential to cause injury or allow an error to occur. For example: **A.** The driver does not buckle her seatbelt. **B.** The driver in the green vehicle enters an intersection with an on-coming red vehicle. **C.** The red vehicle collides into the green vehicle. **D.** The side-curtain airbags in the green vehicle do not deploy and the driver strikes the window with her head.

MVCs) rather than *motor vehicle accidents* (MVAs). However, public use of terminology has changed much more slowly. News reporters still describe persons injured in automobile accidents or accidental shootings. The term *accident* suggests that a person was injured as a result of fate, divine intervention, or bad luck. It implies that the injury was random and, therefore, unavoidable. The use of alternative language is intended to drive people to consider preventability in assessing incidents associated with injury.

It is also important to note that there may be overlap between these two common classifications of injury.[13] For example, a motor vehicle collision may have resulted from a driver attempting to commit suicide. Classifying the incident as a motor vehicle crash alone implies no intent on the part of the driver to harm, whereas knowledge of the suicidal ideation of the driver clearly implies intent to cause the crash or collision.

Scope of the Problem

Injuries are a major health problem worldwide, resulting in close to 5 million deaths annually (**Box 16-1**), with road traffic accidents causing approximately 1.3 million, suicide nearly 800,000, and interpersonal violence around 520,000.[5,14-16] Causes of injury-related deaths vary among countries, both in terms of mechanism and age group impacted. Because of economic, social, and developmental issues, the causes of injury-related death vary from country to country and even from region to region within the same country.

For example, in low-income and middle-income countries of the Western Pacific, the leading injury-related causes of death are road traffic injuries, drowning, and suicide, whereas in Africa the leading causes are road traffic injuries, war, and interpersonal violence. In high-income countries of the Americas, the leading cause of death among people

---

Box 16-1 Worldwide Injury-Related Statistics, 2014 Fact Sheets[5,14,15]

Injury Overall

- The top eight injury-related causes of mortality, in order, were:
  1. Road traffic injuries
  2. Self-inflicted violence
  3. Falls
  4. Interpersonal violence
  5. Drowning
  6. Fire-related burns
  7. Poisonings
  8. War
- Injuries accounted for 9% of the world's deaths and 16% of all disabilities.
- For persons aged 15 to 29 years, three of the top 10 leading causes of death were injury related.
- Road traffic injuries are predicted to become the seventh leading cause of death by 2030.
- Twice as many men die from injury as women; fire-related deaths are the notable exception.
- Males in Africa have the highest injury-related mortality rates.
- About 90% of all injury-related deaths occur in low-income and middle-income countries.
- Injury accounts for 12% of the total years of potential life lost either from premature death or from disability.

Road Traffic Injury

- An estimated 1.25 million people died as a result of road traffic injuries, and as many as 50 million more were injured or disabled.

- Road traffic injury is the leading cause of death for children and youth aged 15 to 29 years.
- Road traffic mortality for males under the age of 25 is almost three times higher than for females.
- Africa accounts for the highest percentage of road traffic injury deaths.

Fire-Related Burns

- An estimated 265,000 deaths every year are caused by burns; the vast majority occur in low- and middle-income countries.
- Females in Southeast Asia have the highest fire-related burn mortality rates.
- Children younger than 5 years of age and elderly persons have the highest fire-related mortality rates.
- The incidence of burn injuries requiring medical care is nearly 20 times higher in the WHO Western Pacific Region than in the WHO Region of the Americas.

Drowning

- In 2015, an estimated 360,000 people died from drowning.
- 97% of drowning deaths occurred in low- and middle-income countries.
- Among the various age groups, children younger than 5 years of age have the highest drowning mortality rates, accounting for more than 50%.
- In the United States of America, drowning is the second leading cause of unintentional injury death in children aged 1 to 14 years.

(continued)

Box 16-1 Worldwide Injury-Related Statistics, 2014 Fact Sheets[5,14,15] (*continued*)

- Males in Africa and the Western Pacific have the highest drowning mortality rates.

Falls
- It is estimated that 424,000 people die as a result of falls annually.
- Over 80% of fall-related fatalities occur in low- and middle-income countries.
- In all regions of the world, adults older than 65 years of age, particularly women, have the highest fall mortality rate.
- Over 80% of fall-related fatalities occur in low- and middle-income countries, with regions of the Western Pacific and South East Asia accounting for more than two-thirds of these deaths.

Poisoning
- According to WHO data, in 2012 an estimated 193,460 people died worldwide from unintentional poisoning.
- It is estimated that deliberate ingestion of pesticides causes 370,000 deaths each year.
- More than 80% of fatal poisonings occurred in low- and middle-income countries.
- The overall poisoning rate among males in Europe is approximately three times higher than the rate in either gender in any other world region.
- The European region accounts for more than one-third of all poisoning deaths worldwide.

- Snakebite is a largely unrecognized public health problem. While reliable data are hard to obtain, it has been estimated that about 5 million snakebites occur each year, resulting in up to 2.5 million envenomations, at least 100,000 deaths, and around three times as many amputations and other permanent disabilities.

Interpersonal Violence
- An estimated 520,000 people died worldwide as a result of interpersonal violence.
- 95% of homicides occurred in low- and middle-income countries.
- The highest interpersonal violence rates are found in the Americas among males aged 15 to 29 years.
- Among females, Africa has the highest mortality rate from interpersonal violence.

Suicide
- Close to 800,000 people worldwide committed suicide.
- 78% of all suicides occurred in low- and middle-income countries.
- While men commit suicide more often than women in most of the rest of the world, women in China are about 40% more likely to commit suicide than men.
- More than 50% of suicides occur in persons aged 15 to 44 years.

Source: Figures compiled from World Health Organization (WHO). 2014 data fact sheets.

between 15 and 29 years of age is road traffic injuries. For this same age group in low-income and middle-income countries of the Americas, the leading cause is interpersonal violence.[6] **Figure 16-3** demonstrates that injury plays a leading role in the global burden of disease.

In 2014, over 33,000 people in the United States died in motor vehicle collisions.[17] Close to 10,000 people were killed in alcohol-related driving crashes, accounting for nearly one-third of all traffic-related deaths in the United States.[18] Nearly 4 million drivers and passengers were treated in the emergency department (ED) after a motor vehicle collision in 2010.[19] In the United States, unintentional injuries are the overall fourth leading cause of death, accounting for approximately 200,000 deaths annually[20] (**Table 16-2**). Injury is an especially serious problem for the youth of America as well as of most industrialized nations of the world. In the United States, injury kills more children and young adults than all diseases combined and remains

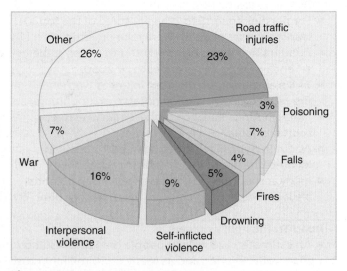

Figure 16-3 Distribution of global injury mortality by cause.

Data from WHO Global Burden of Disease project, 2002, Version 1.

Table 16-2 Ranking of Causes of Injury-Related Deaths by Age Group, 2015

	Age Group										All Ages (number of deaths)
	<1	1-4	5-9	10-14	15-24	25-34	35-44	45-54	55-64	65+	
Unintentional Injury	5th	Leading	Leading	Leading	Leading	Leading	Leading	3rd	3rd	7th	4th (146,571)
Intentional Injury											
Suicide	*	*	*	3rd	2nd	2nd	4th	5th	8th	*	10th (44,193)
Homicide	*	3rd	4th	4th	3rd	3rd	5th	*	*	*	*

*Data not applicable/available or not included in the top 10 causes of death.

Source: Extracted from National Vital Statistics System, National Center for Health Statistics, Centers for Disease Control and Prevention (CDC), Office of Statistics and Programming, National Center for Injury Prevention and Control. Ten leading causes of death by age groups, United States—2010. https://www.cdc.gov/injury/images/lc-charts/leading_causes_of_death_age_group_2015_1050w740h.gif. Accessed September 21, 2017.

the leading cause of death for people 1 to 44 years old.[7] Of the deaths in children under 19 years of age, 65% occur due to unintentional injury.[21]

Unfortunately, deaths from injury are only the tip of the iceberg. The "injury triangle" provides a more complete picture of the **public health impact of injury (Figure 16-4)**. In the United States in 2014 nearly 200,000 individuals died from injury, and another 2.5 million were hospitalized because of nonfatal injuries. Injury also resulted in more than 26.9 million ED visits.[3,4]

The impact can be further realized by examining the number of **years of potential life lost (YPLL)** as a result of injury. YPLL is calculated by subtracting age at death from a fixed age of the group under examination, usually 65 or 70 years or the life expectancy of the group. Injury kills or disables people of all ages, but it disproportionately affects children, youth, and young adults, especially in industrialized nations. Because injury is the leading killer of Americans between 1 and 44 years of age, it is responsible for more YPLL than any other cause of death. In 2015, injury stole an estimated 3.8 million *years* from its victims compared with 1.7 million years for cancer, even though cancer claims more *lives* than injury.[3,22]

A third measure of injury severity can be demonstrated financially. The economics of injury are felt far beyond the patient and the immediate family. The cost of injury is spread across a wide spectrum. All members of society feel the effect because the costs of injury are borne by federal and other agencies, private insurance programs that pass the expense on to other subscribers, and employers as

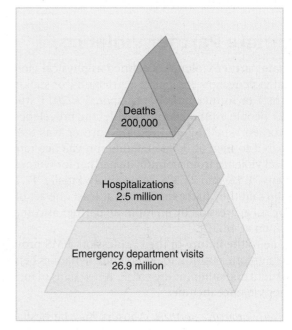

Figure 16-4 Injury triangle.

Data from the US Department of Health and Human Services, Centers for Disease Control and Prevention, National Center for Health Statistics. All injuries. https://www.cdc.gov/nchs/fastats/injury.htm.

Centers for Disease Control and Prevention, National Center for Injury Prevention and Control, Web-based Injury Statistics Query and Reporting System. Nonfatal injury reports, 2000–2015. https://webappa.cdc.gov/sasweb/ncipc/nfirates.html.

well as the patient. As a result, everyone pays when an individual is seriously injured. In 2013, the CDC estimated the cost for injury at $671 billion for direct costs of medical care and indirect costs such as lost earnings.[23] Data from the World Health Organization (WHO) indicate that prevention activities are a good investment:

- Every U.S. dollar invested in motorcycle helmets results in a $32 savings of medical costs.
- Seat belts decrease the risk of ejection and of sustaining serious or fatal injury by 40% to 65% and have saved an estimated 255,000 lives between 1975 and 2008.[24]

The toll of injury in terms of morbidity, mortality, and economic stress is excessive. As stated by Maguire and colleagues:

> Injuries have always been a threat to the public's well-being, but until the mid-twentieth century, infectious diseases overshadowed the terrible contribution injury made to human morbidity and mortality. Public health's success in other areas has left injury as a major public health concern, one that has been termed "the neglected epidemic."[25]

Society is calling on all segments of the medical community to increase its prevention activities. With as many as 840,600 prehospital care providers in the United States alone, according to the American Ambulance Association, EMS systems can make a tremendous contribution to community-based injury prevention efforts.

Intimate Partner Violence

Intimate partner violence is defined as physical violence, sexual violence, psychological aggressions, or stalking by a current or former intimate partner.[26] A 2011 study of 12,727 people estimated that the lifetime prevalence rate for women raped by an intimate partner was 8.8% as compared to men at 0.5%. Lifetime prevalence rates for physical violence from an intimate partner for women and men are 31.5% and 27.5%, respectively. Finally, 47.1% of women said they had experienced at least one act of psychological aggression by an intimate partner as compared with men at 46.5%.[27]

Due to the nature of their profession, EMS providers are in a unique position to observe the dynamics between the patient and others at the scene. A few signs of intimate partner violence include:

- *Overly protective partners.* Abusers may be hesitant to leave their victim alone when they feel their victim might talk about the abuse.
- *Jealous or controlling behavior from the abuser.*
- *Overly timid patient.* You might encounter patients who avoid all eye contact or defer to their partner when asked a question.
- *Unexplained injuries or repeated injuries.* The patient may be unwilling to explain black eyes or bruising to the neck, may present with bruising to the body at various stages of healing, or may have a history of broken bones.

You should report any suspicions of intimate partner violence to the appropriate law enforcement agency. Remember, EMS providers are also in a unique position to become secondary victims on these calls. Pay particularly close attention to your own safety on these calls at all times and maintain a high level of situational awareness.

Injury to EMS Personnel

EMS personnel are exposed to a wide variety of situations that can result in provider injury. Scenes are often unsecured, despite the best efforts of EMS personnel and law enforcement, because these scenes involve people in emotional and physical crisis. There are regular reports of EMS providers being assaulted on the job, shot at, or otherwise targeted. The very nature of the emergency work presents many opportunities for injury. Just driving to the scene can be hazardous. Lifting, exposure to environmental hazards and infectious diseases, sleep deprivation, and the stress of the job also present significant opportunities for injury. The tragic situations encountered often contribute to posttraumatic stress disorder (PTSD), which can have significant physical effects on providers, as well as causing additional psychological stress.

Sleep deprivation is an important factor that clearly affects prehospital care provider performance.[28] The longer a person is awake, the greater the resulting fatigue and drowsiness; the greater the impairment in reaction time, medical decision making, and judgment; and the greater the likelihood of mistakes, injury to self or others, and even fatality.[29] Sleep deprivation has been compared to alcohol intoxication, with no sleep for 18 hours approximating a blood alcohol concentration (BAC) of 0.05 and no sleep for 24 hours approximating a BAC of 0.1.

In addition, sleep deprivation can have profound effects on the health of the prehospital care provider and can interfere with important personal and family relationships. Lack of sleep can lead to irritability, anxiety, and depression.

A study published in 2011 reviewed fatal and nonfatal injuries to EMTs and paramedics during the period from 2003 to 2007.[30] The authors reviewed data from the Bureau of Labor Statistics Census of Fatal Occupational Injuries as well as the occupational portion of the National Electronic Injury Surveillance System. For that time period, they found 99,400 nonfatal injuries and 65 fatalities. Most of the fatalities were transportation related, either motor vehicle collisions (45%) or aircraft crashes (31%). The fatality rate for full-time equivalents EMS workers was 7.0 per 100,000.[31] Among paid EMS personnel in general, the fatality rate was 6.3 per 100,000.[30] In comparison, the fatality rate for fire fighters was 6.1 per 100,000 and for all workers was 4.0 per 100,000 during this same period.[31] The only good news in this report is that the fatality figure is lower than that documented in the report from 10 years prior.

These numbers reveal a disturbing truth. According to Garrison:

> . . . the most dangerous times for EMS personnel are when they are inside their ambulance when it is moving or when they are working at a crash scene near other moving vehicles.[32]

It is critical that EMS personnel know and understand the concepts of injury and injury prevention so that the risks inherent in EMS can be identified and corrected. From the first day of training, students are taught that no one is more important at the scene than the prehospital care provider, so his or her safety must come first. Seat belt use in the ambulance is the first step toward safety.

The National EMS Culture of Safety project was prompted by a recommendation in 2009 from the National Emergency Medical Services Advisory Council (NEMSAC) for the Department of Transportation's National Highway Traffic Safety Administration (NHTSA) to create a strategy for improved safety in EMS. The American College of Emergency Physicians (ACEP) and the EMS for Children (EMSC) program along with other key players from fire and EMS groups were part of the project that agreed on a strategy involving six key elements:

- Just culture, which encourages reporting of mistakes and near-misses, so that errors can be avoided in the future
- Coordinated support and resources among agencies across the nation
- A responder and patient safety data system, allowing for better understanding of the scope of some of these issues
- Evolution of EMS education to include better training on these topics
- Promulgation of safety standards based on good evidence
- Incident reporting and investigation[33]

Prevention as the Solution

The ideal is to prevent an injury from occurring in the first place, thus obviating the need to treat it after it occurs. When injury is prevented, it spares the patient and family from suffering and economic hardship. The National Center for Injury Prevention and Control (NCIPC) of the Centers for Disease Control and Prevention (CDC) estimates the following:

- $1 spent on smoke detectors saves $69.
- $1 spent on bicycle helmets saves $29.
- $1 spent on child safety seats saves $32.
- $1 spent on center and edge lines on roads saves $3 in medical costs alone.
- $1 spent on counseling by pediatricians to prevent injuries saves $10.
- $1 spent on poison control center services saves $7 in medical expenses.[3]

In addition to the NCIPC's findings:

- A CDC-funded evaluation study of a regional trauma care system in Portland, Oregon, found a 35% decrease in the risk of dying for severely injured patients who were treated in the system.[34]
- A smoke detector distribution program in Oklahoma reduced burn-related injuries by 80%.[35]

Because of the variability among the host, agent, and environment at any given time, health care providers cannot always predict or prevent every individual injury. However, it is possible to identify high-risk populations (which include prehospital care providers), high-risk products, and high-risk environments. Prevention efforts focused on high-risk groups or settings influence as wide a range of society as possible. Health care providers can pursue prevention in multiple ways. Some strategies have proven successful across the United States and around the world. However, other strategies work in one region but not in another. Before implementing an injury prevention strategy, efforts must focus on determining whether it will work. Although it is not necessary to "reinvent the wheel," health care providers may need to modify a prevention strategy to improve its chances of success. Methods for doing this are examined in the following section.

Concepts of Injury Prevention

Goal

The goal of injury prevention programs is to bring about a change in knowledge, attitude, and behavior on the part of a previously identified segment of society. Simply providing information to potential victims is not enough to prevent injury. A program must be implemented in a manner that will influence society's attitude and—most important—change behavior. The hope is that any change in behavior will be long term. This task is monumental but not insurmountable.

Opportunities for Intervention

Prevention strategies can be arranged according to their effect on the injury event. They coincide with the temporal phases of the Haddon Matrix. Pre-event interventions, known as primary interventions, strive to prevent the injury from occurring. Actions intended to keep intoxicated drivers off the road, laws to prevent texting while driving, and measures to install traffic lights are designed to prevent crashes from occurring. Event phase interventions are intended to reduce injury severity by softening the blow of injuries that occur. Requiring safety belts, installing cushioned dashboards and air bags in vehicles, and enforcing child safety seat laws are means to reduce the severity of injury sustained in crashes. Postevent interventions provide a means to improve the likelihood of survival for those who are injured. Encouraging physical fitness, designing fuel systems for vehicles that do not explode on impact, and implementing high-quality EMS systems are intended to reduce the recovery time for persons who are injured.

Prehospital systems have traditionally limited their community involvement to the postevent phase. Countless lives have been saved as a result. However, because of the limitations inherent in waiting until injury has occurred, the best results have not been achieved. EMS systems must explore entering the injury cycle earlier. Using the Haddon Matrix, EMS systems can identify opportunities to collaborate with other public health and public safety organizations to prevent injuries from occurring or to soften their blow.

Potential Strategies

No single strategy provides the best approach to injury prevention. The most effective options depend on the type of injury under study. However, Haddon developed a list of 10 generic strategies designed to break the chain of injury-producing events at numerous points (**Table 16-3**). These strategies represent ways that the release of uncontrolled energy can be prevented, or at least reduced, to amounts the body can better tolerate. Table 16-3 also presents countermeasures that can be taken in the pre-event, event, and postevent phases and that are directed toward the host, agent, or environment. This list is not complete and merely serves as a starting point to help determine the most effective options for the particular problem under study.

Most injury prevention strategies are either active or passive. **Passive strategies** require little or no action on the

Table 16-3 Basic Strategies for Injury Countermeasures	
Strategy	**Possible Countermeasures**
Prevent initial creation of the hazard.	Do not produce firecrackers, three-wheeled all-terrain vehicles, or various poisons. Eliminate spearing in high school football.
Reduce amount of energy contained in the hazard.	Limit the horsepower of motor vehicle engines. Package toxic drugs in smaller, safer amounts. **Obey speed limits.** Mandate improved public transportation to reduce the number of privately owned vehicles on the road. **Encourage reduction of temperature on home hot water heaters.** Limit the muzzle velocity of guns. Limit the amount of gunpowder in firecrackers.
Prevent release of a hazard that already exists.	**Store firearms in locked containers or use gun locks.** Close pools and beaches when no lifeguard is on duty. **Encourage use of nonslip surfaces in bathtubs and showers.** **Require childproof containers for all hazardous household drugs and chemicals.** **Limit cell phone use in vehicles, or use hands-free models.** Require safety shields on rotating farm machinery. Improve vehicle handling.
Modify rate or spatial distribution of the hazard.	**Require use of seat belts and child safety seats.** Provide antilock brakes. Encourage use of short cleats on football shoes so feet rotate rather than transmit sudden force to the knees. Require vehicle air bags. Provide hydraulic bumpers on vehicles. Provide safety harnesses to protect workers from falls. **Encourage use of flame-retardant pajamas.**

Table 16-3 Basic Strategies for Injury Countermeasures (*continued*)

Strategy	Possible Countermeasures
Separate in time or space the hazard from that which is to be protected.	Provide pedestrian overpasses at high-volume crossings. Keep roadsides clear of poles and trees. Do not have play areas near unguarded bodies of water. Install bike paths. Spray pesticides at a time when people are not present. Install sidewalks. Route trucks carrying hazardous material along low-density roads. **Encourage use of smoke detectors in the home.**
Separate the hazard from that which is to be protected by a material barrier.	Install fencing around all sides of swimming pools. **Encourage use of protective eyewear for sports and occupational hazards.** Build highway medians. Build protective shields around hazardous machinery. Install guardrails between sidewalks and roads. Install reinforced panels in vehicle doors. **Require health care workers to place used needles directly into a sharps container.** **Require use of helmets for motorcyclists, bicyclists, and high-risk sporting activities.**
Modify basic nature of the hazard.	Provide air bags in motor vehicles. Provide collapsible steering columns. Provide breakaway poles. Make crib slats too narrow to strangle a baby. Adopt breakaway baseball bases. **Remove throw rugs in homes of the elderly.**
Make what is to be protected more resistant to the hazard.	**Encourage calcium intake to reduce osteoporosis.** **Promote campaigns such as Stop the Bleed, hands-only CPR, and other educational events to teach the public how to mitigate emergencies.** Encourage musculoskeletal conditioning in athletes. Prohibit alcohol sales and consumption near recreational water areas. Treat medical conditions such as epilepsy to prevent episodes that can result in burns, drownings, and falls. Check earthquake-resistant building codes in susceptible areas.
Begin to counter the damage already done by the hazard.	**Provide emergency medical care.** **Stock AEDs in public locations such as airports, gyms, and schools.** Employ systems to route injured persons to appropriately trained prehospital care providers. **Develop school protocols for responding to injury emergencies.** **Provide first-aid training to residents.** Install automatic sprinkler systems.
Stabilize, repair, and rehabilitate the object of the damage.	Develop rehabilitation plans at an early stage of injury treatment. Make use of occupational rehabilitation for paraplegic patients.

*The examples listed are for illustrative purposes only and are not necessarily the official recommendations of PHTLS, the National Association of EMTs, or the American College of Surgeons Committee on Trauma.

Bold indicates opportunities for EMS personnel to provide education and leadership.

part of the individual; sprinkler systems and vehicle air bags are examples. **Active strategies** require the cooperation of the person being protected; examples include manual seat belts and choosing to wear a motorcycle or bicycle helmet. Passive measures are generally more effective because people do not need to consciously do anything to take advantage of the protection. Nonetheless, passive strategies are usually more difficult to implement because they can be expensive or require legislative or regulatory action. Sometimes a combination of active and passive strategies is the best option.

Strategy Implementation

Three common approaches to implementing an injury prevention strategy have become known as the Three Es of injury prevention—education, enforcement, and engineering. Each of these elements is described here.

Education

Educational strategies are meant to impart information. The target audience may be individuals who engage in high-risk activities, policy makers who have the authority to enact further prevention legislation or regulation, or prehospital care providers learning to become active participants in injury prevention.

Education once was the primary means of implementing prevention programs because society believed that most injuries were simply the result of human error. Although this assumption is true to a certain extent, many failed to recognize the role that energy and the environment play in causing injury. Education is still often used, however, and is probably the easiest of the three strategies to implement.

Experience has demonstrated that educational strategies have not met with overwhelming success for several reasons. For starters, the target audience may never hear the message. If the message is heard, some may reject it outright or not embrace it enough to alter behavior. Those who embrace it may do so sporadically or with declining enthusiasm over time.[36] However, education still can be particularly useful in reducing injury in the following four areas:

1. *Teaching young children basic safety behaviors and skills that stay with them later in life.* Examples include responding appropriately when a smoke detector sounds an alarm, calling 9-1-1 for help in an emergency, or fastening seat belts.
2. *Teaching about certain types and causes of injuries for certain age groups.* Education may be the only strategy available for these groups.
3. *Altering the public's perception of risk and acceptable risk to change social norms and attitudes.* This approach was used regarding drinking and driving and occurs now regarding wearing a helmet when riding a bicycle, scooter, or skateboard or using rollerblades.
4. *Promoting policy change and educating consumers to demand safer products.*[37]

As a singular approach to injury prevention, educational programs have had disappointing results. Like many drugs, education needs to be "re-dosed" after a period of time in order to have a continued effect. However, when coupled with other forms of implementation strategies, education can be a valuable tool. Education often serves as a starting point to pave the way for enforcement and engineering strategies.

Enforcement

Enforcement seeks to tap the persuasive power of law to compel adherence to simple but effective prevention strategies. Statutory commands can either require or prohibit, and they can be directed at individual behavior (people), products (things), or environmental conditions (places), as follows:

- Legal requirements that apply to people are mandatory seat belt, child restraint, and helmet laws.
- Prohibitions that apply to people are drunk driving laws, speed limits, and assault laws.
- Legal requirements that apply to products include design and performance standards, such as the federal Motor Vehicle Safety Standards.
- Prohibitions that apply to products include restrictions on dangerous animals and flammable fabrics.
- Legal requirements that apply to places include the installation of breakaway signposts along highways and fencing around swimming pools.
- Prohibitions that apply to places include the outlawing of firearms in schools and airport terminals.
- Legal requirements that apply to specific target groups and locations include the federal requirements that public safety and emergency responders wear high-visibility clothing at high-traffic crash sites.[25]

Enforcement is also an active countermeasure because people must obey the law to benefit from it. The target audiences may be less likely to comply if they believe the directive infringes on personal freedom, if they have little chance of getting caught, or if they will not face consequences of violating the law.

Because society as a whole tends to obey laws or at least stay within narrow limits around them, enforcement is often more effective than education. Enforcement in tandem with education appears to produce better results than either initiative alone. Motorcycle helmet laws provide an interesting case study in the role of enforcement in injury prevention. In states in which helmet laws have been repealed for motorcyclists, the rate of serious injuries and fatalities has increased.[38-40]

Engineering

Often the most effective means of injury prevention are those in which destructive energy release is permanently separated from the host. Passive countermeasures accomplish this goal with little or no effort on the part of the individual. Engineering strategies strive to build injury prevention into products or environments so that the host does not have to act differently to be protected. Engineering strategies help the people who actually need them, and they do so every time. Measures such as automatic sprinkler systems in buildings, flotation hulls in boats, and backup alarms on ambulances all are intended to save lives with little or no effort on the part of the host.

Engineering seems to be the perfect answer to injury prevention. It is passive, effective, and usually the least disruptive of the Three Es. Unfortunately, it is often the most expensive to implement. Designing safety into a product usually makes it more expensive and may require legislative or regulatory initiation. The price may be more than the manufacturer is willing to absorb or the customer is willing to pay. Society dictates how much safety it wants built into a product and how much it is willing to support the endeavor financially.

Education initiatives should precede enforcement and engineering strategies. Ultimately, the most effective countermeasures may be those that incorporate all three implementation strategies.

Public Health Approach

Much has been learned about injury and injury prevention. Unfortunately, a wide discrepancy exists between what is known about injury and what is being done about it.[41] Injury is a complex problem in all societies of the world. Unfortunately, a single person or single agency alone will usually have little impact. A public health approach has achieved success in dealing with diseases and is making progress with injury prevention as well. EMS agencies that have joined forces with other public and private organizations have been able to accomplish as much as or more than they could on their own. Partnerships bring together a community's expertise to tackle a complex and perplexing issue.

A public health approach creates a community-based coalition to combat a community-based disease through a four-step process, as follows:

1. Surveillance
2. Risk factor identification
3. Intervention evaluation
4. Implementation

The coalition comprises experts from such diverse fields as epidemiology, the medical community, schools of public health, public health agencies, community advocacy programs, economics, sociology, and criminal justice. EMS systems have an important place in a public health approach to injury prevention. Participating in a coalition to improve playground safety may not have the immediate effect of providing care at the scene of a horrific vehicle crash, but the results will be much more widespread.

Surveillance

Surveillance is the process of collecting data within a community. Collection of population-based data aids in the discovery of an injury's true magnitude and effect on the community. A community can be a neighborhood, city, county, state, or even the ambulance service itself. Support for the program, proper allocation of resources, and even knowing who to include on the interdisciplinary team depend on understanding the scope of the problem.

Sources of information available within a community include the following:

- Mortality data
- Hospital admission and discharge statistics
- Medical records
- Trauma registries
- Police reports
- EMS run sheets
- Insurance reports
- Unique surveillance data collected solely for the study at hand

Risk Factor Identification

After a problem is identified and researched, it is necessary to know who is at risk to direct a prevention strategy at the correct population. "Shotgun" approaches to injury prevention are less successful than targeted ones. Identification of causes and risk factors determines who is injured; what types of injuries are sustained; and where, when, and why those injuries occur.[42] Sometimes a risk factor is obvious, such as the presence of alcohol in fatal vehicle crashes. At other times, research is required to discover the true risk factors involved in injury events. EMS systems can serve as the "eyes and ears" of public health at the scene of injuries to identify risk factors that no one else may be able to uncover. Risk factors can then be charted on a Haddon Matrix as they are properly identified.

Intervention Evaluation

As risk factors become clear, intervention strategies begin to emerge. Haddon's list of 10 injury prevention strategies serves as a starting point (see Table 16-3). Even though communities have different characteristics, with modification, an injury prevention initiative from one community may work in another. Once a potential intervention has been selected, a pilot program using one or more of the Three Es may give indications of the success of full-scale implementation.

Implementation

The final step in the public health approach is implementation and evaluation of the intervention. Detailed implementation procedures are prepared so others interested in implementation of similar programs will have a guide to follow. Collection of evaluation data measures the effectiveness of a program. Answering the following three questions may help determine the success of a program:

1. Have attitudes, skills, or judgment changed?
2. Has behavior changed?
3. Does behavioral change lead to a favorable outcome?[9]

The public health approach provides a proven means to combat a disease such as injury. Through a multidisciplinary, community-based effort, it is possible to identify the "who, what, where, when, and why" of an injury problem and develop a plan of action. EMS systems need to play a much more substantial role in helping to close the gap between what is known about injury and what is being done about it. This approach can be thought of as a continuous loop. Continued surveillance occurs after implementation of an injury control strategy. These data are then used to modify or change the strategy. Successes in injury prevention can be broadened to wider populations at risk.

Evolving Role of EMS in Injury Prevention

Traditionally, the role of the prehospital care provider in health care focuses almost exclusively on postevent, one-on-one treatment of the individual. Little emphasis is placed on understanding the causes of the injuries or what a provider could do to prevent them. As a result, patients may return to the same environment only to be injured again. In addition, information that could aid in the development of a communitywide prevention program to keep others from becoming injured in the first place may not be documented and, therefore, may remain unavailable to other sectors of public health.

The public health approach to injury is more proactive. It works to determine how to alter the host, agent, and environment to prevent injuries. Through coalitions that conduct surveillance and implement interventions, public health works to develop communitywide prevention programs. The Emergency Medical Services Agenda for the Future envisions closer ties between EMS systems and public health that would make both sectors of health care more effective.[8] The practice of community paramedicine is one way that EMS has become more involved in this aspect of injury (and illness) prevention.

Prehospital care providers can take a more active role in the development of communitywide injury prevention programs. EMS systems enjoy a unique position in the community. With approximately 840,600 providers in the United States alone, basic and advanced providers are widely distributed at the community level. Providers enjoy a credible reputation in the community, making them high-profile role models. In addition, they are readily welcomed into homes and businesses. All phases of the public health approach to injury prevention benefit from an EMS presence.

One-on-One Interventions

EMS systems do not have to give up their one-on-one approach to patient care to conduct valuable injury prevention interventions. The one-on-one approach makes EMS systems uniquely able to conduct injury prevention initiatives. Prehospital care providers can bring injury prevention messages directly to high-risk individuals. One indicator of a successful educational program is that the information is received with enough enthusiasm to change behavior. Providers can use their role model status to deliver important prevention messages. Implicitly, people look up to role models, listen to what they have to say, and emulate what they do.

On-scene prevention counseling takes advantage of a "teachable moment." A teachable moment is the time when a patient who does not require critical medical interventions or the patient's family members are in a state that makes them more receptive to what a role model says. The prehospital care provider may think of the on-scene time as wasted when it becomes apparent that little or no medical interventions are necessary. However, this may be the best time to deliver primary prevention.[43]

Not every call allows for injury prevention counseling. Serious and life-threatening calls require concentration on acute care. However, as many as 95% of ambulance calls are not life threatening. A significant proportion of EMS calls require minor, if any, treatment. One-on-one prevention counseling may be appropriate during these noncritical calls.

Patient interactions are typically short encounters, especially those that require little or no treatment. However, they provide enough time to discuss and demonstrate to patients and family members practices that may prevent an injury in the future. Prehospital care providers are in a unique position in that they are the only health care worker who enters the patient's environment, thereby viewing situations that may predispose to injury. A role model who discusses the importance of replacing a burned-out lightbulb and removing a slippery throw rug in a dimly lit hallway may prevent a fall by an elderly resident. Providers have an attentive audience during the ride to a hospital. Prevention is a more valuable topic to discuss than the weather or the local sports team. Teachable moments take 1 to 2 minutes to complete and do not interfere with treatment or transport.

Educational programs have been developed to train prehospital care providers to administer on-scene injury prevention counseling.[44] These types of programs must be further developed and evaluated to discover which are the most valuable and, therefore, worthy of inclusion in the primary education of a provider.

Communitywide Interventions

The public health approach to injury prevention is community based and involves a multidisciplinary team. Prehospital care providers have the expertise to be valuable members of that team. Communitywide prevention strategies depend on data to address properly the "who, what, when, where, and why" of an injury problem. Multiple sources of information, as described previously, provide the needed data. Providers, perhaps more than any other team member, have the opportunity to examine patient interaction with the environment at the time of the injury. This may allow identification of a high-risk individual, high-risk attitude, or high-risk behavior that is not present by the time the patient arrives at the ED.

The prehospital care provider can use documentation acquired en route to a medical facility in the following two ways:

1. Data can be used immediately by emergency personnel who receive the patient. Emergency physicians and nurses are also being called on to improve and increase their role in injury prevention. Their "teachable moment" can reinforce and supplement the provider's on-scene counseling if they know what has already been discussed or demonstrated.

2. Others in public health can use injury data from providers retrospectively to help develop a comprehensive, communitywide injury prevention program.

Prehospital care providers usually do not practice documentation to help support a communitywide prevention program. Knowing what to acquire and when to document information beneficial to the development of communitywide prevention programs requires opening a dialogue with other members of the public health team. Leaders in the EMS system need to build a coalition with others in public health to develop documentation policies that promote complete documentation of injuries.

EMS can be the spearhead for workable, effective injury prevention programs that make a profound impact in a community. Programs have been created out of the desire of a small group of EMS professionals to prevent childhood fatalities.[45,46] Services and individuals in North Carolina, Florida, South Carolina, Oregon, and Virginia have been recognized for their efforts in designing, coordinating, and conducting injury prevention programs through the Nicholas Rosecrans Award for best practices in injury prevention in EMS.[47,48]

While opportunities exist for prehospital care providers to educate patients, one study by Dr. David Jaslow and colleagues suggests that a minority of prehospital providers utilize the teachable moment. They found that only 33% routinely educate their patients on how to modify injury risk behaviors, and only 19% routinely provide instruction about proper use of protective devices.[48]

Injury Prevention for EMS Providers

"Who's the most important person at an incident scene?" EMS students are always asked this question early in their training to make them think about their own safety. Invariably, one or two students will say "the patient," which is what the instructor wanted to hear. This incorrect response provides a teachable moment for the instructor to begin the course-long directive to reinforce the point that self-injury prevention is the most valuable service a prehospital care provider can deliver.

Hostile environments resulting from terrorist activities or hazardous materials spills unfortunately make the news too often. Many terrorist attacks include secondary explosions designed to kill or injure first responders as they are arriving on the scene. However, even the everyday activities of prehospital providers provide sufficient opportunity for injuries that could end a career or life. The Bureau of Labor Statistics paints an accurate picture of the "normal" dangers in EMS:

> EMTs and paramedics work both indoors and outdoors, in all types of weather. They are required to do considerable kneeling, bending, and heavy lifting. These workers risk noise-induced hearing loss from sirens and back injuries from lifting patients. In addition, EMTs and paramedics may be exposed to diseases such as hepatitis-B and AIDS, as well as violence from drug overdose victims or mentally unstable patients. The work is not only physically strenuous but also stressful, involving life-or-death situations and suffering patients.[49]

Prehospital care providers are at substantial risk for injury or death while responding to, managing the patient at, and transporting from an emergency medical call. The risks associated with injury both on scene and in a moving ambulance can be minimized by utilizing proper preventive measures such as seat belts or reflective clothing.

Prehospital care providers can become complacent toward the everyday dangers of the job. Complacency is a feeling of security or safety in the unacknowledged face of potential danger. Compounding the situation are the idealism and invincibility of youth typical of some EMS personnel.[50] Management is needed to create a culture of injury prevention or, better, a culture of safety by instituting prevention policy, maintaining adherence to procedure, and rewarding positive performance. The providers themselves must be equally committed to the principles of injury prevention. Failure in this initiative by either management or providers can have potentially devastating effects.

Other factors to consider are the experience level of personnel and their degree of fatigue. Drivers must be adequately prepared and trained to operate vehicles safely, and EMS personnel must be monitored to ensure they have adequate sleep to maintain safe operations. In a study that looked at common factors in EMS personnel involved in ambulance crashes, the odds were greater that the drivers involved in emergency vehicle crashes would be younger EMS personnel and those EMS personnel reporting sleep problems.[51]

Dr. Neil Stanley of the British Sleep Society noted, "Nobody should be doing anything really important for 15 to 30 minutes after they wake up." This has serious implications for EMS, considering that EMS personnel must respond immediately, no matter what the time of night, whether awake or asleep, and be expected to function "normally."

In a prehospital service, employees are not only the most valuable asset but also the most expensive. The service, community, and, most important, the prehospital care provider benefit when the employee remains uninjured. An in-house injury prevention program is worthwhile on its own merits. Many EMS and law enforcement agencies are realizing the benefits of having athletic trainers on their staff, for immediate treatment and rehab of injuries. Of these agencies, 96% reported that the athletic trainer made an impact on their workers' compensation costs within 1 year, reducing overall medical costs by as much as 50%. The significantly faster return to duty also has a tremendous psychological benefit for the provider.[52,53]

Dr. Janet Kinnane and colleagues mention in-house prevention programs that utilize education, enforcement, and engineering implementation strategies.[43] The wide variability of the programs demonstrates the dangers involved in EMS systems and the need for prevention initiatives. It also demonstrates the variability among EMS communities. Even though all EMS systems are similar, individual services (communities) have different risk factors and different prevention priorities.

As described previously, education programs enhance wellness, prevent back injury, and increase awareness of the potential for violent patients. Enforcement programs introduce mandatory fitness programs and establish protocols to deal with violent patients. Engineering initiatives address increasing seat belt use in the back of the ambulance by evaluating the position of equipment and location of the seat. Preemployment screening and physical strengthening help to reduce back injury.

A small-scale, in-house injury prevention program may reap rewards beyond the most important outcome of improved employee health. Small successes lay the groundwork for participation in larger, more complicated endeavors. They provide a valuable on-the-job learning tool about injury prevention for all employees. In addition, in-house prevention programs provide an introduction of the EMS system to other public health agencies in the community that assist in in-house program implementation and evaluation.

SUMMARY

- The most efficient and effective method to combat injury is to prevent it from happening in the first place.
- Energy exists in five physical forms: mechanical, chemical, thermal, radiation, or electrical.
  - As long as a person's ability to perform a task exceeds the demands of the task, energy is released in a controlled, usable manner.
  - When energy exceeds this threshold, injury results.
- Illness and injury are similar. Both require the presence of the three elements of the epidemiological triad: host, agent, and environment.
- The Haddon Matrix helps predict injury risk by examining the three factors of the epidemiological triad during each event phase—pre-event, event, and postevent.
- According to the Swiss cheese model, every hazard has a trajectory, and a series of failures generally must occur for there to be subsequent harm.
- Injury is classified as intentional or unintentional.
- Because of economic, social, and developmental issues, the causes of injury-related death vary from country to country and even region to region within the same country.
- Injury is the leading killer of Americans between 1 and 44 years of age. It is responsible for more years of potential life lost than any other cause of death.
- Intimate partner violence is defined as physical violence, sexual violence, psychological

SUMMARY (CONTINUED)

aggressions, or stalking by a current or former intimate partner. Providers must report any suspicions of intimate partner violence to the appropriate law enforcement agency.

- Injury prevention programs seek to bring about a change in knowledge, attitude, and behavior on the part of a previously identified segment of society.
- Most injury prevention strategies are either active (requiring the cooperation of the person being protected) or passive (not requiring conscious effort).
- The Three Es of injury prevention are education, enforcement, and engineering.

- A public health approach creates a community-based coalition to combat a community-based disease through a four-step process: (1) surveillance, (2) risk factor identification, (3) intervention evaluation, and (4) implementation.
- Prehospital care providers can take a more active role in the development of communitywide injury prevention programs. They can use their role model status to deliver important prevention messages and should take advantage of "teachable moments."
- Self-injury prevention is the most valuable service a prehospital care provider can provide.

SCENARIO RECAP

You and your partner are on the scene of a motor vehicle collision and are working to rapidly extricate a patient who is overweight from the driver's seat of his vehicle. He was unrestrained in the vehicle during the collision. You and your partner are both wearing approved safety vests over your work gear because you are near the roadway. Law enforcement is on the scene to provide traffic control, and the ambulance is parked to maximize your protection from oncoming vehicles. The patient is packaged properly and secured onto your motorized stretcher, which is being used due to the patient's weight. The motorized stretcher allows you and your partner to lift the patient safely into the ambulance without putting excess strain on your bodies.

Once inside the ambulance, you secure yourself in the rear-facing chair and continue care of the patient while your partner operates the siren and the strobe-flashing lights of the ambulance to attract other drivers' attention. She maneuvers safely into her lane and drives to the hospital. The ambulance arrives safely at the hospital, and you transfer the patient to the care of the emergency department staff.

While completing paperwork after the call, you consider the overall national injury and death statistics for prehospital care providers. You realize that thanks to the careful attention to all aspects of injury prevention that you and your partner demonstrated, the call was concluded safely for everyone involved.

- Is accident prevention a realistic approach in preventing injury and death in motor vehicle collisions and other causes of traumatic injury?
- Is there evidence that compliance with seat belt and safety seat laws has an impact in preventing injury and death?
- As prehospital care providers, what can we do to prevent deaths and injuries from motor vehicle collisions?

SCENARIO SOLUTION

You and your partner remained safe while at the motor vehicle collision scene because you recalled and followed your department's safety protocols. You were aware that flashing or strobe lights are not always sufficient in attracting drivers' attention, so you wore your approved reflective vests to be more visible to other drivers while operating at the scene. You also recalled and followed proper lifting techniques and safety procedures, and you ensured your safety by wearing a seat belt while in the treatment area of the ambulance.

In addition, your department recently updated the reflective chevron design on the rear of the ambulance to enhance the visibility of the ambulance from a distance. To enhance night-time visibility, red and white lights on the exterior of the ambulance were replaced by additional blue lights. These measures have all proven to be very helpful in reducing scene visibility concerns and ensuring crew member safety.

References

1. National Academy of Sciences/National Research Council. *Accidental Death and Disability: The Neglected Disease of Modern Society*. Washington, DC: National Academy of Sciences/National Research Council; 1966.

2. National Center for Health Statistics. *Health, United States, 2000—With Adolescent Health Chartbook*. Hyattsville, MD: National Center for Health Statistics; 2000.

3. National Center for Health Statistics, Centers for Disease Control and Prevention. All injuries. https://www.cdc.gov/nchs/fastats/injury.htm. Updated May 3, 2017. Accessed August 2, 2017.

4. Centers for Disease Control and Prevention, National Center for Injury Prevention and Control, Web-based Injury Statistics Query and Reporting System. Nonfatal injury reports, 2000-2015. https://webappa.cdc.gov/sasweb/ncipc/nfirates.html. Updated February 19, 2017. Accessed August 2, 2017.

5. World Health Organization. Injuries and violence: the facts 2014. Geneva, Switzerland: World Health Organization; 2014. http://apps.who.int/iris/bitstream/10665/149798/1/9789241508018_eng.pdf?ua=1&ua=1&ua=1. Accessed August 2, 2017.

6. Peden M, McGee K, Sharma G. *The Injury Chart Book: A Graphical Overview of the Global Burden of Injuries*. Geneva, Switzerland: World Health Organization; 2002.

7. Centers for Disease Control and Prevention, National Center for Injury Prevention and Control. Ten leading causes of death by age group, United States—2015. https://www.cdc.gov/injury/wisqars/pdf/leading_causes_of_death_by_age_group_2015-a.pdf. Accessed August 2, 2017.

8. National Highway Traffic Safety Administration, U.S. Department of Health and Human Services, Health Resources and Services Administration, Maternal and Child Health Bureau. *Emergency Medical Services Agenda for the Future*. Washington, DC: National Highway Traffic Safety Administration; 1999.

9. Martinez R. Injury control: a primer for physicians. *Ann Emerg Med*. 1990;19:72-77.

10. Waller JA. *Injury Control: A Guide to the Causes and Prevention of Trauma*. Lexington, MA: Lexington Books; 1985.

11. Christoffel T, Gallagher SS. *Injury Prevention and Public Health: Practical Knowledge, Skills, and Strategies*. Gaithersburg, MD: Aspen; 1999.

12. Reason J. Human error: models and management. *BMJ*. 2000;320:768-770.

13. Cohen L, Miller T, Sheppard MA, Gordon E, Gantz T, Atnafou R. Bridging the gap: bringing together intentional and unintentional injury prevention efforts to improve health and well being. *J Safety Res*. 2003;34:473-483.

14. World Health Organization. Road traffic injuries. http://www.who.int/mediacentre/factsheets/fs358/en/. Updated May 2017. Accessed August 2, 2017.

15. World Health Organization. Suicide. http://www.who.int/mediacentre/factsheets/fs398/en/. Updated May 2017. Accessed August 2, 2017.

16. World Health Organization. Interpersonal violence and alcohol. http://www.who.int/violence_injury_prevention/violence/world_report/factsheets/pb_violencealcohol.pdf. Published 2006. Accessed August 2, 2017.

17. Kochanek KD, Murphy SL, Jiaquan X, Tejada-Vera B. Deaths: final data for 2014. *Natl Vital Stat Rep*. 2016;65(4). https://www.cdc.gov/nchs/data/nvsr/nvsr65/nvsr65_04.pdf. Accessed September 23, 2017.

18. Department of Transportation, National Highway Traffic Safety Administration. *Traffic Safety Facts 2014 Data: Alcohol-Impaired Driving*. Washington, DC: National Highway Traffic Safety Administration; 2015.

19. Albert M, McCaig LF, Centers for Disease Control and Prevention, National Center for Health Statistics. Emergency department visits for motor vehicle traffic injuries: United States, 2010-2011. https://www.cdc.gov/nchs/products/databriefs/db185.htm. Updated January 3, 2015. Accessed September 23, 2017.

20. Centers for Disease Control and Prevention, National Center for Injury Prevention and Control. Fatal injury data. Web-based Injury Statistics Query and Reporting System (WISQARS). https://www.cdc.gov/injury/wisqars/fatal.html. Updated January 22, 2017. Accessed September 23, 2017.

21. Daley BJ. Considerations in pediatric trauma: epidemiology. Medscape. http://emedicine.medscape.com/article /435031-overview# aw2aab6b3. Updated November 4, 2015. Accessed September 23, 2017.

22. Centers for Disease Control and Prevention, National Center for Injury Prevention and Control. WISQARS years of potential life lost (YPLL) report, 1981 and 2015. Web-based Injury Statistics Query and Reporting System (WISQARS). https://webappa.cdc.gov/sasweb/ncipc/ypll.html. Updated February 19, 2017. Accessed June 7, 2017.

23. Centers for Disease Control and Prevention, National Center for Injury Prevention and Control. Key injury and violence data. https://www.cdc.gov/injury/wisqars /overview/key_data.html. Updated September 19, 2016. Accessed June 10, 2017.

24. Houry D. Saving lives and protecting people from injuries and violence. *Ann Emerg Med.* 2016 Aug;68(2):230-232.

25. Cristofell T, Gallagher SS. *Injury Prevention and Public Health: Practical Knowledge Skills and Strategies.* Gaithersburg, MD: Aspen; 1999.

26. National Center for Injury Prevention and Control, Division of Violence Prevention. Intimate partner violence: definitions. https://www.cdc.gov/violenceprevention/intimate partnerviolence/definitions.html. Updated August 22, 2017. Accessed September 23, 2017.

27. Breiding MJ, Smith SG, Basile KC, Walters ML, Chen J, Merrick MT, Centers for Disease Control and Prevention. Prevalence and characteristics of sexual violence, stalking, and intimate partner violence victimization—National Intimate Partner and Sexual Violence Survey, United States, 2011. https://www.cdc.gov/mmwr/preview/mmwrhtml /ss6308a1.htm?s_cid=ss6308a1_e. Updated September 5, 2014. Accessed September 23, 2017.

28. VanDale K. Sleep deprivation in EMS. Fire Engineering website. http://www.fireengineering.com/articles /print/volume-166/issue-02/departments/fireems/sleep -deprivation-in-ems.html. Published February 1, 2013. Accessed September 23, 2017.

29. Patterson PD, Weaver MD, Frank RC, et al. Association between poor sleep, fatigue, and safety outcomes in emergency medical services providers. *Prehosp Emerg Care.* 2012;16:86-97.

30. Reichard A, Marsh S, Moore P. Fatal and nonfatal injuries among emergency medical technicians and paramedics. *Prehosp Emerg Care.* 2011;15(4):511-517.

31. Page D. Studies show dangers of working in EMS. *Journal of Emergency Medical Services.* http://www.jems.com/articles /print/volume-36/issue-11/health-and-safety/studies-show -dangers-working-ems.html. Published October 31, 2011. Accessed September 21, 2017.

32. Garrison HG. Keeping rescuers safe. *Ann Emerg Med.* 2002; 40:633-635.

33. Erich J. Creating a culture of safety. http://www.emsworld .com/article/10833708/ems-culture-of-safety-strategy-project. Published November 26, 2012. Accessed June 1, 2017.

34. Mullins RJ, Veum-Stone J, Helfand M, et al. Outcome of hospitalized injured patients after institution of a trauma system in an urban area. *JAMA.* 1994;271(24):1919-1924.

35. Haddix AC, Mallonee S, Waxweiler R, et al. Cost effectiveness analysis of a smoke alarm giveaway program in Oklahoma City, Oklahoma. *Inj Prev.* 2001;7:276-281.

36. National EMS Advisory Council. Strategy for a national EMS culture of safety (draft). http://www.emscultureofsafety .org/wp-content/uploads/2012/12/Strategy-for-a-National -EMS-Culture-of-Safety-NEMSAC-DRAFT.pdf. Accessed September 23, 2017.

37. Maguire BJ, Huntington KL, Smith GS, Levick NR. Occupational fatalities in emergency medical services: a hidden crisis. *Ann Emerg Med.* 2002;40:6.

38. Mertz KJ, Weiss HB. Changes in motorcycle-related head injury deaths, hospitalizations, and hospital charges following repeal of Pennsylvania's mandatory motorcycle helmet law. *Am J Public Health.* 2008;98(8):1464-1467.

39. Bledsoe GH, Li G. Trends in Arkansas motorcycle trauma after helmet law repeal. *South Med J.* 2005;98(4):436-440.

40. Chenier TC, Evans L. Motorcyclist fatalities and the repeal of mandatory helmet wearing laws. *Accid Anal Prev.* 1987; 19(2):133-139.

41. Centers for Disease Control and Prevention. Ambulance crash-related injuries among emergency medical services workers—United States, 1991-2002. *Morb Mortal Wkly Rep.* 2003;52(8):154-156.

42. Todd KH. *Accidents Aren't: Proposal for Evaluation of an Injury Prevention Curriculum for EMS Providers—A Grant Proposal to the National Association of State EMS Directors.* Atlanta, GA: Department of Emergency Medicine, Emory University School of Medicine; 1998.

43. Kinnane JM, Garrison HG, Coben JH, et al. Injury prevention: is there a role for out-of-hospital emergency medical services? *Acad Emerg Med.* 1997;4:306.

44. EPIC Medics. Speaking engagements. http://www.epicmedics .org/Conferences.html. Accessed September 23, 2017.

45. Hawkins ER, Brice JH, Overby BA. Welcome to the world: findings from an emergency medical services pediatric injury prevention program. *Pediatr Emerg Care.* 2007;23(11): 790-795.

46. Griffiths K. Best practices in injury prevention. *J Emerg Med Serv.* 2002;27:8.

47. Krimston J, Griffiths K. Best practices in injury prevention. *J Emerg Med Serv.* 2003;28:9.

48. Jaslow D, Ufberg J, Marsh R. Primary injury prevention in an urban EMS system. *J Emerg Med.* 2003;25(2):167-170.

49. U.S. Department of Labor. Emergency medical technicians and paramedics. In: U.S. Department of Labor, Bureau of Labor Statistics, eds. *Occupational Outlook Handbook,*

2004-2005 Edition. Washington, DC: U.S. Department of Labor; 2004.

50. Federal Emergency Management Agency, U.S. Fire Administration. *EMS Safety: Techniques and Applications*. International Association of Fire Fighters, FEMA contract EMW-91-C-3592. Washington, DC: Federal Emergency Management Agency; 1994.

51. Studnek JR, Fernandez AR. Characteristics of emergency medical technicians involved in ambulance crashes. *Prehosp Disaster Med*. 2008;23(5):432-437.

52. Kilpatrick D. Athletic trainers: a new hope for firefighter recovery. Fire Engineering website. www.fireengineering .com/articles/print/volume-169/issue-12/features/athletic -trainers-a-new-hope-for-firefighter-recovery.html. Published December 1, 2016. Accessed 12 June 2017.

53. Kilpatrick D. The cost efficiency of athletic trainers. Fire-house website. www.firehouse.com/article/12268580/the -cost-efficiency-of-athletic-trainers. Published December 1, 2016. Accessed June 12, 2017.

Suggested Reading

American College of Surgeons Committee on Trauma. *Advanced Trauma Life Support for Doctors, Student Course Manual*. 10th ed. Chicago, IL: American College of Surgeons; 2018.

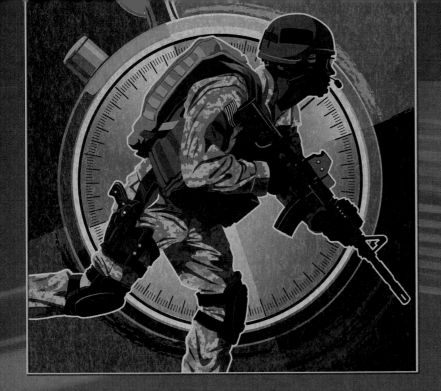

Mass Casualties and Terrorism

CHAPTER 17

© Ralf Hiemisch/Getty Images.

Disaster Management

Lead Editor:
Faizan H. Arshad, MD

CHAPTER OBJECTIVES

At the completion of this chapter, you will be able to do the following:

- Identify the five phases of the disaster cycle.
- Explain the comprehensive emergency management process.
- Discuss common pitfalls encountered during disaster response.
- Understand and discuss the components that constitute the medical response to a disaster.
- Recognize how disaster response may affect the psychological well-being of prehospital care providers.

SCENARIO

You are dispatched to a local high school that has been placed into service as a shelter following community-wide flooding from a large weather event. Your community's mayor and other dignitaries are in attendance at the school to address the community's concerns about closed roads and the lack of electrical power.

While en route to the scene, dispatch updates you that there are multiple reports of many casualties following the structural collapse of elevated bleachers in the gym that were being used as seating during a storm update. Police and fire resources are also en route to the scene but have limited available resources due to other ongoing storm-related public safety incidents.

- What safety and security concerns would you expect to encounter?
- What triage system should be utilized?
- How should the response to this incident be organized?

INTRODUCTION

Disasters, in comparison to traditional emergency response, can be time consuming, may encompass multiple agencies, and include medical and psychosocial challenges. Furthermore, there are phases to disaster response and rebuilding infrastructure that may continue well after the initial response has concluded.

The World Health Organization (WHO) defines a disaster as follows:

> A serious disruption of the functioning of a community or a society causing widespread human, material, economic, or environmental losses which exceed the ability of the affected community or society to cope using its own resources.[1]

This broad definition does not provide specific reference to medical issues or the emergency medical response but is inclusive of the overall community response and sociopolitical response to any disaster of significant magnitude.

From a medical perspective, the definition can be further refined. A disaster is defined as a situation in which the number of patients presenting for medical assistance exceeds the capacity of health care providers with the usual resources at hand and thus requires additional, and sometimes external, assistance.[2] This concept applies to all medical care settings, including hospitals and prehospital settings. This situation is commonly referred to as a **mass-casualty incident (MCI)**. The abbreviation MCI has also been used to refer to "multiple-casualty incidents," which are events that involve more than one casualty but may be handled with standard local resources. In this text, MCI will be used to refer to mass-casualty incidents that overwhelm the community's available resources.

It is important to understand that these definitions describe two key concepts: (1) A disaster is not dependent on a specific number of victims, and (2) the impact of the disaster exceeds the available resources of the medical response and there is typically disruption of infrastructure. Simply stated, all MCIs are a component of a disaster, but not all disasters are MCIs.

It is difficult to predict the time, location, or complexity of the next disaster. Nevertheless, all disasters, regardless of etiology, have similar medical and public health consequences. Disasters differ in the degree to which these consequences occur and the degree to which they disrupt the medical and public health infrastructure of the disaster locale. A guiding principle of disaster response is to do the greatest good for the greatest number of people with the resources available. This objective differs from "conventional" nondisaster-related medical care, which is to do the greatest good for the individual patient.

Natural disasters and human-made disasters, including acts of terror, encompass the spectrum of possible disaster threats. **Weapons of mass destruction (WMDs)**, which

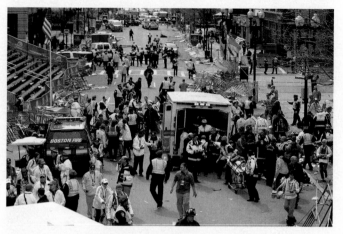

Figure 17-1 Mass-casualty management at the scene of the Boston Marathon bombings.
© Charles Krupa/AP Images.

create large numbers of casualties while possibly also contaminating the environment, represent particularly ominous threats (see the Explosions and Weapons of Mass Destruction chapter).

An approach to disaster management that is consistent, principled, and ideally rehearsed is becoming the accepted practice worldwide. This strategy forms the framework for **mass-casualty incident (MCI) response**. The primary objective of the MCI response is to reduce the morbidity (injury and disease) and mortality (death) caused by the disaster. All prehospital care providers need to incorporate the key principles of MCI response into their training, given the potential complexity and proclivity for disorganization during disaster response (**Figure 17-1**).

The Disaster Cycle

Eric Noji, MD,[3] and others have defined a theoretical framework with which the sequence of events in a disaster can be analyzed. This conceptual description not only provides an overview of the natural history of a disaster but also provides the basis for the development of the response process.[3,4] The five phases of disaster response are described as follows:

1. The **quiescent period**, or **interdisaster period**, represents the time in between disasters or MCIs during which risk assessment and mitigation activities should be undertaken and plans for the response to potential events are developed, tested, and implemented.

2. The next phase is the **prodrome (predisaster) phase**, or **warning phase**. At this point, a specific event has been identified as impending or highly likely to occur. This could reflect a natural weather condition (e.g., hurricane) or the active unfolding of a hostile and potentially violent

situation. During this period, specific steps may be taken to mitigate the effects of the ensuing events. These defensive maneuvers may include such actions as fortifying physical structures, initiating evacuation plans, and mobilizing public health resources to mount a postevent response. It must be noted, however, that not all incidents will have a warning phase. For example, an earthquake may occur without warning.

3. The third phase is the **impact phase**, or the occurrence of the actual event. During this period, there is often little that can be done to alter the impact or outcome of what is occurring.

4. The fourth phase is the **rescue, emergency, or relief phase**, which is the period immediately following the impact during which response occurs and appropriate management and intervention can save lives. The skills of emergency medical responders, prehospital care providers, rescue teams, and medical support services will be brought to bear to maximize the number of survivors of the event.

5. The fifth phase is the **recovery or reconstruction phase**, during which community resources are called upon to endure, emerge from, and rebuild after the effects of the disaster through the coordinated efforts of the medical, public health, and community infrastructure (physical and political). This period is by far the longest, sometimes lasting months, and perhaps years, before a community fully recovers.

Understanding the disaster cycle (**Figure 17-2**) allows prehospital care providers to evaluate the preparations that

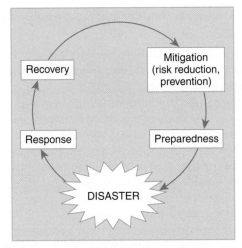

Figure 17-2 The life cycle of a disaster. The quiescent phase is represented by the mitigation and preparedness arrows. The warning phase comes just before the impact of the event. It is followed by the rescue and recovery phases.

© National Association of Emergency Medical Technicians (NAEMT).

have been made in anticipation of the likely hazards and events encountered in their community. After an incident has occurred, there follows an opportunity for critical evaluation of the after-action report and assessment of the provider's individual area of responsibility and response, as well as the response of others, to determine the efficiency and efficacy of the response process and identify areas for future improvement. These concepts apply to all disasters, regardless of size.

The duration of each phase of the disaster life cycle will vary depending upon the frequency with which incidents occur in a given community, the nature of the incident, and the degree to which the community is prepared. For example, the quiescent period in some locations can be extremely long (measured in years), whereas in other communities it may be measured in months or days (e.g., hurricanes). The southeastern states in the United States prepare for hurricanes annually with a quiescent period between events of approximately 6 to 8 months. In contrast, although hurricanes have struck the New England states, they are a rare event with a longer quiescent period. Similarly, the rescue and recovery phases can vary significantly depending on the particular incident. The rescue and recovery from something like a plane crash will be measured in hours, or at most, days, whereas the rescue and recovery from a major flood may take weeks to months or longer.

Comprehensive Emergency Management

Knowledge of the life cycle of disasters can be used to implement the steps involved in **comprehensive emergency management**. Comprehensive emergency management defines the specific steps needed to manage an incident and consists of four components: mitigation, preparedness, response, and recovery.

- **Mitigation**: This component of emergency management generally occurs during the quiescent phase of the disaster cycle. Potential hazards or likely etiologies of MCIs in the community are identified and assessed. Steps are then taken to prevent these hazards from causing an incident or to minimize their effect should something unexpected occur.
- **Preparedness**: This step involves the advance identification of an incident and the specific supplies; the needs of the population, including persons with special needs; equipment; personnel that would be needed to manage the incident; and the specific incident action plan that would be employed if a particular incident occurred.
- **Response**: This phase involves the activation and deployment of the various resources identified in the preparedness phase in order to manage an active incident. Traditional emergency prehospital providers typically operate during this period.

- **Recovery**: This component addresses the actions necessary to return the community to its preincident functional status.

While this process is typically applied to the management of a disaster, these same steps may also be used for the individual emergency preparedness of each emergency responder.

Personal Preparedness

Just as it is vital that each community and agency undertake a comprehensive planning process to be prepared for the challenges of a potential disaster, each prehospital care provider must be ready to face, on a personal and professional level, the many issues the disaster may present.

Prehospital care providers must have a complete understanding of the many potential hazards that may accompany a disaster response in advance of the actual incident and be prepared to take the necessary steps to protect themselves from these dangers. Gaps in knowledge

about such issues as building collapse, hazardous materials incidents, WMDs and their potential effects on patient treatment, appropriate personal protective equipment, and overall incident management should be identified in advance and addressed.

Disasters may extend beyond a typical operating period, and prehospital care providers must discuss with their families their roles, responsibilities, and potentially prolonged absence. This discussion includes preparing their families for what they should do and where they should go during such an event to ensure their safety. Just as the local emergency medical services (EMS) system procures supplies and equipment before a disaster, providers should ensure that adequate supplies are available at home to meet their families' needs (**Box 17-1**, **Box 17-2**, and **Box 17-3**). Providers should plan for who would care for children and pets during an extended tour of duty. Taking these actions will help reassure both the provider and his or her family—allowing the provider to continue operating during a disaster, especially during an extended response.

Box 17-1 Emergency Supply List

All homes should have some basic supplies on hand (at least 3 days' worth) for emergencies. The following is a list of some basic items that emergency supply kits should include. It is important that individuals review this list and consider where they live and the unique needs of their family in order to create an emergency supply kit that will meet their specific needs. Individuals should also consider having at least two emergency supply kits, one full kit at home and smaller portable kits in their workplace, vehicle, or other places where they spend time. Prescription medications are also an important aspect to consider when planning one's emergency kit.

- Water—1 gallon per person and pet, per day (3-day supply for evacuation, 2-week supply for home)
  · Consider storing more water than this for hot climates, for pregnant women, and for persons who are sick.
- Food—nonperishable, easy-to-prepare items, including food for pets (3-day supply for evacuation, 2-week supply for home) (see Box 17-2)
  · Remember, it is better to have extra food that you can share than to run out of food during an emergency.
- Cell phone with chargers
- Battery-powered or hand-cranked radio and a National Oceanic and Atmospheric Administration (NOAA) Weather Radio with tone alert and extra batteries for both

- Flashlight and extra batteries
- First aid kit (see Box 17-3)
- Whistle to signal for help
- Dust mask, to help filter contaminated air, and plastic sheeting and duct tape to shelter in place
- Moist towelettes, garbage bags, and plastic ties for personal sanitation
- Wrench or pliers to turn off utilities
- Can opener for food (if kit contains nonperishable food)
- Local maps

Additional items to consider adding to an emergency supply kit:

- *Items for infants*, including formula, diapers, bottles, pacifiers, powdered milk, and medications not requiring refrigeration
- *Items for seniors, persons with special needs, or anyone with serious allergies*, including special foods, denture items, extra eyeglasses, hearing aid batteries, prescription and nonprescription medications that are regularly used, inhalers, and other essential equipment
- Prescription medications and glasses
- Pet food and extra water for your pet
- Important family documents such as copies of insurance policies, identification, and bank account records in a waterproof, portable container
- Cash or traveler's checks and change

- Emergency reference material such as a first aid book or information from www.ready.gov
- Sleeping bag or warm blanket for each person (Consider additional bedding if you live in a cold-weather climate.)
- Complete change of clothing, including a long-sleeved shirt, long pants, and sturdy shoes (Consider additional clothing if you live in a cold-weather climate.)
- Household chlorine bleach and medicine dropper (When diluted 9 parts water to 1 part bleach, bleach can be used as a disinfectant. In an emergency, you can use it to treat water by using 16 drops of regular household liquid bleach per gallon of water. Do not use bleaches that are scented or color safe or that have added cleaners.)
- Fire extinguisher (A-B-C type)
- Matches in a waterproof container
- Paper and pencil
- Entertainment—including games and books, favorite dolls, and stuffed animals for small children
- Kitchen accessories—a manual can opener; mess kits or disposable cups, plates, and utensils; utility knife; sugar and salt; aluminum foil and plastic wrap; resealable plastic bags; paper towels
- Sanitation and hygiene items—shampoo, deodorant, toothpaste, toothbrushes, comb and brush, lip balm, sunscreen, contact lenses and supplies, any medications regularly used, toilet paper, moist towelettes, soap, hand sanitizer, liquid detergent, feminine supplies, plastic garbage bags (heavy duty) and ties (for personal sanitation uses), medium-sized plastic bucket with tight lid, disinfectant, household chlorine bleach
- Needles and thread
- A map of the area marked with places you could go and their telephone numbers
- An extra set of keys and IDs—including keys for cars and any properties owned and copies of driver's licenses, passports, and work identification badges
- Cash and coins and copies of credit cards
- Copies of medical prescriptions
- A small tent, compass, and shovel

Pack the items in easy-to-carry containers, label the containers clearly, and store them where they would be easily accessible. Duffle bags, backpacks, and covered trash receptacles are good candidates for containers. In a disaster situation, a family may need access to the disaster supply kit quickly—whether sheltering at home or evacuating. Ensuring that family vehicles are filled with gasoline will allow for immediate evacuation to a safe location. Following a disaster, having the right supplies can help a household endure home confinement or evacuation.

Make sure the needs of everyone who would use the kit are covered, including infants, seniors, and pets. It is a good idea to involve whoever may use the kit, including children, in assembling it.

Modified from FEMA: Ready America (www.ready.gov) and the Centers for Disease Control and Prevention: Emergency Preparedness and Response (www.bt.cdc.gov/planning/).

Box 17-2 Food Kit

- Store at least a 3-day supply of nonperishable food.
- Select foods that require no refrigeration, preparation, or cooking and little or no water.
- Pack a manual can opener and eating utensils.
- Avoid salty foods, as they will make you thirsty.
- Choose foods your family will eat.
- Suggested foods include the following:
  · Ready-to-eat canned meats, fruits, and vegetables
  · Protein or fruit bars
  · Dry cereal or granola
  · Peanut butter
  · Dried fruit
  · Nuts
  · Crackers
  · Canned juices
  · Nonperishable pasteurized milk
  · High-energy foods
  · Vitamins
  · Food for infants
  · Comfort/stress foods
- Bring a propane stove or grill for cooking (with extra propane tank).

Data from FEMA: Ready America (www.ready.gov) and the Centers for Disease Control and Prevention: Emergency Preparedness and Response (www.bt.cdc.gov/planning/).

Box 17-3 First Aid Kit

In any emergency, a family member may be cut or burned or may suffer other injuries. An emergency kit should include the following:

- Two pairs of latex gloves or other sterile gloves (if anyone has latex allergies)
- Sterile dressings to stop bleeding
- Cleansing agent/soap and antibiotic towelettes to disinfect
- Antibiotic ointment to prevent infection
- Burn ointment to prevent infection
- Adhesive bandages in a variety of sizes
- Eye wash solution to flush the eyes or to use as a general decontaminant
- Thermometer
- Daily prescription medications such as insulin, cardiac medications, and asthma inhalers (Periodically rotate medicines to account for expiration dates.)
- Prescribed medical supplies such as glucose and blood pressure monitoring equipment and supplies
- Any durable medical equipment like canes or walkers

Other things it may be useful to include:

- Cell phone with charger
- Scissors
- Tweezers
- Tube of petroleum jelly or other lubricant
- Nonprescription medications:
  - Aspirin or nonaspirin pain reliever (acetaminophen)
  - Antidiarrhea medication
  - Antacid (for upset stomach)
  - Laxative

Data from FEMA: Ready America (www.ready.gov) and the Centers for Disease Control and Prevention: Emergency Preparedness and Response (www.bt.cdc.gov/planning/).

An additional resource that provides information about personal and family preparation in the event of a disaster, including how to create a family communication plan, is the Ready campaign sponsored by the Federal Emergency Management Agency (FEMA) and available online at www.ready.gov.

Mass-Casualty Incident Management

An important premise of disaster response is to remember that all disasters are local. The variability of available resources will vary tremendously from urban, to suburban, to rural locales. In general, the severity and diversity of injuries, in addition to the total number of victims, will be major factors in determining whether an MCI requires resources and assistance from outside the impacted community.

Today's complex disasters, especially those involving terrorism and WMDs (chemical, biologic, radiologic, or nuclear), may result in an austere and/or hazardous environment. An **austere environment** is a setting in which resources, supplies, equipment, personnel, transportation, and other aspects of the physical, political, social, and economic environments are limited. As a result of these limitations, constraints on the availability and adequacy of immediate care for the population can be variable, again, depending on one's location and resource infrastructure. Prehospital care providers should anticipate not being able to offer the same level of care provided to an individual sick or injured patient when responding to a disaster and potentially hundreds or thousands of patients. Meaningful interventions provided expediently to patients who meet specific criteria are likely to optimize outcomes for salvageable patients.[5]

Emergency medical concerns related to MCIs include the following five elements:

- *Search and rescue.* This activity involves the process of systematically looking for those individuals who have been impacted by an event and rescuing them from hazardous situations. Depending on the situation, this often requires the use of specially trained teams, particularly when extrication issues are involved.
- *Triage and initial stabilization.* This is the process of systematically evaluating and categorizing each victim according to the seriousness of the injury or illness and providing initial medical care to address immediate life- or limb-threatening problems.
- *Patient tracking.* This is a system by which patients are uniquely identified and followed through their initial contact with search and rescue, evacuation, triage and transport, and ultimately disposition to definitive care.
- *Definitive medical care.* This component involves the provision of the specific medical care needed to treat the patient's specific injuries. This care will usually be provided at hospitals; however, alternate care facilities may be used in major events when hospitals are overwhelmed with casualties or when hospitals have been directly impacted and/or damaged by the incident.
- *Evacuation.* This is the process of transporting disaster victims and injured patients away from the disaster site, either to a safe location or to a definitive care facility.

Public health concerns related to MCIs include the following:

- Water (ensuring a supply of safe, potable water)
- Food (ideally nonperishable and needing no refrigeration or cooking)
- Shelter (a place for cover, protection, and refuge)
- Sanitation (protection from contact with human and animal feces, solid waste, and wastewater)

- Security and safety
- Transportation
- Communication (dissemination of information to the affected population, including information about communicable diseases)
- Endemic and epidemic diseases (Endemic diseases are ones that are always present in a given area or population but that usually occur with low frequency, whereas an epidemic disease is one that develops and spreads rapidly to the population at risk.)

Both medical and public health disaster-response activities are coordinated through one organizational structure: the incident command system.

The National Incident Management System

The National Incident Management System (NIMS) was developed to provide a template for a comprehensive nationwide, systematic approach to managing an incident, regardless of cause, size, location, or complexity. NIMS offers a set of preparedness concepts and principles for all hazards and events. It outlines the essential principles for a common operating structure and interoperability of communications and information management systems. It also provides standardized resource management procedures. NIMS uses the incident command system to oversee the direct response to an incident.

Incident Command System

Many different organizations may participate in the response to a disaster. The **incident command system (ICS)** was created to allow different types of agencies (fire, police, EMS, etc.) and multiple jurisdictions of similar agencies (e.g., city, county, state) to work together effectively, using a common language and organizational structure to manage the response to a disaster or other major incident (**Figure 17-3**) (see the Scene Management chapter). Representatives from the various responding agencies will usually come together in an incident command post to facilitate interagency communications and decision making and work together to unify the command process.

The ICS recognizes that, regardless of the specific nature of the incident (police, fire, or medical), there are a number of functions that must always happen. The ICS is organized around these necessary functions. Its components are:

- Command
  - Safety officer
  - Information officer
  - Liaison officer
- Planning
- Logistics
- Operations
- Finance

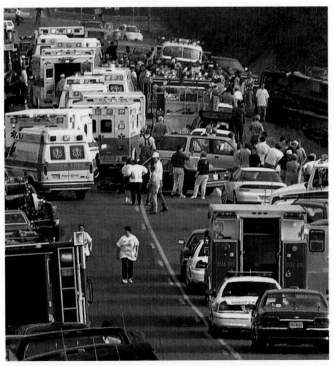

Figure 17-3 The incident command system (ICS) allows integration of fire, police, and EMS assets at a disaster scene.
© David Crigger, Bristol Herald Courier/AP Images.

These functions apply in varying degrees to all incidents and are now used in medical settings of all types, from prehospital to in-hospital, to organize the response to a disaster.

From a medical perspective, several important ICS principles will help during an MCI response:

1. ICS must be established early, preferably upon arrival of the emergency responder to the scene. Establishing command is an important first step for any responder, and it is important to remember command can be transitioned to supervising officers as they arrive on scene.
2. Medical and public health responders, often used to working independently, need to implement the principles of the ICS management structure to better integrate their response with other agencies during an MCI.
3. Using ICS will allow for the integration of the medical response within the overarching response to the incident.

Detailed information and training about the ICS is available on the FEMA website.[6]

Characteristics of the Incident Command System

An ICS provides a standard, professional, organized approach to managing emergency incidents. The use of an ICS enables an emergency response agency to operate more safely and effectively. A standardized approach facilitates and coordinates the use of resources from multiple agencies, working toward common objectives. It also eliminates the need to develop a unique approach for each situation, saving valuable time during an MCI or disaster.

Effective management of incidents requires an organizational structure to provide both a hierarchy of authority and responsibility, as well as to establish formal channels of communications. Through the use of the command structure, the specific responsibilities and authority of everyone in the organization are clearly delineated and predefined, allowing heterogeneous groups to operate together seamlessly.

Jurisdictional Authority

Jurisdictional authority is usually not a problem at an incident with a single focus. Matters can become more complicated when several jurisdictions are involved or multiple agencies within a single jurisdiction have authority for various aspects of the incident. When there are overlapping responsibilities, the ICS may employ a **unified command**. This approach brings representatives of different agencies together to work on one plan and ensures that all actions are fully coordinated. *Command*, although the chosen term of the ICS system, is perhaps misleading. It is important to remember that incidents are managed; personnel are commanded. *Incident command*, whether conducted by an individual or through unified command, is a management and leadership position. It is responsible for setting strategic objectives and maintaining a comprehensive understanding of the impact of an incident as well as identifying the strategies required to manage the scene effectively. The command function is structured in one of two ways: single or unified.

Single command is the most traditional perception of the command function and is the genesis of the term **incident commander**. When an incident occurs within a single jurisdiction, and when there is no jurisdictional or functional agency overlap, a single incident commander should be identified and designated with overall incident management responsibility by the appropriate jurisdictional authority. This does not mean that other agencies do not respond or do not have a role in supporting the management of the incident.

Single command is best used when a single discipline in a single jurisdiction is responsible for the strategic objectives associated with managing the incident. Single command also is appropriate in the later stages of an incident that was initially managed through unified command. Over time, as many incidents stabilize, the strategic objectives become increasingly focused within a single jurisdiction or discipline. In this situation, it is appropriate to transition from unified command to single command.

It is also acceptable, if all agencies and jurisdictions agree, to designate a single incident commander in multiagency and multijurisdictional incidents. In this situation,

however, command personnel should be carefully chosen. The incident commander is responsible for developing the strategic incident objectives on which the **incident action plans (IAPs)** will be based. An IAP is an oral or written plan containing general objectives reflecting the overall strategy for managing an incident. The incident commander is responsible for the IAP and all requests pertaining to the ordering and releasing of incident resources.

When multiple agencies with overlapping jurisdictions or legal responsibilities are involved in the same incident, unified command provides several advantages. In this approach, representatives from each agency cooperate to share command authority. They work together and are directly involved in the decision-making process. Unified command helps ensure cooperation, avoids confusion, and guarantees agreement on goals and objectives.

All-Risk and All-Hazard System

The ICS has evolved into an all-risk, all-hazard system that can be applied to manage resources at fires, floods, tornadoes, plane crashes, earthquakes, hazardous materials incidents, explosions or any other type of emergency situation. This kind of system has also been used to manage many nonemergency events, such as large-scale public events or mass-gathering events, that have similar requirements for command, control, and communications. The flexibility of the ICS enables the management structure to expand as needed, using whichever components are required. The operations of multiple agencies and organizations can be integrated smoothly in the management of the incident.

Everyday Applicability

An ICS can and should be used for everyday operations as well as major incidents. Command should be established at every incident. Regular use of the system ensures familiarity with standard procedures and terminology. It also increases the users' confidence in the system. Frequent use of ICS for routine situations makes it easier to apply to larger incidents.

Unity of Command

Unity of command is a management concept in which each person has only one direct supervisor. All orders and assignments come directly from that supervisor, and all reports are made to the same supervisor. This approach eliminates the confusion that can result when a person receives orders from more than one boss. Unity of command reduces delays in solving problems as well as the potential for life and property losses. By ensuring that each person has only one supervisor, unity of command can increase overall accountability, prevent freelancing, improve the flow of communication, assist with the coordination of operational issues, and enhance the safety of the provider. An ICS is not necessarily a rank-oriented system. The best-qualified person should be assigned to the appropriate level for each situation, even if that means a lower ranking individual is temporarily assigned to a higher level position. This concept is critical for the effective application of the system and must be embraced by all participants. Additionally, a critical component of NIMS will be a national credentialing standard for ICS positions such as command and section chiefs in the operations, planning, logistics, and finance/administration sections.

Span of Control

Span of control refers to the number of subordinates who report to one supervisor at any level within the organization. Span of control relates to all levels of ICS—from the strategic level to the operational/tactical level as well as to the task level.

In most situations, one person can effectively supervise only three to seven people or resources. Because of the dynamic nature of emergency incidents, an individual who has command or supervisory responsibilities in an ICS normally should not directly supervise more than five people. The actual span of control should depend on the complexity of the incident and the nature of the work being performed. For example, in a complex incident involving hazardous materials, the span of control might be only three; during less intense operations, the span of control could be as high as seven.

Modular Organization

The ICS is designed to be flexible and modular. The ICS organizational structure—command, operations, planning, logistics, and finance/administration—is predefined, ready to be staffed and made operational as needed. Indeed, an ICS has often been characterized as an organizational toolbox, where only the tools needed for the specific incident are used. In an ICS, these tools consist of position titles, job descriptions, and an organizational structure that defines the relationships between positions. Some positions and functions are used frequently, whereas others are needed only for complex or unusual situations. Any position can be activated simply by assigning someone to the intended role.

Common Terminology

ICS promotes the use of common terminology both within an organization and among all agencies involved in emergency incidents. Common terminology means that each word has a single definition, and no two words used in managing an emergency incident have the same definition. Everyone uses the same terms to communicate the same thoughts, so everyone understands what is meant. Each job comes with one set of responsibilities, and everyone knows who is responsible for each duty.

Integrated Communications

Integrated communications ensure that everyone at an emergency can communicate with both supervisors and subordinates. The ICS must support communication up and down the chain of command at every level. A message must be able to move efficiently through the system from command down to the lowest level and from the lowest level up to the command level.

Consolidated Incident Action Plans

An ICS ensures that everyone involved in the incident is following one overall plan. Different components of the organization may perform different functions, but all of their efforts contribute to the same overarching goals and objectives. Everything that occurs is coordinated within the overall response. At smaller incidents, command develops an action plan and communicates the incident priorities, objectives, strategies, and tactics to all of the operating units. Representatives from all participating agencies meet regularly to develop and update the plan. In both large and small incidents, those involved in the incident understand what their specific roles are and how they fit into the overall plan.

Designated Incident Facilities

Designated incident facilities are assigned locations where specific functions are always performed. For example, command will always be based at the incident command post. The staging area, rehabilitation area, casualty collection point, treatment area, base of operations, and helispot are all designated areas where particular functions take place. The facilities required for the specific incident are established according to the specific IAP or a predefined ICS plan.

Resource Management

Resource management entails the use of a standard system of assigning and keeping track of the resources involved in the incident. The resource management system of the ICS keeps track of the various resource assignments. At large-scale incidents, units are often dispatched to a **staging area** rather than going directly to the incident location. A staging area is a location close to the incident scene where a number of units can be held in reserve, ready to be assigned if needed.

Organization of the Incident Command System

The ICS structure identifies a full range of duties, responsibilities, and functions that are performed at emergency incidents. Some components are used on almost every incident, whereas others apply to only the largest and most complex situations. The five major components of an ICS organization are command, operations, planning, logistics, and finance/administration.

An ICS organization chart may be basic or add complexity as greater components are needed. Each block on an ICS organization chart refers to a functional area or a job description. Positions are staffed as they are needed by incident command, who decides which additional components are needed for the given situation.

Command

On an ICS organization chart, the first component is **command** (**Figure 17-4**). Command is the only position in the ICS that must always be filled for every incident, as having a clearly defined leader has several advantages to incident management. Command is established when the first unit arrives on the scene and is maintained until the last unit leaves the scene.

In the ICS structure, command (either single or unified) is ultimately responsible for managing an incident and has the necessary authority to direct all activities at the incident scene. Command is directly responsible for the following tasks:

- Determining strategy
- Selecting incident tactics
- Setting the action plan
- Developing the ICS organization
- Managing resources and requesting additional resources
- Coordinating resource activities
- Providing for scene safety
- Releasing information about the incident
- Coordinating with outside agencies

Incident Command Post

The **incident command post (ICP)** is the headquarters for the incident. Command functions are centered in the ICP; thus command and all direct support staff should always be located at the ICP. The location of the ICP should be broadcast to all units as soon as the ICP is established.

Relative to the incident scene, the ICP should be in a protected nearby location. Often, the ICP for a major incident

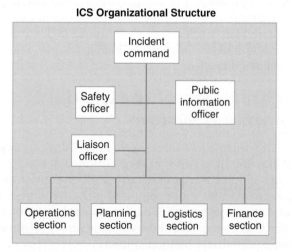

ICS Organizational Structure

Figure 17-4 The ICS organization chart.

is located in a special vehicle or building. This location enables the command staff to function without needless distractions or interruptions. For large incidents that are geographically spread out, the command post may be some distance from the emergency incident.

Command Staff

Individuals on the **command staff** perform functions that report directly to command and cannot be delegated to other major sections of the organization. The safety officer, liaison officer, and public information officer are always part of the command staff. In addition, aides, assistants, and advisors may be assigned to work directly for members of the command staff.

SAFETY OFFICER

The **safety officer** is responsible for ensuring that safety issues are managed effectively at the incident scene. He or she is the eyes and ears of command in terms of safety—identifying and evaluating hazardous conditions, watching out for unsafe practices, and ensuring that safety procedures are followed appropriately. The safety officer is appointed early during an incident. As the incident becomes more complex and the number of resources present at the scene increases, additional qualified personnel can be assigned as assistant safety officers.

LIAISON OFFICER.

The **liaison officer** is a representative of command who serves as a point of contact for representatives from outside agencies. This member of the command staff is responsible for exchanging information with representatives from those agencies. During an active incident, command may not have time to meet directly with everyone who comes to the ICP. The liaison officer functions as the representative of command under these circumstances, obtaining and providing information or directing people to the proper location or authority. The liaison area should be adjacent to, but not inside, the ICP.

PUBLIC INFORMATION OFFICER.

The **public information officer (PIO)** is responsible for gathering and releasing incident information to the news media and other appropriate agencies. At a major incident, communicating with the public and news media is very important for information dissemination. Because command must make managing the incident the top priority, the PIO serves as the contact person for media requests, which frees up command to concentrate on the incident. A media headquarters should be established near—but not within—the ICP. The information presented to the media by the PIO needs to be approved by the incident commander. Employing a PIO also helps disseminate a consistent and coordinated message, especially during a complex event involving multiple agencies.

General Staff Functions

The incident commander has the overall responsibility for the entire incident command organization, although some elements of the incident commander's responsibilities can be handled by the command staff. When the incident is too large or too complex for one person to manage effectively, the incident commander may appoint someone to oversee parts of the operation. Everything that occurs at an emergency incident can be divided among the major functional components within ICS:

- Operations
- Planning
- Logistics
- Finance/administration

The chiefs of these four sections are known as the **ICS general staff**. Command decides which (if any) of these four positions needs to be activated, when to activate it, and who should be placed in each position. Recall that the blocks on the ICS organization chart refer to functional areas or job descriptions, not to positions that must always be staffed.

The four section chiefs on the ICS general staff, when they are assigned, may run their operations from the main ICP, although this structure is not required. At a large incident, the four functional organizations may operate from different locations, but they will always be in direct contact with command.

Operations

The **operations section** is responsible for the management of all actions that are directly related to mitigating the incident. The operations section rescues any trapped individuals, treats any injured patients, and does whatever else is necessary to alleviate the emergency situation.

For smaller incidents, command may directly supervise the functions of the operations section. At complex incidents, a separate **operations section chief** takes on this responsibility so that command can focus on overall strategy while the operations section chief focuses on the tactics that are required to get the job done.

Operations are conducted in accordance with an IAP that outlines what the strategic objectives are and how emergency operations will be conducted. At most incidents, the IAP is relatively simple and can be expressed in a few words or phrases. The IAP for a large-scale incident can be a lengthy document that is regularly updated and used for daily briefings of the command staff.

Planning

The **planning section** is responsible for the collection, evaluation, dissemination, and use of information relevant to the incident. The planning section works with preincident plans, building construction drawings, maps, aerial photographs, diagrams, reference materials, and status boards.

It is also responsible for developing and updating the IAP. The planning section develops what needs to be done by whom and identifies which resources are needed.

Command activates the planning section when information needs to be obtained, managed, and analyzed. The **planning section chief** reports directly to command. Individuals assigned to planning examine the current situation, review available information, predict the probable course of events, and prepare recommendations for strategies and tactics. The planning section also keeps track of resources at large-scale incidents and provides command with regular situation and resource status reports.

Logistics

The **logistics section** is responsible for providing supplies, services, facilities, and materials during the incident. The **logistics section chief** reports directly to command and serves as the supply officer for the incident. Among the responsibilities of this section are keeping vehicles fueled, providing food and refreshments for emergency responders, and arranging for specialized equipment.

Finance/Administration

The **finance/administration section** is the fourth major ICS component managed directly by command. This section is responsible for the accounting and financial aspects of an incident, as well as any legal issues that may arise in its aftermath. This function is not staffed at most incidents, because cost and accounting issues are typically addressed after the incident. Nevertheless, a finance/administration section may be needed at large-scale and long-term incidents that require immediate fiscal management, particularly when outside resources must be procured quickly. A finance/administration section may also be established during a natural disaster or during a hazardous materials incident where reimbursement may come from the shipper, carrier, chemical manufacturer, or insurance company.

Medical Response to Disasters

While there may be multiple simultaneous goals of disaster response, the specific components of medical response, when combined, will help minimize the mortality and morbidity of victims of the event. Although these actions will be discussed sequentially in this chapter, it is important to remember that during an actual disaster many of the actions will occur concurrently (**Box 17-4**). Additionally, it is important to mention that the overall response may depend on the location of the incident and local protocols as well as available resources. The command structure or framework for response may vary considerably for international deployments.

> **Box 17-4** The Basic Steps in Medical Response to Disasters
>
> Medical response to a disaster involves the following basic steps:
>
> 1. Notification and activation of EMS
> 2. Initial response
> 3. EMS response to the scene
> 4. Assessment of the situation
>   a. Cause
>   b. Number of casualties
>   c. Additional resources
>   i. Medical
>   ii. Other
> 5. Communication of the situation and needs
> 6. Activation of the medical community
>   a. Notification of receiving facilities
> 7. Search and rescue
> 8. Triage (treatment of airway and hemorrhage life threats)
> 9. Casualty collection
> 10. Treatment
> 11. Transport
> 12. Retriage

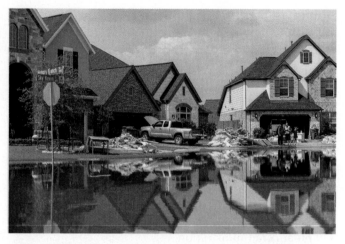

Figure 17-5 Natural disasters, such as hurricanes and floods, result in an influx of calls into local emergency dispatch centers. A view of the storm damage from Hurricane Harvey in Texas in 2017.
© Michelmond/Shutterstock.

Initial Response

The first step is notification and activation of the EMS response system. This is usually performed by witnesses to the event who call the local emergency dispatch center seeking response by appropriate police, fire, and emergency medical agencies (**Figure 17-5**).

The first prehospital care providers to arrive at the scene have a number of important functions to fulfill that will set the stage for the entire emergency medical response to the incident. Most important, these actions do not include initiating care to the most critically injured patients, as would be the case in most non-MCI situations. Before beginning the process of providing emergency medical assistance, the first providers must take the time to perform an overall scene assessment. The goals of this assessment are to evaluate any potential hazards, estimate the potential number of casualties, determine what additional medical resources will be needed at the scene, and evaluate whether any specialized equipment or personnel, such as search-and-rescue teams, will be required. Depending on the incident, providers should also be watchful for signs of a secondary device designed to harm emergency responders.

Once a basic assessment is complete, the information gathered should be efficiently communicated to the dispatch center, which will work to acquire and dispatch the needed resources for a coordinated response. After this,

the prehospital care providers shift their focus to identifying appropriate locations to perform triage, to collect casualties, and to stage incoming ambulances, personnel, and supplies so as not to impede rapid access and egress to the scene or to expose responding assets to potential hazards from the event.

It is also essential that the responding EMS agency notify the likely receiving hospitals in the community regarding the event, communicating the estimated number of casualties and their respective levels of criticality so that the receiving centers may prepare appropriately and consider activating their internal hospital-specific disaster plans. The field component of the disaster response is the first link in the overall chain of survival for the victims of a disaster, and EMS agencies are responsible for the timely notification of receiving centers.

Search and Rescue

At this point, the on-scene process of initiating patient care can begin. Generally, this will start with a search-and-rescue effort to identify and evacuate casualties from the impacted site to a safer location. The local population near a disaster site, as well as survivors themselves if they are able, are often the immediate search-and-rescue resource and may have already begun to search for victims before the arrival of any public safety personnel.[7] Experience has demonstrated that the local community will respond to a disaster site and begin the process of aiding victims.

Many countries and communities have developed formal, specialized search-and-rescue teams as an integral part of their national and local disaster-response plans. Members of these teams receive specialized training in confined-space environments and are activated as needed for a particular event. These search-and-rescue units generally include the following:

- A cadre of medical specialists
- Technical specialists knowledgeable in hazardous materials, structural engineering, heavy equipment operation, and technical search-and-rescue methods (e.g., listening equipment, remote cameras)
- Trained canines and their handlers

Importantly, activation of specialized teams may take time, and in austere environments improvisation is often necessary. For example, at an MCI at a building site, local construction companies may provide valuable search-and-rescue assets including equipment, tools, and materials that can be used at the disaster site to assist in moving heavy debris.

Triage

As patients are identified and evacuated, they are brought to the triage site, where they can be assessed and a triage category assigned. The term *triage* is a French word that means "to sort." From a medical perspective, triage means sorting casualties based on the severity of their injuries. This process was first described in the early 1800s by Baron Dominique Larrey, who was surgeon-in-chief to Napoleon and was most famous for developing the prototype ambulance during the Napoleonic Wars. Larrey stated:

> Those who are dangerously wounded should receive the first attention, without regard to rank or distinction. They who are injured in a less degree may wait until their brethren in arms, who are badly mutilated, have been operated on and dressed, otherwise the latter would not survive many hours; rarely, until the succeeding day.[8]

This concept, which has been further researched and expanded since Larrey, serves to prioritize patients who need immediate medical care and transport to the hospital.

Triage is one of the most important missions of any disaster medical response. As noted previously, the objective of conventional triage in the nondisaster setting is to do the greatest good for the individual patient. This imperative usually means finding and treating the sickest patient. The objective of mass-casualty triage is to do the greatest good for the greatest number of people. Mass-casualty triage in the field should be overseen by a trained triage officer. A **triage officer** should have a wide breadth of clinical experience in the assessment and management of field injuries, as potentially challenging decisions may be made about patients who will be deemed critical versus those who will be classified as mortally wounded or expectant. A paramedic with significant field experience usually meets this requirement. A trained physician with experience in the field may also function in this capacity.[9,10] Nevertheless, all prehospital providers should be able to perform the basic functions of triage and be well rehearsed in the application of an agency-specific triage algorithm.

A number of different methodologies exist for evaluating and assigning the triage category.[11] One method involves a rapid physiologic and mental status evaluation. This triage process is referred to as the **START triage algorithm** (**s**imple **t**riage **a**nd **r**apid **t**reatment). This system evaluates the respiratory status, perfusion status, and mental status of the patient in making a prioritization for initial transfer to definitive care facilities (see Box 5-6 in the Scene Management chapter).[10,12] Other triage systems include the MASS (**m**ove, **a**ssess, **s**ort, **s**end), Smart, JumpStart (pediatric algorithm), and Sacco triage methods.

In an effort to provide national guidance and bring uniformity to the triage process, the Centers for Disease Control and Prevention (CDC) in the United States convened a multidisciplinary group of experts to develop a consensus-based triage system, now known as SALT.[10] (See Box 5-7 in the Scene Management chapter.) This triage system involves **s**orting the patient based on the patient's ability to move, **a**ssessing the patient for the need for **l**ifesaving interventions, performing those interventions, and ultimately **t**reatment and **t**ransport.

Regardless of the exact triage method used, all triage systems ultimately classify patients into one of (usually) four injury-severity categories. The highest priority patients are those who are identified as having critical, but likely survivable, injuries and are usually categorized as *immediate* and color-coded *red*. Patients with moderate injuries (who may be nonambulatory) and can potentially tolerate a short delay in care are categorized as *delayed* patients and color-coded *yellow*. Patients with relatively minor injuries, often referred to as the "walking wounded," are classified as *minimal* victims and color-coded *green*. Patients who have expired on the scene or whose injuries are so severe that death is inevitable are categorized as *dead* or *expectant*, respectively, and color-coded *black*. Of note, some triage systems, particularly SALT, specifically separate those patients classified as mortally wounded from those who are dead, color coding the expectant as *gray*.

All these color codes refer to the use of "disaster tags", at disaster scenes and attached to patients once they have been triaged. The color code provides an immediate visual reference to the patient's triage category. Some triage systems also use a classification system in which immediate, delayed, minimal, and dead or expectant patients are referred to as Class I, Class II, Class III, and Class IV, respectively.

It is important that triage personnel avoid the temptation to pause their triage function in favor of treating a critically injured patient whom they encounter. As mentioned earlier, the primary principle involved in dealing with an MCI is to do the greatest good for the most people. During this initial triage phase, medical interventions are limited to those actions that are performed easily and rapidly and are not labor intensive. Generally, this means performing only procedures such as manual airway opening, needle chest decompression, administration of a chemical antidote, and external hemorrhage control including wound packing and tourniquet deployment. Interventions such as bag-mask ventilation, closed chest compression, establishing IV access, and endotracheal intubation are often deferred during the triage process.

Once patients have been triaged, they are brought together at **casualty collection points** according to their triage priority. Specifically, all of the immediate patients (red) are grouped, as are the delayed (yellow) and minimal (green) patients. Casualty collection points should be located close enough to the disaster site that the victim can be easily carried to them and treatment rapidly provided, but far enough away from the impact site to be safe from any ongoing hazard. Important considerations include the following:

- Proximity to the disaster site
- Safety from hazards and uphill and upwind from contaminated environments
- Protection from climatic conditions (when possible)
- Easy visibility for disaster victims and assigned personnel
- Convenient entry and exit routes for ground, air, and water evacuation
- Safe distance from staging ambulance exhaust fumes

As additional medical staff and resources arrive and become available on scene, medical care and interventions are provided at the casualty collection points according to the triage priority. These are appropriate locations to which physicians responding to the scene may be assigned to further evaluate and treat injured patients.

Finally, as transportation resources become available, patients are transported for definitive care according, once again, to their triage priority (**Figure 17-6**). Immediate patients are not held on scene for the provision of further medical care if transport is available (**Figure 17-7**). Needed medical interventions should be conducted during transport to the definitive care facility.

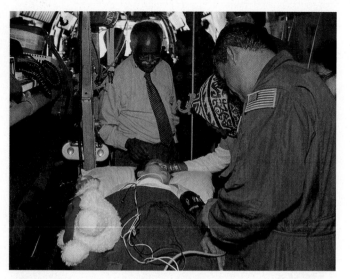

Figure 17-7 Interior of a military transport plane converted for medical evacuation with patient litters.
© Evan Vucci/AP Images.

Because of visible, critical injuries, emergency responders often tend to move individual patients forward for immediate treatment and transport and bypass the triage process. This tendency should be avoided so that all victims can be sorted, reserving treatment for the most severely injured and ill victims first. Nevertheless, bypassing the triage process is indicated in certain situations which include:

1. Risk, as in bad weather
2. Potential impending darkness without the capabilities of lighting resources
3. The continued risk of injury as a result of natural or unnatural events
4. No triage facility or triage officer immediately available
5. Any tactical situation in a law enforcement scenario in which the victims are rapidly moved from the impact site to the collection point for transport[12,13]

Last, triage is not a static process; it is dynamic and ongoing. Once a patient is evaluated and categorized, the patient does not carry that triage category for the remainder of his or her care. Instead, as the patient's condition changes, the triage category may change as well. For example, a patient with a major extremity wound and hemorrhage may initially be categorized as an immediate patient; however, after pressure is applied to the wound and the bleeding is controlled, the patient may be retriaged as delayed. Alternatively, a patient initially categorized as immediate could deteriorate rapidly and subsequently be retriaged as expectant.

Retriage should occur on the scene while patients are waiting for transport resources. In addition, patients will undergo retriage upon arrival at the receiving destination and again as they are prioritized for emergent surgery.

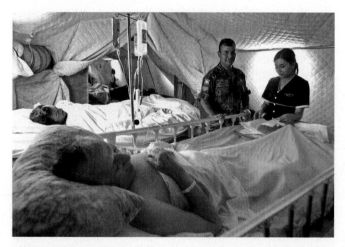

Figure 17-6 Definitive medical care at a U.S. field hospital—Bam, Iran, earthquake, 2005.
© Cristobel Fuentes/AP Images.

Treatment

Because the number of patients will initially exceed the available resources, treatment on the scene is generally limited to manually opening the airway, decompressing tension pneumothoraces, controlling external hemorrhage, and administering chemical agent antidote. Only when adequate resources have arrived on scene or during transport to the hospital will additional interventions be provided, such as intravenous access and splinting of fractures.

Transport

The transport and tracking of patients from an MCI to the receiving hospitals involves a coordinated effort using a variety of transport vehicles. Immediate and delayed patients will be taken to the hospital in ambulances or helicopters (if available and conditions permit). Those incidents that result in huge numbers of patients, particularly patients in the minimal category, may require the use of nontraditional transport vehicles such as buses and vans, and in some cases, patients may be transported to nonhospital sites for evaluation and treatment. It is important to remember, however, that when such alternate transport mechanisms are used, prehospital care providers with adequate supplies and equipment must be assigned to accompany the casualties in that vehicle. Each patient's movement and destination should be accurately recorded on a patient tracking log or via commercially available tracking systems.

Another important issue in effectively responding to an MCI relates to the decision-making process for patient destination once transport is initiated.[14] Recent events have demonstrated that patients with non-life-threatening injuries will often depart the disaster site using any available means of transportation and make their own way to surrounding hospitals.[7] Often this results in large numbers of "walking wounded" arriving at the hospital closest to the disaster site.

Prehospital care providers must understand that the hospital closest to a disaster scene may be overwhelmed with patients even before the arrival of the first transporting ambulance. Before taking a patient to the closest hospital, contact should be made to ascertain the status of the emergency department (ED) and its ability to accept and treat patients transported by ambulance. If the closest hospital is overwhelmed, the EMS system should transport patients to more distant facilities when possible. Although the transport time will be longer, the patient's care will not be complicated by the presence of numerous other patients. Dispersal of patients to multiple institutions will ultimately better preserve the ability of all the receiving hospitals to optimize the patient care that they can provide. Consideration for specialty receiving facilities should also be given due accord, if the patient's condition allows, including trauma, burn, and replantation centers.

Even if the closest medical facility is not overwhelmed with self-transported patients, it is imperative that prehospital care providers do not overwhelm the nearest hospital with patients transported by ambulance. Often, the natural desire is to transport a patient to the closest hospital so that the ambulance and its crew can quickly return to the disaster scene to pick up and transport more patients. Transferring the MCI from the disaster site to the closest hospital will negatively impact the hospital's ability to provide the "most good for the most patients." However, in those communities that have limited numbers of hospitals, EMS may have no option but to transport patients to the nearest hospital. In some municipalities, Disaster Medical Control Centers directly communicate with hospitals to determine their capabilities for handling acutely injured patients.

Medical Assistance Teams

If the disaster is of significant proportion that additional on-scene resources are needed, some hospitals have developed disaster-response teams to help augment the EMS field response and provide on-site care, thus allowing prehospital care providers to be freed from the task of providing medical care at casualty collection points and, instead, performing patient transport. Agencies may have preexisting arrangements with surrounding communities and employ mutual aid to help provide additional prehospital capacity (**Figure 17-8**). Additionally, if outside resources are needed from the state or federal government, other emergency medical response teams are available in many municipalities.

As a result of the Metropolitan Medical Response System (MMRS) in the United States, MMRS task forces or strike teams have been created in many cities. The MMRS was developed and funded by the U.S. Department of Health and Human Services (DHHS) to help respond to terrorist

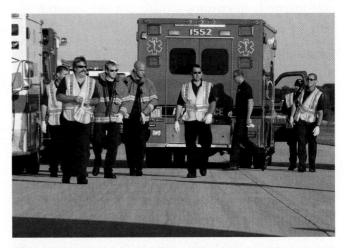

Figure 17-8 Agencies from surrounding communities may provide mutual aid during a large-scale emergency.
© Nancy G Fire Photography, Nancy Greifenhagen/Alamy Stock Photo.

or public health emergencies. The goal is to help integrate the various local response agencies and services together to enhance the response to such an event. These response assets comprise medical personnel from emergency medicine, trauma surgery, surgical subspecialties, and nursing. MMRS task forces can respond with resources that have been purchased through state and federal funds. These strike teams can be used to augment and backfill medical facilities or to staff mobile medical facilities that are established to provide surge capacity and medical care to patients.

On a larger scale basis, the U.S. government has capabilities through the National Disaster Medical System to mobilize disaster medical assistance teams (DMATs). DMATs are able to provide field care as well as create mobile medical facilities, some of which have the capability to perform surgical interventions and meet the critical care needs of patients, when local resources have been overwhelmed. A request for DMATs must come through the appropriate channels, usually from the local emergency manager to the state emergency management authority and the governor's office through the federal government to the DHHS, which houses the National Disaster Medical System's response program.

Threat of Terrorism and Weapons of Mass Destruction

Terrorism may present some of the most challenging MCIs for emergency responders. The spectrum of terrorist threats is limitless, ranging from suicide bombers, to conventional weapons or explosives, to military weapons, to WMDs (chemical, biologic, radiologic, and nuclear). Terrorist events have the greatest potential of all human-made disasters to generate large numbers of casualties and fatalities (see the Explosions and Weapons of Mass Destruction chapter for detailed information about specific weapons).

Terrorists have unfortunately demonstrated remarkable ingenuity in creating civilian casualties. During the terrorist attacks on September 11, 2001, the terrorists used passenger jets replete with fuel to generate massive destruction of life and property.

One of the unique features of a terrorist threat, especially involving WMDs, is that psychological casualties usually predominate. Terrorists do not need to kill a large number of people to achieve their goals; they only need to create a climate of fear and panic to overwhelm the medical infrastructure. In the March 1995 sarin attacks in Tokyo, 5,000 total patients presented to hospitals. Of these, fewer than 1,000 had physical effects from the sarin gas; the remaining presented with psychological stress and desire for physician evaluation. The 2001 anthrax incidents in the United States also dramatically increased the number of individuals presenting to EDs with nonspecific respiratory symptoms that ultimately did not result from actual anthrax infection.

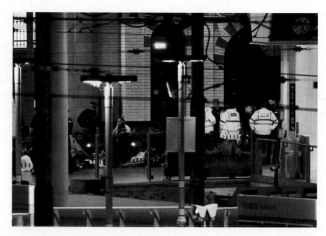

Figure 17-9 Manchester bombing, 2017.
© Dave Thompson/Getty Images News/Getty Images.

Explosions and bombings continue to be the most frequent cause of mass casualties in disasters caused by terrorists worldwide, both as a primary event and when secondary devices are planted to injure or kill emergency responders. The majority of these bombings consist of relatively small explosives that produce low mortality rates. However, when strategically placed in buildings, pipelines, or moving vehicles, their impact can be much greater (**Figure 17-9**). The high morbidity and mortality rates are related not only to the intensity of the blast but also to the subsequent structural damage that leads to the collapse of the targeted buildings. A greater threat will be disasters caused by conventional explosives in combination with a chemical, biologic, or radiologic agent, such as a "dirty bomb" that combines a conventional explosive with radioactive material.

The WMDs that create contaminated environments may prove to be the greatest disaster challenge. Emergency responders will not be able to bring victims into hospitals because of the risk of further contaminating medical facilities. Prehospital care providers must be prepared and equipped to perform triage, not only to determine the extent of the injuries but also to assess the potential for contamination and need for decontamination and initial stabilization. At the same time, providers need to take appropriate steps to protect themselves from potential contamination.

Decontamination

Decontamination is an important consideration for all disasters involving hazardous materials and WMDs (**Figure 17-10**). Terrorist events with large numbers of victims, unknown substances, and multitude of "worried well," significantly increase the specter of contaminated or potentially contaminated casualties (see the Explosions and Weapons of Mass Destruction chapter for additional information). As a general rule, if patients are deemed to be contaminated, decontamination procedures should occur prior to transport to definitive care.

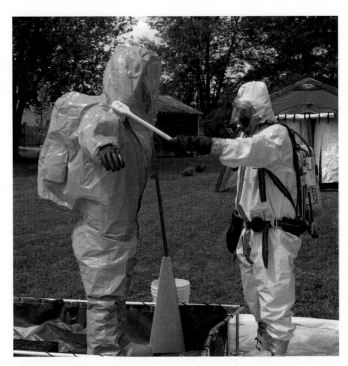

Figure 17-10 Decontamination of personnel in level A personal protective equipment in the "warm zone" by personnel in level B personal protective equipment.
© Jones & Bartlett Learning.

Treatment Area

When responding to a disaster involving hazardous materials and WMDs, it is critical that the triage and casualty collection points be appropriately positioned upwind and uphill of the contaminated area (300 yards [275 meters]).

Psychological Response to Disasters

Psychological trauma and other adverse psychological sequelae are frequently the side effects of events such as natural disasters and unintentional disasters caused by humans.[15] In contrast, one of the objectives of terrorism is to inflict psychological pain, trauma, and disequilibrium. Maintaining good mental health is just as important as maintaining good physical health for all emergency responders.

Characteristics of Disasters That Affect Mental Health

Not all disasters have the same level of psychological impact. Disaster characteristics that seem to have the most significant mental health impact include the following:

- Little or no warning
- Serious threat to personal safety
- Potential unknown health effects

- Uncertain duration of the event
- Human error or malicious intent
- Symbolism related to the terrorist target

Factors Impacting Psychological Response

Everyone who experiences a disaster, either as a victim or as an emergency responder, is affected by it in some fashion. Fortunately, this does not mean that most individuals will develop a mental health disorder. It does mean, however, that all affected individuals, both victims and emergency responders, will have some type of psychological or emotional response to the event.

Similarly, there are both individual and collective reactions that can promote resilience and help communities recover from these extraordinary events. Factors affecting individual response to disasters include the following:

- Physical and psychological proximity to the event
- Exposure to gruesome or grotesque situations
- Diminished health status before or because of the disaster
- Magnitude of loss
- History of previous trauma

Factors impacting collective response to trauma include the following:

- Degree of community disruption
- Predisaster family and community stability
- Community leadership
- Cultural sensitivity of recovery efforts

Psychological Sequelae of Disasters

Postdisaster psychological responses are wide ranging, from mild stress responses to full-blown **posttraumatic stress disorder (PTSD)**, major depression, or acute stress disorder.[15] PTSD is a mental health condition that results from exposure to horrific or terrifying events and leads to flashbacks to the incident, nightmares, anxiety, and uncontrollable thoughts about the incident.

Interventions

A number of relatively simple actions can help individuals to minimize the psychological effects of an event and assist them in returning to normal function.

- Individuals should return to normal activities as soon as possible.
- In persons with no diagnosed mental disorder, it is helpful to provide educational materials that help them understand what they and their families are experiencing.
- Crisis counseling should be provided, followed by referral when treatment is indicated.

- When a mental disorder is diagnosed, therapeutic interventions can be helpful, including cognitive-behavioral therapy and prescription medications.

Emergency Responder Stress

Emergency responders can become secondary victims of stress and other psychological sequelae. These consequences can adversely affect their performance during and after an event. Personal well-being as well as family and professional relationships may be negatively impacted. Supervisory personnel and colleagues should be alert for the development or manifestations of stress and psychological distress in individuals who were involved in an incident response.

A number of intervention strategies are often used in an effort to help prevent and manage stress after an incident. These include debriefing, defusing, and grief management sessions. Collectively, these processes have been referred to as **critical incident stress management (CISM)**. The value of CISM has been questioned in recent years, particularly in those instances where CISM has been a mandated intervention for emergency responders. CISM can be offered as an option to those emergency responders who feel inclined to participate but should never be mandated for all emergency responders as it may actually cause harm in some circumstances. Alternative programs such as Psychological First Aid may address some of the limitations of CISM and provide teams with effective tools for immediate intervention in situations where providers have psychologically related complaints and are amenable to assistance.

Signs of Stress in Workers

Some common signs of stress in emergency responders include physiologic, emotional, cognitive, and behavioral elements.

Physiologic Signs
- Fatigue, even after rest
- Nausea
- Fine motor tremors
- Tics
- **Paresthesias**
- Dizziness
- Gastrointestinal upset
- Heart palpitations
- Choking or smothering sensations

Emotional Signs
- Anxiety
- Irritability
- Feeling overwhelmed
- Unrealistic anticipation of harm to self or others

Cognitive Signs
- Memory loss
- Decision-making difficulties
- Anomia (inability to name common objects or familiar people)
- Concentration problems or distractibility
- Reduced attention span
- Calculation difficulties

Behavioral Signs
- Insomnia
- Hypervigilance
- Crying easily
- Inappropriate humor
- Ritualistic behavior

Managing Stress On-Site

The following on-site interventions can assist in reducing stress:

- Limited exposure to traumatic stimuli
- Reasonable operational hours
- Adequate rest periods (**Figure 17-11**)
- Reasonable diet
- Regular exercise program
- Private time
- Speaking with empathic colleagues
- Monitoring signs of stress

Disaster Education and Training

The development and implementation of a formal educational and training program will improve the prehospital

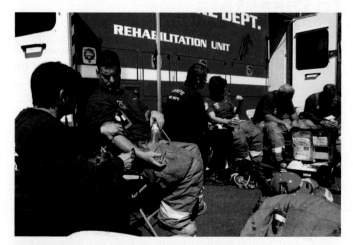

Figure 17-11 Adequate rest periods on scene can help relieve stress.
© Jones & Bartlett Learning, Courtesy of MIEMSS.

care provider's ability to respond efficiently and effectively to an MCI. The provider may fulfill a variety of roles in disaster and mass-casualty management, including mitigation and preparedness, search and rescue, triage, acute medical care, transport, and postevent recovery. Preparedness with regard to education and training can be accomplished in various structured, as well as unstructured, learning environments. Each has its individual advantages and disadvantages, as measured by educational impact and comparative cost.

Independent learning is the foundation of disaster preparedness. A multitude of resources are available through printed literature as well as via the Internet. The CDC, public health agencies, FEMA, the Center for Domestic Preparedness, and the military forces all offer Internet-based learning opportunities and resources to individuals. Courses can be completed on an independent basis on a time-flexible schedule. This modality, however, does not allow for direct hands-on experience.

Group training is directed at specific teams with regard to disaster response. Training programs are broadly available and include understanding incident command structure and WMD preparedness. Numerous professional and paraprofessional organizations have developed training programs and modules specific to their scope of professional practice, including public health, emergency medicine, critical care, and surgical and medical specialties, as well as all levels of prehospital care providers.

Simulations provide a training opportunity that brings together many individuals from varied backgrounds who are essential to the implementation of a disaster response. These exercises come in two specific forms: a tabletop exercise and a fully active field-training exercise. Tabletop exercises are cost-effective and highly useful methods to test and evaluate a disaster response. As the name suggests, these exercises are conducted around a table, with the various participants verbally indicating what the expected response actions would be. Tabletop exercises allow for real-time communications and interaction among multidisciplinary agencies. These activities require direction in the form of an experienced facilitator guiding the participants through the objectives and providing constructive feedback to the group at the conclusion of the exercise.

Field exercises are the most realistic training events, involving the actual execution and performance of the community disaster-response plan. The field exercise allows for a real-time assessment of the physical capacity to meet the objectives as defined in writing. Ideally, the exercises will involve moving victims from the point of impact and injury through the EMS response system and into definitive care at medical facilities. These events, however, are labor intensive, long in duration, and potentially costly.

For optimal learning from educational exercises, it is imperative that interdisciplinary training events be conducted often, and they should include all of the appropriate agencies and participants. In this way, each agency will have the opportunity to learn about and understand the roles, responsibilities, and capabilities of the services with whom they will respond in a disaster.

Common Pitfalls of Disaster Response

Numerous studies performed after significant MCIs have identified several consistent shortcomings in the medical response to these events. Identification of these deficiencies has resulted from subsequent evaluations of the response to these incidents as well as from communities that have performed risk, vulnerability, and needs assessments mandated by the U.S. government in order to receive funding to enhance the disaster-response infrastructure.

Preparedness

As emergency responders in a community, prehospital care providers prepare for the devastation that can occur in a mass-casualty event and plan for such events in a variety of ways. Although a tabletop drill can be a valuable method of preparing, it does not truly test the ability of the providers to perform the necessary duties or the ability of the EMS agency to bring resources and assets to the site in a timely and efficient manner. Realistic functional disaster drills—during which victims are triaged, evaluated, "treated," transported, and tracked through the emergency medical response system to a hospital facility's doors in a realistic fashion—better test the emergency medical response that will be required. The ability to provide for *surge capacity* (the ability to expand services to meet a sudden influx of patients) and for supplying the large number of staff, ambulances, and other equipment needed for victims must be appropriately addressed by the entire medical response community.

Unfortunately, few agencies have actually tested a surge capacity response in real time and, instead, have relied on tabletop drills as a measure of their ability to respond. Communitywide drills that involve multiple agencies more reliably predict an organization's level of preparedness for MCI response. Moreover, MCIs can be highly varied, a response to a large alarm fire is vastly different from a response to an active shooter incident. Agencies should consider use of a hazard vulnerability analysis to identify and prioritize potential MCI or disaster scenarios most likely to affect their specific locale. Hazard vulnerability analysis is a systemic risk assessment approach that facilitates identifying hazards or risks that are most likely to have an impact on the surrounding community (**Box 17-5**).

Communications

Many events have demonstrated that the lack of a unified communication system significantly hinders the ability to mount a coordinated response to an MCI. Individual communication systems are effective, but relying on a single modality for communication is a setup for failure. The use of cellular phones, for example, was no longer possible when the central communication center located in the World Trade Center was destroyed on September 11, 2001. Also, the inability of police, fire, and EMS agencies to communicate with each other because of different radio technologies or frequencies is a limitation that may reduce the ability to effectively respond to MCIs.

Redundancy in the system is paramount, regardless of the chosen source for primary communications. Landlines, hardwired phone systems, cellular phone systems, satellite phone systems, VHF radios, and 800- to 900-MHz frequency systems all have some degree of vulnerability and could be compromised by an incident. Therefore, having multiple communication options is crucial to ensuring ongoing communications.

The following two principles are essential to maintain communications capability:

1. A unified communication system must exist to which all pertinent emergency responders in the community have access.
2. There must be system redundancy such that if one modality of communication fails or is disabled another source can be used efficiently and effectively as a backup.

Another common problem is the use of codes as a form of communication shorthand. Unfortunately, there is no single agreed-upon set of emergency codes for all agencies to use; thus, a responding agency may find itself at a scene with other agencies, all of whom are using codes that may have different meanings. It is for this reason that ICS and NIMS recommend the use of plain English during an incident to avoid any confusion in meaning.

Scene Security

Scene security has become an ever-increasing problem in MCIs. Scene safety and security are important for the following reasons:

1. To protect the emergency response teams from a second incident, resulting in further casualties (e.g., secondary device targeting first responders)
2. To provide for the safe ingress and egress of emergency responders and victims unencumbered by bystanders
3. To protect and facilitate securing the scene and potential physical evidence

Scene security may become a significant challenge during a disaster, because resources may potentially be spread thin due to response to the event. Coordination with local law enforcement leaders is essential for the prehospital and medical community to ensure that security and force protection will be available if necessary.

Self-Dispatched Assistance

In many MCIs, public safety and EMS agencies (as well as medical responders of all types) from adjacent and even distant communities have responded to the scene without any formal request for assistance from the impacted jurisdiction.[5] These "self-dispatched" emergency responders, although well intentioned, often serve only to further complicate and confuse an already chaotic situation. With self-dispatched assistance, coordinated rescue efforts are strained because of the lack of participation in the incident command structure. Communications issues are often made more challenging by incompatible radio systems brought by the self-dispatched emergency responders.

Ideally, public safety and EMS agencies should respond to a disaster site only if they have been specifically requested to do so by the responsible jurisdiction and the incident commander.[16] In addition, it is extremely helpful if access to the scene is controlled and a staging area is established as soon as possible to which all responding units and volunteers can be directed to be credentialed and better incorporated into the incident response.

Supply and Equipment Resources

Most EMS agencies have plans for the routine use of supplies and have purchased supplies based on the expected daily demand. Events of large magnitude will rapidly exhaust

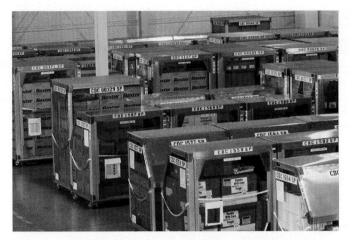

Figure 17-12 In communities that have been designated to receive MMRS funds, community stockpiles of pharmaceuticals have been or are being purchased in preparation for such events.

Strategic National Stockpile Communications Team/Centers for Disease Control and Prevention.

these resources and may disrupt conventional supply lines. Having a seamless backup plan for the reconstitution of supplies during a disaster is essential for the ongoing mission of high-quality patient care. Supplies must be available in a timely fashion, and appropriate mechanisms must be in place for distribution. Distribution plans should not depend on deployed prehospital care providers, as they may be otherwise occupied.

The EMS agency must also have a plan in place for pharmaceutical replenishment. In those communities that have been designated to receive Metropolitan Medical Response System (MMRS) funds, community stockpiles of pharmaceuticals have been or are being purchased in preparation for such events (**Figure 17-12**).

Failure to Notify Hospitals

In the confusion of responding to and assessing an MCI, as well as performing the numerous tasks that must be accomplished in initiating the prehospital medical response to such an event, it is often easy for EMS agencies to overlook the need to contact hospitals and have them activate their internal disaster plans. Numerous actual events have demonstrated that unless hospital notification and activation are integral parts of the EMS agency's MCI plan, hospitals may not be informed or may be informed too late to optimize the influx of patients. It is essential that EMS agencies include hospital notification as part of their MCI plan so that a coordinated seamless transition from field care to hospital care can occur.

In addition, ongoing communication from the field to the hospital and from the hospital to the field is important for monitoring the status of the event and the patient load at hospitals.

Media

The media are often seen as a detriment to the physical and operational process of disaster response. However, EMS agencies are encouraged to partner with the media, including social media, because these outlets can be an asset during a disaster response. The media can help disseminate accurate information to the general population, giving them directions on appropriate actions before, during, or after an event. The media's purpose is to broadcast information to the public, and prehospital agencies have the responsibility to partner with the media to ensure the information provided is timely and accurate as well as helpful to the response process.

Having a designated public information officer (PIO) who is trained to deal with the media and authorized to speak about the incident is an important method of communicating with the various media representatives seeking information about the incident. Of particular importance is the recognition that each responding agency will likely have a PIO present. Under the unified command concept, ideally, one consistent message should be delivered by a single PIO; however, any messages given out by the various agencies' PIOs must be consistent with each other.

SUMMARY

- Disasters result from natural climactic or geologic events; however, they may also result from intentional or unintentional acts of humans.
- Although disasters may be unpredictable, adequate preparation can turn an unthinkable event into a manageable situation.
- The incident command system (ICS) allows different types of agencies (e.g., fire, police, EMS) and multiple jurisdictions of similar agencies (e.g., city, county, state) to work together effectively, using a common language and organizational structure to manage the response to a disaster or other major incident.
- Prehospital care providers must understand the concepts of triage to ensure they can do the greatest good for the greatest number of people with the resources available.
- Transport must take into consideration factors such as whether nearby hospitals have the capacity to meet demands and whether certain patients would benefit from extended transport to a trauma center more capable of meeting their needs.
- Despite the fact that disasters occur in varying sizes and result from many different causes, common pitfalls have been identified that hinder management of such events, including:
  - Inadequate preparedness
  - Communications failures
  - Inadequate scene safety measures
  - Self-dispatched assistance
  - Supply and equipment shortages
  - Poor media relations
- Disaster response may take a heavy psychological toll on those involved, both victims and emergency responders. While critical incident stress management (CISM) is increasingly showing potential harm, agencies should consider voluntary debriefing with affected personnel to help providers maintain good mental health, which is just as important as maintaining good physical health.
- Understanding the disaster cycle is important to preparation and prevention efforts. There are generally five phases in a disaster response: quiescent, or interdisaster, period; prodrome (warning) phase; impact phase; rescue, emergency, or relief phase; and recovery or reconstruction phase.
- The best outcomes in response to MCIs result from the creation of a well-devised disaster plan that has been rehearsed, tested, and critiqued to identify and improve problem areas.

SCENARIO RECAP

You are dispatched to a local high school that has been placed into service as a shelter following community-wide flooding from a large weather event. Your community's mayor and other dignitaries are in attendance at the school to address the community's concerns about closed roads and the lack of electrical power.

While en route to the scene, dispatch updates you that there are multiple reports of many casualties following the structural collapse of elevated bleachers in the gym that were being used as seating during a storm update. Police and fire resources are also en route to the scene but have limited available resources due to other ongoing storm-related public safety incidents.

- What safety and security concerns would you expect to encounter?
- What triage system should be utilized?
- How should the response to this incident be organized?

SCENARIO SOLUTION

While responding to the high school, preplanned mutual aid resources are simultaneously dispatched to assist. The local hospitals are also updated that there is an ongoing MCI. As the first-arriving EMS unit, you report to the incident command post where a unified command structure is being assembled. As practiced, you conduct an overall assessment of the scene and the medical needs and relay that information back to dispatch.

Triage team leaders begin sorting through the casualties. Treatment areas are established a safe distance from the collapse. As casualties arrive at the treatment areas, they are organized by severity of injuries. Prehospital care providers begin appropriate care and secondary triage of the injured. As mutual aid resources arrive at staging areas, they are assigned tasks and placed into service. Transport vehicles arrive, and the injured are transported to hospitals. All patients are tracked and accounted for through each step of this process.

Once all casualties have left the scene, fire services, code inspection services, and police begin to investigate the origin of the collapse.

References

1. World Health Organization. Definitions: emergencies. http://www.who.int/hac/about/definitions/en/index.html. Accessed November 2, 2017.
2. Noji EK. *The Public Health Consequences of Disasters*. New York, NY: Oxford University Press; 1997.
3. Noji EK, Siverston KT. Injury prevention in natural disasters: a theoretical framework. *Disasters*. 1987;11:290.
4. Cuny SC. Introduction to disaster management. Lesson 5: technologies of disaster management. *Prehosp Disaster Med*. 1993;6:372.
5. Phillips SJ, Knebel A, eds. *Mass Medical Care with Scarce Resources: A Community Planning Guide*. Prepared by Health Systems Research, Inc., an Altarum company, under contract No. 290-04-0010. AHRQ Publication No. 07-0001. Rockville, MD: Agency for Healthcare Research and Quality; 2007.
6. Federal Emergency Management Agency. NIMS 2017 learning materials. http://training.fema.gov/EMIWeb/IS/ICSResource/index.htm. Accessed November 2, 2017.
7. Auf der Heide E. The importance of evidence-based disaster planning. *Ann Emerg Med*. 2006;47:34-49.
8. Larrey DJ. *Memoires de Chirurgie Militaire, et Campagnes*. Vols. 1-4. Paris, France: J. Smith, Publisher; 1812-1817.
9. Burkle FM, ed. *Disaster Medicine: Application for the Immediate Management and Triage of Civilian and Military Disaster Victims*. New Hyde Park, NY: Medication Examination Publishing; 1984.
10. Burkle FM, Hogan DE, Burstein JL. *Disaster Medicine*. Philadelphia, PA: Lippincott, Williams & Wilkins; 2002.
11. Lerner EB, Schwartz RB, Coule PL, et al. Mass casualty triage: an evaluation of the data and development of a proposed national guideline. *Disaster Med Public Health Preparedness*. 2008;2(suppl 1):S25-S34.
12. Super G. *START: A Triage Training Module*. Newport Beach, CA: Hoag Memorial Hospital Presbyterian; 1984.
13. Burkle FM, Newland C, Orebaugh S, et al. Emergency medicine in the Persian Gulf. Part II. Triage methodology lessons learned. *Ann Emerg Med*. 1994;23:748.
14. Bloch YH, Schwartz D, Pinkert M, et al. Distribution of casualties in a mass-casualty incident with three local hospitals in the periphery of a densely populated area: lessons learned from the medical management of a terrorist attack. *Prehosp Disast Med*. 2007;22:186-192.
15. Hick JL, Ho JD, Heegaard WG, et al. Emergency medical services response to a major freeway bridge collapse. *Disaster Med Public Health Preparedness*. 2008;2(suppl 1):S17-S24.
16. American College of Emergency Physicians. Unsolicited medical personnel volunteering at disaster scenes. Published June 2002. Reaffirmed October 2008. Accessed November 2, 2017.

Suggested Reading

Briggs SM, Brinsfield KH. *Advanced Disaster Medical Response: Manual for Providers*. Boston, MA: Harvard Medical International; 2003.

De Boer J, Dubouloz M. *Handbook of Disaster Medicine: Emergency Medicine in Mass Casualty Situations*. Utrecht, The Netherlands: Van der Wees; 2000.

Eachempati SR, Flomenbaum N, Barie PS. Biological warfare: current concerns for the health care provider. *J Trauma*. 2002;52:179.

Emerg Med Clin North Am. 1996;14(2) (entire issue).

Feliciano DV, Anderson GV Jr., Rozycki GS, et al. Management of casualties from the bombing at the Centennial Olympics. *Am J Surg*. 1998;176(6):538.

Hirshberg A, Holcomb JB, Mattox KL. Hospital trauma care in multiple-casualty incidents: a critical view. *Ann Emerg Med*. 2001;37(6):647.

Hogan DE, Burstein, JL, eds. *Disaster Medicine*. 2nd ed. Philadelphia, PA: Lippincott, Williams & Wilkins; 2016.

Slater MS, Trunkey DD. Terrorism in America: an evolving threat. *Arch Surg*. 1997;132(10):1059.

Stein M, Hirshberg A. Medical consequences of terrorism: the conventional weapon threat. *Surg Clin North Am*. 1999;79(6):1537.

U.S. Department of Homeland Security, Federal Emergency Management Agency. www.fema.gov. Accessed November 2, 2017.

CHAPTER 18

Explosions and Weapons of Mass Destruction

Lead Editors:
Faizan H. Arshad, MD
Daniel P. Nogee, MD

CHAPTER OBJECTIVES

At the completion of this chapter, the reader will be able to do the following:

- Discuss the essential considerations regarding mitigation of a weapon of mass destruction (WMD) event:
  - Scene assessment
  - Incident command
  - Personal protective equipment
  - Patient triage
  - Principle of decontamination
- Describe the mechanisms of injury, evaluation and management, and transport considerations associated with specific categories of WMD agent:
  - Explosive and incendiary agents
  - Chemical agents
  - Biologic agents
  - Radiologic agents
- Know how to access and utilize resources for further study.

SCENARIO

It is a warm summer evening, and you are dispatched to the scene of a reported explosion outside a popular café. You know this café is usually busy and typically seats patrons inside and outside on the patio. Dispatch informs you the number of victims is not yet known, although they have received multiple emergency calls regarding this incident. Other public safety agencies have also been dispatched to the location.

Upon arrival at the location, you observe you are the first prehospital care provider on scene. No incident command has yet been established. Dozens of people are running away from the cafe. Many are imploring you to assist victims who have obvious bleeding. Other victims are lying on the ground with variable states of consciousness.

- What will you do first?
- What are your priorities as you determine your course of action?
- How will you care for so many people?

INTRODUCTION

Preparing to manage an incident that potentially involves a weapon of mass destruction (WMD) is a challenge for emergency medical services (EMS) systems. Although a number of different mnemonics are used to recall the various types of WMDs, perhaps the easiest to remember is CBRNE, which stands for **c**hemical, **b**iologic, **r**adiologic, **n**uclear, and **e**xplosive.

Recent history has demonstrated these incidents can occur without warning anywhere.

- The 1995 bombing of the Murrah Federal Building in Oklahoma City resulted in 168 deaths and 700 casualties. Eighty percent of the deaths resulted from the collapse of the building rather than the direct effects of the explosive. One-third of the patients brought to one Oklahoma City hospital were transported by EMS. Sixty-four percent of these transported patients required admission to the hospital, whereas only 6% of self-referred patients to the emergency department (ED) required admission.
- The September 11, 2001, World Trade Center attacks in which terrorists used passenger aircraft as flying bombs resulted in over 1,100 injured survivors, with almost one-third of those casualties transported to the hospital by prehospital care providers. Emergency responders accounted for 29% of the casualties.
- The multiple train bombings in Madrid, Spain, in 2004 caused 190 deaths and 2,051 injuries.
- The mass transit attack in London in 2005 in which bombs exploded in three subway trains and one double-decker bus caused 52 deaths and more than 779 injuries.
- The Boston Marathon bombings in 2013 resulted in 3 deaths and approximately 264 injuries.
- The 2015 attacks in Paris, France, perpetrated by both gunmen and suicide bombers, killed 130 people and injured hundreds more.
- In 2016 in Nice, France, a terrorist deliberately drove a large cargo truck through crowds of people who had gathered to celebrate Bastille Day, resulting in 86 deaths and 458 injuries.
- The Manchester Arena bombing in 2017 resulted in 22 deaths and approximately 250 injuries. Many of the victims in this incident were children.
- A 2017 attack in New York City, in which a terrorist deliberately drove a rented work truck through a bicycle path, resulted in the deaths of 8 people and 12 injuries.

Although conventional explosives are the most commonly used and most likely form of WMD event, EMS systems worldwide have also been challenged by chemical and biohazard events. The 1995 sarin gas attack in the Tokyo subway system killed 12, and more than 5,000 people sought medical attention, many of whom were asymptomatic but concerned about possible exposure. The Tokyo Fire Department sent 1,364 fire fighters to the 16 affected subway sites, and 135 emergency responders (10%) were affected by direct or indirect exposure to the nerve agent. Multiple alleged chemical attacks during the Syrian civil war have been investigated by the United Nations, including the use of the potent chemical weapons sarin (2015), chlorine (2014), and sulfur mustard (2015), resulting in many civilian and first responder casualties.

No life-threatening bioterrorism assault in the United States has yielded a large number of casualties, but this does not mean that EMS systems have not been challenged to prepare for bioterrorism threats. During 1998 and 1999, almost 6,000 people across the United States were affected by a series of anthrax-related hoaxes in more than 200 incidents. The letters containing anthrax delivered in the fall of 2001 resulted in only 22 cases of clinical anthrax but generated countless calls for public safety agencies to respond to suspicious packages and powders.

Although not a bioterrorist event, severe acute respiratory syndrome (SARS), a naturally occurring infectious disease outbreak, seriously challenged the Toronto EMS system in 2003. During the epidemic, 526 paramedics had to be quarantined, mostly due to potential unprotected exposure to the virus. This loss of key resources seriously strained Toronto's ability to mitigate the crisis. More recently, natural outbreaks of Ebola virus disease, a viral hemorrhagic fever, in West Africa resulted in over 11,000 deaths from 2013 to 2016, many among health care workers caring for infected patients.

The threat that EMS may one day have to respond to a radiologic WMD event grows, with increasing speculation that terrorists may detonate a radiologic dispersion device ("dirty bomb") that would generate injuries and panic about radioactive contamination.

Weapons of mass destruction, while traditionally thought of as the previously mentioned CBRNE classes, can take on many different forms and shapes. A recently surfaced threat is the "intentional vehicular assault," in which terrorists intentionally drive a wheeled vehicle into a crowd of pedestrians. These attacks have become unfortunately more common in the past several years, likely owing to the ease of obtaining a weapon (vehicle) and a target (crowd) relative to traditional CBRNE attacks.

General Considerations

Scene Assessment

The ability of prehospital care providers to assess the scene properly is crucial to ensuring personal safety and the safety of other emergency responders. WMD events pose significant threats to responding emergency services. In the case of a high-explosives detonation, there may be fire, spilled hazardous materials, power line hazards, and risk of falling debris or *subsidence* (the creation of craters). One emergency responder was killed by falling debris in response to the Oklahoma City bombing.[1] Many emergency responders were killed in the 2001 World Trade Center attack, including 343 fire fighters, 15 emergency medical technicians, and 3 law enforcement officers, when the buildings collapsed.

Chemical attacks potentially expose the prehospital care provider to the offending agent, not only from the primary source—the weapon—but also from secondary exposure to contamination of victims' skin, clothing, and personal belongings. Biologic agents, depending on the form of their delivery, pose a risk of illness from the offending agent (e.g., aerosolized anthrax spores) or from transmission of a communicable disease (e.g., plague or smallpox). A further risk to providers and patients alike is the possibility of additional devices. For example, a second bomb could be placed at the scene of the incident, set to explode after the arrival of emergency responders, with the intention of increasing not only injury but also confusion and panic.

All of these factors must be taken into consideration when prehospital care providers are dispatched to the scene of a possible explosive or WMD event and are evaluating the scene. Before entering any such scene, all responding units from all involved agencies should approach from an upwind and uphill direction and stage at a safe distance from the incident site. Approaching from an upwind direction is important because many of the WMDs, particularly the chemical and biologic agents, pose an inhalation risk, and inadvertent exposure is more likely at a downwind location. An uphill location is chosen to avoid exposure to runoff at an incident involving the release of liquid chemicals.

Prehospital care providers should then conduct a critical evaluation, ideally from a safe distance, of the scene, looking for clues that would warn them of potential hazards. The presence of visible vapors, spilled liquid, or possible ongoing dispersion should be noted; such observations are indicative of an active danger. Looking to see how patients are presenting must be included as part of the scene assessment, with particular attention to the signs and symptoms of patient presentation, such as seizures in multiple casualties, suggesting a possible chemical or biologic agent release. Providers need to communicate their observations through the chain of command so that proper steps can be taken to mount an appropriate and safe response, to increase the protective measures for the emergency responders, and to ensure the effective delivery of care to patients.

Access to and egress from the potentially contaminated site must be controlled. Concerned bystanders and well-meaning volunteers must not be allowed to enter the scene, as they may contribute to the casualty count if they expose themselves to the agent. Victims of the incident must also be contained as they seek to evacuate the scene, since self-transport may further disseminate a dangerous chemical or substance to unsuspecting contacts or hospital EDs. Similar to a hazardous materials incident, scene control zones (hot, warm, cold) should be established with controlled access points and transit corridors to prevent spread of the contaminants and inadvertent exposure and to provide safe areas for patient assessment and management (**Figure 18-1**) (see the Personal Protective Equipment section).

Incident Command System

The incident command system (ICS) offers a management structure that coordinates all available resources to ensure an effective response. The ICS is discussed in detail in the Scene Management chapter and the Disaster Management chapter. All incidents, regardless of size or complexity, will have a designated incident commander, who may be the first responding prehospital care provider until relieved by some other competent authority. It is essential that providers be familiar with and have the opportunity to practice implementation of the ICS, ideally in interagency settings.

Personal Protective Equipment

When responding to WMD events, the proper personal protective equipment (PPE) needs to be worn. Requirements for PPE may range from the standard daily uniform to a fully encapsulated suit with **self-contained breathing apparatus (SCBA)**, depending on the specific agent involved and the specific role and training level of the prehospital care provider. This equipment is designed to protect the emergency responder from exposure to offending agents by providing defined levels of protection of the respiratory tract, skin, and other mucous membranes. When dealing with hazardous substances of any type, PPE has generally been described in terms of the following levels (**Figure 18-2**):

- *Level A.* This level offers the highest amount of respiratory and skin protection. The respiratory tract is protected by an SCBA or **supplied air respirator (SAR)** delivering air to the emergency responder with positive pressure. A chemical-resistant barrier that completely encapsulates the wearer protects the skin and mucous membranes. It takes considerable time to don this protection, thus delaying the provider's ability to access and help patients. Patience on the part of the prehospital care providers responding to the chaos of this type of event is essential. Additional resources also need to be committed to assist emergency responders with donning and doffing this level of protection. The amount of time that a trained emergency responder can spend in level A protection is also limited by both the available air supply and the buildup of heat and humidity within the enclosed suit, as well as specific agency protocols.

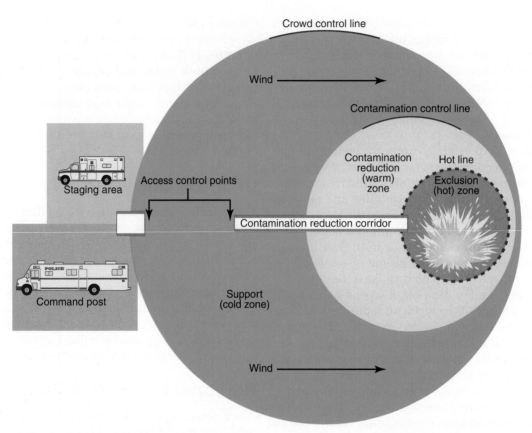

Figure 18-1 The scene of a WMD or hazardous materials incident is generally divided into hot, warm, and cold zones. The command post and staging area should both be located within the cold zone.

© National Association of Emergency Medical Technicians (NAEMT).

- *Level B.* The respiratory tract is protected in the same manner as in Level A protection, with positive-pressure-supplied air. Nonencapsulated chemical-resistant garments, including suit, gloves, and boots, which provide splash protection only, protect the skin and mucous membranes. The highest respiratory protection is afforded, with a lower level of skin protection. Similar to level A protection, level B protection takes time to don and doff, and work time within the suit is limited.
- *Level C.* The respiratory tract is protected by an **air-purifying respirator (APR)**. This may be a **powered air-purifying respirator (PAPR)**, which draws ambient air through a filter canister and delivers it under positive pressure to a face mask or hood, or a nonpowered APR, which relies on the wearer to draw ambient air through a filter canister by breathing through a properly fitted mask. The skin protection is the same as for level B.
- *Level D.* This level represents standard work clothes (i.e., standard uniform for the emergency responder) and may also include a gown, gloves, and surgical mask. Level D provides minimal respiratory protection and minimal skin protection.

It might be concluded that the best protective posture for a prehospital care provider is always to respond in the highest level of protection, level A, regardless of the threat. This is, however, not a reasonable response. Level

A protection is cumbersome, often making manual tasks difficult to perform. Significant training and experience are required when using an SCBA. Level A protection puts the wearer at risk for heat stress and physical exhaustion. It can make communication between emergency responders and victims difficult. Appropriate PPE must be selected based on the presumed threat, the level of training, and the operational responsibilities of the provider. Most important, the provider must be trained and practiced in the use of the PPE selected.

Control Zones

PPE is selected based on the known (or suspected) hazards of the environment and proximity to the threat. Proximity to the threat has often been described in terms of the following control zones:

- The *hot zone* is the area where there is immediate threat to health and life. This includes an environment contaminated with a hazardous gas, vapor, aerosol, liquid, or powder. PPE adequate to protect the emergency responder is determined based on potential routes of exposure to the substance and the likely agent. Level A protection is most often used in the hot zone.
- The *warm zone* is characterized as an area where the concentration of the offending agent is limited. In

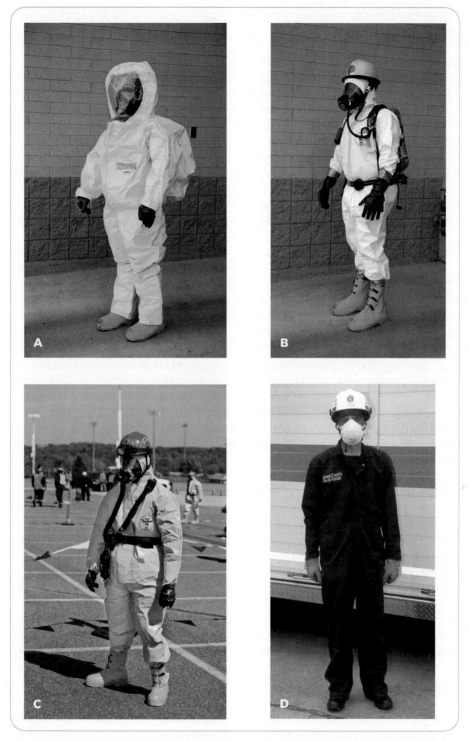

Figure 18-2 Personal protective equipment. **A.** Level A. **B.** Level B. **C.** Level C. **D.** Level D.

A-C: Courtesy of Rick Brady; **D:** © Jones & Bartlett Learning. Courtesy of MIEMSS.

the case of a WMD scene, this is the area to which victims are brought from the hot zone and where decontamination takes place. The prehospital care provider is still at risk for exposure if working in this area as the agent is carried from the hot zone on victims, emergency responders, and equipment. PPE is recommended based on potential routes of exposure to the substance.

- The *cold zone* is the area outside the hot and warm zones that is not contaminated, where there is no risk of exposure, and thus no specific level of PPE is required beyond standard universal precautions.

It is important to note that it is often difficult to define these control zones and that they may be dynamic rather than static. Factors that contribute to the dynamics of the control zones include the activity of the victims and emergency responders and ambient conditions. For example, unless completely incapacitated, contaminated victims might walk toward prehospital care providers in the cold zone or leave the scene completely, either in panic or with the intention of seeking medical aid at a nearby hospital. By design, warm zones and cold zones are designated upwind of the hot zone, but if wind direction changes, providers would be at risk of exposure if they were unable to don the proper PPE or to rapidly retreat. These contingencies must be anticipated when planning for or responding to a WMD event.

Patient Triage

Prehospital care providers will potentially face a large and overwhelming number of victims who will require evaluation and treatment after a WMD event. Every EMS system should identify and rehearse a mechanism for rapidly triaging victims. The objective of patient triage in a WMD incident is to do the greatest good for the greatest number of victims.

Field triage is typically based on easily measurable physiologic criteria that assign patients to severity categories in order to identify those victims who require treatment and transport to a medical treatment facility most urgently.[2] Several triage schemes and criteria are available.[3] Triage systems include the START (**s**imple **t**riage **a**nd **r**apid **t**reatment) system, the MASS (**m**ove, **a**ssess, **s**ort, **s**end) system, and the SALT (**s**ort by ability to move, **a**ssess need for **l**ifesaving interventions, **t**riage and **t**ransport) system advocated by the Centers for Disease Control and Prevention (CDC).[4] (For more information about triage, see the Disaster Management chapter.)

Whatever patient triage system is used, it must be employed in routine EMS operations to promote familiarity and to ensure recognition among prehospital care providers at all levels of care, including the hospital or trauma center.

Principles of Decontamination

Patients and prehospital care providers alike may require decontamination after exposure to agents that may pose a risk to health. These individuals should have decontamination procedures performed in the field in a designated decontamination area. Decontamination areas are typically upwind and uphill of the affected area when conditions allow. Known exposure to only vapor or gases does not require decontamination to prevent secondary contamination, although the victim's clothing should be removed.

Decontamination is a two-step process that first involves removal of all clothing, jewelry, and shoes, which are bagged, tagged, and secured for later identification. These items may serve as evidence in incident investigation and may be returned to the owner if successfully decontaminated. The simple act of removing clothing achieves removal of the majority of contamination. Any remaining solid contaminant should be carefully brushed away, and any liquid contamination should be blotted off. The second step involves washing the skin surfaces with water or water and a mild detergent to ensure removal of all substances from the skin. Avoid using harsh detergents or bleach solutions on skin, and scrub gently. Chemically or physically aggravating the skin may contribute to increased absorption of the offending agent. When washing, skin folds, axillae, groin, buttocks, and feet must receive special attention because contaminants can collect in these areas and may be overlooked. Decontamination during a radiologic event is almost always dry, as washing may lead to contaminated runoff and is largely effective in removing secondary contamination.

Recently developed specialized decontamination agents, including the Reactive Skin Decontamination Lotion system, Fuller's earth, and various other products, contain active ingredients that may neutralize hazardous chemical agents before they can be fully absorbed through the skin. The exact mechanism of action and application procedures vary by product, but in general they are incorporated as part of the skin decontamination process and are used in place of or in addition to traditionally used soap-and-water or diluted sodium hypochlorite (bleach) solutions. Lab and animal models have suggested usage of these specialized decontamination agents can reduce systemic toxicity and improve survival.[5-6] Individual EMS agencies should consider adding one or more of these products to their decontamination setup; the U.S. Department of Health and Human Services maintains the "Chemical Hazards Emergency Medical Management" website, which contains a helpful database of medical countermeasures and links to supporting research.[7]

Decontamination should be performed in a systematic manner to avoid missing areas of contaminated skin. Contact lenses should be removed from the eyes, and the mucous membranes should be irrigated with copious amounts of water or saline, especially if the patient is symptomatic. Ambulatory patients should be able to perform their own decontamination under instruction from prehospital care providers. Nonambulatory patients will require the assistance of emergency responders properly outfitted with appropriate PPE to decontaminate patients on litters.

Expeditious decontamination may be warranted in the effort to decrease exposure time to various life-threatening substances. All prehospital care providers need to be familiar with a hasty decontamination procedure that may be executed even before arrival of the formal hazardous materials/decontamination team, to minimize exposure time for both patients and emergency responders.

When planning for and setting up a decontamination area, the issues to consider include the following:

- Offering privacy for males and females required to disrobe
- Having warm water available when possible for irrigation and showering
- Providing a suitable substitute for clothing at the completion of decontamination
- Ensuring victims that their personal belongings will be secure until a final disposition is made regarding their return or necessary disposal
- Appropriately disposing of waste water, if practical

After the victim has been decontaminated, there must be a method in place for documenting that the patient has undergone decontamination. At this point, the victim is not released but is instead observed for a period to note whether signs of toxicity occur or reoccur, indicating incomplete removal of the offending agent and the need for repeat washing and treatment.

Explosions, Explosives, and Incendiary Agents

Understanding injury from explosives is essential for all prehospital care providers in both civilian and military settings. Providers need to understand the pathophysiology of injury resulting from unintentional and industrial explosive devices and from the wide range of antipersonnel explosive devices such as letter bombs, shaped warheads from rocket-propelled grenades, antipersonnel land mines, aerial-delivered cluster bombs, enhanced blast weapons, and improvised explosive devices (IEDs). A study of the 36,110 bombing incidents in the United States reported by the Bureau of Alcohol, Tobacco, and Firearms (ATF) between 1983 and 2002 concluded that "the U.S. experience reveals that materials used for bombings are readily available [and] healthcare providers . . . need to be prepared."[8]

Explosions occur in homes (primarily due to gas leaks or fires) and are an occupational hazard of many industries, including mining, demolition, chemical manufacturing, or the handling of fuel or dust-producing substances such as grain. Industrial explosions result from chemical spills, fires, faulty equipment maintenance, or electrical/machinery malfunctions, and they may produce fires, toxic fumes, building collapse, secondary explosions, falling debris, and large numbers of casualties. Another common cause of explosion is the rupture of a pressurized containment vessel, such as a boiler, when the internal pressure exceeds the capability of the container to withstand the elevated pressure. Analyses of workplace-associated fatalities from 1995 to 2010 identified 2,373 incidents of unintentional fires and explosions causing at least one fatality, with fewer than 12% of incidents causing multiple fatalities.[9]

Terrorists worldwide are increasingly using bombs, especially IEDs, against civilian targets. These devices are inexpensive, are made from easily obtained materials, and result in the devastating havoc that focuses international exposure on their efforts. An emergency responder is much more likely to encounter injury from conventional explosives than from a chemical, biologic, or nuclear attack. Globally, over 58,000 terrorist attacks involving the use of explosive devices were identified between 1970 and 2014, with a significant increase in the number of terrorist explosions occurring annually starting in the early 2000s. Of these attacks, approximately 5% were suicide bombings and were associated with significantly increased numbers of fatalities and injuries per attack.[10]

Because both civilian and military emergency responders may be called upon during a bomb attack on civilian populations, all prehospital care providers need to be familiar with their roles during these increasingly frequent occurrences.

At present, although the United States is not typically exposed to as many bomb attacks as other countries, explosive incidents (including intentional bombings, accidental explosions, and incidents of undetermined intent) totaled 912 in 2014; these incidents resulted in 473 injuries and 41 fatalities.[11]

Categories of Explosives

Prehospital care providers need to consider the type of explosive device and its location when evaluating casualties of terrorist blast incidents.[12] Explosives fall into one of two categories based on the velocity of detonation: high explosives and low explosives.

High Explosives

High explosives react almost instantaneously. Because they are designed to detonate and release their energy very quickly, high explosives are capable of producing a shock wave, or **overpressure phenomenon**, which can result in primary blast injury. The initial explosion creates an instantaneous rise in pressure, creating a *shock wave* that travels outward at supersonic speed (1,400–9,000 miles per second, or 2,250–14,500 kilometers (km) per second).[13] Overpressures from high explosions can exceed 4 million pounds per square inch (psi), compared with 14.7 psi ambient pressure. The shock wave is the leading front and an integral component of the *blast wave*, which is created on the rapid release of enormous amounts of energy, with subsequent propulsion of fragments, generation of environmental debris, and often intense thermal radiation (**Box 18-1**). The shock wave, or pressure wave, propagates from the point of origin, rapidly dissipating as the distance from the point of detonation increases. This wave is not to be confused with wind generated by a blast.

Box 18-1 Explosion Terminology

- *Blast wave.* A blast wave results from the sudden conversion of a high explosive from a solid (or liquid) to a gas. This event produces an almost instantaneous rise in atmospheric pressure in the area around the detonation, resulting in highly compressed air molecules that travel faster than the speed of sound. This wave will dissipate rapidly over time and distance.
- *Shock wave.* The leading edge of a blast wave is the shock wave. This high-velocity wave travels at supersonic speeds (10,000–26,000 feet per second [ft/sec], or 3,000–8,000 meters per second [m/sec]). The shock wave carries energy that will strike and pass through objects in its path, causing damage.
- *Stress wave.* Stress waves are high-frequency, supersonic, longitudinal pressure waves that create high local forces with small, rapid distortions of tissue. Longitudinal waves are waves in which the particle displacement occurs in the same direction as the wave is traveling. They cause microvascular injury and are reinforced/reflected at tissue interfaces, thereby enhancing injury potential, especially in gas-filled organs such as the lungs, ears, and intestines. They cause injury via pressure

differentials across delicate structures such as alveoli, rapid compression/reexpansion of gas-filled structures, and reflection of the tension wave (a component of the compressive stress wave) at the tissue–gas interface.
- *Shear wave.* Shear waves are low-frequency, transverse waves with a lower velocity and longer duration than stress waves. Transverse waves are waves in which the displaced particles move perpendicular to the direction in which the wave is traveling. They cause asynchronous movement of tissues. The degree of damage depends on the extent to which the asynchronous motions overcome inherent tissue elasticity, resulting in tearing of tissue and possible disruption of organ attachments.
- *Blast wind.* After the detonation of a high explosive, the force of the explosion pushes all of the air out of the area immediately around the detonation site, creating a sudden vacuum. Once the force of the explosion has been spent, all of the air that was pushed out comes rushing back in response to the vacuum. The result is a powerful wind that can cause objects and debris to be sucked back in toward the site of the explosion.

Common examples of high explosives are 2,4,6-trinitrotoluene (TNT), nitroglycerin, dynamite, ammonium nitrate–fuel oil, and the more recent polymer-bonded explosives that have 1.5 times the power of TNT, such as gelignite and the plastic explosive Semtex. High explosives have a sharp, shattering effect (*brisance*) that can pulverize bone and soft tissue, create blast overpressure injuries (*barotrauma*), and propel debris at ballistic speeds (*fragmentation*). It is also important to note that a high explosive may result in a low-order explosion, particularly if the explosive has deteriorated as a result of age (Semtex) or, in some cases, has become wet (dynamite). The reverse, however, is not true; a low explosive cannot produce a high-order explosion.

Low Explosives

Low explosives (e.g., gunpowder), when activated, change relatively slowly from a solid to a gaseous state (in an action more characteristic of burning than of detonation), generally creating a blast wave that moves less than 6,500 ft/sec (2,000 m/sec). Examples of low explosives include pipe bombs, gunpowder, and pure petroleum-based bombs such as Molotov cocktails.[14] Explosions resulting from container rupture and ignition of volatile compounds fall into this category as well. Because they release their

energy much more slowly, low explosives are not capable of producing overpressure.

The type and amount of explosive will determine the size of the blast associated with detonation of the device. This fact makes the approach to the scene and the location for staging emergency responders and equipment a critical decision. When responding to a scene that involves either a suspicious device or a potential secondary device, all emergency responders must stage at a safe distance from the site in the event of a second detonation (see the Scene Management chapter). **Figure 18-3** provides guidelines for safe distances depending on the possible size of the explosion.

Mechanisms of Injury

Traumatic injury after explosions has generally been divided into three categories: primary, secondary, and tertiary blast injury.[15] In addition to the injuries that result directly from the blast, additional categories of injuries classified as quaternary and quinary have been described and result from complications or toxic effects that are related to the explosive or contaminants. Although these injuries are described separately, they may occur in combination in victims of explosions. **Table 18-1** lists the effects of explosions on the human body.

BOMB THREAT STAND-OFF CHART

Threat Description Improvised Explosive Device (IED)	Explosives Capacity[1] (TNT Equivalent)	Building Evacuation Distance[2]	Outdoor Evacuation Distance[3]
Pipe Bomb	5 LBS	70 FT	1200 FT
Suicide Bomber	20 LBS	110 FT	1700 FT
Briefcase/Suitcase	50 LBS	150 FT	1850 FT
Car	500 LBS	320 FT	1500 FT
SUV/Van	1,000 LBS	400 FT	2400 FT
Small Moving Van/ Delivery Truck	4,000 LBS	640 FT	3800 FT
Moving Van/ Water Truck	10,000 LBS	860 FT	5100 FT
Semi-Trailer	60,000 LBS	1570 FT	9300 FT

1. These capacities are based on the maximum weight of explosive material that could reasonably fit in a container of similar size.
2. Personnel in buildings are provided a high degree of protection from death or serious injury; however, glass breakage and building debris may still cause some injuries. Unstrengthened buildings can be expected to sustain damage that approximates five percent of their replacement cost.
3. If personnel cannot enter a building to seek shelter they must evacuate to the minimum distance recommended by Outdoor Evacuation Distance. These distance is governed by the greater hazard of fragmentation distance, glass breakage or threshold for ear drum rupture.

Figure 18-3 Explosives safe distance stand-off chart.

Courtesy of U.S. Department of Homeland Security.

Table 18-1 Blast Injury Categories			
Effect	**Impact**	**Mechanism of Injury**	**Typical Injuries**
Primary	Direct blast effects (over- and under-pressurization)	■ Contact of blast shockwave with body ■ Stress and shear waves occurring in tissues ■ Waves reinforced/reflected at tissue density interfaces ■ Impact with gas-filled organs (lungs, ears, etc.), which are at particular risk	■ Tympanic membrane rupture ■ Blast lung ■ Eye injuries ■ Concussion
Secondary	Projectiles propelled by explosion	Ballistic wounds produced by: ■ Primary fragments (pieces of exploding weapon) ■ Secondary fragments (environmental fragments [e.g., glass])	■ Penetrating injuries ■ Traumatic amputations ■ Lacerations ■ Concussion

(continued)

Table 18-1 Blast Injury Categories (*continued*)

Effect	Impact	Mechanism of Injury	Typical Injuries
Tertiary	Propulsion of body onto hard surface or object or propulsion of objects onto individuals	▪ Whole-body movement ▪ Crush injuries caused by structural damage and building collapse	▪ Blunt injuries ▪ Crush syndrome ▪ Compartment syndrome ▪ Concussion
Quaternary	Heat and/or combustion fumes	▪ Burns and toxidromes from fuel and metals ▪ Septic syndromes from soil and environmental contamination of wounds	▪ Burns ▪ Inhalation injury ▪ Asphyxiation
Quinary	Additives such as radiation or chemicals (e.g., dirty bombs)	Contamination of tissue from: ▪ Bacteria, radiation, or chemical agents ▪ Bone fragments from other victims	▪ Variety of health effects, depending on agent

Data from Department of Defense Directive: Medical Research for Prevention, Mitigation, and Treatment of Blast Injuries. Number 6025.21E. http://www.dtic.mil/whs/directives/corres/pdf/602521p.pdf. Accessed April 19, 2014.

Primary Blast Injury

Primary blast injury results from high-order explosive detonation and the interaction of the blast overpressure wave with the body or tissue to produce stress and shear waves. **Stress waves** are supersonic, longitudinal pressure waves that (1) create high local forces with small, rapid distortions; (2) produce microvascular injury; and (3) are reinforced and reflected at tissue interfaces, thereby enhancing injury potential, especially in gas-filled organs such as the lungs, ears, and intestines. Injuries from the stress waves are caused by (1) pressure differentials across delicate structures such as the alveoli of the lung, (2) rapid compression of and subsequent reexpansion of gas-filled structures, and (3) reflection of the wave at the tissue–gas interface.

Shear waves are transverse waves with a lower velocity and longer duration that cause asynchronous movement of tissues. The degree of damage depends on the extent to which the asynchronous motions overcome inherent tissue elasticity, resulting in tearing of tissue and possible disruption of attachments. However, muscle, bone, and solid-organ injury are much more likely to result from the tertiary and quaternary effects of the explosion than from the shock wave alone.[16,17]

Depending on the proximity of the victim to the explosion, as well as shielding from or augmentation to the shock wave if the explosion occurs in a closed space, a victim may suffer primary blast injury.

Primary blast injury occurs in gas-filled organs such as the lung, bowel, and middle ear. The injury to the tissue occurs at the gas–fluid interface, presumably from a rapid compression of the gas in the organ, causing violent collapse of that organ, followed by an equally rapid and violent expansion, resulting in tissue injury. Damage to the lung manifests as pulmonary contusions, or possibly *hemopneumothoraces*, resulting in hypoxemia if the patient does not immediately succumb to the injuries (**Box 18-2**). The alveolar–capillary interface can also become disrupted, resulting in arterial gas emboli, which may cause cerebral or cardiac embolic complications. Damage to the bowel may include hematomas of the bowel wall or even perforation of the bowel. Tympanic membrane rupture or disruption of the middle ear ossicles also may occur. Loss of hearing is common after an explosion and may be temporary or permanent.

Evidence of primary blast injury to the lung (or BLI) is found more often in patients who die minutes after the explosion from associated injuries than those who survive; however, pulmonary primary blast injury has been noted with greater frequency among surviving victims of confined-space explosions.[18-20] Primary blast injury has also been associated with other severe injuries and is indicative of increased mortality risk in survivors of the initial event. After an open-air explosion in Beirut, only 0.6% of survivors had evidence of primary blast injury, and 11% of those died.[21] In a confined-space explosion in Jerusalem,

Box 18-2 Blast Lung Injury: What Prehospital Care Providers Need to Know

Current patterns in worldwide terrorist activity have increased the potential for casualties related to explosions, yet few civilian prehospital care providers in the United States have experience treating patients with explosion-related injuries. **Blast lung injury (BLI)** presents unique triage, diagnostic, and management challenges and is a direct consequence of the blast wave from high-explosive detonations upon the body. Persons in enclosed space explosions or those in close proximity to the explosion are at a higher risk. BLI is a clinical diagnosis characterized by respiratory difficulty and hypoxia. BLI can occur, although rarely, without obvious external injury to the chest. It is often not an immediate manifestation but develops over several hours during the overall course of resuscitation.

Clinical Presentation

- Symptoms may include dyspnea, hemoptysis, cough, and chest pain.
- Signs may include tachypnea, hypoxia, cyanosis, apnea, wheezing, decreased breath sounds, and hemodynamic instability.
- Victims with greater than 10% body surface area burns, skull fractures, and penetrating torso or head injuries may be more likely to have BLI.
- Hemothoraces or pneumothoraces may occur.
- Due to tearing of the pulmonary and vascular tree, air may enter the arterial circulation (*air emboli*) and result in embolic events involving the central nervous system, retinal arteries, or coronary arteries, resulting in stroke-like symptoms.
- Clinical evidence of BLI is often present at the time of initial evaluation; however, it more typically presents several hours after initial injury during the course of resuscitation and has been reported to occur as late as 24 to 48 hours after an explosion.
- Other injuries may often be present.

Prehospital Management Considerations

While scene safety is always a major consideration for prehospital care providers, incidents such as these often require emergency responders of all types to enter the scene before it can be declared completely secure. Providers must remain aware of their surroundings, be observant for possible additional devices, and consider other hazards that may have resulted as a consequence of the primary explosion.

Patient assessment and management steps are as follows, assuming direct and indirect threat potential has been mitigated and providers have a safe operating environment consistent with the instruction in tactical combat casualty care (TCCC) and tactical emergency casualty care (TECC):

- Initial triage, trauma resuscitation, and transport of patients should follow standard protocols for multiple injured patients or mass casualties, including assessment and treatment of the XABCDEs (exsanguinating hemorrhage, airway, breathing, circulation, disability, and expose/environment) and immediate control of exsanguinating hemorrhage.
- Note the patient's location and the surrounding environment. Explosions in a confined space result in a higher incidence of primary blast injury, including lung injury.
- All patients with suspected or confirmed BLI should receive supplemental high-flow oxygen sufficient to prevent hypoxemia.
- Impending airway compromise requires immediate intervention.
- If ventilatory failure is imminent or occurs, patients should be intubated; however, prehospital care providers must realize that mechanical ventilation and positive pressure may increase the risk of alveolar rupture, pneumothorax, and air embolism in BLI patients.
- High-flow oxygen should be administered if air embolism is suspected, and the patient should be placed in a semi-left lateral or left lateral position.
- Clinical evidence of or suspicion for a hemothorax or pneumothorax warrants close observation. Chest decompression should be performed for patients clinically presenting with a tension pneumothorax. Close observation is warranted for any patient with suspicion of BLI who is transported by air.
- Fluids should be administered judiciously, as overzealous fluid administration in the patient with BLI may result in volume overload and the worsening of pulmonary status.
- Patients with BLI should be transported rapidly to the nearest appropriate facility, in accordance with community response plans for mass-casualty events.

Data from Centers for Disease Control and Prevention, Atlanta.

38% of survivors had evidence of primary blast injury, with a similar mortality rate of approximately 9%.[22] Similarly, two of the three bombs that were detonated in the London subway system exploded in wide tunnels, resulting in 6 and 7 fatalities, respectively. The third device detonated in the subway system was exploded in a narrow tunnel, causing 26 fatalities. This difference in mortality between open- and closed-space bombings results from the reflection of the blast wave back onto the victims rather than the dispersal of the blast wave into the surrounding area.

Secondary Blast Injury

Secondary blast injury is caused by flying debris and bomb fragments. Secondary blast injury is the most common category of injury in terrorist bombings and low explosions. These projectiles may be components of the bomb itself, as in military weapons designed to fragment, or they may be parts of improvised bombs augmented with nails, screws, and bolts. Secondary blast injury is also caused by debris that is carried by the *blast wind* (Box 18-1). The force required to create enough overpressure to rupture 50% of exposed tympanic membranes (approximately 5 psi) can briefly generate blast winds of 145 miles per hour (233 km per hour). Blast winds associated with an overpressure resulting in significant primary blast injury may exceed 831 miles per hour (1,337 km per hour).[16] Although brief in duration, these blast winds can propel debris with great force and for great distances, causing both penetrating and blunt trauma.

Tertiary Blast Injury

Tertiary blast injury is caused by the blast wind throwing the victim's body, resulting in tumbling and collision with stationary objects. This can result in the whole spectrum of injuries associated with blunt trauma and even penetrating trauma, such as an impalement.

Quaternary and Quinary Effects

Following the blast itself, **quaternary effects** may be seen.[15] These injuries include burns and toxicities from fuel, metals, trauma from structural collapse, and septic syndromes from soil and environmental contamination of wounds.

The increasing threat of radiation-, chemical-, or biologic-enhanced explosives (i.e., dirty bombs) has given rise to a fifth (*quinary*) category of effects, which includes injuries caused by radiation, chemicals, or biologic agents and projectiles such as bone fragments of a suicide bomber.[23,24]

Injury Patterns

The prehospital care provider will be confronted with a combination of familiar penetrating, blunt, and thermal injuries and possibly survivors with primary blast injury.[25] The numbers and types of injuries will depend on multiple factors, including explosion magnitude, composition,

environment, and location and number of potential victims at risk.

Various mortality rates have been associated with different types of bombings. One study that examined terrorist bombings showed that 1 of 4 victims died immediately after structural-collapse bombings, 1 of 12 died immediately in closed-space bombings, and 1 of 25 died immediately after open-space bombings.[13,26] Additional studies have found that mortality is higher when an explosion occurs in an enclosed space.[27,28] Soft-tissue injuries, orthopedic trauma, and traumatic brain injury are predominant among survivors (**Box 18-3**).

For example, of 592 survivors of the Oklahoma City bombing, 85% had soft-tissue injuries (lacerations, puncture wounds, abrasions, contusions), 25% had sprains, 14% had head injuries, 10% had fractures/dislocations, 10% had ocular injuries (9 with ruptured globes), and 2% had burns.[29] The most common location for soft-tissue injury was the extremities (74%), followed by head and neck (48%), face (45%), and chest (35%). Eighteen survivors had severe soft-tissue injuries, including carotid artery and jugular vein lacerations; facial and popliteal artery lacerations; and severed nerves, tendons, and ligaments. Seventeen survivors had serious internal organ injury, including partial bowel transection; lacerated kidney, spleen, and liver; pneumothorax; and pulmonary contusion. Of patients with fractures, 37% had multiple fractures. Of those diagnosed with a head injury, 44% required admission to the hospital.[28]

Evaluation and Management

The general evaluation and management of trauma victims are applicable to the casualty from a WMD and are addressed in other chapters. Unique to this patient population, however, is the possibility of primary blast injury.

Primary blast injuries might increase the likelihood that prehospital care providers will encounter patients with hemoptysis and pulmonary contusions, pneumothorax or tension pneumothorax, or even arterial gas embolism. Among survivors of primary blast injury, clinical manifestations may be present immediately[30,31] or may have a delayed onset of 24 to 48 hours.[32] Intrapulmonary hemorrhage and focal alveolar edema result in frothy bloody secretions and lead to ventilation–perfusion mismatch, increased intrapulmonary shunting, and decreased compliance. Hypoxia results, with increased work of breathing. This is similar in pathophysiology to pulmonary contusions induced by other mechanisms of nonpenetrating thoracic trauma.[33] The presence of rib fractures should increase suspicion of tertiary or quaternary injury to the thorax.

Primary blast injuries are not immediately apparent, and, therefore, care at the scene should include (1) monitoring for frothy secretions and respiratory distress, (2) sequential oxygen saturation (SpO_2) measurements, and (3) provision of oxygen. Decreased SpO_2 is a "red flag" for early BLI even before symptoms begin. Fluid administration must be carefully managed, with care taken to avoid fluid overload.[1]

The likelihood of multisystem trauma is increased in bomb victims.[34] The management principles for these patients are similar to those for trauma from other mechanisms.

Transport Considerations

Patients requiring transport must be brought to an appropriate medical treatment facility for further evaluation and management. These patients often require the services of a designated trauma center. Prehospital care providers should be aware of the epidemiology of patient transport after an explosives event. Patient arrival at hospitals is usually *bimodal*, with ambulatory patients arriving first and more critically ill patients arriving later by ambulance.

This bimodal patient transport was demonstrated in the Oklahoma City bombing. Patients began to arrive in the EDs 5 to 30 minutes after the bombing, with patients who were more seriously injured taking longer to arrive. Also, the geographically closest hospitals in Oklahoma City received the majority of victims, as seen with other disasters. Nearby hospitals that are overwhelmed by the first wave of patients may experience some difficulty managing the critically ill patients that arrive in the second wave. In Oklahoma City, the aggregate peak arrival rate of patients to EDs was 220 per hour at 60 to 90 minutes; 64% of patients visited EDs within a 1.5-mile radius of the event. Prehospital care providers should consider this latter fact when determining the destination of patients transported by ambulance from the bomb scene.[1]

Incendiary Agents

Incendiary agents are typically encountered in the military and are used to burn equipment, vehicles, and structures.

Terrorists may use them to increase the lethality of improvised explosive devices. The three incendiary agents most often recognized are thermite, magnesium, and white phosphorus. All three are highly flammable compounds that burn at extremely high temperatures.

Thermite

Thermite is powdered aluminum and iron oxide that burns furiously at 3,600°F (1,982°C) and scatters molten iron.[35] Its primary mechanism of injury is partial-thickness or full-thickness burns. The primary and secondary surveys are performed with intervention directed at treating burns. Thermite wounds can be irrigated with copious amounts of water and any residual particles or material subsequently removed.

Magnesium

Magnesium is also a metal in powdered or solid form that burns furiously hot. In addition to its ability to cause partial-thickness or full-thickness burns, magnesium can react with tissue fluid and cause alkali burns. The same chemical reaction produces hydrogen gas, which can cause the wound to bubble or can result in subcutaneous emphysema. Inhalation of magnesium dust can produce respiratory symptoms, including cough, tachypnea, hypoxia, wheeze, pneumonitis, and airway burns. Residual magnesium particles in a wound will react with water, so irrigation is discouraged until the wounds can be debrided and the particulates removed. If irrigation is required for other reasons, such as decontamination of another suspected material, care should be taken to ensure flushing or removal of magnesium particles from the wound.[35]

White Phosphorus

White phosphorus (WP) is a solid that spontaneously ignites when exposed to air, causing a yellow flame and white smoke. WP that comes in contact with skin can quickly result in partial-thickness or full-thickness burns. WP can become embedded in the skin, propelled by the blast of WP munitions. The substance will continue to burn in the skin if exposed to air. Prehospital care providers can decrease the likelihood of combustion in the skin by immersing the affected areas in water or applying saline-soaked dressings to the area. Oily or greasy dressings are avoided in these patients because WP is lipid soluble, and application of these dressings may increase the likelihood of systemic absorption and toxicity. Systemic absorption can lead to lethal heart, liver, and kidney injury. Contaminated clothing should be removed, as it may catch fire if the WP re-ignites. WP fluoresces under ultraviolet light, which can be used to ensure thorough decontamination. Copper sulfate has historically been used to neutralize WP and facilitate its removal because the reaction results in a black compound, which is easier to identify in the skin.

Copper sulfate has fallen out of favor, however, because of complications from its use—specifically, intravascular hemolysis (breakdown or rupture of red blood cells within blood vessels); topical application of silver nitrate may be safer and more effective in decontaminating WP embedded in skin and wounds.[36]

Chemical Agents

Many scenarios could expose the prehospital care provider to chemical agents, including an industrial complex accident, a spilled tanker truck or railway car, unearthed military ordnance, or a terrorist attack (**Box 18-4**). The 1984 Union Carbide industrial accident in Bhopal, India, and the sarin gas attack in Tokyo in 1995 are examples of such incidents.

Physical Properties of Chemical Agents

The physical properties of a substance are affected by its chemical structure, the environmental temperature, and ambient pressure. These factors will determine whether a substance exists as a solid, liquid, or gas. Understanding the physical state of a chemical agent is important for the prehospital care provider because it gives clues about the likely route of exposure and the potential for transmission and contamination.

A solid is in a state of matter that has a fixed volume and shape; a powder is an example of a solid. When heated to its melting point, solids become liquids. Liquids that are heated to their boiling point become a gas. Solid particles and liquid particles can become suspended in the air, similar to a dust particle or a liquid mist. This is considered

---

Box 18-4 Classification of Chemical Agents

- Cyanides (blood agents or asphyxiants)
  · Hydrogen cyanide, cyanogen chloride
- Nerve agents
  · Tabun (GA), sarin (GB), soman (GD), cyclosarin (GF), VX, some agricultural pesticides
- Lung toxicants (choking or pulmonary agents)
  · Chlorine, phosgene, diphosgene, ammonia
- Vesicants (blistering agents)
  · Sulfur mustard, lewisite
- Incapacitating agents
  · BZ (3-quinuclidinyl benzilate)
- Lacrimating agents (riot control agents)
  · CN and CS (tear gas agents), oleoresin capsicum (OC or pepper spray)
- Vomiting agents
  · Adamsite

---

an **aerosol**. A **vapor** is simply a solid or liquid that is in a gaseous state but technically would be expected to be found as a solid or liquid at standard temperature and pressure, defined as 32°F (0°C) and normal atmospheric pressure (1 atmosphere, 14.7 psi). Some solids and liquids can, therefore, emit vapors at room temperature. The process of solids emitting vapors, bypassing the liquid state, is called **sublimation**. The likelihood that solids or liquids vaporize into a gaseous form at room temperature is defined as the **volatility** of the substance. Highly volatile substances easily convert into a gas at room temperature.

These physical properties have implications for primary and secondary contamination and possible routes of exposure. **Primary contamination** is defined as exposure to the chemical agent at its point of release. For example, primary contamination occurs, by definition, in the hot zone. Gases, vapors, liquids, solids, and aerosols can all play a role in primary contamination.

Secondary contamination is defined as exposure to a chemical agent after it has been carried away from the point of origin, whether by a victim, an emergency responder, or a piece of contaminated equipment or debris. Secondary contamination generally occurs in the warm zone, although it may happen at more remote locations if the exposed victim is able to self-evacuate. Solids and liquids (and sometimes aerosols) generally contribute to secondary contamination. Gases and vapors do not typically play a role in secondary contamination because they cause injury by inhalation of the substance and do not deposit on skin. However, vapors can become trapped in clothing and then off-gas to potentially expose others to the hazard.

Volatility plays a significant role in the risk of secondary contamination. More volatile substances are considered "less persistent," meaning that because they vaporize, the likelihood of long-lasting physical contamination is unlikely. These chemical agents will readily disperse and be carried away by the wind. Less volatile substances are considered "more persistent." These substances do not vaporize, or do so at a very slow rate, thereby remaining on exposed surfaces for a long time, increasing the risk of secondary contamination. For example, the nerve agent sarin is a nonpersistent agent, whereas the nerve agent VX is a persistent agent.[37]

Personal Protective Equipment

PPE is selected based on the threat of exposure to the chemical agent. Level A is appropriate for emergency responders entering the hot zone, until specific agents in use and their concentrations are known. Once the agent has been identified, incident command may make the decision to move to lower levels of PPE (B or C), particularly for responders tasked with carrying out decontamination or working in the "warm zone." Of note, agency-specific protocols should always determine the zone in which responders are able to operate safely.

Evaluation and Management

After ensuring the safety of the scene, the prehospital care provider must first confirm that victims are undergoing decontamination. Patients with likely skin exposure to the liquid form of a chemical will require decontamination with water. If available, soap may be used as well, but showering with copious amounts of water will generally suffice. Exposure to a gas does not mandate decontamination by shower, but it does mandate removal from any ongoing exposure and removal of any clothing that may have trapped residual vapors, which can subsequently off-gas and pose a hazard to care providers in the field or in the hospital.

Once the victim has been properly decontaminated, the prehospital care provider will likely encounter patients with signs and symptoms of exposure to a hazardous substance that has not yet been specifically identified. Victims of chemical agents can manifest signs and symptoms of exposure that affect the following areas:

- The respiratory system, affecting oxygenation and ventilation
- The mucous membranes, causing eye and upper airway injury
- The nervous system, resulting in seizures or coma and altered levels of consciousness
- The gastrointestinal (GI) tract, causing vomiting or diarrhea
- The skin, causing burning and blistering

It is important to evaluate the presenting signs and symptoms and whether they are improving or progressing. Patients with worsening clinical findings likely had incomplete cleansing of the contaminant and should undergo repeat decontamination to assure complete removal.

Patients require a primary survey to determine what lifesaving intervention may be immediately required. A secondary survey may then assist in the identification of symptom constellations that might indicate the nature of the chemical agent and suggest a specific antidote. This constellation of clinical signs and symptoms suggesting exposure to a certain class of chemical or toxin is called a **toxidrome**.[38]

The *irritant gas toxidrome* includes mucous membrane burning and inflammation, coughing, and difficulty breathing. Agents responsible might include chlorine, phosgene, or ammonia.

The *asphyxiant toxidrome* is caused by cellular oxygen deprivation. This can result from inadequate oxygen availability, as in an oxygen-poor atmosphere; inadequate oxygen delivery to the cells, as in carbon monoxide poisoning; or inability to utilize oxygen at the cellular level, as in cyanide poisoning. Signs and symptoms include shortness of breath, chest pain, dysrhythmias, syncope, seizures, coma, and death.

The *cholinergic toxidrome* is characterized by rhinorrhea, respiratory secretions, difficulty breathing, nausea, vomiting, diarrhea, profuse sweating, pinpoint pupils, possible altered mental status, seizures, and coma. Pesticides and nerve agents can cause these cholinergic signs and symptoms.[39,40]

Most often, prehospital care providers will initiate supportive therapy without knowing the specific chemical cause of the injury. If the offending agent is properly identified, or if its identity is suggested by the toxidrome or clinical presentation, therapy specific to the agent may be delivered. Cyanide and nerve agent victims are examples of patients who can benefit from agent-specific antidote therapy.

Transport Considerations

Contaminated patients should not be transported until they have been decontaminated. Transporting contaminated patients results in cross-contamination of the transporting vehicle and personnel, thus taking them out of service until they have been decontaminated. This leads to compromise of the response capability of the ambulance service and may prolong the scene time and management of ill or injured patients. This same concern about not transporting contaminated patients applies to air-medical services.

Patients must be brought to an appropriate medical treatment facility for further evaluation and management. Transporting to the optimal facility is particularly important because some chemical toxic effects may not become apparent for 8 to 24 hours. Communities may identify preferred hospitals for the management of chemical casualties. These facilities may be more capable of managing these patients by virtue of specialized training or availability of critical care services and specific antidotes. Considerations similar to those previously noted for explosive incidents regarding transport epidemiology also apply to these patients.

Nearby EDs may become overwhelmed by ambulatory, self-evacuated, self-transported patients. Of the 640 patients presenting to one hospital in Tokyo after the sarin incident, 541 arrived without EMS assistance.[41] Hospitals closest to the event will likely receive the largest number of ambulatory patients. These factors should be considered in determining the destination of patients transported via ambulance.

Selected Specific Chemical Agents

Cyanides

Prehospital care providers encounter cyanides most commonly when responding to a fire in which certain plastics or textiles are burning or to certain industrial complexes, where they may be found in large quantities. Cyanides are used in chemical syntheses, electroplating, mineral extraction, dyeing, printing, photography, agriculture, and the manufacture of paper, textiles, and plastics. However, cyanide also has been inventoried in military stockpiles, and some terrorist websites have provided instructions for making a cyanide dispersal device.

Hydrogen cyanide is a highly volatile liquid and, thus, will most often be encountered as a vapor or gas. Therefore, it has greater potential for mass casualties in a confined space with poor ventilation than if released outdoors. Although a smell of bitter almonds has been associated with this agent, this is not a reliable indicator of hydrogen cyanide exposure. It is estimated that up to half of the general population is incapable of detecting the odor of cyanide.

Cyanide's mechanism of action is arrest of metabolism or respiration at the cellular level, quickly resulting in cell death. Cyanide binds in the mitochondria of cells, preventing oxygen usage in cellular metabolism. Victims of cyanide poisoning actually are able to inhale and absorb oxygen into the blood but are unable to use it at the cellular level. Thus, patients who are ventilating will present with evidence of acyanotic hypoxia.

The organs most affected are the central nervous system (CNS) and the heart. Symptoms of mild cyanide poisoning include headache, dizziness, drowsiness, nausea, vomiting, and mucosal irritation. Severe cyanide poisoning includes alteration of consciousness, dysrhythmias, hypotension, seizures, and death. Death can occur within a few minutes after inhalation of high levels of cyanide gas.

Management

Supportive therapy is important, including high-concentration oxygen delivery, correction of hypotension with fluids or vasopressors, and management of seizures. Cyanide antidote kits are available for patients with known or suspected cyanide poisoning.

Hydroxocobalamin (pro-vitamin B_{12}) is the preferred field antidote for cyanide poisoning because it is easy to use, it involves a single medication administration instead of two, and it does not create an intermediate chemical that is itself a poison. Modern cyanide antidote kits contain IV hydroxocobalamin, which binds with cyanide to form cyanocobalamin (vitamin B_{12}), which is nontoxic.

The traditional, now antiquated, cyanide antidote treatment kit involved treatment with two medications, a nitrite followed by thiosulfate. The administration of inhaled amyl nitrite, or preferably intravenous (IV) sodium nitrite, creates methemoglobin (itself a poison that in high enough concentrations can kill), which binds cyanide in the bloodstream, making it less available to poison the patient's cellular respiration. The nitrite is followed by IV administration of sodium thiosulfate to assist the body in the conversion of cyanide to harmless thiocyanate, which is excreted by the kidneys.

Nerve Agents

Nerve agents were originally developed as insecticides, but once their effects on humans were recognized, numerous different types were developed in the early to mid-1900s. These deadly chemicals can be found in the military stockpiles of many nations. Nerve agents have also been produced and used by terrorist organizations, the most notorious releases occurring in Matsumoto, Japan, in 1994 and in the Tokyo, Japan, subway system in 1995. More recently, United Nations inspectors confirmed the use of the nerve agent sarin against civilians in the Syrian civil war in 2013, resulting in multiple casualties, including first responders.[42] Commonly available pesticides (e.g., malathion, carbaryl [Sevin]) and common therapeutic medications (e.g., physostigmine, pyridostigmine) share properties with nerve agents, causing similar clinical effects.

Nerve agents are usually liquids at room temperature. Sarin is the most volatile of the group. VX is the least volatile and is found as an oily liquid. The main routes of intoxication are through inhalation of the vapor (usually the volatile or nonpersistent agents) and absorption through the skin (usually VX). Nerve agents can injure or kill at very low doses. A single small drop the size of a pinhead of VX, the most potent nerve agent developed, placed on the skin could kill a victim. Because nerve agents are liquids, they pose a risk for secondary contamination from contact with contaminated clothes, skin, and other objects.

The mechanism of action of nerve agents is inhibition of the enzyme acetylcholinesterase, an enzyme required to break down acetylcholine. **Acetylcholine** is a neurotransmitter that stimulates cholinergic receptors. Acetylcholine receptors are found in smooth muscles, skeletal muscles, the CNS, and most exocrine (secretory) glands. Some of these cholinergic receptors are termed **muscarinic sites** (because experimentally they are stimulated by muscarine) and are mostly found in smooth muscles and glands. Others are termed **nicotinic sites** (because experimentally they are stimulated by nicotine) and are mostly found in skeletal muscle. The mnemonic **DUMBELS** (**d**iarrhea, **u**rination, **m**iosis, **b**radycardia, **b**ronchorrhea, **b**ronchospasm, **e**mesis, **l**acrimation, **s**alivation, **s**weating) represents the constellation of symptoms associated with the muscarinic effects of nerve agent toxicity. The mnemonic **MTWHF** (**m**ydriasis [rarely seen], **t**achycardia, **w**eakness, **h**ypertension, **h**yperglycemia, **f**asciculations) represents the constellation of symptoms associated with stimulation of nicotinic receptors (**Box 18-5**). The CNS effects, a result of both muscarinic and nicotinic receptors, include confusion, convulsions, and coma.

The clinical effects depend on the dose and route of nerve agent exposure (inhalation or dermal) and whether the muscarinic or nicotinic effects predominate. Small amounts of vapor exposure primarily cause irritation to eyes, nose, and airways. Large amounts of vapor exposure can quickly lead to loss of consciousness, seizures, apnea, and muscular flaccidity. *Miosis* (constricted pupils) is the most sensitive marker of exposure to vapor. Symptoms of dermal exposure also vary according to dose and time of onset. Small doses may not result in symptoms for up to 18 hours. Fasciculations of the underlying muscles and localized sweating at the site of the skin exposure may occur, followed by GI symptoms, nausea, vomiting, and diarrhea. Large dermal doses will result in onset of symptoms in minutes, with effects similar to a large vapor exposure.

Clinical symptoms of nerve agents include *rhinorrhea* (runny nose), chest tightness, miosis (pupil is pinpoint, and patient complains of blurry or dim vision), shortness of breath, excessive salivation and sweating, nausea, vomiting, abdominal cramps, involuntary urination and defecation, muscle fasciculations, confusion, seizures, flaccid paralysis, coma, respiratory failure, and death.

Management

Management of nerve agent poisoning includes decontamination (**Figure 18-4**), a primary survey, administration of antidotes, and supportive therapy. Ventilation and oxygenation of the patient may be difficult because of bronchoconstriction and copious secretions. The patient will likely require frequent suctioning. These symptoms improve after the antidote is administered. The three therapeutic medications for the management of nerve agent poisoning are atropine, pralidoxime chloride, and benzodiazepines.

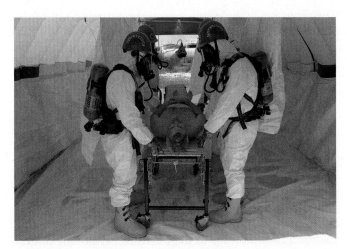

Figure 18-4 Decontamination from nerve agents.
© Jones & Bartlett Learning. Photographed by Glen E. Ellman.

Atropine is an anticholinergic medication that reverses most of the muscarinic effects of the nerve agent via competitive antagonism at the receptor site, although it has little effect on the nicotinic sites. Atropine is indicated for exposed victims with pulmonary complaints. Miosis alone is not an indication for atropine, and furthermore, atropine will not correct the ocular abnormalities. Atropine is given according to local system protocols. It is titrated until the patient's ability to breathe or ventilate is improved or there is drying of pulmonary secretions. In moderate to severe exposures, it is not unusual to start with an initial dose of 4 to 6 milligrams (mg) and give as much as 10 to 20 mg of atropine over a few hours.

Pralidoxime chloride (2-PAM chloride) is an oxime. Pralidoxime works by uncoupling the bond between the nerve agent and acetylcholinesterase, thereby reactivating the enzyme and helping to reduce the effects of the nerve agent, primarily on nicotinic receptors. The oxime therapy needs to be initiated within minutes to a few hours of the exposure to be effective, depending on the nerve agent released; otherwise, the bond between acetylcholinesterase and the nerve agent will become permanent ("aging"), delaying recovery of the patient.

Benzodiazepine therapy is initiated to manage the seizures and help to reduce the brain injury and other life-threatening effects associated with status epilepticus. They are recommended for all patients with signs of severe nerve agent poisoning whether or not they have begun to seize. Midazolam (Versed) is the preferred benzodiazepine medication, due to its rapid, high bioavailability after intramuscular or intravenous injection. Evidence from animal models suggests the seizure-terminating and neuroprotective effects are lessened if administration is delayed after the initial poisoning.[43] If midazolam is unavailable, diazepam (Valium) or lorazepam (Ativan) are alternative agents, but they may be less effective than midazolam.[44,45]

Atropine and pralidoxime come packaged together in a single autoinjector called DuoDote (**Figure 18-5**). The dose of atropine is 2.1 mg, and the dose of pralidoxime is 600 mg. This autoinjector is intended for rapid intramuscular injection in the event of a nerve agent exposure. Total dosage is determined by protocol and titration of these medications to effect. In the past, the atropine and pralidoxime were supplied in individual autoinjectors marketed as the Mark-1 kit. These kits have largely been supplanted by the single autoinjector containing both antidotes. Midazolam and diazepam for seizures are also available as autoinjectors.

Lung Toxicants

Lung toxicants, including chlorine, phosgene, ammonia, sulfur dioxide, and nitrogen dioxide, are present in numerous industrial manufacturing applications. Phosgene has been stockpiled for military applications and was the most lethal chemical warfare agent used in World War I.

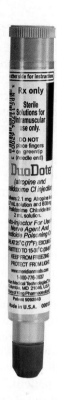

Figure 18-5 DuoDote.
Courtesy of Pfizer, Inc.

United Nations investigators researching chemical attacks during the Syrian civil war suspected, but could not absolutely confirm, that chlorine was used as a weapon in multiple incidents.[46]

Lung toxicants that are chemical pulmonary agents may be gases, vapors, aerosolized liquids, or solids. The properties of the agent influence its ability to cause injury. For example, aerosolized particles of 2 micrometers (μm) or smaller readily access the alveoli of the lung, causing injury there, whereas larger particles are filtered out before reaching the alveoli. Water solubility of an agent also affects the injury pattern. Ammonia and sulfur dioxide, which are highly water soluble, cause irritation and injury to the eyes, mucous membranes, and upper airways. Phosgene and nitrogen oxides, which have low water solubility, tend to cause less immediate irritation and injury to the eyes, mucous membranes, and upper airways, thus providing little warning to the victim and allowing for prolonged exposure to these agents. Prolonged exposure makes it more likely that the alveoli will be injured, resulting not only in upper-airway injury, but also in alveolar collapse and noncardiogenic pulmonary edema. Moderately water-soluble agents, such as chlorine, can cause both upper airway and alveolar irritation.

The mechanisms of injury vary among the lung toxicants. Ammonia, for example, combines with the water in the mucous membranes to form a strong base, ammonium hydroxide. Chlorine and phosgene, when combined with water, produce hydrochloric acid, causing injury to the tissues. Lung toxicants are not systemically absorbed but compromise the victim by damaging components of the pulmonary system, from the upper airway to the alveoli.

The agents with high water solubility cause burning of the eyes, nose, and mouth. Tearing, rhinorrhea, coughing, dyspnea, and respiratory distress secondary to glottic irritation or laryngospasm are possible. Bronchospasm can result in coughing, wheezing, and dyspnea. Agents with low water solubility, causing injury to the alveoli, can immediately injure the alveolar epithelium in the case of a large exposure, leading to death from acute respiratory failure, or, with less massive exposure, can result in a delayed onset (24 to 48 hours) of respiratory distress, secondary to development of mild noncardiogenic pulmonary edema to fulminant acute respiratory distress syndrome, depending on the dose.

Management

Management of lung toxicants includes removal of the patient from the offending agent, decontamination with copious irrigation (if solid, liquid, or aerosol exposure, especially for ammonia), primary survey, and supportive therapy, which will likely require interventions to maximize ventilation and oxygenation. Eye irritation can be managed with copious irrigation using normal saline. Contact lenses should be removed. Expect to manage profuse airway secretions, which will require suctioning. Bronchospasm may respond to inhaled beta-adrenergic agonists. Hypoxia will require correction with high-flow oxygen and possibly intubation with positive-pressure ventilation. Prehospital care providers need to be prepared to encounter difficult airway management secondary to copious secretions, inflammation of glottic structures, and laryngeal spasm. All victims exposed to phosgene should be transported for evaluation because of the likelihood of delayed symptoms.

Vesicant Agents

The vesicants include sulfur mustard, nitrogen mustards, and lewisite. These agents have been stockpiled for military operations by many countries. Sulfur mustard was first introduced to the battlefield in World War I. It was reportedly used by Iraq against its Kurdish population and also in its conflict with Iran in 1980. More recently it is suspected to have been used in warfare in Syria. It is relatively easy and inexpensive to manufacture.

Sulfur mustard is an oily, clear to yellow-brown liquid that can be aerosolized by a bomb blast or a sprayer. Its volatility is low, allowing it to persist on surfaces for a week or more. This persistence allows for easy secondary contamination. The agent is absorbed through the skin and mucous membranes, resulting in direct cellular damage within 3 to 5 minutes of the exposure, although clinical symptoms and signs may take 1 to 12 hours (usually 4 to

6 hours) after exposure to develop. The delayed onset of symptoms often makes it difficult for the victim to recognize that the exposure occurred and, therefore, increases the potential for secondary contamination. Warm, moist skin increases the likelihood of skin absorption, making the groin and axillary regions particularly susceptible. The eyes, skin, and upper airways can develop a range of findings, from erythema and edema to vesicle development to full-thickness necrosis. Upper airway involvement can result in cough and bronchospasm. High-dose exposures can result in nausea and vomiting, as well as bone marrow suppression.

Management for sulfur mustard involves decontamination using soap and water, primary survey, and supportive therapy; no antidote exists for the effects of mustard agents. In fact, it is important to note that because the cellular damage from sulfur mustard occurs within several minutes of the exposure, decontamination will not change the clinical course of the exposed patient. It is primarily intended to prevent inadvertent cross-contamination. Eyes and skin should be decontaminated with copious amounts of water as soon as exposure is recognized to minimize further absorption of the agent and prevent secondary contamination. The fluid in resulting vesicles and blisters is not a source of secondary contamination. Pulmonary bronchoconstriction may benefit from nebulized beta-agonists. Skin wounds should be treated as burns, with regard to local wound care.

Lewisite has a similar constellation of symptoms, but the onset of action is much quicker than with sulfur mustard, resulting in immediate pain and irritation to the eyes, skin, and respiratory tract. Unlike sulfur mustard, lewisite does not cause bone marrow suppression. Also unique to this agent is "lewisite shock," the result of intravascular volume depletion secondary to capillary leakage.

As with sulfur mustard, prehospital management of these exposed patients involves decontamination, primary survey, and supportive care. British anti-lewisite is an antidote available for the in-hospital treatment of lewisite-exposed patients. It is administered intravenously for patients with hypovolemic shock or pulmonary symptoms. Applied topically, British anti-lewisite ointment has been reported to prevent mucous membrane and skin injury. Care providers should be careful to avoid coming in contact with the fluid inside skin blisters caused by lewisite, as it may contain toxic arsenic compounds and active lewisite or dangerous breakdown products.[47]

Biologic Agents

Biologic agents in the form of contagious disease exposure represent a threat to prehospital care providers on a daily basis (**Box 18-6**). Proper infection control procedures must be in place to prevent the contraction or transmission of

---

Box 18-6 Classification of Biologic WMD Agents

- Bacterial agents
  - Anthrax
  - Brucellosis
  - Glanders
  - Plague
  - Q fever
  - Tularemia
- Viral agents
  - Smallpox
  - Venezuelan equine encephalitis
  - Ebola virus (viral hemorrhagic fevers)
- Biologic toxins
  - Botulinum
  - Ricin
  - Staphylococcal enterotoxin B
  - T-2 mycotoxins

---

tuberculosis, influenza, human immunodeficiency virus (HIV), methicillin-resistant *Staphylococcus aureus* (MRSA), SARS, meningococcus, and myriad other organisms.

Preparing for bioterrorist events increases the complexity of EMS system preparation. An intentional terrorist act might include delivery of a biologic agent with the potential to cause disease or illness, such as aerosolized spores, aerosolized live organisms, or an aerosolized biologic toxin. Patients with pathogens not typically seen by prehospital care providers, such as plague, anthrax, and smallpox, might be encountered, requiring appropriate PPE and precautions. Familiar infection control procedures will be effective in the safe management of these potentially contagious patients. If the provider is responding to an overt release event, appropriate precautions regarding decontamination of victims and PPE are required, similar to other hazardous materials events. However, this entire process becomes much more complicated in the context of delayed presentation. Variability in incubation periods makes determination of sources of contamination and control of spread more difficult to achieve.

Concentrated Biohazard Agent Versus Infected Patient

Prehospital care providers can experience bioterrorism in two ways. The first scenario involves the overt release of a material that is either identified as, or thought to be, a biologic agent. The anthrax hoaxes of 1998 and 1999 and the anthrax letters of 2001 are good examples. Providers responded on countless occasions to individuals covered in "white powder" or suspected anthrax. In this situation, the provider will encounter an environment or a patient contaminated with a suspicious substance. EMS systems may be summoned to suspicious activity, such as a device delivering an unknown aerosol agent. The nature of the threat at these events is usually unknown, and precautions for personal safety should always be paramount. These incidents must be respected and treated as a WMD incident until proven otherwise. If the suspicious substance is in fact a concentrated aerosol of an infectious organism or toxin, PPE appropriate for the biologic agent and decontamination are required.

In this situation, prehospital care providers will be caring for victims contaminated with a suspected biologic agent on their skin or clothing. Any person, patient, or provider coming in direct physical contact with a suspected biologic agent should remove all exposed articles of clothing and perform a thorough washing of exposed skin with soap and water.[48] Clinically significant re-aerosolization of material from victims' skin or clothing is unlikely, and the risk to the provider is negligible.[49] However, as a matter of routine practice, potentially contaminated clothing normally removed by pulling the item over the face and head should instead be cut off to minimize any risk of inadvertent inhalation of contaminant. Decontamination may then proceed using water or soap and water. Consultation with appropriate public health and law enforcement officials will then determine the need for antibiotic prophylaxis.

The second scenario involves a response to a patient who is a victim of a remote, covert bioterrorist event. Perhaps the patient inhaled anthrax spores after a covert attack at work and now, several days later, is manifesting signs of pulmonary anthrax. Perhaps a terrorist has inoculated himself or herself with smallpox, and you are summoned to assist the victim with a suspicious rash. In these cases, personal and public safety can be ensured by knowledge of proper infection control procedures and the proper donning and removal of PPE appropriate for the biohazard (**Box 18-7** and **Box 18-8**). Decontamination of the patient in this scenario is not necessary because the exposure occurred several days in the past.

All prehospital care providers should be familiar with PPE for infection-control purposes. Different types of PPE are recommended, depending on the potential for transmission and the likely route of transmission. **Transmission-based PPE** is used in addition to the standard precautions, which are used in the care of all patients. These include contact, droplet, and aerosol precautions.

Contact Precautions

This level of protection is recommended to reduce the likelihood of transmission of microorganisms by direct or indirect contact. Contact precautions include the use of gloves and a gown.

Commonly encountered organisms that require contact precautions include viral conjunctivitis, MRSA, scabies,

---

Box 18-7 Sequence for Donning PPE

The type of PPE used will vary based on the level of precautions required (e.g., standard precautions and contact, droplet, or airborne infection isolation).

1. Gown
   · Fully cover torso from neck to knees, arms to end of wrists, and wrap around the back.
   · Fasten in back of neck and waist.
2. Mask or respirator
   · Secure ties or elastic bands at middle of head and neck.
   · Fit flexible band to nose bridge.
   · Fit snug to face and below chin.
   · Fit/check respirator.
3. Goggles or face shield
   · Place over face and eyes and adjust to fit.
4. Gloves
   · Extend to cover wrist of isolation gown.

Use safe work practices to protect yourself and limit the spread of contamination:

■ Keep hands away from face.
■ Limit surfaces touched.
■ Change gloves when torn or heavily contaminated.
■ Perform hand hygiene.

From Centers for Disease Control and Prevention, Atlanta.

---

and herpes simplex or zoster virus. Organisms that require strict contact precautions that might be encountered as a result of bioterrorism include bubonic plague or the viral hemorrhagic fevers, such as Marburg or Ebola, as long as the patient does not have pulmonary symptoms or profuse vomiting and diarrhea, in which case airborne precautions should also be taken.

Droplet Precautions

This level of protection is recommended to reduce the likelihood of transmission of microorganisms that are known to be transmitted by large droplet nuclei (greater than 5 μm) expelled by an infected person in the course of talking, sneezing, or coughing or during routine procedures, such as suctioning. These droplets infect by landing on the exposed mucous membranes of the eyes, nose, and mouth. Because the droplets are large, they do not remain suspended in air, and therefore, contact must be in close proximity, usually defined as 3 ft (0.9 m) or less. Droplet precautions include the contact precautions of gloves and gown and add eye protection and a surgical mask. Because the droplets do not remain suspended in air, no additional respiratory protection or air filtration is required.

Box 18-8 Sequence for Removing PPE

Except for the respirator, remove PPE at the doorway or in an anteroom of the involved room. Remove the respirator after leaving the contaminated room and closing the door.

1. Gloves
   - The outside of the glove is contaminated!
     - Grasp outside of glove with opposite gloved hand; peel off.
     - Hold removed glove in gloved hand.
     - Slide fingers of ungloved hand under remaining glove at wrist.
     - Peel glove off over first glove.
     - Discard gloves in waste container.
2. Goggles
   - The outside of the goggles or face shield is contaminated!
     - To remove, handle by headband or ear pieces.
     - Place in designated receptacle for reprocessing or in waste container.
3. Gown
   - The gown front and sleeves are contaminated!
     - Unfasten gown ties.
     - Pull away from neck and shoulders, touching inside of gown only.
     - Turn gown inside out.
     - Fold or roll into a bundle and discard.
4. Mask or respirator
   - The front of the mask/respirator is contaminated—do not touch!
     - Grasp bottom, then top ties or elastics, and remove.
     - Discard in waste container.

Once PPE is removed, wash hands.

From Centers for Disease Control and Prevention, Atlanta.

Typically encountered organisms in this category include influenza, *Mycoplasma pneumoniae*, and invasive *Haemophilus influenzae* or *Neisseria meningitidis*, causing sepsis or meningitis. Pneumonic plague is an example of a possible agent encountered as a result of a bioterrorist event.

Aerosol Precautions

This level of protection is recommended to reduce the likelihood of transmission of microorganisms by the airborne route. Some organisms can become suspended in the air attached to small droplet nuclei (less than 5 µm) or attached to dust particles. In this case, microorganisms can become widely dispersed by air currents immediately around the source or more distant from the source, depending on environmental conditions. To avoid such dispersion, these

Box 18-9 Biologic Agent Precautions

Note that many illnesses associated with biologic events require no additional protection beyond standard precautions, provided there is no risk of exposure to a concentrated agent. Examples include patients with inhalational anthrax or a biologic toxin such as botulinum. However, in most cases, the specific biologic agent will likely not be identified for several days. Although some agents, such as anthrax, are not spread from person to person, prehospital care providers must assume the worst—that the biologic agent is contagious—and use all available precautions, including aerosol precautions.

patients are kept in negative-pressure isolation rooms in a hospital in which the exhaust ventilation can be filtered.

Aerosol precautions include gloves, gown, eye protection, and a fit-tested high-efficiency particulate air (HEPA) filter mask, such as the N95 (**Box 18-9**). Examples of illnesses typically encountered that would require aerosol precautions include tuberculosis, measles, chickenpox, and SARS. Smallpox and viral hemorrhagic fever with pulmonary symptoms are examples that could possibly be related to a bioterrorist event.

Selected Agents

Anthrax

Anthrax is a disease caused by the bacterium *Bacillus anthracis*. *B. anthracis* is a spore-forming bacterium and, thus, can exist as either a vegetative cell or as a spore. The vegetative cell lives well in a host organism but cannot survive long outside the body, unlike the spore, which can remain viable in the environment for decades.

The disease is naturally occurring, contracted most often by persons in contact with infected animals or anthrax-contaminated animal products resulting in the cutaneous form of the disease. The spores have been weaponized and are known to be inventoried in several nations' military stockpiles. The accidental release of aerosolized anthrax spores from a Soviet military facility at Sverdlovsk in 1979 resulted in approximately 79 cases of pulmonary anthrax with 68 reported deaths. Letters contaminated with anthrax spores were sent through the U.S. Postal Service in 2001 to prominent legislators and media outlets. Although only 22 cases (11 pulmonary, 11 cutaneous) and 5 deaths resulted, thousands of people required prophylaxis with antibiotics. A hypothetical release of 220 pounds (100 kilograms [kg]) of anthrax spores over Washington, DC, is estimated to be capable of causing 130,000 to 3 million deaths.[50]

Routes of exposure to anthrax include the respiratory tract, the GI tract, and breaks in the skin. Exposure to anthrax through the respiratory tract leads to inhalational or pulmonary anthrax. Exposure through the GI tract causes gastrointestinal anthrax, and skin infection causes cutaneous anthrax.

Gastrointestinal anthrax is rare and would result from ingesting food substances contaminated with spores. Patients have nonspecific symptoms of nausea, vomiting, malaise, bloody diarrhea, and acute abdomen; mortality is approximately 50%. Cutaneous anthrax follows deposition of spores or organisms into a break in the skin. This results in a papule, which subsequently ulcerates and causes a dry, black eschar with local edema. If not treated with antibiotics, mortality approaches 20%; with antibiotics, mortality is rare.[51]

For maximal effectiveness in a terrorist attack, anthrax would likely be disseminated in its spore form. Anthrax spores are approximately 1 to 5 μm in size, which allows the spores to be suspended in air as an aerosol. Aerosolized spores can be inhaled into the lungs and deposited in the alveoli. They are then consumed by macrophages and carried to the mediastinal lymph nodes, where they germinate, manufacture toxins, and cause *acute hemorrhagic mediastinitis* (bleeding into the lymph nodes in the middle of the chest cavity) and often death. The onset of symptoms after inhalation of spores varies, with most victims developing symptoms within 1 to 7 days, although there may be a latency period of as long as 60 days. Symptoms initially are nonspecific, including fever, chills, dyspnea, cough, chest pain, headache, and vomiting. After a few days, symptoms improve, followed by a rapidly deteriorating course of fever, dyspnea, diaphoresis, shock, and death.[48,51,52] Before the 2001 anthrax attacks, mortality from inhalational anthrax was thought to be 90%, but outcomes from those incidents suggest that with early antibiotic therapy and critical care services, mortality may be significantly lower.[51]

Inhalational anthrax is not contagious and does not pose a risk to the prehospital care provider. Only exposure to aerosolized spores poses a risk of infectivity. Caring for patients known to be infected with inhalational anthrax requires only standard precautions; however, if the specific agent is unknown, aerosol precautions are warranted. The provider should provide supportive therapy and transport ill patients to facilities in which critical care services are available.

Management

Anthrax spores are extremely difficult to destroy and can be easily transported on victims' skin or clothes, presenting an infectious hazard to providers. Victims of known or suspected anthrax releases (e.g., letters containing suspicious white powders) should be decontaminated on scene by responders wearing level A PPE, in order to avoid contamination of transport equipment or infection of providers by anthrax spores carried on victims' skin or clothes.

Prophylaxis with antibiotics is required only for individuals who have been exposed to spores. Local public health officials will determine the appropriate antibiotic and length of prophylactic treatment. The latest recommendations suggest 60 days of therapy with oral ciprofloxacin or doxycycline and postexposure vaccination.[53]

An anthrax vaccine does exist, and an immunization program for U.S. military forces was instituted in 1998. The current regimen requires a series of six initial shots and annual boosters. It is currently recommended only for military personnel and for laboratory and industrial workers at high risk for exposure to spores. The CDC has purchased tens of thousands of doses of the anthrax vaccine for the Strategic National Stockpile that would be made available to emergency responders in the event of an anthrax incident with risk of exposure.

Plague

Plague is a disease caused by the bacterium *Yersinia pestis*. It is naturally occurring, found in fleas and rodents. If an infected flea bites a human, the person can develop *bubonic plague*. If this local infection goes untreated, the patient can become systemically ill, resulting in septicemia and death. A number of patients may proceed to develop pulmonary symptoms (*pneumonic plague*). Plague was responsible for the Black Death of 1346, which killed 20 to 30 million people in Europe, approximately one-third of its population at that time. *Y. pestis* has been weaponized for military stockpiles with techniques developed to aerosolize the organism directly, bypassing the animal vector. The World Health Organization reports that in a worst-case scenario, 110 pounds (50 kg) of *Y. pestis*, released as an aerosol over a city of 5 million, would result in 150,000 cases of pneumonic plague and 36,000 deaths.[54]

Naturally occurring plague, resulting from the bite of an infected flea, causes symptoms in 2 to 8 days, with onset of fever, chills, weakness, and acutely swollen lymph nodes (buboes) in the neck, groin, or axilla. Untreated patients can deteriorate to systemic illness and death. Twelve percent have been described as developing pneumonic plague, with complaints of chest pain, dyspnea, cough, and hemoptysis, and these patients can also succumb from systemic illness.

Plague occurring from terrorist deployment of a weapon would likely result from aerosolized organisms, and thus, it would clinically present as the pneumonic form of the disease. Inhalation of *Y. pestis* aerosol would result in symptoms in 1 to 6 days. Patients will present with fever, cough, and dyspnea, with bloody or watery sputum. They may also develop nausea, vomiting, diarrhea, and abdominal pain. Buboes are not typically present. Without antibiotics, death occurs in 2 to 6 days after the development of respiratory symptoms.[55]

Currently, no vaccine is available to protect from pneumonic plague. Treatment of the disease includes antimicrobial and supportive therapy, often requiring critical care services. Antibiotic regimens are also recommended for individuals with unprotected close exposure to patients with known pneumonic plague.

Patients with plague represent a communicable disease risk. If patients present with only cutaneous signs and symptoms (bubonic plague), contact precautions are adequate to protect the prehospital care provider. If patients present with pulmonary signs of plague (pneumonic plague), a more likely scenario after a terrorist attack, providers must wear PPE suitable for respiratory droplet protection. Droplet precautions include a surgical mask, eye protection, gloves, and a gown. Responders to the scene of an overt *Y. pestis* aerosol delivery, which would not likely be a recognized event, would require level A PPE suitable for a hazardous environment if entering the hot zone or warm zone.

Management

Plague victims are treated in the field with supportive therapy. Communication with the receiving facility is vital before arrival to ensure that the pneumonic plague patient can be properly isolated in the ED and that staff are prepared with the appropriate PPE. Asking the patient to wear a surgical mask, if tolerated, may decrease the likelihood of secondary transmission.

Decontamination of the vehicle and equipment is similar to that required after transport of any patient with communicable disease. Contact surfaces should be wiped down with disinfectant approved by the Environmental Protection Agency (EPA) or 1:1,000 diluted bleach solution. There is no evidence to suggest that *Y. pestis* poses a long-term environmental threat after dissolution of the primary aerosol.[55] The organism is sensitive to heat and sunlight and does not last long outside the living host. *Y. pestis* does not form spores.

Smallpox

Smallpox is also known as *variola major* and *variola minor*, depending on the severity of the illness. This naturally occurring viral disease was eradicated in 1977 but still exists in at least two laboratories—Russia's Institute of Virus Preparations and the CDC. It was alleged that the Soviet government began a program in 1980 to produce large quantities of smallpox virus for use in bombs and missiles, as well as to develop more virulent strains of the virus for military purposes. There is concern that smallpox virus may have changed hands after the dissolution of the Soviet Union.[56]

The smallpox virus infects its victim by entering the mucous membranes of the oropharynx or respiratory mucosa. After a 12- to 14-day incubation period, the patient develops fever, malaise, headache, and backache. The patient then develops a **maculopapular rash** that starts on the oral mucosa and quickly progresses to a

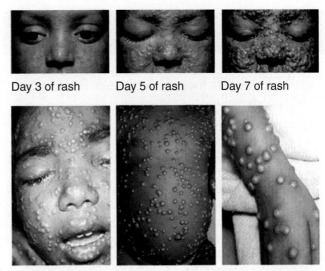

Day 3 of rash   Day 5 of rash   Day 7 of rash

On any part of the body, all lesions are in the same stage of development.

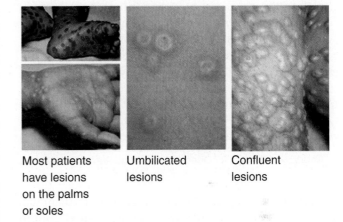

Most patients   Umbilicated   Confluent
have lesions   lesions   lesions
on the palms
or soles

Figure 18-6 Smallpox.
Courtesy of Centers for Disease Control and Prevention, Atlanta.

generalized skin rash with characteristic round, tense vesicles and pustules. The rash tends to affect the head and extremities more densely than the trunk (centrifugal), with the stage of the lesions appearing uniform (**Figure 18-6**). This presentation distinguishes smallpox from *varicella*, or chickenpox (**Box 18-10**), which begins on and is denser on the trunk (centripetal) and has lesions at various stages of development (new lesions appear with older, crusted lesions) (**Figure 18-7**). Mortality from naturally occurring smallpox was approximately 30%.[56] Little is known about the natural course of the disease in immunocompromised patients, such as those with HIV.

Smallpox is a contagious disease that is primarily spread by droplet nuclei projected from the oropharynx of infected patients and by direct contact. Contaminated clothing and bed linens can also spread the virus. Patients are contagious beginning slightly before the onset of the rash, although this might not always be obvious if the rash

Box 18-10 Differentiating Chickenpox From Smallpox

Chickenpox (varicella) is the most likely condition to be confused with smallpox. Characteristics of chickenpox include the following:

- There is no prodrome or mild prodrome.
- Lesions are superficial vesicles: "dewdrop on a rose petal."
- Lesions appear in crops; on any one part of the body, there are lesions in different stages (papules, vesicles, crusts).
- Distribution is centripetal, with the greatest concentration of lesions on the trunk, and the fewest lesions on distal extremities. Lesions may involve the face/scalp; occasionally, the entire body is equally affected.
- First lesions appear on the face or trunk.
- Patients are rarely toxic or moribund.
- Lesions evolve rapidly, from macules to papules to vesicles to crusts (less than 24 hours).
- Palms and soles are rarely involved.
- Patient lacks a reliable history of varicella or varicella vaccination.
- Of these patients, 50% to 80% recall an exposure to chickenpox or shingles 10 to 21 days before rash onset.

Courtesy of Centers for Disease Control and Prevention, Atlanta.

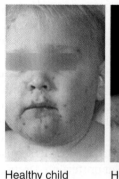
Healthy child with varicella

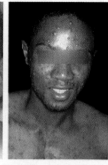
Healthy adult with varicella

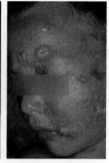
Bacterial super-infection of lesions

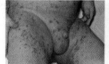
Note centripetal distribution of rash

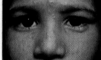
Day 3 of rash

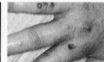
Lesions are in different stages of development

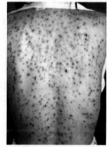
Healthy adult with varicella

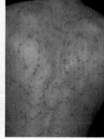
Healthy adult with varicella

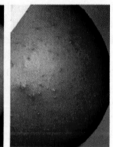
Pregnant woman with varicella

Figure 18-7 Chickenpox.
Courtesy of Centers for Disease Control and Prevention, Atlanta.

is subtle in the oropharynx. When managing a patient with smallpox, prehospital care providers must wear PPE appropriate for contact and aerosol precautions. This includes an N95 mask, eye protection, goggles, and gown. Ideally, persons managing patients with smallpox will have been immunized.[57]

The smallpox vaccination program in the United States was stopped in 1972. The residual immunity provided by this vaccination program is unknown, and it is suggested that individuals whose last immunization was 40 years ago will likely now be susceptible to contracting smallpox.[56] Vaccination for the smallpox virus is available to certain U.S. Department of Defense and State Department members. It was also made available under a Department of Health and Human Services program to develop public health Smallpox Response Teams. It is currently available to the general public only for participants in clinical trials. In case of a public health emergency, the United States has stockpiles of vaccine that can be released for mass immunization of the public. Vaccination within 4 days of the exposure has been shown to offer some protection against contracting the illness and substantial protection against a fatal outcome.[56]

Management

To manage a patient with smallpox, prehospital care providers provide supportive care. The recommended PPE must be worn at all times, and it is imperative that there is no breach in infection-control procedures. Hospitals with the appropriate isolation facilities and properly trained staff should be identified in the community. The receiving facility must be contacted to inform the staff of the intention to transport the confirmed or suspected case of smallpox to their facility so that proper precautions can be taken to prevent transmission of the virus. The identification of a patient with smallpox would be considered a public health emergency of enormous significance.

Proper removal of PPE without breach in infection control procedures is important for the safety of the prehospital care provider. All contaminated disposable medical waste must be properly bagged, labeled, and disposed of as other regulated medical waste. Reusable medical equipment must be cleaned after use according to standard protocol, either by autoclaving or by subjecting the equipment to high-level disinfection. Environmental surfaces need to be cleaned by an approved EPA-registered detergent-disinfectant. Air decontamination or fumigation of the emergency vehicle is not required.[58]

Ebola Virus and Viral Hemorrhagic Fevers

Viral hemorrhagic fevers (VHFs) are a clinical syndrome caused by several different viruses and typified by the clinical presentation of fever, malaise, and hemorrhagic symptoms, including coagulopathy, bleeding from venipuncture sites and mucous membranes, petechiae, and ecchymoses in the most severe cases. Case fatality rates, defined as the percentage of infected who die from the infection, vary significantly among different VHF viruses and even among outbreaks of the same virus but can exceed 90%. Examples of viruses that cause VHFs include Ebola virus, Marburg virus, yellow fever virus, and Lassa virus.[59] There is some evidence to suggest that the former Soviet Union conducted research on weaponized VHF viruses, and currently terrorist organizations may be developing their own programs to exploit VHFs.[60]

Ebola virus is a type of filovirus (named for the filament-like shape of viral particles in this family), first isolated and identified in 1976 from patients in two outbreaks of VHFs near the borders of current-day South Sudan and the Democratic Republic of the Congo. The name *Ebola* comes from the name of a small river near the latter outbreak. Later scientific work identified several separate strains of Ebola viruses responsible for different outbreaks, including Reston Ebola virus, which caused an outbreak among research monkeys housed in a quarantine facility in Reston, Virginia, in 1989. Unlike smallpox, Ebola virus is thought to have a natural reservoir in animals, most likely bats, meaning new outbreaks could occur at any time.[59,61] Ebola virus gained worldwide attention in 2014 when an outbreak spread throughout West Africa causing over 11,000 deaths among over 28,000 reported cases between 2013 and 2016, including several in the United States and other Western countries.[62]

Clinically, infection with Ebola virus causes Ebola virus disease (EVD), a VHF, which initially manifests after a 2- to 21-day incubation period with fevers, chills, generalized malaise, and muscle aches, and progresses to GI symptoms with abdominal pain, vomiting, and diarrhea, as well as neurologic symptoms, including headache and confusion, and respiratory symptoms including cough, chest pain, and shortness of breath. At the peak of illness, severe cases may develop hemorrhagic symptoms and generalized coagulopathy. Death occurs from multiorgan failure, sepsis, electrolyte abnormalities, and hypovolemic shock, primarily from gastrointestinal volume loss.[61] While the case fatality rate varies significantly among strains and different outbreaks, the 2013–2016 West African outbreak had a final case fatality rate of below 40%, versus around 75% at the start of the outbreak, and over 90% in some prior outbreaks. It is suspected that the improvement in this rate was due to improvements in caring for patients with EVD, primarily aggressive replacement of gastrointestinal volume and electrolyte losses.[63]

Management

Transport of suspected EVD victims poses a significant risk to EMS personnel, due to the highly infectious nature of the virus. Body fluids from symptomatic patients contain extremely large amounts of active virus, and only a small exposure is needed to infect an individual. Review of the West African outbreak showed that 3.9% of cases were among health care workers who became infected while caring for EVD patients.[63] The CDC has published specific guidelines on PPE use for transporting EVD patients, based on the best currently available evidence; in short, the CDC recommends skin protection with multiple layers (disposable scrubs, impermeable gown, over-apron, multiple layers of gloves, and boot covers) and respiratory/mucous membrane protection with a preference for a PAPR and hood over N95 mask and eye protection, analogous to OSHA level C. These recommendations may be updated if another outbreak occurs.[64] Extensive training on EVD PPE and direct supervision of donning/doffing procedures by experienced observers are strongly recommended.

EMS agencies affiliated with Grady Hospital in Atlanta, Georgia, and Nebraska Medical Center in Omaha, Nebraska, developed equipment and plans for transporting critically ill patients with highly contagious disease prior to the 2013–2016 EVD outbreak and afterward published reports on their experiences treating and transporting actual and suspected EVD patients. These reports made many specific and helpful recommendations for transporting EVD patients, including the following:

- Use of appropriate PPE (with strict attention paid to donning/doffing procedure and recommendation for a PAPR over negative-pressure mask for better provider protection and comfort during long transports)
- Isolation of the driver compartment of the ambulance from the patient compartment with an improvised positive-pressure system
- Covering of all equipment and surfaces within the patient compartment of the ambulance with thick plastic sheets to limit contamination
- Further isolation of patients within a contamination-limiting suit or capsule

- Careful decontamination of ambulance and equipment afterward with use of disinfectant wipes (as opposed to spraying down surfaces with pressurized water, which could aerosolize virus particles)[65,66]

Based on experience gained in the 2013–2016 outbreak, medical management of EVD patients now focuses primarily on symptom control and oral repletion of GI fluids and electrolyte losses. There are multiple new therapies that may improve survival rates, including antiviral and immunomodulatory medications and vaccines, but their efficacy is still under investigation. Advance supportive care interventions, such as IV fluids, lab monitoring of electrolytes, cell counts, and viral levels, antibiotics, and intubation/ventilation may also be helpful, but these measures significantly increase the risk of infection to health care providers.[63]

Botulinum Toxin

Botulinum toxin is produced by the bacterium *Clostridium botulinum* and is the most poisonous substance known. It is 15,000 times more toxic than the nerve agent VX and 100,000 times more toxic than sarin.[67] Botulinum toxin has been weaponized for military use by the United States; the former Soviet Union; Iraq; and probably Iran, Syria, and North Korea.[68] The Aum Shinrikyo cult, responsible for the Tokyo subway sarin attack, attempted, without success, to deliver an aerosol of botulinum toxin in 1995. Despite the reported difficulty of concentrating and stabilizing the toxin for dissemination, it is estimated that a terrorist point-source delivery of botulinum aerosol could incapacitate or kill 10% of persons downwind 0.3 mile (0.5 km).[68] The toxin could also be introduced into the food supply in an attempt to poison large numbers of people.

Three forms of botulism exist naturally. *Wound botulism* occurs when toxins are absorbed from a dirty wound, often with devitalized tissue, in which *C. botulinum* is present. *Foodborne botulism* occurs when improperly prepared or home-canned foods allow the bacteria to grow and produce toxin, which is ingested by the victim. *Intestinal botulism* occurs when toxin is produced and absorbed within the GI tract. In addition to these three naturally occurring forms, a man-made form of botulism, called *inhalational botulism*, can occur as a result of aerosolized botulinum toxin.

Regardless of the route, botulinum toxin is carried to the neuromuscular junction where it binds irreversibly, preventing normal release of the neurotransmitter acetylcholine and causing a descending flaccid paralysis. Onset of symptoms is several hours to a few days. All patients will present with diplopia (double vision) and multiple cranial nerve deficits, causing difficulty with sight, speech, and swallowing. The extent and rapidity of the descending paralysis depend on the dose of the toxin. Patients become fatigued, lose the ability to control the muscles of the head and neck, may lose their gag reflex, or may progress to paralysis of the muscles of respiration and develop respiratory failure, requiring intubation and months of mechanical ventilation. Untreated patients usually die of mechanical upper airway obstruction or inadequate ventilation. The classic triad of botulinum toxicity is (1) descending symmetric flaccid paralysis with cranial nerve deficits, (2) lack of fever, and (3) a clear sensorium. After weeks to months, patients may recover as new axon buds develop to innervate the denervated muscles.

Management

Care for the patient with botulism is supportive, with administration of antitoxin in the hospital. Early use of antitoxin will minimize further deterioration but cannot reverse existing paralysis. This antitoxin is available from the CDC.

Prehospital care providers caring for victims of botulism would need to be vigilant about airway compromise and insufficient ventilation. Patients may not be able to manage their secretions or maintain a patent airway. Because of diaphragm paralysis, patients may not be able to generate an adequate tidal volume. This may be exacerbated by having the patient in a supine or semi-recumbent position. Patients experiencing respiratory difficulty should be intubated and adequately ventilated.

Standard precautions are adequate for the management of patients experiencing the effects of botulinum toxicity because it is not a contagious disease. Botulism aerosols degrade readily in the environment, and it is anticipated that after delivery in a terrorist incident, substantial inactivation will occur after 2 days. Responders to an overt aerosol dissemination event would require level A PPE suitable for a hazardous environment if working in the hot zone or warm zone.

Because the aerosol can persist for approximately 2 days under average weather conditions, victims who have been exposed to botulinum aerosol require decontamination by clothing removal and washing with soap and water. Equipment can be decontaminated using a 0.1% hypochlorite bleach solution.[68] Patients will not require isolation after arrival at the hospital, but critical care services may be needed for patients requiring mechanical ventilation.

Radiologic Disasters

Since the terrorist attacks of September 11, 2001, new consideration has been given to the likelihood of EMS systems needing to manage a radiologic emergency. Historically, planning has focused on civil-defense preparation for a strategic exchange of military nuclear weapons or the rare occurrence of a nuclear power plant accident. Currently, however, there is increasing awareness of the possibility that terrorists could deploy an improvised nuclear detonation device, or perhaps more likely, a radiologic dispersion device, that uses conventional explosives to disseminate radioactive material into the environment. While the large-scale nuclear exchanges feared during the Cold War seem less likely today, the proliferation of nuclear weapons in the past few decades among smaller nations has led to concerns of rogue states or terrorist groups obtaining nuclear weapons and using them to attack civilian populations.

Although radiologic accidents are rare, there have been 243 radiation accidents since 1944 in the United States, with 1,342 casualties that met criteria for significant exposure. Worldwide, 403 accidents have occurred, with 133,617 victims, 2,965 with significant exposure, and 120 fatalities. The Chernobyl disaster of 1986 was responsible for 116,500 to 125,000 exposed casualties and close to 50 deaths as of 2005, although it is estimated that the total number of deaths could reach as many as 4,000 as additional cancer victims succumb.[69,70] In the 1987 Goiania, Brazil, incident, a canister of cesium-137, a highly radioactive isotope used for medical radiation therapy, was broken open and the radioactive material inside disseminated. Of the 129 people who were contaminated, 20 were hospitalized and 4 died; approximately 125,000 people were screened for radiation contamination. The release of the radioactive isotope was not realized until 16 days after the canister was opened, when victims presented to local hospitals with symptoms of radiation poisoning; this delay in recognition likely increased the number of victims contaminated.[71] The Fukushima nuclear power plant in Japan was seriously damaged after a nearby earthquake and tsunami in 2011, resulting in the destruction of several reactors and the release of radiation into the environment. It will take years and even decades before the health impact of this incident on the surrounding population and environment can be fully evaluated.

Radiation disasters can generate fear and confusion in both victims and emergency responders. Familiarization with the hazard and management principles will help to ensure an appropriate response and help to reduce panic and disorder (**Box 18-11**).

Exposure to ionizing radiation and radioactive contamination may result from several different scenarios: (1) detonation of a nuclear weapon, whether high grade or an improvised low-yield device; (2) detonation of a dirty bomb or radiologic dispersion device, in which there is no nuclear detonation, but rather conventional explosives are detonated to disperse a *radionuclide* (radioactive material); (3) sabotage or accident at a nuclear reactor site; and (4) mishandled nuclear waste.

Medical Effects of Radiation Catastrophes

The injuries and risks associated with a radiologic catastrophe would be multifactorial. In the case of a nuclear detonation, casualties would be produced by the explosion,

---

Box 18-11 Principles of Management of a Radiologic Disaster

1. Assess the scene for safety.
2. All patients should be medically stabilized from their traumatic injuries before radiation injuries are considered. Patients are then evaluated for their external radiation exposure and contamination.
3. An external source of radiation, if great enough, can cause tissue injury, but it does not make the patient radioactive. Patients with even lethal exposures to external radiation are not a threat to prehospital care providers.
4. Patients can become contaminated with radioactive material deposited on their skin or clothing. More than 90% of surface contamination can be removed by removal of clothing.[71] The remainder can be washed off with soap and water.
5. Prehospital care providers should protect themselves from radioactive contamination by observing, at a minimum, standard precautions, including protective clothing, gloves, and a mask.
6. Patients who develop nausea, vomiting, or skin erythema within 4 hours of exposure have likely received a high external radiation exposure.
7. Radioactive contamination in wounds should be treated as dirt and irrigated as soon as possible. Avoid handling any metallic foreign body.
8. Potassium iodide (KI) is of value only if there has been a release of radioactive iodine. KI is not a general radiation antidote.
9. The concept of time/distance/shielding is key in the prevention of untoward effects from radiation exposure. Radiation exposure is minimized by decreasing time in the affected area, increasing distance from a radiation source, and using metal or concrete shielding.

Modified from Department of Homeland Security Working Group on Radiological Dispersion Device Preparedness/ Medical Preparedness and Response Subgroup, 2004.

---

resulting in primary, secondary, and tertiary blast injuries, thermal injury, and structural collapse. Victims may be further subjected to radiation injury from *irradiation*, in which radiation passes through the body causing damage but does not result in contamination (similar to getting an x-ray); from external radioactive contamination, which can be deposited on skin and clothing from fallout; or from internal radiation through radioactive particulate contamination, which victims may inhale, ingest, or have deposited in wounds.

Accidents at nuclear reactors could generate large doses of ionizing radiation, without a nuclear detonation, especially under circumstances in which the reactor reaches a point of "criticality." Explosions, fire, and gas release could also result in radioactive gas or particulate matter, which could expose emergency responders to the risk of exposure to contamination with radioactive particles.

Radiologic dispersion devices (RDDs) typically would not deliver enough radiation to cause immediate injury. However, RDDs would complicate management for prehospital care providers by distributing radioactive particulates that could contaminate victims and emergency responders and make it difficult to manage the injuries caused by the conventional explosive. RDDs could cause confusion and panic in the public and among emergency responders concerned about radioactivity, hindering efforts to assist victims.

Ionizing radiation causes injury to cells by interacting with atoms and depositing energy. This interaction results in **ionization**, which can damage the cell nucleus either directly, causing cell death or malfunction, or indirectly, damaging cell components by interacting with water in the body and producing toxic molecules. Acute exposure to large doses of penetrating ionizing radiation (irradiation with gamma rays and neutrons) in a short time can result in acute radiation illness. Types of ionizing radiation include alpha particles, beta particles, gamma rays, and neutrons.

Alpha particles are relatively large and cannot penetrate even a few layers of the skin. Intact skin or a uniform offers adequate protection from external contamination emitting alpha particles. Ionizing radiation from alpha particles is a concern only if it is internalized by inhaling or ingesting alpha-particle emitters. When internalized, alpha-particle radiation can cause significant local cellular injury to adjacent cells.

Beta particles are small charged particles that can penetrate more deeply than alpha particles and can affect deeper layers of the skin with the ability to injure the base of the skin, causing a *beta burn*. Beta-particle radiation is found most frequently in nuclear fallout. Beta particles also result in local radiation injury.

Gamma rays are similar to x-rays and can easily penetrate tissue. Gamma rays are emitted with a nuclear detonation and with fallout. They also could be emitted from some radionuclides that might be present in an RDD. Gamma radiation can result in what is termed *whole-body exposure*. Whole-body exposure can result in acute and chronic radiation illnesses (**Box 18-12, Table 18-2,** and **Table 18-3**).

Neutrons can penetrate tissue easily, with 20 times the destructive energy of gamma rays, disrupting the atomic structure of cells. Neutrons are released during a nuclear detonation but are not a fallout risk. Neutrons also contribute to whole-body radiation exposure and can result in acute radiation illness. Neutrons can convert stable metals into radioactive isotopes. This ability has significance in

Box 18-12 Terrorism With Ionizing Radiation: General Guide

Diagnosis
Be alert to the following:

1. The acute radiation syndrome follows a predictable pattern after substantial exposure or catastrophic events (Table 18-2).
2. Individuals may become ill from contaminated sources in the community and may be identified over much longer periods based on specific syndromes (Table 18-3).
3. Specific syndromes of concern, especially with a 2- to 3-week prior history of nausea and vomiting, are:
   - Thermal burn-like skin effects without documented thermal exposure
   - Immunologic dysfunction with secondary infections
   - Tendency to bleed (epistaxis, gingival bleeding, petechiae)
   - Marrow suppression (neutropenia, lymphopenia, and thrombocytopenia)
   - Epilation (hair loss)

Understanding Exposure
Exposure may be known and recognized or clandestine and may occur by the following means:

1. Large recognized exposures, such as a nuclear bomb or damage to a nuclear power station
2. Small radiation source emitting continuous gamma radiation, producing group or individual chronic intermittent exposures (e.g., radiologic sources from medical treatment devices, environmental water or food pollution)
3. Internal radiation from absorbed, inhaled, or ingested radioactive material (internal contamination)

This information is not meant to be complete and is intended as a quick guide only; please consult other references and expert opinion.

Modified from Department of Veterans Affairs pocket guide produced by Employee Education System for Office of Public Health and Environmental Hazards. This information is not meant to be complete but to be a quick guide; please consult other references and expert opinion.

patients with metal hardware or those in possession of metal objects at the time of exposure.

Whole-body exposure is measured in terms of the *gray* (Gy). The *rad* (radiation absorbed dose) was a familiar dose unit that was replaced by the gray; 1 Gy equals 100 rad. The rem (radiation equivalent–man) describes the dose in rad multiplied by a "quality factor," which takes into account

Table 18-2 Acute Radiation Syndrome

Feature	Effects of Whole-Body Irradiation or Internal Absorption, by Dose Range in rad (1 rad = 1 centigray; 100 rad = 1 gray)					
	0–100 (0–1 Gy)	100–200 (1–2 Gy)	200–600 (2–6 Gy)	600–800 (6–8 Gy)	800–3,000 (8–30 Gy)	> 3,000 (> 30 Gy)
Prodromal Phase of Syndrome						
Nausea, vomiting	None	5–50%	50–100%	75–100%	90–100%	100%
Time of onset	—	3–6 hr	2–4 hr	1–2 hr	< 1 hr	N/A
Duration	—	< 24 hr	< 24 hr	< 48 hr	48 hr	N/A
Lymphocyte count	Unaffected	Minimally decreased	< 1,000 at 24 hr	< 500 at 24 hr	Decreases within hours	Decreases within hours
CNS function	No impairment	No impairment	Routine task performance Cognitive impairment for 6–20 hr	Simple, routine task performance Cognitive impairment for > 24 hr	Rapid incapacitation; may have a lucid interval of several hours	
Latent Phase of Syndrome						
No symptoms	> 2 wk	7–15 d	0–7 d	0–2 d	None	None
Manifest Illness						
Signs/ symptoms	None	Moderate leukopenia	Severe leukopenia, purpura, hemorrhage, pneumonia, hair loss after 300 rad		Diarrhea, fever, electrolyte disturbance	Convulsions, ataxia, tremor, lethargy
Time of onset	—	> 2 wk	2 d to 4 wk	2 d to 4 wk	1–3 d	1–3 d
Critical period	—	None	4–6 wk; greatest potential for effective medical intervention		2–14 d	1–46 hr
Organ system	None	—	Hematopoietic; respiratory (mucosal) systems		GI tract Mucosal systems	CNS
Hospitalization duration	0%	< 5% 45–60 d	90% 60–90 d	100% 100+ d	100% Weeks to months	100% Days to weeks
Mortality	None	Minimal	Low with aggressive therapy	High	Very high; significant neurologic symptoms indicate lethal dose	

CNS, central nervous system; d, day(s); hr, hour(s); N/A, not available; wk, week(s).

Modified from Armed Forces Radiobiology Research Institute. Medical management of radiological casualties. Bethesda, MD, 2003.

Table 18-3 Symptom Clusters as Delayed Effects After Radiation

1	2	3	4
Headache	Anorexia	Partial-thickness and full-thickness skin damage	Lymphopenia
Fatigue	Nausea	Epilation (hair loss)	Neutropenia
Weakness	Vomiting	Ulceration	Thrombocytopenia
	Diarrhea		Purpura
			Opportunistic infections

Modified from Armed Forces Radiobiology Institute. Medical management of radiological casualties. Bethesda, MD, 2003.

the intrinsic special deposition pattern of different types of radiation. The rem has been replaced with the *sievert* (Sv); 1 Sv equals 100 rem.

Radiation affects rapidly dividing cells most readily, resulting in injury to the bone marrow and GI tract where high cell turnover rates occur. Higher doses can affect the CNS directly. The dose of whole-body exposure determines the medical consequences of the exposure. Patients receiving up to 1 Gy of whole-body irradiation would typically not exhibit signs of injury. At 1 to 2 Gy, less than half of patients will develop nausea and vomiting, many will subsequently develop *leukopenia* (decreased white blood cell count), and deaths will be minimal. Most victims receiving greater than 2 Gy will become ill and require hospitalization; at greater than 6 Gy, mortality becomes high. At doses greater than 30 Gy, neurologic signs are manifest, and death is most likely.[17]

Acute radiation syndrome generally follows a defined progression that first manifests in a prodromal phase characterized by malaise, nausea, and vomiting. This is followed by a latent phase, in which the patient is essentially asymptomatic. The length of the latent phase depends on the total absorbed dose of radiation. The greater the dose of radiation, the shorter the latent phase. The latent phase is followed by the subsequent illness phase, manifested by the organ system that has been injured. Damage to the bone marrow occurs with total doses of 0.7 to 4.0 Gy and results in decreasing levels of white blood cells and decreased immunity to infection over several days to weeks. Decreased platelets can result in easy bruising and bleeding. Decreased red blood cells will result in anemia. At 6 to 8 Gy, the GI tract will be affected, resulting in diarrhea, volume loss, and hematochezia (bloody stools). Above 30 Gy, the patient will manifest symptoms of the neurovascular syndrome, experiencing the prodromal phase of nausea and vomiting, a short latent phase lasting only a few hours, followed by a rapid deterioration of mental status, coma, and death, sometimes accompanied

by hemodynamic instability. Doses this high can occur after a nuclear detonation, but the victim will most likely have been killed by injuries associated with the blast. Victims could also be exposed to these high doses at a nuclear power facility where no blast has occurred, but a reactor core has reached criticality.[17]

Not all radiation accidents or terrorist events will result in high-dose radiation exposure. Low-dose radiation exposure, as would most likely occur after an RDD detonation, probably would not produce acute injury secondary to radiation. Dependent on dose, the patient may have an increased future risk of developing cancer. The acute effects of RDD detonation, besides the effects of the detonation of the conventional explosive, will likely be psychological, including stress reactions, fear, acute depression, and psychosomatic complaints, which would significantly strain the EMS agencies and medical infrastructure.

Patients can become contaminated with material that emits alpha, beta, and even gamma radiation, but the most common contaminants will emit alpha and beta radiation. Only gamma radiation contributes to whole-body irradiation, as previously described. Alpha and beta radiation have limited ability to penetrate, but still can cause local tissue injury. Patients can easily be decontaminated by clothing removal and washing with water or soap and water. It is impossible for a patient to be so contaminated as to be a radiologic hazard to prehospital care providers caring for the individual, so management of traumatic life-threatening injury is an immediate priority and should not be delayed pending decontamination.[17]

As described, radioactive particles can be inhaled, ingested, or absorbed through the skin or contaminated wounds. This type of exposure to radiation will not result in acute effects of radiation exposure but can result in delayed effects. Any victims or emergency responders who operate in an area at risk for airborne radioactive particles without the benefit of respiratory protection would require subsequent evaluation to identify internal contamination, which could require medical intervention to dilute or block the effects of the inhaled radionuclide.

Personal Protective Equipment

Prehospital care providers would be operating in an environment with risk of exposure to ionizing radiation after a radiologic disaster. The radiation risk would depend greatly on the type of radiologic event.

The PPE available to prehospital care providers for use in chemical and biologic hazards will offer some protection from radioactive particulate contamination. However, it will not provide protection from high-energy radiation sources, such as a damaged reactor or nuclear blast at ground zero.

Radioactivity can be present in gases, aerosols, solids, or liquids. If radioactive gases are present, SCBA will offer the highest protection. If aerosols are present, an APR may be adequate to prevent internal contamination caused by inhalation of contaminated particles. An N95 mask will offer some protection from inhaled particulates. A standard splash-resistant suit will protect against particulates that emit alpha radiation and will offer some protection from beta radiation but will provide no protection from gamma radiation or neutrons. This type of barrier protection will assist in the decontamination of particulate matter from an individual, but it does not protect against the risks of acute radiation illness when the person is exposed to high-energy sources of external radiation.

None of the typical PPE carried by prehospital care providers protects from a high-energy point source of radiation. This type of radiation is encountered during the first minute of a nuclear detonation, in a critical reactor core, or with a high-energy radiation source such as cesium-137, which may be dispersed in an RDD. The best protection from these sources is decreased time of exposure, increased distance from the source, and shielding. New materials that may offer some protection from low-level gamma radiation for emergency responder PPE are under investigation.

Unlike insufficient PPE worn to protect against chemical agents, the inhalation, ingestion, or skin absorption of radiation-emitting gas or particulate will not immediately incapacitate a prehospital care provider or victim. All providers who operated in an environment potentially contaminated with radioactive material would have to undergo a radiation survey to determine if internal contamination had occurred and undergo active management if warranted.

Dose rate meters or alarms should be worn if available. Standards exist for acceptable doses of ionizing radiation in the occupational environment under normal and emergency conditions.[18] Dose rates of ionizing radiation can be measured to prevent emergency responders from putting themselves at risk for acute radiation illness or an unacceptably higher incidence of cancer. The incident commander should be approached for guidance on radiation-exposure readings and limits.

Assessment and Management

Patients who have been injured in a radiologic catastrophe should receive primary and secondary surveys as dictated by the mechanism of injury. Prehospital care providers can expect to evaluate patients who have sustained blast injury and thermal injury in the case of a nuclear detonation or from the conventional high-explosive detonation of an RDD (**Box 18-13**). Priority should be given to management of traumatic injuries with the radiologic aspects of the case receiving secondary consideration. Decontamination of the victim is recommended to eliminate radioactive particulate contamination but should not delay the care of patients requiring immediate intervention for their traumatic

---

Box 18-13 Treatment and Decontamination Considerations for Radiation Exposure

Treatment Considerations
- If trauma is present, treat.
- If external radioactive contaminants are present, decontaminate (after treatment of life-threatening problems).
- If radioiodine (e.g., reactor accident) is present, consider giving prophylactic potassium iodide (Lugol's solution) within first 24 hours only (ineffective later).
- See www.usuhs.edu/afrri or www.orau.gov/reacts/guidance.htm.

Decontamination Considerations
- Exposure without contamination requires no decontamination.
- Exposure with contamination requires standard (universal) precautions, removal of patient clothing, and decontamination with water.
- Internal contamination will be determined at the hospital.
- Treating contaminated patients before decontamination may contaminate the facility; plan for decontamination before arrival.
- For a patient with a life-threatening condition, *treat*, then decontaminate.
- For a patient with a non-life-threatening condition, *decontaminate*, then treat.

Modified from Armed Forces Radiobiology Institute: Medical management of radiological casualties, Bethesda, MD, 2003.

injuries. If the patient does not show signs of serious injury requiring immediate intervention, the patient can be decontaminated first.

If radioiodine is present in the environment, as might be encountered in a nuclear reactor, following a spent fuel rod accident, or following detonation of a nuclear device, then giving potassium iodide to emergency responders and victims may help prevent accumulation of radioiodine in the thyroid, where it can increase the likelihood of cancer. Other *blocking* and *decorporation therapy* may be recommended by the hospital or federal assistance agencies when more information about the catastrophe is available. Blocking therapy is designed to interfere with the effects of the radiologic agent, whereas decorporation treatment is targeted at removing the agent from the body using medications that combine with the agent and allow for its elimination.

Transport Considerations

Patients should be transported to the nearest appropriate medical center that is capable of managing trauma and radiation injuries. All hospitals are required to have a plan for management of a radiologic emergency, but communities may have identified institutions that have decontamination facilities, are capable of managing trauma, and have staff trained to deal effectively with possible external or internal radioactive contamination, as well as the complications of whole-body exposure to ionizing radiation.

SUMMARY

- Weapons of mass destruction manufactured by terrorist regimes pose a significant threat to civilized society.
- Prehospital care providers may come in contact with explosions and with chemical and radiologic material as the result of industrial mishaps.
- The safety of prehospital care providers is paramount. They should possess a working knowledge of levels of personal protective equipment and the fundamentals of decontamination.
- Explosive agents have predominated in recent terrorist attacks. High explosives produce primary blast injuries in survivors who are in close proximity to the blast, and secondary injuries result from flying debris.
- Not only may chemical agents injure the skin and pulmonary system, but they may also result in systemic illness, manifesting as a specific toxidrome that yields clues to the agent. Antidotes are used for some of these agents.
- Biologic agents can be highly virulent bacteria or viruses or toxins produced by living organisms. The types of protective precautions used by providers vary with the specific agents.
- Several types of radiation exist. Exposure to these agents may result in acute radiation illness, which is typically a function of the type of radiation and the length of exposure.

SCENARIO RECAP

It is a warm summer evening, and you are dispatched to the scene of a reported explosion outside a popular café. You know this café is usually busy and typically seats patrons inside and outside on the patio. Dispatch informs you the number of victims is not yet known, although they have received multiple emergency calls regarding this incident. Other public safety agencies have also been dispatched to the location.

Upon arrival at the location, you observe you are the first prehospital care provider on scene. No incident command has yet been established. Dozens of people are running away from the cafe. Many are imploring you to assist victims who have obvious bleeding. Other victims are lying on the ground with variable states of consciousness.

- What will you do first?
- What are your priorities as you determine your course of action?
- How will you care for so many people?

SCENARIO SOLUTION

As always, the first priority is safety. Assess the scene. Look for evidence of a secondary device that may pose a threat to emergency responders. Are there other hazards? Look for hanging debris, downed or exposed power lines, or hazardous materials spills.

Communicate with your chain of command, and use the incident command system (ICS). Because you are the first emergency responder to the scene, the communications center will be relying on you for information. Describe pertinent details of the scene, observed hazards, numbers of victims, and likely number of resources required to manage the scene and victims. Carefully observe the crowd for evidence of a toxidrome. Is there an unusually high proportion of respiratory difficulty? Are victims vomiting and seizing? Is there evidence of agent dispersal in addition to the explosive blast? Based on your observations, the communications center and the on-duty supervisor can apprise other units and agencies of your situation and dispatch the necessary resources. A predefined disaster response plan may be activated.

Once the personal safety of all emergency responders has been ensured and information has been communicated, prepare to serve as the incident commander until relieved by another competent authority.

As soon as is feasible, don PPE appropriate for the incident, and then approach the victims with the intention of triaging them for treatment and transport using the START algorithm. Without engaging in the medical management of victims initially, sort the victims into immediate, urgent, delayed, and expectant categories. Remember, blast victims may not be able to hear directions or questions from emergency responders. As other assistance arrives, direct personnel to assume roles of the ICS until supervisory personnel arrive to assume command and control functions.

References

1. Hogan DE, Waeckerle JF, Dire DJ, et al. Emergency department impact of the Oklahoma City terrorist bombing. *Ann Emerg Med*. 1999;34:160.
2. Kennedy K, Aghababian R, Gans L, et al. Triage: techniques and applications in decision making. *Ann Emerg Med*. 1996;28(2):136.
3. Garner A, Lee A, Harrison K. Comparative analysis of multiple-casualty incident triage algorithms. *Ann Emerg Med*. 2001;38:541.
4. Lerner EB, Schwartz RB, Coule PL, et al. Mass casualty triage: an evaluation of the data and development of a proposed national guideline. *Disaster Med Public Health Preparedness*. 2008;2(suppl 1):S25-S34.
5. Thors L, Koch M, Wigenstam E, Koch B, Hägglund L, Bucht A. Comparison of skin decontamination efficacy of commercial decontamination products following exposure to VX on human skin. *Chem Biol Interact*. 2017;273:82-89.
6. Taysse L, Daulon S, Delamanche S, Bellier B, Breton P. Skin decontamination of mustards and organophosphates: comparative efficiency of RSDL and Fuller's earth in domestic swine. *Hum Exp Toxicol*. 2007;26(2):135-41.
7. U.S. Department of Health and Human Services. Medical Countermeasures Database. Chemical Hazards Emergency Medical Management website. https://chemm.nlm.nih.gov/medical_countermeasures.htm. Updated September 29, 2017. Accessed March 16, 2018.
8. Kapur GB, Hutson HR, Davis MA, Rice PL. The United States twenty-year experience with bombing incidents: implications for terrorism preparedness and medical response. *J Trauma*. 2005;59:1436-1444.
9. Pierce B. How rare are large, multiple-fatality work-related incidents? *Accid Anal Prev*. 2016;96:88-100.
10. Edwards DS, Mcmenemy L, Stapley SA, Patel HD, Clasper JC. 40 years of terrorist bombings - A meta-analysis of the casualty and injury profile. *Injury*. 2016;47(3):646-652.
11. U.S. Bomb Data Center. *Explosive Incident Report (EIR)—2014*. Redstone Arsenal, AL: U.S. Bomb Data Center; 2016.
12. Arnold J, Halpern P, Tsai M. Mass casualty terrorist bombings: a comparison of outcomes by bombing type. *Ann Emerg Med*. 2004;43:263.
13. DePalma RG, Burris DG, Champion HR, et al. Blast injuries. *N Engl J Med*. 2005;352(13):1335-1342.
14. Explosions and blast injuries: a primer for clinicians. Centers for Disease Control and Prevention website. https://www.cdc.gov/masstrauma/preparedness/primer.pdf. Updated May 9, 2003. Accessed November 4, 2017.
15. Wightman JM, Gladish JL. Explosions and blast injuries. *Ann Emerg Med*. 2001;37:664.
16. Armed Forces Radiobiology Research Institute (AFRRI). *Medical Management of Radiological Casualties*. Bethesda, MD: AFRRI; 2003.

17. U.S. Department of Veterans Affairs. Department of Homeland Security Working Group on Radiological Dispersion Device Preparedness/Medical Preparedness and Response Subgroup. American College of Radiology website. https://www.acr.org/~/media/ACR/Documents/PDF/Membership/Legal-Business/Disaster-Preparedness/Counter-Measures.pdf. Published May 1, 2003. Accessed November 4, 2017.

18. Almogy G, Mintz Y, Zamir G, et al. Suicide bombing attacks: can external signs predict internal injuries? *Ann Surg.* 2006;243(4):541-546.

19. Garner MJ, Brett SJ. Mechanisms of injury by explosive devices. *Anesthesiol Clin.* 2007;25(1):147-160.

20. Avidan V, Hersch M, Armon Y, et al. Blast lung injury: clinical manifestations, treatment, and outcome. *Am J Surg.* 2005;190(6):927-931.

21. Frykberg ER, Tepas JJ, Alexander RH. The 1983 Beirut Airport terrorist bombing: injury patterns and implications for disaster management. *Am Surg.* 1989;55:134.

22. Katz E, Ofek B, Adler J, et al. Primary blast injury after a bomb explosion in a civilian bus. *Ann Surg.* 1989;209:484.

23. Kluger Y, Nimrod A, Biderman P, et al. Case report: the quinary pattern of blast injury. *J Emerg Mgmt.* 2006;4(1):51-55.

24. Sorkine P, Nimrod A, Biderman P, et al. The quinary (Vth) injury pattern of blast (Abstract). *J Trauma.* 2007;56(1):232.

25. Nelson TJ, Wall DB, Stedje-Larsen ET, et al. Predictors of mortality in close proximity blast injuries during Operation Iraqi Freedom. *J Am Coll Surg.* 2006;202(3):418-422.

26. Mallonee S, Shariat S, Stennies G, et al. Physical injuries and fatalities resulting from the Oklahoma City bombing. *JAMA.* 1996;276:382.

27. Arnold JL, Tsai MC, Halpern P, et al. Mass-casualty, terrorist bombings: epidemiological outcomes, resource utilization, and time course of emergency needs (Part I). *Prehosp Disaster Med.* 2003;18(3):220-234.

28. Halpern P, Tsai MC, Arnold JL, et al. Mass-casualty, terrorist bombings: implications for emergency department and hospital emergency response (Part II). *Prehosp Disaster Med.* 2003;18(3):235-241.

29. U.S. Bomb Data Center. Explosive incidents 2007. 2007 USBDC explosives statistics. Washington, DC: U.S. Bomb Data Center; 2007.

30. Caseby NG, Porter MF. Blast injury to the lungs: clinical presentation, management and course. *Injury.* 1976;8:1.

31. Leibovici D, Gofrit ON, Shapira SC. Eardrum perforation in explosion survivors: is it a marker of pulmonary blast injury? *Ann Emerg Med.* 1999;34:168.

32. Coppel DL. Blast injuries of the lungs. *Br J Surg.* 1976;63:735.

33. Cohn SM. Pulmonary contusion: review of the clinical entity. *J Trauma.* 1997;42:973.

34. Peleg K, Limor A, Stein M, et al. Gunshot and explosion injuries: characteristics, outcomes, and implications for care of terror-related injuries in Israel. *Ann Surg.* 2004;239(3):311.

35. Tappan J. Magnesium and thermite poisoning. Medscape website. http://emedicine.medscape.com/article/833495-overview. Updated September 8, 2015. Accessed November 4, 2017.

36. Irizarry L. White phosphorus exposure. Medscape website. http://emedicine.medscape.com/article/833585-overview. Updated April 17, 2017. Accessed March 16, 2018.

37. Sidell FR, Takafuji ET, Franz DR, eds. *Medical Aspects of Chemical and Biological Warfare, TMM Series. Part 1: Warfare, Weaponry and the Casualty.* Washington, DC: Office of the Surgeon General, TMM Publications; 1997.

38. Walter FG, ed. *Advanced HAZMAT Life Support.* 2nd ed. Tucson, AZ: Arizona Board of Regents; 2000.

39. U.S. Army, Medical Research Institute of Chemical Defense. *Medical Management of Chemical Casualties Handbook.* 3rd ed. Aberdeen Proving Ground, MD: U.S. Army Research Institute; 2000.

40. Greenfield RA, Brown BR, Hutchins JB, et al. Microbiological, biological and chemical weapons of warfare and terrorism. *Am J Med Sci.* 2002;323(6):326.

41. Okumura T, Takasu N, Ishimatsu S, et al. Report on 640 victims of the Tokyo subway sarin attack. *Ann Emerg Med.* 1996;28(2):129.

42. Sellstrom A, Cairns S, Barbeschi M. Report of United Nations Mission to Investigate Allegations of the Use of Chemical Weapons in the Syrian Arab Republic on the Alleged Use of Chemical Weapons in the Ghouta Area of Damascus on 21 August 2013. United Nations website. http://undocs.org/A/67/997. Published September 16, 2013. Accessed June 3, 2017.

43. Reddy SD, Reddy DS. Midazolam as an anticonvulsant antidote for organophosphate intoxication—a pharmacotherapeutic appraisal. *Epilepsia.* 2015;56(6):813-821.

44. Rotenberg JS, Newmark J. Nerve-agent attacks on children: diagnosis and management. *Pediatrics.* 2003;112:648.

45. McDonough JH, Capacio BR, Shih TM. Treatment of nerve-agent-induced status epilepticus in the nonhuman primate. In: *U.S. Army Medical Defense—Bioscience Review, June 2–7.* Hunt Valley, MD: U.S. Army Medical Research Institute; 2002.

46. United Nations, Security Council. Organization for the Prohibition of Chemical Weapons-United Nations Joint Investigative Mechanism. Fourth report of the Organization for the Prohibition of Chemical Weapons-United Nations Joint Investigative Mechanism. United Nations website. http://undocs.org/S/2016/888. Published October 21, 2016. Accessed June 3, 2017.

47. Tuorinsky SD. *Textbooks of Military Medicine: Medical Aspects of Chemical Warfare.* Washington, DC: Borden Institute, Walter Reed Army Medical Center; 2008.

48. Ingelsby TV, Henderson DA, Bartlett JG, et al. Anthrax as a biological weapon: medical and public health management. *JAMA.* 1999;281(18):1735.

49. Keim M, Kaufmann AF. Principles for emergency response to bioterrorism. *Ann Emerg Med.* 1999;34(2):177.

50. U.S. Congress, Office of Technology Assessment. Proliferation of weapons of mass destruction, Pub. No. OTA-ISC-559. Washington, DC: U.S. Government Printing Office; 1993.

51. Inglesby TV, O'Toole T, Henderson DA, et al. Anthrax as a biological weapon, 2002: updated recommendations for management. *JAMA.* 2002;287:2236-2252.

52. Kman NE, Nelson RN. Infectious agents of bioterrorism: a review for emergency physicians. *Emerg Med Clin North Am.* 2008;26:517-547.

53. Stern EJ, Uhde KB, Shadomy SV, Messonnier N. Conference report on public health and clinical guidelines for anthrax. *Emerging Infect Dis.* 2008;14(4).

54. World Health Organization. *Health Aspects of Chemical and Biological Weapons*. Geneva, Switzerland: World Health Organization; 1970.

55. Inglesby TV, Dennis DT, Henderson DA. Plague as a biological weapon: medical and public health management. *JAMA*. 2000;283(17):2281.

56. Henderson DA, Inglesby TV, Bartlett JG. Smallpox as a biological weapon: medical and public health management. *JAMA*. 1999;281(22):2127.

57. Centers for Disease Control and Prevention. *Smallpox Response Plan and Guidelines*. Version 3.0, Guide C, Part 1. Atlanta, GA: Centers for Disease Control and Prevention; 2008:1-13.

58. Centers for Disease Control and Prevention. *Smallpox Response Plan and Guidelines*. Version 3.0, Guide F. Atlanta, GA: Centers for Disease Control and Prevention; 2003:1-10.

59. Basler CF. Molecular pathogenesis of viral hemorrhagic fever. *Semin Immunopathol*. 2017;39(5):551-561.

60. Cenciarelli O, Gabbarini V, Pietropaoli S, et al. Viral bioterrorism: learning the lesson of Ebola virus in West Africa 2013–2015. *Virus Res*. 2015;210:318-326.

61. Feldmann H, Geisbert TW. Ebola haemorrhagic fever. *Lancet*. 2011;377(9768):849-862.

62. Coltart CE, Lindsey B, Ghinai I, Johnson AM, Heymann DL. The Ebola outbreak, 2013–2016: old lessons for new epidemics. *Philos Trans R Soc Lond B Biol Sci*. 2017;372(1721):20160297.

63. Duraffour S, Malvy D, Sissoko D. How to treat Ebola virus infections? A lesson from the field. *Curr Opin Virol*. 2017;24:9-15.

64. Guidance on personal protective equipment (PPE) to be used by healthcare workers during management of patients with confirmed Ebola or persons under investigation (PUIs) for Ebola who are clinically unstable or have bleeding, vomiting, or diarrhea in U.S. hospitals, including procedures for donning and doffing PPE. Centers for Disease Control and Prevention, National Center for Emerging and Zoonotic Infectious Diseases, Division of Healthcare Quality Promotion website. https://www.cdc.gov/vhf/ebola/healthcare-us/ppe/guidance.html. Updated November 17, 2015. Accessed June 7, 2017.

65. Lowe JJ, Jelden KC, Schenarts PJ, et al. Considerations for safe EMS transport of patients infected with Ebola virus. *Prehosp Emerg Care*. 2015;19(2):179-183.

66. Isakov A, Miles W, Gibbs S, Lowe J, Jamison A, Swansiger R. Transport and management of patients with confirmed or suspected Ebola virus disease. *Ann Emerg Med*. 2015;66(3):297-305.

67. Franz DR, Jahrling PB, Friedlander AM, et al. Clinical recognition and management of patients exposed to biological warfare agents. *JAMA*. 1997;278(5):399.

68. Arnon SS, Schechter R, Inglesby TV, et al. Botulinum toxin as a biological weapon. Medical and public health management. *JAMA*. 2001;285:1059-1070.

69. Hogan DE, Kellison T. Nuclear terrorism. *Am J Med Sci*. 2002;323(6):341.

70. World Health Organization, International Atomic Energy Agency, United Nations Development Programme. Chernobyl: the true scale of the accident. World Health Organization website. http://www.who.int/mediacentre/news/releases/2005/pr38/en/index.html. Published September 5, 2005. Accessed November 5, 2017.

71. Flynn DF, Goans RE. Nuclear terrorism: triage and medical management of radiation and combined-injury casualties. *Surg Clin North Am*. 2006;86(3):601-636.

Suggested Reading

Centers for Disease Control and Prevention. Emergency Preparedness and Response. https://emergency.cdc.gov/.

U.S. Army Medical Research Institute of Infectious Diseases. USAMRIID: Biodefense Solutions to Protect Our Nation. http://www.usamriid.army.mil/.

Army Public Health Center. https://phc.amedd.army.mil/Pages/default.aspx.

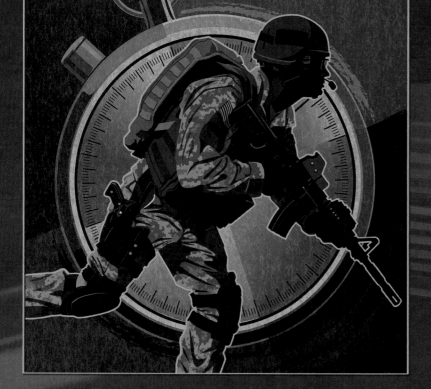

Special Considerations

CHAPTER **19**

Environmental Trauma I: Heat and Cold

Lead Editors:
Seth Hawkins, MD
R. Bryan Simon, RN, MSc, DiMM, FAWM

CHAPTER OBJECTIVES

At the completion of this chapter, you will be able to do the following:

- Explain why heatstroke is considered an emergent life-threatening condition.
- Identify the similarities and differences between heatstroke and exercise-associated hyponatremia.
- Describe the two most effective and rapid cooling procedures for heatstroke.
- List the five factors that place prehospital care providers at risk for heat illness.
- Discuss the fluid hydration guidelines and how they can be applied to prevent dehydration in warm or cold environments.
- Identify the differences in the management of mild hypothermia from that of severe hypothermia.
- List the signs of mild, moderate, and severe frostbite and discuss how to prevent its progression.
- Explain reasons for actively warming hypothermic patients in cardiopulmonary arrest.

SCENARIO

It is a hot summer afternoon with temperatures reaching 102°F (38.9°C). Over the past 30 days, it has been very humid, with temperatures reaching over 100°F (37.8°C) daily. The ambient temperature has resulted in many heat-related injuries that have required emergency medical services (EMS) personnel to transport numerous patients to the emergency departments (EDs) of the inner city.

At 1700 hours, your ambulance unit responds to a dispatch for an unresponsive male patient in a vehicle. As your ambulance unit arrives on scene, you observe a 76-year-old man who appears to be unconscious and uninjured in a vehicle parked outside of a department store. Your rapid assessment of the patient's airway, breathing, and circulation (ABCs) and level of consciousness reveals that the patient is verbal, but he is saying things that are illogical and irrational.

- What are the potential causes for this patient's decreased level of consciousness?
- What hallmark signs support a heat-related diagnosis?
- How would you emergently manage this patient at the scene and en route to the emergency department?

INTRODUCTION

This chapter focuses on recognizing and treating exposure to both hot and cold temperatures (**Box 19-1**). The most significant morbidity and mortality in the United States from all environmental traumas are caused by thermal trauma.[1-5]

Environmental extremes of heat and cold have a common outcome of injuries and potential death that can affect many individuals during the peak summer and winter months. It is critical to know that mortality increases significantly when a traumatized patient presents in the hospital with either hypothermia (core body temperature less than 95°F [35°C]) or with a heat-related illness (hyperthermia) with core body temperatures usually greater than 101°F [38.5°C]).[6,7] Individuals who are especially susceptible to both highs and lows of temperature are very young persons, the older adult population, people living in urban areas and in poverty, individuals who take specific medications, patients with chronic illnesses, and persons with alcoholism.[3-5,8-11] Most EMS responses in the United States for heat and cold injuries are for patients with hyperthermia or hypothermia in an urban setting. For this reason, these topics are not simply considered "wilderness medicine" and cannot be used to define a call as wilderness EMS. All EMS providers need to be familiar with these topics (**Box 19-2**).[12] Additionally, expanding interest in recreational and high-risk adventure activities in the wilderness backcountry during periods of environmental extremes places more individuals in wilderness areas at risk for heat-related and cold-related injuries and fatalities.[6,13-15]

Box 19-1 Frostbite Prevention

For those traveling to or responding in remote or austere environments, the Wilderness Medical Society has detailed practice guidelines on the prevention and care of frostbite, which can be found on their website.

Box 19-2 Prehospital Versus Out-of-Hospital

While this text focuses on prehospital care, the term *prehospital* is not accurate in all scenarios. Studies have demonstrated that most of the people cared for in wilderness and other remote outdoor environments are not transferred to a hospital, given that typically a hospital is not immediately accessible. Thus, some organizations refer to medical care provided in such environments as *out-of-hospital* care.

Epidemiology

Heat-Related Illness

Approximately 618 people die each year in the United States from conditions relating to extreme heat.[3] The year 2016 was the warmest documented year in recorded history (since 1880) and the third record-setting year in a row. Global surface temperatures have trended upward over the past 35 years, with 16 of the 17 warmest years on record occurring since 2001.[16] More deaths were caused by heat stress than by hurricanes, lightning, tornadoes, floods, and earthquakes combined. Of the 11,457 deaths, 6,068 (53%) were related directly to high ambient temperatures.[2,17] Furthermore, morbidity and mortality can be extremely high when periodic seasonal heat waves occur (more than three consecutive days of air temperatures 90°F [32.2°C] or higher). The Centers for Disease Control and Prevention (CDC) reported a total of 3,442 deaths (1999 to 2003) resulting from exposure to extreme heat (annual mean = 688).[17]

Cold-Related Illness

Mild to severe cold weather conditions cause an average of 774 deaths per year in the United States.[4,18] Almost one-half of these deaths occurred in persons 65 years of age and older.[4,16] When adjusted for age, death from hypothermia occurred approximately 2.5 times more often in men than in women. The incidence of hypothermia-related deaths progressively increases with age, and it is three times higher in males than in females after age 15 years. Major contributing factors for accidental hypothermia are urban poverty, socioeconomic conditions, alcohol intake, malnutrition, and age (very young and older adults).[4,9]

While hypothermia is typically associated with cool or colder weather, it may occur in conditions that one would ordinarily not consider cold but that allow the body's temperature to fall below 96°F (35.6°C). For example, the elderly and infants may develop hypothermia in summertime if the air conditioning in their home is too cold for their limited adaptive mechanisms. Swimmers and surfers can become hypothermic in the summer when exposed to water that is cooler than body temperature, and the combination of low, but not freezing, temperatures, along with high winds and rain, can result in conditions conducive to hypothermia.[19] Thus hypothermia is not just a cold weather disease.

Anatomy

The Skin

The skin, the largest organ of the body, interfaces with the external environment and serves as a layer of protection. It

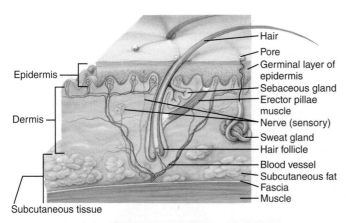

Figure 19-1 The skin is composed of three tissue layers—epidermis, dermis, and subcutaneous tissue—and associated muscle. Some layers contain structures such as glands, hair follicles, blood vessels, and nerves. All of these structures are interrelated with the maintenance, loss, and gain of body temperature.

prevents the invasion of microorganisms, maintains fluid balance, and regulates temperature. Skin is composed of three tissue layers: the epidermis, dermis, and subcutaneous tissue (**Figure 19-1**). The outermost layer, the epidermis, is made up entirely of epithelial cells, with no blood vessels. Underlying the epidermis is the thicker dermis. The dermis is 20 to 30 times thicker than the epidermis. It is made up of a framework of connective tissues that contain blood vessels, blood products, nerves, sebaceous glands, and sweat glands. The innermost layer, the subcutaneous layer, is a combination of elastic and fibrous tissue as well as fatty deposits. Below this layer is skeletal muscle. The skin, nerves, blood vessels, and other underlying anatomic structures have major roles in regulating body temperature.

Physiology

Thermoregulation and Temperature Balance

Humans are considered **homeotherms**, or warm-blooded animals. A key feature of homeotherms is that they can regulate their own internal body temperature at a constant level, often above the level of their environment, and independent of varying environmental temperatures.

The human body is essentially divided into a warmer inner core and an outer shell. The brain and the thoracic and abdominal organs are included in the inner core, and the skin and subcutaneous layer make up the outer shell. The outer shell plays a critical role in the regulation of the body's **core temperature**. The core temperature is regulated through a balance of heat-production and

heat-dissipation mechanisms. The temperature of the skin's surface and the "thickness" of the outer shell depend on the **environmental temperature**. The outer shell becomes "thicker" in colder temperatures and "thinner" in warmer temperatures based on the shunting of blood away from or to the skin, respectively. This outer shell, or tissue insulation, as induced by vasoconstriction, has been estimated to offer about the same level of protection as wearing a light business suit.

Metabolic heat production will vary based on activity levels. Independent of the variation of external temperature, the body normally functions within a narrow temperature range, known as **environmental temperature**, of about 1°F (0.6°C) on either side of 98.6°F (37°C ± 0.6°C). Normal body temperature is maintained in a narrow range by homeostatic mechanisms regulated in the brain's hypothalamus. The **hypothalamus** is known as the **thermoregulatory center** and functions as the body's thermostat to control neurologic and hormonal regulation of body temperature. Trauma to the brain can disrupt the hypothalamus, which in turn causes an imbalance in the regulation of body temperature.

Humans have two systems to regulate body temperature: **behavioral regulation** and **physiologic thermoregulation**. Behavioral regulation is governed by the individual's thermal sensation and comfort, and the distinguishing feature is the conscious effort to reduce thermal discomfort (e.g., adding or shedding clothing, seeking shelter in cold environments). The processing of sensory feedback to the brain of thermal information in behavioral regulation is not well understood, but the feedback of thermal sensation and comfort responds more quickly than physiologic responses to changes in environmental temperature.[20]

Heat Production and Thermal Balance

Basal metabolic rate is the heat produced primarily as a by-product of metabolism, mostly from the large organs of the core and from skeletal muscle contraction. The heat generated is transferred throughout the body by blood in the circulatory system. Heat transfer and its dissipation from the body by the cardiopulmonary system are important in the assessment and management of heat illness, as discussed later in the chapter.

Shivering increases the metabolic rate by increasing muscle tension, which leads to repeated bouts of muscular contraction and relaxation, and it is the most powerful of the body's heat production mechanisms. Although shivering can occur due to skin cooling at core temperatures measuring 98.6°F (37°C), typically shivering begins when the core temperature drops to between 94°F and 97°F (34.4°C to 36.1°C) and continues until the core temperature is 86°F (30°C).[7] With maximal shivering, heat production is increased by five to six times the resting level.[21,22]

The physiologic thermoregulation systems that control heat production and heat loss responses are well documented.[20,22,23] Two principles in thermoregulation are key to understanding how the body regulates core temperature: **thermal gradient** and **thermal equilibrium**. A thermal gradient is the difference in temperature (high vs. low temperature) between two objects. Thermal equilibrium is the state at which two objects in contact with one another are at the same temperature; it is achieved by the transfer of heat from a warmer object to a colder object until the objects are the same temperature.

When body temperature rises, the normal physiologic response is to increase skin blood flow and to begin sweating. Most body heat is transferred to the environment at the skin surface by conduction, convection, radiation, and evaporation. Because heat is transferred from greater temperature to lower temperature, the human body can gain heat by radiation and conduction during hot weather conditions.

Methods to maintain and dissipate body heat are important concepts for prehospital care providers. They must understand how both heat and cold are transferred to and from the body so that they can effectively manage a patient who has hyperthermia or hypothermia (**Figure 19-2**). The methods of heat and cold transfer are described as follows:

- **Radiation** is the loss or gain of heat in the form of electromagnetic energy; it is the transfer of energy from a warm object to a cooler one. A patient with heat illness can acquire additional body heat directly from the sun. Sources of radiant heat must be eliminated by the prehospital care provider when assessing and treating the patient, as they will impede interventions to cool or warm a patient.
- **Conduction** is the transfer of heat between two objects in direct contact with each other, such as a patient lying on a frozen lawn after a fall. A patient will generally lose heat faster when lying on the cold ground than when exposed to cold air. Therefore, prehospital care providers need to protect and insulate the patient from colder ground temperatures rather than merely covering the patient with a blanket.
- **Convection** is the transfer of heat from a solid object to a medium that moves across that solid object, such as air or water over the body. The movement of cool air or water across the warmer skin provides for the continuous transfer of heat from the body. The body will lose heat 25 times faster in water than in air of the same temperature. A patient with wet clothing will lose body heat rapidly in mild to cold temperatures, so prehospital care providers should remove wet clothing and keep a patient dry to maintain body heat. When prehospital care providers effectively manage a patient with heat illness, they use the principle of convective

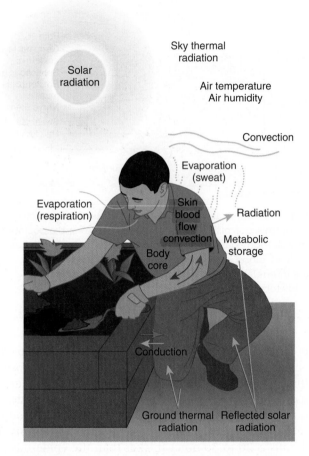

Figure 19-2 How humans exchange thermal energy with the environment.

© National Association of Emergency Medical Technicians (NAEMT).

heat loss by moistening and fanning the patient to dissipate body heat quickly.

- **Evaporation** of sweat from a liquid to a vapor is an extremely effective method of producing heat loss from the body, depending on the relative humidity or moisture in the air. A **basal level** of both water and accompanying heat loss from exhaled air, skin, and mucous membranes is called **insensible loss** and is caused by evaporation. This insensible loss is normally about 10% of basal heat production, but when the body temperature rises, this process becomes more active (sensible), and sweat is produced. Evaporative heat loss increases in cool, dry, and windy conditions such as deserts. Collectively, convection and evaporation are more important than other methods of heat transfer because they are regulated by the body to control core temperature.[5]

Increases (hyperthermia) and decreases (hypothermia) in body temperature beyond the steady-state range (98.6°F ± 1°F [37°C ± 0.6°C]) can result from different internal and external causes, and return to steady-state temperature can occur without complications.[24] Hyperthermia occurs primarily in one of three ways:

- As a normal response to sustained exercise, in which the heat produced elevates core temperature and is the stimulus for heat-dissipating responses (e.g., sweating, increased blood flow to the skin)
- When the sum of heat production and heat gained from the environment is greater than the body's heat dissipation capability
- From a fever

Unlike the first two ways, fever usually occurs in response to inflammation because of a change in the *thermoregulatory set point* (body temperature setting) of the brain, and the body responds by elevating body temperature to a higher value (100°F to 106°F [37.8°C to 41.1°C]). Heat production increases temporarily to achieve a new thermoregulatory set point temperature in an attempt to make the environment less hospitable for the invading infection.[23]

Homeostasis

These anatomic structures and physiologic systems are designed to interact in such a way that the body functions appropriately when exposed to temperature changes. The body is in a constant state of neurologic feedback from peripheral and internal regions to the thermoregulatory center and other regions in the brain and consequent responses. All of these systems interact to maintain constant, stable internal conditions, called homeostasis, in the body. However, at times, homeostasis is not achieved. For example, an imbalance may occur in the cardiovascular and thermoregulatory adjustments to eliminate excessive body heat, one outcome of which is the loss of excessive body fluid through sweating that causes acute dehydration and may lead to signs and symptoms of heat illness.

Risk Factors in Heat Illness

Numerous studies on humans have demonstrated large individual differences in tolerance to hot environments.[24] These differences can be partially explained by both physical characteristics and medical conditions that are associated with an increased risk for heat illness (**Box 19-3**). It is important to realize that any situation in which heat production exceeds the body's ability to dissipate heat may result in heat injury.

Key risk factors that contribute to the onset of heat illness are alcohol consumption, medications, dehydration, higher body mass index, obesity, inadequate diet,

---

Box 19-3 Heat Illness Risk Factors[19,25-27]

Factors That Increase Internal Heat Production
Physical exertion
Response to infection (fever)
Hyperthyroidism
Agitated and tremulous states (Parkinson, psychosis, mania, drug withdrawal—opiate and alcohol)
Drug overdoses (such as cocaine, caffeine, LSD, phencyclidine hydrochloride, methamphetamine, ecstasy)

Factors That Interfere with Heat Dissipation
High ambient temperature
High humidity
Obesity (insulation effect, less efficient dissipation)
Impaired vasodilation
Diabetes
Alcoholism
Medications: diuretics, tranquilizers, beta-blockers, antihistamines, phenothiazines, antidepressants
Impaired ability to sweat (cystic fibrosis, skin diseases, healed burns)
Heavy or tight clothing

Factors That Impair the Body's Response to Heat Stress Dehydration (including recent GI or respiratory infections)
Prior episode of heatstroke
Hypokalemia
Cardiovascular disease)

Abbreviations: GI, gastrointestinal; LSD, lysergic acid diethylamide

---

improper clothing, low fitness, sleep loss, extremes of age, cardiovascular disease, skin injuries, previous heat-related illness, sickle cell trait, cystic fibrosis, sunburn, viral illness, and exercise during the hottest hours of day.[18,19,25,26,28,29] Transient conditions include those affecting individuals who travel from cooler climates and are not heat-acclimatized to warmer climates on arrival. Other transient factors that place individuals at risk for heat illness are common illnesses, including colds and other conditions that cause fever, vomiting, and diarrhea, along with poor dietary and fluid intake.[30,31] Cumulative exposure is also a known risk factor for members of the military or fire fighters, with risk increasing with additional days of exposure unless relieved.[32]

Factors considered to be chronic conditions that place individuals at greater risk for heat illness are fitness level, body size, age, medical condition, and medication use.

Obesity, Fitness, and Body Mass Index

Obesity and low levels of physical fitness caused by genetic factors or a sedentary lifestyle with inadequate daily physical activity will reduce tolerance to heat exposure. Physical fitness provides a cardiovascular reserve to maintain cardiac output as needed to sustain thermoregulation, and it allows individuals to acclimatize more quickly through sustained tolerance for physical activity and increased sweat production while hyperthermic.[27,33,34] Individuals who are overweight have a normal response to heat exposure—vasodilation of skin blood vessels and increased sweating. However, the combination of low fitness, lack of heat acclimatization, increased thermal insulation, and altered sweat gland distribution increases the energy cost of movement and places them at greater risk for heat illness.

Age

Thermoregulatory capacity and tolerance to heat diminish with age, particularly in those individuals aged 65 years or older. These individuals can improve their heat tolerance by maintaining a low body weight and attaining an improved level of physical fitness.

Special consideration must be given for infants and young children because their body surface area makes up a much greater proportion of their overall weight compared to that of an adult, causing them to face a much greater risk of heat-related illness. Furthermore, infants have an immature thermoregulatory capacity that does not allow them to adequately maintain body temperature when exposed to high heat.

Medical Conditions

Underlying medical conditions such as diabetes mellitus, thyroid disorders, and renal disease can increase the risk for heat intolerance and heat illness. Cardiovascular disease and circulatory problems that increase cutaneous blood flow and circulatory demand are aggravated by heat exposure. In these extreme environmental conditions, heart disease and pulmonary diseases may be the presenting signs and symptoms aggravated by high ambient temperatures. A mild form of heat illness seen in individuals is miliaria rubia (prickly heat, heat rash, sweat rash), which has been shown to cause reduced heat tolerance through blocked or inflamed sweat pores.[19,33]

Medications

The use of specific prescription or over-the-counter medications can place individuals at a greater risk for heat illness (see Box 19-3). Certain medications can increase metabolic heat production, suppress body cooling and thirst, reduce cardiac reserve, and alter renal electrolyte and fluid balance.[6,33] Sedative and narcotic drugs affect mental status and can affect logical reasoning and judgment, potentially suppressing decision-making ability when the individual is exposed to heat.

Dehydration

Total body water (TBW) is the largest component of the human body, representing 50% to 70% of body weight.[35] For example, a 165-pound (lb; 75-kilogram [kg]) man contains approximately 45 liters of water, representing 60% of body weight. Excessive changes in the normal body water balance (*euhydration*) resulting from either overconsumption of water (*hyperhydration*) or fluid deficit (*hypohydration*) alter homeostasis, producing specific signs and symptoms. Dehydration, defined as the hypotonic hypovolemia caused by a net loss of hypotonic body fluids, can be a serious outcome of both heat and cold exposure, and it is also seen as a dangerous side effect of diarrhea, vomiting, and fever.[35]

Dehydration is a common finding in both cases of heat illness occurring over many days, as seen in geriatric patients, or during physical activity, as seen with profuse sweating in athletes, members of the military, and fire fighters. In the elderly, dehydration is often due to low fluid consumption, whereas athletes, military personnel, and fire fighters consume inadequate volumes of fluid during daily activities and thus do not replace depleted TBW. Children (younger than 15 years) and persons older than 65 years are particularly susceptible to dehydration.

Body water is lost daily through sweat, tears, urine, and stool. Normally, drinking fluids and eating foods that contain water replace these losses. When a person becomes sick with fever, diarrhea, or vomiting, or an individual is exposed to heat, dehydration occurs. Occasionally, drugs that deplete body fluids and electrolytes, such as diuretics, can cause dehydration.

During heat exposure, body water is primarily lost as sweat, as this is the primary means of heat removal from the body. Individuals can sweat 0.8 to 1.4 liters per hour (liters/hour), and it has been reported that some elite athletes who are heat-acclimatized can sweat up to 3.7 liters/hour during competition in hot environments.[36] The keys to avoiding the onset of heat illness are to maintain a body fluid balance and to minimize dehydration during daily activities, particularly during any physical activity in moderate to high heat exposure. Signs and symptoms of dehydration are nonspecific and at times difficult to identify.

With mild to moderate levels of acute dehydration (2% to 6% body weight), individuals experience thirst, weakness, fatigue, headache, light-headedness, irritability, decreased heat tolerance, dark odorous urine, diminished urine output, and cognitive deterioration, along with reductions in strength and aerobic physical capacity.[33,35,37,38] Severely dehydrated patients will present with signs and symptoms similar to those of hypovolemic shock: rapid pulse, pale, sweaty skin, weakness, and nausea.[33]

When individuals are encouraged to drink fluids frequently during heat exposure, the rate at which fluids can be replaced by mouth is limited by the rate of gastric emptying and the rate of fluid absorption in the small intestine.[39] Fluids empty from the stomach to the small intestine, where absorption occurs into the bloodstream, at a maximal rate of approximately 1 to 1.2 liters/hour.[38] Furthermore, gastric emptying rates are decreased approximately 20% to 25% when sweat-induced weight loss causes dehydration of 5% of total body weight (e.g., 5% of a 200-lb male = 10-lb weight loss [5% of a 100-kg male = a 5-kg weight loss).[40] Various hydration strategies and considerations are discussed in more detail later in this chapter.

Signs and Symptoms of Dehydration[33,35]

The following are the most common signs and symptoms of dehydration in infants, children, and adults, although people may experience different symptoms:

- Less frequent urination and dark color urine
- Thirst
- Dry skin
- Fatigue
- Light-headedness
- Headache
- Dizziness

- Confusion
- Dry mouth and mucous membranes
- Increased heart rate and breathing

In infants and children, additional symptoms may include the following:

- Dry mouth and tongue
- No tears when crying
- No wet diapers for more than 3 hours
- Sunken abdomen, eyes, or cheeks
- High fever
- Listlessness
- Irritability
- Skin that does not flatten when pinched and released (*skin tenting*)

Injuries Caused by Heat

Heat-related disorders can range from minor to severe in patients with heat illness.[29,41] It is important to note that prehospital care providers may or may not see a progression of signs and symptoms, starting with minor syndromes (e.g., miliaria rubra, exercise-associated muscle cramps) and advancing to major heat-related illness (e.g., heatstroke). In most heat exposures, the patient can dissipate core body heat adequately and maintain core temperature within the normal range. However, when heat-related conditions result in a call for EMS assistance, the minor heat-related conditions may be apparent to the prehospital care provider during patient assessment, along with signs and symptoms of a major heat illness (**Table 19-1**).

Table 19-1 Common Heat-Related Disorders			
Disorder	**Cause/Problem**	**Signs/Symptoms**	**Treatment**
Exercise-associated muscle (heat) cramps	Failure to replace fluids and electrolytes lost through sweating; electrolyte and muscle problems	Painful, spasmodic muscle cramps, usually in heavily exercised muscles such as calves, thighs, and abdominals	Move to cool place; rest; encourage drinking sport drinks or drinks with NaCl (e.g., tomato juice). Transport those with signs or symptoms listed for the following conditions.
Dehydration	Failure to replace sweat loss with fluids	Thirst, nausea, excessive fatigue, headache, hypovolemia, decreased thermoregulation; reduced physical and mental capacity	Replace sweat loss with lightly salted fluids; rest in cool place until body weight and water losses are restored. In some patients, IV rehydration is necessary.

(continued)

Table 19-1 Common Heat-Related Disorders (*continued*)

Disorder	Cause/Problem	Signs/Symptoms	Treatment
Heat exhaustion	Excessive heat strain with inadequate water intake; cardiovascular problems with venous pooling, decreased cardiac filling time, reduced cardiac output; untreated, may progress to heatstroke	Low urine output, tachycardia, tachypnea, weakness, malaise, unstable gait, extreme fatigue, pale/cool/clammy skin, headache, dizziness (fainting possible), nausea/vomiting, temperature normal or mildly elevated, sweating	Stop exertion, remove from heat stress, and place patient in prone position in cooler location; remove restrictive clothing; cool body with water and fanning; encourage drinking lightly salty fluids (e.g., sport drinks); administer intravenous (IV) 0.9% NaCl or lactated Ringer solution.
Heatstroke	High core temperatures > 105°F (40.5°C); cellular disruption; dysfunction of multiple organ systems common; neurologic disorder with thermoregulatory center failure	Mental status changes, including confusion, irrational behavior, or delirium; possible shivering; tachycardia initially, then bradycardia late; hypotension; rapid and shallow breathing; dry or wet, hot skin; loss of consciousness; seizures and coma	Emergency: Apply rapid, immediate cooling by water immersion or wetting patient, or wrap patient in cool, wet sheets and fan vigorously. Apply ice packs in axillae, groin, chest wall. Continue until core temperature is < 102°F (38.9°C). Treat for shock if necessary once core temperature is lowered. Protect the airway and immediately transport to ED.
Exercise-associated hyponatremia	Low plasma sodium concentration (< 135 mmol/liter); typically seen in individuals during prolonged activity in hot environments; drinking water (> 1.5 liters/hour) or that exceeds sweat rate; inappropriate arginine vasopressin secretion; failure to replace sodium loss in sweat	Headache, nausea, vomiting, malaise, dizziness, ataxia, altered mental status, polyuria, pulmonary edema, signs of intracranial pressure, seizures, coma; core temperature < 102°F (38.9°C); mimics signs of heat exhaustion and dehydration	Restrict hypotonic and isotonic fluid intake; give salty foods/saline. Unresponsive patients receive standard resuscitative care, 15 liters/min oxygen by nonrebreathing mask. If serum sodium levels can be measured and are below 130 mmol/liter, provide IV hypertonic saline, 100-ml bolus of 3% hypertonic saline, every 10-minutes for three doses or until neurologic symptoms end. Transport immediately with alert patient in sitting position or left-lateral position if unresponsive.

Source: Modified from Schimelpfenig T, Richards G, Tartar S. Management of heat illnesses. In Hawkins SC, ed. *Wilderness EMS*. Philadelphia, PA: Wolters Kluwer, 2018; Bennett BL, Hew-Butler T, Hoffman MD, Rogers IR, Rosner MH. Wilderness Medical Society Practice guidelines for treatment of exercise-associated hyponatremia: 2014 update. *Wilderness Environ Med.* 2014;25:s30-s42.

Minor Heat-Related Disorders

The minor heat-related disorders include miliaria rubra, heat edema, exercise-induced muscle (heat) cramps, and heat syncope. These are not life-threatening problems, but they do require assessment and treatment.

Miliaria Rubra

Miliaria rubra, also known as "prickly heat" and "heat rash," is a red, *pruritic* (itchy), *papular* (raised bumps) rash normally seen on the skin in areas of restrictive clothing and heavy sweating (**Figure 19-3**). This condition is caused by inflammation of the sweat glands that blocks the sweat ducts. As a result, affected areas cannot sweat, putting individuals at increased risk of heat illness, depending on the amount of skin surface involved.[13,19,25,27]

Management

Treatment begins by cooling and drying the affected area(s) and by preventing further conditions that cause sweat in these areas. For example, get the patient out of the heat and humidity and into a cooler, dryer environment. A cool shower and "dab" drying the area will help resolve these rashes. Antihistamines may be administered to relieve itching.[13,19,25,27]

Heat Edema

Heat edema is a mild, dependent edema in the hands, feet, and ankles seen during early stages of heat acclimatization when plasma volume is expanding to compensate for the increased need for thermoregulatory blood flow. This form of edema does not indicate excessive fluid intake or cardiac, renal, or hepatic disease. In the absence of other diseases, this condition is of no clinical significance and is self-limited. Heat edema is observed more often in females.

Management

Treatment consists of loosening any constricting clothing, removing any tight or constricting jewelry, and elevating the legs. Diuretics are not indicated and may increase the risk of heat illness.

Exercise-Associated Muscle (Heat) Cramps

Exercise-associated muscle cramps can occur at any temperature and are not related specifically to elevated body temperature. They manifest as short-term, painful muscle contractions frequently seen in the calf (gastrocnemius) muscles, but also in the voluntary muscles of the abdomen and extremities, and are commonly observed following prolonged physical activity, often in warm to hot temperatures. These cramps occur in individuals during exercise that produces profuse sweating or during the exercise-recovery period. Smooth muscle, cardiac, diaphragm, and *bulbar* muscles (muscles involved with speech, chewing, and swallowing) are not involved. Muscle cramps can occur alone or in association with heat exhaustion.

The cause of muscle cramping is unknown, but it is believed to be related to a combination of neuromuscular fatigue along with body water loss and sodium and other electrolyte losses. It is more commonly seen when individuals exercise in hot, humid environments without proper heat acclimatization, exercise beyond their physical fitness level, or experience profuse sweating.[13,27,33]

Management

Treatment consists of rest in a cool environment, prolonged stretching of the affected muscle, massage, and consuming oral fluids and food containing sodium chloride (e.g., ⅛ to ¼ teaspoon of table salt added to 10 to 16 ounces [oz; 300 to 500 milliliters (ml)] of fluids or sport drinks, 1 to 2 salt tablets with 10 to 16 oz [300 to 500 ml] of fluid, or salty snacks). Intravenous (IV) fluids are rarely needed, but prolonged and severe diffuse muscle cramps can be resolved more rapidly with IV normal saline (NS). Avoid the use of salt tablets by themselves because they can cause gastrointestinal (GI) distress.[13,27,33]

Heat Syncope

Heat syncope is seen with prolonged standing in warm environments and is caused by low blood pressure that results in dizziness, weakness, or brief and transient loss of consciousness. Heat exposure causes peripheral vasodilation and orthostatic venous blood pooling in the legs, causing low blood pressure. Heat syncope often occurs to soldiers in formation or during a parade and can be seen in athletes after completion of a long duration exercise. Another common name for heat syncope is heat-associated postural hypotension.[27,33]

Management

Remove from the heat stress to a cool environment, and rest the patient in a recumbent position. Loosen or remove

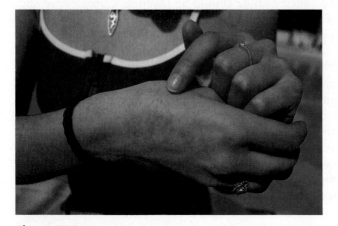

Figure 19-3 Heat rash.
© Ian west/Alamy Stock Photo.

constrictive clothing, and if dehydration is suspected, provide oral or IV rehydration. If a fall occurred, patients should be thoroughly evaluated for injury. Patients with a significant history of cardiac or neurologic disorders need further evaluation for the cause of their syncopal episode. Monitoring of vital signs and the electrocardiogram (ECG) during transport is essential.[27,33]

Major Heat-Related Disorders

The major heat-related disorders include exercise-associated collapse, heat exhaustion, and heatstroke (classic and exertional forms) and may pose a life threat if allowed to progress.

Exercise-Associated Collapse

This disorder occurs when an individual collapses after strenuous exercise.[42-48] During exercise, contraction of the muscles of the lower extremities assists in augmenting venous blood return to the heart. When exercise stops, such as at the end of a jog, the muscle contraction that assisted blood return to the heart slows significantly. This in turn causes venous blood return to the heart to decrease, resulting in a decreased cardiac output to the brain. This disorder is often seen at the completion of marathons, ultramarathons, and triathlons.[49]

Assessment

Signs and symptoms include difficulty standing and walking, nausea, light-headedness, dizziness, or syncope. Patients may feel better when lying down but become light-headed when they attempt to stand or sit (*orthostatic hypotension*). Profuse sweating is not unusual. Ventilation and pulse rates may be rapid. The patient's core body temperature may be normal or slightly elevated. It is difficult to rule out dehydration, but this type of postexercise collapse is not from hypovolemia. In contrast, collapse that occurs during exercise requires immediate evaluation for other causes (e.g., cardiovascular).

Management

The patient is removed to a cool environment to rest in a recumbent position with legs elevated. IV rehydration is provided if truly needed for moderate to severe dehydration; otherwise provide cool fluids by mouth. Because many of these patients experienced collapse because of the decreased venous return at the end of exercise and not from dehydration, it is highly recommended to withhold IV therapy until further assessment is completed and passive "cooldown." As with any form of collapse, further evaluation is necessary to rule out other disorders (e.g., heatstroke, exercise-associated hyponatremia, cardiac or neurologic causes). Monitoring of vital signs and ECG during transport is essential to detect cardiac dysrhythmias.

Heat Exhaustion

Heat exhaustion is the most common heat-related disorder seen by prehospital care providers. This condition can develop over days of exposure (often seen in elderly persons) or acutely (often seen in athletes). Heat exhaustion results from cardiac output that is insufficient to support the increased circulatory load caused by competing demands of thermoregulatory heat dissipation, increased skin blood flow, reduced plasma volume, reduced venous return to the heart from vasodilation, and sweat-induced depletion of salt and water.[31] Heat exhaustion often occurs to older adults due to a combination of high temperatures, medication use (e.g., diuretics), inadequate water intake, and preexisting cardiac insufficiency.[13,33]

Distinguishing severe heat exhaustion from heatstroke often may be difficult, but a quick mental status assessment will determine the level of neurologic involvement. If heat exhaustion is not effectively treated, it may lead to heatstroke, a life-threatening form of heat illness. Heat exhaustion is a *diagnosis of exclusion* when there is no evidence of heatstroke. These patients will need further physical and laboratory evaluation in the ED.

Assessment

Signs and symptoms of heat exhaustion are neither specific nor sensitive. They include fatigue, dizziness, headache, vomiting, malaise, hypotension, and tachycardia. Core body temperatures measure from 101.3°F to 104°F (38.5°C to 40°C).[13] During the acute stage of heat exhaustion, the blood pressure is low, and the pulse and ventilatory rates are rapid. The radial pulse may feel thready. The patient generally appears sweaty, pale, and ashen. The patient's core body temperature may be either normal or slightly elevated but generally is below 104°F (40°C).

It is important to obtain a good history of prior heat illness and the current heat exposure incident because these patients may display signs and symptoms of other conditions of fluid and sodium loss (e.g., hyponatremia; see later discussion). Reassessment is critical because heat exhaustion may progress to heatstroke. Continuously look for any changes in mentation and personality (i.e., confusion, disorientation, irrational or unusual behavior). Any such change should be taken as a progressive sign of hyperthermia indicating heatstroke—*an immediately life-threatening condition!*

Management

Immediately remove the patient from the hot environment (e.g., sun, hot pavement, hot vehicle) to a cooler location either in the shade or air-conditioned space (i.e., ambulance). Place the patient in a recumbent position. Remove clothing and anything restricting heat dissipation, such as a hat or any excess clothing. Assess the patient's heart rate, blood pressure, ventilatory rate, and rectal temperature (if a thermometer is available and conditions permit), and be alert particularly for central nervous system (CNS) status changes as an early indicator of life-threatening heatstroke.

Oral rehydration with electrolytes should be considered for any patient who can take fluids by mouth and who is not at risk of aspirating. Sport drinks are the ideal choice, but the drinks should be diluted to half-strength due to their high sugar content when undiluted. Large amounts of oral fluids may increase bloating, nausea, and vomiting. Normally IV fluids are not needed if blood pressure, pulse, and rectal temperature are normal. However, in patients who are not able to consume fluids by mouth, IV fluids provide rapid recovery from heat exhaustion.[29] If IV fluids are needed, lactated Ringer (LR) solution or NS should be used. IV solutions produce more rapid fluid recovery than do fluids by mouth due to delays in gastric emptying and absorption in the small intestine caused by dehydration.

In exertional heat exhaustion, most exercising patients recover with recumbent rest and oral fluids. Before making any decision regarding IV therapy for these patients, the prehospital care provider needs to conduct a thorough assessment for signs and symptoms of dehydration, *orthostatic* (postural) pulse, blood pressure changes, and the ability to ingest oral fluids. Ongoing mental status changes should prompt further evaluation for heatstroke, hyponatremia, hypoglycemia, and other medical problems. In the exertional heat exhaustion patient, the recommended IV fluids are NS or 5% dextrose in NS for patients who are mildly hypoglycemic. However, providers must exercise caution to ensure that large amounts of IV fluids are not administered to a patient who has been participating in prolonged exercise (greater than 4 hours), especially individuals who do not have obvious clinical signs of dehydration, or in a collapsed athlete with suspected heat exhaustion who has been drinking a large amount of water. This type of patient may have exercise-associated hyponatremia (low serum sodium level), and providing oral and/or IV fluids will cause further *dilutional hyponatremia*, potentially precipitating a life-threatening condition.[50,51] See the discussion on exercise-associated hyponatremia for information on how best to correctly assess the patient for heat-related illness or exercise-associated hyponatremia.

Because heat exhaustion may be difficult to distinguish from heatstroke and because patients with heatstroke should be cooled rapidly to reduce core temperature, the best course of action is to provide some active cooling procedures to all patients with heat exhaustion. Active cooling can be done simply and quickly by wetting the head and upper torso with water or a wet cloth and then fanning or positioning the patient into the wind to increase convective body heat dissipation. Body-cooling procedures will also improve mental status. Rapidly transport all patients who are unconscious, or who do not recover rapidly, as this is a sign of an immediately life-threatening heatstroke condition. Proper environmental temperature control and monitoring of vital signs and mental status are essential during transport.

Heatstroke

Heatstroke is considered the most emergent and life-threatening form of heat illness and is one of the most time-sensitive life-threatening conditions that prehospital care providers encounter. Heatstroke is a form of hyperthermia resulting in failure of the thermoregulatory system—a failure of the body's physiologic systems to dissipate heat and cool down. Heatstroke is characterized by an elevated core temperature of 104°F (40°C) or greater and CNS dysfunction, resulting in delirium, convulsions, or coma.[40,44,52]

The most significant difference in heatstroke compared with heat exhaustion is neurologic disability, which presents to the prehospital care provider as mental status changes. Pathophysiologic changes often result in multiple organ failure.[41,53] These pathophysiologic changes occur when organ tissue temperatures rise above a critical level. Cell membranes are damaged, leading to disruption in cell volume, metabolism, acid–base balance, and membrane permeability that causes cellular and a whole-organ dysfunction with ultimate cell death and organ failure.[29] The degree of complications in patients with heatstroke is not entirely related to the magnitude of core temperature elevation.

This whole-body pathophysiologic dysfunction is the underlying reason for the need for early heatstroke recognition by prehospital care providers. With early recognition, aggressive whole-body cooling to rapidly reduce core temperature and decrease the associated heatstroke morbidity and mortality is possible.

Morbidity and mortality are directly associated with the duration of elevated core temperature, and a positive patient outcome is directly related to how fast the core temperature can be decreased below 102°F (38.9°C). Even with aggressive prehospital intervention and in-hospital management, heatstroke is often fatal, and many patients who survive have permanent neurologic disability.

Heatstroke has two different clinical presentations: classic heatstroke and exertional heatstroke (**Table 19-2**).

Classic heatstroke is a disorder most commonly seen in infants, febrile children, people who are homeless or cannot afford adequate air conditioning, older adults, people with alcoholism, and patients with chronic illnesses. It may be compounded by the risk factors listed in Box 19-3 (e.g., medications). A classic presentation is a patient who is exposed to elevated humidity and high room temperatures over several days without air conditioning, leading to dehydration and high core temperature. Often this patient's sweating mechanism has stopped, known as **anhidrosis**. This is especially common in large cities during summer heat waves, when effective home ventilation is either not possible or not used.[54] Scene assessment will provide information helpful in the identification of classic heatstroke.

Exertional heatstroke (EHS) is a preventable disorder often seen when people who lack the requisite physical

Table 19-2 Classic Versus Exertional Heatstroke		
	Classic	**Exertional**
Patient characteristics	Elderly	Men (15 to 45 years)
Health status	Chronically ill	Healthy
Concurrent activity	Sedentary	Strenuous exercise
Drug use	Diuretics, antidepressants, antihypertensives, anticholinergics, antipsychotics	Usually none
Sweating	May be absent	Usually present
Lactic acidosis	Usually absent; poor prognosis if present	Common
Hyperkalemia	Usually absent	Often present
Hypocalcemia	Uncommon	Frequent
Hypoglycemia	Uncommon	Common
Creatine	Mildly elevated	Greatly elevated
Rhabdomyolysis	Mild	Frequently severe

Source: Modified from Knochel JP, Reed G. Disorders of heat regulation. In: Kleeman CR, Maxwell MH, Narin RG, eds. *Clinical Disorders of Fluid and Electrolyte Metabolism.* New York, NY: McGraw-Hill; 1987.

Box 19-4 Common Causes of Death From Exertional Heatstroke (EHS)

1. *Inaccurate temperature assessment or misdiagnosis.* This is often due to the inability to rule out other similar medical conditions. Oral, axillary, and tympanic temperature measurements may underestimate the degree of temperature elevation; therefore, prehospital care providers should rely only on the rectal temperature to determine the degree of hyperthermia and maintain a high index of suspicion in high-risk patients.
2. *No care or a treatment delay.* Failing to recognize the potential for EHS and delaying the response to provide effective care can have disastrous results.
3. *Inefficient whole-body cooling techniques.* Rapid reduction of core temperature to below 104°F (40°C) within 30 minutes is critical. This goal is recognized as the "golden half-hour" of heatstroke management and is the standard to meet with rapid whole-body cooling.
4. *Immediate transport.* With EHS, it is critical to begin whole-body cooling to reduce the core temperature at the scene and not to transport until this treatment has begun. Cooling should continue during transport with rectal temperature assessment to ensure core temperature drops below 104°F (40°C).

Some of the common reasons that death from EHS may occur are listed in **Box 19-4**.[42-44] The motto to "cool first, transport second" is meant to avoid any delays in initiating the lowering of core temperature.

Assessment

The appearance of signs and symptoms depends on the degree and duration of hyperthermia.[36] Patients with heatstroke typically present with hot, flushed skin. They may or may not be sweating, depending on where they are found and whether they have classic or exertional heatstroke. Blood pressure may be elevated or diminished, and the radial pulse is usually tachycardic and thready; 25% of these patients are hypotensive. The patient's level of consciousness can range from confused to unconscious, and seizure activity may also be present, particularly during cooling.[55] As confirmed in hospitals, rectal temperature may range from 104°F to 116°F (40°C to 46.7°C), but patients can have heatstroke with body temperatures lower than 104°F (40°C).[41,55,56]

The key to distinguishing heatstroke from one of the other heat-related conditions is altered mental status.

fitness or heat acclimatization engage in short-term, strenuous physical activity (e.g., industrial workers, athletes, military recruits, fire fighters, and other public safety personnel) in a hot, humid environment. These conditions can rapidly elevate internal heat production and limit the body's ability to dissipate heat. Almost all EHS patients exhibit sweat-soaked and pale skin at the time of collapse as compared to dry, hot, and flushed skin in the classic heatstroke patient.[29] Even though drinking fluids can slow the rate of dehydration during strenuous activity and reduce the rate at which core temperature rises, hyperthermia and EHS may still occur in the absence of significant dehydration.

With aggressive treatment, no one should die from EHS if prompt care begins within 10 minutes of collapse.

Temperature is usually elevated and often is quite high. Any patient who is warm to the touch with an altered mental status (confused, disoriented, combative, or unconscious) should be presumed to have heatstroke and managed immediately and aggressively to reduce core temperature.

Management

Heatstroke is a true time-sensitive emergency. Immediately remove the patient from the source of heat. Cooling the patient should begin immediately in the field by one prehospital care provider while another provider assesses and stabilizes the patient's ABCs. Cooling of the patient begins immediately with whatever means are available (e.g., garden hose, bottled water, IV saline liter bags), even before removing clothing. Application of ice and cold-water immersion are the fastest two methods of cooling, but these approaches may be limited in the prehospital setting.[43,57-59]

Since the late 1950s, it has been thought that cold- or ice-water immersion will cause vasoconstriction sufficient to decrease heat loss from the body and cause the onset of shivering so that internal heat is produced, thus limiting the exchange of heat. Current empirical evidence refutes the concern that cooling rates in these patients would be blunted. Therefore, this form of cooling, if available, should not be withheld from a patient with heatstroke.[47] Many protocols and curricula recommend that temperature not be actively dropped below 102°F (40°C) to avoid rebound shivering (increasing body temperature) or "overshoot" or "afterdrop," causing the patient to become hypothermic.[46,59] However, the evidence-based Wilderness Medical Society practice guidelines for hyperthermia management note that there is no evidence to support a risk of either of these theoretical concerns and imply that normal body temperature is a reasonable goal.[27]

If cold water and ice are not immediately available, remove the patient's excess clothing, wet down the patient from head to toe, and provide continuous fanning of the skin. It is essential that this procedure begin immediately and not be delayed before preparing to transport the patient from the scene to the ambulance. Patient wetting and fanning are the next most effective cooling techniques, causing evaporation and convective heat loss.[57] Individuals who rapidly become lucid during whole-body cooling usually have the best prognosis. The most important intervention prehospital care providers can deliver to a patient with heatstroke (along with management of ABCs) is immediate and rapid whole-body cooling to reduce core temperature.

During transport, the patient should be placed in a prepared, air-conditioned ambulance. It is an error to place a patient with heatstroke into a hot internal cabin of an ambulance, even if transfer time to the hospital is short. Remove any additional clothing, cover the patient with a sheet, and wet down the sheet with irrigation fluids along with providing continuous fanning, ideally by powered fans from the cabin overhead. Ice packs, if available and time allows, can be placed in the groin area, in the axillae, and around the anterior-lateral neck because blood vessels are closest to the skin surface in these areas. The widespread recommendation of using ice packs alone is a much less effective core cooling technique. Ice packs alone are insufficient to rapidly lower core body temperature unless they cover the entire body and should be considered only as an extra cooling method and not a priority in patient care.[4,27,55,57]

If possible, the patient's rectal temperature should be measured every 5 to 10 minutes during transport to ensure effective cooling. Other means to assess the patient's temperature (e.g., oral, skin, axillary) should not be used for treatment decisions because they do not adequately reflect the patient's core temperature.[29]

Provide high-flow oxygen, support ventilations with a bag-mask device as needed, and monitor the patient's cardiac rhythm.

Patients with heatstroke generally do not require extensive fluid resuscitation and typically are initially given IV fluids consisting of 1.0 to 1.5 liters of NS. Provide a 500-ml fluid challenge and assess vital signs. Fluid volume should not exceed 1 to 2 liters in the first hour, or follow local medical protocol. Monitor blood glucose because these patients are frequently hypoglycemic and may require a bolus of 50% dextrose IV. Seizures can be managed with 5 to 10 milligrams (mg) of diazepam or other benzodiazepines as per local protocol. Transport the patient in a right or left lateral recumbent position to maintain an open airway and to avoid aspiration.

Exercise-Associated Hyponatremia

Exercise-associated hyponatremia (EAH), also known as water intoxication, is a life-threatening condition that has been increasingly described after prolonged physical exertion in recreational hikers, climbers, marathoners, ultra-marathoners, triathletes, adventure racers, and military infantry personnel.[49,60-64] With the increasing popularity of these outdoor activities, the incidence of mild to severe EAH has steadily increased since it was first reported in the mid-1980s.[63] It is now known to be one of the most severe medical complications of endurance activities and is an important cause of event-related fatalities.[50,51]

EAH is commonly associated with excessive consumption of water (1.5 quarts [qt; 1.4 liters] or greater per hour) during prolonged activities.[64] Two major pathogenic mechanisms largely account for the development of EAH: (1) excessive fluid intake and (2) impaired urinary water excretion due largely to persistent secretion of *arginine vasopressin (AVP)*, also referred to as antidiuretic hormone (ADH).[50,51] EAH can take two forms, mild or severe, depending on presenting symptoms.

In the severe form, low plasma sodium concentration disturbs the osmotic balance across the blood–brain barrier, resulting in the rapid influx of water into the brain, which causes cerebral edema.[49-51,63,64] In similar fashion to the signs and symptoms of increased intracranial pressure in head trauma (see the Head Trauma chapter), a progression of neurologic symptoms from hyponatremia will occur, including headache, vomiting, malaise, confusion, and seizures, progressing to coma, permanent brain damage, brain stem herniation, and death.[50,51,63] These individuals are said to have **exercise-associated hyponatremic encephalopathy (EAHE)**.[50,51,63]

Symptomatic EAHE patients generally have a serum sodium concentration below 126 milliequivalents (mEq)/liter (normal range, 135 to 145 mEq/liter) with rapidly developing (less than 48 hours) hyponatremia, as seen frequently in prolonged endurance activities.[50,51,60,64] Alternatively, the milder form of EAH generally presents with isolated serum sodium levels of 135 to 128 mEq/liter, without easily discernable symptoms (i.e., weakness, nausea/vomiting, headache, or no symptoms), and is self-limiting with rest, food, and electrolyte fluids. Even with the initial presenting mild signs and symptoms of EAH, a patient can progress into EAHE. It has been suggested that there is an acute drop in serum sodium concentration at the end of an endurance event caused by the absorption of water retained in the GI tract.[50,51] This may account for a transient lucid period after finishing an endurance activity followed by the acute development of clinic signs of EAHE within about 30 minutes following the cessation of the activity.

Studies have reported that 18% to 23% of ultramarathoners and 29% of the Hawaiian Ironman Triathlete finishers had EAH.[46,53-68] In 2003, 32 cases of EAH were reported in hikers in the Grand Canyon National Park (GCNP), and 19% of all nonfatal heat-related incidents in GCNP from 2004 to 2009 were attributed to hyponatremia.[69-71]

EAH can occur in the following situations:

1. Excessive sodium and water loss in sweat throughout an endurance event, resulting in dehydration and sodium depletion
2. Overhydration solely with water while maintaining plasma sodium, creating a dilution of sodium concentration
3. Combination of excessive sodium and fluid loss in sweat and an excessive overhydration with water only

The evidence indicates that EAH is a result of fluid retention in the extracellular space (*dilutional*) rather than fluid remaining unabsorbed in the intestine.[60] Typically, these patients have not consumed sport electrolyte drinks, have consumed energy food supplements containing no salt, or have consumed salt in insufficient quantity to balance the loss of sodium in sweat or the dilution from excessive water intake.

The following are a few key risk factors that have been linked to the development of EAH[42,43,49,72]:

1. Activity or exercise duration (greater than 4 hours) or slow running/exercise pace
2. Female gender (may be explained by lower body weight)
3. Low or high body mass index
4. Excessive drinking (greater than 1.5 liters/hour) during an event or activity
5. Use of nonsteroidal anti-inflammatory drugs, which decrease renal filtration

EAH has been described as the "other heat-related illness" because the symptoms are nonspecific and are similar to those exhibited in minor and major heat-related disorders.[69] Many endurance events and multiday adventure activities are conducted in warm to hot environments; therefore, it is assumed that the signs and symptoms of EAH are some form of heat illness, and patients are managed with standard protocols that address the presumed hypovolemia and excessive body heat. Standard protocols that provide body cooling and IV fluid challenge to correct hyperthermia, sweat-induced dehydration, and mental status changes can complicate the dilutional hyponatremia and place the patient at further risk for seizure and coma. Treating a patient with EAH with fluids and rest will worsen the patient's condition, unlike the heat exhaustion patient.

This "other heat-related disorder" is becoming more widely recognized and correctly treated today by EMS and ED personnel, largely because of an increased effort to educate medical personnel and the public in its prevention, early recognition, and management (**Box 19-5**). Prehospital care providers directly supporting or responding to calls at physical endurance events in urban or wilderness settings need to be aware that EAH is more frequently reported today. It is important to remember that, in general, dehydration is more common in prolonged exertional activities and that it can lead to impaired performance during exercise or work-related tasks and to serious heat illness; however, symptomatic hyponatremia brought on by overdrinking is more dangerous and potentially a life-threatening illness.[72] This distinction illustrates a tension in hydration strategies: Waiting for thirst as an indicator to hydrate may predispose individuals to mild dehydration, while set regimens for hydration regardless of thirst risk may predispose individuals to overhydration

---

Box 19-5 Guidelines for Managing EAH and EAHE

Recently, the Wilderness Medical Society published practice guidelines for managing EAH and EAHE, with an emphasis on how patients competing in endurance events should be managed in the prehospital environment by a medical director and staff or by responding EMS personnel.[49,56,73]

and EAH. See the Hydration section later in this chapter for further discussion of this issue.

Assessment

A wide range of signs and symptoms may be found in the endurance-athlete population with hyponatremia (see Table 19-1). Core temperature is usually normal but can be low or slightly elevated, depending on the ambient temperature, body heat dissipation, and recent exercise intensity at assessment. Heart rate and blood pressure can be low, normal, or elevated, depending on core temperature, exercise intensity, hypovolemia, or shock. Ventilatory rate ranges from within normal limits to slightly elevated. Hyperventilation observed with EAH can account for vision

disturbances, dizziness, tingling in hands, and paresthesias in the extremities. The hallmark assessment and findings are mental status changes, fatigue, malaise, headache, and nausea. Other forms of neurologic changes include slowed speech, ataxia, and cognitive changes, including irrational behavior, combativeness, and fear. These patients often report that they have a sense of "impending doom."

Management

The first step in treatment is recognizing the disorder and determining the severity. Management is based on the severity of EAH and what portable diagnostic tools are available to measure serum sodium.[73] **Figure 19-4** provides an algorithm for assessing patients to determine whether

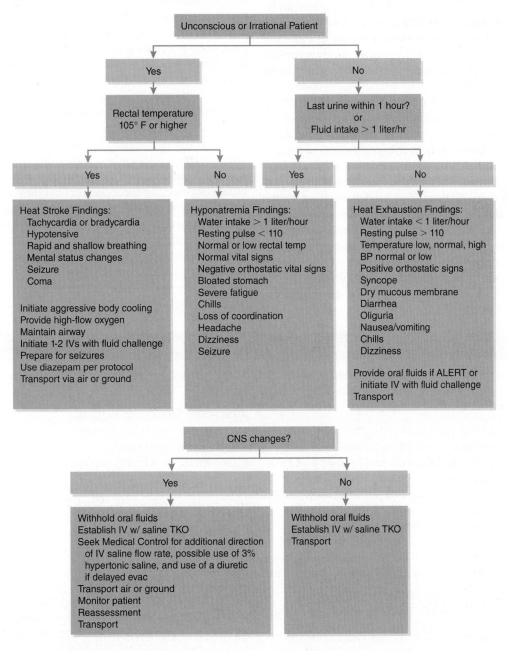

Figure 19-4 Treatment algorithm for heat exhaustion, heatstroke, and hyponatremia.
© National Association of Emergency Medical Technicians (NAEMT).

EAH or a heat-related illness is present. Mild symptoms should be managed conservatively by observing the patient to ensure no further progression to EAHE and waiting for normal diuresis of excessive fluid.

Place symptomatic patients in an upright position to maintain their airway and to minimize any positional effect on intracranial pressure. These patients are known to have projectile vomiting when transported. Place unconscious patients in the left lateral recumbent position, anticipate vomiting, and consider active airway management. Provide high-flow oxygen, establish IV access at the keep vein open (KVO) rate, and monitor for seizures.

As needed, administer anticonvulsant therapy (e.g., titrate benzodiazepines IV, per medical protocol). Check with medical control for volume of NS fluid, if any, to be administered, depending on patient severity and transport time to the hospital. Because these patients are already fluid overloaded, infusion of IV hypotonic fluids is contra-indicated, as this can worsen the degree of hyponatremia and fluid overload.[74]

Patients with extensive signs and symptoms of EAHE (i.e., cerebral edema and pulmonary edema) need to have their plasma sodium concentration increased. The current consensus for management in the prehospital setting is to provide a 100-ml bolus infusion of 3% hypertonic saline over 10 minutes to acutely reduce brain edema. Each dose will raise sodium by 2 to 3 mEq/liter, if this solution is available.[56,74] If no clinical improvement is noted, up to two additional 100-ml, 3% bolus infusions can be given per medical protocol.[73,74] These severe cases of EAHE have a poor outcome if patients do not receive hypertonic saline.[75] Keep the patient calm while en route to the ED, and continue to monitor for mental status changes or seizures.

Prevention of Heat-Related Illness

Because heat stress is a significant public health factor in the United States, methods for preventing heat illness are vital to any community, particularly for those individuals who must work in high-heat occupational settings. For example, from 2006 to 2015, a total of 1,000 fire fighters (including volunteer, career, and wildland fire fighters) were killed in the line of duty in the United States,[76] for a yearly average of 100 fire fighter deaths. In 2015, 90 fire fighters were killed in the line of duty, with 60 (66.7%) deaths occurring at the scene due to stress or overexertion; heat illness is included as a cause of death in this category.[76]

Prehospital care providers and their EMS agencies are a good resource as partners for community education on heat stress prevention strategies in many different formats, including workshops, educational handouts, agency website or newsletter, community presentations, and local newspaper.

As with the general public, heat-related illness in prehospital care providers represents an occupational risk; therefore, EMS and other public safety personnel need to use prevention strategies and prepare for exposure to high ambient temperature when appropriate and relevant. These strategies, which include administrative policies, proce-dures, engineering controls, use of equipment, and medical surveillance programs, are designed to help minimize the overall impact from acute or chronic heat exposure. The implementation of simple preventive procedures can have a dramatic impact on lowering the incidence of heat illness. **Box 19-6** provides an overview of heat stress prevention strategies for prehospital care providers, fire fighters, and other public safety personnel.[77]

Box 19-6 Prevention of Heat-Related Disorders in Prehospital Care Providers

You can prevent the serious consequences of heat disorders by improving your level of fitness and becoming acclimated to the heat.

Maintaining a high level of aerobic fitness is one of the best ways to protect yourself against heat stress. The fit prehospital care provider has a well-developed circulatory system and increased blood volume. Both are important to regulate body temperature. Fit providers start to sweat sooner, so they work with a lower heart rate and body temperature. They adjust to the heat twice as fast as unfit providers. They lose acclimatization more slowly and regain it quickly.

The time required for heat acclimatization varies depending on timing and frequency of exposure, and it has been shown to occur within 10 to 14 days of heat exposure as the body changes in the following ways[13,78-80]:

- Increases sweat production
- Improves blood distribution
- Decreases heart rate
- Lowers skin and body temperatures

As a prehospital care provider, you can acclimatize by gradually increasing work time in the heat, taking care to replace fluids, and resting as needed. Acclimatization is maintained with periodic work or exercise in a hot environment.

On the Job
The heat stress index (see Figure 19-5) illustrates how temperature and humidity combine to create moderate-heat or high-heat stress conditions. Be alert for heat stress when radiant heat from the sun or nearby

flames is high, when the air is still, or when working hard and therefore creating large amounts of metabolic heat. The heat stress index does not consider the effects of long hours of hard work, dehydration, or the impact of personal protective clothing and equipment.

When heat stress conditions exist, you must modify the way you work or exercise. Pace yourself. There are individual differences in fitness, acclimatization, and heat tolerance. Push too hard and you will become a candidate for a heat-related illness.

When possible, you should do the following:

- Avoid working close to heat sources.
- Do harder work during cooler morning and evening hours.
- Change tools or tasks to minimize fatigue.
- Take frequent rest breaks.
- Most important, maintain hydration by replacing lost fluids.

Hydration

Maintaining body fluids is essential for sweating and the removal of internal heat generated during physical activities. To minimize dehydration and the risk of heat illness, you must hydrate before, during, and after exercise or physical work. The Wilderness Medical Society now recommends *ad libitum* (drink to thirst) fluid intake to ensure proper hydration while preventing excessive fluid intake and onset of EAH. Prehospital care providers must monitor their own level of thirst throughout the day and drink fluids in an amount necessary to prevent a loss of body weight greater than 2%.[49,56] Individual characteristics (e.g., body weight, genetic predisposition, heat acclimatization state, and metabolic state) will influence sweat rate for a given activity. These factors will result in large individual sweat rates and total sweat loss. For example, long-distance running is known to cause an average sweat rate of 1.5 to 2 qt (1.4 to 1.9 liters) per hour in summer months, whereas football players (large body mass and wearing protective gear) are known to sweat on average over 2 qt (1.9 liters) per hour and up to 9 qt (8.5 liters) per day.[60] A commitment to frequent hydration breaks is required to ensure dehydration does not exceed greater than 2% of body weight (based on preactivity nude body weight) throughout the duration of physical activity.

Before work, you should take extra fluids to prepare for the heat. Drink 8 to 16 oz (0.2 to 0.5 liters) of water, juice, or a sport drink before work. Avoid excess caffeine; it hastens fluid loss in the urine. There is no physiologic advantage to excessively consuming large amounts of fluid prior to physical activity. The American College of Sports Medicine now recommends prehydrating slowly for several hours before a physical activity and consuming 0.16 to 0.24 oz (approximately 5 to 7 ml) per kg of body weight.[35] The goal is to produce urine output that is clear to straw color in appearance and prevent starting an activity in a dehydrated state.

While working, take several fluid breaks every hour based on recognition of thirst. Individual sweat rates will vary, as will the amount of water needed to be consumed per hour. Caution should be used to prevent consumption of excessive fluids greater than 1.5 qt/hour (1.4 liters/hour) for prolonged periods unless you have determined your individualized sweat loss rate per hour. The American College of Sports Medicine now recommends a starting point of 14 to 28 oz (0.4 to 0.8 liters) on average per hour for exercise activities (e.g., marathon running) and adjusting the amount consumed based on individual lower or higher sweat rates for activities in cool or warm temperature conditions and for lighter or heavier individuals.[60]

Water is the body's greatest need during work in the heat. Studies show that workers drink more when lightly flavored beverages are available. Providing a portion of fluid replacement with a carbohydrate/electrolyte sport beverage will help to retain fluids and maintain energy and electrolyte levels. Unfortunately, many sport drinks contain large amounts of sugar, which can actually slow absorption of ingested fluid.

After work, you need to continue drinking to replace fluid losses. To achieve rapid and complete recovery for activities resulting is large sweat loss (i.e., firefighting), drink approximately 24 oz for each pound of body weight loss (1.5 liters for each kilogram of body weight loss).[60] Rehydration is enhanced when fluids contain sodium and potassium or when foods with these electrolytes are consumed along with the fluid.

Make potassium-rich foods such as potatoes, prune juice, carrot juice, bananas, and citrus fruits a regular part of your diet, and vary your intake of fluids to include lemonade, orange juice, or tomato juice. Limit the amount of caffeine drinks such as coffee and colas because caffeine increases fluid loss in the urine, although moderate amounts have no negative effect.[49] Avoid alcoholic drinks because they also cause dehydration. To avoid common viruses, avoid sharing water bottles except in emergencies.

Hydration can be reassessed by observing your urine's volume, color, and concentration. Low volumes of dark,

(continued)

Box 19-6 Prevention of Heat-Related Disorders in Prehospital Care Providers (*continued*)

concentrated urine and painful urination indicate a serious need for rehydration. Other signs of dehydration include a rapid heart rate, weakness, excessive fatigue, and dizziness. Rapid loss of several pounds of body weight is a certain sign of dehydration. Rehydrate before returning to work. Continuing to work in a dehydrated state can lead to serious consequences, including heatstroke, muscle breakdown, and kidney failure.

Clothing
Personal protective clothing strikes a balance between protection and comfort. Australian researchers have concluded that the task for personnel wearing personal protective equipment (PPE) is not to keep heat out, but to let it out. About 70% of the heat load comes from within, from metabolic heat generated during hard work. Only 30% comes from the environment. Wear loose-fitting garments to enhance air movement. Wear cotton T-shirts and underwear to help sweat evaporate in hot environments. Avoid extra layers of clothing that insulate, restrict air movement, and contribute to heat stress.

Individual Differences
Individuals differ in their response to heat. Some emergency responders, such as fire fighters, are at greater risk for heat disorders due to their environment and gear requirements. Other reasons include inherited differences in heat tolerance and sweat rate; excess body weight, which raises metabolic heat production; and illness, illicit drugs, and medications, which can also influence the body's response to work in a hot environment. Check with your physician or pharmacist if you are using prescription or over-the-counter medications, or if you have a medical condition.

You should always train and work with a partner who can help in the event of a problem. Remind each

other to drink fluids, and watch each other. If your partner develops a heat disorder, begin treatment immediately.

Summary
Prevention
- Improve or maintain aerobic fitness.
- Acclimate to the heat.

On the job
- Be aware of conditions (temperature, humidity, air movement).
- Take frequent rest breaks and drink fluids regularly to relieve thirst.
- Avoid extra layers of clothing.
- Maintain a steady pace.

Hydrate
- The hydration goal is to prevent dehydration (sweat loss) of greater than 2% of nude body weight.
- Before work, drink several cups of water, juice, or a sport drink.
- During work, take frequent fluid breaks.
- After work, keep drinking to ensure rehydration.
- Remember, "Only you can prevent dehydration."

Partners
- Always work or train with a partner.

Drinks
- Sport drinks with carbohydrates (5% to 10%) and electrolytes (e.g., sodium 20 to 30 mEq/liter and potassium 2 to 5 mEq/liter) encourage fluid intake, provide energy, and diminish urinary water loss. The carbohydrates also help maintain immune function and mental performance during prolonged, arduous work. Drinks with caffeine and alcohol interfere with rehydration by increasing urine production.

Modified from U.S. Department of Agriculture, US Forest Service: Heat stress brochure, http://www.fs.usda.gov/fire/safety/fitness/heat_stress/hs_pg1.html. See also: American College of Sports Medicine Position Stand: Exercise and Fluid Replacement. *Med Sci Sports Exerc.* 39(2):377, 2007.

A complex interaction of factors that combine to exceed the tolerance limits for individual heat exposure can eventually lead to the onset of signs and symptoms of heat-related illness. The capacity of humans to work in moderate to hot environments can be maximized through advanced preparation of physical fitness, heat acclimatization, living and working conditions, personal hygiene, and use of food and beverages to maintain and replace electrolytes and water in the body. Environment, fluid

hydration, physical fitness, and heat acclimatization are essential factors to understand.

Environment

Prehospital care providers and other public safety personnel are subjected to high heat environments as part of their occupational requirements. During training or an emergency response, many personnel will encounter high levels of heat

Temperature (°F) versus Relative Humidity (%)

°F	90%	80%	70%	60%	50%	40%
80	85	84	82	81	80	79
85	101	96	92	90	86	84
90	121	113	105	99	94	90
95		133	122	113	105	98
100			142	129	118	109
105				148	133	121
110						135

High	Possible Heat Disorder
80°F - 90°F	Fatigue possible with prolonged exposure and physical activity.
90°F - 105°F	Sunstroke, heat cramps, and heat exhaustion possible.
105°F - 130°F	Sunstroke, heat cramps, and heat exhaustion likely, and heat stroke possible.
130°F or greater	Heat stroke highly likely with continued exposure.

Due to the nature of the heat index calculation, the values in the tables have an error +/− 1.3° F.

Figure 19-5 Heat stress index.

Courtesy of the National Weather Service, Pueblo, Colorado (http://www.crh.noaa.gov/pub/heat.htm).

stress while working in PPE (impermeable clothing), such as turnout gear, hazardous material suit, or chemical/biologic protective garment. This heat stress is further compounded by the need to enter poorly ventilated or confined spaces or to work on a multivehicle crash in the sun on a hot, humid day.

PPE compromises the body's ability to dissipate body heat and prevents the evaporation of sweat during a heavy workload. With high sweat rates from internal heat production during physically demanding tasks and the external heat exposure, personnel are at a high risk of dehydration and heat illness. Thus, the use of PPE diminishes the physiologic advantage gained through heat acclimatization and physical fitness.

These risks can be minimized by measuring the environmental heat conditions and, when applicable, following the recommended work/rest and hydration guidelines for work in highly thermal environments.[24,81]

One traditional tool for measuring the thermal load is the **heat stress index** (**Figure 19-5**). This index uses the combination of ambient temperature (read on a thermometer) and relative humidity. This is a better method of predicting potential systemic heat injury than the ambient temperature alone. If working in direct sunlight, near surfaces that radiate large amounts of heat, or in heavy protective clothing, 10°F (~5.5°C) should be added to the value in the table.

A more widely used method for measurement of environmental heat strain used in many industrial and military settings is the *wet-bulb globe temperature (WBGT) index*[24,82] (**Table 19-3**). This index uses the combination of a dry bulb for ambient temperature, wet bulb for humidity measurement, black globe for radiant heat, and air movement to provide a more accurate impact of the environmental conditions. Integrated in the five-level WBGT index range of temperatures are hourly work/rest (minutes) and hydration (quarts) guidelines. A color flag (no flag, green, yellow, red, or black) represents each of the five WBGT ranges of temperatures. The WBGT can be monitored hourly and the corresponding color flag placed on a flagpole outdoors for all personnel to see throughout the day. When applicable, the appropriate adjustments of clothing, physical activity, work/rest cycles, and fluid intake can then be made based on these WBGT conditions. This integrated WBGT system and related policies can easily be developed at various public safety locations and training sites to ensure that effective heat illness prevention programs are in use to reduce fatigue, injuries, and heat illness.

Hydration

If the WBGT flag system is not used to provide guidelines for hydration, another excellent resource is published by the American College of Sports Medicine, based on years of research.[72] These guidelines are easily applied to any individual engaged in physical activity. Hydration guidelines should be established within an agency to prevent excessive dehydration (greater than 2% body weight loss) by creating easy access to water and sport electrolyte drinks, particularly during activity in warm environments and when the individual feels thirsty (**Box 19-7**). Ideally, fluid-replacement programs should be customized based on individualized sweat rate loss, body mass, and exercise intensity as determined from a pre- or post-physical activity nude body weight loss measurement.

Table 19-3 Fluid Replacement Guidelines for Warm-Weather Training

Heat Category	WBGT Index (°F)	Easy Work		Moderate Work		Hard Work	
		Work/Rest (minutes)	Water Intake (qt/hour)	Work/Rest (minutes)	Water Intake (qt/hour)	Work/Rest (minutes)	Water Intake (qt/hour)
1	78 to 81.9	NL	1/2	NL	3/4	40/20	3/4
2	82 to 84.9	NL	1/2	50/10	3/4	30/30	1
3	85 to 87.9	NL	3/4	40/20	3/4	30/30	1
4	88 to 89.9	NL	3/4	30/30	3/4	20/40	1
5	> 90	50/10	1	20/40	1	10/50	1

		Easy Work	Moderate Work	Hard Work
		Walking on hard surface at 2.5 miles/hour (mph; 4 kilometers/hour [kph]), less than 31-lb (14 kg) load	Walking on hard surface at 3.5 mph (5 kph), less than 40-lb (19 kg) load Walking in loose sand at 2.5 mph (4 kph), no load; calisthenics	Walking on hard surface at 3.5 mph (6 kph), greater than 40-lb (18 kg) load Walking in loose sand at 2.5 mph (4 kph) with load

Note: lb, pound; mph, miles per hour; NL, no limit to work time; WBGT, wet-bulb globe temperature.

The work/rest times and fluid replacement volumes will sustain performance and hydration for at least 4 hours of work in the specified heat category. Individual water needs will vary. Rest means minimal physical activity (sitting or standing), accomplished in shade if possible.

Caution: Hourly fluid intake should not exceed 1.5 qt (1.4 liters). Daily fluid intake should not exceed 12 qt (11.4 liters). When wearing body armor: Add 5°F (~2.75°C) to WBGT index in humid climates. When wearing PPE over garment: Add 10°F (~5.5°C) to WBGT index for easy work and 20°F (~11°C) for moderate and hard work.

Current version of WBGT, hydration, and work/rest guidelines as updated by U.S. Army Research Institute for Environmental Medicine (USARIEM) and published by Montain SJ, Latzka WA, Sawka MN: *Mil Med.* 164:502, 1999.

Fitness

To increase heat tolerance effectively in high-heat conditions, prehospital care providers should increase their aerobic fitness through individualized programs (e.g., walking, jogging, biking, swimming, stair stepping, using elliptical exercise machines).[82] These programs will provide the cardiac reserve to sustain the cardiac output required to meet the competing demands of physical (muscular) work and heat dissipation mechanisms (thermoregulation) in a high-temperature environment.[83,84] The American College of Sports Medicine, American Heart Association, and Department of Health and Human Services have collaborated to establish updated nationwide physical activity recommendations to maintain health and well-being.[84]

Heat Acclimatization

A policy and protocol for heat acclimatization should be provided within a public safety organization.[85] Heat acclimatization can be achieved with 60 to 120 minutes of heat-exposed exertion per day for approximately 8 to 14 days.[35,49,86] The benefits of heat acclimatization are increased work performance, heat tolerance, and reduced physiologic strain. These adjustments include increased blood volume, increased stroke volume, decreased heart rate at a given activity level, reduced sodium concentration in sweat, sodium conserved in the body, earlier onset of sweating, and increased sweat volume rate (**Box 19-8**). These changes improve the transfer of body heat from the core to the skin in an effort to increase the heat transfer from the skin to the environment. Although heat tolerance is

Box 19-7 Hydration Guidelines to Minimize Dehydration

General Principles

It is important to maintain hydration, especially when exercising or performing activities that involve heavy physical exertion. A person's hydration needs will differ depending on how heavily the person sweats. General principles to remember include:

1. Drink before and during exertion and when thirsty.
2. Use water and electrolyte drinks to replace lost fluids.
3. Note your weight before and after exertion to help track whether your fluid intake is sufficient, deficient, or excessive.

Make sure you drink sufficiently even when not exercising. If you postpone drinking during your regular day, your body may dehydrate more quickly once you exert yourself.

Weight

Weight is a factor used to determine hydration (or dehydration). It is important to replace fluid lost during physical exertion. If a person does not replace this fluid, he or she will weigh less after exertion. Conversely, if a person drinks excessive amounts during physical exertion, he or she may gain weight due to the fluid intake. Ideally, a person will weigh approximately the same before and after exercise; this indicates that the person maintained the appropriate fluid level.

When you do not drink enough during exertion, be sure to replenish fluids afterward. Do not use dehydration as a weight-loss technique.

Type of Drink

In addition to remembering to drink sufficient amounts, it is important to know what type of fluid to drink. Drinking only water during heavy exertion can lead to electrolyte imbalance. Sport electrolyte drinks are designed to replace electrolytes lost through sweat. However, most commercial sport drinks have excessive carbohydrates; oral hydration solutions should not have more than 6% carbohydrate content.[56] During exercise, stay alert for swelling of the hands and feet, headache, and bloating, which could indicate hyponatremia.

In addition, if you are an athlete or work in a profession that requires heavy exertion, include a moderate amount of salt in your diet to help fulfill your body's increased need for sodium chloride.

Fluid Intake Recommendations

Recommendations for replacing fluid (with water and sport electrolyte drinks) are as follows (**Table 19-4**):

Table 19-4 Fluid Intake Recommendations

Time Frame	Quantity
4 hours before exercise	16–20 oz (0.5–0.6 liters)
10–15 minutes before exercise	8–12 oz (0.2–0.4 liters)
During exercise for less than 60 minutes	3–8 oz (0.1–0.2 liters) every 15–20 minutes
During exercise for greater than 60 minutes	3–8 oz (0.1–0.2 liters) of a sport beverage every 15–20 minutes
Post exercise (within 2 hours)	20–24 oz (0.6–0.7 liters) every 1 lb (0.5 kg) lost

Source: Data from American College of Sports Medicine. Selecting and Effectively Using Hydration for Fitness. https://www.acsm.org/docs/brochures/selecting-and-effectively-using-hydration-for-fitness.pdf. Accessed April 10, 2018.

improved in these individuals (e.g., endurance athletes, military infantry personnel) and is considered desirable, the greater sweat-volume production 1.1 to 2.1 qt/hour (1 to 2 liters/hour) results in large fluid losses, leading to dehydration. Consequently, the greater volume of sweat loss in heat-acclimatized individuals increases the hydration requirements during heat exposure, particularly when the person does not adhere to a rigorous oral hydration schedule. **Box 19-9** provides an overview of heat acclimatization guidelines.

Box 19-8 Benefits of Heat Acclimatization

1. Thermal comfort: improved
2. Core temperature: reduced
3. Skin blood flow: earlier
4. Heart rate: lowered
5. Salt losses (sweat and urine): reduced
6. Exercise performance: improved
7. Sweating: earlier and greater
8. Body heat production: lower
9. Thirst: improved
10. Organ protection: improved

From the Heat Acclimatization Guide, Ranger and Airborne School Students, 2003, www.usariem.army.mil/ download/heatacclimatizationguide.pdf.

Emergency Incident Rehabilitation

Even when taking appropriate precautions (e.g., hydration, heat acclimatization) while working in extremely hot settings, EMS practitioners will sometimes be pushed to their physical limits. Fire fighters, in particular, may wear a wide range of PPE, depending on the capacity in which they are working. This PPE is often heavy and restrictive and can add greatly to the heat stress experienced on scene.[87] Rehabilitation must occur before the point of overexertion, not after.

Rehabilitation involves the following principles[87]:

*   Relief from extreme climatic conditions
*   Rest and recovery

Box 19-9 Heat Acclimatization Guidelines

The following is a modified version of the heat acclimatization guidelines designed for healthy and physically fit infantry personnel in preparation for physical activity in hot environments.

Should You Be Concerned About Hot Weather?
If you are used to working in cool or temperate climates, exposure to hot weather will make it much more difficult to complete your work. Hot weather will make you feel fatigued, make it more difficult to recover, and increase your risk of heat illness. Individuals with the same abilities but who are used to working in hot weather will have a greater heat tolerance and physical ability during heat exposure.

What Is Heat Acclimatization?
Heat acclimatization refers to biologic adaptations that reduce physiologic strain (e.g., heart rate, body temperature), improve physical work capabilities, improve comfort, and protect vital organs (brain, liver, kidneys, muscles) from heat injury. The most important biologic adaptation from heat acclimatization is an earlier and greater sweating response, and for this response to improve, it needs to be invoked.

Heat acclimatization is specific to the climate and physical activity level. Individuals who perform only light or brief physical work will achieve the level of heat acclimatization needed to perform that task. If they attempt a more strenuous or prolonged task, additional acclimatization and improved physical fitness will be needed to perform that task successfully in the heat.

How Do You Become Heat Acclimatized?
Heat acclimatization occurs when repeated heat exposures are sufficiently stressful to elevate body temperature and provoke profuse sweating. Resting in the heat, with physical activity limited to that required for existence, results in only partial acclimatization. Physical exercise in the heat is required to achieve optimal heat acclimatization for that exercise intensity in a given hot environment.

Generally, about 8 to 14 days of daily heat exposure is needed to induce heat acclimatization. Heat acclimatization requires a minimum daily heat exposure of 1 to 2 hours (can be broken into two 1-hour exposures) combined with physical exercise that requires cardiovascular endurance (e.g., jogging) rather than strength training. Gradually increase the exercise intensity or duration each day. Work up to an appropriate physical training schedule adapted to the required physical activity.

The benefits of heat acclimatization will be retained for about 1 week and then decay, with about 75% lost by about 3 weeks, once heat exposure ends. One or 2 days of intervening cool weather will not interfere with acclimatization to hot weather.

How Quickly Can You Become Heat Acclimatized?
For the average individual, heat acclimatization requires about 8 to 14 days of heat exposure and progressive increases in physical work. By the second day of acclimatization, significant reductions in physiologic strain are observed. By the end of the first week and second week, greater than 60% and greater than 80% of the physiologic

adaptations are complete, respectively. Less fit individuals or those unusually susceptible to heat exposure may require several additional days or weeks to fully acclimatize.

Physically fit individuals should be able to achieve heat acclimatization in about 1 week. However, several weeks of living and working in the heat (seasoning) may be required to maximize tolerance to high body temperatures.

What Are the Best Heat Acclimatization Strategies?

1. Maximize physical fitness and heat acclimatization before hot weather exposure. Maintain physical fitness with maintenance programs tailored to the environment, such as physical training in the cooler morning or evening hours.
2. Integrate training and heat acclimatization. Train in the coolest part of the day, and acclimatize in the heat of the day. Start slowly by reducing your usual training intensity and duration (compared to what you could achieve in temperate climates). Increase training and heat exposure volume as your heat tolerance permits. Use interval training to modify your activity level.
3. If the new climate is much hotter than what you are accustomed to, recreational activities may be appropriate for the first 2 days with periods of run/walk. By the third day, you should be able to integrate training runs (20 to 40 minutes) at a reduced pace.
4. Consume sufficient water to replace sweat losses. Sweat rates of more than 1 qt (0.9 liter) per hour are common. Heat acclimatization increases the sweating rate and, therefore, increases water requirements. As a result, heat-acclimatized individuals will dehydrate faster if they do not consume fluids. Dehydration negates many of the thermoregulatory advantages conferred by heat acclimatization and high physical fitness.

Source: Sawka MN, Kolka MA, Montain SJ. *Ranger and Airborne School Students' Heat Acclimatization Guide.* Natick, MA: U.S. Army Research Institute of Environmental Medicine; 2003.

- Cooling or rewarming (as needed)
- Rehydration (fluid replacement)
- Calorie and electrolyte replacement
- Medical monitoring
- Tracking team members (accountability)

Injuries Produced by Cold

Dehydration

Dehydration occurs very easily in the cold, particularly with increased physical activity. This occurs for three primary reasons:

- Evaporation of sweat
- Increased respiratory heat and fluid losses caused by the dryness of cold air
- Cold-induced diuresis

Cold-induced diuresis is a normal physiologic response resulting from skin vasoconstriction from prolonged cold exposure. This is the body's response to reduce body heat loss by shunting blood away from the colder periphery to deeper veins within the body. This response causes a central blood volume expansion, which results in a rise in the mean arterial pressure, stroke volume, and cardiac output.[88] The expanded blood volume can produce a diuresis, manifested by frequent urination. Cold-induced diuresis can reduce plasma volume by 7% to 15%, resulting in hemoconcentration and acute dehydration from an almost twofold fluid loss over normal.

As with exposure to heat, adherence to fluid hydration guidelines and access to liquids when thirsty while working in cold environments are necessary to minimize dehydration along with the associated fatigue and physical and cognitive changes. Because thirst is suppressed in cold environments, dehydration is a significant risk.

Minor Cold-Related Disorders

Contact Freeze Injury

When cold material contacts unprotected skin, it can produce local **frostbite** immediately. Do not touch any metal surface, alcohol, gasoline, antifreeze, ice, or snow with the hands; see the Frostbite section for assessment and management.

Frostnip

Frostnip is often a precursor to frostbite and produces reversible signs of skin blanching and numbness in localized tissue. It is typically seen on the cheeks, nose, and earlobes. Frostnip is a self-limited and nonfreezing tissue injury as long as cold exposure does not continue; it does not require prehospital care provider intervention and transport.

Cold Urticaria

Cold urticaria ("hives") is a disorder characterized by the rapid onset (within minutes) of itchiness, redness, and swelling of the skin after exposure to cold. The sensation of burning may be a prominent feature. This condition, caused by a local release of histamine, is sometimes observed when ice is applied directly to the skin during cold therapy for sprains and strains. Individuals with a history of cold urticaria are advised to avoid cold-water immersion, which could potentially cause death from systemic anaphylaxis. Treatment includes avoiding the cold and possibly taking antihistamines.

Chilblains (Pernio)

Chilblains are a nonfreezing cold injury that presents as small skin lesions that are itchy and tender, appearing as bluish red bumps that occur on the extensor skin surface of the finger or any skin surface (most commonly the feet, hands, legs, and thighs) from chronic cold exposure. Chilblains occur several hours after exposure to the cold in temperate humid climates. They are sometimes aggravated by sun exposure. Cold causes constriction of the small arteries and veins in the skin, and rewarming results in leakage of blood into the tissues and swelling of the skin.

Chilblains are more likely to develop in those with poor peripheral circulation. Some contributing factors are a familial tendency, peripheral vascular disease caused by diabetes, smoking, hyperlipidemia (increased serum lipid levels), poor nutrition (e.g., anorexia nervosa), connective tissue disease, and bone marrow disorders. Each chilblain comes up over a few hours as an itchy, bluish red swelling and subsides over the next 7 to 14 days. In severe cases, blistering, pustules, scabs, and ulceration can occur. Occasionally the lesions may be ring shaped. They may become thickened and persist for months.

Symptoms will subside with removal of the individual from the cold. Management involves protection from cold with appropriate gloves and clothing.

Solar Keratitis (Snow Blindness)

Without protection from dry air and from exposure to bright reflections on snow, the risk of ultraviolet burns to skin and eyes increases. This risk is greatly enhanced at higher altitudes. **Solar keratitis** is insidious during the exposure phase, with corneal and conjunctival epithelium burns occurring in as little as 2 hours but not becoming apparent until 6 to 12 hours after exposure.[19]

Management of snow blindness is based on symptoms, which include excessive tearing, severe pain, redness, swollen eyelids, pain when looking at light, headache, a gritty sensation in the eyes, and decreased (hazy) vision. Prehospital care providers need to consider patching affected eyes if there is no other method to prevent further ultraviolet exposure (e.g., sunglasses) and then transport the patient. Topical ophthalmic anesthetic drops, if available, may be used to provide symptomatic relief. Medical attention is required to determine the level of severity and the need for antibiotics and analgesics.[89]

Major Cold-Related Disorders

Localized Cutaneous Cold Injury

Cold injuries occur at peripheral sites on the body and are classified as either freezing (e.g., frostbite) or nonfreezing (e.g., frostnip, chilblains, immersion foot) injuries. Localized cold injuries are preventable with proper preparation for cold exposure, early recognition of cold injury, and effective medical care. However, frostbite, the most serious form of freezing injury because of the risk of limb loss, is the primary injury of concern in this section.

Prevention of cold injury through an understanding of the contributing factors is key. Nicotine, alcohol intoxication, homelessness, and major psychiatric disorders remain important predisposing factors.[90] Tight or constricting clothes, too many socks, and tight-fitting footwear are predictable factors in the onset of frostbite. With an increase in adventure sports and other recreational activities conducted in the winter season, localized cold injuries are seen more often.

Prehospital care providers need to prevent body heat loss and protect exposed skin from frostbite in patients during prolonged exposure to cold conditions. For example, in patients needing vehicular extrication, in scenarios resulting in the inability to move the patient, and in patients in cold environments with soft-tissue swelling, impaired circulation can lead to an increased incidence of localized cold injury. The priority of care for all patients presenting with frostbite or other cold injuries is to protect them from further exposure to the elements and focus on hypothermia prevention and treatment.

Nonfreezing Cold Injury

Nonfreezing cold injury (NFCI) is a syndrome that causes damage to tissues in cold, but not freezing, temperatures. Most often associated with immersion foot and trench foot, this syndrome can affect any extremity. NFCI results from damage to peripheral tissues caused by prolonged (hours to days) wet/cold exposure, does not involve freezing of tissue, but may coexist with a freezing injury such as frostbite.[91-94] This syndrome primarily involves the feet and is reflected in two types of NFCI. While the following injuries are clinically identical, they are caused by different environmental conditions. **Trench foot** occurs primarily in military personnel during infantry operations and is related to the combined effects of prolonged cold exposure and restricted circulation in the feet; it does not involve immersion in water.[90] **Immersion foot** is caused by prolonged immersion of extremities in moisture that is cool to cold. Prehospital care providers may see immersion foot in persons who are homeless, persons with alcoholism, or elderly persons; in hikers and hunters; in multiday adventure sport athletes; and in ocean survivors.[91,95,96] Frequently, this syndrome goes unrecognized during assessment of individuals who have been exposed to cold or wet conditions because of failure to remove boots or shoes and examine the feet and because of the lack of formal medical training in NFCI.[91] Immersion foot may extend to the knees and above, depending on the depth of immersion.[94]

This syndrome occurs as a result of many hours of cooling of the lower extremities in temperatures ranging from 32°F to 59°F (0°C to 15°C).[97] Soft-tissue injury occurs to the skin of the feet, known as **maceration**. The breakdown of the skin predisposes individuals to infection. The greatest injury is seen to the peripheral nerves and blood vessels, caused by secondary ischemic injury. Mild NFCI is self-limited initially, but with continued prolonged cold exposure, it becomes irreversible. When the feet are wet and cold, they are at increased risk, and the injury's course is accelerated because wet socks insulate poorly and water cools more effectively than air at the same temperature. Any factors that reduce circulation to the extremities will contribute to the injury, such as constrictive clothing, boots, prolonged immobility, hypothermia, and crouched posture.

NFCI is classified in four degrees of severity, as follows:

- *Minimal.* Hyperemia or engorgement caused by an increase in blood flow to the feet and slight sensory change will remain 2 to 3 days after injury. The condition is self-limited, and no signs of injury remain after 7 days. Occasionally, cold sensitivity will remain.
- *Mild.* Edema, hyperemia, and slight sensory change remain 2 to 3 days after injury. Seven days after injury, anesthesia is found on the plantar surface of the foot and tips of the toes and lasts 4 to 9 weeks. Blisters and skin loss are not observed. Ambulation is possible when walking does not cause pain.
- *Moderate.* Edema, hyperemia, blisters, and mottling are present 2 to 3 days after injury. At 7 days, anesthesia to touch is present to both dorsal and plantar surfaces and toes. Edema persists 2 to 3 weeks, and pain and hyperemia last up to 14 weeks. Some blister sloughing occurs but no loss of deep tissue. Some patients will have permanent injury.
- *Severe.* Severe edema, blood forced into surrounding tissues (*extravasation*), and gangrene are present 2 to 3 days after injury. Complete anesthesia of the entire foot remains at 7 days, with paralysis and muscle wasting in the affected extremities. The injury goes beyond the foot into the lower leg. This severe injury produces significant tissue loss, resulting in *autoamputation* (nonsurgical amputation of dead tissue). Gangrene is a constant risk until tissue loss is complete. The patient is expected to have prolonged convalescence and a permanent disability.[91]

ASSESSMENT

Because the patient has experienced mild or moderate cold exposure, it is essential to rule out hypothermia and assess for dehydration. Even though this is not a freezing injury, NCFI still is an insidious and potentially disabling injury; the common finding with these two localized cold injuries is that the extremity is cooled to the point of anesthesia or numbness while the injury is occurring.

The key to management of NFCI is detection and recognition during assessment. During the primary assessment, injured tissue appears macerated, edematous, pale/yellowish white, anesthetized, pulseless, and immobile but not frozen. Patients complain of clumsiness and stumbling when attempting to walk. After removal from cold, and during or after rewarming, peripheral blood flow increases as reperfusion of ischemic tissue begins. Extremities change color from white to mottled pale blue while remaining cold and numb. The diagnosis of trench foot or immersion foot is generally made when these signs have not changed after passive rewarming of the feet. From 24 to 36 hours after rewarming, a marked hyperemia develops, along with severe burning pain and reappearance of sensation proximally but not distally. This is caused by venous vasodilation. Edema and blisters develop in the injured areas as perfusion increases. Skin will remain poorly perfused after hyperemia appears, and the skin is likely to slough as the injury evolves. Any pulselessness after 48 hours in the injured extremity suggests severe, deep injury and a greater chance of substantial tissue loss and the development of gangrene.

MANAGEMENT

Once a possible NFCI is detected, the priorities are to eliminate any further cooling of the patient or the extremity, prevent further trauma at the site of injury, and transport the patient. Do not allow the patient to walk on an injured extremity. Carefully remove the footwear and socks. Note: Do not remove boots and socks and initiate the process of rewarming unless you are confident that you will be able to prevent refreezing of the extremity and achieve timely transport to the hospital. Cover the injured part or extremity with a loose, dry, sterile dressing; protect it from the cold; and begin passive rewarming of injured tissue during transport. The affected area may be aggravated by the weight of a blanket. No active rewarming is necessary. Do not massage the affected area because doing so may cause further tissue damage. As needed, treat the patient for dehydration with a bolus of IV fluids, and reassess. Depending on length of transport, severe pain may develop during passive rewarming as tissues begin to reperfuse.

Freezing Cold Injury

On the continuum of further peripheral cold tissue exposure beginning with frostnip (no tissue loss), frostbite ranges from mild to severe tissue destruction and possibly the loss of tissue due to intense vasoconstriction.[9,10,14] The most susceptible body parts for frostbite are those tissues with large surface-to-mass ratios, such as the ears and nose or areas farthest from the body's core, such as the hands, fingers, feet, toes, and male genitalia. The feet and toes are the most commonly affected areas.[97] These structures are most susceptible to cold injury because they contain many arteriovenous capillary **anastomoses** (connections) that easily shunt blood away during vasoconstriction. The body's normal response to lower-than-desirable temperatures is to reduce blood flow to the skin surface to reduce heat exchange with the environment. The body accomplishes this by vasoconstriction of peripheral blood vessels to shunt warm blood to the body's core to maintain a normal body temperature. Reduction of this blood flow greatly reduces the amount of heat delivered to the distal extremities.

The longer the period of exposure to the cold, the more the blood flow is reduced to the periphery. The body conserves core temperature at the expense of extremity and skin temperature. The heat loss from the tissue becomes greater than the heat supplied to that area.

When an extremity is cooled to 59°F (15°C), maximal vasoconstriction and minimal blood flow occur. If cooling continues to 50°F (10°C), vasoconstriction is interrupted by periods of **cold-induced vasodilation (CIVD)** and an associated increase in tissue temperature caused by an increase in blood flow. CIVD recurs in 5- to 10-minute cycles to provide some protection from the cold. Individuals show differences in susceptibility to frostbite when exposed to the same cold conditions, which may be explained by the amount of CIVD.

Tissue does not freeze at 32°F (0°C) because cells contain electrolytes and other solutes that prevent tissue from freezing until skin temperature reaches approximately 28°F (−2.2°C). In cases of below-freezing temperatures, when the extremities are left unprotected, the intracellular and extracellular fluids can freeze. This results in the formation of ice crystals. As the ice crystals form, they expand and cause damage to local tissues. Blood clots may form, further impairing circulation to the injured area.

The type and duration of cold exposure are the two most important factors in determining the extent of freezing injury. Frostbite is classified by depth of injury and clinical presentation.[14] The degree of injury in many cases will not be known for at least 24 to 72 hours after thawing, except in very minor or severe exposures. Skin exposure to cold that is short but intense will create a superficial injury, whereas severe frostbite to a whole extremity can occur during prolonged exposures. Direct cold injury is usually reversible, but permanent tissue damage occurs during rewarming. In more severe cases, even with appropriate rewarming of tissue, microvascular thrombosis can develop, leading to early signs of gangrene and necrosis. If the injured site freezes, thaws, and then refreezes, the second freezing causes a greater amount of severe thrombosis and vascular damage and tissue loss. For this reason, prehospital care providers need to prevent any frozen tissue that thaws during initial field treatment from refreezing.

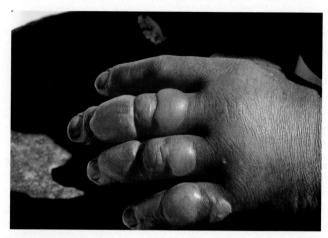

Figure 19-6 Edema and blister formation 24 hours after frostbite injury.
© ANT Photo Library/Science Source.

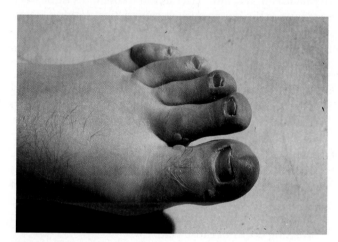

Figure 19-7 Deep second-degree and third-degree frostbite with hemorrhagic blebs, one day after thawing.
© ANT Photo Library/Science Source.

Traditional methods of frostbite classification present four degrees of injury (similar to burns) based on initial physical findings after freezing and advanced imaging in the hospital after rewarming (**Figure 19-6** and **Figure 19-7**), as follows:

- **First-degree frostbite.** This epidermal injury is limited to skin that has brief contact with cold air or metal. The skin appears white or as yellowish plaque at the site of injury. There is no blister or tissue loss. Skin thaws quickly, feels numb, and appears red with surrounding edema; healing occurs in 7 to 10 days.
- **Second-degree frostbite.** This degree of injury involves all of the epidermis and superficial dermis. It initially appears similar to first-degree injury; however, frozen tissues are deeper. Tissue feels stiff to the touch, but tissue beneath gives way to pressure. Thawing is rapid; after thawing, superficial skin blister or vesiculation occurs, with clear or milky fluid after several hours,

surrounded by erythema and edema. There is no permanent loss of tissue. Healing occurs in 3 to 4 weeks.

- **Third-degree frostbite.** This degree of injury involves the epidermis and dermis layers. Frozen skin is stiff, with restricted mobility. After tissue thaws, skin swells along with a blood-filled blister (*hemorrhagic bulla*), indicating vascular trauma to deep tissues; swelling restricts mobility. Skin loss occurs slowly, leading to mummification and sloughing. Healing is slow.
- **Fourth-degree frostbite.** At this level, frozen tissue involves full thickness completely through the dermis, with muscle and bone involvement. There is no mobility when frozen and passive movement when thawed, with no intrinsic muscle function. Skin perfusion is poor, and blisters and edema do not develop. Early signs of necrotic tissue are evident. A slow mummification process will occur along with sloughing of tissue and autoamputation of nonviable tissue.

Although traditional classification of frostbite is by the four degrees of injury, it is easiest for providers in the prehospital setting to classify as either superficial or deep.[98-100] **Superficial frostbite** (first and second degree) affects the skin and subcutaneous tissues, resulting in clear blisters when rewarmed. **Deep frostbite** (third and fourth degree) affects skin, muscle, and bone, and the skin has hemorrhagic blisters when rewarmed. The level of severity and anticipated tissue loss may vary within a single extremity.[101] An additional classification method has been introduced that examines the frozen tissue after rewarming in an effort to identify amputation risk.[102]

In certain situations, frostbite may occur rapidly, and prehospital care providers may respond to the following:

- Hydrocarbon fluid spills on skin (e.g., gasoline, butane, propane) will cause rapid evaporation and conduction in below-freezing temperatures)
- Touching extremely cold metal with warm skin
- Intense windchill on exposed skin caused by rotary wind from a medical helicopter

ASSESSMENT

On arrival, assess scene safety and then the patient for ABCs. Remove the patient from the cold, and place him or her in an area protected from moisture, cold, and wind to prevent further cooling. Many frostbite victims may have additional associated medical conditions, such as dehydration, hypovolemia, hypothermia, hypoglycemia, and traumatic injury. Remove any wet clothing to minimize further body heat loss. *When in doubt, treat hypothermia first.* Superficial frostbite is usually assessed through a combination of recognizing the environmental conditions, locating the patient's chief complaint of pain or numbness, and observing discolored skin in the same area. The environmental conditions during exposure must be below freezing.

Frostbite injuries are insidious because the patient may have no pain at the injury site when skin is frozen and covered by a glove or footwear. Detection of the affected area requires direct visual inspection of highly suspect body regions, as previously listed. Gentle palpation of the area can determine if the underlying tissue is compliant or hard. Ensure that the patient or prehospital care provider does not rub or massage the affected skin, because this will cause further cellular damage to frozen tissues. The patient with superficial freezing will usually complain of discomfort during the manipulation of the frostbitten area. In patients with deep frostbite, the frozen tissue will be hard and usually is not painful when touched. After inspection of the affected area, a decision is necessary about the method of rewarming, which is usually based on transport time to the ED.

The state of Alaska EMS protocol for frostbite rewarming in the prehospital phase states the following[103]:

1. If transport time is short (1 to 2 hours at most), then the risks posed by improper rewarming or refreezing in the prehospital phase outweigh the risks for delaying treatment for deep frostbite.
2. If transport time will be prolonged (more than 1 to 2 hours), frostbite will often thaw spontaneously. It is more important to prevent hypothermia than to rewarm frostbite rapidly in warm water. This does not mean that a frostbitten extremity should be kept in the cold to prevent spontaneous rewarming. Anticipate that frostbitten areas will rewarm as a consequence of keeping the patient warm; protect them from refreezing at all costs.

MANAGEMENT

Patients with superficial frostnip or frostbite should be placed with the affected area against a warm body surface, such as covering the patient's ears with warm hands or placing affected fingers into armpits, axillae, or groin regions. Superficial frostbite only needs to be warmed at normal body temperatures.

Management of deep frostbite in the prehospital setting includes first assessing and treating the patient for hypothermia, if present.[101,104] Provide supportive care and appropriate shelter for the patient and the affected part to minimize heat loss. Do not allow the patient to walk on affected feet. Protect fragile tissues from further trauma during patient movement. Assess the frostbite area. Remove any clothing and jewelry from the affected area, and check for loss of sensation.

If there is frostbite distal to a fracture, attempt to align the limb unless there is resistance. Splint the fracture in a manner that does not compromise distal circulation.

Air dry the affected area, and do not rub the tissues. Cover the affected area with a loose, dry, bulky sterile dressing that is noncompressive and nonadherent. Fingers and toes should be individually separated by and protected with sterile cotton gauze. Do not drain any blisters. Hands and feet should be splinted and elevated to reduce edema.

Analgesics may be required for pain relief and should be initiated before the tissues have thawed. Initiate IV NS with a 250-ml bolus to treat dehydration and reduce blood viscosity and capillary sludging. Ensure early transport to an appropriate facility.

Attempts to begin rewarming of deep frostbite patients in the field can be hazardous to the patient's eventual recovery and are not recommended unless prolonged transport times (over 2 hours) are involved. If prolonged transport is involved, thaw the affected part in a warm water bath at a temperature no greater than 98.6°F to 102.2°F (37°C to 39°C) on the affected area until the area becomes soft and pliable to the touch (~30 min).[97,104] If refreezing is a concern, do not thaw. Protect the injured extremity while thawing by preventing any area from touching the sides or bottom of the water bath as sensation is diminished or absent in frostbitten tissue and additional damage can occur.[19]

Administer ibuprofen (12 mg/kg up to 800 mg) or aspirin (75–81 mg) if available and permissible given local protocols.[102] Nonsteroidal medications such as ibuprofen help decrease inflammation and pain and inhibit the production of substances that cause vasoconstriction.

During transport, hydrate the patient by providing something warm (and nonalcoholic) if it is available, depending on the patient's level of consciousness and other injuries. Tobacco use (smoking, chewing, using nicotine patches) should be discouraged because nicotine causes further vasoconstriction.

Accidental Hypothermia

Hypothermia is defined as the condition in which the core body temperature is 95°F (35°C) or below, as measured by a rectal thermometer probe placed at least 6 inches (15 cm) into the rectum.[15,49] Hypothermia can be viewed as a decrease in core temperature that renders a patient unable to generate sufficient heat production to return to homeostasis or normal body functions.

Hypothermia can occur in many different situations, resulting from cold ambient air, cold-water immersion, or cold-water submersion, and can be intentionally induced during surgery.[15,105,106] Immersion ("head out") hypothermia typically occurs when an individual is accidentally placed into a cold environment without preparation or planning. For example, a person who has fallen into ice water is immediately in danger of submersion injury, resulting from cold shock gasp reflex, loss of motor skills, hypothermia, and drowning. These unique aspects of submersion incidents can lead to hypoxemia and hypothermia (see later discussion and the chapter titled Environmental Trauma II: Drowning, Lightning, Diving, and Altitude).

The progression of hypothermia in cold air or cold water can be delayed if the metabolic heat production can match the loss of heat. Surviving an overwhelming cold exposure is possible, with many reported cases of survival at sea and in other extreme situations.[107,108] Many factors are known to affect survival after cold exposure, including age, gender, body composition (e.g., body surface area to body mass ratio), onset and intensity of shivering, level of physical fitness, nutritional state, and alcohol consumption.

Hypoglycemia can occur during progressive phases of hypothermia and may be more common in immersion hypothermia. This occurs due to the rapid depletion of the fuel sources blood glucose and muscle glycogen by the contracting muscles during the shivering process. As the blood glucose stores are depleted through shivering, the brain's hypothalamus, which acts as the body's thermoregulatory center, is deprived its primary fuel. Consequently, a person who has consumed alcohol is at greater risk for hypothermia since alcohol blocks the production of glucose in the body and inhibits maximal shivering for heat production.[15] Thus, rapid assessment and effective management of low blood glucose in the patient with hypothermia are essential to achieve effective increase in metabolism and shivering during rewarming.

Unlike frostbite, hypothermia leading to death can occur in environments with temperatures well above freezing. **Primary hypothermia** generally occurs when healthy individuals are in adverse weather conditions, they are unprepared for overwhelming acute or chronic cold exposure, and there is an involuntary drop of core temperature (below 95°F [35°C]). Deaths by primary hypothermia are a direct result of cold exposure and are documented by the medical examiner as accident, homicide, or suicide.[14]

Secondary hypothermia is considered a normal consequence of a patient's systemic disorders, including hypothyroidism, hypoadrenalism, trauma, carcinoma, and sepsis. See **Box 19-10** for a wide variety of medical conditions associated with secondary hypothermia. If unrecognized or improperly treated, this type of hypothermia can be fatal, in some cases within 2 hours. Death in patients with secondary hypothermia is often caused by the underlying disease and is potentiated by hypothermia. Mortality is greater than 50% in cases of secondary hypothermia caused by complications of other injuries and in severe cases in which the core body temperature is below 89.6°F (32°C).[15]

The prehospital care provider must rapidly act to prevent further body heat loss in the traumatic patient, as mild hypothermia is very common following injury in all weather conditions.

Hypothermia and the Trauma Patient

It is all too common to receive patients with hypothermia arriving at a trauma center and to have further body heat loss occur during the primary assessment.[109,110] The

Box 19-10 Conditions Associated With Secondary Hypothermia

Impaired Thermoregulation
- Central failure
- Anorexia nervosa
- Cerebrovascular accident
- CNS trauma
- Hypothalamic dysfunction
- Metabolic failure
- Neoplasm
- Parkinson disease
- Pharmacologic effects
- Subarachnoid hemorrhage
- Toxins
- Peripheral failure
- Acute spinal cord transection
- Decreased heat production
- Neuropathy
- Endocrinologic failure
- Alcoholic or diabetic ketoacidosis
- Hypoadrenalism
- Hypopituitarism
- Lactic acidosis
- Insufficient energy
- Extreme physical exertion
- Hypoglycemia
- Malnutrition
- Neuromuscular compromise
- Recent birth and advanced age with inactivity
- Impaired shivering

Increased Heat Loss
- Dermatologic disorder
- Burns
- Medications and toxins
- Iatrogenic cause
- Emergency childbirth
- Cold infusions
- Heatstroke treatment
- Other associated clinical states
- Carcinomatosis
- Cardiopulmonary disease
- Major infection (bacterial, viral, parasitic)
- Multisystem trauma
- Shock

Data from the 2005 Cardiopulmonary Resuscitation and Emergency Cardiovascular Care Guidelines and 2010 American Heart Association Guidelines for cardiopulmonary resuscitation and emergency cardiovascular care. *Circulation.* 2005;112(24):IVI-203. American Heart Association. 2010 guidelines for cardiopulmonary resuscitation and emergency cardiovascular care. *Circulation.* 2010;122:S640-S656.

development of hypothermia that begins in the prehospital setting is related to the effect of trauma on thermoregulation and the inhibition of shivering as a primary mechanism for heat production.[111] In many patients, heat loss continues after arrival at the hospital due to a multitude of reasons: an exposed patient in a cold ED or trauma center, administration of cool resuscitation fluids, open abdominal or thoracic cavities, the use of anesthetic and neuromuscular blocking agents that prevent heat-producing shivering, and cold exposure in an operating room environment.[112,113]

In the prehospital setting, the trauma patient should be moved off of cold ground as soon as possible and placed in a warm ambulance. The temperature in the ambulance should be adjusted to minimize heat loss from the patient and maximize performance of prehospital care providers, whose work may be impaired by too hot an ambient work environment. The Wilderness Medical Society recommends an in-compartment ambulance temperature of 75°F (24°C) as an ideal balance of these two considerations.[7] Warmed (100°F to 108°F [37.8°C to 42.2°C]) IV fluids will also help to maintain the patient's body temperature.

One cause of higher mortality in hypothermic trauma patients is related to the lethal combination of *hypothermia, acidosis,* and *coagulopathy* (inability of blood to clot normally). This is known as the *lethal triad* in trauma patients.[114] It is essential to assess and treat patients for both trauma and hypothermia because the coagulopathy is reversible with patient rewarming.[110] In one study, 57% of the trauma patients admitted to a level I trauma center were hypothermic at some point in the continuum of care. The mortality rate has been reported to range from 40% to 100% when core temperature falls below 90°F (32.2°C) in a trauma patient. This rate contrasts with a mortality of 20% in a primary hypothermic (nontraumatic) patient at moderate core temperature levels (82°F to 90°F [27.8°C to 32.2°C]).[113] Consequently, the mortality rate associated with hypothermia in the trauma victim is very significant, such that some researchers have created a special trauma hypothermia classification beyond the standard definition of mild, moderate, and severe hypothermia (**Table 19-5**).[114,115]

This relationship of trauma, hypothermia, and increased mortality has been reported for decades, including recently in combat casualty patients.[116] However, recent clinical studies have reported that hypothermia is not an independent risk factor for mortality in trauma patients but is more closely related to injury severity or multiple organ dysfunction syndrome.[117-120] One study reported that certain prehospital care practices can influence the severity of hypothermia in trauma patients. These practices include anticipating hypothermia, avoiding undressing patients, taking frequent temperature measurements, maintaining warm mobile cabin temperatures, and maintaining and providing only warm IV fluids.[119] The potential therapeutic benefits of intentionally induced hypothermia are currently under study (**Box 19-11**).

Table 19-5 Classifications of Hypothermia

Classification	Core Body Temperature
Mild hypothermia	95–89.6°F (35–32°C)
Moderate hypothermia	89.5–82.4°F (32–28°C)
Severe hypothermia	82.3–75.2°F (28–24°C)
Profound hypothermia	75.2°F (< 24°C)

Data from: Zafren K, Giesbrecht GG, Danzl DF, et al. Wilderness Medical Society practice guidelines for the out-of-hospital evaluation and treatment of accidental hypothermia. *Wilderness Environ Med.* 2014;25:426.

Immersion Hypothermia

During immersion, if there is no heat gain or heat loss by the body, water temperature is considered *thermoneutral*. Thermoneutral water temperature is 91.4°F to 95°F (33°C to 35°C), at which temperatures a naked individual passively standing in neck-level water can maintain a nearly constant core temperature for at least 1 hour.[113,128,129] Individuals in thermoneutral water are at almost no risk for the initial immersion cold shock and hypothermia experienced in sudden cold-water exposure.[130]

When immersion occurs in water temperature colder than the lower thermoneutral limit, the immediate physiologic changes are a rapid decline in skin temperature, peripheral vasoconstriction resulting in shivering, and increased metabolism, ventilation, heart rate, cardiac output, and mean arterial pressure. To offset any heat loss in water, heat production must occur by increasing physical activity, shivering, or both. If not, core temperature continues to fall and shivering ceases, and these physiologic responses decrease proportionally with the fall in core temperature.[106]

The greatest risk of immersion hypothermia usually begins in water temperature less than 77°F (25°C).[129] Because the heat dissipation capacity of water is 25 times greater than that of air, individuals are at risk for more rapid hypothermia in water. However, continued physical activity (i.e., swimming to keep warm) in cold water will eventually become a detriment by increasing convective heat loss to the colder water surrounding the body, resulting in a faster onset of hypothermia. This understanding has led to the recommendation for individuals to minimize heat loss during cold-water immersion by using the *heat escape lessening posture* (HELP) or the *huddle position* when multiple immersion victims are together (**Figure 19-8**).[129]

The lowest recorded core temperature for an infant with an intact neurologic recovery from accidental hypothermia is 59°F (15°C).[123] In an adult, 56.6°F (13.7°C)

Box 19-11 Therapeutic Hypothermia

It is well established that the detrimental *lethal triad* in trauma victims increases mortality. However, there is some developing early evidence to suggest that intentionally induced hypothermia may have a beneficial role in select circumstances of shock, organ transplantation, nontraumatic cardiac arrest, and control of intracranial pressure from traumatic brain injury.[115,121]

Although the value of initiating therapeutic hypothermia (TH) in the prehospital setting has not been demonstrated, the fastest growing application of this therapy is for victims of sudden nontraumatic cardiac arrest.[115,122,123] It is well known that the outcome following cardiac arrest is very poor, with only 3% to 27% of all cardiac arrest patients surviving to discharge. However, there is a growing amount of evidence for increased survival rate with TH following nontraumatic cardiac arrest. These statements recommended intentional cooling of the patient to 89.6°F to 93.2°F (32°C to 34°C) for 12 to 24 hours in unconscious adults with spontaneous circulation after nontraumatic (often fibrillatory) cardiac arrest with evidence of subsequent neurologic compromise.[121,123,124]

Currently, evidence regarding TH in the multiple trauma patient is conflicting. Preclinical studies suggest that TH may be useful in hypotensive penetrating trauma patients. There is potential for TH to be used in cases of blunt trauma, but it has not been well studied. Clinical trials have conflicting results, or results with uncertain clinical significance, in the case of traumatic brain injury (TBI)[125,126] and spinal cord injuries. TH cannot be definitively recommended for general trauma patients until better clinical research is available.[127] There is presently no role for TH in the prehospital setting for survivors of traumatic cardiac arrest or for trauma patients.

is the lowest recorded core temperature for a survivor of accidental hypothermia. This occurred in a 29-year-old female who struggled to self-rescue for more than 40 minutes before symptoms of severe hypothermia affected muscular contraction.[108] She was immersed for more than 80 minutes before a rescue team arrived and cardiopulmonary resuscitation (CPR) was initiated during transport to a local hospital. After 3 hours of continuous rewarming, her core temperature returned to normal, and she survived with normal physiologic function.

Because vital signs may have decreased to a nearly imperceptible level, the initial impression of hypothermic

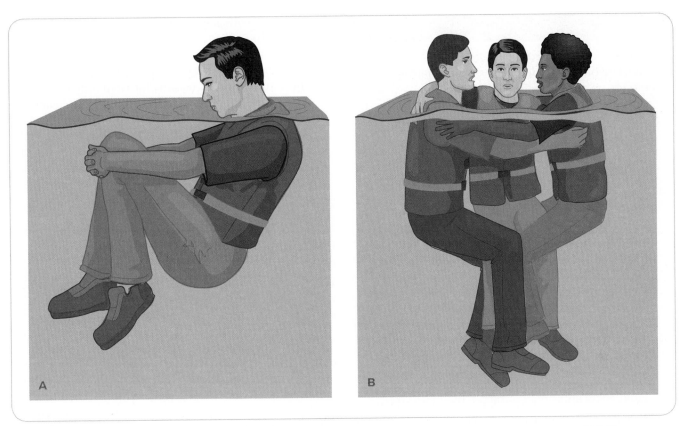

Figure 19-8 Techniques for decreasing cooling rates of survivors in cold water. **A.** Heat escape lessening posture (HELP). **B.** Huddle technique.

© National Association of Emergency Medical Technicians (NAEMT).

patients may be that they are dead. Prehospital care providers managing patients with hypothermia should not stop treatment interventions and declare the patient dead until the patient has been rewarmed to over 95°F (35°C) and still has no evidence of cardiorespiratory and neurologic function, or signs of nonsurvivability are present (ice in airway, frozen chest wall, etc.). The 29-year-old hypothermia survivor is just one example of a patient being discharged from the hospital with full neurologic function after prolonged CPR in the field. The lesson from this case, and others with a similar outcome, is that although the initial impression of a hypothermic patient may be that he or she is dead, this impression is not sufficient justification to withhold basic or advanced life support. Keep the following phrase in mind: *Patients are not dead until they are warm and dead.*

Whether intentional or unintentional, cold-water immersion (head out) occurs throughout the year in the United States because of recreational and commercial activities, as well as from accidents. If individuals survive the initial submersion incident without fatally drowning, they are at risk for hypothermia, depending on the water temperature. It is important to note that the public generally underestimates the amount of time required to become hypothermic in very cold water, believing that it occurs

rapidly, with a short time until death. However, rapid death from immersion often is the result of panic or cold shock response leading to aspiration of water or transient muscular paralysis/dysfunction and fatal drowning, not hypothermia. The key points to understand are that (1) cold shock is initially the greatest threat and (2) patients should focus more on controlling the gasp reflex and their breathing to survive this initial physiologic response (**Box 19-12**). The body's responses to cold-water immersion can be divided into four phases, leading to death. It is important to note that deaths have been reported as occurring in all four of the following phases[129]:

- *First phase—cold shock response.* This phase begins with a cardiovascular reflex known as *cold shock response* that occurs quickly (within 1 to 2 minutes) after immersion (may occur in water colder than 68°F [20°C]). It begins with rapid skin cooling, peripheral vasoconstriction, a gasp reflex and the inability to breath-hold, hyperventilation, and tachycardia.[90,105,129] The gasp response may lead to aspiration and drowning, depending on the individual's head location above or below water. These responses can lead to immediate sudden death or death within minutes following immersion because

When a person becomes immersed in ice-cold water, the onset of cold shock or hypothermia depends on several factors, including body size, water temperature, and the amount of the person's body that is immersed. Generally speaking, however, the physiologic response to cold water immersion can be described by the 1-10-1 principle.

- *1 minute:* The threat of cold shock will pass in about 1 minute. The person should avoid panicking and focus on gaining control of his or her breathing and keeping the airway clear.
- *10 minutes:* After about 10 minutes, a person will not be able to move his or her arms, legs, and other body parts. The person should use this time to self-rescue, if possible, or establish a survivable position until rescuers arrive.
- *1 hour:* A person has up to 1 hour before becoming unconscious from hypothermia. Panicking or struggling unnecessarily will reduce this time. Wearing a personal flotation device could allow another hour before the heart stops beating.

of several conditions, including syncope or convulsions resulting in drowning, vagal arrest, and ventricular fibrillation.[106,129,131-133]

- *Second phase—cold incapacitation.* If a victim survives the cold shock phase, significant cooling of peripheral tissues, especially in the extremities, occurs over the next 5 to 15 minutes of immersion. This cooling has a deleterious effect on gross and fine motor skills of the extremities, causing finger stiffness, poor coordination, and loss of muscle power, making it nearly impossible to swim, grasp a rescue line, or perform other survival motor skills.[106,129]
- *Third phase—onset of hypothermia.* Surviving the first two phases without drowning places an individual at risk of hypothermia from continued heat loss and core temperature reduction from immersion longer than 30 minutes.[129] If the victim is not able to remain above the water surface because of fatigue and hypothermia, he or she is at risk of becoming a submersion casualty, leading to aspiration and drowning.[90,109] How long an individual can survive in cold water depends on many factors. It has been estimated that a submersion victim cannot survive for more than 1 hour at a water temperature of 32°F (0°C); and at a water temperature of 59°F (15°C), survival is uncommon after 6 hours.[134]
- *Fourth phase—circumrescue collapse.* In this phase, fatalities have been observed during all periods of survivor rescue (before, during, and after) despite the apparent

stable and conscious condition. Symptoms range from fainting to cardiac arrest and have been referred to as rewarming shock or postrescue collapse, with deaths occurring at any stage after rescue, up to 24 hours. The three proposed reasons for circumrescue collapse are (1) afterdrop of core temperature, (2) collapse of arterial blood pressure, and (3) changes in hypoxia, acidosis, or rapid changes in pH that induce ventricular fibrillation. It is noted that up to 20% of those who are recovered alive during the fourth phase will die due to circumrescue collapse.[129]

For more information about surviving cold-water immersion, see **Box 19-13** and **Box 19-14**.

Pathophysiologic Effects of Hypothermia on the Body

Whether from exposure to a cold environment or immersion, the influence of hypothermia on the body affects all major organ systems, particularly the cardiac, renal, and central nervous systems. As the body's core temperature decreases to 95°F (35°C), maximal rate of vasoconstriction, shivering, and metabolic rate occurs, with increases in heart rate, respiration, and blood pressure. Cerebral metabolism oxygen demand decreases by 6% to 10% per 1.8°F (~1°C) drop in core temperature, and cerebral metabolism is preserved.

When core temperature falls to between 86°F (30°C) and 95°F (35°C), cognitive function, cardiac function, metabolic rate, ventilatory rate, and shivering rate are all significantly decreased or completely inhibited. At this point, the limited physiologic defensive mechanisms to prevent heat loss from the body are overwhelmed, and core temperature falls rapidly.

At a core temperature of 85°F (29.4°C), cardiac output and metabolic rate are reduced approximately 50%. Ventilation and perfusion are inadequate and do not keep up with the metabolic demand, causing cellular hypoxia,

The U.S. Coast Guard and other search-and-rescue (SAR) organizations use guidelines to assist in estimating how long individuals can survive in cold water. These guidelines are mathematical models that estimate core temperature cooling rate based on the influence of the following variables:

- Water temperature and sea state
- Clothing insulation
- Body composition (amount of fat, muscle, and bone)
- Amount of the body immersed in water
- Behavior (e.g., excessive movement) and posture (e.g., HELP, huddle) of the body in the water
- Shivering thermogenesis[135-137]

Box 19-14 Self-Rescue

Early studies in the 1960s to 1970s suggested that during accidental immersion in cold water, it was a better option not to self-rescue by attempting to distance-swim to safety but to stay in place, float still in lifejackets, or hang on to wreckage and not swim around to keep warm. More recent research has suggested that self-rescue swimming during accidental immersion in cold water (50°F to 57°F [10°C to 13.9°C]) is a viable option based on the following conditions:

- The victim has initially survived the cold-shock phase within the first few minutes of cold-water exposure.
- The victim has decided early to attempt self-rescue or wait for rescue since decision-making ability will become impaired as hypothermia progresses. After 30 minutes of submersion, the likelihood of success is significantly lower.
- There is a low probability for rescue by emergency responders in the area.
- The victim can reach shore within 45 minutes of swimming based on his or her fitness level and swimming ability.[129]
- On average, a cold-water immersion victim wearing a personal flotation device should be able to swim approximately a half mile (800 m) in 50°F (10°C) water before incapacitation due to muscle cooling and fatigue of the arms, rather than general hypothermia, occurs.
- Cold-water swim distance is about one-third of the distance covered in warmer water.[138]

increased lactic acid, and, eventually, metabolic and respiratory acidosis. Oxygenation and blood flow are maintained in the core and brain.

Bradycardia occurs in a large percentage of patients as a direct effect of cold on the depolarization of cardiac pacemaker cells and their slower propagation through the conduction system. It is important to note that the use of atropine, as well as other cardiac medications, is often ineffective to increase the heart rate when the myocardium is cold.[9] When core temperature falls below 86°F (30°C), the myocardium becomes irritable. The PR, QRS, and QTC intervals are prolonged. ST-segment and T-wave changes and J (or Osborn) waves may be present and may mimic other ECG abnormalities, such as an acute myocardial infarction. The J waves are a striking ECG feature in hypothermic patients and are seen in approximately one-third of moderate to severe hypothermia patients (less than 90°F [32.2°C]). The J wave is described as a "humplike" deflection between the QRS complex and the early part of the ST segment.[129,139] The J wave is best viewed in the aVL, aVF, and left precordial leads (**Figure 19-9**).

Atrial fibrillation and extreme bradycardia develop and may continue between 83°F and 90°F (28.3°C to 32.2°C). When the core temperature reaches 80°F to 82°F (26.7°C to 27.8°C), any physical stimulation of the heart can cause ventricular fibrillation (VF). CPR or rough handling (patient assessment and movement) of the patient could be sufficient to cause VF. At these extremely low core temperatures, pulse and blood pressure are not detectable, the joints are stiff, and the pupils become fixed and dilated. Remember, a patient should not be assumed to be dead until he or she is rewarmed and still has no signs of life (ECG, pulse, ventilation, and CNS function).

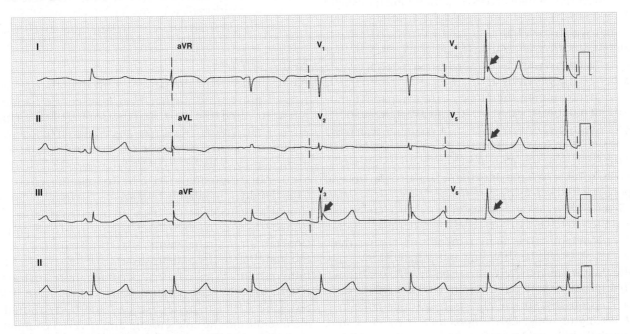

Figure 19-9 Osborn or J wave in hypothermic patient.

From 12-Lead ECG: The Art of Interpretation, courtesy of Tomas B. Garcia, MD.

With acute cold exposure, renal blood flow increases because of the shunting of blood during vasoconstriction. This may result in a phenomenon known as *cold diuresis* in which patients produce more urine and may, as a result, become dehydrated. At 80.6°F to 86°F (27°C to 30°C), renal blood flow is depressed by 50%. At this moderate to severe hypothermic level, the decrease in cardiac output causes a fall in renal blood flow and glomerular filtration rate, which in turn results in acute kidney failure.[129]

Assessment

It is imperative to assess scene safety on arrival. All emergency responders need to maximize their safety and protection from cold exposure while working in this environment. There should be a high suspicion for hypothermia even when the environmental conditions are not highly suggestive (e.g., wind, moisture, temperature).

Protect patients from further cooling, either by carefully moving them to shelter or by insulating them in place from the elements. Doing so prevents further heat loss. Assess the patient's ABCs. Take up to 60 seconds to carefully evaluate the patient's pulse, which may present as very weak or absent in a patient with moderate to severe hypothermia. Some patients who are alert may present with vague complaints of fatigue, lethargy, nausea, and dizziness. Neurologic function is assessed and monitored frequently. Patients with severe hypothermia generally present with bradypnea, stupor, and coma.

To accurately measure hypothermic temperatures, a low-range rectal thermometer is often necessary. However, rectal temperatures are not usually assessed in the field or widely used as a vital sign in most prehospital systems. Ambulances that do have access to a thermometer usually carry a standard-range oral or rectal (for infants) thermometer with a lower limit of 96°F (35.6°C). Electronic thermometers are not useful in hypothermic situations for accurate readings. Tympanic membrane infrared temperature measurement is generally accurate if careful technique is used to assure aiming the probe at the tympanic membrane and not the ear canal, which can affect the reading. In addition, the ear must be clear of cerumen (ear wax) and blood. Therefore, prehospital care providers need to rely on scene size-up, patient mental status, skin vitals, and ABCS. **Table 19-6** provides the anticipated physiologic responses with decreasing core temperature.

Signs of shivering and mental status change are important in the assessment of suspected hypothermia. Patients with mild hypothermia (core temperature greater than 90°F [32.2°C]) will be shivering and usually show signs of altered level of consciousness (e.g., apathy, confusion, slurred speech, altered gait, clumsiness). They will be slow in their actions and are usually found in a nonambulatory state, sitting or lying. Law enforcement personnel and prehospital care providers may misinterpret this condition

as drug or alcohol intoxication or, in geriatric patients, as cerebrovascular accident (stroke). However, a patient's level of consciousness is not a reliable indicator of the degree of hypothermia; some patients have remained conscious at core temperature below 80°F (26.7°C).

When the patient's core temperature falls below 90°F (32.2°C), moderate hypothermia is present, and the patient will probably not complain of feeling cold. Shivering may be absent, and the patient's level of consciousness will be greatly decreased, possibly to the point of unconsciousness. The patient's pupils will react slowly or may be dilated and fixed. The patient's palpable pulses may be diminished or absent, and the patient will have mild to moderate hypotension. The patient's ventilations may have slowed to as few as 2 breaths/minute. An ECG may show atrial fibrillation, the most common dysrhythmia. Other arrhythmias may be present with prolonged PR, QR, and QTC intervals. J (Osborn) waves may be present. As the myocardium becomes progressively colder and more irritable at about 82°F (27.8°C), VF is observed more often.

Because of the changes in cerebral metabolism, evidence of *paradoxical undressing* may be observed before the patient loses consciousness. This is an attempt by the patient to remove the clothing while in the cold environment, and it is thought to represent a response to an impending thermoregulatory failure.

The clinical management of hypothermia is based on the following three ranges of rectal body temperature as presented by the Wilderness Medical Society[129,149]:

- *Mild hypothermia* is above 95°F to below 89.6°F (35°C to 32°C).
- *Moderate hypothermia* is 89.6° to 82.4°F (32°C to 28°C).
- *Severe hypothermia* is below 82.4°F (below 28°C).
- *Profound hypothermia* is below 68°F (below 20°C).

Management

Prehospital care of the patient with hypothermia consists of preventing further heat loss, gentle handling, initiating rapid transport, and rewarming. This includes moving the patient away from any cold source to a warm ambulance or to a warm shelter if transportation is not immediately available (see the Prolonged Transport section). After assessing pulse and finding no signs of life, CPR should immediately be started.[140] Any wet clothing should be removed by cutting with trauma shears to avoid unnecessary movement and agitation of the patient. Concern for initiating ventricular dysrhythmia based on the handling of the patient should not delay any critical interventions. This concern becomes more realistic in severe hypothermia patients (core temperature below 86°F [30°C]). The patient's head and body should be insulated from the cold ground and covered completely with warm blankets or sleeping bags, followed by an

Table 19-6 Characteristics of Hypothermia

Classification	Core Body Temperature	Physiologic Response
Mild hypothermia	95–89.6°F (35–32°C)	Shivering, foot stamping
		Constricted blood vessels
		Increased respiratory rate
		Flat affect
		Dysarthria
		Ataxia
		Cold diuresis
Moderate hypothermia	89.5–82.4°F (32–28°C)	Shivering ceases; progressively weaker and stiffer muscles with loss of coordination
		Slowed respiratory rate
		Slow pulse
		Profound hypoventilation
		Decline in protective airway reflexes
		Oxygen consumption decreases by half
		Confusion
		Lethargy
Severe hypothermia	82.3–75.2°F (28–24°C)	Decrease in minute volume
		Increase in tracheobronchial secretions
		Bronchospasm may occur
		Weak pulse
		Dysrhythmia
		Slow respirations
		Coma
Profound hypothermia	< 75.2°F (< 24°C)	Apparent death
		Cardiac arrest

outer windproof layer to prevent conductive, convective, and evaporative heat loss.

If the patient is conscious and alert, he or she should avoid drinks containing alcohol or caffeine. Anticipate hypoglycemia, and assess the patient's blood glucose level. For the patient with mild hypothermia with normal glucose levels, provide warm, high-caloric or glucose-containing fluids. For patients with moderate hypothermia with low blood glucose concentration, establish IV fluids and administer dextrose IV per local medical protocol, and repeat glucose determination every 5 minutes to determine the need for an additional dextrose bolus.

Hypothermic patients need high-flow oxygen because they have decreased oxygen delivery to the tissues; the oxyhemoglobin dissociation curve shifts to the left with a decrease in core temperature. High-flow oxygen should be delivered using a nonrebreathing mask or bag-mask device. Ideally, the patient may benefit more if the oxygen can be warmed and humidified (108°F to 115°F [42.2°C to 46.1°C]). If possible, warmed oxygen administered before movement may prevent VF during transport.

In unresponsive hypothermic patients, passive rewarming will be insufficient to increase core temperature.

These patients will need an airway adjunct to protect the airway, and this should be initiated depending on jaw rigidity. The prehospital care provider should not hesitate to definitively support the airway since there is a low risk of triggering a fatal dysrhythmia during an advanced airway procedure.[109] If endotracheal intubation cannot be successfully achieved without rough handling, continue ventilation with a bag-mask device, and consider another advanced airway device (e.g., King supraglottic airway, laryngeal mask airway, nasal intubation). At a minimum, use an oral or nasal pharyngeal airway with bag-mask ventilation.

Intravenous NS, ideally with 5% dextrose, should be warmed to 109°F (42.8°C) and administered without agitating the patient. The patient with hypothermia should not be given "cold" (room-temperature) fluids because this could make the patient colder or could delay rewarming. When NS and dextrose solutions are unavailable, any warm crystalloid solution is satisfactory. Provide a fluid challenge of 500 to 1,000 ml, and prevent the solution from freezing or becoming colder by placing the IV bag under the patient to infuse warm fluids under pressure. The rewarming effect of warmed IV fluids is minimal at best, and the prehospital care provider should use good judgment to decide whether fluids (orally or IV) are worth the risks of aspiration, coughing, and painful stimuli to the patient. Hot packs or massaging of the patient's extremities is not recommended.[7]

Typically, active external rewarming occurs only to the thoracic region, with no active rewarming of the extremities. This approach will prevent increased peripheral circulation, which can cause an increased amount of colder blood to return from the extremities to the thorax before central core rewarming. Increased return of peripheral blood can increase acidosis and hyperkalemia and can decrease the core temperature ("afterdrop"). This complicates resuscitation and may precipitate VF.

2015 American Heart Association Guidelines for Cardiopulmonary Resuscitation and Emergency Cardiovascular Care Science

Cardiac Arrest in Special Situations—Accidental Hypothermia

Guidelines for resuscitation of a patient with hypothermia have evolved over many decades. The most recent revision of the emergency cardiovascular care guidelines by the American Heart Association (AHA) were published by the AHA in the journal *Circulation* in 2015. These guidelines did not change those published for cardiac arrest secondary to accidental hypothermia in 2010.[140,141]

The victim with hypothermia can present many challenges to the prehospital care provider, particularly the unconscious patient with moderate to severe hypothermia. Because severe hypothermia is defined by a core temperature of less than 86°F (30°C), the patient can present as clinically dead with no detectable pulse or respiration because of the reduced cardiac output and decreased arterial pressure. Historically, the challenge has been to determine whether to initiate basic life support (BLS) or advanced life support (ALS) interventions on these patients based on the viability of the patient. Furthermore, it may be difficult to determine from bystanders whether these patients had a primary hypothermic exposure or a medical event or traumatic injury that preceded the hypothermia. Other concerns for a prehospital care provider are protecting the hypothermic patient with a potential irritable myocardium from any rough handling and initiating chest compression for the patient with nondetectable pulse, in whom both these interventions may initiate VF.[140]

Independent of any scenario that created the primary or secondary hypothermia, lifesaving procedures should generally not be withheld on the basis of clinical presentation, whether in an urban setting with short transport distances or in the backcountry environment with potentially significant delays in transport, in which scenario, extended patient care may be necessary (see later discussion).

Basic Life Support Guidelines for Treatment of Mild to Severe Hypothermia

Patients with hypothermia should be kept in a horizontal position when possible, and certainly during initial care, to avoid aggravating hypotension and afterdrop.[7] These patients are often volume depleted from cold diuresis. It may be difficult to feel or detect respiration and a pulse in the patient with hypothermia. Therefore, it is recommended initially to assess for breathing and then check for a pulse for up to 60 seconds to confirm one of the following:

- Respiratory arrest
- Pulseless cardiac arrest (asystole, ventricular tachycardia, VF)
- Bradycardia (requiring CPR)

If the patient is not breathing, start rescue breathing immediately unless the victim is obviously dead (e.g., decapitation, rigor mortis). Start chest compressions immediately in any patient with hypothermia who is pulseless and has no detectable signs of circulation.[140] If there is a doubt about detecting a pulse, begin compressions. Never withhold BLS interventions until the patient is rewarmed. If the patient is determined to be in cardiac arrest, use the current BLS guidelines.

An automated external defibrillator (AED) should be used if pulseless ventricular tachycardia or VF is present. The current emergency cardiovascular care guidelines (see

Figure 19-10) recommend that these patients be treated by providing up to five cycles (2 minutes) of CPR (one cycle is 30 compressions to 2 breaths) before checking the ECG rhythm and attempting to shock when an AED arrives.[142] If a shockable rhythm is determined, give one shock, and then continue five cycles of CPR. If the patient with hypothermia does not respond to one shock with a detectable pulse, further attempts to defibrillate the patient should be

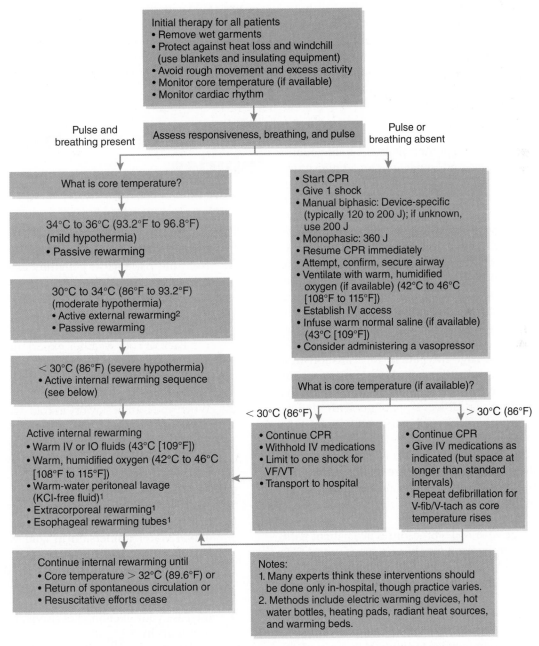

Figure 19-10 Modified from American Heart Association (AHA) hypothermia algorithm from the 2010 Cardiopulmonary Resuscitation and Emergency Cardiovascular Care guidelines. Note: Peritoneal lavage, extracorporeal rewarming, and esophageal rewarming tubes are usually hospital-only procedures.

Data from: American Heart Association: Handbook of Emergency Cardiovascular Care for Healthcare Providers, Chicago, 2006, AHA.

deferred and efforts directed toward effective CPR with an emphasis on rewarming the patient to above 86°F (30°C) before attempting further defibrillation.[142]

When performing chest compressions in a patient with hypothermia, a greater force is required because chest wall elasticity is decreased when cold.[143] If core temperature is below 86°F (30°C), the conversion to normal sinus rhythm does not normally occur until rewarming above this core temperature is accomplished.[144]

The importance of not declaring a patient dead until the patient has been rewarmed and remains unresponsive cannot be overemphasized. Studies of victims of hypothermia indicate that cold exerts a protective effect on the vital organs.[144,145]

Advanced Cardiac Life Support Guidelines for Treatment of Hypothermia

The treatment of severe hypothermia in the field remains controversial.[140] However, the guidelines for administering advanced cardiovascular life support (ACLS) procedures are different from those with a normothermic patient. Unconscious patients with hypothermia need a protected airway and should be intubated. Do not delay airway management based on the concern of initiating VF. As noted earlier, if a shockable rhythm is detected, defibrillate once at 120 to 200 biphasic joules or 360 monophasic joules, resume CPR, and then defer cardiac drugs and subsequent defibrillation attempts until core temperature is above 86°F (30°C). If possible, initiate active rewarming procedures with warm, humidified oxygen and warm IV solutions, and package the patient for transport in a way that will prevent further heat loss. It is important to note that passive rewarming is adequate for patients with mild hypothermia. However, patients with moderate to severe hypothermia need active rewarming that is generally limited to procedures performed in an ED, operating room, or critical care unit. Passive rewarming procedures alone for these patients are totally inadequate to increase core temperature in the prehospital setting, and EMS personnel should focus on effective techniques in preventing further heat loss.[15]

The challenge with ACLS procedures in a patient with hypothermia is that the heart may be unresponsive to ACLS drugs, pacing, and defibrillation.[146] Furthermore, ACLS drugs (e.g., epinephrine, amiodarone, lidocaine, procainamide) can accumulate to toxic levels in the circulation with repeated administration in the patient with severe hypothermia, particularly when the patient rewarms.[140] Consequently, it is recommended to withhold IV medications in patients with a core temperature below 86°F (30°C). If

a patient with hypothermia initially presents with a core temperature above 86°F (30°C), or if a patient with severe hypothermia has been rewarmed above this temperature, IV medications may be administered. However, longer intervals between drug administration are recommended than with standard drug intervals in ACLS.[140] The use of repeated defibrillation is indicated if the core temperature continues to rise above 86°F (30°C), consistent with the current ACLS guidelines.[142]

Finally, BLS/ACLS procedures performed in the field should be withheld only if the patient's injuries are incompatible with life, if the body is frozen such that chest compressions are impossible, or if the mouth and nose are blocked with ice.[15,140] Figure 19-10 provides an algorithm of mild, moderate, and severe hypothermia guidelines for both patients with a pulse and pulseless patients.[119]

Prevention of Cold-Related Injuries

The prevention of cold injuries in patients, yourself, and other prehospital care providers is vital when on the scene. Recommendations to prevent cold-related injuries include the following:

1. Note the risk factors generally associated with cold injury:
   - Fatigue
   - Dehydration
   - Undernutrition
   - Lack of cold weather experience
   - African ancestry
   - Tobacco use
   - Windchill
2. When you cannot stay dry in cold, wet, and windy conditions, seek shelter as soon as possible.
3. Remember that individuals with a history of cold injury are at a greater risk of a subsequent cold injury.
4. Avoid dehydration.
5. Avoid alcohol in cold environments.
6. Use the huddle technique with others if accidental water immersion in cold water occurs. You are more likely to survive if you remain still in cold water less than 68°F (20°C) and do not attempt to swim to shore unless it is nearby (< 45 minutes away).
7. Increase your likelihood of survival in cold environments by:
   - Maintaining a will to survive
   - Being adaptable and improvising

- Staying optimistic and believing that the event is only a temporary situation
- Maintaining a calm outlook and even a sense of humor

8. Use body heat to warm extremities that are cold or nearly frozen by placing fingers in the armpits or groin area. Toes and feet can be placed on another person's stomach.

9. Keep protective cold weather clothing (e.g., boots, socks, gloves, winter hat, insulated pants and jacket, windproof outer shell) in your car for unexpected car emergencies during cold weather months. Avoid clothing that absorbs moisture, as wet clothing will exacerbate heat loss (e.g., use wool or fleece).

10. Always wear gloves. Frostbite can occur rapidly when touching metal objects in the cold with your bare hands. Mittens are more effective than gloves at trapping warm air around all fingers.

11. Understand that the windchill index (**Figure 19-11**) is composed of wind speed and air temperature,

and dress for extreme cold with insulated clothing and a windproof garment.

12. Keep feet dry with socks that transfer moisture from your feet to footwear.

13. Do not walk through snow with low-cut shoes. If you lack appropriate shoes and protective clothes, attempt to stay in a protected area.

14. Do not lie or rest directly on snow. Insulate with tree boughs, a sleeping pad, a poncho, or any material available. Use a sleeping bag outdoors.

15. Do not wear clothing that will absorb and retain sweat; any sweat retained in your clothes will increase heat loss and cause shivering.

16. When using lotion, use oil-based products (e.g., ChapStick, Vaseline). Water-based lotions on the face, hands, and ears will increase the risk for frostnip and frostbite.

17. When protecting the lower extremities from cold weather, be sure to protect the genital region. Use sweatpants, long underwear, Lycra tights, Gore-Tex pants, or any combination of these garments.

Wind Chill Chart

Temperature (°F)

Calm	40	35	30	25	20	15	10	5	0	−5	−10	−15	−20	−25	−30	−35	−40	−45
5	36	31	25	19	13	7	1	−5	−11	−16	−22	−28	−34	−40	−46	−52	−57	−63
10	34	27	21	15	9	3	−4	−10	−16	−22	28	−35	−41	−47	−53	−59	−66	−72
15	32	25	19	13	6	0	−7	−13	−19	−26	−32	−39	−45	−51	−58	−64	−71	−77
20	30	24	17	11	4	−2	−9	−15	−22	−29	−35	−42	−48	−55	−61	−68	−74	−81
25	29	23	16	9	3	−4	−11	−17	−24	−31	−37	−44	−51	−58	−64	−71	−78	−84
30	28	22	15	8	1	−5	−12	−19	−26	−33	−39	−46	−53	−60	−67	−73	−80	−87
35	28	21	14	7	0	−7	−14	−21	−27	−34	−41	−48	−55	−62	−69	−76	−82	−89
40	27	20	13	6	−1	−8	−15	−22	−29	−36	−43	−50	−57	−64	−71	−78	−84	−91
45	26	19	12	5	−2	−9	−16	−23	−30	−37	−44	−51	−58	−65	−72	−79	−86	−93
50	26	19	12	4	−3	−10	−17	−24	−31	−38	−45	−52	−60	−67	−74	−81	−88	−95
55	25	18	11	4	−3	−11	−18	−25	−32	−39	−46	−54	−61	−68	−75	−82	−89	−97
60	25	17	10	3	−4	−11	−19	−26	−33	−40	−48	−55	−62	−69	−76	−84	−91	−98

Wind (MPH)

Frostbite Times: ☐ 30 minutes ☐ 10 minutes ■ 5 minutes

Wind Chill (°F) = 35.74 $0.6215T - 35.75(V^{0.16}) + 0.4275T(V^{0.16})$
Where, T = Air temperature (°F) and V = Wind speed (mph)

Figure 19-11 Windchill index.
Courtesy National Weather Service.

18. To prevent frostbite:
- Do not wear tight clothing, gloves, or boots that restrict circulation.
- Exercise fingers, toes, and face periodically to keep them warm and to detect numb areas.
- Work or exercise with a partner, who watches for warning signs of cold injury and hypothermia.
- Wear properly insulated clothing, and keep it dry; always carry extra undergarments, socks, and shoes.
- Watch for numbness and tingling.[147]

Prolonged Transport

At times, the location of a patient will result in a delay in transport or a prolonged transport to an appropriate facility, necessitating extended prehospital care. Consequently, providers may need to consider management options beyond what would be used with a rapid transport. How the patient is managed will depend on the time to definitive care, approved medical protocols, equipment and supplies on hand, additional personnel and resources, and location of the patient and severity of the injuries.

Some extended care considerations for moderately to severely injured patients from each of the environments discussed in this chapter are provided here. As with all patient care, it is understood that the first priorities are scene safety, XABCDEs (exsanguinating hemorrhage, airway, breathing, circulation, disability, expose/environment), and the use of standard assessment and management procedures appropriate to these environments. Specific attention must be paid to removal of the environmental stress (heat or cold). If medical control is available, always obtain a consult early, and communicate routinely throughout the extended care period. Any of the procedures listed that fall outside an individual's scope of practice are to be used only by other, credentialed medical providers.

It is important to know that all agencies have established guidelines for discontinuation of CPR. The AHA published a discussion on the ethical issues arising from withholding or withdrawing BLS or ALS resuscitation efforts.[142] The Wilderness Medical Society recommends that once CPR is initiated, it should be continued until resuscitation is successful with an awake patient, until rescuers are exhausted, until rescuers are placed in danger, until the patient is turned over to more definitive care, or until the patient does not respond to prolonged (30 minutes) resuscitative efforts.[148] The National Association of EMS Physicians also provides guidelines for the termination of CPR in the out-of-hospital environment (see the Patient Assessment and Management chapter).[149] If medical control is available, begin patient consult early, if possible, for consideration of CPR termination after a total time of 20 minutes, depending on special patient circumstances (see the Environmental Trauma II: Drowning, Lightning, Diving, and Altitude chapter for additional situations [e.g., cold water submersion, lightning strike] in which CPR may be extended longer than 20 to 30 minutes).[149]

Heat-Related Illness

Heatstroke

Provide whole-body cooling as quickly as possible. Consider using any available access to water. Immerse the body to neck level in cool water (maintain body control and protect the airway), or spray the whole body with water (e.g., IV fluids, saline, water bottles, water from hydration backpacks), and provide a source of continuous wind current (e.g., natural wind current, fanning with towel, fire ventilation fans). When possible, stay in contact with medical control to keep them informed of the patient's status and to receive further medical directions. Stop body cooling when rectal temperature reaches 102°F (38.9°C). Then protect the patient from shivering and hypothermia. If an athletic trainer has already instituted treatment with an ice bath prior to EMS arrival, consider continuation of the ice bath until the patient's rectal temperature reaches 102°F (38.9°C), and advise medical control of the situation.

As you are cooling the patient, manage the airway in unresponsive patients, and initiate good ventilation with a bag-mask device with high-flow oxygen. Insert an IV line, provide a 500-ml NS fluid challenge, and assess vital signs. Patients should have vital signs assessed after every 500 ml. Total fluid volume should not exceed 1 to 2 liters in the first hour. An additional liter can be considered during the second hour if prehospital care is extended.

The next priorities are to manage any seizure activity and hypoglycemia per medical protocol with diazepam and dextrose, respectively. Place the patient in the recovery position, and continue the assessment to include level of consciousness, vital signs, rectal temperature, and blood glucose. Provide supportive care and basic bodily needs throughout the remaining extended care period.

Exercise-Associated Hyponatremia

Correct the presumed low blood sodium concentration. If the patient can take food by mouth and if such food is available, provide potato chips, pretzels, or other salty food or a sport electrolyte or other sodium-containing beverage. An oral sodium solution has been demonstrated to be an appropriate hypertonic saline treatment.[150] In the field, this solution could be prepared by dissolving three to four bouillon cubes in a half cup of water (125 ml) (~9% saline). Salt tablets given alone are not recommended; additional fluid must accompany the tablets, and there is the risk of increasing sodium levels too much.

Next, establish an IV line and start NS with a flow rate set to KVO. Check with medical control to consider a flow rate of 250 or greater ml/hour based on the estimated delay in transporting the patient to the hospital or the presence of severe dehydration or **rhabdomyolysis**. Do not use hypotonic IV fluids because they will exacerbate cerebral edema and could potentiate the condition, leading to seizure, coma, and death. In a patient with severe signs or symptoms (seizure or coma), consider administration of furosemide (a diuretic, if available) to reduce extracellular body water content while providing some sodium by infusing NS, 250 to 500 ml/hour IV.

Assess cerebral edema and increased intracranial pressure. Establish a baseline Glasgow Coma Scale score, and reassess every 10 minutes as an indicator of progressive cerebral edema and increased intracranial pressure (manage per recommendations for cerebral edema; see the Head Trauma chapter).

Be prepared to manage nausea and projectile vomiting. Take one side of a large trash bag and make a hole for the patient's head about 12 inches (30 centimeters) below the rim of the bag. Place the patient's head through the hole so that the patient can look down into the center of the bag. Also be prepared to manage urine when diuresis begins. Use a large trash bag as a diaper or use a bucket or other container.

Give supplemental oxygen (2 to 4 liters/minute by nasal cannula) if the patient shows signs of pulmonary distress or for lethargic or obtunded patients. Manage the airway of unresponsive patients, and initiate good ventilation with a bag-mask device (no hyperventilation; see the Head Trauma chapter), with oxygen at 10 breaths/minute.

Assess the patient's blood glucose level, and provide IV dextrose per protocol to hypoglycemic patients. Monitor for seizures, and administer an anticonvulsant (e.g., diazepam, initially 2 to 5 mg IV/intramuscular, and titrate per medical protocol). Place unconscious patients in a left lateral recumbent position. Continue ongoing assessment of the patient.

Cold-Related Illness

Frostbite

Protect and treat the patient for hypothermia, if present. Start IV fluid hydration, or at least establish an IV, before initiation of rewarming procedures. If a vein cannot be accessed, the intraosseous route is an alternative. In a situation of significant transport delay, active rewarming should be considered. Rapid, active rewarming can reverse the direct injury of ice crystals in tissues, but it may not change the injury severity. It is critical to keep the thawed tissue from refreezing because this significantly worsens the outcome compared with passive thawing. When and where to begin active rewarming are key considerations, if active rewarming is to be done at all.

A standard rewarming procedure is to immerse the affected extremity in circulating water warmed to a temperature between 98.6°F and 102.2°F (37°C and 39°C) in a large enough container to accommodate the frostbitten tissues without their touching the sides or bottom of the container.[102,103] Water should feel warm, but not hot, to the normal hand. (Note that the temperature range given here is lower than that previously recommended; this temperature range decreases pain for the patient while only slightly slowing the rewarming phase.) If available, an oral or rectal thermometer should be used to measure water temperature. A temperature below that recommended will thaw tissue but is less beneficial for rapid thawing and for tissue survival. Any greater temperature will cause greater pain and may cause a burn injury. Do not rewarm with intense sources of dry heat (e.g., placing near campfire). Continue immersion until tissue is soft and pliable, which may take up to 30 to 60 minutes. Active motion of the extremity during immersion is beneficial, without direct rubbing or massaging of the affected part. If immersion warming is not available, the affected parts may be wrapped in loose, bulky sterile dressings with sterile cotton gauze placed between fingers or toes to avoid further tissue damage. Blisters should not be ruptured.[104]

Extreme pain is experienced during rapid thawing. Treat with IV analgesics and titrate as needed and based on local protocols. (Aspirin is contraindicated in pediatric patients because of the risk of Reye's syndrome.)

The return of normal skin color, warmth, and sensation in the affected part are all favorable signs. Dry all affected parts with warm air (do not towel dry affected parts), and ideally, apply topical aloe vera on skin, place sterile gauze between toes or fingers, bandage, splint, and elevate the extremity. Cover any extremity with insulating material, and wrap a windproof and waterproof material (e.g., trash bag) as the outer layer, particularly if continuing patient extraction outdoors to a transport location.

Hypothermia

Start active rewarming procedures. The key point is to prevent further heat loss by insulating from the environment and removing wet clothing, replacing with dry. Administer heated IV fluids (104°F to 107.6°F [40°C to 42°C]).

Shivering is the single best way for rewarming patients with mild hypothermia in the prehospital setting compared with external methods of rewarming. Patients with hypothermia who are able to shiver maximally can increase their core temperature by up to 6°F to 8°F (~3°C to 4°C) per hour. External heat sources are often used but may provide only minimal benefit.[91] For the patient with moderate to severe hypothermia, these heat sources remain important considerations in the extended-care situation when used in combination with the hypothermia insulation wrap (described later). Some considerations regarding external heat sources include the following:

- Warmed (maximum 108°F [42.2°C]), humidified oxygen by mask can prevent heat loss during ventilation and provide some heat transfer to the chest from the respiratory tract.
- Body-to-body contact has merit for heat transfer, but many studies fail to show any advantage except in patients with mild hypothermia.
- Electric and portable heating pads provide no additional advantage.
- Forced-air warming has some benefit in minimizing postcooling core temperature ("afterdrop"); it provides an effective warming rate comparable to shivering for patients with mild hypothermia.

Insulate all patients with hypothermia in the remote setting to minimize heat loss. Prepare a multilayer hypothermia wrap. Place a large, waterproof plastic sheet on the floor or ground. Add an insulation layer of a sleeping pad, blankets, or a sleeping bag on top of the waterproof layer. Lay the patient on top of the insulation layer along with any external heat sources. Add a second insulating layer on top of the patient. The left side of the hypothermia wrap is folded over the patient first, then the right side. The patient's head is covered to prevent heat loss, keeping an opening at the face to allow patient assessment.[19,151]

Assess the patient for hypoglycemia. Providing dextrose will ensure that adequate fuel (sugar) is available for muscular metabolism during shivering and will prevent further hypoglycemia. Alert patients can consume warm, sugary fluids by mouth.

SUMMARY

- Prehospital care providers will inevitably be faced with environmental encounters such as those described in this chapter.
- To provide rapid assessment and treatment in the prehospital setting, providers must possess basic knowledge of common environmental emergencies. They must also understand how the body regulates temperature, including the role of the skin and the thermoregulatory mechanisms in the brain.
- Methods to maintain and dissipate body heat are important concepts for prehospital care providers. Providers must understand how both heat and cold are transferred to and from the body (i.e., radiation, conduction, convection, evaporation) so that they can effectively manage a patient who has hyperthermia or hypothermia.
- For heat-related illness, providers should treat patients with heatstroke with effective, rapid, whole-body cooling to reduce core temperature quickly.
- For cold-related illness, providers should manage all patients with moderate to severe hypothermia

gently, taking the time to remove them from the cold environment, and begin passive rewarming while monitoring core temperature. The key is to prevent further body heat loss.
- Providers must remember that drugs and defibrillation are generally ineffective when core temperature is less than 86°F (30°C).
- Patients are not dead until they are warm and dead, unless signs are present of obvious futility of resuscitation (e.g., frozen chest, decapitation, ice in airway).
- Providers must know how to protect themselves from heat- and cold-related injuries and how to advocate for the safety of others. Important prevention concepts include hydration, physical fitness, heat acclimatization, adequate clothing for cold weather, and avoidance of risk factors.
- Remember that you must maintain your own safety to be an effective rescuer. In too many cases, providers have lost their lives while attempting a rescue.

SCENARIO RECAP

It is a hot summer afternoon with temperatures reaching 102°F (38.9°C). Over the past 30 days, it has been very humid, with temperatures reaching over 100°F (37.8°C) daily. The ambient temperature has resulted in many heat-related injuries that have required EMS personnel to transport numerous patients to the EDs of the inner city.

At 1700 hours, your ambulance unit responds to a dispatch for an unresponsive male patient in a vehicle. As your ambulance unit arrives on scene, you observe a 76-year-old man who appears to be unconscious in a vehicle parked outside of a department store. Your rapid assessment of the patient's ABCs and level of consciousness reveals that the patient is verbal, but he is saying things that are illogical and irrational.

· What are the potential causes for this patient's decreased level of consciousness?
· What hallmark signs support a heat-related diagnosis?
· How would you emergently manage this patient at the scene and en route to the ED?

SCENARIO SOLUTION

This 76-year-old man has been waiting in his car for his spouse to return from the shopping center. He has been exposed to high heat without effective hydration to offset fluid loss (sweat) and is dehydrated. The patient has a body mass index over 30, placing him at greater risk of heat-related illness because of obesity.

On the wife's return, she provided additional history indicating that he is taking a diuretic for hypertension, a beta-blocker for coronary heart disease, and an anticholinergic for Parkinson disease. All three medications are known risk factors for heat-related illness. This patient needs quick assessment of his ABCs and level of consciousness using the AVPU (**a**lert, responds to **v**erbal stimulus, responds to **p**ainful stimulus, **u**nresponsive) scale, as he was found in a non-air-conditioned car. Due to his irrational and illogical verbal statements, his age, and the location, you have a high suspicion for heatstroke.

You rapidly assess for blunt or penetrating trauma and find none. Next, geriatric patients must be assessed for exacerbation of any underlying medical disease, such as cardiac disease or a neurologic disorder (e.g., stroke). All three of his medical conditions are known to be made worse with hyperthermia, thereby increasing his mortality risk. It is essential that this patient receive whole-body cooling immediately.

You move the patient out of the direct sunlight on the front seat and remove any excess clothing. You use the saline water bottles from the trauma bag to begin wetting him down from his head to toes. You have your partner start the fan and place the air conditioning on high to increase airflow across the patient's body to increase convective heat transfer. The stretcher is readied to transfer the patient to the ambulance. Ice water and cool moist towels are readied in the back of the ambulance for this patient with hyperthermia.

You quickly transfer the patient from his vehicle to the ambulance. As transport is initiated, the patient's whole body is wetted down with cold wet towels, and the overhead fans are directed at the patient. The patient is placed on high-flow oxygen, ECG is monitored, and an IV is established at a KVO rate initially. You are prepared to evaluate rectal temperature to confirm hyperthermia (greater than or equal to 104°F [40°C]). If confirmed, you will provide a 500-ml saline IV bolus. You take a set of vital signs and inform medical control to prepare for a 76-year-old male patient with heatstroke.

References

1. Centers for Disease Control and Prevention/National Center for Health Statistics. Compressed mortality file. https://www.cdc.gov/nchs/data_access/cmf.htm. Updated February 21, 2017. Accessed November 13, 2017.

2. Centers for Disease Control and Prevention. Heat-related deaths—Chicago, Illinois, 1996–2001, and United States, 1979–1999. *Morb Mortal Wkly Rep.* 2003;52(26):610.

3. National Center for Environmental Health (NCEH)/Agency for Toxic Substances and Disease Registry (ATSDR), Coordinating Center for Environmental Health and Injury Prevention (CCEHIP). Natural disasters and severe weather: extreme heat. https://www.cdc.gov/disasters/extremeheat/index.html. Updated June 19, 2017. Accessed November 13, 2017.

4. Meiman J, Anderson H, Tomasallo C. Hypothermia-related deaths—Wisconsin, 2014, and United States, 2003-2013. *Morb Mortal Wkly Rep.* 2015;64(6):141-143.

5. Centers for Disease Control and Prevention. Hypothermia-related deaths—United States, 2003. *Morb Mortal Wkly Rep.* 2004;53(8);172.

6. O'Brien KK, Leon LR, Kenefick RW. Clinical management of heat-related illnesses. In: Auerbach PS, ed. *Auerbach's Wilderness Medicine.* 7th ed. St. Louis, MO: Mosby Elsevier; 2017.

7. Zafren K, Giesbrecht GG, Danzl DF, et al. Wilderness Medical Society practice guidelines for the out-of-hospital evaluation and treatment of accidental hypothermia. *Wilderness Environ Med.* 2014;25:s66-s85.

8. Lugo-Amador NM, Rothenhaus T, Moyer P. Heat-related illness. *Emerg Med Clin North Am.* 2004;22:315.

9. Ulrich AS, Rathlev NK. Hypothermia and localized injuries. *Emerg Med Clin North Am.* 2004;22:281.

10. Centers for Disease Control and Prevention. Hypothermia-related deaths—United States, 2003. *Morb Mortal Wkly Rep.* 2004;53(8):172.

11. Brown DJA, Brugger H, Boyd J, et al. Accidental hypothermia. *N Engl J Med.* 2012;367(20);1930.

12. Hawkins SC. Wilderness EMS systems. In: Hawkins SC, ed. *Wilderness EMS.* Philadelphia, PA: Wolters Kluwer; 2018.

13. Leon LR, Kenefick RW. Pathophysiology of heat-related illnesses. In: Auerbach PS, ed. *Auerbach's Wilderness Medicine.* 7th ed. St. Louis, MO: Mosby Elsevier; 2017.

14. Freer L, Handford C, Imray CHE. Frostbite. In: Auerbach PS, ed. *Auerbach's Wilderness Medicine.* 7th ed. St. Louis, MO: Mosby Elsevier; 2017.

15. Danzl DF, Huecker MR. Accidental hypothermia. In: Auerbach PS, ed. *Auerbach's Wilderness Medicine.* 7th ed. St. Louis, MO: Mosby Elsevier; 2017.

16. National Aeronautics and Space Administration. NASA, NOAA data show 2016 warmest year on record globally. https://www.nasa.gov/press-release/nasa-noaa-data-show-2016-warmest-year-on-record-globally. Published January 18, 2017. Accessed September 19, 2017.

17. Centers for Disease Control and Prevention. Heat-related deaths—United States, 1999–2003. *Morb Mortal Wkly Rep.* 2006;55(29):796.

18. Centers for Disease Control and Prevention. Hypothermia-related deaths—United States, 1999–2002 and 2005. *Morb Mortal Wkly Rep.* 2006;55(10):282-284.

19. Hawkins SC, Simon RB, Beissinger JP, Simon D. *Vertical Aid: Essential Wilderness Medicine for Climbers, Trekkers, and Mountaineers.* New York, NY: The Countryman Press; 2017.

20. Hardy JD. Thermal comfort: skin temperature and physiological thermoregulation. In: Hardy JD, Gagge AP, Stolwijk JAJ, eds. *Physiological and Behavioral Temperature Regulation.* Springfield, IL: Charles C. Thomas; 1970.

21. Pozos RS, Danzl DF. Human physiological responses to cold stress and hypothermia. In: Pandolf KB, Burr RE, eds. *Medical Aspects of Harsh Environments.* Vol 1. Washington, DC: Office of the Surgeon General, Borden Institute/TMM Publications; 2001:351-382.

22. Stocks JM, Taylor NAS, Tipton MJ, Greenleaf JE. Human physiological responses to cold exposure. *Aviat Space Environ Med.* 2004;75:444.

23. Wenger CB. The regulation of body temperature. In: Rhoades RA, Tanner GA, eds. *Medical Physiology.* Boston, MA: Little, Brown; 1995.

24. Nunnelely SA, Reardon MJ. Prevention of heat illness. In: Pandolf KB, Burr RE, eds. *Medical Aspects of Harsh Environments.* Vol 1. Washington, DC: Office of the Surgeon General, Borden Institute/TMM Publications; 2001:209-230.

25. Hall B, Hall J. *Sauer's Manual of Skin Diseases.* 10th ed. Philadelphia, PA: Lippincott Williams & Wilkins; 2010.

26. Krakowski A, Goldenberg A. Exposure to radiation from the sun. In: Auerbach PS, ed. *Auerbach's Wilderness Medicine.* 7th ed. Philadelphia, PA: Mosby Elsevier; 2017.

27. Lipman GS, Eifling KP, Ellis MA, Gaudio FG, Otten EM, Grissom CK. Wilderness Medical Society practice guidelines for the prevention and treatment of heat-related illness: 2014 update. *Wilderness Environ Med.* 2014;25:S55-S65.

28. Yeo T. Heat stroke: a comprehensive review. *AACN Clin Issues.* 2004;15:280.

29. Wenger CB. Section I: human adaption to hot environments. In: Pandolf KB, Burr RE, eds. *Medical Aspects of Harsh Environments.* Vol 1. Washington, DC: Office of the Surgeon General, Borden Institute/TMM Publications; 2001:51-86.

30. Sonna LA. Practical medical aspects of military operations in the heat. In: Pandolf KB, Burr RE, eds. *Medical Aspects of Harsh Environments.* Vol 1. Washington, DC: Office of the Surgeon General, Borden Institute/TMM Publications; 2001: 293-309.

31. Tek D, Olshaker JS. Heat illness. *Emerg Med Clin North Am.* 1992;10(2):299.

32. Wallace RF, Kriebel D, Punnett L, et al. The effects of continuous hot weather training on risk of exertional heat illness. *Med Sci Sports Exerc.* 2005;37(1):84-90.

33. Schimelpfenig T, Richards G, Tartar S. Management of heat illnesses. In: Hawkins SC, ed. *Wilderness EMS.* Philadelphia, PA: Wolters Kluwer; 2018.

34. Bedno SA, Li Y, Han W, et al. Exertional heat illness among over-weight U.S. Army recruits in basic training. *Aviat Space Environ Med.* 2010;81(2):107-111.

35. Kenefick RW, Cheuvront SN, Leon LR, O'Brien KK. Dehydration and rehydration. In: Auerbach PS, ed. *Auerbach's Wilderness Medicine.* 7th ed. Philadelphia, PA: Mosby Elsevier; 2017.

36. Armstrong LE, Hubbard RW, Jones BH, Daniels JT. Preparing Alberto Salazar for the heat of the 1984 Olympic marathon. *Phys Sportsmed*. 1986;14:73.

37. Johnson RF, Kobrick JL. Psychological aspects of military performance in hot environments. In: Pandolf KB, Burr RE, eds. *Medical Aspects of Harsh Environments*. Vol 1. Washington, DC: Office of the Surgeon General, Borden Institute/TMM Publications; 2001.

38. Sawka MN, Pandolf KB. Physical exercise in hot climates: physiology, performance, and biomedical issues. In: Pandolf KB, Burr RE, eds. *Medical Aspects of Harsh Environments*. Vol 1. Washington, DC: Office of the Surgeon General, Borden Institute/TMM Publications; 2001.

39. Dutchman SM, Ryan AJ, Schedl HP, et al. Upper limits of intestinal absorption of dilute glucose solution in men at rest. *Med Sci Sport Exerc*. 1997;29:482.

40. Neufer PD, Young AJ, Sawka MN. Gastric emptying during exercise: effects of heat stress and hypohydration. *Eur J Appl Physiol*. 1989;58:433.

41. Bouchama A, Knochel JP. Medical progress: heatstroke. *N Engl J Med*. 2002;346(25):1978-1988.

42. Adams T, Stacey E, Stacey S, Martin D. Exertional heat stroke. *Br J Hosp Med (London)*. 2012;73(2):72-78.

43. Case DJ, Armstrong LE, Kenny GP, O'Connor FG, Huggins RA. Exertional heat stroke: new concepts regarding cause and care. *Curr Sports Med Rep*. 2012;11(3):115-123.

44. Casa DJ, McDermott BP, Lee E, Yeargin SW, Armstrong LE, Maresh CM. Cold-water immersion: the gold standard for exertional heat stroke treatment. *Exerc Sport Rev*. 2007;35(3):141-149.

45. Holtzhausen LM, Noakes TD. Collapsed ultra-endurance athlete: proposed mechanisms and an approach to management. *Clin J Sport Med*. 1997;7(4):292.

46. Gardner JW, Kark JA. Clinical diagnosis, management and surveillance of exertional heat illness. In: Pandolf KB, Burr RE, eds. *Medical Aspects of Harsh Environments*. Vol 1. Washington, DC: Office of the Surgeon General, Borden Institute/TMM Publications; 2001:231-279.

47. Asplune CA, O'Connor FG, Noakes TD. Exercise-associated collapse: an evidence-based review and primer for clinicians. *Br J Sports Med*. 2011;45:1157-1162.

48. Nichols AW. Heat-related illness in sports and exercise. *Curr Rev Musculoskelet Med*. 2014;7:355-365.

49. Bennett BL, Hew-Butler T, Hoffman MD, Rogers IR, Rosner MH. Wilderness Medical Society practice guidelines for treatment of exercise-associated hyponatremia: 2014 update. *Wilderness Environ Med*. 2014;25:s30-s42.

50. Rosner MH. Exercise-associated hyponatremia. *Semin Nephrol*. 2009;29(3):271-281.

51. Rosner M, Bennett B, Hoffman M, Hew-Butler T. Exercise induced hyponatremia. In: Simon E, ed. *Hyponatremia: Evaluation and Treatment*. New York, NY: Springer; 2013.

52. Leon LR, Helwig BG. Heat stroke: role of the systemic inflammatory response. *J Appl Physiol*. 2010;109(6):1980-1988.

53. Gaffin SL, Hubbard RW. Pathophysiology of heatstroke. In: Pandolf KB, Burr RE, eds. *Medical Aspects of Harsh Environments*. Vol 1. Washington, DC: Office of the Surgeon General, Borden Institute/TMM Publications; 2001:161-208.

54. Semenza JC, Rubin CH, Flater KH, et al. Heat-related deaths during the July 1995 heat wave in Chicago. *N Engl J Med*. 1996;335(2):84.

55. Knochel JP, Reed G. Disorders of heat regulation. In: Narins RE, ed. *Maxwell and Kleenman's Clinical Disorders of Fluid and Electrolyte Metabolism*. 5th ed. New York, NY: McGraw-Hill; 1994.

56. Hawkins SC. Environmental emergencies. In: Pollak AN, ed. *Caroline's Emergency Care in the Streets*. 8th ed. Burlington, MA: Jones & Bartlett Learning; 2018.

57. Armstrong LE, Crago AE, Adams R, et al. Whole-body cooling of hyperthermic runners: comparison of two field therapies. *Am J Emerg Med*. 1996;14:335.

58. Costrini A. Emergency treatment of exertional heatstroke and comparison of whole-body cooling techniques. *Med Sci Sports Exerc*. 1984;22:15.

59. Gaffin SL, Gardner J, Flinn S. Current cooling method for exertional heatstroke. *Ann Intern Med*. 2000;132:678.

60. Speedy DB, Noakes TD. Exercise-associated hyponatremia: a review. *Emerg Med*. 2001;13:17.

61. Backer HD, Shopes E, Collins SL, Barkan H. Exertional heat illness and hyponatremia in hikers. *Am J Emerg Med*. 1999;17(6):532.

62. Gardner JW. Death by water intoxication. *Mil Med*. 2002;164(3):432.

63. Noakes TD, Goodwin N, Rayner BL, et al. Water intoxication: a possible complication during endurance exercise. *Med Sci Sports Exerc*. 1985;17:370.

64. Rosner MH, Kirven J. Exercise-associated hyponatremia. *Clin J Am Soc Nephrol*. 2007;2:151.

65. Adrogue HJ, Madias NE. Hyponatremia. *N Engl J Med*. 2000;342(21):1581.

66. Hiller WDB. Dehydration and hyponatremia during triathlons. *Med Sci Sports Exerc*. 1989;21:S219.

67. Speedy DB, Noakes TD, Rodgers IR. Hyponatremia in ultra-distance triathletes. *Med Sci Sports Exerc*. 1999;31:809.

68. Laird RH. Medical care at ultra-endurance triathlons. *Med Sci Sports Exerc*. 1989;21:S222.

69. Collins S, Reynolds B. The other heat-related emergency. *JEMS*. 2004;29(7):74-88.

70. Backer HD, Shopes E, Collins SL, Barkan H. Exertional heat illness and hyponatremia in hikers. *Am J Emerg Med*. 1999;17:532-539.

71. Noe RS, Choudhary E, Cheng-Dobson J, Wolkin AF, Newman SB. Exertional heat-related illnesses at the Grand Canyon National Park, 2004–2009. *Wilderness Environ Med*. 2013;24:422-428.

72. American College of Sports Medicine. Position stand on exercise and fluid replacement. *Med Sci Sports Exerc*. 2007;39(2):377.

73. Bennett BL, Hew-Butler T, Hoffman M, Rogers I, Rosner M. Wilderness Medicine Society practice guidelines for treatment of exercise-associated hyponatremia. *Wilderness Environ Med*. 2013;24(3):228-240.

74. Hew-Butler T, Ayus JC, Kipps C, et al. Statement of Second International Exercise-Associated Hyponatremia Consensus Development Conference, New Zealand, 2007. *Clin J Sport Med*. 2008;18:111.

75. Ayus JC, Arieff A, Moritz ML. Hyponatremia in marathon runners. *N Engl J Med*. 2005;353:427.

76. U.S. Fire Administration. Firefighter fatalities in the United States in 2015. Federal Emergency Management Agency. https://www.usfa.fema.gov/downloads/pdf/publications /ff_fat15.pdf. Published October 2016. Accessed November 14, 2017.

77. U.S. Department of Agriculture, U.S. Forest Service. Heat stress brochure. http://www.fs.fed.us/fire/safety/fitness /heat_stress/hs_pg1.html. Accessed November 15, 2017.

78. Brazaitis M, Skurvydas A. Heat acclimation does not reduce the impact of hyperthermia on central fatigue. *Eur J Appl Physiol.* 2010;109:771-778.

79. Cheung SS, McLellan TM. Heat acclimation, aerobic fitness, and hydration effects on tolerance during uncompensable heat stress. *J Appl Physiol.* 1998;84:1731-1739.

80. Garrett AT, Goosens NG, Rehrer NJ, Patterson MJ, Cotter JD. Induction and decay of short-term heat acclimation. *Eur J Appl Physiol.* 2009;107:659-670.

81. Montain SJ, Latzka WA, Sawka MN. Fluid replacement recommendations for training in hot weather. *Mil Med.* 1999;164(7):502.

82. Parson KC. International standards for the assessment of the risk of thermal strain on clothed workers in hot environments. *Ann Occup Hyg.* 1999;43(5):297.

83. American College of Sports Medicine. Position stand on the recommended quantity and quality of exercise for developing and maintaining cardiorespiratory and muscular fitness, and flexibility in adults. *Med Sci Sports Exerc.* 1998;30(6):975.

84. Haskell WL, Lee IM, Pate RR, et al. Physical activity and public health: updated recommendation for adults from the American College of Sports Medicine and the American Heart Association. *Med Sci Sports Exerc.* 2007;39(8):1423.

85. Sawka MN, Kolka MA, Montain SJ. *Ranger and Airborne School Students' Heat Acclimatization Guide.* Natick, MA: U.S. Army Research Institute of Environmental Medicine; 2003.

86. Eichna LW, Park CR, Nelson N, et al. Thermal regulation during acclimatization in a hot, dry (desert type) environment. *J Appl Physiol.* 1950;163:585.

87. Federal Emergency Management System, U.S. Fire Administration. Emergency Incident Rehabilitation. http://www .usfa.fema.gov/downloads/pdf/publications/fa_314.pdf. Published February 2008. Accessed January 24, 2014.

88. Hostler D. First responder rehab: good, better, best. *JEMS.* 2007;32(12):98-112; quiz 114.

89. Paterson R, Drake B, Tabin G, Butler FK Jr, Cushing T. Wilderness Medical Society practice guidelines for treatment of eye injuries and illnesses in the wilderness: 2014 update. *Wilderness Environ Med.* 2014;25:S19-S29.

90. Ulrich AS, Rathlev NK. Hypothermia and localized injuries. *Emerg Med Clin North Am.* 2004;22:281.

91. Thomas JR, Oakley EHN. Nonfreezing cold injury. In: Pandolf KB, Burr RE, eds. *Medical Aspects of Harsh Environments.* Vol 1. Washington, DC: Office of the Surgeon General, Borden Institute/TMM Publications; 2001:467-490.

92. Montgomery H. Experimental immersion foot: review of the physiopathology. *Physiol Rev.* 1954;34:127.

93. Francis TJR. Nonfreezing cold injury: a historical review. *J R Nav Med Serv.* 1984;70:134.

94. Imray CHE, Handford C, Thomas OD, Castellani JW. Nonfreezing cold-induced injuries. In: Auerbach PS, ed.

Auerbach's Wilderness Medicine. 7th ed. Philadelphia, PA: Mosby Elsevier; 2017.

95. Wrenn K. Immersion foot: a problem of the homeless in the 1990s. *Arch Intern Med.* 1991;151:785.

96. Ramstead KD, Hughes RB, Webb AJ. Recent cases of trench foot. *Postgrad Med J.* 1980;56:879.

97. Laskowski-Jones L, Jones L. Management of cold injuries. In: Hawkins SC, ed. *Wilderness EMS.* Philadelphia, PA: Wolters Kluwer, 2018.

98. Biem J, Koehncke N, Classen D, Dosman J. Out of cold: management of hypothermia and frostbite. *Can Med Assoc J.* 2003;168(3):305.

99. Vogel JE, Dellon AL. Frostbite injuries of the hand. *Clin Plast Surg.* 1989;16:565.

100. Mills WJ. Clinical aspects of freezing injury. In: Pandolf KB, Burr RE, eds. *Medical Aspects of Harsh Environments.* Vol 1. Washington, DC: Office of the Surgeon General, Borden Institute/TMM Publications; 2001.

101. McIntosh SE, Hamonko M, Freer L, et al. Wilderness Medical Society Practice guidelines of the prevention and treatment of frostbite. *Wilderness Environ Med.* 2011;22;156-166.

102. Cauchy E, Davis CB, Pasquier M, Meyer EF, Hackett PH. A new proposal for management of severe frostbite in the austere environment. *Wilderness Environ Med.* 2016;27:92-99.

103. Gilbertson J, Mandsager R. State of Alaska cold injuries guidelines. Department of Health and Social Services, Juneau, Alaska. dhss.alaska.gov/dph/Emergency/Documents/ems /assets/Downloads/AKColdInj2005.pdf. Revised January 2005. Accessed November 15, 2017.

104. McIntosh SE, Opacic M, Freer L, Grissom CK, Auerbach PS, et al. Wilderness Medical Society practice guidelines for the prevention and treatment of frostbite: 2014 update. *Wilderness Environ Med.* 2014;25:s43-s54.

105. Sessler DI. Mild preoperative hypothermia. *N Engl J Med.* 1997;336:1730.

106. Giesbrecht GG. Cold stress, near drowning and accidental hypothermia: a review. *Aviat Space Environ Med.* 2000;71:733.

107. Stocks JM, Taylor NAS, Tipton MJ, Greenleaf JE. Human physiological responses to cold exposure. *Aviat Space Environ Med.* 2004;75:444.

108. Gilbert M, Busund R, Skagseth A, et al. Resuscitation from accidental hypothermia of 13.7°C with circulatory arrest. *Lancet.* 2000;355:375.

109. Danzl DF, Pozos RS, Auerbach PS. Multicenter hypothermia survey. *Ann Emerg Med.* 1987;16:1042.

110. Tsuei BJ, Kearney PA. Hypothermia in the trauma patient. *Injury Int J Care Injured.* 2004;35:7.

111. Stoner HB. Effects of injury on the responses to thermal stimulation of the hypothalamus. *J Appl Physiol.* 1972;33:665.

112. Ferrara A, MacArthur J, Wright H. Hypothermia and acidosis worsen coagulopathy in the patient requiring massive transfusion. *Am J Surg.* 1990;160:515.

113. Epstein M. Renal effects of head-out immersion in man: implications for understanding volume homeostasis. *Physiol Rev.* 1978;58:529.

114. Jurkovich G. Hypothermia in the trauma patient. *Adv Trauma.* 1989;4:111.

115. Jurkovich GJ. Environmental cold-induced injury. *Surg Clin N Am.* 2007;87:247.

116. Arthurs Z, Cuadrado D, Beekley A, Grathwohl K. The impact of hypothermia on trauma care at the 31st combat support hospital. *Am J Surg*. 2006;191(5):610-614.

117. Beilman GJ, Blondett JJ, Nelson AB. Early hypothermia in severely injured trauma patients is a significant risk factor of multiple organ dysfunction syndrome but not mortality. *Ann Surg*. 2009;249:845-850.

118. Mommsen P, Andruszkow H, Fromke C, et al. Effects of accidental hypothermia on posttraumatic complications and outcome in multiple trauma patients. *Injury*. 2013;44(1):86-90.

119. Lapostolle F, Sebbah JL, Couvreur J. Risk factors for the onset of hypothermia in trauma victims: the Hypotrauma study. *Crit Care*. 2012;16(4):R142.

120. Trentzsch H, Huber-Wagner S, Hildebrand F, et al. Hypothermia for prediction of death in severely injured blunt trauma patients. *Shock*. 2012;37(2):131.

121. Nolan JP, Morley PT, Vanden Hoek TL, et al. Therapeutic hypothermia after cardiac arrest. An advisory statement by the Advance Life Support Task Force of the International Liaison Committee on Resuscitation. *Circulation*. 2003;108:118.

122. Alzaga AG, Cerdan M, Varon J. Therapeutic hypothermia. *Resuscitation*. 2006;70:369.

123. Nolan JP, Neumar RW, Adrie C, et al. Post-cardiac arrest syndrome: epidemiology, pathophysiology, treatment, and prognostication. A scientific statement from the International Liaison Committee on Resuscitation; the American Heart Association Emergency Cardiovascular Care Committee; the Council on Cardiovascular Surgery and Anesthesia; the Council on Cardiopulmonary, Perioperative, and Critical Care; the Council on Clinical Cardiology; the Council on Stroke. *Resuscitation*. 2008;79:350.

124. Nolan JP, Hazinski MF, Billi JE, et al. Part 1: executive summary: 2010 International Consensus on Cardiopulmonary Resuscitation and Emergency Cardiovascular Care Science With Treatment Recommendations. *Resuscitation*. 2010;81S:e1-e25.

125. Crompton EM, Lubomirova I, Cotlarciuc I, Han T, Sharma SD, Sharma P. Meta-analysis of therapeutic hypothermia for traumatic brain injury in adult and pediatric patients. *Crit Care Med*. 2017;45(4):575-583.

126. Andres PJD, Sinclair HL, Rodriguez A, et al. Hypothermia for intracranial hypertension after traumatic brain injury. *N Engl J Med*. 2015;373:2403-2412.

127. Finkelstein RA, Alam HB. Induced hypothermia for trauma: current research and practice. *J Intensive Care Med*. 2010;25(4):205-206.

128. Carlson LD. Immersion in cold water and body tissue insulation. *Aerospace Med*. 1958;29:145.

129. Giesbrecht GG, Steinman AM. Immersion into cold water. In: Auerbach PS, ed. *Auerbach's Wilderness Medicine*. 7th ed. St. Louis, MO: Mosby Elsevier; 2017.

130. Wittmers LE, Savage M. Cold water immersion. In: Pandolf KB, Burr RE, eds. *Medical Aspects of Harsh Environments*. Vol 1. Washington, DC: Office of the Surgeon General, Borden Institute/TMM Publications; 2001:531–552.

131. Tipton MJ. The initial responses to cold-water immersion in man. *Clin Sci*. 1989;77:581.

132. Keatinge WR, McIlroy MB, Goldfien A. Cardiovascular responses to ice-cold showers. *J Appl Physiol*. 1964;19:1145.

133. Mekjavic IB, La Prairie A, Burke W, Lindborg B. Respiratory drive during sudden cold water immersion. *Respir Physiol*. 1987;70:21.

134. Sempsrott J, Schmidt AC, Hawkins SC, Cushing TA. Drowning and submersion injuries. In: Auerbach PS. *Auerbach's Wilderness Medicine*. 7th ed. St. Louis, MO: Mosby Elsevier; 2017.

135. Wissler EH. Probability of surviving during accidental immersion in cold water. *Aviat Space Environ Med*. 2003;74:47.

136. Tikuisis P. Predicting survival time at sea based on observed body cooling rates. *Aviat Space Environ Med*. 1997;68:441.

137. Hayward JS, Errickson JD, Collis ML. Thermal balance and survival time prediction of man in cold water. *Can J Physiol Pharmacol*. 1975;53:21.

138. Ducharme MB, Lounsbury DS. Self-rescue swimming in cold water: the latest advice. *Appl Physiol Nutr Metab*. 2007;32:799.

139. Van Mieghem C, Sabbe M, Knockaert D. The clinical vales of the ECG in noncardiac conditions. *Chest*. 2004;125:1561.

140. Vanden Hoek TL, Morrison LJ, Shuster M, et al. Part 12.9: cardiac arrest in special situations: accidental hypothermia. In: *2010 American Heart Association Guidelines for Cardiopulmonary Resuscitation and Emergency Cardiovascular Care. Circulation*. 2010;122:S829-S861.

141. Lavonas EJ, Drennan IR, Gabrielli, et al. Part 10: special circumstances of resuscitation. 2015 American Heart Association guidelines update for cardiopulmonary resuscitation and emergency cardiovascular care. *Circulation*. 2015;132:S501-S518.

142. Morrison LJ, Kierzek G, Diekema DS, et al. Part 3: Ethics. In: *2010 American Heart Association Guidelines for Cardiopulmonary Resuscitation and Emergency Cardiovascular Care. Circulation*. 2010;122:S665-S675.

143. Danzl DF, Lloyd EL. Treatment of accidental hypothermia. In: Pandolf KB, Burr RE, eds. *Medical Aspects of Harsh Environments*. Vol 1. Washington, DC: Office of the Surgeon General, Borden Institute/TMM Publications; 2001:491-529.

144. Southwick FS, Dalglish PH. Recovery after prolonged asystolic cardiac arrest in profound hypothermia: a case report and literature review. *JAMA*. 1980;243:1250.

145. Bernard MB, Gray TW, Buist MD, et al. Treatment of comatose survivors of out-of-hospital cardiac arrest with induced hypothermia. *N Engl J Med*. 2002;346(8):557.

146. Reuler JB. Hypothermia: pathophysiology, clinical setting, and management. *Ann Intern Med*. 1978;89:519.

147. Armstrong LE. Cold, windchill, and water immersion. In: Armstrong, *Performing in Extreme Environments*. Champaign, IL: Human Kinetics; 2000.

148. Wilderness Medical Society. Myocardial infarction, acute coronary syndromes, and CPR. In: Forgey WW, ed. *Practice Guidelines for Wilderness Emergency Care*. 5th ed. Guilford, CT: Globe Pequot Press; 2006.

149. Position paper of the National Association of EMS Physicians: termination of resuscitation in nontraumatic cardiac arrest. *Prehosp Emerg Care*. 2011;15:545.

150. Siegel AJ, d'Hemecourt P, Adner MM, Shirey T, Brown JL, Lewandrowski KB. Exertional dysnatremia in collapsed marathon runners: a critical role for point-of-care testing to guide appropriate therapy. *Am J Clin Pathol*. 2009;132(3):336-340.

151. Auerbach PS, Constance BB, Freer L. *Field Guide to Wilderness Medicine*. 4th ed. Philadelphia, PA: Mosby Elsevier; 2013.

Suggested Reading

Auerbach PS, ed. *Auerbach's Wilderness Medicine*. 7th ed. Philadelphia, PA: Mosby Elsevier; 2017.

Hawkins SC, Simon RB, Beissinger JP, Simon D. *Vertical Aid: Essential Wilderness Medicine for Climbers, Trekkers, and Mountaineers*. New York, NY: The Countryman Press; 2017.

Hawkins SC. *Wilderness EMS*. Philadelphia, PA: Wolters Kluwer; 2017.

Pandolf KB, Burr RE, eds. *Medical Aspects of Harsh Environments*. Vol 1. Washington, DC: Office of the Surgeon General, Borden Institute/TMM Publications; 2001.

CHAPTER **20**

Environmental Trauma II: Lightning, Drowning, Diving, and Altitude

Lead Editor:
Seth Hawkins, MD

CHAPTER OBJECTIVES

At the completion of this chapter, you will be able to do the following:

- Explain safety hazards associated with outdoor lightning strikes.
- Describe the use of "reverse" triage for multiple lightning casualties.
- Identify the key risk factors for high-altitude illness.
- Explain appropriate initial ABC (airway, breathing, and circulation) management of a drowning incident.
- Describe three signs or symptoms that can occur in a patient after a drowning incident.

- Identify five methods for preventing a drowning incident.
- Contrast the signs and symptoms of type I and type II decompression sickness.
- Describe two primary treatment interventions for type II decompression sickness and arterial gas embolism.
- Discuss the similarities and differences between acute mountain sickness and high-altitude cerebral edema.

SCENARIO

In a coastal town, a family of four was strolling on the beach with their dog during a chilly winter day. The son tossed a rubber ball toward the water's edge, and the dog gave chase. In an instant, a large shore-breaking wave swallowed up the dog in the rough surf. The 17-year-old son was first into the water to attempt to save the dog, only to be overtaken by the water. He was seen struggling in the rough, surging surf by his parents and sister.

The boy's father and mother grabbed a nearby flotation device stationed on the beachfront and followed him into the surf to help. Their 19-year-old daughter remained on shore and called for help on her cell phone. The dog eventually made it back to the shore. The parents pulled their son out of the cold water after finding him submerged and unresponsive. Your paramedic unit arrives to the scene within 7 minutes of the daughter's call.

As you exit the ambulance, you observe an unconscious teenage boy lying partially prone with his face rotated to the side in sand with surging water close by. He is still in the surf zone and could be submersed by a wave. You join with arriving fire department emergency responders to approach the victim.

- How should you approach the patient in this setting?
- If the patient has no pulse or respirations, what is the next immediate intervention?
- What other concerns do you have for the patient that need to be addressed on scene?

INTRODUCTION

Each year worldwide, significant morbidity and mortality are caused by a variety of environmental conditions, including lightning strikes, submersion incidents, recreational scuba diving, and high-altitude climbing. (See the Environmental Trauma I: Heat and Cold chapter for heat and cold conditions.) Prehospital care providers must know the disorders associated with each type of environment; understand the anatomy, physiology, and pathophysiology involved; and know how to rapidly perform patient assessment and management. At the same time, they must know how to prevent injury to themselves and other public safety personnel.

Lightning-Related Injuries

Lightning is the most widespread threat to people and property during the thunderstorm season and is second only to floods in causing storm-related death in the United States since 1959.[1] Over 50,000 thunderstorms occur daily in the world, with lightning striking the earth more than 100 times each second.[2] Lightning is reported to start approximately 75,000 forest fires annually and starts 40% of all fires.[3] The most destructive form of lightning is the cloud-to-ground strike (**Figure 20-1**). Based on real-time lightning-detection systems in the United States, it is estimated that cloud-to-ground lightning strikes occur approximately 20 million times per year, with as many as 50,000 flashes per hour during a summer afternoon.[4,5] In the United States, lightning occurs most frequently from June through August but occurs in Florida and along the southeastern coast of the Gulf of Mexico throughout the year, with Florida and Texas accounting for 25% of lightning deaths.[6,7] Worldwide, rural populations are at the greatest risk due to the lack of lightning-safe structures and prevention education. Consequently, it is estimated that 24,000 fatalities occur annually and lightning causes about 10 times more injuries than deaths worldwide.[7,8]

Since the 1950s, the number of deaths from lightning in the United States has decreased, possibly because of fewer people working outdoors in rural areas, improved warning systems for approaching storms, increased public education on lightning safety, and improved medical care.[9] While the early part of the 20th century saw as many as 400 annual deaths from lightning, the average number of annual deaths from 1968 to 2010 was 79, and the latest reports indicate that lightning now kills only about 30 individuals each year and injures about 400.[3,7,10-12]

The greatest threats from lightning strikes are neurologic and cardiopulmonary injuries. Practice guidelines from the Wilderness Medical Society (WMS) are available for the prevention and treatment of lightning injuries for prehospital and in-hospital care.[13] These recommendations for medical management are graded based on the quality of the supporting evidence. (See the chapter titled Golden Principles, Preferences, and Critical Thinking.)

Epidemiology

Based on National Oceanic and Atmospheric Administration (NOAA) data, in the decade from 2007 to 2016, there were 305 deaths (an average of 30 deaths per year) due to lightning. Of these fatalities, 79% were male.[12] **Figure 20-2** shows the number of lightning fatalities by sex from 2008 to 2017.[10]

Cranial or leg burn involvement indicates a greater risk for death, and some analyses show that about 74% of lightning strike survivors have permanent disabilities.[14]

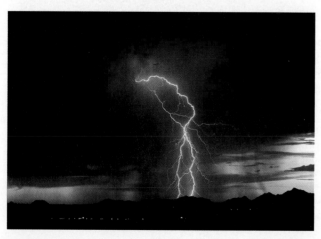

Figure 20-1 A cloud-to-ground lightning strike, with streak lightning pattern.

© Jhaz Photography/Shutterstock.

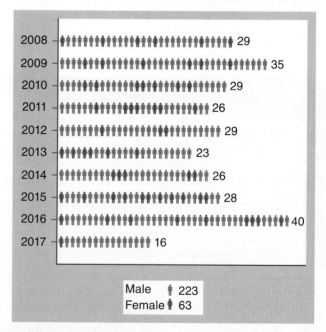

Figure 20-2 The number of lightning fatalities by sex in the United States from 2008 to 2017.

Data from National Weather Service. U.S. lightning deaths in 2017. www.lightningsafety.noaa.gov/fatalities.shtml. Accessed April 11, 2017.

However, this finding is controversial, with other studies reporting much less permanent injury.[11,15] Of the individuals who died from a lightning strike, 52% were outside (25% of whom were at work). Death occurred within 1 hour in 63% of the lightning victims in one review of Florida lightning incidents.[9]

Mechanism of Injury

Injury from lightning can result from the following six mechanisms:[11,13,14]

- *Direct strike* occurs when a person is in an open environment unable to find shelter. It accounts for only 3% to 5% of lightning strikes involving people.[7]
- *Side flash* or *splash contact* occurs when lightning hits an object (e.g., ground, building, tree) and splashes onto a victim or multiple victims. The current will jump from the primary strike object and can splash over to a person. Splashes occur from person to person, tree to person, and even indoors from telephone wire to a person talking on the phone (this can sometimes be direct rather than splash contact, depending on phone and wire proximity to face).
- *Contact* occurs when a person is in direct contact with an object that is struck directly or by a splash. It accounts for one-third of all lightning injuries. For rescue personnel who may have metal gear on their body (such as carabiners) or who are tied into a rescue system such as a belay during a climbing rescue that could involve a thunderstorm, the WMS and climbing medicine experts recommend tying off individually. Also, metal objects such as carabiners, ice tools, or hiking/ski poles should be isolated and direct contact avoided.[7,13]
- *Step voltage* occurs when lightning hits the ground or a nearby object and the current spreads outward radially, passing through a person's body in the process. Human tissue provides less resistance than the ground, and the current will travel, for example, up one leg and down the other, following the path of least resistance. Ground current accounts for the majority of lightning injuries. Step voltage is also known as *stride voltage* or *ground current*.
- *Upward streamer* occurs when current passes up from the ground and through the victim but does not connect with the downward lightning streamer. The energy in this streamer is less, compared to a full lightning strike, and accounts for approximately 1% to 15% of lightning injuries. Upward streamer is a more recently identified form of lightning contact.
- *Blast injury* or other blunt trauma can occur from a shock wave produced by lightning, which can propel a person up to 30 feet (9.1 meters [m]). In addition, injuries can result from lightning that causes forest fires, building fires, and explosions.[3,16,17]

There are six known factors that determine the injury severity from electrical and lightning current:

- Type of circuit
- Duration of exposure
- Voltage
- Amperage
- Resistance of tissue
- Current pathway

Once lightning or another high-voltage electrical source contacts the human body, the heat generated within the body is directly proportional to the amount of current, tissue resistance, and duration of contact. As resistance of various tissues increases (e.g., nerve < blood < muscle < skin < fat < bone), so does the heat generated by the passage of current.

It is easy to assume that lightning injuries are like high-voltage electrical injuries. However, significant differences exist between the two mechanisms of injury. A lightning strike is direct current (DC) as opposed to alternating current (AC), which is responsible for industrial and household electrical injuries. Lightning produces millions of volts of electrical charge, with currents ranging from 30,000 to 50,000 amperes, and the duration of exposure to the body is instantaneous (10 to 100 milliseconds). The temperature of lightning varies with the diameter, but the average temperature is approximately 14,430°F (8,000°C).[10] In comparison, high-voltage electrical exposure tends to be a much lower voltage than lightning. However, the key factor that distinguishes lightning injury from high-voltage electrical injury is the duration of current exposure within the body.[16] **Table 20-1** lists differences between lightning and generator-produced, high-voltage electrical injuries.

At times, lightning can show injury patterns like those seen with high-voltage electricity because of a rare lightning pattern that produces a prolonged strike lasting up to 0.5 second. This type of lightning, called *hot lightning*, can cause deep burns to human tissue, exploding trees, and setting fires. Lightning can show entry and exit wounds on the body, but a more common pathway of lightning once it strikes a victim is to pass over the body. This is referred to as a *flashover* current. A flashover current can also enter the eyes, ears, nose, and mouth. It is theorized that the flashover current flow is the reason why many victims survive lightning strikes. It is also known that a flashover current may vaporize moisture on skin or blast a part of clothing or shoes off a victim. The immense flashover current generates large magnetic fields, which can, in turn, induce secondary electric currents within the body and are thought to cause cardiac arrest and other internal injuries.[18,19]

Injuries From Lightning

Lightning injuries range from minor superficial wounds to major multisystem trauma and death. **Table 20-2** lists

Table 20-1 Comparison of Lightning and High-Voltage Electrical Injuries		
Factor	**Lightning**	**High Voltage**
Energy level	30 million volts; 50,000 amperes	Usually much lower
Time of exposure	Brief, instantaneous	Prolonged
Pathway	Flashover, orifice	Deep, internal
Burns	Superficial, minor	Deep, internal
Cardiac	Primary and secondary arrest, asystole	Ventricular fibrillation
Renal	Rare myoglobinuria or hemoglobinuria	Myoglobinuric renal failure common
Fasciotomy	Rarely, if ever, necessary	Common, early, and extensive
Blunt injury	Explosive thunder effect	Falls, being thrown

Modified from Cooper MA, Andrews CJ, Holle RL, Blumenthal R, Aldana NN. Lightning-related injuries and safety. In: Auerbach PS, ed. *Auerbach's Wilderness Medicine*. 7th ed. Philadelphia, PA: Mosby Elsevier; 2017.

common signs and symptoms of lightning injury. As a tool to determine the likely recovery or prognosis from lightning strikes, victims can be placed in one of three injury categories: minor, moderate, and severe.[13,20]

Minor Injury

Patients with minor injury are awake and report an unpleasant and abnormal sensation (*dysesthesia*) in the affected extremity or extremities. In a more serious lightning strike, victims report they have been hit in the head or state that an explosion hit them, because they are unsure of the source. A patient may present at the scene with the following:

- Confusion (short term or hours to days)
- Amnesia (short term or hours to days)
- Temporary deafness
- Blindness
- Temporary unconsciousness
- Temporary paresthesia
- Muscular pain
- Cutaneous burns (rare)
- Transient paralysis

Victims present with normal vital signs or with mild, transient hypertension, and recovery is usually gradual and complete.

Moderate Injury

Victims with moderate injury have progressive single or multisystem injuries, some of which are life threatening.

Table 20-2 Lightning Injury: Common Signs, Symptoms, and Treatment		
Injuries	**Signs/Symptoms**	**Treatment**
Minor	Feeling of strange sensation in extremity; confusion; amnesia; temporary unconsciousness, deafness, or blindness; tympanic membrane rupture	Scene safety; XABCDEs; medical history and secondary survey; monitor ECG; give oxygen and transport all patients with mild injuries.
Moderate	Disorientation, combativeness, paralysis, fractures, blunt trauma, absent pulses in lower extremities, spinal shock, seizures, temporary cardiorespiratory arrest, comatose	Scene safety; XABCDEs; medical history and secondary survey; monitor ECG; CPR (CAB) early when needed; give oxygen and transport all patients.
Severe	Any of the above, otorrhea (fluid leak) in ear canal, cardiac fibrillation or cardiac asystole	CPR (CAB) and advanced lifesaving procedures; use "reverse" triage with multiple patients.

Note: CAB, circulation, airway, breathing; CPR, cardiopulmonary resuscitation; ECG, electrocardiogram; XABCDE, exsanguinating hemorrhage, airway, breathing, circulation, disability, expose/environment.

Data from O'Keefe GM, Zane RD. Lightning injuries. *Emerg Med Clin North Am.* 2004;22:369; and Cooper MA, Andrews CJ, Holle RL, Blumenthal R, Aldana NN. Lightning-related injuries and safety. In: Auerbach PS, ed. *Auerbach's Wilderness Medicine*. 7th ed. Philadelphia, PA: Mosby Elsevier; 2017.

Some patients in this category can have a permanent disability. Patients may present at the scene with the following:

- Immediate effects
    - Neurologic signs
    - Seizures
    - Deafness
    - Cardiac arrest and cardiac injuries
    - Pulmonary injuries
    - Confusion, amnesia
    - Blindness
    - Dizziness
    - Contusion from shockwave
    - Blunt trauma (e.g., fractures)
    - Chest pain, muscle aches
    - Tympanic membrane rupture
    - Headache, nausea, postconcussion syndrome
- Delayed effects
    - Neurologic symptoms and signs
    - Memory deficits
    - Attention deficits
    - Neuropsychological changes
    - Coding and retrieval problems
    - Distractibility
    - Personality changes
    - Irritability
    - Chronic pain
    - Seizures

Depending on the location of the lightning strike, a strike affecting the respiratory center of the brain can result in prolonged respiratory arrest that may lead to secondary cardiac arrest as a result of hypoxemia.[14] Victims in this category may experience immediate cardiopulmonary arrest, although the inherent automaticity of the heart may produce a spontaneous return to normal sinus rhythm.[14] Because immediate cardiopulmonary arrest is the greatest threat, prehospital care providers need to address immediate life threats in a CAB (circulation, airway, breathing) sequence immediately for all lightning strike victims and continuously monitor the electrocardiogram (ECG) for secondary cardiac events, which may occur as far out as 3 days after the incident.[13]

Severe Injury

The mechanism for sudden death from lightning strike is simultaneous cardiac and respiratory arrest. Victims with severe injury from a direct lightning strike (cardiovascular or neurologic injuries) or delays in cardiopulmonary resuscitation (CPR) have a poor prognosis. On arrival at the scene, the prehospital care provider may find the patient in cardiac arrest with asystole or ventricular fibrillation. Lightning causes a massive DC countershock, which simultaneously depolarizes the entire myocardium.[18] The American Heart Association (AHA) recommends vigorous resuscitation measures

for those who appear dead on initial evaluation. This is based on many reports of excellent recovery after lightning-induced cardiac arrest and on the fact that victims in this category are typically young and without heart disease.[17] Data published in 1980 suggested that only 23% of lightning strike patients receiving CPR survived[14]; this statistic is still shared in contemporary medical literature but may not account for more recent innovations in CPR-based resuscitation. Of all causes of cardiopulmonary arrest, lightning may have one of the most promising prognoses for recovery, since the initial insult is temporary and may be reversible.

It is not uncommon to observe the initial cardiac arrest with spontaneous recovery of electrical activity following the lightning strike, but any ongoing respiratory arrest due to a paralyzed medullary respiratory center may cause secondary hypoxemic cardiac arrest.[17,21] If prolonged cardiac and neurologic ischemia has occurred, it may be very difficult to resuscitate these patients.[10] Other common findings are tympanic membrane rupture with cerebrospinal fluid and blood in the ear canal, ocular injuries, and various forms of blunt trauma from falls, including soft-tissue contusions and fractures of the skull, ribs, extremities, and spine. Many patients in this category have no evidence of burns. In those patients presenting with cutaneous burns caused by lightning, it is generally reported to be less than 20% total body surface area.

Injury to the central nervous system (CNS) is common in a lightning victim and has been classified into four groups of CNS injuries[14]:

- *Group 1 CNS effects* (immediate and transient): Loss of consciousness (75%); paresthesias (80%); weakness (80%); confusion, amnesia, and headaches
- *Group 2 CNS effects* (immediate and prolonged): Hypoxic ischemic neuropathy; intracranial hemorrhage; postarrest cerebral infarction
- *Group 3 CNS effects* (possible delayed neurologic syndromes): Motor neuron diseases and movement disorders
- *Group 4 CNS effects* (trauma from fall or blast): Subdural and epidural hematomas and subarachnoid hemorrhage

Assessment

On arrival at the scene, as with any other call, the priority is the safety of the prehospital care providers and other public safety personnel. Emergency responders must determine whether there is still a chance of lightning in the area. As a storm approaches or has passed, there still is a source of danger that is not always apparent since lightning remains a very real threat as far as 10 to 15 miles away from the main storm cell—hence its nickname, the "bolt from the blue." Indeed, this reality is one source of the popular saying "out of the blue" or "out of the clear blue sky" for an unexpected event.[7,14]

The mechanism of injury may be unclear without a witness because lightning can strike during a sunny day. When in doubt about the mechanism of injury, immediately assess for XABCDEs (exsanguinating hemorrhage, airway management, breathing, circulation, disability, expose/environment) and any life-threatening conditions, as for any emergency. Patients who were struck by lightning (as opposed to those electrocuted as a result of other mechanisms) do not carry an electrical charge, and touching them poses no risk in providing patient care. Assess the victim's heart rhythm with the ECG. It is common to see nonspecific ST-segment and T-wave changes such as QT interval prolongation and transient T-wave inversions, but more specific evidence of myocardial infarction with Q-wave or ST-segment elevation is rarely seen.[22]

Once the patient is stable, a detailed head-to-toe assessment is necessary to identify the wide range of injuries that can occur with this type of trauma. Assess the patient's situational awareness and the neurologic function of all extremities because the upper and lower extremities may experience transient paralysis (known as *keraunoparalysis*). Lightning victims are known to have an autonomic dysfunction causing dilated pupils, which will mimic head trauma.[21] Assess the eyes because more than half of victims have some form of ocular injury. Look for blood and cerebrospinal fluid in the ear canals; half of these victims will have one or two ruptured tympanic membranes. All victims of lightning injury have a high probability of blunt trauma from being thrown against a solid object or being struck by falling objects or other musculoskeletal injury such as dislocation from muscle spasm. Possibility of spinal injury should be considered during the assessment, and corresponding management steps implemented as determined by local protocol.

Assess the skin for signs of burns, ranging from superficial to full thickness. Lightning burns may or may not be apparent in the field because they develop within the first few hours. Burns occur in less the one-half of lightning survivors and in most cases are superficial.[13,14] It is common to see a feathering appearance in the skin, known as **Lichtenberg's figures**, but these patterns are not burns and resolve in 24 hours (**Figure 20-3**). It is more common to see burns secondary to igniting of clothes and heating of jewelry or other objects.

If the incident involves multiple victims, the principles of triage should be implemented immediately. The normal rules of triage are to focus limited personnel and resources on patients with moderate and severe injuries and quickly bypass those patients without respiration and circulation. However, with multiple lightning strike patients, the rule changes to use "reverse" triage and "resuscitate the dead," because these patients are either in respiratory arrest or cardiac arrest and have a high probability of recovery if managed expeditiously.[7,10,11,14,23] In contrast, other patients who have survived a lightning strike have little likelihood

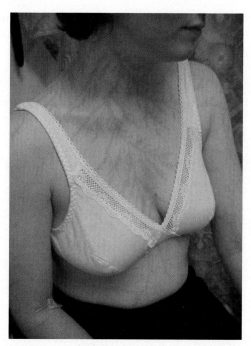

Figure 20-3 Lichtenberg's figures.
© British Association of Plastic, Reconstructive and Aesthetic Surgeons.

of deteriorating, unless there is associated trauma and occult hemorrhage.[10]

Management

The priorities for managing a lightning victim are to ensure scene safety for yourself and your crew and to assess any victim for XABCDE. If spontaneous respiration or circulation is absent, initiate effective CPR up to five cycles (2 minutes), and evaluate the heart rhythm with an automated external defibrillator (AED) or cardiac monitor based on current guidelines.[17] AEDs have proven helpful in some documented cases.[10] Use advanced life support (ALS) measures to manage lightning-induced cardiopulmonary arrest based on current AHA guidelines for advanced cardiovascular life support (ACLS) and pediatric advanced life support (PALS), as discussed elsewhere.[17] Evaluate and treat for shock and hypothermia. Apply high-flow oxygen for all moderately and severely injured patients. Intravenous fluids should be started at a keep vein open (KVO) rate since patients who have been injured by lightning, unlike conventional high-voltage electrical-injured patients, do not have massive tissue destruction and burns requiring a larger amount of fluids. Patients who show unstable vital signs or who have sustained associated trauma may have their fluids titrated as appropriate.

Stabilize any fractures, and package the blunt trauma patient considering spinal cord protection. Lightning strike victims with minor to severe injuries need to be transported to an emergency department (ED) for further evaluation and observation. Transport the patient by either ground or air, as determined by availability, distance, and time to the hospital and overall risk to the flight crew and benefit to the patient.

As mentioned previously, lightning strike victims have a higher probability of a positive outcome from early and effective resuscitation. However, there is little evidence to suggest that these patients can regain a pulse from prolonged basic life support (BLS) or ALS procedures lasting longer than 20 to 30 minutes.[3] Before terminating resuscitation, all efforts should be made to stabilize the patient by establishing an airway, supporting ventilation, and correcting any hypovolemia, hypothermia, and acidemia.

Prevention

With numerous thunderstorms throughout the year, lightning ground strikes are common. Both prehospital care providers and the general public must be educated about prevention and the many lightning myths and misconceptions (**Box 20-1**). Numerous lightning-prevention resources are provided by agencies such as the National Weather Service/NOAA, National Lightning Safety Institute, American Red Cross, and Federal Emergency Management Agency.[24-26]

Official guidelines are published for lightning-injury prevention and treatment by both national and international medical commissions and organizations, including the WMS, the AHA, the International Commission for Mountain Emergency Medicine, and the medical commission of the International Climbing and Mountaineering Federation (**Box 20-2**).[13,17,27]

Prehospital care providers and other public safety personnel should establish procedures for a severe weather watch that provides storm warnings and is updated throughout the day as one method of prevention. There is no place that is 100% safe outdoors. The ambulance is the safest shelter if the providers are near it when no large building is available.

One public education motto used is, "If you see it, flee it; if you hear it, clear it." Another useful rule is the "30–30 rule." When the time between seeing lightning and hearing thunder is 30 seconds or less, individuals are in danger and need to seek appropriate shelter. Following this rule, it is recommended to resume outdoor activity only after 30 minutes following the last lightning or thunder, because a passing thunderstorm still is a threat and lightning can strike up to 10 to 15 miles after the storm passes.[7,26,28] Another measure of lightning proximity is the "flash-to-bang" rule, which states that 5 seconds = 1 mile (1.6 kilometers [km]); that is, following lightning, for every 5 seconds until the sound of thunder, the lightning is 1 mile (1.6 km) away. Note that some erroneous teaching of the 30–30 rule suggests that 30 minutes following the last thunderclap, the storm cell is 30 miles or more away. As the "flash-to-bang" rule explains, when the time between

the flash and the boom is 30 seconds or less, the storm is only 6 miles (9.7 km) away, well within the 10- to 15-mile (16.1–24.1 km) distance for lightning strike outside the main storm cell.[7]

For more information about preventing lightning strike, see **Box 20-3**. See **Box 20-4** for information about support for lightning strike survivors.

Box 20-1 Myths and Misconceptions About Lightning

General Myths

All of the following common beliefs about lightning are *false:*

- Lightning strikes are invariably fatal.
- A major cause of death is burns.
- A victim struck by lightning bursts into flames or is reduced to ashes.
- Victims remain charged or electrified after they are struck.
- Individuals are only at risk for being struck when there are storm clouds overhead.
- Occupying a building during the storm affords 100% protection from lightning.
- Lightning never strikes the same place twice.
- Wearing rubber-soled shoes and a raincoat will protect a person.
- Rubber tires in a vehicle are what protect a person from injury.
- Wearing metal jewelry increases the risk of attracting lightning.
- Lightning always hits the highest object.
- There is no danger from lightning unless it is raining.
- Lightning can occur without thunder.

Misconceptions Regarding Patient Care

Some myths and misconceptions held by prehospital care providers can adversely affect the care and outcome of their patients.

- If the victim is not killed by lightning, he or she will be okay.
- If the victim has no outward signs of injury, the damage cannot be that serious.
- Lightning injuries should be treated similar to other high-voltage electrical injuries.
- Lightning victims who undergo resuscitation efforts for several hours might still recover successfully.

Modified from O'Keefe GM, Zane RD. Lightning injuries. *Emerg Med Clin North Am.* 2004;22:369; and Cooper MA, Andrews CJ, Holle RL, Blumenthal R, Aldana NN. Lightning-related injuries and safety. In: Auerbach PS, ed. *Auerbach's Wilderness Medicine.* 7th ed. Philadelphia, PA: Mosby Elsevier; 2017.

Box 20-2 Prevention Guidelines for Prehospital Care Providers in Mountainous Regions

Prehospital care providers servicing mountainous regions are at greater risk for lightning strike, especially those who serve as park rangers, search and rescue members, and other public safety personnel in high-altitude and remote areas. Some general prevention guidelines for these providers include the following:

- Take note of the weather forecast since thunder and lightning in the mountains occur mainly during summer months in the late afternoons and night. Thus, the saying, "Up by noon and down by 2:00 p.m." is used to remind individuals to return to lower elevations by the middle to late afternoon to decrease the risk for lightning strike.
- The best place to get out of a lightning storm in the mountains is a hut or mountain refuge. Stay away from open doors and windows.
- Tents do not provide any protection from lightning strike, and tent poles may act as lightning rods.
- Larger caves and valleys are protective, but small caves provide little protection if the person is near the opening and sidewalls.

- Wet stream beds are more dangerous than open areas.
- Stay off mountain ridges and summits, power lines, and ski lifts.
- Stay clear of the base of taller trees since lightning will travel down the trunk to the base. In a forest, it is best to get into a cluster of smaller trees.
- If caught in the open, do not sit or lie flat. It is best to crouch down with feet or knees together and keep contact with as small an area of the ground as possible to minimize injury from ground current. Prehospital care providers should try to use some insulation between themselves and the ground, such as a dry pack on which to kneel or sit.
- If in a group, stay apart from each other, but within sight, to reduce the number of people injured by ground current or side flashes between persons.
- Consider the use of small, portable lightning detectors so that advance warning is received and prevention steps can be implemented before the storm arrives.

Box 20-3 Lightning Safety Guidelines

The following are guidelines for lightning safety as a storm develops:

- Find a lightning-safe vehicle or a lightning-safe structure.[24,28]
  - An automobile that is a fully enclosed metal vehicle is a lightning-safe shelter. Other all-metal mobile transportation-related vehicles such as airplanes, buses, vans, and construction equipment with enclosed mostly metal cabs are also safe. A cautionary note, however, will emphasize that the "outer metal shield" of a vehicle should not be compromised. This means:
    – Windows need to be rolled up.
    – Contact must not be made with any interior objects such as radio dials, metal door handles, two-way radio microphones, etc., that connect with external objects.
  - All other objects that penetrate from inside to outside should be avoided.
  - Unsafe vehicles include those made of fiberglass and other plastics, plus small riding machinery or vehicles without enclosed canopies, such as motorcycles, farm tractors, golf carts, and all-terrain vehicles.

  - Metal buildings are lightning-safe places. So, too, are large permanent structures made of masonry and wood. Once again, the caveat is to not become part of the pathway conducting lightning. This means avoiding all electrical circuits, switches, powered equipment, metal doors and windows, hand rails, and so on. Small post-supported structures, such as bus stops, picnic shelters, or baseball field dugouts are not safe.

The following are guidelines for lightning safety when indoors:

- Stay away from windows, open doors, fireplaces, bath and shower, and metal objects such as sinks and appliances.
- Turn off the radio and computer and avoid hardwired telephones; use a telephone only in an emergency.
- Turn off all faucets, electrical appliances, and devices before a storm arrives.

The following are guidelines for lightning safety when outdoors:

- Avoid using handheld radios, cell phones, or other electronic signal/communication devices if possible.

- Avoid metal objects such as bikes, tractors, and fences.
- Avoid tall objects such as trees, and make yourself small.
- Avoid areas near pipelines, power lines, and ski lifts.
- Avoid open fields.
- Avoid open shelters (e.g., carport, bus shelter), depending on overall size, because side flashes or ground strikes can occur.
- Drop ski poles and golf clubs, which may attract lightning.
- In large public outdoor events, seek out nearby buses or minivans.

- Seek to make the smallest contact with ground, if possible, to minimize ground contact. In the "lightning position," the individual squats with the feet together, hands covering the ears; a ground pad, backpack, or some insulation material is placed under the feet. An alternative position of comfort is to kneel or sit cross-legged.
- Do not stand, hug, squat, or huddle near tall trees; seek out a low area of lower trees or saplings.
- Seek out ditches unless there is contact with water.
- If on water, seek shore immediately and move inland, away from the water. Avoid swimming, boating, or being near the tallest object on water.[1,10]

Box 20-4 Survivors of Lightning Injury

Support for survivors of lightning injury is available from Lightning Strike and Electric Shock Survivors International, Inc. (LS&ESSI, Inc.). This nonprofit support group comprises survivors, their families, and other interested parties. There are members throughout the United States and in more than 13 other countries (www.lightning-strike.org).

Drowning

Drowning incidents that lead to injury are all too common in the United States, accounting for over 4,000 deaths annually.[29] It is the third leading cause of unintentional death worldwide.[29,30] Drowning remains a leading cause of preventable death across all age groups but is an epidemic in children.[30-33] The World Health Organization estimates that approximately 400,000 deaths occur annually from unintentional submersion incidents.[34] This statistic likely underestimates the actual worldwide burden of drowning deaths, as it does not include deaths from drowning due to floods, suicide, or homicide; furthermore, in many middle- and low-income countries, patients may die from drowning and never reach a hospital.[29,34]

The terminology describing these patients continues to evolve. In the 20th century, *drowning* was defined as the process by which air-breathing mammals succumb on submersion in a liquid. Multiple modifier terms were used in this century, including *dry drowning, wet drowning, secondary drowning, delayed drowning,* and *near-drowning.*[29] None of these terms had a universal definition, but the term *delayed* or *secondary drowning* was sometimes used to describe patients who recovered initially from a submersion injury, but then died from respiratory failure secondary to submersion. *Near-drowning* sometimes referred to nonfatal drowning, and *dry drowning* sometimes referred to the

phenomenon that a small proportion of people who died from drowning had no demonstrable water in their lungs during autopsy and were presumed to have died due to laryngospasm.[29,35,36] However, in the 21st century, based on the 2002 World Congress on Drowning consensus agreement, none of these terms is now considered medically acceptable.[37] This position—maintaining that there is no role in modern medicine for terms like dry drowning, secondary drowning, and near-drowning—has also been adopted by the World Health Organization, the International Liaison Committee on Resuscitation, the WMS, the U.S. Centers for Disease Control and Prevention (CDC), the AHA, the American Red Cross, and the American College of Emergency Physicians.[37,38]

The more accepted definition adopted by the 2002 World Congress on Drowning, which has been subsequently accepted by the above organizations, is that drowning is the *process* of experiencing respiratory impairment from submersion/immersion in a liquid.[39,40] The patient may live or die after this process, but all incidents of this sort are defined as drownings. The drowning process begins with respiratory impairment as the person's airway goes below the surface of the water (submersion) or water splashes over the face (immersion, with injury through aspiration).[41] The drowning process has only three outcomes or modifiers: fatal drownings (the patient dies), nonfatal drownings with morbidity (the patient lives but sustains injury or illness), and nonfatal drownings without morbidity (there is no death or apparent significant injury or illness).[29,39,42] Further considerations involving the classification of drowning include the following:

- Incidents involving patients who experience a submersion or immersion incident without evidence of respiratory impairment but who require retrieval from the water should be considered a water rescue and not a drowning. Another example of submersion injury that is not a type of drowning is infectious conditions such as brain infection by *Naegleria fowleri* (sustained due to inhalation of this amoeba through the nose while swimming). These situations will not be addressed further in this chapter, which is focused specifically on drowning prevention and treatment.

- As with lightning, the WMS has developed consensus-derived practice guidelines for drowning that are helpful in evaluating the most current recommendations and their evidence within the wilderness medicine community.[43]

Epidemiology

Death by unintentional drowning is the fifth leading cause of unintentional injury death for all ages in the United States, but it overwhelmingly affects younger age groups.[29,44] Excluding birth defects, drowning is the leading cause of death by unintentional injury for ages 1 to 4 years, the second leading cause of death for ages 5 to 9 years, and the sixth leading cause of injury death for ages 15 to 24 years.[29] It is the third leading cause of death of infants (less than 1 year of age), who are often at risk for drowning in bathtubs, buckets, and toilets.[31,45] The CDC reported that from 2005 to 2009 there were an average of 3,880 cases of unintentional fatal drownings in the United States each year, and an estimated 5,789 cases were treated in U.S. hospital EDs each year for nonfatal drowning (**Table 20-3**).[31,32] An additional 347 people died each year from drowning in boating-related incidents.[31]

Statistics demonstrate that for every child who fatally drowns, four others experience nonfatal drowning and require emergency care; many of those who survive suffer irreversible brain injury.[29,33,44,45]

Devastating neurologic injury is the most feared outcome for drowning survivors of all ages and demonstrates the axiom that drowning is truly a neurologic disease with a pulmonary pathway. The major determinant of survival and long-term functionality following drowning is the extent of CNS injury.[29]

The CDC reported an average of 9,669 submersion casualties (fatal and nonfatal) annually from 2005 to 2009.[31] Of these, fatal incidents occurred in bathtubs (10%), pools (18%), and natural water settings such as lakes, rivers, and oceans (51%). In comparison, unintentional nonfatal drownings treated in EDs in the United States were highest for pools (58%), with natural water settings accounting for 25% and bathtubs 10%. The nonfatal and fatal injury rates were the highest for children 4 years of age or younger and for males of all ages. The nonfatal rate for males was almost twice that of females, and 80% of fatal drowning patients are males.[44]

Risk Factors for Drowning

Specific factors place individuals at an increased risk for drowning.[29,35,45-47] Recognizing these factors will increase

Table 20-3 Unintentional Drowning—United States, 2005–2009

Characteristic	Nonfatal*	Fatal*
Age (in years)		
Newborn to 4	3,057	513
5 to 14	1,012	252
≥ 15	1,718	3,107
Unknown	2	9
Gender		
Male	3,486	3,057
Female	2,301	823
Location		
Bathtub	534	403
Pool	3,341	683
Natural water (ocean, lakes, rivers)	1,460	1,982
Other	484	813
Disposition		
Treated/released	2,540	—
Hospitalized	2,908	—
Other	340	—
Total	5,789	3,880

*Estimated number.

Data from Centers for Disease Control and Prevention: Annual average Nonfatal and fatal drownings in recreational water settings—United States, 2005–2009. *MMWR.* 61(19):345, 2012.

awareness and assist in the creation of preventive strategies and policies to minimize these occurrences. For infants and young children, the major risk factor is inadequate supervision; for adolescents and adults, it is risky behavior and use of drugs or alcohol.[45]

Drowning risk factors include the following:

- *Breathing behaviors leading to hypoxic blackout.* To increase their underwater swim distance, some swimmers will intentionally hyperventilate immediately before going underwater, lowering their partial pressure of arterial carbon dioxide ($Paco_2$). Because the body's carbon dioxide level provides the stimulus to breathe in patients without chronic obstructive pulmonary disease,[48] a decrease in $Paco_2$ decreases the feedback to the respiratory center in the hypothalamus to take a breath during breath holding. However, these swimmers are at risk of drowning because the partial pressure of arterial oxygen (Pao_2) does not change significantly with hyperventilation. As the individual continues to swim underwater, Pao_2 will decrease significantly and cause a possible loss of consciousness and cerebral hypoxia. This condition has also been called shallow water blackout,[49,50] hypoxia of ascent (in a diving context), surface blackout, and static apnea blackout,[51] although most recent references and consensus dialogues suggest that "hypoxic blackout" is the preferred term for this condition.[52-54]

- *Accidental cold-water immersion leading to cold shock.* Another situation that places individuals at greater risk of drowning is cold-water immersion (*head out*). The physiologic changes that occur with cold-water immersion can have either a disastrous outcome or a protective effect on the body, depending on many circumstances.[29] Adverse outcomes are more common, resulting from both cardiovascular collapse and sudden death within minutes of cold-water immersion, a condition known as "cold shock." (See the Environmental Trauma I: Heat and Cold chapter for more information.)

- *Age.* Drowning is recognized as a young person's disease epidemic, with toddlers as the largest group, based on their inquisitive nature and a lack of parental supervision. Children under 1 year of age have the highest drowning rate.[31,55]

- *Gender.* Males account for 80% of submersion victims, with two age-related peak incidences.[44] The first peak incidence occurs in males at age 2 years, decreases until age 10 years, and then rises rapidly to peak again at age 18 years. Older males may be more at risk for drowning because of higher exposure rates to aquatic activities, higher alcohol consumption while at the waterfront, and more risk-taking behavior.[29,56]

- *Race.* Due to the history of segregation in the United States, many older African Americans were denied access to pools and swimming lessons. If a grandparent or parent does not swim, swimming lessons for children may become a lower priority for the family. Today, African American children drown more often than white children. African American children tend to drown in ponds, lakes, and other natural sources of water.[30] However, when drowning is in a swimming pool, African American children from age 5 to 19 years fatally drown 5.5 times more often than white children, with the greatest disparity in the 11- to 12-year-old subset, where African American children drown 10 times more often than white children.[44] Overall, the drowning rate of African American male children has been estimated to be as high as three times that of white males, and in the military, African American soldiers drown 62% more often than white soldiers.[57,58]

- *Location.* Submersion incidents typically occur in backyard swimming pools and in natural areas such as lakes, ponds, and the ocean, but they also occur in buckets and bathtubs.[29,35] Houses in rural areas with open wells increase the risk of a young child drowning sevenfold.[29] Other hazardous locations are water barrels, fountains, and underground cisterns.

- *Alcohol and drugs.* Alcohol is the primary drug associated with submersion incidents,[29,59,60] most likely because it causes a loss of sound judgment.[46] As many as 20% to 30% of adult boating fatalities and submersion incidents involve alcohol use in which the occupants used poor judgment, were speeding, failed to wear life jackets, or handled the watercraft recklessly.[29,61]

- *Underlying disease or trauma.* The onset of illness from underlying disease can account for submersion victims. Hypoglycemia, myocardial infarction, cardiac dysrhythmia, depression and suicidal thoughts, and syncope predispose individuals to drowning incidents.[45] A study reported that the risk of drowning in people with epilepsy is raised 15- to 19-fold compared to people in the general population.[62] Cervical spine injuries and head trauma should be suspected in all unwitnessed incidents and injuries involving body surfers, board surfers, and victims diving in shallow water or water with submerged objects such as rocks or trees. Note that long backboard immobilization in or out of water is no longer recommended by leading lifeguard organizations or wilderness EMS authorities, although backboards may be useful as a transportation tool in moving patients.[63-67] (See the Spinal Trauma chapter for a detailed discussion of spinal protection.)

- *Child abuse.* A high incidence of child abuse from submersion incidents is reported, particularly in bathtubs. A study of children sustaining bathtub submersion between 1982 and 1992 found that 67% had historical or physical findings compatible with a diagnosis of abuse or neglect.[47] Consequently, it is highly recommended that any suspicious child-submersion bathtub incident be reported to local social services for appropriate investigation.

- *Hypothermia.* Drowning may result directly from prolonged immersion leading to hypothermia. (See the Cold-Related Disorders section in the Environmental Trauma I: Heat and Cold chapter for further discussion of accidental hypothermia.) Hypothermia is defined as a core (central) body temperature less than 95°F

(35°C). Immersion into water allows for rapid loss of body heat into the usually cooler water, thus precipitating hypothermia, although most deaths in cold water are due directly to drowning, not secondary to hypothermia. Any time boating or other nonswimming activities are done in cold water, a personal flotation device (PFD) must be available and ideally should be worn during any operation that could lead to immersion or submersion.

- Interestingly, *ability to swim* is not a consistent risk factor for drowning.[29] This may be because nonswimmers may avoid water, while highly talented swimmers (like surfers or military personnel routinely deployed in aquatic environments) might take higher risks. White males have a higher incidence of drowning than white females, even though they are reported to have better swimming ability.[29] On the other hand, one study reported that nonswimmers or beginners accounted for 73% of drownings in home swimming pools and 82% of incidents in canals, lakes, and ponds.[68] While statistically speaking, the ability to swim might not correlate with a reduced risk of drowning, swimming instruction is nonetheless recommended and encouraged as a preventive measure against drowning. One study suggests that children ages 1 to 4 years old with some formal swim instruction are more than eight times less likely to die by drowning than matched controls.[69] However, for young children, far more protective than swimming lessons is vigilant parental supervision.[29] In addition, in many nontechnical water exposures (e.g., not surf or whitewater), survival ability may be linked to one's ability to stay afloat, not swim, emphasizing the importance of PFDs or other flotation devices, as well as directing educational opportunities for those seeking survival skills (flotation) rather than true swimming skills.

Mechanism of Injury

A common scenario of *head-out immersion* in water or a whole-body submersion incident begins with a situation that creates a panic response, leading to breath holding, air hunger, and increased physical activity in effort to stay or get above the water surface. According to most bystander reports, submersion victims are rarely seen screaming and waving for assistance while struggling to stay above the surface of the water. Rather, they are seen either floating on the surface or in a motionless position, or they dive underwater and fail to come up. As the submersion incident continues, a reflex inspiratory effort draws water into the pharynx and larynx, causing a choking response. Previously, many authorities have cited suspected laryngospasm. The onset of laryngospasm could represent the first step in suffocation and brain hypoxia, which in turn causes the victim to lose consciousness and submerge

underwater even farther.[41] This is also part of much erroneous dialogue in the popular press about "dry drowning." Drowning experts now believe that laryngospasm is much rarer than previously thought, probably occurring in only 3% to 5% of cases or less.[41,64] In the vast majority of cases, it is water aspiration and subsequent hypoxemia that causes unconsciousness.[41]

As noted earlier, archaic and historical dialogues about the pathophysiology of drowning persist in modern medicine, mostly concerning differences between drowning in freshwater versus saltwater and whether water entered or did not enter the lungs.[35,39,45] It has been definitively shown that these distinctions are not medically helpful.

As discussed earlier, in the 20th century, approximately 15% of drownings were termed *dry drowning* at autopsy, in which the severe laryngospasm prevents the aspiration of fluid into the lungs. The remaining 85% of drownings were considered *wet drownings*, in which the laryngospasm relaxes, the glottis opens, and the victim aspirates water into the lungs.[70] We now know laryngospasm is much less prevalent, and it is not clear that this theoretical distinction makes any difference to field management of a drowning patient.

Theoretically, there also could be different effects on the pulmonary system when freshwater (hypotonic) versus saltwater (hypertonic) versus chlorinated water enters the lung. In freshwater drowning, the hypotonic fluid enters the lung and then moves across the alveolus into the intravascular space, causing a volume overload and dilutional effect on serum electrolytes and other serum components. Conversely, in saltwater aspiration, the hypertonic fluid enters the lung, which in turn causes additional fluid from the intravascular space to enter the lung across the alveolus, causing pulmonary edema and hypertonicity of serum electrolytes.

Despite these theoretical distinctions, it has been shown that no real differences exist between wet and dry drowning and freshwater and saltwater aspiration.[45,71,72] For prehospital care providers, the common denominator in any of these four submersion scenarios is brain hypoxia caused by either laryngospasm or water aspiration. Whether hypoxemia results from laryngospasm or water aspiration is not meaningful to patient management or outcome. Also, it has been demonstrated that the aspiration volume causing electrolyte shifts in saltwater drowning is higher than the volume that is fatal, removing electrolyte concentration as a factor in drowning in seawater.[29] The whole drowning process from immersion or submersion to hypoxemia, apnea, loss of consciousness that leads to cardiac arrest, pulseless electrical activity, and asystole usually occurs in seconds to a few minutes.[41] For those victims who survive, the scene management should be aimed at quickly reversing hypoxemia and subsequent tissue hypoxia (especially in the brain) in drowning patients, thereby preventing cardiac arrest or brain damage.

Surviving Cold-Water Immersion or Submersion

There are four phases that describe the body's responses and mechanisms of death during cold-water immersion. These phases correlate to the 1-10-1 principle[73]:

1. *Initial immersion and the cold shock response.* The victim has 1 minute to get his or her breathing rate under control.
2. *Short-term immersion and the loss of performance.* The victim has 10 minutes of meaningful movement to get out of the water.
3. *Long-term immersion and the onset of hypothermia.* The victim has up to 1 hour until he or she become unconscious from hypothermia.
4. *Circumrescue collapse just before, during, or after rescue.* If the victim survives the first three phases, up to 20% may experience this type of collapse during rescue.

In each of these phases, there is wide individual variation due to body size, water temperature, and the amount of the body that is immersed. Each phase is accompanied by specific survival hazards for the immersion victim that originate from or are influenced by a variety of pathophysiologic mechanisms. Deaths have occurred during all four phases of immersion.

In rare cases of prolonged submersion—one case for as long as 66 minutes—patients have presented to the hospital with severe hypothermia and recovered with either partial or full neurologic function.[74,75] In these submersion incidents, the lowest recorded core temperature of a survivor is 56.6°F (13.7°C) in an adult female.[76] In another case, a child survived fully intact after submersion in ice water for 40 minutes, with a core temperature of 75°F (23.9°C). After 1 hour of resuscitation, spontaneous circulation returned.[77] While this case is noteworthy as an exceptional outlier, the survivor demonstrated that from a population-based perspective, the only variable that can predict outcome is submersion time (longer submersion time equates to a lower chance of survival).[78]

No definitive explanation exists for such cases, but hypothermia is thought to be protective. Immersion in cold water may lead to hypothermia within an hour depending on many factors, as listed below, because of increased surface heat loss and core cooling. In addition, swallowing or aspiration of cold water may contribute to rapid cooling. Rapid onset of hypothermia during freshwater drowning may result from core cooling caused by pulmonary aspiration and rapid absorption of cold water and subsequent brain cooling.

Another factor that may explain why some young children survive is the mammalian diving reflex (**Box 20-5**). The **mammalian diving reflex** slows heart rate and shunts blood to the brain. Recent evidence suggests that the diving

reflex present in various mammals is active in only 15% to 30% of human subjects, so while it cannot be considered the lone explanation of why some children survive, it still may explain part of this phenomenon.[29]

Every submersion patient should receive full resuscitation efforts, regardless of the presence or absence of any of these factors. The following factors appear to influence the outcome of a drowning patient.

- *Age.* Many successful infant and child resuscitations have been documented in the United States and Europe. This success is likely because the smaller mass of a child's body cools faster than an adult's body, thus permitting fewer harmful by-products of anaerobic metabolism to form and causing less irreversible damage. (See the Shock: Pathophysiology of Life and Death chapter.)
- *Submersion time.* The shorter the duration of submersion, the lower the risk for cellular damage caused by hypoxia. Accurate information concerning submersion time needs to be obtained. Submersion longer than 60 minutes is probably fatal. Therefore, a reasonable approach to resuscitation of a submersion victim is that efforts should be initiated if the duration of submersion is less than 1 hour.
- *Water temperature.* While any water temperature below 95°F (35°C) is capable of inducing hypothermia based on exposure time, water temperatures of 70°F (21.1°C) and below are most commonly seen inducing hypothermia. While in rare cases hypothermia appears to be protective during prolonged submersion, in general, cold water is a risk factor for drowning due to the effects of hypothermia on survival mechanisms.
- *Struggle.* Submersion victims who struggle less may have a better chance of resuscitation (unless their struggling efforts are successful in avoiding drowning).

Less struggling means less hormonal release (e.g., adrenaline, the hormonal equivalent of epinephrine) and less muscle activity; this translates to less heat (energy) production and less vasodilatation. These factors in turn cause decreased muscular oxygen demand, which results in smaller muscle oxygen deficit, and less carbon dioxide and lactic acid production. Thus, the rate of cooling of the patient is increased, which may improve resuscitation chances.

- *Cleanliness of water*. Patients generally have increased survival after resuscitation if they were submerged in clean rather than muddy or contaminated water.
- *Quality of CPR and resuscitative efforts*. Patients receiving adequate and effective CPR, combined with proper rewarming and ALS measures, generally do better than patients receiving one or more substandard measures. Immediate initiation of CPR is felt to be a key factor for submersion-hypothermia patients. Past and current studies of cardiac arrest resuscitations overall reveal that poor CPR technique is directly related to poor resuscitation outcome.[79,80] See the current treatment guidelines as outlined in the AHA recommendations for the treatment of accidental hypothermia algorithm.[81]
- *Associated injuries or illness*. Patients with an existing injury or illness, or who become ill or injured in combination with the submersion, do not fare as well as otherwise healthy individuals. Particularly risky comorbid conditions include seizure and cardiac disorders.[29]

Water Rescue

Many water safety organizations recommend the use of highly skilled professionals who regularly train for water rescue, retrieval, and resuscitation. If no professional water rescue teams are available, however, prehospital care providers must consider their own safety and the safety of all emergency responders before attempting an in-water rescue. The following guidelines are recommended to safely rescue a victim out of the water. All of these steps follow an initial, top-priority attempt to provide flotation to the victim; in most aquatic rescue scenarios, this intervention potentially interrupts the drowning process and buys time to plan further rescue interventions.

- *Reach*. Attempt to perform the water rescue by reaching out with a pole, stick, paddle, or anything so that the rescuer stays on land or on a boat. Use caution to avoid being inadvertently pulled into the water.
- *Throw*. When reaching is not possible, throw something to a victim, such as a life preserver or rope so that it floats to the victim.
- *Tow*. Once the victim has a rescue line, tow the victim to safety.

- *Row*. If water entry is necessary, it is preferable to use a boat or paddleboard to reach the victim and to wear a PFD.[29]
- *Go (Don't Go)*. The riskiest technique is to deploy a rescue swimmer. Some wilderness EMS texts describe this risk by naming this step "Go (Don't Go)," indicating that the "Go" step should be initiated only following proper training and a complete risk–benefit analysis suggesting the benefit exceeds the risk.[43,65,82] Rescuers should wear a PFD if entering the water and ideally be leashed to a belay system capable of self-release for swift-water environments.[29,64,65,82]
- *Helo*. In some parts of the country, a helicopter may be equipped to assist with flood or swift-water water rescue and is thus labeled in this algorithm.[65] Helicopter rescue is listed as the final step because helicopters tend to introduce a level of complexity and risk to an operation and require additional risk–benefit analysis. Helicopter rescue is rarely available for rapid deployment and is usually part of a longer rescue operation where immediate fatal drowning risk has been contained.

Swimming rescues are not recommended unless the prehospital care provider has been trained appropriately to manage a victim who can rapidly turn violent from panic, creating a potential double drowning. Too many well-intentioned emergency responders have become victims because their own safety was not the priority; some studies from other countries suggest as many as 5% of drowning fatalities are would-be rescuers.[83,84] See **Figure 20-4** for a few options for in-water rescue systems, equipment for a submersion and/or trauma victim, and movement when in deep water.

Predictors of Survival

The following are important facts and predictors of outcome in resuscitation of a person who has drowned.[41]

1. Early BLS is crucial. For cardiac arrest patients or unresponsive drowning patients, early application of oxygen and rescue breathing or CPR as indicated is critically important to outcome.
2. During drowning, a reduction of brain temperature by 10°C (~18°F) decreases adenosine triphosphate (ATP) consumption by 50%, doubling the duration of time a brain can survive.
3. The greater the duration of submersion, the greater the risk of death or severe neurologic impairment after hospital discharge:
   - 0 to 5 minutes = 10%
   - 6 to 10 minutes = 56%
   - 11 to 25 minutes = 88%
   - Greater than 25 minutes = 100%
4. Signs of brain stem injury predict death or severe neurologic impairment and deficits.

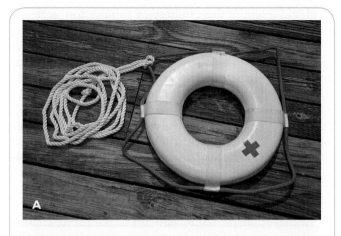

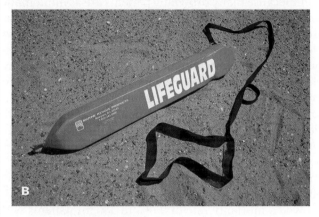

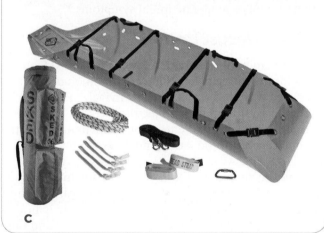

Figure 20-4 Options for in-water rescue equipment and patient packaging. **A.** Rescue throw lines. **B.** Tow device. **C.** In-water patient packaging equipment.

Courtesy of Rick Brady.

Assessment

The initial priorities for any drowning patient include the following[29,41]:

1. Prevent injuries to the patient and emergency responders, ensuring access to flotation devices for all individuals in the water.

2. Initiate plans early for water extraction, availability of at least BLS-level EMS management, and rapid transport to the ED.

3. Conduct a safe water rescue (consider a possible diving-related cause and the need for spinal cord protection).

4. Due to hypoxemia, assess the ABCs (airway, breathing, circulation) using the traditional approach, not CAB (circulation, airway, breathing).

5. Reverse hypoxemia and acidemia with five rescue breaths initially, followed by 30 chest compressions, and continue with two breaths thereafter (30:2). Watch for regurgitation, which is the most common complication during rescue breathing and during CPR.

6. CPR with only chest compression is not advised in persons who have drowned.

7. Restore or maintain cardiovascular stability.

8. Prevent further loss of body heat and initiate rewarming efforts in hypothermic patients, bearing in mind previous discussion that therapeutic hypothermia temperatures might be considered in postarrest patients.

Initially, it is safest to presume that the submersion patient is hypoxemic and hypothermic until proved otherwise. Consequently, efforts should be made to establish effective respirations during water rescue since cardiac arrest from drowning is the result primarily of lack of oxygen. Submersion patients in respiratory arrest usually respond after a few rescue breaths. Attempts to provide chest compressions when in the water are ineffective, so taking time to assess for the presence of a pulse is meaningless and will only delay getting the patient to land.

Remove the patient from the water safely. Once on land, the patient should be placed in a supine position with the trunk and head in the same position, which is usually parallel (on sloping beaches or banks) to the shore. Check for responsiveness, and continue rescue breathing as needed.

If the patient is breathing, place the patient in the recovery position, and monitor for effective respirations and pulse. Quickly assess the patient for any other life threats, and evaluate for head trauma and cervical spine injuries, particularly if there is suspicion of trauma associated with the submersion incident (e.g., falls, boat accidents, diving into water with underwater hazards). However, it has been shown that the typical submersion casualty has a low chance of traumatic injury, unless it is known that the victim dove into the water.[85] Acquire the vital signs, and assess all lung fields of submersion patients because they present with a wide range of pulmonary distress, including shortness of breath, rales, rhonchi, and wheezing. Drowning patients can present with minimal symptoms initially and then deteriorate rapidly with signs of pulmonary edema. However, there has never been a case published in the medical literature of a patient who was initially completely asymptomatic on clinical examination who then died hours later of abrupt, late-onset symptoms.[37]

Assess the patient's oxygen saturation with pulse oximetry, and monitor the end-tidal carbon dioxide ($ETCO_2$) levels. Assess for cardiac rhythm disturbances, because submersion patients often have dysrhythmias secondary to hypoxia and hypothermia. Assess for altered mental status and neurologic function of all extremities because many submersion patients develop sustained neurologic damage. Determine the patient's blood glucose level, as hypoglycemia may have been the cause for the submersion incident. Acquire a baseline Glasgow Coma Scale (GCS) score, and continue to assess for trends. Always suspect hypothermia, and minimize further heat loss. Remove all wet clothing and assess temperature (if the appropriate thermometers are available and the situation permits) to determine the level of hypothermia, and initiate steps to minimize further heat loss. (See the Environmental Trauma I: Heat and Cold chapter for management of hypothermia.)

The following variables are predictive of a more favorable outcome in nonfatal drownings:

- Children age 5 years and older
- Female sex
- Water temperature less than 50°F (10°C)
- Duration of submersion less than 10 minutes
- No aspiration
- Time to effective BLS less than 10 minutes
- Rapid return of spontaneous circulation
- Spontaneous cardiac output on arrival in ED
- Core temperature less than 95°F (35°C)
- No coma on arrival and GCS score greater than 6
- Pupillary responses present
- Arterial pH > 7.10[29]
- Initial blood glucose < 200 mg/dL[86]

Management

Figure 20-5 presents a management tool for persons who have drowned based on a six-grade classification system and a guide for medical intervention for each grade.[41] A patient who has experienced some form of submersion incident, but who is not presenting with any signs or symptoms at the time of the primary survey, still needs follow-up care in a hospital after assessment at the scene due to the potential for delayed onset of symptoms. Many asymptomatic patients (Grade 2) are released in 6 to 8 hours, depending on clinical findings in the hospital. In one study of 52 swimmers who experienced a submersion incident and were all initially asymptomatic immediately after the incident, 21 (40%) went on to develop shortness of breath and respiratory distress due to hypoxemia within 4 hours.[87] In general, all symptomatic patients are admitted to the hospital for at least 24 hours for supportive care and observation because the initial clinical assessment can be misleading. It is critical to obtain a good history of the

incident, detailing the estimate of submersion time and any past medical history.

All suspected submersion patients should receive high-flow oxygen (15 liters/minute) independent of their initial breathing status or oxygen saturation, based on the concern for delayed pulmonary distress, particularly if the patient develops shortness of breath. Monitor and maintain the patient's oxygen saturation greater than 90%. Apply and monitor the ECG, particularly for pulseless electrical activity or asystole. Obtain intravenous (IV) access, and provide normal saline (NS) or lactated Ringer (LR) solution at a KVO rate unless the patient is hypotensive. Then provide a 500-milliliter (ml) fluid bolus, and reassess vital signs.

Transport all drowning patients to the ED for evaluation. Because many drowning patients are asymptomatic, some may refuse transport because they have no immediate chief complaint. If so, take the time necessary to provide good patient education about the delayed signs and symptoms in a drowning incident, explaining that some victims develop secondary complications from pulmonary injury. Firm and persistent persuasion is needed for them to agree to be transported or for them to report to the closest ED for further evaluation and observation. If the patient is adamant about refusing care, the patient must be informed of the potential ramifications of refusing care, and a signed refusal of care against medical advice must be obtained. The largest study of drowning patients to date showed a mortality rate of 0.6% to 5% for patients with only minimal or moderate initial symptoms.[88]

Patient Resuscitation

Rapid initiation of effective BLS and standard ALS procedures for drowning patients in cardiopulmonary arrest is associated with the best chance of survival.[35] Patients may present in asystole, pulseless electrical activity, or pulseless ventricular tachycardia/ventricular fibrillation. Follow the current version of the AHA guidelines for pediatric and adult ALS and ACLS for managing these rhythms. It is currently recommended to use therapeutic hypothermia (TH) in patients who remain in a coma from cardiac arrest caused by ventricular fibrillation. (This topic is briefly presented in the Environmental Trauma I: Heat and Cold chapter.) It might be equally effective for other causes of cardiac arrest, but it has not been proven beneficial to induce hypothermia for submersion patients.[89] For drowning patients who are already hypothermic, hypothetical arguments could be made that they should be warmed only to standard TH temperature, per local protocol, although this recommendation is based on hypothetical benefit without strong underlying science to defend or refute it.[29,43,64] The WMS Practice Guidelines for Drowning, with a recommendation grade of 2C, state, "There is insufficient evidence to either support or discourage induction or maintenance of TH in drowning patients."[43]

A symptomatic patient with a history of immersion or submersion who presents with signs of distress (e.g.,

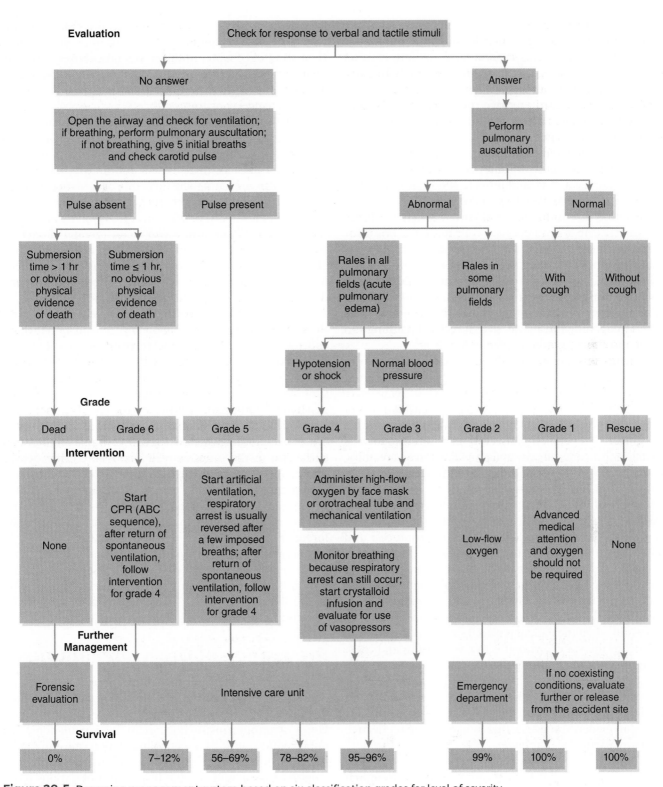

Figure 20-5 Drowning management system based on six classification grades for level of severity.

Szpilman D, Bierens JLM, Handley A, Orlowshi JP. Drowning. *New Engl J Med.* 2012;366:2102-2110.

anxiety, rapid respirations, difficulty breathing, coughing) is considered to have a drowning pulmonary injury until hospital evaluation has proved otherwise. Emphasis should be placed on correcting hypoxemia, acidemia, and hypothermia. Provide spinal cord restriction in all suspected trauma patients. In unresponsive patients, use suction to clear the airway and keep the airway open with an airway adjunct. Hypoxemia and acidemia can be corrected with effective ventilation support. Patients who are apneic should be supported with bag-mask ventilation. Intubation should be considered early to protect the airway in patients who are apneic or cyanotic or who have decreased mental status, because drowning patients swallow large amounts of water and are at risk of vomiting and aspirating stomach contents. If ventilations are impaired, the amount of pressure applied should be modified to improve the ease of ventilation. Monitor the ECG for rate and rhythm disturbances, and investigate for evidence of a cardiac event that might have preceded or followed the submersion incident. Provide 100% oxygen (15 liters/minute) with a nonrebreathing mask. Obtain IV access, and provide NS or LR solution at a KVO rate. Provide transport to the local ED.

Routine attention to spinal cord restriction during in-water rescue is not necessary unless the reasons leading to the submersion indicate that trauma is likely (e.g., diving, use of water slide, signs of injury, alcohol use).[89] When these indicators are not present, spinal injury is unlikely. Routine cervical stabilization and other means to immobilize the spine during a water rescue can cause delays in opening the airway so that rescue breathing can begin and should not be implemented.[64,65,82]

The use of compressions during in-water rescue is not recommended for many reasons.[43] First, the depth of chest compressions is ineffective in water. Besides delaying effective CPR out of water, attempting to provide CPR in water puts rescuers at risk from fatigue, cold water, wave, surge, and current dangers. Emphasis should be directed toward establishing an open airway and providing rescue breathing for patients who are apneic as soon as possible. In-water resuscitation is a recognized technique that provides for rescue breathing while a patient is in water. However, it has been shown to be effective only when implemented by trained providers under specific circumstances, and should be attempted only by those trained to perform it.[43]

When rescue from a beach (or other location) involves sloping terrain, it is no longer recommended to place a patient in a head-down (or head-up) position to drain the airway.[82] Resuscitation efforts are shown to be more successful when the patient is placed supine on the ground, parallel to the water, with effective ventilation and chest compressions. Maintaining a level position on the ground will prevent a decrease in forward blood flow during chest compressions in the head-up position or an increase in intracranial pressure in the head-down position. Furthermore, no evidence suggests that lung drainage is effective with any particular maneuver.

The Heimlich maneuver has been previously suggested for use in submersion patients. However, the Heimlich maneuver is designed for airway obstruction and does not remove water from the airway or lungs. Rather, it may induce vomiting in submersion patients and place them at greater risk for aspiration. Currently, the AHA, the WMS, and the Institute of Medicine advise against the Heimlich maneuver except when the airway is blocked with foreign material.[43,90] If the patient recovers with spontaneous breathing, he or she should be placed in a lateral recumbent position to reduce the risk of aspiration if the patient vomits. (The Environmental Trauma I: Heat and Cold chapter outlines ALS procedures regarding resuscitation of a hypothermic patient. These guidelines are the same for all hypothermic patients regardless of the source of cold exposure.)

Use the regional EMS medical protocol for established guidelines that determine the criteria for an obviously dead individual. Acceptable guidelines for an obviously dead patient are pulselessness, apnea, and normothermia in a patient who presents with rigor mortis or other findings clearly incompatible with life such as transection, decapitation, ice in the airway, or a frozen chest wall. A patient who has been recovered from warm water (greater than 43°F [6.1°C]) without vital signs or unsuccessful resuscitative efforts lasting 30 minutes or who has been recovered after known submersion over 60 minutes in water less than 43°F (6.1°C), may be considered dead on the scene.[29,43,91] Patients with hypothermia may need to be warmed unless there are other signs of obvious death. Consult local medical control early for any individual recovered from cold-water submersion. As stated previously, at least one individual has recovered from more than 60 minutes of cold-water submersion. These submersion patients should be managed as a hypothermic patient, based on the rectal temperature.

Most drowning patients have copious froth coming out of the mouth, which is a result of water mixing with surfactant in the lungs as well as possibly other debris. There is no benefit to suctioning this froth, and, in fact, time spent trying to clear the airway of this material is time lost in establishing oxygenation for the patient. The froth can be breathed back into the lungs after any large, solid foreign bodies are removed from the airway.[29,64]

Because of the critical nature of oxygenation and ventilation in drowning patients in cardiac arrest, the preference would be to intubate cardiac arrest drownings as soon as possible. Supraglottic airway devices are of unproven benefit in drowning due to high airway resistance.[92-94]

Prevention of Drowning Injuries

Prevention strategies are vital in the effort to lower the rates of drowning incidents in the United States. It is estimated that 85% of all cases of drowning can be prevented by supervision, swimming instruction, technology regulations, and public education.[41] Many education programs emphasize the reduction of unintentional water entry of infants and children by encouraging the installation of various types of barriers around pools (e.g., isolation fences, pool covers, alarms) and the use of PFDs such as life vests.[46] Furthermore, CPR initiated by a bystander before the arrival of prehospital care personnel is associated with improved patient prognosis, so community CPR training can certainly be considered a preventive intervention for drowning.[95]

Prehospital care providers have great opportunities to be advocates of water safety and education in their respective communities, with an emphasis on communication of the risk factor areas previously identified. Furthermore, prevention should be emphasized to providers and other public safety personnel who arrive on the scene so that they do not become additional submersion victims. A panicked and struggling victim can be a danger to an unprepared in-water rescuer, potentially resulting in a double drowning. Providers need to assess the problem quickly, control the scene to prevent bystanders from entering the water, and ensure their own safety.

Community education regarding submersion incidents should include the following recommendations:

- Beaches
  - Always swim near a lifeguard.
  - Ask a lifeguard about a safe place to swim.
  - Always swim with others.
  - Do not overestimate your swimming capability.
  - Always watch your children.
  - Swim away from piers, rocks, and stakes.
  - Avoid drinking alcohol.
  - Take lost children to the nearest lifeguard tower.
  - Be aware that the majority of ocean drownings occur in rip currents.
  - Know the weather conditions before going into water.
  - Never try to rescue someone without knowing what you are doing; many people have died in such attempts.
  - If you are fishing on rocks, be cautious with waves that may sweep you into the ocean.
  - Always enter shallow water feetfirst.
  - Do not dive in shallow water; injury to the cervical spine could result.
  - Keep away from marine animals.
  - Read and heed signs and flags posted on the beach.
- Residential pools and other water sources
  - Adult supervision is necessary, closely observing all children.
  - Set rules for water safety.
  - Never leave a child alone near a pool or a source of water, such as a bathtub or bucket.
  - Install a four-sided fence that is at least 4 ft (1.2 m) tall around the pool with a self-closing and self-latching gate.
  - Do not allow children to use arm buoys or other air-filled swim aids.
  - Know how to use an approved life jacket.
  - Avoid toys that will attract children around pools.
  - Use two drains 3 ft (9 m) apart and anti-hair covers, or turn off pump filters when using pools.
  - Use cordless or mobile phones near pool to prevent leaving the poolside to answer the telephone elsewhere.
  - Keep rescue equipment (e.g., shepherd's hook, life preserver) and a telephone by the pool.
  - Do not try or allow hyperventilation to increase underwater swim time.
  - Do not dive in shallow water.
  - Provide swimming lessons for all children by age 4 years but not before 1 year of age.[29,96]
  - After the children have finished swimming, secure the pool so they cannot return (locks or audible alarms on gates are recommended).
  - All family members and others watching children should learn water safety, first aid, and CPR.[14]

Last, communities can help prevent drownings by educating the public about the dangers of driving through floodwaters. As intense flood-causing storms become more common, this message is becoming increasingly important. If drivers do find themselves in a submerged vehicle, they will need to know how to promptly, safely free themselves (**Box 20-6**).

Box 20-6 Drowning in Submerged Vehicles

Studies suggest that as many as 10% of drownings occur in submerging vehicles and that 10% of motor vehicle–related deaths during disasters are due to submerging vehicles.[29,97,98] Many erroneous strategies have been shared in the media about how to escape a vehicle filling with water, including waiting for it to fill with water before trying to escape so that the doors will open, breathing trapped air, or kicking out the windshield.[64,98] However, recent thorough investigations of these strategies have proven them to be dangerous and ineffective and have resulted in a more evidence-based set of instructions for escaping a submerging vehicle.[99]

Vehicles float for about 30 to 120 seconds before sinking. During this time, the windows should be rolled down and the vehicle exited as rapidly as possible. Studies have shown that three adults can escape a vehicle in this way, while also releasing a child manikin in a back seat, within 51 seconds.[99] Emergency medical dispatchers in particular should be aware of advising callers to escape a submerging vehicle before further action is taken, especially in light of numerous drowning deaths from submerging vehicles while callers were on the phone with a dispatcher.[100] The series of actions that should be taken by an individual in a submerging vehicle, or by someone attempting a rescue of individuals in a submerging vehicle, are as follows[29]:

1. *Seat belts:* Unfasten
2. *Windows:* Open
3. *Children:* If present, release from restraints and bring close to an adult who can assist in their escape
4. *Out:* Children should be pushed out the window first and then be followed immediately

Recreational Scuba-Related Injuries

Recreational diving using **self-contained underwater breathing apparatus (scuba)** is a common activity enjoyed by many age groups. The popularity of this activity continues to grow, with more than 400,000 new certified divers each year, now totaling nearly 4 million recreational scuba divers in the United States.[101,102] Relative to the increasing number of new divers each year, the injury rate is low, but the concern for medical fitness to dive has increased because of the diversity of divers, increasing age, low physical fitness, and underlying medical conditions. Water is an unforgiving environment when problems occur. Currently, there are medical guidelines that indicate relative and temporary health risks and absolute contraindications for scuba diving.[102-107]

Injuries to divers occur from many underwater hazards (e.g., shipwrecks, coral reefs) or from handling hazardous marine life. However, more often, prehospital care providers respond to scuba-related injuries and fatalities caused by **dysbarism**, or altered environmental pressure, which accounts for most serious diving medical disorders. The mechanism of injury is based on the principles of gas laws when breathing compressed gases (e.g., oxygen, carbon dioxide, nitrogen) at varying underwater depths and pressures, as will be described in detail in subsequent sections.

The associated causes for diving fatalities have not changed significantly in recent history. The most frequently cited problem is insufficient gas (air) or running out of gas. Other common factors included entrapment or entanglement, buoyancy control, equipment misuse or problems, rough water, and emergency ascent. The principal injuries or causes of death included drowning or asphyxia due to inhalation of water, air embolism, and cardiac events. Older divers were at greater risk of cardiac events, with men at higher risk than women, although the risks were equal at age 65 years.[108]

Most scuba-related injuries caused by dysbarism present with signs (e.g., ear squeeze on descent) and symptoms either immediately or within 60 minutes after surfacing, but some symptoms are delayed up to 48 hours after individuals depart the dive site and return home. Consequently, with the increasing number of scuba divers today flying to and from popular dive sites in the United States, Caribbean, and other remote locations, there is a greater possibility of responding to diving-related injuries at locations distant from the actual dive site. Prehospital care providers need to recognize these scuba-related disorders, provide initial treatment, and initiate plans early for transport to the local ED or for treatment at the closest recompression chamber.[105]

Epidemiology

Divers Alert Network (DAN) compiles an extensive morbidity and mortality database based on casualty data provided from participating recompression chambers in North America. Diving-associated death rates peaked in the 1970s, with annual rates as high as 150, but since then have remained stable at much lower annual death rates ranging from 77 to 91.[102,108] DAN publishes these data in annual reports, which can be found on their website.[109] In 2016, the most recent year for which data are available, scuba-related diving injuries in the United States and North American occurred most frequently from April to October, with October as the peak month. However, a single year of data can be misleading. Measured over a longer period, the number of U.S. fatalities reported to DAN usually increases as summer approaches, peaks around July, and then diminishes as winter approaches. North America has the most reported diving deaths, with Europe coming in a distant second. Three to four times more male divers are injured than female divers.

The primary cause of diving-related injury is decompression sickness. Males account for 81% of deaths, with most of the deaths in divers 40 to 59 years of age. Drowning was the most common cause of death. Cardiovascular disease was the second most common cause of death and the most common cause of disabling injury. Both these causes were significantly more common as causes of death and disabling injury than arterial gas embolism (AGE), the third most common condition.[109] Even though drowning was the leading cause of fatalities, it is unclear what led to the drowning, such as equipment issues, lack of air, entanglement, narcosis, panic, disorientation, hypothermia, heart attack, or AGE. Many drowning deaths during scuba diving are actually arterial gas emboli leading to drowning.[108]

Mechanical Effects of Pressure

Scuba-related diving injuries incurred by the changing atmospheric pressure, or dysbarism, can be separated into two types: (1) the conditions when a change in pressure from the underwater environment results in tissue trauma or barotrauma in closed air spaces in the body (e.g., ears, sinuses, intestines, lungs) and (2) the problems that occur from breathing compressed gases at elevated partial pressure, such as decompression sickness.

Barotrauma associated with scuba diving relates directly to the pressure effects of air and water on the diver. When standing at sea level, the atmospheric pressure is 760 torr, which is essentially the same as 760 millimeters of mercury [mm Hg]) or 14.7 pounds per square inch (psi) on the body. This amount of pressure is also known as 1 atmosphere (1 atm). As a diver descends deeper in water,

Table 20-4 Common Units of Pressure in Underwater Environment

Depth (FSW)	PSIA	ATA	Torr or mm Hg (absolute)
Sea level	14.7	1	760
33	29.4	2	1,520
66	44.1	3	2,280
99	58.8	4	3,040
132	73.5	5	3,800
165	88.2	6	4,560
198	102.9	7	5,320

Note: ATA, atmosphere absolute; FSW, feet seawater; mm Hg, millimeters of mercury; PSIA, pounds per square inch absolute.

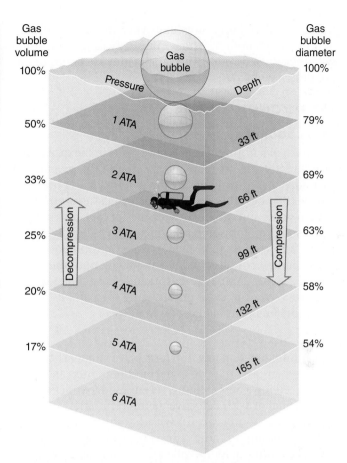

Figure 20-6 Boyle's law. The volume of a given quantity of gas at constant temperature varies inversely with pressure.
© Jones & Bartlett Learning.

the absolute pressure increases 1 atm for every 33 ft (10 m) of seawater. Consequently, a depth of 33 ft of seawater is equivalent to 2 atm (air [1 atm] and 33 ft of water [1 atm]) of pressure on the body. **Table 20-4** lists common units of pressure in the underwater environment.

When a diver descends under the increasing pressure of seawater, the effect of the forces exerted on the body differs depending on the tissue compartments. The force applied to solid tissue acts in similar fashion to a fluid medium, and the diver is generally unaware of compressive force. In the air-containing spaces of the body, however, gases are compressed as the diver descends. Conversely, these gases expand as the diver ascends toward the surface. Boyle's law and Henry's law explain the effects of pressure on the body when underwater.

Boyle's Law

Boyle's law states that the volume of a given mass of gas is inversely proportional to the absolute pressure found in that environment. Stated another way, as a diver descends in the water to a greater depth, the pressure increases and the volume of the gas (e.g., the volume in the lung or ear) decreases. The reverse is also true, the volume of the gas (e.g., in the lung or ear) increases in size when the diver returns toward the surface. This is the principle behind the effects of barotrauma and AGE in the body. **Figure 20-6** shows the effects of pressure on the volume and diameter of a gas bubble.

Henry's Law

At a constant temperature, the amount of gas that will dissolve in a liquid is directly proportional to the partial

pressure of that gas outside the liquid. Henry's law is fundamental in the understanding of how gas from a compressed air cylinder (scuba tank) behaves in the body as the diver descends in the water. For example, the increasing partial pressure of nitrogen will cause it to dissolve in the fluids of the body's tissues as the pressure increases during descent. On return toward the surface, nitrogen will "bubble out" of the fluid solution in the tissues. Henry's law describes the principle that explains why decompression sickness occurs.

Barotrauma

Barotrauma, also known as *squeeze*, is the most common form of scuba-related diving injury.[110] Although many forms of barotraumas cause pain, most resolve spontaneously and do not require EMS involvement or recompression chamber therapy. However, some pulmonary overpressurization injuries are very serious. During scuba diving, barotrauma occurs within noncompressible, gas-filled body cavities (e.g., sinuses). If the pressure in these spaces cannot equalize during a dive as ambient pressure increases, vascular engorgement, hemorrhage, and mucosal edema result from decreasing air volume when the diver descends, and tissue disruption results from increasing air volume when the diver ascends. The various forms of barotraumas are described next.

Barotrauma of Descent

Mask Squeeze

This form of barotrauma generally occurs in inexperienced or inattentive divers who fail to equalize the pressure in their face mask by increasing the external water pressure during their descents. Examine the soft tissue around the patient's eyes and conjunctival tissues for capillary rupture. Signs and symptoms of mask squeeze include skin ecchymoses and conjunctival hemorrhage. Mask barotrauma is self-limited, and treatment is no diving until the tissue damage clears. Management includes providing a cold compress over the eyes, encouraging the patient to rest, and providing pain medication as needed.

Tooth Squeeze

A very infrequent finding, this form of barotrauma occurs in divers when gas is trapped in the interior portion of a tooth after receiving a dental filling, recent tooth extractions, or a root canal or with defective dental restorations. During descent, the tooth can fill with blood or can implode with increasing external pressure. During ascent, any air forced into the tooth will expand, causing either pain or explosion of the tooth. To prevent tooth squeeze, it is recommended that divers do not dive for 24 hours after any dental treatment.

Examine the affected tooth to see if it is intact. Signs and symptoms of tooth squeeze include pain and a fractured tooth. Refer the patient for dental evaluation, and give pain medication as needed.

Middle-Ear Squeeze

This type of squeeze occurs in 40% of scuba divers and is considered the most common diving injury.[111] Ear squeeze occurs near the surface of the water, when the greatest changes in pressure occur as the diver descends. Divers need to begin equalizing their middle ear early as they start to descend so a pressure differential across the tympanic membrane (TM) leading to rupture of the eardrum does not occur. The diver will experience pain and vertigo if the TM ruptures, allowing water to enter the middle ear. Divers with upper respiratory infection or allergies may have difficulty equalizing their middle ear during a dive.

Examine the ear canal for blood caused by ruptured TM. Signs and symptoms of middle-ear squeeze include pain, vertigo, conductive hearing losses with TM rupture, and vomiting.

No pressure changes are permitted (e.g., diving or flying) in patients with middle-ear squeeze. Patients may need decongestants if the TM has not ruptured to open up the eustachian tube and allow the pressure to equalize.

Antiemetics such as prochlorperazine (Compazine) or ondansetron (Zofran) may be necessary for vertigo and vomiting. Transport the patient in an upright position or position of comfort. Antibiotics may be prescribed with ruptured TM to prevent infection. The patient should be referred for audiometric evaluation to assess possible hearing loss.

Sinus Squeeze

Normally, pressure in the sinuses equalizes easily as the diver is descending and ascending. Pressure develops by the same mechanism as the middle ear squeeze, but sinus squeeze is not as common. As a diver descends, there is an inability to maintain pressure in the sinuses, and a vacuum develops in the sinus cavity, causing intense pain, mucosal wall trauma, and bleeding in the sinus cavity. This squeeze may be caused by congestion, sinusitis, *mucosal hypertrophy* (enlargement or thickening), rhinitis, or nasal poyps.[110] A reverse sinus squeeze during ascent can occur as well (see later discussion on Sinus Barotrauma).

Examine the patient's nose for discharge. Signs and symptoms of sinus squeeze include severe pain over the affected sinus or bloody discharge, usually from frontal sinuses.

No specific management is needed at the scene unless extensive bleeding is observed, in which case, treat the patient for epistaxis (nosebleed) by pinching firmly on the fleshy part of the patient's nostrils just below the nasal bones. Transport in a position of comfort.

Internal-Ear Barotrauma

Although much less common than middle-ear squeeze, this is the most serious form of ear barotrauma because it may lead to permanent deafness.[111] Internal-ear barotrauma occurs when a diver descends and has failed attempts to equalize the middle ear. Further forceful attempts can result in a large rise in middle-ear pressure and can rupture the round window structure.

Examine the ear canal for any discharge. Signs and symptoms include roaring tinnitus, vertigo, hearing loss, a feeling of fullness or "blockage" in the affected ear, nausea, vomiting, pallor, diaphoresis (sweating), disorientation, and ataxia (loss of muscular coordination).

The patient should avoid strenuous activities and loud noises, with no pressure changes (e.g., diving or flying). Transport the patient in an upright position. Early medical consultation with DAN or an ED is recommended because it may be difficult to determine if this is inner-ear decompression sickness and if there is an immediate need for recompression chamber therapy.

Barotrauma of Ascent (Reverse Squeeze)

Alternobaric Vertigo

This is an unusual form of barotrauma in that it occurs as expanding gas moves through the eustachian tube and unequal pressure develops in the middle ear, which can cause vertigo. Although the symptoms are brief, vertigo can trigger panic in divers, leading to other forms of injury caused by a rapid ascent to the surface (e.g., air embolism, drowning).

Examine the ear canal for any discharge; assess any hearing loss. Signs and symptoms of alternobaric vertigo are short in duration, resulting in transient vertigo, pressure in the affected ear, tinnitus, and hearing loss.

No specific intervention is required; diving is not recommended until any lost hearing returns. Provide decongestants as needed and according to the EMS system's policies and procedures. No transport to the ED is needed if symptoms resolve quickly, and the patient may follow up with his or her primary care provider. If symptoms persist, transport for evaluation is appropriate.

Sinus Barotrauma

This form of sinus squeeze can occur on ascent when any form of blockage in the sinus openings prevents expanding gas from escaping. The expanding gas puts pressure on the mucosal lining of the sinus, causing pain with hemorrhage. Sinus barotrauma occurs in divers with upper respiratory infections or allergies. It is common for divers to take a decongestant before a dive as a preventive measure to help equalize the middle ear when diving. However, the vasoconstrictive benefits can wear off at depth, causing mucosal tissue expansion and forming a sinus blockage of expanding gas during the return to the surface.

Examine the nose for discharge. Signs and symptoms of sinus barotrauma include severe pain over the affected sinus and bloody discharge, usually from the frontal sinuses.

No specific management is needed at the scene unless extensive bleeding is observed, in which case treat for epistaxis by pinching firmly on the fleshy part of the patient's nostrils, just below the nasal bones. Transport the patient in a position of comfort.

Gastrointestinal Squeeze

This type of barotrauma occurs when expanding gas in the gut becomes trapped as the diver surfaces. Gastrointestinal (GI) barotrauma occurs in novice divers who frequently perform Valsalva maneuvers in the head-down position, which forces air into the stomach. It can also occur in divers who chew gum when diving or who have consumed carbonated beverages or other gas-producing foods before diving.

Examine the abdominal quadrants. Signs and symptoms of GI squeeze include abdominal fullness, belching, and flatulence.

GI squeeze normally resolves on its own and rarely needs medical attention. If the pain and fullness do not resolve, transport for evaluation is appropriate. Only in severe cases is recompression chamber therapy needed.

Pulmonary Overinflation Barotrauma

Pulmonary overinflation is a serious form of barotrauma resulting from the expansion of gas in the lungs during ascent. Normally the diver eliminates expanding gas with normal exhalations when returning to the surface. If the expanding gas does not escape, alveoli will rupture. This causes any one of several forms of injuries, depending on the amount of air that escapes outside the lung and its final location. A common scenario is a diver who has a rapid and uncontrollable ascent to the surface caused by running out of air, panic, or a dropped weight belt. These types of injuries are collectively called "pulmonary over-pressurization syndrome" (POPS), or *burst lung*.

The five forms of POPS are as follows:

1. Overdistension with local injury
2. Mediastinal emphysema
3. Subcutaneous emphysema
4. Pneumothorax
5. AGE

OVERDISTENSION WITH LOCAL INJURY

This is the mildest form of POPS, with only a small, isolated lung barotrauma. Auscultate the lung fields for diminished breath sounds. Chest pain may or may not be present. Blood is often seen in the sputum (hemoptysis).

Ensure that the patient rests in a position of comfort, and treat the patient's symptoms as needed. Monitor the patient's vital signs and oxygen saturation with pulse oximetry; provide oxygen at 2 to 4 liters/minute with nasal cannula. Transport the patient in position of comfort. The patient needs further medical evaluation to rule out a more severe form of POPS and should avoid further pressure exposure (e.g., diving or commercial flying).

MEDIASTINAL EMPHYSEMA

This is the most common form of POPS, caused by escaping gas from ruptured alveoli entering the interstitial space to the mediastinum. This condition is usually benign. Examine the lung fields for diminished breath sounds. Signs and symptoms include hoarseness, neck fullness, and minor substernal chest pain; often a dull ache or tightness is present that worsens with breathing and coughing. Examine the patient's chest and neck for subcutaneous emphysema. In severe cases, the diver presents with chest pain, dyspnea, and difficulty swallowing.

Ensure that the patient rests in a position of comfort. Monitor the patient's vital signs and oxygen saturation with pulse oximetry; provide oxygen at 2 to 4 liters/minute with nasal cannula. Usually, mediastinal emphysema requires no specific treatment or recompression therapy. However, patients may need to be medically evaluated to rule out other causes of chest pain and severe forms of POPS. Transport the patient in a supine position. The patient should avoid further pressure exposure (e.g., diving or commercial flying).

SUBCUTANEOUS EMPHYSEMA

With subcutaneous emphysema, air escaping from ruptured alveoli continues to move superiorly into the neck and clavicle regions of the chest. Examine the lung fields for diminished breath sounds. Signs and symptoms of subcutaneous emphysema include swelling, crepitus, hoarseness, sore throat, and difficulty swallowing.

No specific treatment is required besides rest. Monitor the patient's vital signs and oxygen saturation with pulse oximetry, and provide oxygen by nasal cannula at 2 to 4 liters/minute. The patient needs further medical evaluation to rule out more severe forms of POPS. Transport the patient in the supine position. The patient should avoid further pressure exposure (e.g., diving or commercial flying).

PNEUMOTHORAX

Pneumothorax is seen in less than 10% of POPS cases because air must escape through the visceral pleura around the lung, which presents greater resistance than air escaping through the interstitial space between the lung and visceral pleura. If the diver is at depth when a pulmonary rupture occurs, a tension pneumothorax can result as the volume of escaping gas expands as the diver continues toward the surface. Examine the lung fields for diminished breath sounds. Signs and symptoms will vary based on the size of the pneumothorax and include sharp chest pain, diminished breath sounds, breathlessness, subcutaneous emphysema, and dyspnea.

Provide ongoing assessment to monitor for conversion from simple to tension pneumothorax. Ensure rest in a position of comfort. Monitor the patient's vital signs and oxygen saturation with pulse oximetry, and provide oxygen by nasal cannula at 2 to 4 liters/minute. Provide standard ALS management of tension pneumothorax with 14-gauge needle thoracostomy as necessary. Transport the patient in a position of comfort. The patient needs further medical evaluation to rule out more severe forms of POPS and should avoid further pressure exposure (e.g., diving or commercial flying). Recompression therapy is generally not necessary.

ARTERIAL GAS EMBOLISM

This is the most feared complication of POPS and, after drowning, is a leading cause of death in divers, accounting for about 30% of fatalities.[112] AGE can occur from any of the four POPS conditions previously presented as a result of air escaping and forming an air embolism. AGE typically occurs in divers who have an uncontrolled ascent to the surface without appropriate exhalation, causing an overinflation pulmonary injury. However, AGE can occur in divers who surface slowly without underlying lung pathology. During ascent, once the pulmonary overinflation bursts alveoli, air enters the pulmonary venous capillary circulation; the gas bubbles enter the left atrium and left ventricle, then exit the heart through the aorta, and are distributed to the cerebral, coronary, and other systemic vasculature. Gas bubbles can enter the coronary circulation, causing an occlusion resulting in cardiac dysrhythmia, cardiac arrest, or myocardial infarction.[113] If gas bubbles enter the cerebral circulation, the diver presents with signs and symptoms similar to an acute stroke.

Unlike decompression sickness, which can present with delayed symptoms hours after diving, symptoms of AGE appear either immediately at the water surface or typically within 2 minutes. Any loss of consciousness once a diver surfaces must be presumed to be AGE until proved otherwise.[113] The primary treatment for AGE is recompression chamber (hyperbaric) therapy.

Historically, it was recommended that patients with AGE be placed in the Trendelenburg position for transport, based on the belief that this would help keep bubbles from circulating in the systemic vasculature. However, evidence has shown that the head-down position does not prevent systemic circulation of nitrogen bubbles, makes it more difficult to oxygenate the patient, and may worsen cerebral edema.[114] Currently, it is recommended that all AGE patients be placed in a supine position in the field and during transport. The supine position also provides a greater rate of nitrogen bubble washout.[115,116]

Decompression Sickness

Decompression sickness (DCS) is directly related to Henry's law. When scuba divers breathe compressed air containing oxygen (21%), carbon dioxide (0.03%), and nitrogen (79%), the amount of gas that will be dissolved in liquid is directly proportional to the partial pressure of gas in contact with liquid. Oxygen is used in the body for tissue metabolism when in solution and does not form gas bubbles during ascent from depth.

Nitrogen, an inert gas not used for metabolism, is the primary source of concern in DCS. Nitrogen is five times more soluble in fat than in water and becomes dissolved in tissue proportionately to the increasing ambient pressure. Consequently, the deeper underwater the diver goes and the longer the diver stays at depth, the greater the amount of nitrogen that dissolves into tissue. As the diver ascends toward the surface, the absorbed nitrogen must be eliminated. If there is inadequate time to eliminate nitrogen during ascent, nitrogen comes out of solution in the tissues in the form of intravascular gas bubbles, causing obstruction of the vascular and lymphatic systems and tissue distension, and activating inflammatory responses.[117]

Most divers experience DCS within the first hour after surfacing, although some will present with symptoms up to 6 hours after surfacing. Traditionally, symptoms of DCS are categorized as type I, a mild form involving cutaneous, lymphatic, and musculoskeletal systems, or type II, a severe form involving neurologic and cardiopulmonary systems (**Box 20-7**). Mild symptoms of DCS include fatigue and malaise. However, mild symptoms can be precursors to more severe signs and symptoms, such as numbness, weakness, and paralysis.

Studies now suggest that it is more important clinically to describe DCS by the region of the body affected and not as type I or type II.[102] This suggestion is applicable for prehospital care providers to ensure that even patients with mild DCS symptoms are treated aggressively with 100% oxygen and an early consult for recompression therapy. Many divers with the mild form of DCS will not have a medical evaluation. Divers may delay up to 32 hours before seeking medical care for DCS because denial of DCS is a common finding in the scuba diving population.[120]

Several factors predispose a diver to DCS.[121,122] Some risk factors are known to enhance the uptake of nitrogen in tissues during descent and slow the release of nitrogen during ascent. Certain host and environmental factors, as well as equipment failures and improper technique, increase the risk for DCS.

Limb Pain (Type I DCS)

This form of DCS results from bubble formation in the musculoskeletal system, typically occurring in one or more joints. The most common joints involved are the shoulder and elbow, followed by the knee, hip, wrist, hand, and ankle.[101] This pain is described as a severe tendonitis—joint pain with a grating sensation on movement. The pain starts gradually, presenting as a deep, dull ache of mild to severe intensity. Victims often attempt to relieve their pain by flexion of their joints, hence the common name for this condition—the *bends*. Although this form of DCS is not life threatening, it indicates that bubbles are present in the venous circulation. It can lead to more severe forms if left untreated.

Cutaneous and Lymphatic (Type I DCS)

This form of DCS is uncommon. It represents inadequate elimination of bubbles forming in the skin or lymphatic systems. Cutaneous *skin bends* are uncommon and usually not serious, but signs of mottling and marbling are considered precursors of delayed neurologic problems.[80] Symptoms include an intense rash that progresses to a red patchy or bluish discoloration of the skin.[115] Lymphatic obstruction can result in swelling and an orange-peel appearance (*peau d'orange*).

Cardiopulmonary (Type II DCS)

This severe form of DCS is referred to as the *chokes* and results when venous bubbles overwhelm the pulmonary capillary system. Hypotension can occur from a massive venous air embolism in the lung. Symptoms include nonproductive cough, substernal chest pain, cyanosis, dyspnea, shock, and cardiopulmonary arrest. This disorder resembles acute respiratory distress syndrome.[123] (See the Airway and Ventilation chapter for further information.)

Spinal Cord (Type II DCS)

The white matter of the spinal cord is vulnerable to bubble formation, and nitrogen is highly soluble in spinal cord tissue (*myelin*). The most common site for this form of DCS is the lower thoracic spine, followed by the lumbar/sacral and cervical regions.[120] Common signs and symptoms include low back pain and "heaviness" in the legs. With this form of DCS, the patient often gives a vague statement in an effort to describe "strange sensations," or paresthesia, which can progress to weakness, numbness, and paralysis. Bowel and bladder dysfunction, leading to urinary retention, also has been reported.[124]

Assessment of AGE and DCS

A standardized approach for patients with AGE and DCS is provided to ensure that consistent care is given. It is recommended that all patients with scuba-related diving injuries be examined for signs and symptoms of AGE and DCS because the primary and essential lifesaving treatment is recompression chamber therapy, which requires specific planning and logistics to access.[51]

Arterial Gas Embolism

About 5% of all AGE patients present with immediate apnea, unconsciousness, and cardiac arrest. Others present with signs and symptoms similar to acute stroke, with loss of consciousness, stupor, confusion, hemiparesis, seizure, vertigo, visual changes, sensory changes, and headache.

Decompression Sickness

Type I DCS is characterized by deep pain in a joint, including minor forms of cutaneous pruritus (severe itching) and obstruction of lymph vessels (lymphedema). Type II DCS is characterized by symptoms involving the CNS, ranging from weakness and numbness to paralysis.

Obtain a dive profile and medical history of the events that led to the diving-related injury from a fellow diver, including:

- Time of onset of signs and symptoms
- Source of breathing medium (e.g., air or mixed gases; heliox)
- Dive profile (dive activity, depth, duration, dive frequency, surface interval, interval between dives)

- Dive location and water conditions
- Dive risk factors
- Underwater medical and equipment problems on ascent and descent
- Whether the diver was attempting a no-decompression dive or a decompression dive
- Rate of ascent
- Decompression stop(s)
- Post-dive activity level
- Post-dive aircraft travel, with type and duration
- Past and present medical history (especially a history of previous DCS)
- Medication use
- Current use of alcohol or illicit drugs[125]

Management

Ensure the ABCs, protect the patient's airway, and initiate BLS or ALS procedures as required. Initiate 100% oxygen at 12 to 15 liters/minute, and give NS or LR (no dextrose) IV fluid therapy (1 to 2 ml/kg/hour). Monitor the patient's vital signs, pulse oximetry, and ECG. Check and treat the patient's blood glucose as required. Control any seizures. Protect the patient from hypothermia, and consult early with local medical control or DAN for the closest recompression chamber (primary treatment). Note that recompression chambers capable of accepting divers are rare—for example, in the entire state of Florida there are only four—meaning that specific planning, and ideally preplanning before an incident, is needed to ensure rapid transport to the closest appropriate facility.[51] See **Box 20-8** for DAN contact information. Standard recompression therapy with 100% hyperbaric oxygen is given according to the U.S. Navy treatment tables.[126] Transport the patient in a supine position. For any scuba-related diving injury, if air evacuation is provided by helicopter or other nonpressurized aircraft, it is recommended to fly as low as possible (e.g., 500 ft [150 m]), and certainly not to exceed 1,000 ft (300 m), to minimize further expansion of air bubbles (Boyle's law) and further dysbarism trauma.[51,102,107,116]

Definitive treatment for specific barotraumas, including AGE and DCS, is to administer 100% oxygen by mask at two to three times the atmospheric pressure at sea level in a recompression chamber.[126] For further discussion of recompression chamber treatment methods for scuba-related diving injuries, see the *U.S. Navy Diving Manual* or other sources.[102,126] The patient immediately benefits, based on the principles of Boyle's law, by increasing the ambient pressure and decreasing the size of bubbles formed and increasing the oxygen concentration in tissues. **Box 20-9** describes recompression and hyperbaric oxygen therapy.

For the transporting prehospital team, it is critical to ensure that the receiving ED or other facility knows that diving-related conditions such as DCS and AGE are true emergencies and that a detailed examination, including a neurologic examination, will need to be completed as soon as possible by a facility-based emergency clinician. There are additional reading resources that describe techniques for optimizing team-to-team communication and hand-offs of this sort. See the Patient Assessment and Management chapter for more details on the patient hand-off process.

Table 20-5 summarizes signs and symptoms of barotrauma and its treatment. **Table 20-6** summarizes signs and symptoms of DCS and its treatment.

Prevention of Scuba-Related Diving Injuries

Millions of certified scuba divers need frequent skill refresher training to prevent and recognize scuba-related dive injuries. Many scuba professionals in the United States, such as lifeguards, fire and law enforcement personnel, search and rescue members, Coast Guard members, and Department of Defense employees, depend on local prehospital care providers to provide initial and follow-up medical care and transport to local hospitals or recompression chambers. Collaboration among dive teams and local EMS agencies to develop medical scenarios during dive training is strongly encouraged.[51] This should include frequent scuba training in varying underwater conditions and locations, along with in-water rescue scenarios and initial medical care, which are paramount to responding safely and effectively for in-water swimmer/diver rescues and recoveries. Scuba training coordination among medical dive team members and local providers will ensure effective communication and appropriate continuity of field care. This training should include scenario-based consults with local medical control and DAN.

Box 20-8 Divers Alert Network (DAN) Contact Information

Diving Emergencies (Remember: Call local EMS first, then DAN!)
1-919-684-9111

Nonemergency Medical Questions
1-800-446-2671 or 1-919-684-2948
Monday–Friday, 8:30 a.m. to 5:00 p.m. (EST)

All Other Inquiries
1-800-446-2671 or 1-919-684-2948
1-919-490-6630 (fax)

Contact Information to Send a Letter
Divers Alert Network

6 West Colony Place

Durham, NC 27705 USA

Data courtesy of Divers Alert Network® (DAN®).

Box 20-9 Recompression Therapy for Scuba-Related Diving Injuries

The goals of recompression therapy for scuba-related diving injuries caused by pulmonary overinflation barotrauma and DCS are to compress the bubbles and increase oxygen delivery to tissues. Recompression therapy includes the following mechanisms:

- Reduces volume of the bubbles where they are circulated to the pulmonary capillaries and filtered out
- Promotes reabsorption of bubbles in solution
- Increases oxygen delivery to the tissues
- Corrects hypoxia
- Provides an increased diffusion gradient for nitrogen
- Reduces edema
- Reduces blood vessel permeability

All divers with AGE and DCS must be considered early for recompression in a hyperbaric treatment facility because the treatment is more successful if started within 6 hours after the onset of symptoms. Divers are not always near a recompression chamber when symptoms occur, and there can be considerable delays getting to a chamber by ground or by arranging for air transport. Contact the Diver's Alert Network to consult for diving medical assistance and to determine the closest recompression chamber.

In the meantime, place the patient in a supine position. Nitrogen washout can be increased by providing 100% oxygen by mask and by starting an IV fluid line with normal saline or lactated Ringer solution at 1 to 2 ml/kg/hr to ensure adequate intravascular volume and capillary perfusion. During recompression treatment, patients with AGE or DCS normally will receive recompression treatment at 2.5 to 3.0 atm for 2 to 4 hours while breathing 100% oxygen. Longer and repeated treatment will be necessary if the patient has no clinical improvement of symptoms.

Recompression treatment principles include the following:

- Any painful or neurologic signs or symptoms occurring within 24 hours of a dive are caused by DCS until proved otherwise.
- Any painful or neurologic signs or symptoms occurring within 48 hours of flying after diving are caused by DCS until proved otherwise.
- Contact the DAN 24-hour emergency hotline for consultation at 919-684-9111.
- Every diver with signs or symptoms of DCS should receive recompression treatment.
- Never fail to treat cases when in doubt about the diagnosis.
- Early treatment improves outcomes, whereas delayed treatment worsens outcomes.
- Long delays should never preclude treatment because divers respond to recompression therapy days to weeks after injury.
- Monitor the patient closely for signs of relief from or progression of symptoms.
- Inadequate treatment can lead to a recurrence.
- Continue to treat until clinical plateau.

Modified from Tibbles PM, Edelsberg JS: Hyperbaric oxygen therapy. *N Engl J Med* 334(25):1642, 1996; Barratt DM, Harch PG, Van Meter K: Decompression illness in divers: A review of the literature. *Neurologist* 8:186, 2002; and Van Hoesen KB, Bird NH: Diving medicine. In Auerbach PS: *Wilderness Medicine*, ed 6, St. Louis, 2012, Mosby Elsevier.

Medical Fitness to Dive

Prehospital care providers responding to diving-related incidents must assess divers, in all age groups, not only for primary diving disorders related to a submersion incident (e.g., DCS, AGE) but also for underlying medical conditions (e.g., cardiac, pulmonary, neurologic, endocrine, psychiatric, or a combination of both medical and dysbaric disorders). Ideally, all new divers should be cleared medically before the start of scuba training. Five general medical screening recommendations for identifying individuals who are at an increased risk for a diving-related problem are listed below. These recommendations are based on the consensus of medical diving specialists.[102,107,127] Also refer to **Table 20-7** for the severe risk (absolute contraindications), relative risk, and temporary risk conditions of concern for scuba diving.[102,107] Recommendations include the following:

- Inability to equalize pressure in one or more of the body's air spaces increases the risk for barotrauma.
- Medical or psychiatric conditions may manifest underwater or at a remote diving site and can endanger the diver's life because of the condition itself, because it occurs in the water, or because adequate medical help is not available.
- Impaired tissue perfusion or diffusion of inert gases increases the risk of DCS.
- Poor physical condition increases the risk of DCS or exertion-related medical problems. The factors compromising physical condition may be physiologic or pharmacologic.
- In women who are pregnant, the fetus may be at increased risk of dysbaric injury.

For many years, people with diabetes have questioned the diving medical experts about scuba diving waivers for

Table 20-5 Barotrauma: Common Signs, Symptoms, and Treatment

Type	Signs/Symptoms	Treatment*
Mask squeeze	Corneal injection, conjunctival hemorrhage	Self-limited; rest, cold compresses, pain medication
Sinus squeeze	Pain, bloody nasal discharge	Pain medication, decongestants, antihistamines
Middle-ear squeeze	Pain, vertigo, tympanic membrane rupture, hearing loss, vomiting	Decongestants, antihistamines, pain medication; may need antibiotics; avoid diving and flying
Internal-ear barotraumas	Tinnitus, vertigo, ataxia, hearing loss	Bed rest; elevate head; avoid loud noises; stool softeners; avoid strenuous activity; no diving or flying for months
External-ear barotraumas	Difficulty with Valsalva maneuver, earache, bloody discharge, possible tympanic membrane rupture	Maintain dry ear canal; antibiotics may be needed for infection
Tooth squeeze	Tooth pain while diving	Self-limited; pain medication
Alternobaric vertigo	Pressure, pain in affected ear, vertigo, tinnitus	Usually short lived; decongestants; prohibit diving until resolution with normal hearing
Pulmonary barotraumas	Substernal pain, voice change, dyspnea, subcutaneous emphysema	Assess ABCs, neurologic functions; 100% oxygen 12 to 15 liters/minute nonrebreathing mask; transport patient lying supine; need to rule out AGE
Subcutaneous emphysema	Substernal pain and crepitus, brassy voice, neck swelling, dyspnea, bloody sputum	Rest; avoid diving and flying; oxygen and recompression therapy only in severe cases
Pneumothorax	Sharp chest pain, dyspnea, diminished breath sounds	100% oxygen 12 to 15 liters/minute nonrebreathing mask; monitor pulse oximetry; transport in position of comfort; assess for tension pneumothorax
Tension pneumothorax	Cyanosis, distended neck veins, tracheal deviation	14-gauge needle thoracentesis; 100% oxygen 12 to 15 liters/minute nonrebreathing mask; monitor pulse oximetry
AGE	Unresponsiveness, confusion, headache, visual disturbances, seizure	Assess ABCs, neurologic functions; initiate BLS/ALS; control seizures; 100% oxygen 12 to 15 liters/minute nonrebreathing mask; transport patient lying supine; glucose-free IV fluid therapy (1 to 2 ml/kg/hr); monitor ECG; consult DAN (919-684-9111) for closest recompression chamber (primary treatment)

*Good patient education on scene for minor barotrauma injuries is important because some of these injuries are self-limiting and others need physician evaluation; others need patient referral to the family physician or ED and will not necessitate EMS transport.

Note: ABCs, airway, breathing, circulation; AGE, arterial gas embolism; ALS, advanced life support; BLS, basic life support; DAN, Divers Alert Network; ECG, electrocardiogram.

Modified from Clenney TL, Lassen LF: Recreational scuba diving injuries. *Am Fam Physician* 53(5):1761, 1996; Salahuddin M, James LA, Bass ES. SCUBA medicine: A first-responder's guide to diving injuries. *Curr Sports Med Reports.* 10(3):134-139, 2011; and Van Hoesen KB, Bird NH: Diving medicine. In Auerbach PS: *Wilderness Medicine*, ed 6, St. Louis, 2012, Mosby Elsevier.

Table 20-6 Decompression Sickness: Common Signs, Symptoms, and Treatment

Condition	Signs/Symptoms	Treatment
DCS Type I		
Skin bends	Intense itching (pruritus); red rash patches over shoulders and upper chest; skin marbling may precede burning sensation and itching over shoulders and torso; localized cyanosis and pitting edema.	Self-limiting; resolves on its own; observe for delayed signs of limb-pain DCS.
Limb-pain DCS	Large joint tenderness; mild to severe joint or extremity pain; pain is usually steady but may throb and present in 75% of cases; grating sensation on joint motion; worse with movement. DCS type I may progress to DCS type II.	Mild pain only often resolves on its own; observe 24 hours; moderate to severe pain. Start with 100% oxygen, 12 to 15 liters/minute nonrebreathing mask; transport all patients in supine position; glucose-free IV fluid therapy (1 to 2 ml/kg/hr); early consult DAN (919-684-9111) for closest recompression chamber for definitive treatment.
DCS Type II		
Cardiopulmonary "chokes"	Substernal pain, mild cough, dyspnea, nonproductive cough, cyanosis, tachypnea, tachycardia, shock and cardiac arrest	ABCs; 100% oxygen, 12 to 15 liters/minute nonrebreathing mask; BLS or ALS as needed; glucose-free IV fluid therapy (1 to 2 ml/kg/hr); transport all patients in supine position; early consult DAN (919-684-9111) for closest recompression chamber for definitive treatment.
Neurologic		
Brain	Many visual changes, headache, confusion, disorientation, nausea and vomiting	
Spinal cord	Back pain, heaviness or weakness, numbness, paralysis, urine retention, fecal incontinence	
Inner ear	Vertigo, ataxia	

Note: ABCs, airway, breathing, circulation; ALS, advanced life support; BLS, basic life support; DAN, Divers Alert Network; DCS, decompression sickness; IV, intravenous.

Modified from Barratt DM, Harch PG, Van Meter K: Decompression illness in divers: A review of the literature. *Neurologist.* 8:186, 2002; and Van Hoesen KB, Bird NH: Diving medicine. In Auerbach PS: *Wilderness Medicine,* ed 6, St. Louis, 2012, Mosby Elsevier.

individuals who have control of their blood glucose. In June 2005, an international workshop was held in the United States that was jointly sponsored by the Undersea and Hyperbaric Medical Society (UHMS) and DAN. They brought together over 50 medical and research experts from around the world to develop guidelines for recreational divers with diabetes.[128] The panel indicated that dive candidates who use medication (oral hypoglycemic agents or insulin) to treat diabetes but who are otherwise qualified to dive may undertake recreational scuba diving. However, they stated that strict criteria need to be met before diving. The panel agreed that people with diabetes who are using

dietary control will easily meet the new guidelines. The consensus guidelines (**Box 20-10**) consist of 19 points, under the categories of selection and surveillance, scope of diving, and glucose management on the day of diving.

Flying After Diving

Because diving is conducted at many popular dive locations in the United States and at remote locations outside the United States, persons may dive the day before flying. Because of Boyle's principle, flying too soon after a dive can increase the risk of DCS during flight or after arriving at the

Table 20-7 Fitness to Dive: Guidelines for Medical Clearance for Recreational Diving

System	Severe Risk Conditions	Relative Risk Conditions	Temporary Risk Conditions
Neurologic	Seizures Transient ischemic attack or cerebrovascular accident Serious decompression sickness with residual deficits	Complicated migraine Head injury with sequelae Herniated disc Peripheral neuropathy Multiple sclerosis Spinal cord or brain injury Intracranial tumor or aneurysm	Arterial gas embolism without residual, in which pulmonary air trapping has been excluded and probability of recurrence is low
Cardiovascular	Intracardiac right-to-left shunt (atrial septal defect) Hypertrophic cardiomyopathy Valvular stenosis	Coronary artery bypass grafting Percutaneous transluminal coronary angioplasty or coronary artery disease History of myocardial infarction Congestive heart failure Hypertension Dysrhythmias Valvular regurgitation	Pacemaker: if problem necessitating pacing does not preclude diving; pacemakers must be certified by manufacturer to withstand pressure
Pulmonary	Spontaneous pneumothorax Impaired exercise performance due to respiratory disease	Asthma or reactive airway disease Exercise-induced bronchospasm Solid, cystic, or cavitating lesions Pneumothorax caused by surgery, trauma, previous overinflation Immersion pulmonary edema Interstitial lung disease	
Gastrointestinal	Gastric outlet obstruction Chronic or recurrent small bowel obstruction Severe gastroesophageal reflux Paraesophageal hernia	Inflammatory bowel disease Functional bowel disorders	Unrepaired hernias of the abdominal wall Peptic ulcer disease associated with obstruction or severe reflux
Metabolic and endocrine	Pregnancy	Type 1 or type 2 diabetes mellitus	
Otolaryngologic	Open tympanic membrane perforation Tube myringotomy Middle ear or inner ear surgery Tracheostomy	Recurrent otitis externa, otitis media, or sinusitis Eustachian tube dysfunction History of tympanic membrane perforation, tympanoplasty, or mastoidectomy Significant conductive or sensorineural hearing loss History of round or oval window rupture	Acute upper respiratory infection Acute sinusitis Acute otitis media

System	Severe Risk Conditions	Relative Risk Conditions	Temporary Risk Conditions
Orthopedic		Amputation Scoliosis with impact on respiratory performance Aseptic necrosis	Back pain
Hematologic		Sickle cell disease Leukemia Hemophilia Polycythemia vera	
Behavioral health	Inappropriate motivation to dive Claustrophobia Acute psychosis Untreated panic disorder	Use of psychotropic medications Previous psychotic episodes	

From Van Hoesen KB, Bird NH: Diving medicine. This article was published in *Wilderness Medicine*, 6e, Auerbach PS, Copyright Mosby Elsevier 2012.

Box 20-10 Guidelines for Recreational Diving With Diabetes

Selection and Surveillance
- Individual must be at least 18 years of age (16 years if in special training program).
- Diving will be delayed after starting/changing medication, as follows:
  · Three months with oral hypoglycemic agents
  · One year after initiation of insulin therapy
- There must be no episodes of hypoglycemia or hyperglycemia requiring intervention from a third party within at least 1 year.
- There must be no history of hypoglycemia unawareness.
- A glycated hemoglobin (HbA1c) test result of ≤ 9% must be recorded no more than 1 month prior to initial assessment and at each annual review.
  · Values > 9% indicate the need for further evaluation and possible modification of therapy.
- There must be no significant secondary complications from diabetes.
- A physician/diabetologist should carry out an annual review and determine that the diver has a good understanding of the disease and the effect of exercise in consultation with an expert in diving medicine, as required.

- An evaluation for silent cardiac ischemia for candidates older than 40 years of age must be performed.
  · After initial evaluation, periodic surveillance for silent cardiac ischemia can be in accordance with accepted local/national guidelines for the evaluation of diabetics.
- Candidate must document intent to follow protocol for divers with diabetes and to cease diving and seek medical review for any adverse events during diving possibly related to diabetes.

Scope of Diving
- Diving should be planned to avoid:
  · Depths > 100 ft (30 m) seawater
  · Durations > 60 minutes
  · Compulsory decompression stops
  · Overhead environments (e.g., cave, wreck penetration)
  · Situations that may exacerbate hypoglycemia (e.g., prolonged cold and arduous dives)
- Individuals must have a dive buddy/leader informed of diver's condition and steps to follow in case of problem.
  · Dive buddy should not have diabetes.

(continued)

Box 20-10 Guidelines for Recreational Diving With Diabetes (*continued*)

Glucose Management on the Day of Diving

- Individuals should perform a general self-assessment of fitness to dive.
- Blood glucose must be ≥ 150 mg/dl (8.3 mmol/l), stable or rising, before entering the water.
  - Complete a minimum of three predive blood glucose tests to evaluate trends at 60 minutes, 30 minutes, and immediately prior to diving.
  - Alterations in dosage of oral hypoglycemic agent or insulin on evening prior or day of diving may help.
- Delay dive if blood glucose is:
  - < 150 mg/dl (8.3 mmol/l)
  - > 300 mg/dl (16.7 mmol/l)

- Rescue medication considerations include:
  - Carry readily accessible oral glucose during all dives.
  - Have parenteral glucagon available at the surface.
- If hypoglycemia is noticed underwater, the diver should surface (with buddy), establish positive buoyancy, ingest glucose, and leave the water.
- Check blood glucose frequently for 12 to 15 hours after diving.
- Ensure adequate hydration on days of diving.
- Log all dives, including blood glucose test results and all information pertinent to diabetes management.

Data courtesy of Divers Alert Network® (DAN®).

Box 20-11 Current Guidelines Recommended by Diver's Alert Network for Flying Safely After Diving

The following guidelines are the consensus of attendees at the 2002 Flying After Diving Workshop. They apply to dives followed by flights at cabin altitudes of 2,000 to 8,000 ft (610 to 2,440 m) for divers who do not have symptoms of DCS. The recommended preflight surface intervals do not guarantee avoidance of DCS. Longer surface intervals will reduce DCS risk further.

- For a single no-decompression dive, a minimum preflight surface interval of 12 hours is suggested.
- For multiple dives per day or multiple days of diving, a minimum preflight surface interval of 18 hours is suggested.

For dives requiring decompression stops, there is little evidence on which to base a recommendation, and a preflight surface interval substantially longer than 18 hours appears prudent.

Data courtesy of Divers Alert Network® (DAN®).

destination because of the reduced atmospheric pressure in either a pressurized or a nonpressurized commercial aircraft. **Box 20-11** lists the current guidelines recommended by DAN for flying safely after diving.[102]

High-Altitude Illness

In the United States, more than 40 million people each year travel above 8,200 ft (2,500 m) without acclimatization to participate in activities that include snowboarding, alpine skiing, hiking, camping, festivals, climbing, work, and many others. Thus, many people are at risk for altitude-related illness, which can develop within hours to days after they arrive at altitude.[129] Prehospital care providers and ED staff need to become familiar with the predisposing factors, signs and symptoms, medical management, and education and prevention techniques to reduce the morbidity and mortality of high-altitude illness.

This section presents three medical conditions directly caused by high-altitude environments and highlights specific underlying medical conditions that worsen as a result of high-altitude–induced hypoxia (altitude-exacerbated preexisting medical conditions).

Epidemiology

High-altitude illness is a term that encompasses cerebral and pulmonary syndromes: (1) acute mountain sickness (AMS), (2) high-altitude cerebral edema (HACE), and (3) high-altitude pulmonary edema (HAPE). AMS and HACE are mild and severe ends of a spectrum, while HAPE involves separate processes. Even though the risks of acquiring high-altitude illness are low, once it develops, progression can be fatal.[130,131]

Acute mountain sickness (AMS) is a mild form of high-altitude illness, rarely experienced at altitudes below 6,540 ft (2,000 m), but the incidence increases to 1.4% to 25% with increasing altitudes of 6,750 to 8,000 ft (2,060 to 2,440 m).[132,133] AMS develops in 20% to 25% of cases above 8,200 ft (2,500 m) and in 40% to 50% of cases at 14,000 ft (4,270 m). The incidence of AMS is greater than 90% when the rate of ascent to approximately 14,000 ft (4,270 m) occurs over hours versus days.[134] Furthermore, a small number of AMS cases (5% to 10%) progress from mild symptoms to become high-altitude cerebral edema, a severe form of AMS.[131]

High-altitude cerebral edema (HACE) is a severe neurologic form of high-altitude illness. It has a low incidence rate (0.01%) in the general population at an altitude above 8,200 ft (2,500 m); this rate increases to 1% to 2% in more physically active individuals and is even higher above 13,120 ft (4,000 m) with rapid ascent.[129]

High-altitude pulmonary edema (HAPE) is generally rare outside of certain high-altitude operations but accounts for the most deaths from high-altitude illness and is easily reversed if recognized early and managed correctly. HAPE typically presents within 2 to 5 days after arrival at altitude.[131] The incidence rate for HAPE is 0.01% to 0.1% at 8,200 ft (2,500 m) in the general population and increases to 2% or more in climbers at an altitude of 13,120 ft (4,000 m).

Hypobaric Hypoxia

There are three defined levels of altitude. **High altitude** is defined as an elevation of 5,000 to 11,480 ft (1,500 to 3,500 m). This is a common altitude in the western mountain ranges of the United States, where high-altitude illness is reported with greater frequency than in other regions, and whose ski areas are generally higher than in areas such as the European Alps.[135] **Very high altitude** is defined as an elevation of 11,480 to 18,045 ft (3,500 to 5,500 m) and is the more common altitude for serious forms of high-altitude illness.[136] **Extreme altitude** is defined as elevations higher than 18,045 ft (5,500 m).[131] With a progressive increase in altitude, the environment becomes very hostile to any person who is not acclimatized to the decreased

availability of oxygen, causing a condition known as **hypobaric hypoxia**. However, hypobaric hypoxia occurs at all altitudes to differing degrees.

High altitude is a unique environment because there is a decreased availability of oxygen for respiration, which results in cellular hypoxia. Even though the concentration of oxygen remains at 21% at all altitudes, decreased atmospheric pressure at higher altitude results in a decreased partial pressure of oxygen (Po_2). For example, Po_2 is 160 mm Hg at sea level (1 atm) and 80 mm Hg at 18,045 ft (0.5 atm at 5,500 m), resulting in less oxygen available during respiration. **Table 20-8** shows that as altitude increases from sea level to extreme altitude, there is a proportional decrease in barometric pressure, arterial blood gases, and arterial oxygen saturation (Sao_2). It is worth noting that Sao_2 remains, on average, above 91% in healthy, acclimatizing adults until reaching an altitude above 9,200 ft (2,800 m).

This relationship between increasing altitude and progressive hypoxia forms the basis for the acute physiologic adjustments in ventilatory rate and cardiac output and biochemical changes.[137] Consequently, it is the hypobaric hypoxia and hypoxemia that set up nonacclimatized individuals for high-altitude illness.[130]

Factors Related to High-Altitude Illness

The development of high-altitude illness depends on many factors specific to each high-altitude exposure, but key factors include rapid ascent, individual acclimatization rate, physical exertion at altitude, young age, and history

Table 20-8 Relationship of Altitude, Barometric Pressure (Pb), Arterial Blood Gases, and Oxygen Saturation*

Altitude (meters)	Altitude (feet)	Pb (mm Hg)	Pao₂ (mm Hg)	Sao₂ (%)	Paco₂ (mm Hg)
Sea level	Sea level	760	100	98.0	40.0
1,646	5,400	630	73.0	95.1	35.6
2,810	9,200	543	60.0	91.0	33.9
3,660	12,020	489	47.6	84.5	29.5
4,700	15,440	429	44.6	78.0	27.1
5,340	17,500	401	43.1	76.2	25.7
6,140	20,140	356	35.0	65.6	22.0

*Data are mean values for subjects ages 20 to 40 years.

Note: $Paco_2$, arterial carbon dioxide partial pressure; Pao_2, arterial oxygen partial pressure; Sao_2, arterial oxygen saturation.

Modified from Hackett PH, Roach RC: High-altitude medicine. In Auerbach PS: *Wilderness Medicine*, ed 6, St. Louis, 2012, Mosby Elsevier.

of prior altitude illness.[138] Additional factors include the following:

- *Increased altitude and ascent rate.* The incidence and severity of high-altitude illness are primarily related to the speed of ascent, altitude reached, and length of stay (in shorter durations; longer duration at altitude after a certain period of time equates to less risk), because these three factors increase the hypoxic stress in the body.[129,136]

- *Previous history of high-altitude illness.* A documented history of high-altitude illness is a valuable predictor of who is susceptible for subsequent high-altitude illness when returning to the same altitude at the same ascent rate.[139] Incidence rates for HAPE increase from 10% to 60% for those with a previous history of HAPE who abruptly ascend to an altitude of 14,960 ft (4,560 m).[140]

- *Preacclimatization.* Having a permanent residence above 2,950 ft (900 m) provides some preacclimatization and is associated with a lower rate of and severity of high-altitude illness when ascending to higher altitudes. However, this protection is limited if the ascent rate is rapid or reaches an extreme altitude.[135,136]

- *Age and gender.* Age, but not gender, is a factor in developing AMS; the incidence is lower in those older than 50 years. HAPE occurs more frequently and with greater severity in children and young adults and is reported in equal proportions of males and females in these age groups.[130,141]

- *Physical fitness and exertion.* The onset and severity of high-altitude illness are independent of physical fitness; fitness does not accelerate altitude acclimatization. A high level of fitness does allow individuals to exert themselves more, but vigorous exertion on arrival at high altitude further exacerbates hypoxemia and hastens the onset of high-altitude illness.[135,142]

- *Medications and intoxicants.* Any substance that depresses ventilation and disrupts sleep patterns at altitude should be avoided because this will further exacerbate altitude-induced hypoxemia. These substances include alcohol, barbiturates, and opioids.[131,143]

- *Cold.* Exposure to cold ambient temperatures increases the risk for HAPE because cold increases the pulmonary arterial pressure.[144,145]

Preexisting medical conditions are another factor related to high-altitude illness. It is important to note that when clinical studies are used to determine effective dose of medication for AMS and HACE, they generally include only healthy individuals without underlying medical problems. However, today many more high-altitude travelers and those who move their residence to higher altitudes have underlying diseases such as diabetes, hypertension, heart disease, or depression. The current medication recommendations for managing altitude illness may not

be appropriate for these patients due to the potential for drug interactions and for those patients with renal and/or hepatic insufficiencies. A discussion of these issues can be found in a review article of the medications for the prevention and treatment of altitude illness (i.e., AMS, HAPE, and HACE) for healthy individuals and the drug selection and dosing for patients with underlying medical conditions.[145]

Table 20-9 lists conditions that increase the likelihood of developing high-altitude illness. Additionally, specific

Table 20-9 Risk Categories of High-Altitude Illness	
Risk Category	**Description**
Low	▪ Individuals with no prior history of altitude illness and ascending to < 9,200 ft (2,800 m) ▪ Individuals taking ≥ 2 days to arrive at 8,200 to 10,000 ft (2,500 to 3,000 m) with subsequent increases in sleeping elevation of less than 1,600 ft (500 m) per day
Moderate	▪ Individuals with prior history of AMS and ascending to 8,200 to 9,100 ft (2,500 to 2,800 m) in 1 day ▪ No history of AMS but ascending to > 9,100 ft (2,800 m) in 1 day ▪ All individuals ascending > 1,600 ft (500 m) per day at altitudes above 10,000 ft (3,000 m)
High	▪ History of AMS and ascending to ≥ 9,100 ft (2,800 m) in 1 day ▪ All individuals with prior history of HAPE or HACE ▪ All individuals ascending to > 11,500 ft (3,500 m) in 1 day ▪ All individuals ascending > 1,600 ft (500 m) per day at altitudes above 11,500 ft (3,500 m) ▪ Very rapid ascents

Note: AMS, acute mountain sickness; HACE, high-altitude cerebral edema; HAPE, high-altitude pulmonary edema.

Modified from Luk AM, McIntosh SE, Grissom et al. Wilderness Medical Society consensus guidelines for the prevention and treatment of acute altitude illness. *Wilderness Environ Med.* 21:146-55;2010.

medical conditions known to increase susceptibility to high-altitude illness include the following:

- Cardiopulmonary congenital abnormalities: absent pulmonary artery, primary pulmonary hypertension, congenital heart defects
- Carotid artery surgery: irradiation or abolishing carotid bodies

Acute Mountain Sickness

AMS is a self-limited, nonspecific symptom complex that can be easily mistaken for a number of other conditions because of common symptoms, including influenza, hangover, exhaustion, and dehydration. A consensus panel defined AMS as the presence of headache in an unacclimatized person who has recently arrived at an altitude above 8,200 ft (2,500 m) and has one or more symptoms of AMS.[146] However, AMS can occur at levels as low as 6,600 ft (2,000 m). HACE is viewed as a severe form of AMS.[147,148] The majority of AMS cases do not progress to more severe forms of high-altitude illness.

The hallmark symptom of AMS is a mild to severe protracted headache believed to be caused by hypoxia-induced cerebral vasodilation.[149] Patients describe their headache as throbbing, as located in the occipital or temporal regions, and as worsening at night or on awakening. Other symptoms include nausea, vomiting, insomnia, dizziness, *lassitude* (weariness), fatigue, and difficulty sleeping. Malaise and lack of appetite may be present along with a decrease in urine output. It is important to recognize early symptoms of AMS so that continued ascent does not cause a preventable condition to progress into a severe form of HACE.

The onset of symptoms in AMS can occur as early as 1 hour after arriving at high altitude but typically occurs after 6 to 10 hours of exposure. Symptoms usually peak in 24 to 72 hours and subside in 3 to 7 days. If the onset of symptoms occurs beyond 3 days after arriving at altitude and does not include headache, and if oxygen therapy provides no benefit, the condition is probably not AMS.[130]

As with lightning and drowning management, the WMS has a consensus-derived set of practice guidelines regarding AMS. These guidelines are available online and should help providers determine evidence-based current best practices.[138]

Assessment

If patients are alert, the key is to obtain a good medical history, including the onset and severity of symptoms, rate of ascent, duration of exposure, use of medications that may cause dehydration, use of alcohol, and level of physical exertion. Obtain vital signs, including pulse oximetry. Also, assess the status of any underlying medical condition, as determined by the medical history.

Because a headache is the most common finding with AMS, assess for location and quality. Periodic breathing is a common finding in individuals who have ascended above about 10,000 ft (about 3,000 m). Assess neurologic function, and assess specifically for ataxia and excessive lethargy, as these symptoms are indicative of HACE.

Management

Descending 1,600 to 3,300 ft (500 to 1,000 m) will provide the quickest resolution of symptoms. Mild AMS will usually resolve on its own, but patients should avoid further ascent and any exertion until symptoms resolve. Provide analgesics for headache and antiemetics for nausea per local protocols. For moderate symptoms, descend to lower altitude. Assess pulse oximetry for SpO_2 greater than 90%. If lower than 90%, titrate oxygen by 1 to 2 liters/minute and reassess. However, this is altitude related; at 14,100 ft (4,300 m), a normal SpO_2 is in the mid-80s. Unexpectedly low SpO_2 might represent HACE, but SpO_2 readings are generally not very helpful in diagnosing AMS. For patients with neurologic symptoms, see management of HACE. Patients with underlying medical problems exacerbated by altitude should be transported on oxygen for medical evaluation of their primary illness and the secondary development of high-altitude illness.

See **Table 20-10** for a summary of the signs and symptoms, management, and prevention of AMS. See **Table 20-11** for dosing recommendations for children with AMS.

High-Altitude Cerebral Edema

HACE is a very serious neurologic syndrome that can develop in individuals with AMS or HAPE or that can develop on its own without relation to the other altitude illnesses. At altitudes above 8,000 ft (2,440 m), cerebral blood flow increases as a result of hypoxia-induced vasodilation. The mechanism of injury appears to be related to a combination of sustained cerebral vasodilation, increased capillary permeability across the blood–brain barrier, and the inability to compensate sufficiently for the excess cerebral edema.[150]

HACE can occur at any time within 3 to 5 days after arrival at 9,000 ft (2,750 m), but generally it occurs at altitudes above 12,000 ft (3,600 m), with an onset of symptoms within hours. Some symptoms of AMS may be present, but the hallmark features of HACE are altered level of consciousness and ataxia, along with drowsiness, stupor, and confusion progressing to coma. Death results from brain herniation.[151]

Assessment

If the patient is alert, as with AMS, the key is to obtain a good medical history, including the onset and severity of symptoms, rate of ascent, duration of exposure, and level of physical exertion. Obtain the patient's vital signs, including pulse oximetry. Also, assess the status of any underlying

Table 20-10 High-Altitude Illness (AMS, HACE, HAPE): Signs, Symptoms, Treatment, and Prevention

Signs/Symptoms	Treatment	Prevention
Acute Mountain Sickness (AMS)		
Mild: Headache, nausea, dizziness, and fatigue in first 12 hours	Oxygen 1 to 2 liters/minute by nasal cannula, and/or descend 1,600 to 3,300 ft (500 to 1,000 m); avoid further ascent until symptoms resolve; consider acetazolamide (250 mg PO bid) to speed acclimatization; give analgesics and antiemetics as needed	Ascend at slow rate; spend night at intermediate altitude; avoid overexertion; avoid direct transport above 9,840 ft (3,000 m) Consider acetazolamide 125 mg PO bid, starting day before ascent and continued for 2 days at maximum altitude Early AMS treatment may prevent subsequent complications
Moderate: Moderate to severe headache, marked nausea, vomiting, decreased appetite, dizziness, insomnia, fluid retention for ≥ 12 hours	Descend, consider dexamethasone* (4 mg PO/IM every 6 hours) and/or acetazolamide (250 mg PO bid); if unable to descend, vigilant observation for deterioration; oxygen (1 to 2 liters/minute) and/or portable hyperbaric therapy (2 to 4 psi) for a few hours, if available	Same as listed above. Dexamethasone 2 mg every 6 hours, or 4 mg every 12 hours PO, starting day of ascent and discontinued cautiously after 2 days at maximum altitude, may be considered but should be used only if there is a high-risk ascent and acetazolamide is contraindicated
High-Altitude Cerebral Edema (HACE)		
AMS for ≥ 24 hours, ataxia, confusion, bizarre behavior, severe lassitude; usually symptoms of AMS also present with HACE	Immediately descend or evacuate ≥ 3,300 ft (1,000 m); give oxygen 2 to 4 liters/minute; titrate to maintain Spo_2 ≥ 90%; dexamethasone (8 mg IV/IM/ PO initially, then 4 mg every 6 hours); hyperbaric therapy if cannot descend	As listed above for AMS
High-Altitude Pulmonary Edema (HAPE)		
Dyspnea at rest, cough, crackles, severe exercise limitation, cyanosis, drowsiness, tachycardia, tachypnea, desaturation	Start oxygen 4 to 6 liters/minute, then titrate to maintain SpO_2 ≥ 90%; minimize exertion; keep warm; descend or evacuate 1,700 to 3,300 ft (500 to 1,000 m); consider nifedipine (30 mg sustained-release PO every 12 hours or 20 mg of sustained-release every 8 hours) if no HACE; consider inhaled beta-agonists (salmeterol, 125 mcg inhaled every 12 hours, or albuterol) in high-risk patients only; dexamethasone only if HACE develops	Ascend at a slow rate; avoid overexertion; consider nifedipine (30-mg sustained-release dose every 12 hours bid PO or 20 mg sustained-release every 8 hours) in person with repeated episodes of HAPE; start 1 day prior to ascent and continue for 2 days at maximum altitude

Note: bid, twice daily; EPAP, expiratory positive airway pressure; IM, intramuscular; IV, intravascular; m, meter; mcg, microgram; mg, milligram; PO, by mouth; psi, pounds per square inch; Sao₂, arterial oxygen saturation.

*Dexamethasone should be used only if no further ascent is contemplated; if for some operational reason the individual must ascend farther, dexamethasone is relatively contraindicated.

Modified from Luk AM, McIntosh SE, Grissom et al. Wilderness Medical Society consensus guidelines for the prevention and treatment of acute altitude illness. *Wilderness Environ Med.* 21:146-55;2010.

Table 20-11 Drug Dosing for Children With Altitude Illness[138]	
In 2001, the International Society for Mountain Medicine published a consensus statement recommending that adult treatment algorithms (for AMS, HACE, and HAPE) be followed with adjustments for pediatric drug dosages.	
AMS	Acetazolamide 2.5 mg/kg/dose PO q 12 hours (maximum 250 mg per dose)
	Dexamethasone 0.15 mg/kg/dose PO q 6 hours up to 4 mg
HACE	Acetazolamide 2.5 mg/kg/dose PO q 12 hours (maximum 250 mg per dose)
	Dexamethasone 0.3 mg/kg per dose
HAPE	Dexamethasone 0.15 mg/kg/dose PO q 6 hours up to 4 mg

Note: kg, kilogram; mg, milligram; PO, by mouth; q, every.

Modified from Pollard AJ, Niermeyer S, Barry PB, Bartsch P, Berghold F, Bishop RA, et al: Children at high altitude: An international consensus statement by an ad hoc committee of the International Society for Mountain Medicine. *High Alt Med Biol.* 2001:2; 389–401; Luk AM, McIntosh SE, Grissom et al. Wilderness Medical Society consensus guidelines for the prevention and treatment of acute altitude illness. *Wilderness Environ Med.* 21:1146-55;2010.

medical condition, as determined by the patient's medical history. It may be helpful to assess the patient's lung sounds and level of neurologic function because a strong association exists between HACE and HAPE. However, although they are often found together, HAPE will manifest with dyspnea at rest, cough, and a low Spo_2, while HAPE can occur without crackles.

Management

Do not delay planning for treatment and evacuation at the first signs or symptoms of HACE. The highest priority for any patient with HACE is immediate descent, along with initiation of high-flow oxygen (15 liters/minute) by nonrebreathing mask and monitoring of Spo_2 until 90% or greater. Unconscious patients should be managed as a patient with head injury (see the Airway and Ventilation chapter and the Head Trauma chapter), including intubation and other ALS procedures.[143] Dexamethasone should be administered, and a portable hyperbaric chamber may be used if supplemental oxygen is limited or absent.

See Table 20-10 for a summary of the signs and symptoms, management, and prevention of HACE. See Table 20-11 for dosing recommendations for children with HACE.

High-Altitude Pulmonary Edema

The onset of HAPE follows a pattern like that seen with AMS and HACE, occurring in unacclimatized individuals after a rapid ascent to high altitude. This high-altitude illness has a different mechanism of injury than AMS and HACE, however, because HAPE is induced by hypobaric hypoxia. HAPE is a form of noncardiogenic pulmonary edema associated with pulmonary hypertension and elevated capillary pressure.[139] More than 50% of patients with HAPE have AMS, and 14% have HACE.[152] The signs and symptoms most often appear in the morning after the second night (onset of 1 to 3 days) and rarely occur 4 days after arriving at a given altitude.[153] The development of HAPE and the rate of progression are hastened by cold exposure, vigorous exertion, and continued ascent. Compared with the other two high-altitude illnesses, HAPE accounts for the greatest number of fatalities.

Assessment

Patient assessment, including vital signs, lung sounds, and medical history, are vital in the determination of HAPE, which is defined by at least two or more symptoms (e.g., dyspnea at rest, cough, weakness, or decreased performance during exertion; chest tightness or congestion) and at least two signs (e.g., crackles or wheezing, central cyanosis or low Spo_2, tachypnea, or tachycardia).[154] Crackles are generally present in the lung fields, starting in the right axilla and eventually becoming bilateral. Assess the patient for fever; low fever may be seen with HAPE, while high fever might be suggestive of other conditions such as pneumonia. Late findings as HAPE progresses are resting tachycardia, tachypnea, and blood-tinged sputum. If treatment interventions are not provided, symptoms will progress over hours to days to include audible gurgling, respiratory distress, and eventually death.

Management

Descending or evacuating to a lower altitude by at least 1,700 to 3,300 ft (500 to 1,000 m) provides the fastest recovery, but initially patients show good improvement with rest and oxygen or hyperbaric treatment. Keep patients warm, and prevent any exertion. These patients need to improve their arterial oxygenation, so start oxygen at 4 to 6 liters/minute or titrate oxygen flow until Sao_2 is 90% or greater. Reassess the patient's vital signs after starting oxygen because improved arterial oxygenation decreases the tachycardia and tachypnea. As HAPE is a form of noncardiogenic pulmonary edema, diuretics have not been shown to be helpful. Anecdotal case reports have suggested favorable results with the use of continuous positive airway pressure (CPAP) for serious cases of HAPE, and the WMS suggests it can be considered as an adjunct to supplemental oxygen.[139,155,156]

See Table 20-10 for a summary of the signs and symptoms, management, and prevention of HAPE. See Table 20-11 for dosing recommendations for children with HAPE.

Prevention

Acute high-altitude illness in unacclimatized individuals is preventable. The common factor for the onset of AMS, HACE, and HAPE is the rate of ascent to higher altitude. Altitude illness may be experienced by skiers who travel by commercial airlines and take an early morning flight from continental American cities at sea level, arrive at high altitude around noon, and begin skiing by early afternoon at about 7,000 to 14,000 ft (2,100 to 4,500 m). Another scenario with risk of high-altitude illness is a call for mutual aid to various public safety personnel living below 3,300 ft (1,000 m). They assemble quickly and then arrive at 9,000 ft (2,750 m) or higher to assist local volunteer search-and-rescue teams trekking to higher altitudes in search of a missing backcountry hiker. Prehospital care personnel, whether ground crew or flight crew, who have responsibilities at high altitude for patient transfer to another hospital or for medical evacuation from the backcountry need to possess the knowledge to minimize the risk of high-altitude illness for their own safety and the safety of coworkers (**Box 20-12** and **Box 20-13**).

Medications as Prophylaxis for High-Altitude Illness

In all cases, gradual ascent with specific logistical strategies for mitigation (such as "climb high and sleep low") are recommended for prevention of high-altitude illnesses of all types.[132,139,157-160]

AMS/HACE Pharmacologic Prevention

For the prevention of AMS and HACE, individuals traveling from sea level to over 9,850 ft (3,000 m) as their sleeping altitude in 1 day or individuals who have a history of AMS should consider prophylactic treatment. The WMS practice guidelines stratify risk, and the corresponding importance of prophylactic treatment, based on ascent plans

---

Box 20-12 Altitude Acclimatization Procedures

The following are key points for acclimatizing to high altitude:

- Ascend high enough to induce adaptions but not so high as to develop altitude illness.
- Unacclimatized individuals should ascend slowly and cautiously above 9,000 ft (2,800 m).
- Avoid heavy exertion for the first 3 days.
- Keep well hydrated with water.
- Avoid alcohol, sleeping pills, and other sedatives.
- Eat a high-carbohydrate diet.
- Avoid overexertion.
- Avoid smoking.
- Physical training is not preventive for high-altitude illness.

Box 20-13 Golden Rules of High-Altitude Illness

The "golden rules" of high-altitude illness are as follows:

1. If you are ill at altitude, your symptoms are caused by the altitude until proved otherwise.
2. If you have altitude symptoms, do not go any higher.
3. If you are feeling ill or are getting worse, or if you cannot walk heel to toe in a straight line, descend immediately.
4. A person ill with altitude illness must always be accompanied by a responsible companion who can accomplish or arrange for descent should it become necessary.[137]

---

and past medical history.[139] If pharmacologic prophylaxis is determined to be desirable, the drug of choice is oral acetazolamide (Diamox), 125 mg twice daily, beginning 1 day before ascent and continuing for 2 days at maximum altitude or when starting descent.[139,157] An alternative drug is dexamethasone (Decadron), 4 mg orally or intramuscularly (IM) every 6 hours and continuing for 2 days at maximum altitude (this dosing assumes active ascent with physical exertion).[157] The combination of both drugs may be more effective than either drug alone,[144,146] but the WMS and wilderness EMS experts recommend that this combination be restricted to emergency situations that mandate very rapid ascent.[139,158] Aspirin (325 mg) taken every 4 hours for three doses reduced the incidence of headache from 50% to 7% in one study.[148]

Two studies suggest a benefit from prophylactic use of ibuprofen 600 mg three times per day beginning 6 hours before ascending from 4,100 ft (1,250 m) up to 12,570 ft (3,800 m) as compared to a placebo treatment.[161,162] Lipman et al. reported that 43% of the participants in the ibuprofen group reported the development of AMS compared with 69% in the placebo group. Also, the placebo group reported that the severity of AMS was worse than reported in the ibuprofen group.[161] The benefit for using ibuprofen is that it provides a second-choice medication and can be taken the same day of ascent with no or low side effects when compared to the traditional use of acetazolamide for the prevention of AMS.[161] However, the drawback is that ibuprofen does not seem to speed acclimatization.[157] At least one wilderness EMS reference textbook argues that ibuprofen should not be recommended instead of acetazolamide until more data become available.[157] In addition, a single trial specifically comparing acetazolamide and ibuprofen found equal incidence of high-altitude headache and AMS in both groups.[163]

HAPE Pharmacologic Prevention

For the prevention of HAPE in individuals with a history of repeated episodes, prophylaxis with oral nifedipine, 60 mg daily divided into 2 or 3 doses (extended-release formulation), is recommended as a first-line intervention.[139,157] Salmeterol may also be considered as a supplement to nifedipine, at a dose of 125 mcg inhaled twice daily, but only in high-risk individuals with a clear history of recurrent HAPE.[139,157] Other medications being studied for HAPE prevention that show potential promise include sildenafil, tadalafil, and dexamethasone,[132] but further research is needed before they can be recommended for wilderness EMS purposes.[157]

Currently, prophylactic treatment should be avoided as a method to prevent altitude illness in children because of insufficient clinical studies.[164]

Prolonged Transport

Because environmental trauma often occurs in remote locations or in settings that do not easily accommodate ambulances, delivery of the patient to the nearest appropriate trauma center may be delayed. Prehospital care providers may need to continue managing the patient for an extended period while driving to the nearest hospital or waiting for helicopter arrival.

Drowning

Minimally symptomatic patients can become more symptomatic in an extended-care situation with a delay of

4 hours before worsening of symptoms. However, there is no case in the medical literature of a drowning patient presenting as initially completely asymptomatic and then deteriorating or dying hours or days later.[37] Initiate CPR for a drowning victim with five continuous breaths using the traditional ABC approach, not CAB, to begin correcting hypoxemia. Obtain a pulse oximetry reading before and after administration of oxygen. Provide high-flow oxygen via a nonrebreathing mask at 15 liters/minute.

Any patient with pulse oximetry values less than 92% (especially those with this level after initiation of oxygen), altered mental status, apnea, or coma may require early invasive airway management to protect from aspiration. Any patient who continues to be hypoxemic with pulse oximetry readings less than 92% after administration of high-flow oxygen is a candidate for CPAP or rapid-sequence intubation protocol. Use care with suction through the endotracheal tube as this may compromise oxygenation, although it may be needed if secretions are compromising ventilation. Consult with medical control, if available, to sedate and paralyze the patient (if permitted by protocols) to ensure successful intubation, oxygenation, and effective ventilation.

Another effective method to ensure effective oxygenation and ventilation is the use of positive end-expiratory pressure (PEEP) for respiratory assistance.[29,45] PEEP recruits collapsed alveoli, improving the ventilatory–perfusion ratio and arterial oxygenation.

Determine the patient's GCS score, and assess routinely for trends because it is predictive of patient outcome. Monitor for hypothermia and hypoglycemia. Any comatose patient should have his or her blood glucose measured or, if unable, receive IV dextrose. The placement of a nasogastric tube may be needed to reduce gastric content and water swallowed during submersion after a secure airway is achieved.

Lightning Injury

Victims of lightning may be in respiratory arrest, cardiac arrest, or both. Following CAB assessment, initiate CPR rapidly. When in an extended-care situation with multiple victims, use *reverse triage*, and first resuscitate those who appear dead. However, prolonged (multiple hours) CPR on these victims has a poor patient outcome, and there is little benefit from CPR or ACLS procedures lasting longer than 20 to 30 minutes. All measures to stabilize the patient to correct for hypoxemia, hypovolemia, hypothermia, and acidosis should be attempted before terminating resuscitative efforts.[3]

Assess the patient for cerebral edema and increased intracranial pressure (ICP). Establish a baseline GCS score, and reassess the patient every 10 minutes as an indicator of progressive cerebral edema and increased ICP (manage per recommendation for cerebral edema; see the Head Trauma chapter).

Recreational Scuba-Related Diving Injuries

The standard treatment protocol for scuba-related injuries causing pulmonary overpressurization syndrome (e.g., AGE, DCS) is to provide high-flow oxygen (15 liters/minute via nonrebreathing mask) at the scene and continue oxygen therapy during transport of the patient to the closest recompression chamber for hyperbaric oxygen therapy. Conduct an extensive neurologic evaluation, and reassess the patient frequently for progression of signs and symptoms. Use analgesics for pain control per local protocols. Also consider giving aspirin (325 or 650 mg) for its antiplatelet activity.[103]

Use DAN and local medical control for the closest location of a functional recompression chamber. Before transporting a patient for hyperbaric oxygen therapy, contact the chamber directly because the status of chamber readiness can change without notification. When transporting by air, use aircraft that can preferably maintain sea-level atmosphere during flight. Any nonpressurized aircraft should maintain an altitude below 1,000 ft (300 m) en route to the chamber site.

High-Altitude Illness

Mild to moderate AMS can be managed with low-volume oxygen at 2 to 4 liters/minute by nasal cannula, titrated by 1 to 2 liters/minute (greater than 90% SpO_2), with a combination of analgesics (e.g., aspirin, 650 mg; acetaminophen, 650 to 1,000 mg; ibuprofen, 600 mg) for headache and prochlorperazine (5 to 10 mg IM) or ondansetron (4 mg orally dissolving tablet or IM) for nausea. Other medications used for treating mild to moderate AMS include oral acetazolamide (250 mg twice daily) and dexamethasone (4 mg orally [PO] or IM every 6 hours) until symptoms resolve (although note that dexamethasone would be dangerous if contemplating further ascent).

Treat HACE with immediate descent, oxygen by nasal cannula to maintain greater than 90% SpO_2 (usually 2 to 4 liters/minute), and dexamethasone (8 mg PO, IV, or IM initially, then 4 mg every 6 hours). Consider using oral acetazolamide (250 mg twice daily) with prolonged delays to descent. Consider use of a hyperbaric chamber if descent is delayed. If a severe form of HACE develops and the patient is comatose, manage according to recommendations for cerebral edema (see the Shock: Pathophysiology of Life and Death chapter).

Prolonged management of HAPE primarily consists of administering oxygen at 4 to 6 liters/minute by nasal cannula (greater than 90% SpO_2) until improvement of symptoms, then 2 to 4 liters/minute for conserving oxygen, or use a hyperbaric chamber. If oxygen is not available, give oral nifedipine (10 mg initially, then 30 mg extended-release dose every 12 to 24 hours). Consider CPAP. If the patient acquires HACE, add dexamethasone (8 mg PO or IM every 6 hours).

Use of portable hyperbaric chambers, such as the Gamow bag (Altitude Technologies), Portable Altitude Chamber (PAC), or Certec, has been successful for treating high-altitude illness.[132] These lightweight, fabric pressure bags simulate descending to a lower altitude with or without the use of supplemental oxygen or medication (e.g., acetazolamide, dexamethasone, nifedipine). They inflate with manual pumps up to 2 psi, which is equivalent to descending a variable distance depending on the initial altitude and severity of HAPE. The use of these chambers for 2 to 3 hours can effectively improve symptoms. This is an ideal use of technology while waiting for transportation to definitive care, and sometimes a chamber represents the definitive care itself if the patient's symptoms resolve.

SUMMARY

- Basic knowledge of common environmental emergencies is necessary so that rapid assessment and treatment in the prehospital setting can be provided.
- Lightning
  - Lightning injuries range from minor superficial wounds to major multisystem trauma and death.
  - The mechanism for sudden death from lightning strike is simultaneous cardiac and respiratory arrest.

- The priorities for managing a lightning victim are to ensure scene safety and to assess the XABCDEs, ensuring cardiac function, which will typically involve CPR and possibly defibrillation.
- Drowning
  - Prehospital care providers must understand the pathophysiologic process of drowning. The major determinant of survival and long-term functionality following drowning is the extent of CNS injury.
  - When managing submersion victims, all patients receive high-flow oxygen. Generally,

SUMMARY (CONTINUED)

management involves IV access and fluid administration (normal saline or lactated Ringer solution), and transport to the ED for evaluation.

- Rapid initiation of effective BLS and standard ALS procedures for drowning patients in cardiopulmonary arrest is associated with the best chance of survival.
- Drowning prevention efforts that prehospital care providers can encourage in their communities include installing barriers around pools, monitoring children when near water, using personal flotation devices such as life vests, initiating CPR by bystanders before the arrival of prehospital care, and avoiding high-risk behaviors such as alcohol consumption when participating in water-related activities.

■ Recreational diving
- The type of recreational diving injury to which providers will most commonly respond is scuba-related injury or fatality caused by dysbarism (altered environmental pressure).
- Barotrauma can result in various types of pressure injuries. Examples of descent-related injuries include mask squeeze, tooth squeeze, middle-ear squeeze (most common), sinus squeeze, and internal-ear barotrauma. Ascent-related injuries include alternobaric vertigo, sinus barotrauma, and pulmonary

overpressurization syndrome (POPS). Providers must be prepared to recognize these injuries to effectively evaluate and manage them.
- Management of diving injuries involves assessing the ABCs, protecting the patient's airway, and initiating BLS or ALS.

■ High-altitude illness
- High-altitude illness is a term that encompasses cerebral and pulmonary syndromes: (1) acute mountain sickness (AMS), (2) high-altitude cerebral edema (HACE), and (3) high-altitude pulmonary edema (HAPE).
- Prehospital care providers and ED staff need to become familiar with the predisposing factors, signs and symptoms, medical management, and education and prevention techniques to reduce the morbidity and mortality of high-altitude illness.
- Prehospital management for these conditions generally involves descent from high elevation, oxygen administration, and possible pharmacologic intervention (as indicated).

■ Due to the possibility of prolonged transport often relating to environmental trauma, prehospital care providers must be prepared to deliver ongoing patient management in the ambulance.

SCENARIO RECAP

In a coastal town, a family of four was strolling on the beach with their dog during a chilly winter day. The son tossed a rubber ball toward the water's edge, and the dog gave chase. In an instant, a large shore-breaking wave swallowed up the dog in the rough surf. The 17-year-old son was first into the water to attempt to save the dog, only to be overtaken by the water. He was seen struggling in the rough, surging surf by his parents and sister.

The boy's father and mother grabbed a nearby flotation device stationed on the beachfront and followed him into the surf to help. Their 19-year-old daughter remained on shore and called for help on her cell phone. The dog eventually made it back to the shore. The parents pulled their son out of the cold water after finding him submerged and unresponsive. Your paramedic unit arrives to the scene within 7 minutes of the daughter's call.

As you exit the ambulance, you observe an unconscious teenage boy lying partially prone with his face rotated to the side in sand with surging water close by. He is still in the surf zone and could be submersed by a wave. You join up with arriving fire department emergency responders to approach the victim.

- How should you approach the patient in this setting?
- If the patient has no pulse or respirations, what is the next immediate intervention?
- What other concerns do you have for the patient that need to be addressed on scene?

SCENARIO SOLUTION

Your plan is to have one fire fighter, equipped with a PFD, serve as a lookout for a threat of oncoming surf and for you, your partner, and two other fire fighters to approach the victim to pick him up by all four extremities and quickly carry him away from the surging waves. All individuals near or entering the water will have PFDs.

As the lead prehospital care provider, you direct the team to place the victim supine, parallel to the shore, so that the head and trunk are at the same level and then immediately check for responsiveness. The other emergency responders begin staging the emergency medical gear near the victim as you check the ABCs, remembering that in this case, an XABCDE sequence would be inappropriate. The patient may be apneic and need only rescue breathing or may need full CPR. In either situation, you know that the recommendation for drowning is now to provide five rescue breaths initially followed by 30 chest compressions and then to continue two breaths and 30 compressions until signs of life appear or resuscitation is terminated as futile.

The initial approach to the ABCs in drowning victims is essential to address the hypoxemia. High-flow oxygen is provided using a bag-mask device. You start an IV with crystalloids. In this case, spinal immobilization is not needed since there was no mechanism of injury to suspect spinal trauma. Early intubation or assisted mechanical ventilation, such as CPAP, may be indicated if the victim shows signs of deterioration with SpO_2 less than 92%. You transport the patient and his parents to the hospital for continued treatment and evaluation. During the transport, you discuss water rescue with the family. The son's decision to enter the water without a flotation device and without known water rescue training put him significantly at risk; as noted in the chapter, in some studies, 5% of drownings are from would-be rescuers. Such dialogue with the family better prepares them, and those they talk about this experience with, for any future water rescues and drowning care.

References

1. Curran EB, Holle RL, Lopez RE. Lightning fatalities, injuries and damage reports in the United States, 1959–1994. NOAA Tech Memo NWS SR-193, 1997.

2. Centers for Disease Control and Prevention. QuickStats: number of deaths from lightning among males and females—National Vital Statistics System, United States, 1968–2010. *Morb Mortal Wkly Rep.* http://www.cdc.gov/mmwr/preview/mmwrhtml/mm6228a6.htm. Updated July 19, 2013. Accessed October 19, 2017.

3. Gatewood MO, Zane RD. Lightning injuries. *Emerg Med Clin North Am.* 2004;22:369.

4. Huffins GR, Orville RE. Lightning ground flash density and thunderstorm duration in the contiguous United States. *J Appl Meteorol.* 1999;38:1013.

5. Cummins KL, Krider EP, Malone MD. A combined TOA/MDF technology upgrade of the U.S. National Lightning Detection Network. *J Geophys Res.* 1998;103:9035.

6. MacGorman, DR, Rust WD. Lightning strike density for the contiguous United States from thunderstorm duration records, Pub No NUREG/CR03759. Washington, DC: Office of Nuclear Regulatory Research; 1984.

7. Hawkins SC, Simon RB, Beissinger JP, Simon D. *Vertical Aid: Essential Wilderness Medicine for Climbers, Trekkers, and Mountaineers.* New York, NY: The Countryman Press; 2017.

8. Cherington M, Walker J, Boyson M, Glancy R, Hedegaard H, Clark S. Closing the gap on the actual numbers of lightning casualties and deaths. 11th Conference on Applied Climatology. Dallas, TX: American Meteorological Society; 1999:379-380.

9. Dulcos PJ, Sanderson LM, Klontz KC. Lightning-related mortality and morbidity in Florida. *Pub Health Rep.* 1990;105:276.

10. Cooper MA, Andrews CJ, Holle RL, Blumenthal R, Aldana NN. Lightning-related injuries and safety. In: Auerbach PS, ed. *Auerbach's Wilderness Medicine.* 7th ed. Philadelphia, PA: Mosby Elsevier; 2017.

11. Nelson RD, McGinnis H. Lightning injuries and severe storms. In: Hawkins SC, ed. *Wilderness EMS.* Philadelphia, PA: Wolters Kluwer; 2018.

12. National Oceanic and Atmospheric Administration. U.S. lightning fatalities 2007–2017. http://www.lightningsafety.noaa.gov/fatalities.shtml. Published 2017. Accessed August 6, 2017.

13. Davis C, Engeln A, Johnson E, et al. Wilderness Medical Society practice guidelines for the prevention and treatment of lightning injuries: 2014 update. *Wilderness Environ Med.* 2014;25(4):S86-S95.

14. Cooper MA. Lightning injuries: prognostic signs of death. *Ann Emerg Med.* 1980;9:134.

15. Cooper MA, Edlich RF. Lightning injuries. Medscape website. http://emedicine.medscape.com/article/770642-overview. Updated December 8, 2016. Accessed August 6, 2017.

16. Andrews CJ, Darveniza M, Mackerras D. Lightning injury: a review of the clinical aspects, pathophysiology and treatment. *Adv Trauma.* 1989;4:241.

17. Lavonas EJ, Drennan IR, Gabrielli A, et al. 2015 American Heart Association guidelines update for cardiopulmonary resuscitation and emergency cardiovascular care: cardiac arrest associated with electric shock and lightning strikes (2010 update, Part 12.2). *Circulation*. 2015;132(18):S2.

18. Ritenour AE, Morton MJ, McManus JG, Barillo DJ, Cancio LC. Lightning injury: a review. *Burns*. 2008;34:585.

19. Beir M, Chen W, Bodnar E, Lee RC. Biophysical injury mechanisms associated with lightning injury. *Neurorehabilitation*. 2005;20(1):53.

20. Cooper MA. Electrical and lightning injuries. *Emerg Med Clin North Am*. 1984;2:489.

21. Casten JA, Kytilla J. Eye symptoms caused by lightning. *Acta Ophthalmol*. 1963;41:139.

22. Kleiner JP, Wilkin JH. Cardiac effects of lightning stroke. *JAMA*. 1978;240:2757.

23. Taussig HB. Death from lightning and the possibility of living again. *Ann Intern Med*. 1968;68:1345.

24. Zimmerman C, Cooper MA, Holle RL. Lightning safety guidelines. *Ann Emerg Med*. 2002;39:660.

25. National Lightning Safety Institute. Personal lightning safety. http://www.lightningsafety.com/nlsi_pls.html. Accessed August 6, 2017.

26. National Weather Service. Lightning risk reduction outdoors. http://www.lightningsafety.noaa.gov/outdoors.shtml. Accessed August 6, 2017.

27. Zafren K, Durrer B, Henry JP, Brugger H. Lightning injuries: prevention and on-site treatment in mountains and remote areas—official guidelines of the International Commission for Mountain Emergency Medicine and Medical Commission of the International Mountaineering and Climbing Federation (ICAR and UIAA MEDCOM). *Resuscitation*. 2005;65:369.

28. National Oceanic and Atmospheric Administration. Lightning myths and truths. http://www.lightningsafety.noaa.gov/myths.shtml. Accessed August 6, 2017.

29. Sempsrott J, Schmidt AC, Hawkins SC, Cushing TA. Drowning and submersion injuries. In: Auerbach PS, ed. *Auerbach's Wilderness Medicine*. 7th ed. Philadelphia, PA: Mosby Elsevier; 2017.

30. Peden M, Oyegbite K, Ozanne-Smith J, et al., eds. World report on child injury prevention. Geneva, Switzerland: World Health Organization; 2008.

31. Centers for Disease Control and Prevention. Nonfatal and fatal drowning in recreational water settings—United States, 2005–2009. *Morb Mortal Wkly Rep*. 2012;61(19):345.

32. Centers for Disease Control and Prevention. Drowning—United States, 2005–2009. *Morb Mortal Wkly Rep*. 2012;61(19);344-347.

33. Zuckerman GB, Conway EE Jr. Drowning and near-drowning. *Pediatr Ann*. 2000;29:6.

34. World Health Organization. Facts about injuries: drowning. http://www.who.int/violence_injury_prevention/publications/other_injury/en/drowning_factsheet.pdf. Accessed August 6, 2017.

35. DeNicola LK, Falk JL, Swanson ME, Kissoon N. Submersion injuries in children and adults. *Crit Care Clin*. 1997;13(3):477.

36. Olshaker JS. Near-drowning. *Emerg Med Clin North Am*. 1992;10(2):339.

37. Hawkins SC, Sempsrott J, Schmidt A. Drowning in a sea of misinformation: dry drowning and secondary drowning. *Emerg Med News*. 2017;39(8):1,39-40.

38. American College of Emergency Physicians. Death after swimming is extremely rare—and is NOT "dry drowning." http://newsroom.acep.org/2017-07-11-Death-After-Swimming-Is-Extremely-Rare-And-Is-NOT-Dry-Drowning. Published July 11, 2017. Accessed August 6, 2017.

39. Van Beeck EF, Branche CM, Szpilman D, et al. A new definition of drowning: towards documentation and prevention of a global public health program. *Bull World Health Organ*. 2005;83:853-856.

40. van Beeck EF, Branche CM, Szpilman D, et al. Definition of drowning. In: Bierens JLM, ed. *Handbook on Drowning: Prevention, Rescue, Treatment*. Berlin, Germany: Springer; 2006.

41. Szpilman D, Bierens JLM, Handley A, Orlowshi JP. Drowning. *N Engl J Med*. 2012;366:2102-2110.

42. World Health Organization. Global report on drowning: preventing a leading killer. http://www.who.int/violence_injury_prevention/publications/drowning_global_report/Final_report_full_web.pdf. Published 2014. Accessed October 19, 2017.

43. Schmidt AC, Sempsrott JR, Hawkins SC, Arastu AS, Cushing TA, Auerbach PS. Wilderness Medical Society practice guidelines for the prevention and treatment of drowning. *Wilderness Environ Med*. 2016;27(2):236-251.

44. Centers for Disease Control and Prevention. Unintentional drowning: get the facts. https://www.cdc.gov/homeandrecreationalsafety/water-safety/waterinjuries-factsheet.html. Updated April 28, 2016. Accessed August 6, 2017.

45. Olshaker JS. Submersion. *Emerg Med Clin North Am*. 2004;22:357.

46. Moran K, Quan L, Franklin R, Bennett E. Where the evidence and expert opinion meet: a review of the open-water recreational safety messages. *Int J Aquatic Res Educ*. 2011;5:251-270.

47. Lavelle JM. Ten-year review of pediatric bathtub near-drownings: evaluation for child abuse and neglect. *Ann Emerg Med*. 1995;25:344.

48. Craig AB Jr. Underwater swimming and loss of consciousness. *JAMA*. 1961;176:255.

49. Dickinson P. Shallow water blackout. In: Bierens JJLM, ed. *Drowning: Prevention, Rescue, Treatment*. 2nd ed. Berlin, Germany: Springer; 2014.

50. International Life Saving Federation. Medical Position Statement—MPS 16: shallow water blackout. International Life Saving Federation position statements. http://ilsf.org/about/position-statements. Accessed August 11, 2017.

51. Chimiak JM, Buzzacott P. Management of diving injuries. In: Hawkins SC, ed. *Wilderness EMS*. Philadelphia, PA: Wolters Kluwer; 2018.

52. United States Lifesaving Association. *Open Water Lifesaving: The United States Lifesaving Association Manual*. 3rd ed. Boston, MA: Pearson; 2017.

53. Pearn JH, Franklin RC, Peden AE. Hypoxic blackout: diagnosis, risks, and prevention. *Int J Aquatic Res Educ*. 2015;9:342-347.

54. Royal Life Saving Society. Fact Sheet No. 23: hypoxic blackout. https://www.royallifesaving.com.au/__data/assets/pdf_file/0009/4005/RLS_FactSheet_23HR_updated07Sep16.pdf. Accessed October 19, 2017.

55. Jensen LR, Williams SD, Thurman DJ, Keller PA. Submersion injuries in children younger than 5 years in urban Utah. *West J Med*. 1992;157:641.

56. Howland J, Smith GS, Mangione TW, et al. Why are most drowning victims men? Sex differences, aquatic skills and behaviors. *Am J Public Health*. 1996;86:93.

57. Schuman SH, Rowe JR, Glazer HM, et al. The iceberg phenomenon of near-drowning. *Crit Care Med*. 1976;4:127.

58. Bell NS, Amoros PJ, Yore MM, et al. Alcohol and other risk factors for drowning among male active duty U.S. army soldiers. *Aviat Space Environ Med*. 2001;72(12):1086-1095.

59. Howland J, Mangione T, Hingson R, et al. Alcohol as a risk factor for drowning and other aquatic injuries. In: Watson RR, ed. *Alcohol and Accidents: Drug and Alcohol Abuse Reviews*. Vol 7. Totowa, NJ: Humana Press; 1995.

60. Howland J, Hingson R. Alcohol as a risk factor for drownings: a review of the literature (1950–1985). *Accid Anal Prev*. 1988;20(1):19-25.

61. Howland J, Smith GS, Mangione T, et al. Missing the boat on drinking and boating. *JAMA*. 1993;270:91.

62. Bell GS, Gaitatzis A, Bell CL, Johnson AL, Sander JW. Drowning in people with epilepsy. *Neurology*. 2008;71:578.

63. White J. *StarGuard: Best Practices for Lifeguards*. 5th ed. Champaign, IL: Human Kinetics; 2017.

64. Sempsrott J. Management of drowning. In: Hawkins SC, ed. *Wilderness EMS*. Philadelphia, PA: Wolters Kluwer; 2018.

65. Padgett J. Technical rescue interface: swiftwater rescue. In: Hawkins SC, ed. *Wilderness EMS*. Philadelphia, PA: Wolters Kluwer; 2018.

66. Smith B, Bledsoe B, Nicolazzo P. General management of trauma in the wilderness environment. In: Hawkins SC, ed. *Wilderness EMS*. Philadelphia, PA: Wolters Kluwer; 2018.

67. Smith W. Technical rescue interface introduction: principles of basic technical rescue, patient care integration, and packaging. In: Hawkins SC, ed. *Wilderness EMS*. Philadelphia, PA: Wolters Kluwer; 2018.

68. Rowe MI, Arango A, Allington G. Profile of pediatric drowning victims in a water-oriented society. *J Trauma*. 1977;17:587.

69. Brenner RA, Taneja GS, Haynie DL, et al. Association between swimming lessons and drowning in childhood: a case-control study. *Arch Pediatr Adolesc Med*. 2009; 163:203.

70. Karch KB. Pathology of the lung in near-drowning. *Am J Emerg Med*. 1986;4(1):4.

71. Orlowski JP. Drowning, near-drowning, and ice water submersion. *Pediatr Clin North Am*. 1987;34(1):75.

72. Modell JH, Moya F. Effects of volume of aspirated fluid during chlorinated fresh-water drowning. *Anesthesiology*. 1966;27:663.

73. Giesbrecht GG, Steinman AM. Immersion into cold water. In: Auerbach PS, ed. *Wilderness Medicine*. 6th ed. St. Louis, MO: Mosby Elsevier; 2012.

74. Bolte RG, Black PG, Bowers RS. The use of extracorporeal rewarming in a child submerged for 66 minutes. *JAMA*. 1988;260:377.

75. Lloyd EL. Accidental hypothermia. *Resuscitation*. 1996;32:111.

76. Gilbert M, Busund R, Skagseth A. Resuscitation from accidental hypothermia of 13.7°C with circulatory arrest. *Lancet*. 2000;355:375.

77. Siebke H, Breivik H, Rod T, et al. Survival after 40 minutes submersion without cerebral sequelae. *Lancet*. 1975;1:1275.

78. Quan L, Mack CD, Schiff MA. Association of water temperature and submersion duration and drowning outcome. *Resuscitation*. 2014;85(9):1304.

79. Abella BS, Alvarado JP, Myklebust H, et al. Quality of cardiopulmonary resuscitation during in-hospital cardiac arrest. *JAMA*. 2005;293(3):305.

80. Wik L, Kramer-Johansen J, Myklebust H, et al. Quality of cardiopulmonary resuscitation during pre-hospital cardiac arrest. *JAMA*. 2005;293(3):299.

81. American Heart Association. Part 10: Special Circumstances of Resuscitation: Cardiac Arrest in Accidental Hypothermia. Web-based Integrated 2010 & 2015 American Heart Association Guidelines for Cardiopulmonary Resuscitation and Emergency Cardiovascular Care. https://eccguidelines.heart.org/index.php/circulation/cpr-ecc-guidelines-2/part-10-special-circumstances-of-resuscitation/. Accessed April 6, 2018.

82. Schmidt A, Sempsrott J, Abo B. Technical rescue interface: open water rescue. In: Hawkins SC, ed. *Wilderness EMS*. Philadelphia, PA: Wolters Kluwer; 2018.

83. James Cook University. Drowning researchers look for help. Media Release, July 12, 2017. https://www.jcu.edu.au/news/releases/2017/july/drowning-researchers-look-for-help. Published July 12, 2017. Accessed October 19, 2017.

84. Zhu Y, Jiang X, Li H, et al. Mortality among drowning rescuers in China, 2013: a review of 225 rescue incidents from the press. *BMC Pub Health*. 2015;15:631.

85. Hwang V, Frances S, Durbin D, et al. Prevalence of traumatic injuries in drowning and near-drowning in children and adolescents. *Arch Pediatr Adolesc Med*. 2003;157(1):50-53.

86. Graf WD, Cummings P, Quan L, et al. Predicting outcome in pediatric submersion victims. *Ann Emerg Med*. 1995;26(3):312-319.

87. Pratt FD, Haynes BE. Incidence of "secondary drowning" after saltwater submersion. *Ann Emerg Med*. 1986;15(9):1084.

88. Szpilman D. Near-drowning and drowning classification: a proposal to stratify mortality based on the analysis of 1,831 cases. *Chest*. 1997;112:660.

89. American Heart Association. Part 5: Adult Basic Life Support and Cardiopulmonary Resuscitation Quality. Web-based Integrated 2010 & 2015 American Heart Association Guidelines for Cardiopulmonary Resuscitation and Emergency Cardiovascular Care. https://eccguidelines.heart.org/index.php/circulation/cpr-ecc-guidelines-2/part-5-adult-basic-life-support-and-cardiopulmonary-resuscitation-quality/. Accessed April 22, 2018.

90. Rosen P, Stoto M, Harley J. The use of the Heimlich maneuver in near-drowning: Institute of Medicine report. *J Emerg Med*. 1995;13:397.

91. Wilderness Medical Society. Submersion injuries. In: Forgey WW. *Practice Guidelines for Wilderness Emergency Care*. 5th ed. Helena, MT: Globe Pequot Press; 2006.

92. Moran K, Quan L, Franklin R, Bennett E. Where the evidence and expert opinion meet: a review of open-water recreational safety messages. *Int J Aquatic Res Educ*. 2011;5(3):5.

93. Baker PA, Webber JB. Failure to ventilate with supraglottic airways after drowning. *Anaesth Intensive Care*. 2011;39:675-677.

94. Smith T, ed. *Clinical Procedures and Guidelines: Comprehensive Edition, 2016–2018*. Guideline 10.4: Drowning. http://www.rgpn.org.nz/Network/media/documents/St%20John%20CPGs%202016-18/St-J-ohn-CPGs,-comprehensive-edition,-2016-2018.pdf. Accessed October 19, 2017.

95. Kyriacou DN, Arcinue EL, Peek C, Kraus JF. Effect of immediate resuscitation on children with submersion injury. *Pediatrics*. 1994;94:137.

96. American Academy of Pediatrics. AAP gives updated advice on drowning prevention. http://www.aap.org/en-us /about-the-aap/aap-press-room/Pages/AAP-Gives-Updated -Advice-on-Drowning-Prevention.aspx. Published May 24, 2010. Accessed August 6, 2017.

97. Wintemute GJ, Kraus JF, Teret SP, Wright MA. Death resulting from motor vehicle immersions: the nature of the injuries, personal and environmental contributing factors, and potential interventions. *Am J Public Health.* 1990;80:1068.

98. Hawkins SC. Submerged vehicles. *Wilderness Medicine Magazine.* www.wildernessmedicinemagazine.com/1137 /drowning-submerged-vehicles. Published February 26, 2015. Accessed August 6, 2017.

99. McDonald GK, Giesbrecht GG. Vehicle submersion: a review of the problem, associated risks, and survival information. *Aviat Space Environ Med.* 2013;84:498-510.

100. Hawkins SC. Setting the record straight to reduce fatalities in sinking vehicles. *Emerg Med News.* 2015;37:5B.

101. Melamed Y, Shupak A, Bitterman H. Medical problems associated with underwater diving. *N Engl J Med.* 1992;326:30.

102. Van Hoesen KB, Lang MA. Diving medicine. In: Auerbach PS, ed. *Auerbach's Wilderness Medicine.* 7th ed. Philadelphia, PA: Mosby Elsevier; 2017.

103. Salahuddin M, James LA, Bass ES. SCUBA medicine: a first-responder's guide to diving injuries. *Curr Sports Med Rep.* 2011;10(3):134-139.

104. Lynch JA, Bove AA. Diving medicine: a review of the current evidence. *J Am Board Fam Med.* 2009;22:399-407.

105. Strauss MB, Borer RC Jr. Diving medicine: contemporary topics and their controversies. *Am J Emerg Med.* 2001; 19:232.

106. Morgan WP. Anxiety and panic in recreational scuba divers. *Sports Med.* 1995;20(6):398.

107. Della-Giustina D, Ingebretsen R. *Advanced Wilderness Life Support.* Salt Lake City, Utah: AdventureMed; 2013.

108. Divers Alert Network (DAN). Eleven-year trends (1987–1997) in diving activity: the DAN annual review of recreational SCUBA diving injuries and fatalities based on 2000 data. In: *Report on Decompression Illness, Diving Fatalities and Project Dive Exploration.* Durham, NC: Divers Alert Network; 2000:17-29.

109. Divers Alert Network (DAN). *Report on Diving Fatalities: 2016 Edition.* Durham, NC: Divers Alert Network; 2017.

110. Hardy KR. Diving-related emergencies. *Emerg Med Clin North Am.* 1997;15(1):223.

111. Green SM. Incidence and severity of middle-ear barotraumas in recreational scuba diving. *J Wilderness Med.* 1993;4:270.

112. Kizer KW. Dysbaric cerebral air embolism in Hawaii. *Ann Emerg Med.* 1987;16:535.

113. Cales RH, Humphreys N, Pilmanis AA, Heilig RW. Cardiac arrest from gas embolism in scuba diving. *Ann Emerg Med.* 1981;10(11):589.

114. Butler BD, Laine GA, Leiman BC, et al. Effect of Trendelenburg position on the distribution of arterial air emboli in dogs. *Ann Thorac Surg.* 1988;45(2):198.

115. Moon RE. Treatment of diving emergencies. *Crit Care Clin.* 1999;15:429.

116. Van Meter K. Medical field management of the injured diver. *Respir Care Clin North Am.* 1997;5(1):137.

117. Francis TJ, Dutka AJ, Hallenbeck JM. Pathophysiology of decompression sickness. In: Bove AA, Davis JC, eds. *Diving Medicine.* 2nd ed. Philadelphia, PA: Saunders; 1990.

118. Neuman TS. DCI/DCS: does it matter whether the emperor wears clothes? *Undersea Hyperb Med.* 1997;24:2.

119. Bove AA. Nomenclature of pressure disorders. *Undersea Hyperb Med.* 1997;24:1.

120. Spira A. Diving and marine medicine review. Part II. Diving diseases. *J Travel Med.* 1999;6:180.

121. Clenney TL, Lassen LF. Recreational scuba diving injuries. *Am Fam Physician.* 1996;53(5):1761.

122. Kizer KW. Women and diving. *Physician Sportsmed.* 1981; 9(2):84.

123. Francis TJ, Dutka AJ, Hallenbeck JM. Pathophysiology of decompression sickness. In: Bove AA, Davis JC, eds. *Diving Medicine.* 2nd ed. Philadelphia, PA: Saunders; 1990.

124. Greer HD, Massey EW. Neurologic injury from undersea diving. *Neurol Clin.* 1992;10(4):1031.

125. Kizer KW. Management of dysbaric diving casualties. *Emerg Med Clin North Am.* 1983;1:659.

126. Department of the Navy. *U.S. Navy Diving Manual.* Vol 1, Rev 4. Washington, DC: U.S. Government Printing Office; 1999.

127. Davis JC. Hyperbaric medicine: critical care aspects. In: Shoemaker WC, ed. *Critical Care: State of the Art.* Aliso Viejo, CA: Society of Critical Care Medicine; 1984.

128. Pollock NW, Uguccioni DM, Dear GdeL, eds. Diabetes and recreational diving: guidelines for the future. Proceedings of the Undersea and Hyperbaric Medical Society/Divers Alert Network. June 19, 2005, Workshop. Durham, NC: Divers Alert Network; 2005.

129. Gallagher SA, Hackett PH. High-altitude illness. *Emerg Med Clin North Am.* 2004;22:329.

130. Hackett PH, Roach RC. High-altitude illness. *N Engl J Med.* 2001;345(2):107.

131. Hackett PH, Luks AM, Lawley JS, Roach RC. High-altitude medicine and pathophysiology. In: Auerbach PS, ed. *Wilderness Medicine.* 7th ed. Philadelphia, PA: Mosby Elsevier; 2017.

132. Houston CS. High-altitude illness disease with protean manifestations. *JAMA.* 1976;236:2193.

133. Montgomery AB, Mills J, Luce JM. Incidence of acute mountain sickness at intermediate altitude. *JAMA.* 1989; 261:732.

134. Gertsch JH, Seto TB, Mor J, Onopa J. Ginkgo biloba for the prevention of severe acute mountain sickness (AMS) starting day one before rapid ascent. *High Alt Med Biol.* 2002; 3(1):29.

135. Honigman B, Theis MK, Koziol-McLain J, et al. Acute mountain sickness in a general tourist population at moderate altitudes. *Ann Intern Med.* 1993;118(8):587.

136. Zafren K, Honigman B. High-altitude medicine. *Emerg Clin North Am.* 1997;15(1):191.

137. Hultgren HN. *High-Altitude Medicine.* Stanford, CA: Hultgren Publications; 1997.

138. Luks AM, McIntosh SE, Grissom CK, et al. Wilderness Medical Society consensus guidelines for the prevention and treatment of acute altitude illness: 2014 update. *Wilderness Environ Med.* 2014;25:S4-S14.

139. Schneider M, Bernasch D, Weymann J, et al. Acute mountain sickness: influence of susceptibility, pre-exposure, and ascent rate. *Med Sci Sports Exerc.* 2002;34(12):1886.

140. Bartsch P. High-altitude pulmonary edema. *Med Sci Sports Exerc.* 1999;31(suppl 1):S23.

141. Roach RC, Houston CS, Honigman B. How well do older persons tolerate moderate altitude? *West J Med.* 1995;162(1):32.

142. Roach RC, Maes D, Sandoval D, et al. Exercise exacerbates acute mountain sickness at simulated high altitude. *J Appl Physiol*. 2000;88(2):581.

143. Roeggla G, Roeggla H, Roeggla M, et al. Effect of alcohol on acute ventilation adaptation to mild hypoxia at moderate altitude. *Ann Intern Med*. 1995;122:925.

144. Reeves JWJ, Zafren K, Honigman B, Schoene R. Seasonal variation in barometric pressure and temperature in Summit County: effect on altitude illness. In: Sutton JHC, Coates G, eds. *Hypoxia and Molecular Medicine*. Burlington, VT: Charles S. Houston; 1993:272-274.

145. Luks AM, Swenson ER. Medication and dosage considerations in the prophylaxis and treatment of high-altitude illness. *Chest*. 2008;133:744.

146. Roach RC, Bartcsh P, Oelz O, Hackett PH, Lake Louise Scoring Committee. The Lake Louise Acute Mountain Sickness Scoring System. In: Sutton JR, Houston CS, Coates G, eds. *Hypoxia and Molecular Medicine*. Burlington, VT: Charles S. Houston; 1993.

147. Muza SR, Lyons TP, Rock PB. Effect of altitude on exposure on brain volume and development of acute mountain sickness (AMS). In: Roach RC, Wagner PD, Hackett PH, eds. *Hypoxia: Into the Next Millennium: Advances in Experimental Medicine and Biology*. Vol 474. New York, NY: Kluwer Academic/Plenum; 1999.

148. Hacket PH. High-altitude cerebral edema and acute mountain sickness: a pathological update. In: Roach RC, Wagner PD, Hackett PH, eds. *Hypoxia: Into the Next Millennium: Advances in Experimental Medicine and Biology*. Vol 474. New York, NY: Kluwer Academic/Plenum; 1999.

149. Sanchez del Rio M, Moskkowitz MA. High-altitude headache: lessons from aches at sea level. In: Roach RC, Wagner PD, Hackett PH, eds. *Hypoxia: Into the Next Millennium: Advances in Experimental Medicine and Biology*. Vol 474. New York, NY: Kluwer Academic/Plenum; 1999.

150. Hackett PH. The cerebral etiology of high-altitude cerebral edema and acute mountain sickness. *Wilderness Environ Med*. 1999;10(2):97.

151. Yarnell PR, Heit J, Hackett PH. High-altitude cerebral edema (HACE): the Denver/Front Range experience. *Semin Neurol*. 2000;20(2):209.

152. Hultgren HN, Honigman B, Theis K, Nicholas D. High-altitude pulmonary edema at ski resort. *West J Med*. 1996;164:222.

153. Stenmark KR, Frid M, Nemenoff R, et al. Hypoxia induces cell-specific changes in gene expression in vascular wall cells: implications for pulmonary hypertension. In: Roach RC, Wagner PD, Hackett PH, eds. *Hypoxia: Into the Next Millennium: Advances in Experimental Medicine and Biology*. Vol 474. New York, NY: Kluwer Academic/Plenum; 1999.

154. The Lake Louise consensus on the definition and quantification of altitude illness. In: Sutton JR, Coates G, Houston C, eds. *Hypoxia and Mountain Medicine*. Burlington, VT: Queen City Press; 1992.

155. Luks AM. Do we have a "best practice" for treating high-altitude pulmonary edema? *High Alt Med Biol*. 2008;9: 111-114.

156. Koch RO, Burtscher M. Do we have a "best practice" for treating high-altitude pulmonary edema? [Letter to the Editor]. *High Alt Med Biol*. 2008;9:343-344.

157. Zafren K. Management of altitude illnesses. In: Hawkins SC, ed. *Wilderness EMS*. Philadelphia, PA: Wolters Kluwer; 2018.

158. Hackett PH, Rennie D, Levine HD. The incidence, importance, and prophylaxis of acute mountain sickness. *Lancet*. 1976;2:1149-1155.

159. Bartsch P, Maggiorini M, Mairbaurl H, et al. Pulmonary extravascular fluid accumulation in climbers. *Lancet*. 2002;360:571.

160. Singh I, Kapila CC, Khanna PK, et al. High-altitude pulmonary oedema. *Lancet*. 1965;191:229-234.

161. Lipman GS, Kanaan NC, Holck PS, et al. Ibuprofen prevents altitude illness: randomized controlled trial for prevention of altitude illness with nonsteroidal anti-inflammatories. *Ann Emerg Med*. 2012;59(6):484-490.

162. Gertsch JH, Corbett B, Holck PS, et al. Altitude sickness in climbers and efficacy of NSAIDs trial (ASCENT): randomized, controlled trial of ibuprofen versus placebo for prevention of altitude illness. *Wilderness Environ Med*. 2012;23:307-315.

163. Gertsch JH, Lipman GS, Holck PS, et al. Prospective, double-blind, randomized, placebo-controlled comparison of acetazolamide versus ibuprofen for prophylaxis against high altitude headache: the headache evaluation at altitude trial (HEAT). *Wilderness Environ Med*. 2010;21:236-243.

164. Pollard AJ, Niermeyer S, Barry PB, et al. Children at high altitude: an international consensus statement by an ad hoc committee of the International Society for Mountain Medicine. *High Alt Med Biol*. 2001;2:389.

Suggested Reading

Auerbach PS, ed. *Auerbach's Wilderness Medicine*. 7th ed. Philadelphia, PA: Mosby Elsevier; 2017.

Bechdel L, Ray S. *River Rescue: A Manual for Whitewater Safety*. 4th ed. Asheville, NC: CFS Press; 2009.

Bennett P, Elliott D. *Bennett and Elliots' Physiology and Medicine of Diving*. 5th ed. London: Saunders; 2003.

Bierens JJLM. *Drowning: Prevention, Rescue, Treatment*. 2nd ed. Berlin, Germany: Springer; 2014.

Bove AA. *Bove and Davis' Diving Medicine*. 5th ed. Philadelphia, PA: Saunders; 2003.

Hawkins SC, ed. *Wilderness EMS*. Philadelphia, PA: Wolters Kluwer; 2018.

Hawkins SC, Simon RB, Beissinger JP, Simon D. *Vertical Aid: Essential Wilderness Medicine for Climbers, Trekkers, and Mountaineers*. New York, NY: The Countryman Press; 2017.

Rodway GW, Weber DC, McIntosh SE. *Mountain Medicine and Technical Rescue*. Herefordshire, UK: Carreg; 2016.

Sutton JR, Coates G, Remmers JE, eds. *Hypoxia: The Adaptations*. Philadelphia, PA: BC Dekker; 1990.

United States Lifesaving Association. *Open Water Lifesaving—The United States Lifesaving Association Manual*. 3rd ed. Boston, MA: Pearson; 2017.

CHAPTER 21

Wilderness Trauma Care

Lead Editors:
Will Smith, MD, Paramedic
John Trentini, MD, PhD, FAWM

CHAPTER OBJECTIVES

At the completion of this chapter, you will be able to do the following:

- Explain the four principles of the LATE acronym, representing a simplified approach to wilderness emergency medical services (EMS) operations and trauma care.
- Identify levels of wilderness EMS care providers and how they should interface with the standard patient care continuum from the point of injury/illness to the hospital.
- Discuss the reasons for the dictum, "Every wilderness patient is hypothermic, hypoglycemic, and hypovolemic until proven otherwise."

- Describe escalating ways to manage bleeding wounds in the wilderness, in what situations to start with a tourniquet, and when to consider a tourniquet conversion (removal).
- Discuss the signs and symptoms of common bites and stings and medical management in the wilderness.
- Describe several operationally specific (expanded scope of practice) protocols that should be considered in wilderness trauma care.

SCENARIO

You are the medical and team leader for the local search and rescue team and have been dispatched to a popular canyoneering site in your jurisdiction. The only information you have is a GPS location from a distress signal broadcast via an emergency satellite beacon. The time is about 1800 hours, and current temperature is 74°F (23°C). The weather forecast shows some building thunderstorms throughout the evening and an overnight low of 36°F (2°C). The team begins to plan the response using the LATE acronym: *l*ocate, *a*ccess, *t*reat, *e*xtricate.

Your team assembles the necessary gear, including the still-/swift-water and high-angle rescue kits, their own personal protective equipment, and the standard medical kit and begins responding to the location. As the team leader, you interface with the incident commander and develop a communication plan with a staged team member to enable a communication relay from the top of the canyon back to the incident command post.

(continued)

SCENARIO (CONTINUED)

- What are the essential items for a team and individual medical kit to handle the most severe and most likely injuries for this type of rescue scenario?
- What operationally specific (expanded scope of practice) protocols would you want in place to care for patients in remote and/or prolonged care settings? Do you have standing orders, as you are expecting limited communication options?
- What safety concerns should you be considering for your rescue team? How do situational factors such as time of day, location of patient, and experience and training of your team affect safety?

You *locate* the GPS position and find a slot canyon with three known separate 100-foot (ft; 30-meter [m]) rappels. You attempt to yell and try to make contact but are unable to get any response. When you blow your whistle, you are able to hear a faint whistle blast in return. You and your team safely make your way toward the location. At the top of the second rappel, you find the two members of the party that set off the emergency beacon. They tell you one of their team members sustained an approximately 50-ft (15-m) fall deeper in the canyon at 1300 hours. They had to climb back up from the location to get a signal out on their emergency beacon. Another friend rappelled down to assess the victim and stated the injuries appear to be an angulated open femur fracture, with a lot of pooled blood. He also stated that the patient appeared confused. The patient did not lose consciousness or show any other signs of head trauma. He was wearing a helmet. The friend has been holding pressure on a "pumper" with some continued bleeding.

You continue down the next rappel and establish verbal communication with the friend who is attending to the patient. You direct him to place an improvised tourniquet with 1-inch tubular webbing proximal to the wound that is continuing to bleed. You direct him to tighten the webbing by twisting a spare carabiner until the bleeding is stopped and to then secure it in place with another carabiner. The friend reports that the bleeding has been controlled.

Once your additional equipment reaches your location, you begin your final rappel to *access* the patient. Upon reaching the patient, you find a 25-year-old otherwise healthy man awake and now more alert with an obvious open deformed right femur fracture. The friend has tried to get extra clothing around the patient, but he is in a shallow pool of cold water and has wet clothing and is shivering. You begin planning and implementing the *treat* portion of your mission, but because it is getting dark, your team will have to wait until morning to *extricate* the patient.

- How can you direct others to provide care in a wilderness setting? Are you familiar with how dispatchers use emergency medical dispatch to assist with prearrival instructions during a 9-1-1 call, and can you remotely direct someone to provide initial care? What else would you direct the friend to perform if you have an additional delay in reaching the patient?
- What are your priorities of care in assessment and intervention? What are the prolonged patient care considerations?
- What is your plan to get this patient packaged and extricated?

Wilderness EMS Defined

Many terms are used to describe areas far from civilization (**Figure 21-1**), including wilderness, remote, backcountry, isolated, and austere. Emergency medical services (EMS) personnel tend to lump these terms together under the heading "wilderness." According to the dictionary, the following are definitions of *wilderness*[1]:

- A tract or region uncultivated and uninhabited by human beings

- An area essentially undisturbed by human activity together with its naturally developed life community
- An empty or pathless area or region

Because EMS is focused on patient care, the definition of *wilderness EMS* diverges slightly from the preceding definitions of wilderness. The *wilderness EMS* definition is really the application of medical care to patients in the wilderness. This chapter on wilderness trauma care provides guidance on questions such as, "When and where do we encounter wilderness EMS?" That is, "When should we think and

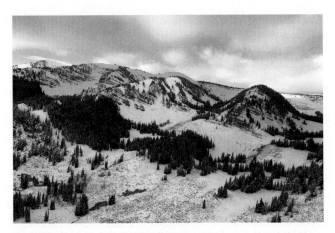

Figure 21-1 Wilderness is traditionally thought of as areas far from civilization, but similar surroundings may also occur in the street EMS settings when disasters or other resource-constrained events occur (e.g., mass-casualty incident).

Courtesy of Will Smith.

work differently from the way we do in the traditional front country or street EMS settings?" The answer to this question goes beyond simple geography and involves many of the following considerations:

- Access to the scene
- Weather
- Daylight
- Terrain and elevation
- Special transport and handling needs
- Access and transport times
- Available personnel
- Communications
- Hazards present
- Medical and rescue equipment available
- Injury patterns for the specific environment

Numerous examples exist that expand the traditional view of wilderness EMS. For example:

1. In a city after an earthquake, it may be difficult to access those who are injured or trapped, there may be no roads for transport, and local EMS systems may be incapacitated and/or overwhelmed. In this situation, patients are likely to remain in their location for a considerable amount of time. They will have the same care requirements as a hiker who has fallen in the mountains and is hours or days away from a hospital.
2. A person who has fallen in a large suburban park late in the evening during an ice storm is at risk from the same factors as a patient suffering the same type of fall in the wilderness. The patient may need a rescue team with ropes, crampons, and prehospital care providers who can anticipate and manage issues such as hypothermia, packaging, wound management, and difficult patient extrication.

Wilderness EMS Versus Traditional Street EMS

We often talk of how *wilderness* EMS differs from the traditional *street* EMS, but in reality, all aspects of EMS exist on a spectrum. At one end of the spectrum is an incident half a block from a level I trauma center, and at the other end of the spectrum is an incident in the deepest part of the Wind-Ice Cave system in western Wyoming (**Figure 21-2**). Wilderness EMS even goes beyond the rural and frontier EMS settings.[2] In the final analysis, where does the *street* end and the *wilderness* begin? The answer is, "It depends." It depends on the distance from the ambulance to the emergency department (ED). It depends on the weather. It depends on the terrain. It depends on the resources available and whether they remain intact and functional. Even more important, it depends on the nature of the injury and the capabilities of the EMS and rescue personnel on scene.

In recognizing these situational EMS variations, it is clear that wilderness EMS should be considered as part of the overall medical system, from the point of injury, to the definitive care provided at the trauma center, to the rehabilitation facility or home, until the patient has returned to baseline function. Documentation, quality

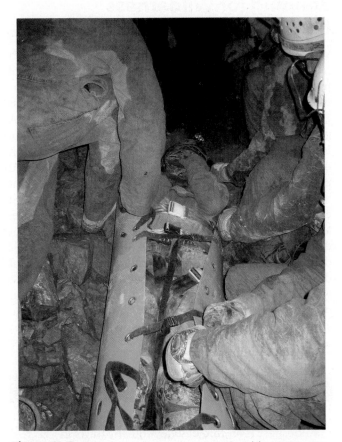

Figure 21-2 Patient care in a cave unquestionably represents wilderness EMS.

Courtesy of Will Smith.

assurance, medical oversight, protocols, skills validation, and other factors, all of which are mainstays of any traditional street EMS system, should also be components of a wilderness EMS system.

Wilderness EMS System

Several issues are critical for optimal wilderness patient care and are common problems for which management is different from on the street. This chapter provides an overview of the many issues involved in wilderness medical emergencies. Prehospital care providers who function in a formal capacity in the wilderness setting as wilderness medical providers should obtain specific training (**Box 21-1**).[3,4] In addition, oversight direction by a knowledgeable physician should be an integral component of wilderness medical activities.[5-7] In many regions of the United States, there is no medical oversight for wilderness medical providers on many search and rescue (SAR) teams.[8] While this is a suboptimal arrangement, there is a growing recognition that the best practice of providing medical oversight is essential for all prehospital EMS providers, including those who operate in wilderness and other austere settings.[6-8]

Training for Wilderness EMS Providers

Wilderness EMS providers traditionally have been set apart from traditional EMS. Some have viewed them as first aid providers and thus not under the scope of EMS regulations. Some states have even excluded certain wilderness EMS providers, such as ski patrol, from EMS regulation. A growing realization is that any care provided at the point of injury/illness should be integrated into the overall system of care. This integration should start with prevention, and it should encompass immediate responders at the point of injury, who are probably providing traditional first aid care, to the traditional EMS and definitive hospital care. Wilderness-specific responders are generally trained at designated levels, although some of the traditional wilderness EMS training programs and certifications do not directly align with traditional street EMS models.[9] The National Association of EMS Physicians (NAEMSP) and other organizations have begun to help standardize the scope of practice of these providers, which in turn helps

to standardize wilderness EMS operations to ensure best practices in training and patient care.[10]

Common wilderness EMS certifications include the following[3,4,11,12]:

- *Wilderness First Aid (WFA)*. The basic level of wilderness EMS training. It is generally a 16- to 20-hour course.[4,13]
- *Wilderness Advanced First Aid (WAFA)*. Training that builds on the WFA curriculum. It is generally a 36- to 40-hour course.
- *Wilderness Emergency Medical Responder (WEMR)/Wilderness First Responder (WFR)*. The most common level of wilderness EMS provider. Many SAR teams as well as mountain and other guide services have individuals trained at this level. Some education models pair this with the national registry of EMTs (NREMT) scope of practice to meet the emergency medical responder (EMR) certification to make a nationally recognized EMS standard. This is generally a 70- to 80-hour course. Some online and blended learning programs are being developed as well. This course focuses on the medical decision making needed in remote care environments, critical skills and patient care interventions, when to evacuate, and how to work safely.[4,14-16]
- *Wilderness EMT (WEMT)*. A course that often consists of modules added to a traditional emergency medical technician (EMT) course, including WEMR/WFR decision making, skills, and wilderness protocols.
- *Outdoor Emergency Care (OEC)*. A basic life support (BLS) course that is commonly taught by the National Ski Patrol and is generally 80 to 100 hours.[17] It has many similarities to a traditional EMT and WEMT training, but there remain some differences.[18,19] In many settings, ski patrollers interface with SAR teams, with both groups providing wilderness EMS care (**Figure 21-3**).

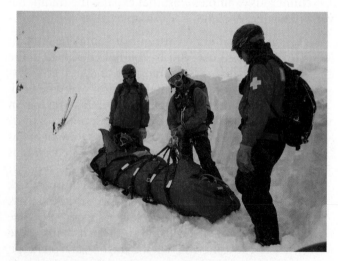

Figure 21-3 Ski patrollers and SAR teams often interface in wilderness EMS settings to provide optimal patient care.
Courtesy of Will Smith.

Box 21-1 Wilderness EMS Training

Prehospital care providers who may provide wilderness EMS care or who regularly travel in the backcountry are advised to take a specialized course or courses.

- *ParkMedic.* Generally an advanced emergency medical technician (AEMT)-level course with additional focused wilderness EMS skill sets required for optimal patient care in many of the remote National Park Service (NPS) locations.[20,21] The NPS has been training wilderness EMS providers for many years to this certification. It has been taught every other year in January at the University of California, San Francisco (UCSF)–Fresno Emergency Medicine program since the 1970s.
- *Wilderness AEMT, Wilderness Paramedic.* Generally training that is similar to the traditional EMS programs, followed by augmented training, through local and national conferences and courses, for advanced life support (ALS) providers.
- *Wilderness Physician Assistant (PA), Wilderness Advanced Practice Registered Nurse (APRN).* Training provided for those who may be involved with wilderness care and/or serve in formal roles in wilderness EMS systems. Many locations in the United States are staffed with PAs or APRNs, especially in remote or rural areas.
- *Wilderness Physician.* Training for physicians who are ordinarily identified by their primary and/or subspecialty board certification (e.g., emergency medicine, surgery, family practice, etc.) but who, by chance, are exposed to caring for patients in the wilderness (i.e., on a good Samaritan basis), or who, in some cases, are members and medical directors for dedicated wilderness EMS teams. They not only give medical oversight to a team or agency but often provide direct patient care. Other allied health professionals (e.g., veterinarians, dentists) can also be involved in wilderness medical care, with the appropriate training and experience. There are multiple programs and organizations that provide this kind of education for physicians, from formal academic fellowships to other training programs.[4,22]

Wilderness EMS Medical Oversight

In this chapter, *front country* refers to any area in which conventional EMS can be delivered; it stands in contrast to *backcountry*, which refers to remote, often austere, locations. Just as front country EMS systems have medical oversight, so should wilderness EMS systems. In some regards, it is even more important as the complex medical decision making and prolonged patient care virtually all require standing orders. Medical directors providing this oversight must be knowledgeable in the variables that affect care in these settings. They also must understand the scope of practice and limitations of their providers. In some settings, the medical director may even be providing direct medical oversight in the field and sometimes even direct patient care. If they enter the field, they must be fully trained and competent to manage themselves safely in these settings.[7,8,11,23,24]

Wilderness EMS Agencies

There are many agencies that practice wilderness EMS care. Examples of wilderness EMS agencies include the following[12,25,26]:

- SAR teams
- National, state, and local parks
- Ski patrols
- Expedition medical teams
- Specialized military teams

The Wilderness EMS Context

Key Wilderness EMS/SAR Principles: Locate, Access, Treat, Extricate (LATE)

In wilderness EMS, which is a common component of many SAR operations, a few key principles can help simplify the overall mission or callout. As discussed in the opening scenario, the acronym LATE can help organize the response—*l*ocate, *a*ccess, *t*reat, *e*xtricate.[25] Generally, every wilderness EMS operation will have some component of each (**Box 21-2**).

Locate is the first step in any event or callout. You have to find the patient before you can begin care. In some

---

Box 21-2 LATE

The acronym LATE (*l*ocate, *a*ccess, *t*reat, *e*xtricate) represents simplified principles in SAR and other wilderness EMS operations[25]:

- *Locate.* This is generally the first step in any wilderness EMS event. The patient must be located before the next steps of a rescue can be undertaken.
- *Access.* After a patient is located, the wilderness EMS provider must be able to access the location in order to begin patient care.
- *Treat.* This is the main function of the wilderness EMS provider, but in some settings, extrication may become a higher priority, delaying care until the patient arrives at a safe location.
- *Extricate.* This is the final step of an SAR or other wilderness EMS operation. It involves removing the patient from the technical environment and transporting toward definitive care.

Modified from: Smith WR. Principles of basic technical rescue, packaging, and patient care integration. Hawkins SC, ed. *Wilderness EMS.* Philadelphia, PA: Wolters Kluwer; 2018.

situations, this may be easy if a 9-1-1 call was made and you know the exact patient location. In other situations, this may be more difficult, and you will need to perform an extensive search operation.

Access can be a technical challenge. For example, a patient may be found but is on the opposite shore of a raging river. This type of situation is what distinguishes traditional street EMS from wilderness EMS.

Treat is often the phase in which the real definition of wilderness EMS care becomes clear. While some care may be identical to that performed in the street EMS setting, medical decision making, such as when to apply different treatment interventions, may be different in crucial ways. These decisions can dramatically change the duration of the next stage of the rescue, as well as the risk to the patient and rescuers.

Extricate is the last step in these simplified rescue principles. While some of these principles can overlap, some may take priority over others. Just like in a hazardous materials or tactical situation, extrication may be a higher priority than standard treatment options, such as starting an intravenous (IV) line.

Technical Rescue Interface

Wilderness EMS providers must not only deliver appropriate care, but they must also be able to access patients in technical terrain safely. This means they must be able to navigate through the *technical rescue interface*.[25] This problem or interface is what often helps to define the wilderness EMS setting. While rescue group structures can be quite varied, some examples of how wilderness EMS care is provided include the following:

- Self-rescue
- Companion rescue
- Bystander rescue
- Organized small group/strike team rescue (i.e., specialized SAR team)
- Ski patrol
- Organized large-group rescue
- Fire department technical rescue teams
- Industrial site rescue teams
- Military systems (e.g., Air Force pararescue)
- Multigroup/interagency rescue coordinating a complex response

Wilderness EMS Realms

There are many realms to wilderness EMS. A few potential scenarios are listed here, each with specific patient care considerations, patient access limitations, and other individual factors that often must be mitigated or overcome.[25-27]

- Space
- High angle (cliff/near vertical)
- Steep angle (side of a road on a mountain pass)

- Low angle
- Avalanche
- Cave, confined space, canyoneering
- Helicopter operations (long line, short haul)
- Still water, swift water, open water
- All-terrain vehicle, off-road vehicle, snowmobile, mountain bike
- Helicopter, fixed-wing rescue
- Snow, glaciated, crevasse rescue
- Mountaineering, climbing
- High altitude
- Diving

Wilderness Injury Patterns

Death from trauma has a trimodal (three-phase) distribution, as mentioned in the PHTLS: Past, Present, and Future chapter. The **first phase of death** is within seconds to minutes of injury. Deaths occurring during this first phase are usually caused by injuries to the brain, brain stem, high spinal cord, heart, aorta, or other large vessels and can best be managed by preventive measures such as helmets. Only a few of these patients can be saved, and then generally only in large urban areas where rapid emergency transport is available.

The **second phase of death** occurs within minutes to a few hours after injury. Rapid assessment and resuscitation are carried out to reduce this second phase of trauma deaths. Deaths occurring during this phase are usually caused by subdural and epidural hematomas, hemopneumothoraces, ruptured spleen, lacerations of the liver, pelvic fractures, or multiple injuries associated with significant blood loss. The fundamental principles of trauma care (hemorrhage control, airway management, balanced fluid resuscitation, and transport to an appropriate facility) can best be applied to these patients. The **third phase of death** occurs several days or weeks after the initial injury and is almost always caused by sepsis and organ failure.

Prehospital care providers focus mostly on saving patients from the second phase. In the wilderness, most of those who survive to be rescued have already passed the first phase of death and usually most of the second. However, the presence of medically trained individuals on an SAR team may be able to prevent deaths related to the second phase.[28,29] Often, this wilderness care focuses on, "What can we do *now* that will keep the patient from dying or having major complications later?" Wilderness EMS providers need to make sure the patient does not develop problems such as kidney failure from dehydration, overwhelming infection from poor resistance due to starvation, severe hypothermia, and skin necrosis from decubitus ulcers from unnecessary immobilization.

Preventive SAR programs have become an important focus to limit and decrease wilderness EMS encounters.

Helmets and other safety features at ski areas have decreased the morbidity and mortality of users. The National Park Service and other programs, such as Back Country Zero, in partnership with Teton County SAR in Jackson, Wyoming, have extensive programs that promote education and prevention.

Safety

In the wilderness, even more so than on the street, scene safety is a critical consideration.[30] An injured or dead wilderness EMS provider distracts from the care of the patient and limits the possibility of a successful rescue mission. Street scene safety considerations apply even in the wilderness. In the wilderness, scene dangers can be less obvious than on the street, especially if the provider is not properly trained to function in the given environment.

The wilderness EMS provider and patient will be exposed to the environment and changes in weather. An incoming cold front with freezing rain, for example, may complicate the operation or even injure or kill the wilderness medicine provider and patient. If a rescue lasts for hours or days, the lack of food and water may cause debilitation. The wilderness terrain is often rugged, and dangerous technical terrain may complicate patient care and extrication (**Figure 21-4**). Wilderness EMS providers need to be aware of dangers specific to the environment, such as rockfall, avalanche risk, rising waters, high altitudes or altitude exposure, and recirculating eddies at the base of waterfalls.

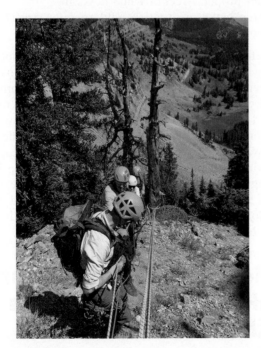

Figure 21-4 Steep slopes, cliffs, rockfall, and uneven footing are dangerous in wilderness rescue.
Courtesy of Will Smith.

Each member of the SAR team must take appropriate preparations and precautions to ensure the safety, health, and well-being of the SAR team collectively. All members must be educated about the hazards and dangers of the specific environment in which they will be working. They must know their limitations and not exceed their capabilities trying to rescue an injured patient. Each member of the SAR team must be appropriately prepared with the necessary clothing and personal protective equipment (PPE) for the environmental conditions and rescue at hand. Last, ensuring that the medical needs of the SAR team are met must be an integral component of the response effort. Appropriate supplies to address potential illness or injury of an SAR team member as well as enforcement of work–rest cycles will help maintain a well-functioning SAR team.

Proper Care Depends on Context

Our medical knowledge, understanding, and technology change as we make advances in medicine; however, some basic principles of medical care change little over the years and are independent of the patient's location. Prehospital Trauma Life Support (PHTLS) has long advocated that the critically injured patient be transported as quickly as possible to an appropriate destination, sometimes without detailed physical examination and treatment of noncritical conditions. However, *proper* care is somewhat context dependent. The definition of *detailed physical examination* and *noncritical conditions* may be different on an urban street than when deep in the wilderness (**Figure 21-5**). The situation, knowledge level, skill, scene conditions, and equipment available may alter medical decision making and management of the trauma patient.[20] (This concept is introduced in the Golden Principles, Preferences, and Critical Thinking chapter.)

Ideal to Real Care

In wilderness EMS, complex medical decisions sometimes must be made based on an "ideal to real" care concept.[31] This decision-making process is what sets apart a wilderness EMS provider from a traditional street EMS provider.

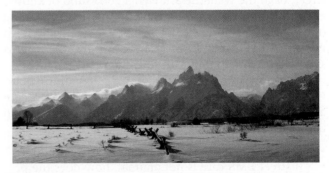

Figure 21-5 Wilderness terrain.
Courtesy of Will Smith.

The ability to improvise is almost the standard in most wilderness EMS situations, and EMS providers must take the traditional ideal care protocol or treatment and adapt/improvise to meet the reality of the setting in which they find themselves.

Consider a patient with a complex fracture–dislocation of the shoulder. What is the proper care in the operating room (OR)? In many cases, it involves an open reduction and internal fixation (ORIF). However, proper care in the OR may not be proper care in the ED, where it would not be proper to attempt an open reduction. In the ED, x-ray films are taken to evaluate the fracture–dislocation, a short-acting pain medication is given, and a closed reduction of the dislocation is performed to reduce pain and swelling, to realign the bones grossly, and to decrease pressure on nerves and blood vessels. The definitive ORIF will occur later, in the OR.

Likewise, proper care in the ED may not be proper care in the street EMS setting. The prehospital care providers may not have the advantage of a large, warm, dry area to perform an assessment and provide treatment. They may be working in the rain, where the patient is hanging upside down inside a crushed vehicle while a rescue crew uses power tools to cut and remove metal to reach the patient. Once the patient is free, the prehospital care provider will assess the patient for other injuries, check the distal neurovascular status in the arm, immobilize the patient's shoulder, provide pain medication, and transport the patient rapidly to the ED. Similarly, on the street, it might not be proper care to attempt a closed or open reduction to reduce the fracture–dislocation (based on local protocols).

Finally, proper care on the street may not be proper care in the wilderness. What protocols may need to be modified for a patient who, following a motor vehicle crash, is trapped in a car that is in the middle of a flowing river or that is submerged (**Figure 21-6**)? In this case, swift-water rescue skills, techniques, and modified priorities must be performed in addition to patient care.[32] Examples such as this are why wilderness EMS protocols may require an operationally specific scope of practice for best patient care.[6,12]

For most conditions, however, proper care is proper care whether it is performed in the OR, in the ED, on the street, or in the wilderness. Given a good fund of knowledge, critical-thinking skills, training, and understanding of key principles, prehospital care providers can perform medical decision making in the field to reflect the various situations in which they will encounter patients.

For a small but significant number of situations, noteworthy differences exist between proper street EMS care and proper wilderness EMS care. Such situations bring up the following important questions:

- Is street EMS care always optimal in the wilderness?
- If street EMS care is not optimal, how does the prehospital care provider know what the optimal care is? Is this established in local protocols?

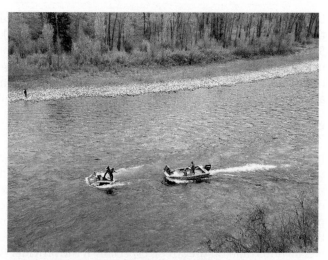

Figure 21-6 A patient trapped in a vehicle in the middle of a flowing river after a motor vehicle crash may need to be treated by modified protocols. Trauma care in the wilderness is often hampered by adverse environmental conditions, water, mud, underbrush, and confined spaces.
Courtesy of Brian Coe.

- How does the prehospital care provider deal with situations in the field when unsure precisely what the patient's injury might be? For example, how does the wilderness medical provider determine that a fracture–dislocation is present when examining a patient who is hanging upside down from a rope deep within a cave?
- How does the prehospital care provider decide, for a particular patient in a particular situation, which is *more* proper, street or wilderness care?
- What makes a situation wilderness or street? What about all the in-between cases?

Definitive answers to all of these questions cannot easily be provided here. As stated previously, often the answer is "it depends." However, at least good background information can be provided so that prehospital care providers may, as needed in a particular patient care situation, answer the questions in their respective setting. The PHTLS philosophy has always been that, given a good fund of knowledge and key principles, prehospital care providers are capable of making reasoned decisions regarding patient care. In the end, it is providing *real care* to the patient—based on the situation and resources at hand and based on the *ideal care*—that represents the standard in that setting.

Wilderness EMS Decision Making: Balancing Risks and Benefits

Experienced physicians, nurses, and prehospital care providers know that procedures such as airway management and wound management are the easy part of medicine.

The difficult part is in knowing *when* to do *what*: critical thinking. Even more often than on the street, in the wilderness one risk needs to be weighed carefully against another and against the potential benefits. For *this* particular patient, in *this* particular setting, and with *these* particular resources, and with *this* particular likelihood of *this* particular help arriving at *this* particular time in the future, what are the potential risks? What are the potential benefits? Wilderness EMS is largely the art of compromise: balancing the particular risks and benefits for each patient.

TCCC and TECC Principles Applied in Wilderness Trauma Care

The importance of considering the incident's context is evident in the combat and tactical settings of the Iraq and Afghanistan conflicts. Development and implementation of Tactical Combat Casualty Care (TCCC) guidelines have been clearly linked to improved casualty survivor rates.[33-37] Many of the concepts learned in the combat setting can be applied to the wilderness context. An entire preconference session was held on this topic at the Seventh World Congress of Wilderness Medicine in 2016 (Telluride, Colorado) and resulted in a publication: *Special Edition: Tactical Combat Casualty Care; Transitioning Battlefield Lessons Learned to Other Austere Environments.*[38] While the sources of danger may not be the same (e.g., caring for a gunshot wound sustained in combat versus one sustained while hunting, or injuries from improvised explosive devices [IEDs] versus an avalanche), many of the same injury patterns and care priorities are shared by both rescuers and patients.[39]

Patient care priorities extrapolated from TCCC to wilderness settings have been widely adopted by many organizations. The NPS has a unique challenge in providing care in extremely diverse remote care settings (**Figure 21-7**). NPS rangers care for patients in remote, austere wilderness settings using both tactical and wilderness protocols.[20,21,40]

Further development of the TCCC tactical guidelines has been adapted by the Committee on Tactical Emergency Casualty Care (TECC) for civilian and federal use.[41] TECC applies similar TCCC concepts across multiple all-hazard risk areas (tactical, hazardous materials, etc.) and to expanded populations (children, older adults, etc.). Many agencies have begun providing care based on TECC guidelines and have formalized rescue task force programs to blend this care into tactical and other hazardous situations (including wilderness and remote trauma care).[21,42]

See further discussion on TCCC/TECC and patient care priorities in tactical settings in the Civilian Tactical Emergency Medical Support (TEMS) chapter.

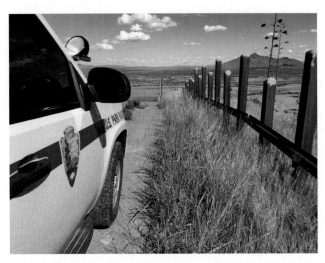

Figure 21-7 National Park Service ranger on patrol at the United States–Mexico border, a remote environment with the possibility of trauma-related injuries.
Courtesy of Will Smith.

Principles of Basic Patient Packaging

Patient packaging becomes a paramount issue in wilderness EMS care, as ultimately the patient needs to be extricated from the remote environment to definitive care. Sometimes this can be an easy task when managing an isolated injury. For example, an upper extremity injury can be splinted, and the patient can walk or be assisted out. However, other minor injuries, such as a lower extremity sprain or fracture, may require the patient to be carried out. More critical or life-threatening injuries always require some degree of patient packaging and more intensive extrication. Different rescue systems can be used to evacuate a nonambulatory patient in technical situations. **Figure 21-8** shows a patient packaged in a wheeled litter, a common rescue tool used to move patients when they are unable to walk. In overwater operations, care must be taken to ensure proper flotation for the patient (e.g., personal flotation device), in addition to the extrication capability (**Figure 21-9**). All of these factors must be considered when packaging patients in a wilderness EMS situation. Often patient packaging must employ more padding than usual and ongoing efforts to ensure a position of comfort for the patient, as the rescues are frequently prolonged.

Physiologic Splinting

Physiologic splinting is a concept that can be applied to virtually any injury in any EMS setting, not just the wilderness. It uses the premise of establishing normal physiologic alignment to the injured area and then immobilizing or supporting in that position. The same concepts of immobilizing the joint above and below a long-bone injury and the

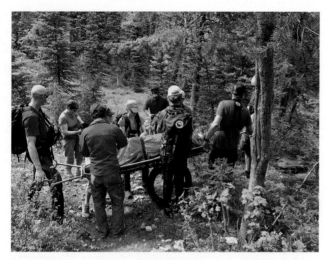

Figure 21-8 A wheeled litter is being used to transport an injured patient after a mountain bike crash. While easier than directly carrying a nonambulatory patient, it still requires considerable resources.

Courtesy of Will Smith.

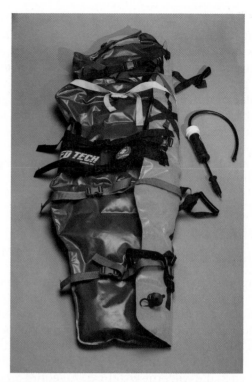

Figure 21-10 A full-body vacuum mattress used in physiologic splinting of the entire body.

Courtesy of David Bowers.

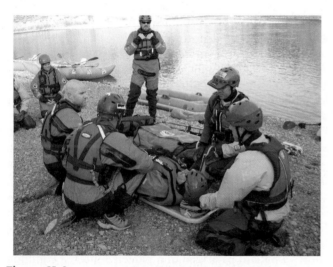

Figure 21-9 A personal flotation device is a mandatory packaging adjunct whenever you transport a patient over water.

Courtesy of Will Smith.

bone above and below a joint injury are incorporated.[12,25] Distal circulation, sensory, and motor assessments should be performed before and after any splinting and then continuously reassessed.

Wilderness application of *physiologic splinting* usually requires a great deal more padding than traditional EMS application. This is due mostly to the prolonged transport times to extract a patient from the remote setting. It is also important to make sure the patient packaging and physiologic splinting are done correctly at the outset. More padding not only reduces overall discomfort but also promotes normal neurovascular function and allows for expedited rescue operations. A hurried patient packaging without

appropriate physiologic splinting and ample padding may lead to delays in the rescue if a patient must be repackaged.

The vacuum mattress (**Figure 21-10**) has become the standard of care for wilderness *EMS* patients requiring whole-body immobilization (including *spinal motion restriction/immobilization*). As with any specialized tool, it must be brought to the rescue scene; however, it is often more portable than the urban alternatives.[25] Smaller vacuum splints can be used for isolated extremity injuries. However, as with much of wilderness EMS, the ideal tools may not be available, and improvisation may be required to achieve the same patient care objective. This situation is another example of the *ideal* to *real* care concept, as previously discussed.

Airway Considerations

Airway management has been the utmost priority in EMS care, leading to the long-standing ABC (airway, breathing, circulation) mantra. Wilderness EMS care must also consider airway management, but sometimes to an even higher degree. During extrication of an immobilized patient, especially if he or she is supine, the wilderness EMS provider may have a limited ability to monitor the airway and access the patient. Airway considerations with the potential for vomiting and airway compromise are of paramount concern. Elements of technical rescue and evacuation must be balanced with patient packaging and

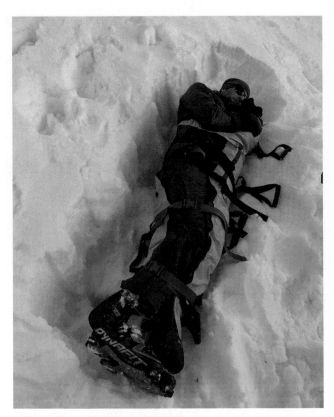

Figure 21-11 A patient packaged in a vacuum mattress in a lateral position to achieve physiologic splinting as well as help to maintain an open airway.

Courtesy of Will Smith.

physiologic splinting. Lateral packaging is an option with the vacuum mattress. This option would allow fluids and vomit to be more likely to drain from the airway based on gravity (**Figure 21-11**). Other considerations in prolonged patient care include anticipating potential problems, such as pretreating a patient with an antiemetic when there is a concern for vomiting. One easily administered option is ondansetron (Zofran) as an orally dissolving tablet. Typical antiemetic options such as promethazine (Phenergan) and atypical agents such as diphenhydramine (Benadryl) can be considered and have an additive effect. As always, medications should be managed by EMS providers at the appropriate skill level and are beyond the scope of this text.

Spinal Injuries and Spinal Motion Restriction

Much debate has occurred since the birth of EMS over the best care of both actual spine injuries and suspected injuries. Patients with a true spinal cord injury and obvious neurologic deficit have a relatively clear treatment pathway. They need to be packaged in the prehospital setting to limit further spinal motion until they reach definitive medical care. Ideally, in the context of prolonged transport times,

that is with a vacuum mattress or other device that conforms to the shape of the spine rather than a rigid flat backboard.

The bigger dilemma occurs in wilderness trauma care when no clear neurologic deficit is present but there is a concern for a possible spine injury. For many years, patients have been immobilized based on mechanism of injury alone, in anticipation that an unstable injury might lead to an actual spinal cord injury and long-term deficits. Treating for this concern of a possible spine injury became a mainstay of EMS training. The application of spinal motion restriction (also called spinal immobilization or spinal stabilization) was a hallmark feature of traditional EMS care. Many patients were immobilized over the years with the traditional hard backboard along with rigid cervical collars.

Numerous studies over the past few decades have led to revised treatment paradigms (e.g., National Emergency X-Radiography Utilization Study [NEXUS] criteria,[43] Canadian Cervical-Spine Rule [CCR],[44] and others discussed in the Spinal Trauma chapter), limiting the number of patients immobilized for "possible spine injury." Research revealed that the rigid backboard and cervical collar were often harming patients without providing the intended benefits. Studies have shown moderate pain even in healthy volunteers at 30 minutes and severe pain after about 45 minutes.[45] Other more concerning problems develop with prolonged immobilization, such as airway compromise, aspiration risk, and pressure sores. Rigid cervical collars can be associated with complications of increased intracranial pressure, decreased cerebral outflow, and cervical distraction in the context of incorrect application.[46-48] These complications become compounded by the additional factors encountered in prolonged care settings. For this reason, wilderness EMS systems and providers became early adopters of the limited use of spinal motion restriction.

Spinal motion restriction in the wilderness/remote care settings has dramatic implications on transport decisions, technical rescue risks, and other dynamics. This increase in risk to the patient and rescuers must be balanced with the small risk of a possible spinal cord injury (in many cases well under 1% with a normal neurologic exam).[49] To illustrate the wilderness EMS decision-making process, consider the following example:

A healthy 22-year-old woman was rock climbing along a river gorge when she fell 65 ft (20 m). Her anchors were placed in the cracks of the cliff and came out, one by one, slowing her fall slightly. But ultimately, she impacted the ground. She was wearing a helmet and did strike her head, experiencing a brief loss of consciousness. After an hour-long hike up the river gorge from where the ambulance could be parked, a wilderness EMS provider reaches the patient. She is now conscious and alert, complaining of only a mild headache, with a normal neurologic examination and a normal physical examination. Friends had encouraged her to remain still and not move. It is late fall, it is getting dark, the nearest helicopter landing zone is back at the road an hour away, and the forecast is for a blizzard to start tonight. Does the patient need to undergo spinal motion restriction? Can she walk out assisted if she is able? Does the wilderness EMS provider need to call for an SAR team with a Stokes litter and proceed with a prolonged rescue lasting hours into the night? Do you have protocols to assess and treat patients in situations similar to this?

A number of trauma experts now maintain that rigid boards have no requisite role in wilderness EMS operations, even in cases of suspected spinal injury.[25,39] Vacuum mattresses, which have been used outside the United States for some time, are becoming the standard of care when spinal motion restriction is indicated. These devices are malleable and contour to the spine; they also can be used to limit motion of the head without a rigid cervical collar.

A patient with no detectable deficit but severe back pain after high-energy trauma may have an occult unstable spinal injury that is at risk. In general in the wilderness setting, if the patient is able to walk, it is safe to do so. Patients who are unable to walk should not be forced to do so.

An example of a death caused by spinal motion restriction occurred in Cornish, New Hampshire, in 2006. A patient who had tripped and injured her ankle was immobilized on a rigid backboard based on the concern of a possible head/spine injury and then transported on a rescue boat. When the boat sank, the patient died from the rescue and not her minor injuries.[50] Cases like this must remind wilderness EMS providers that the real risk of the rescue decisions and the potential risk from possible spine injury and blindly following rigid protocols must be balanced.[25] In general, if a patient is able to self-ambulate out of a technical wilderness situation with minimal pain and no neurologic symptoms, that is one of the safest options to be considered.

Wilderness Extrication Options

Carrying patients in the wilderness is an extremely difficult, time-consuming, and potentially dangerous activity for both the patient and those doing the carrying. Those with no SAR experience generally underestimate the time and difficulty of a wilderness evacuation by at least half, or sometimes up to a factor of five for more difficult evacuations, especially cave rescues. In some cases, helicopter evacuation may provide the most appropriate evacuation from remote or technical locations (**Figure 21-12**).[51]

If someone with no SAR experience says, "It'll take us about 2 hours to get the patient out of here," the time frame is likely much, much longer. Wilderness EMS providers should expect it to take even longer if the patient is in a cave or other confined space, if the SAR team is short on people, if the terrain is particularly difficult, or if the weather is bad. This is especially important to remember if darkness is approaching or the weather is deteriorating.

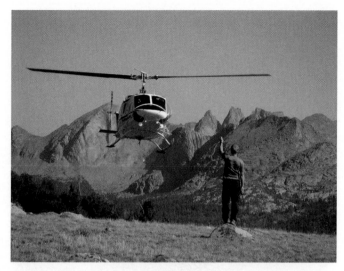

Figure 21-12 Helicopters can be used to balance the risk of exposing many rescuers to technical terrain for longer periods by using a potentially higher risk tool for a very short time. This balance of risk must constantly be evaluated for all wilderness extrications.
Courtesy of Will Smith.

Walking a patient out, even with several people helping, is almost always much faster. If the patient is able to and starts moving now, rather than waiting for a litter or SAR team, the evacuation will be much, much faster and completed much earlier. If the patient cannot walk (e.g., because of an ankle fracture), it may be possible to use a piggyback carry or to make an improvised stretcher out of sticks and rope.

Other Wilderness EMS Patient Care Considerations

Principles of Patient Assessment

While patient assessment is not unique in wilderness EMS settings, providers are generally with a patient for a much longer time. Vital sign trends, and especially mental status changes, give the prolonged care provider much better insight into how treatments are affecting the patient's condition. Mental status is considered the most important vital sign; it ensures that the three main critical systems (circulatory, respiratory, nervous) are functioning. Other traditional vital signs, such as blood pressure, may be completely impractical in some wilderness settings. Training to interpret a normal mental status and rate and presence of a radial pulse may offer all the details needed for a wilderness patient assessment.

MARCH PAWS

Initial patient assessment is the same regardless of the environment. The priority of attention is based on the major life threats that can be mitigated immediately at the point of injury. A systematic approach that is in accordance with PHTLS could follow the MARCH PAWS mnemonic, developed by the military. This approach has been gaining recognition in many military medicine settings.[52] Adaptations to MARCH PAWS for climbers and climbing rescue providers have also been published.[53]

M—*Massive hemorrhage.* At the point of injury, the initial priority of care should be to identify and stop any massive hemorrhage. This is identified by doing an initial blood sweep of the extremities and proximal junctional hemorrhage sites (axilla and groin). A pelvic assessment is then performed with consideration of placement of a pelvic binder early if the pelvis is unstable.

A—*Airway.* A simple assessment of the airway in conscious patients is accomplished by asking their name and to describe the situation. For unconscious patients, a simple jaw thrust can alleviate an obstructed airway. A nasopharyngeal airway is lightweight and can be placed for airway protection. In the case of severe maxillofacial trauma, a nasopharyngeal airway should be avoided. Sometimes lateral recumbent positioning may be all that is needed for a temporizing airway maneuver. Rapid sequence induction followed by intubation should be performed only by highly experienced and trained practitioners who have practiced intubation in austere environments. A surgical cricothyrotomy can be considered as an airway protection skill, by the appropriately trained provider but should be performed early if deemed clinically indicated and essential.

R—*Respirations.* The assessment of respirations can be accomplished with traditional street EMS tools such as a stethoscope and pulse oximetry device, but in some wilderness settings, other patient assessment skills, such as physical palpation of the chest, may be needed. Secondary findings such as subcutaneous emphysema or crepitus associated with a rib fracture may lead to a clinical diagnosis of pneumothorax.

C—*Circulation.* A major goal of circulation assessment is to evaluate whether a patient is showing signs of shock. An overall assessment of the patient's circulatory status should be determined based on mentation and general appearance. An altered or confused patient should be considered to have signs of shock and treated accordingly. Careful attention should be made to assess and trend the presence of central (carotid, femoral) and distal (radial, posterior tibial, dorsalis pedis) pulses.

H—*Head/Hypothermia.* An initial gross neurologic examination should be conducted to assess the patient's level of consciousness. A patient can be described as Alert, responds to Verbal, responds to Pain, or is Unresponsive (AVPU). In the case of a suspected moderately or severely head-injured patient, the priority of care is to prevent hypoxia, hypotension, and hypoglycemia. During this phase of the assessment, the patient should be exposed for a full assessment. Wet clothes should be removed, and attention should be directed to prevent hypothermia by placing the patient in warm, dry clothes and off the ground using a sleeping pad or other barrier.

P—*Pain.* After the initial lifesaving interventions are completed in the MARCH assessment, you should next attend to managing the patient's pain. In an awake and alert patient, this can be accomplished by offering a dose of acetaminophen (Tylenol/Paracetamol) initially. Nonsteroidal anti-inflammatories (NSAIDs) such as ibuprofen or naproxen should be avoided if there is a concern for hemorrhage, due to their antiplatelet effects. Meloxicam (Mobic) is an alternative long-acting NSAID that does not affect bleeding time and may be more safely used in trauma. Advanced practitioners who carry controlled substances such as fentanyl or ketamine should adhere to their local protocols for dosing and administrative guidance.

A—*Antibiotics.* Early antibiotics, ideally within 12 to 24 hours of a traumatic injury, may be indicated. A broad-spectrum antibiotic that covers the most likely pathogens for traumatic injuries should be used. Doxycycline is an excellent choice for travelers to carry, as it can be used to treat many conditions, including skin, respiratory, and gastrointestinal (GI) infections. Advanced providers who are providing point-of-injury care may administer ertapenem (Invanz) either intramuscularly or intravenously. If only one antibiotic is to be carried by an EMS team, some wilderness EMS infectious disease authorities recommend the use of ceftriaxone (Rocephin).[54] Providers must always check for known drug allergies prior to administering any medications to reduce the risk of inducing anaphylaxis and thus further complicating the patient's condition and creating new care challenges.

W—*Wounds.* Irrigation and wound care should be accomplished prior to packaging and transporting a patient. A general rule is that as long as the water is potable, it is clean enough for wound irrigation. Gross decontamination and debris removal followed by copious volume irrigation should occur, and a sterile or clean dressing should be applied to the wound.

S—Splinting. Application of a modified splint provides immense pain relief for a patient with a fracture or severe soft-tissue injury. Simple immobilization, such as buttoning a wrist button to the chest for a shoulder dislocation or padding and immobilizing an ankle fracture using trekking poles for splints, can greatly improve pain control and ease transport of a casualty.

Prolonged Patient Care Considerations

As mentioned previously, wilderness EMS occurs in a wide variety of remote rescue settings that may be similar to military and other austere settings. With military theaters changing from Iraq and Afghanistan to other more remote areas of the world (e.g., Africa, the Pacific), the Prolonged Field Care (PFC) working group has been established to help focus on medical and trauma care in extended patient care settings ranging from hours to days. The group has identified 10 essential PFC capabilities to help focus training for these prolonged care settings (**Table 21-1**).[55] Virtually all patient care lessons learned can be bridged between the wilderness EMS provider and the military PFC settings.

Elimination (Urination/Defecation) Needs

The truth described in a popular children's book, *Everyone Poops*,[56] applies to wilderness patients as well. Given the relatively short transport times in an urban setting, most patients do not have an elimination need. Trauma patients almost never defecate during their prehospital and ED care. However, if you are caring for a patient who has been in the wilderness for a day or more and it takes you several hours to get to the patient, it is much more likely that the patient will need to urinate or defecate, especially if there is a prolonged evacuation.

Having patient care supplies that include *blue pads* (Chux) for placing under the patient, having some sanitary wipes, carrying adult-type diapers that can be replaced after the patient has voided or defecated, or even stopping to let the patient urinate or defecate are all reasonable measures (**Figure 21-13**). It is possible for men and women to urinate even while immobilized in a Stokes litter (**Figure 21-14**) with a full-body vacuum splint, if packaging is planned carefully and the litter is tipped up on the foot end. For women, a small funnel device, often carried by women when backpacking, will be needed to assist in elimination.

Table 21-1 The 10 Core Capabilities as Identified by Prolonged Field Care in Austere Locations			
PFC Tasks	**Minimum**	**Better**	**Best**
1. Monitor the patient to create a useful vital sign trend	Blood pressure cuff, stethoscope, pulse oximetry, Foley catheter (measure urine output), mental status, and understanding of vital sign interpretation	Add capnometry	Vital sign monitor to provide hands-free vital sign data at regular intervals
2. Resuscitate the patient beyond crystalloid or colloid infusion	Field fresh whole-blood (FWB) transfusion kits	Maintenance crystalloids also prepared for a major burn and/or closed-head injury resuscitation (2 to 3 cases of lactated Ringer solution or PlasmaLyte A; hypertonic saline); consider adding lyophilized plasma as available; fluid warmer	Maintain a stock of packed red blood cells and fresh frozen plasma and have type-specific donors identified for immediate FWB draw

Table 21-1 The 10 Core Capabilities as Identified by Prolonged Field Care in Austere Locations (*continued*)

PFC Tasks	Minimum	Better	Best
3. Ventilate/ Oxygenate the patient	Provide positive end-expiratory pressure (PEEP) via bag-valve mask (you cannot ventilate a patient in the PFC setting [prolonged ventilation] without PEEP or he or she will be at risk of developing acute respiratory distress syndrome)	Provide supplemental oxygen (O_2) via an oxygen concentrator	Portable ventilator (e.g., Eagle Impact ventilator, Zoll Medical Corp, http://www.impact instrumentation.com; or similar) with supplemental O_2
4. Gain definitive control of the patient's airway with an inflated cuff in the trachea (and keep the patient comfortable)	Medic is prepared for a ketamine cricothyrotomy	Add ability to provide long-duration sedation	Add a responsible rapid-sequence intubation capability with subsequent airway maintenance skills, in addition to providing long-term sedation (to include suction and paralysis with adequate sedation)
5. Use sedation/ pain control to accomplish the above tasks	Provide opiate analgesics titrated intravenously	Have training to sedate with ketamine (and adjunctive midazolam as needed)	Experienced with and maintains currency in long-term sedation practice using intravenous morphine, ketamine, midazolam, fentanyl, and so forth
6. Use physical examination/ diagnostic measures to gain awareness of potential problems	Uses physical examination without advanced diagnostics, maintain awareness of potential unseen injuries (e.g., abdominal bleed, head injury)	Have training to use advanced diagnostics such as ultrasound, point-of-care laboratory testing, and so forth	Experienced in both
7. Provide nursing, hygiene, and comfort measures	Ensure the patient is clean, warm, dry, padded, and catheterized, and provide basic wound care	Elevate head of bed, debride wounds, perform washouts, wet-to-dry dressings, decompress stomach	Experienced in both
8. Perform advanced surgical interventions	Chest tube, cricothyrotomy	Perform fasciotomy, wound debridement, amputation, and so forth	Experienced in both
9. Perform telemedicine consult	Make reliable communications, present patient, pass trends of key vital signs	Add laboratory findings and ultrasound images	Video teleconference
10. Prepare the patient for flight	Be familiar with physiologic stressors of flight	Have training in critical care transport	Experienced in critical care transport

Keenan S, Riesberg JC. Prolonged field care: beyond the "Golden Hour." Wilderness Environ Med. 2017;28(2S):S138.

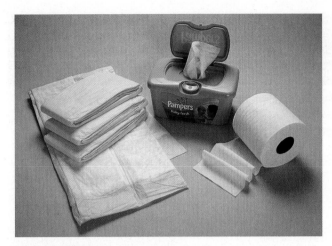

Figure 21-13 Elimination supplies.
© National Association of Emergency Medical Technicians (NAEMT).

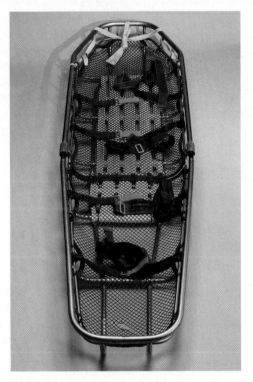

Figure 21-14 Stokes litter. Some models are made of titanium for lightweight transport and split into two sections.
Courtesy of David Bowers.

In some rescue teams, a Foley catheter may even be used with the proper training.

Patients who are lying on their backs for a long time tend to develop decubitus ulcers. These sores may end up requiring surgery or debridement, resulting in a longer hospital stays. Some patients will die from infection and other complications of the sores. Lying in one's own urine and feces for a long time (just hours, not even days) may make decubitus ulcers more likely. If patient care occurs for only a few minutes during a short transport, urine and feces are not a major issue. However, if a wilderness medicine provider has been taking care of a patient for several hours and delivers the patient to the ED lying in his or her own feces, the likelihood of decubitus ulcers and resulting sepsis is much greater.

Food and Water Needs

Every wilderness patient should be considered to be cold, hungry, and thirsty; that is, he or she should be considered hypothermic, starved, and dehydrated—or at a slight expense of accuracy, *hypothermic, hypoglycemic,* and *hypovolemic.*

Starvation is much more than just hypoglycemia (low blood glucose), and not all starving patients are significantly hypoglycemic. Dehydration is more than just hypovolemia, which refers only to intravascular volume within the blood vascular system. Patients who are dehydrated have also lost water from their cells and the interstitial spaces between the cells.

On the street, water and food are generally not given to patients. There are many reasons not to feed patients during street EMS care. If the patient needs to go to the OR, having food or fluid in the stomach is potentially harmful; it increases the likelihood of vomiting or, more likely, passive regurgitation leading to possible aspiration during induction of anesthesia. Also a patient will not starve or dehydrate in the time it takes to get to the hospital.

In the wilderness, if a rescued patient needs to go to the OR, it will take time to transport the patient to the hospital, to be evaluated in the ED, and to be prepared for the OR. With wilderness patients, the focus is to ensure that the patient maintains caloric intake and hydration, as transport times are generally delayed. Because the stomach is ideally fasted for several hours before anesthesia, the wilderness medical provider may provide food and water to any reasonably alert wilderness patient who can safely swallow.[57,58] Even if a helicopter can quickly expedite an otherwise prolonged rescue, hospitals are capable of taking care of patients with "full" stomachs; for example, people involved in a vehicle crash are not necessarily fasting.

Vomiting and aspiration are always a danger, and careful attention to the patient's airway is always important (e.g., positioning on the side for long transports, even if the patient needs full-body immobilization). Wilderness EMS providers may still attempt to provide food and water for their patients, even though they have vomited once or twice. Frequent small sips in many settings can keep a patient hydrated. This concept has transformed many pediatric centers where IV hydration, once the mainstay of treatment for vomiting children, is being replaced with oral hydration. This is good news for wilderness EMS patient care.

When building medical kits, consider adding oral rehydration salts for balanced hydration. Also consider high-calorie, low-volume snacks in the form of gel. Foods high in sugar content can be readily absorbed and provide significant high-yield energy for a casualty during evacuation.

Suspension Syndrome

Suspension syndrome has been called by many names, including suspension trauma, harness-induced death, orthostatic intolerance, and harness hang syndrome. *Suspension syndrome* has been established as a better term than these alternatives, as there is little to no direct trauma, and a harness is not needed to cause the condition.[53] The real pathophysiology is a cascade of events that correlates to a syndrome, ultimately culminating as a state of shock caused by blood pooling in dependent lower extremities while the body is held upright without any movement for a prolonged time.[53,59] While uncommon, it remains a real concern for many wilderness-related activities.

Many types of recreationalists (e.g., climbers, cavers) who wear a harness and can have their legs become immobile in a dependent position are susceptible to this syndrome. Other cohorts of individuals such as industrial workers, military service members (parachutists), circus performers, and stunt actors who can become suspended vertically as part of their occupation may be exposed to similar pathophysiology. Wilderness EMS providers need to be proficient in high-angle terrain to extricate and care for these kinds of patients (**Figure 21-15**).

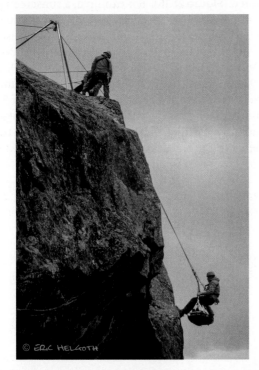

Figure 21-15 Technical proficiency in high-angle terrain is essential for wilderness EMS providers. It allows them to take care of patients with potential suspension syndrome as well as prevent it from occurring in rescuers.

Courtesy of Eric Helgoth.

Suspension syndrome can be worsened by other conditions, such as hypovolemia (e.g., hemorrhage, dehydration), vasodilation (e.g., heat, infection), or any other factors that alter the body's ability to maintain homeostasis (e.g., illicit or prescribed drugs, alcohol). Soldiers standing at attention are trained to make small flexing movements of their calf muscles. This action acts as a pump to accentuate venous return to the heart. By contracting these muscles and the one-way valves in the lower extremity veins, blood is assisted back into the central circulation. Without this venous pump mechanism, suspension syndrome can develop in a matter of minutes and potentially result in death in as little as 10 minutes if the patient remains suspended upright. Mortimer's landmark 2011 publication in *Wilderness and Environmental Medicine* provides one of the best-case report summaries of suspension syndrome.[60]

Whenever a patient experiences a passive hanging situation, blood pools in the lower extremities. Although no blood is lost, a relative hypovolemic state is induced. Some estimate that as much as 60% of the body's blood volume can collect in the lower extremities. This dramatically reduces the preload for the heart, rendering it unable to pump sufficient blood forward with subsequent contractions. Due to this decreased blood flow, the brain quickly becomes affected, and the patient will lose consciousness. This is often called postural syncope, and in most normal and unencumbered settings, the patient will fall to the ground and become horizontal, restoring blood supply to the brain. However, in the technical rescue environment, the patient is often suspended upright and the body's protective mechanisms are thwarted, often leading to death if not quickly reversed.[53]

In addition to venous pooling and decreased cardiac preload, it is thought that additional maladaptive responses contribute to the hemodynamic collapse in suspension syndrome. Hyperkalemia and acidemic blood are thought to contribute to the morbidity and mortality as patients are resuscitated. Pooled blood may have become relatively hypothermic and may cause a systemic cooling when reintroduced to the central circulation. There is some speculation that overlapping problems of asphyxia from certain harnesses causing chest constriction or patient positioning and airway compromise may accelerate the mental status changes and likelihood of death in these patients. While these additional factors may play a role, there are still some pathophysiologic parameters that remain unclear.[60]

Treatment recommendations for suspension syndrome focus on extricating the patient as soon as possible to a supine position. After this critical step, wilderness EMS providers can begin traditional BLS and ALS care and rapid transport of the patient to definitive care. Concern has arisen about case studies of "rescue death,"[53,60] where patients experienced cardiac arrest immediately after being extricated from their prolonged suspension. Prior recommendations suggested that a delayed extrication and slow removal of the harness would result in lower morbidity and mortality; however, this is no longer recommended. Mortimer and others have demonstrated that immediate extrication to a supine position provides the best chance for the patient to restore circulation to the heart and brain.[60-62] Standard treatments for crush syndrome and other rhabdomyolysis conditions suggest that IV hydration and possibly even alkalization of the urine with sodium bicarbonate added to IV fluids may be beneficial. These advanced discussions are beyond the scope of this text.

Patients with possible suspension syndrome, even if no clear outward symptoms are present, should be evaluated by a medical professional. Signs and symptoms of delayed rhabdomyolysis (muscle breakdown) and renal failure could develop during rescue or at a later time.

If a patient or rescuer becomes trapped in a suspended vertical position for any period of time, he or she should immediately call for help, attempt to self-rescue, and self-extricate from the situation. If self-rescue is not possible or the victim becomes exhausted, an attempt should be made to support, raise, or move the legs to decrease the dependent pooling of blood. Another preemptive measure would be to engage the body's normal venous pump mechanism by contracting the calf and leg muscles to help return blood to the central circulation. Pushing up against a rock wall or using a set of Purcell Prusiks (rope lanyards) to provide something to push against may delay the progression of suspension syndrome.

While this life-threatening condition has been reported in the literature, only recently has a better understanding of the pathophysiology and updated treatment recommendations emerged. In summary, the best care for suspension syndrome is to extricate the patient as soon as possible to a supine position and restore blood flow to the vital organs and then continue standard resuscitation protocols.

Eye/Head Protection

During evacuation, pay close attention to ensure you are protecting your patient from iatrogenic injuries, as well as making sure that all the rescuers have the PPE (e.g., helmet, safety glasses) appropriate to the setting. A minor head injury can be made worse by repeated concussion should your patient slip and fall or impact his or her head on a rock during evacuation. Carrying a person through brush and trees, or having unnoticed debris fall onto your patient can lead to potential eye injuries. As a result, keep your patient in a helmet with goggles or safety glasses for protection. Rescue litters sometimes include a face and head shield.

Sun Protection

Sunlight is essential for the synthesis of vitamin D in the human body, and it also has beneficial effects on mood. However, the ultraviolet (UV) rays of the sun can damage the skin. Acute injury can include superficial, partial-thickness, and full-thickness sunburns seen in some severe cases of exposure. In extreme cases, solar burns may even contribute to shock or death, especially with other comorbid conditions and trauma. Avoiding exposure to direct sunlight, especially from 1000 to 1500 hours, when UV radiation from the sun is strongest, decreases but does not eliminate the risk of sunburn and long-term damage (photoaging and skin cancers).

Topical sunscreens usually contain combinations of organic chemicals and/or inorganic filters that absorb various wavelengths of UV light. Zinc oxide and titanium dioxide are common examples of inorganic filters. Both types of sunscreens aim to block UV light exposure at two specific frequencies, A and B (UVA and UVB). UVA was once thought to be harmless, but we now know that it works synergistically with UVB to cause sunburn. UVB is responsible for most of the *erythema* (redness) of sunburn. UVA has been implicated in the development of phototoxicity and photoaging.[63] Thus, sun-blocking materials or creams must block both UVA and UVB to be effective. Look for the term *broad-spectrum* sun protection factor (SPF) on the product label to ensure coverage for both UVA and UVB.

The SPF is a numeric measure of how much the clothing or cream increases the minimum dose of UV light to make the skin red (**Figure 21-16**). For example, a sunscreen lotion with a rating of SPF 45 provides protection from sunburn for about 45 times longer than without the sunscreen. An SPF of 10 blocks 90% of UVB radiation, an SPF of 15 blocks 93%, an SPF of 30 blocks 97%, and an SPF of 50 blocks 98%. Since 2012, the Food and Drug Administration has restricted sunscreen products to an SPF of 50 due to the limited additional protective benefit. The degree of protection against UVA is hard to quantify and is usually much less than protection against UVB.[64,65]

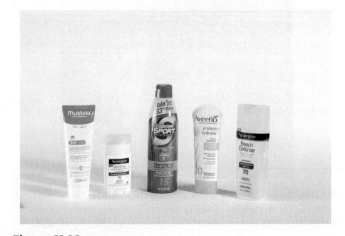

Figure 21-16 Sunscreen.
© Jones & Bartlett Learning. Photographed by Darren Stahlman.

It is advisable to wear protective clothing, such as wide-brimmed hats, pants, and long-sleeved shirts, and to apply sunscreen to exposed skin. Several factors of clothing contribute to the ultraviolet protection factor (UPF), and many outdoor clothing brands now provide a UPF rating. Factors that contribute to the UPF rating of a fabric include the following[66]:

- Composition of the yarns (e.g., cotton, polyester)
- Tightness of the weave or knit (tighter improves the rating; the tightness of the weave probably contributes more than other factors to the UPF of a garment[67])
- Color (darker colors are generally better)
- Stretch (more stretch lowers the rating)
- Moisture (many fabrics have lower ratings when wet)
- Condition (worn and faded garments may have reduced ratings)
- Finishing (some fabrics are treated with UV-absorbing materials)

Protective lotions with a minimum SPF of 15 should be applied to exposed skin to minimize the potential injury from sun exposure. For prolonged evacuations, lotion with an SPF of 30 should be used, but little benefit can be claimed with an SPF 30 alone unless it is reapplied every 90 minutes. Ideally, sunscreens should be applied 15 to 30 minutes before going out into the sun. Most people do not apply a thick enough layer to achieve the claimed SPF. A minimum of 1 ounce (30 milliliters [ml]; about a shot glass full) should be used on all exposed areas for the average adult at the beach. With profuse sweating or water immersion, sunscreen should be reapplied frequently depending on the product label. Generally, water-resistant sunscreen will be effective for up to 40 or 80 minutes, per product description. Further considerations regarding the application of sunscreen are included in **Box 21-3** and **Box 21-4**.

Box 21-3 Factors That Decrease SPF Effectiveness

Wind, heat, humidity, and altitude can all decrease the effective sun protection factor (SPF) of a sunscreen. The combined application of sunscreen and insect repellents that contain DEET (N,N-diethyl-meta-toluamide) also decreases SPF effectiveness.[63]

Box 21-4 Allergic Reactions From Sunscreens

Some patients may have an acute allergic reaction if the lotion contains para-amino benzoic acid (PABA); therefore PABA-free products are recommended.

Box 21-5 Sunburn Treatment

Prevention
Best prevented with sunscreen SPF > 30, wearing sun-protective clothing.

Pain relief
Nonsteroidal anti-inflammatory drugs (NSAIDs) (e.g., ibuprofen, naproxen, aspirin, indomethacin)
Analgesics: acetaminophen

Immunomodifiers
Corticosteroids – topical or systemic (prednisone)

Skincare
Cool compresses soaked with water or aluminum acetate solution (Burrow solution)
Aloe vera
Topical anesthetics
Fluid resuscitation (oral or rarely IV) as needed

© National Association of Emergency Medical Technicians (NAEMT).

Sunburn is treated as any other burn, and the care is essentially the same in the wilderness as on the street (**Box 21-5**).[64] The only major difference is that in the wilderness, the prehospital care provider needs to be aware of and treat the potential delayed infection, fluid loss, dehydration, or sometimes even shock and to recognize that patients with sunburn are at higher risk for hypothermia.

Specifics of Wilderness EMS

This section reviews a few of the most important situations in which proper wilderness trauma care differs from care on the street. Areas covered where operationally specific (expanded scope of practice) protocols could be beneficial include wound management, joint dislocations, cardiopulmonary arrest, and bites and stings.

Wound Management

Wound management encompasses the following:

- *Hemostasis* (stopping bleeding)
- *Antisepsis* (preventing infection)
- Restoration of function (returning the skin to its protective function and restoring a limb or other body part to normal function)
- *Cosmesis* (ensuring pleasant appearance)

In the wilderness, prevention of infection and restoration of function assume great importance.

Hemostasis

Control of bleeding is part of the primary survey. On the street, arterial bleeding can kill. In the wilderness, even venous bleeding can kill if it continues for a sufficient amount of time. Remember, every red blood cell counts. Bleeding control, including standard measures such as direct pressure, is as important or more important in the wilderness. Unless medical personnel are part of the actual injured party's group, severe bleeding that is not stopped will probably result in the patient's demise prior to the SAR team's arrival (**Box 21-6**).

Training programs for those venturing into wilderness situations should address these lifesaving skills:

* Tourniquets should be the first option for severe life-threatening bleeding.[21,39,41,53,68] In some situations in the wilderness, multiple patients and limited resources (e.g., at a mass-casualty incident) make it difficult or impossible to apply direct pressure to wounds; a similar challenge exists in a technical situation (e.g., side of a cliff) when extraction is the next critical step and maintaining direct pressure is not feasible. In some situations, a tourniquet that has been in place for less than 6 hours[50] may be converted (i.e., removed and replaced with a different means of bleeding control) to a bandage if there is no longer life-threatening bleeding and hemorrhage can be controlled by other means.[69,70] Specific protocols should be in place for responders to care for patients in these types of settings.
* Well-aimed direct pressure should be applied for 10 to 15 minutes directly on the bleeding site followed by a pressure bandage.
* Hemostatic agents may be useful in wilderness care in the control of severe bleeding. Wilderness medicine providers may encounter injured patients who have had hemostatic agents already applied by others in their group. Many of these agents are available for sale to the general public; however, training on how to effectively apply them is still recommended. It is important

---

Box 21-6 Updated Hemorrhage Control Principles

Recently, an international consensus panel, convened by the American Heart Association, updated first aid skills, including hemorrhage control principles.[68] It is now recommended to control severe bleeding by manual direct pressure, gauze and a pressure dressing, hemostatic agents, and a tourniquet. The traditional methods of using pressure points and extremity elevation are no longer recommended because of the lack of evidence supporting their effectiveness.

Box 21-7 Tourniquet Mistakes to Avoid

* Not using one when the injury indicates it should be used (life-threatening or uncontrolled bleeding)
* Waiting too long to apply the tourniquet (Apply tourniquet first for obvious life-threatening bleeding.)
* Taking it off when the patient is in shock or has a short transport time (less than 1 to 2 hours) to the hospital
* Not taking it off when indicated (i.e., not converting) if applied less than 6 hours
* Not making it tight enough (The tourniquet should eliminate the distal pulse.)
* Not using a second tourniquet if needed (immediately adjacent to the first)
* Periodically loosening the tourniquet to allow blood flow to the injured extremity
* Using a tourniquet for minimal bleeding (when direct pressure/bandaging can be applied successfully)

Modified from the Department Defense Lessons Learned from the Committee on Tactical Combat Casualty Care. See Chapter 27 in the eighth edition of PHTLS: Prehospital Trauma Life Support, Military Edition

---

to remember that even if hemostatic agents are used, direct pressure on the wound remains a critical part of the treatment process.

In the wilderness situation when prolonged application (greater than 2 hours) is anticipated, the tourniquet should be applied above the wound but as close to the wound as possible (**Box 21-7**). (For more about hemostatic agents, tourniquets, and other hemorrhage control principles and preferences, see the Shock: Pathophysiology of Life and Death chapter.)

Improvised Tourniquets

In many wilderness situations, responders may have to improvise the tools they use to provide care. Tourniquet improvisation using an available product, such as a belt or clothing article, is a vital skill in the wilderness setting. While manufactured tourniquets are generally quicker to apply and are likely to achieve hemostasis faster,[51] a manufactured tourniquet is not always available in wilderness trauma care.

The U.S. Army Institute of Surgical Research identified key features of a successful tourniquet when evaluating tourniquets for the Iraq and Afghanistan conflicts.[71] These features should be present in the tourniquet supplied in an EMS agency's medical kit and should be the basis for an improvised device[52]:

- At least 1 inch (25 millimeters [mm]) wide (e.g., climbing webbing or belt)
- Windlass or cam to achieve tightening of band
- Ability to capture the tightness
- Easy application (less than 60 seconds to self-apply)
- Adjustable
- Nonslip

Prevention of Infection

After injury in the wilderness, it may be a long time before the wound receives definitive treatment in an ED. Routine wound care in the ED includes appropriate cleaning to prevent infection. Wounds contaminated by dirt or caused by penetration from a dirty object are cleaned with high-pressure irrigation. Uncontaminated wounds are cleaned with low-pressure irrigation.

High-pressure irrigation may cause swelling of wounds, but in the case of contaminated wounds full of dirt and bacteria, the benefit of removing bacteria outweighs the risks from wound swelling.[54,72,73] Infection may set in quickly. After a wound has been open for about 8 hours, bacteria have spread from the skin deep into the wound, and suturing a wound is likely to create a deep wound infection. Deep wound infections develop pressure, which keeps out white blood cells, the body's normal defense mechanism against infection.

Routine wound care in street EMS does not include cleansing the wound because it makes sense to delay wound cleansing for a few minutes until the patient reaches the ED, which is better suited for cleansing and evaluating the patient's wound. The ED can determine if the patient has a tendon or nerve laceration, an associated fracture, a spleen laceration, or a subdural hematoma in the head.

Delaying wound care does not make sense in wilderness EMS care. If it will take hours to get to the ED, the wound should be cleaned. In extremely remote areas, the wound could even become infected before the patient arrives at the ED several days later.

Studies have shown that early irrigation is essential to removing bacteria and reducing wound infections.[74-76] It is not necessary or practical to carry sterile solutions for wound irrigation. There is no need to add an antiseptic to the water.[77] Water that is good enough to drink is good enough to irrigate a wound. Water from streams or melted snow can be treated with any standard wilderness drinking water treatment and used to cleanse a wound.[72,78-82]

If the wound is contaminated, it must be irrigated with enough pressure to clean out the bacteria. The original studies showed that a 35-ml syringe with an 18-gauge needle provided an appropriate amount of pressure (5 to 15 pounds per square inch [psi]).[83-85] Squirt the water, at high pressure, throughout the wound. Squirting clean water from a drinking-water bottle or a hydration bladder-backpack system will also work.[86] This procedure, however, causes a major bloodborne pathogen risk to the rescuer; protection from the spray of blood with a gown or a clean trash bag or rain poncho when irrigating is necessary. Eye protection and gloves are essential when caring for these patients.

Sometimes it is necessary to debride the wound of gross dirt and/or foreign material. Wound debridement should be performed with as little trauma to the wound as possible, possibly using a gauze pad or clean cloth, forceps/tweezers, or even gloved fingers. The patient's pain may need to be treated before the wound can be cleaned. Lidocaine applied topically to the wound or injected subcutaneously for local anesthesia can provide relief in most cases. Conversely, narcotic analgesics may impair the patient's ability to ambulate and thus delay the evacuation. Once the irrigation is complete, dress and bandage the wound. Reapply a clean dressing at least daily or more often if the bandage becomes wet or soiled.

If the wound is gaping open, a wet dressing will prevent tissue damage as a result of drying out; change or at least rewet the dressing with clean water several times per day. However, because the wound will be mostly closed by bandaging, a dry dressing can be used in most cases.

Early antibiotic administration is commonly used upon arrival at the ED for patients with significant trauma. Antibiotics are not given in most civilian prehospital emergency medical systems because of the short transport times encountered in the urban environment. Definitive care may be significantly delayed in wilderness settings due to the longer distances to be covered and rescue considerations in rugged terrain, and early antibiotic use may be appropriate in this environment.[54]

Antibiotics must be given as soon as possible after injury to maximize their ability to prevent wound infections. Intramuscular benzylpenicillin begun within 1 hour of injury was found to be effective in preventing streptococcal infections in a swine model of wound infection. If administration was delayed until 6 hours after injury, the medication was not effective.[87]

A recent military review of antibiotic use on the battlefield recommended that antibiotics be used if arrival at a medical treatment facility was anticipated to be 3 hours or longer.[88] The U.S. Department of Defense's TCCC course advocates the early administration of antibiotics for any open wounds at the point of wounding. TCCC cites multiple case studies where no wound infections developed when service men and women received battlefield antibiotics. TCCC further recommends that oral antibiotics be given to casualties once per day if the casualty has the ability to swallow. Although no comparable studies have been done in the civilian setting, these recommendations make sense for application in the wilderness environment if the physician medical director agrees.

Restoration of Function and Cosmesis: Delayed Closure of Wilderness Wounds

Because of the lack of good lighting, appropriate and clean/sterile supplies, and a warm, dry place to work, in most cases it does not make sense to perform definitive wound closure in the wilderness. It is recommended to simply cleanse and irrigate the wound, dress and bandage, ensure ongoing routine wound care, and then have a **delayed primary closure** performed by the appropriate medical provider. As long as the wound is not infected, it is safe to suture the wound several days later as if it had just occurred. Although bacteria move into the wound soon after injury, eventually enough of the body's defenses (e.g., white blood cells) have entered the wound to make it safe to close. If a physician or someone else experienced at wound closure is present, the wound may be closed at the scene. However, it is still reasonable to simply cleanse, dress, and bandage the wound and allow closure to occur later.

Closing a wilderness wound may be important in one situation: when bleeding cannot be controlled in any other way. These situations are uncommon and usually involve a scalp laceration. For this reason, some wilderness medicine providers are trained to use disposable surgical staplers to repair scalp wounds. However, wound repair is complex and should not be attempted without sufficient training and experience.[89]

Pain Management

Appropriate pain management in wilderness EMS care can dramatically change the patient's tolerance of the extrication and rescue. The ideal goal is to reduce the pain, and sometimes anxiety along with it, to a tolerable level while ensuring that the patient maintains normal or near normal physiologic function. Oligoanalgesia, the undertreatment of acute pain, can have short-term complications, can delay the rescue, and can potentially cause longer term complications such as increasing the risk of posttraumatic stress disorder. Alternate pain control strategies are emerging that use ketamine and other shorter acting narcotics such as fentanyl.[90]

Novel delivery strategies are becoming useful and are being adopted for use in the wilderness EMS environment. Transmucosal delivery of fentanyl has had great success in these settings (e.g., military, ski patrol, SAR). Intranasal administration (ketamine, fentanyl, versed) has become a much more frequent route of administration for pain medications during a rescue. NSAIDs, such as ibuprofen, as well as acetaminophen are great nonnarcotic options that can provide adequate pain management with few side effects. Some injuries require an expanded pain control regimen, and in those cases narcotics and other pain medications (e.g., ketamine, nitrous oxide, methoxyflurane [Penthrane]) can be administered. A hybrid pain control strategy may decrease the total amount of narcotic medication required, as well as decrease dose-related side effects. For example, administering 50 milligrams (mg) of ketamine and 50 micrograms (mcg) of fentanyl intranasally may provide better analgesia than higher doses of either medication alone. As with any medication, the wilderness EMS provider must balance the risk versus benefit of the single agent chosen with the polypharmacy approach. In many rescue settings, the ability to closely monitor a patient can be difficult. A finger pulse oximetry probe may be the only monitoring device that is available, but with appropriate training it may provide sufficient data. **Figure 21-17** shows a wilderness EMS medical kit being used to treat a fractured femur on a backcountry rescue. Choosing an individualized pain control plan for a specific patient, and not using a generic algorithm, is important, as often monitoring the patient can be challenging. Deep procedural sedation, as performed in the hospital, is difficult to perform in the wilderness. Appropriate training, as with other advanced care practices, is essential for administration of many of these advanced medications.

Pain management, however, needs to be approached in a much broader sense and not just in regard to a specific medication that a wilderness EMS provider can give. It encompasses much more, including psychological reassurance, physiologic splinting, and medication support. Psychological first aid is an expanding concept and can be a useful tactic in any pain control strategy.[91] A wilderness EMS provider must balance all of these options to provide optimal patient care. The Wilderness Medical Society practice guidelines for the treatment of acute pain

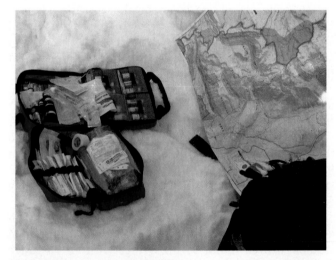

Figure 21-17 Advanced life support medical kit being used on a wilderness rescue of a patient with a femur fracture. Pain management options are crucial for treatment of patients in austere settings.
Courtesy of Will Smith.

in remote environments gives a good summary of treatment options, that begins with comfort care and PRICE (protection, rest, ice, compression, elevation) therapy and builds with more advanced treatments up to intravenous and intraosseous medications.[25,90]

Dislocations

A healthy 20-year-old man was kayaking along a white-water stream when the top of his kayak paddle hit a low-hanging tree branch and caused indirect trauma to his shoulder. Now his right shoulder is deformed and painful. He cannot bring his right arm across his chest or bring his elbow to his side. Distal pulses, capillary refill, sensation, and movement are intact. From the ambulance, the wilderness EMS provider hikes a mile through the woods to get to the stream. Should the shoulder be "splinted as it lies," or should the provider try to reduce what looks like an anterior shoulder dislocation?

The common practice for fractures and dislocations on the street is to splint them as they lie and transport for definitive treatment. The only exception is the patient whose distal pulse is not palpable, in which case the extremity is realigned anatomically in an effort to restore circulation.

Although "splint it as it lies" is a good general rule for the street, "make it look normal" with physiologic splinting is a better general rule for the wilderness patient. It is certainly appropriate for both fractures and dislocations when transport is delayed, although local scopes of practice must also be considered. In some jurisdictions, front country EMS protocols are beginning to allow reduction techniques for some dislocations.[72]

There are many types of dislocations—finger, toe, shoulder, patella, knee, elbow, hip, ankle, and jaw—and all have been successfully reduced in the wilderness, some more easily than others. It is usually easy to reduce dislocations of the ankle (which are almost always fracture–dislocations), patella, toe, or finger, except the proximal interphalangeal joint of the index finger in some cases. Elbow, knee, and hip dislocations are usually quite difficult. All are much easier with training and practice; in particular, it takes training or experience to know, without a radiograph, when a joint is likely dislocated and to attempt reduction.

Traditional street EMS training courses seldom provide training in dislocation reduction. However, because wilderness dislocations are so common, dislocation reduction of a digit, patella, or shoulder is covered in almost all wilderness EMS training or at orthopedic workshops at wilderness medicine conferences. Those who might provide EMS in the wilderness or who regularly travel in the backcountry are advised to take one of these courses. However, even though the education has been gained, the provider must also be certified and credentialed to perform these skills, just like with any other patient care

skill.[9,26] In addition, when considering scope of practice, dislocation reduction is one of the circumstances where an EMS physician deployed as part of the field team may be particularly helpful.[39,92,93]

Cardiopulmonary Resuscitation in the Wilderness

Traumatic cardiac arrest on the street has a poor prognosis, even if the scene is within minutes of a level I trauma center. No person survives more than a few minutes of cardiopulmonary resuscitation (CPR) after traumatic arrest.[94-97] This reality is recognized in many street EMS protocols. For traumatic cardiac arrest, consider initiating CPR in the following situations:

1. Cardiac arrest occurs in the presence of EMS personnel.
2. A victim of penetrating trauma had signs of life within 15 minutes of the arrival of EMS personnel.

Wilderness Traumatic Arrest

The following signs can be uniformly equated with nonsurvivability:

- Decapitation
- Transection of the torso
- Patient is frozen so hard that the patient's chest cannot be compressed
- Patient's rectal temperature is very cold and the same as the environment
- Well-progressed decomposition

The following presumptive signs of death may be of use to wilderness medicine providers, although no one sign by itself is reliable:

- **Rigor mortis.** Postmortem rigidity is well known but not always present, and similar rigidity is often observed in hypothermic patients.
- **Dependent lividity.** This finding is common in corpses but can also be found, along with pressure necrosis and frostbite, in some patients exposed to the elements for a long time.
- **Decomposition.** This finding is usually self-evident.
- *Lack of presumptive signs of life.* Hypothermia can mimic death, in that pulses may not be palpable, respirations may be undetectable, and pupils may be dilated and unreactive with no signs of consciousness. However, severely hypothermic patients have occasionally been resuscitated, with full neurologic recovery.

Therefore, in the wilderness context, CPR is inappropriate for most cases of traumatic arrest. It is appropriate for wilderness medicine providers and the SAR team members to examine the patient and then gently but firmly tell the companions that the victim is dead and there is no reason to initiate/continue resuscitation. Although it is often difficult to use the word *dead*, euphemisms often lead to misunderstanding and misinterpretation of what is actually being said.

Wilderness Medical Arrest

The term *medical cardiac arrest* applies to a patient who has a contributing underlying medical condition or suffers an acute medical condition (e.g., chest pain, shortness of breath, diabetes) and then sustains a cardiac arrest. Again, in the wilderness context, the chances of survival are poor or nonexistent when the patient is more than a few minutes from CPR or defibrillation.[98-104] It is possible that a SAR team might need to respond to a sudden cardiac arrest—whether sustained by the patient or even a team member. Lightweight defibrillators are now available, and some SAR teams carry them or at least have them at their incident command posts or forward staging locations.[53] As with all medical and other equipment, the weight-to-need-for-use ratio must be examined closely.

There are a variety of other causes of cardiac arrest in the wilderness, such as ventricular fibrillation (VF) cardiac arrest secondary to hypothermia or cardiac arrest secondary to pulmonary embolism. For such cardiac arrests, survival is even less likely than with a cardiac arrest secondary to a myocardial infarction. However, nontraumatic wilderness cardiac arrest might be survivable in the following situations:

- Hypothermia[104,105]
- Cold-water submersion[106-109]
- Lightning strike[110,111]
- Electrocution
- Drug overdose
- Avalanche burial[112,113]

In all of these cases, a patient may appear to be in cardiac arrest but still might be resuscitated by basic CPR. For hypothermia in particular, there is a saying that "Nobody is dead until he or she is warm and dead." (See the Environmental Trauma I: Heat and Cold chapter.) A significant minority of those who appear dead from these mechanisms can be resuscitated. There are special considerations for each of these situations—for example, scene safety for those who have been electrocuted and are still attached to a power line, or the fact that external cardiac compression can actually induce a VF cardiac arrest in a hypothermic patient whose heart is beating just enough to keep the patient alive.[114-117] Although appropriate in a wilderness EMS course, detailed discussion of these topics is beyond the scope of this chapter (see the Environmental Trauma I: Heat and Cold and the Environmental Trauma II: Drowning, Lightning, Diving, and Altitude chapters).

Two simple and standard wilderness CPR recommendations are as follows[11,31,118]:

- If the patient appears to be in cardiac arrest from causes other than trauma, attempt CPR for 15 to 30 minutes; if, at the end of this time, the patient has not been resuscitated, stop CPR and consider the patient dead.
- Do not start CPR if it will put rescuers at risk and decrease their chances of retreating from the scene safely, given concerns about daylight, terrain, weather, and available nearby shelter.

The NAEMSP's position statement, "Termination of Resuscitation of Nontraumatic Cardiopulmonary Arrest," available on the NAEMSP website, can provide guidance on when to consider termination of a cardiac arrest resuscitation effort.[103]

Bites and Stings

Bites and stings are common wilderness problems. The exact type of bite or sting likely in a wilderness area depends on the specific locale. Local knowledge and resources are important to help guide the care of these patients, but routine patient care guidelines are still necessary.

Insect Bite and Stings

Many insects may become a nuisance in the wilderness settings (e.g., biting flies, mosquitoes) but do not transmit disease. Most people who are bitten or stung by an insect develop only a minor local reaction. While painful, and generally associated with significant anxiety, there are generally no life-threatening issues. However, mosquito-borne diseases, such as West Nile virus and the Zika virus, have prompted high-profile concerns recently. In addition, people traveling to tropical areas must be aware of a host of other vector-transmitted diseases (e.g., malaria, dengue).

Allergic reactions occur on a spectrum from localized signs and symptoms to life-threatening anaphylaxis. The time from the sting to onset of maximal symptoms can be variable, but most severe symptoms usually occur within an hour of the sting. More significant systemic reactions can peak at 48 or more hours, and in some delayed-type hypersensitivities, it may be even longer. Anaphylaxis is reported in 0.3% to 8% of stings.[119-123] At least 40 identified deaths are reported annually in the United States.[122,124,125]

A wilderness EMS provider must be able to identify the severity of the reaction from the anxiety often associated with the event. Not all patients who have had a severe allergic reaction before will develop an equally severe reaction upon a second exposure, but they may, or it could be worse. For this reason, it can be extremely difficult to predict who will have a less severe overall reaction, and the provider should err on the side of treatment and/or early evacuation.

Some individuals who are stung will progress within a few minutes to a generalized allergic reaction. This reaction may range from *urticarial* (hives) to a full-blown anaphylactic reaction. Although the exact spectrum of generalized allergic reaction depends on the contents of the injected toxin (which varies among the many species of bees and wasps) and the allergic history of the patient, one or more of the following are usually seen:

- Urticaria (hives) (**Figure 21-18**)
- Lip and/or facial swelling
- Hoarseness or stridor
- Wheezing and/or shortness of breath
- Abdominal cramping, vomiting, or diarrhea
- Tachycardia or bradycardia
- Hypotension
- Syncope and/or altered mental status

A patient with mild localized or sometimes even diffuse urticaria after a sting will probably do well. If a patient with hives after a bite or sting progresses to real anaphylaxis, however, the most telling early sign is hoarseness and hypotension. The major cause of death after bee sting allergic reaction is airway obstruction from swelling in the airway, and hoarseness is usually the first sign of airway swelling. Any patient with a generalized reaction to an insect bite or sting needs treatment immediately.

Honeybee stingers usually remain in the skin when the insect leaves because the stinger is barbed. Venom from the stinger and venom sac will continue to enter the skin for 45 to 60 seconds if the stinger is not removed; thus it is important to remove the stinger quickly. There has been a great deal of discussion about the proper way to remove a bee stinger, but recent information indicates it really does not matter how it gets out as long as it is removed as soon as possible. Fingernails, a knife blade edge, or a credit card edge are all effective tools for removing an embedded stinger. If a stinger is removed within 15 seconds of the sting, the severity of the sting is reduced. Other insects such as wasps can cause an allergic reaction, and they can sting a patient multiple times without embedding a stinger.

BLS interventions generally involve keeping the patient sitting in a position of comfort, performing standard airway management, and providing oxygen.

The main medications used to treat allergic reactions to insect bites or stings include the following:

1. *Epinephrine (adrenalin).* Although epinephrine acts for only a few minutes, it can be lifesaving. Repeated dosing may be required in severe cases.
2. *Antihistamines.* Both histamine-1 (e.g., diphenhydramine [Benadryl]) and histamine-2 (e.g., famotidine [Pepcid]) blockers are used. Anyone who requires epinephrine for a bee sting allergy should also receive an antihistamine.
3. *Steroids* (e.g., prednisone, dexamethasone [Decadron]). Most people who require epinephrine should also receive a steroid to suppress the longer term allergic response.

The most important drug is epinephrine, which acts rapidly to reverse the acute reaction. Epinephrine is available as a pen-sized autoinjector (e.g., EpiPen), which is often prescribed to any patient who has had a generalized allergy to bee stings (**Box 21-8**). These autoinjectors are found in many wilderness first-aid kits. The Wilderness Medical Society has published a practice guideline on the use of epinephrine in the wilderness.[126] This guideline recommends the administration of epinephrine by wilderness EMS providers who are trained to recognize acute anaphylaxis and to give epinephrine.

Some wilderness SAR teams carry drugs for allergic reactions in their medical kits, and the wilderness EMS

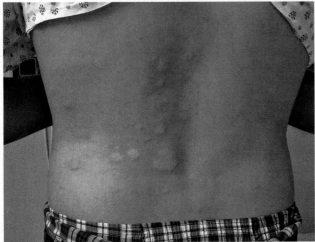

Figure 21-18 Allergic urticaria.
© Chuck Stewart, MD, EMDM, MPH.

Box 21-8 Autoinjectors

Warning: There is another autoinjector medication on the market that has the appearance of an EpiPen autoinjector. The drug is Alsuma, a sumatriptan autoinjector prescribed to treat migraines. This autoinjector could be used by mistake on an anaphylactic patient because there is no warning that it is not epinephrine and has the identical size, color, and cap appearance as the EpiPen released in 2010.[127]

providers have special training in their use. Often, people with a history of severe allergy will carry these medications in their personal first-aid kits.

While this chapter focuses on wilderness trauma care, which can involve insect bites and stings, responders must keep in mind that a patient may develop a severe allergy from other exposures and foods, and the same patient evaluation and treatment would apply.

Snakebite

There are approximately 3,000 species of snakes, of which some 600 are poisonous, but only 200 are considered to be medically significant venomous types.[128,129] Few are found in northern latitudes. Most reside naturally in tropical areas, and many are deadly. Although many snakes have venom glands, there are only two types of native snakes in North America with venom strong enough to cause more than minor irritation to humans. All snakebites have the potential to cause infection and other local tissue damage and should be managed like other puncture wounds.

Coral snakes are small snakes found in the southern parts of North America. They have venom that is neurotoxic and causes paralysis (**Figure 21-19**). These snakes are small, have small front fangs, cannot open their mouths very far compared to larger snakes, and are rather timid compared to certain other crotalids; therefore, serious envenomations are not common. Of the North American coral snakes, the Eastern, or Floridian, has the most toxic venom. The popular rhyme used to identify coral snakes based on colored bands only works for certain North American species and should not be relied on to identify the snake. Signs of envenomation may be delayed up to 15 hours, come on rapidly, and begin with central paralysis (ptosis, double vision, disconjugate gaze, trouble managing oral secretions).[130]

Pit vipers, often called crotalids, are found throughout large portions of North America and include *rattlesnakes* of various types (**Figure 21-20**), *copperheads* (**Figure 21-21**), and *water moccasins*, or *cottonmouths* (**Figure 21-22**). The majority of pit viper bites do not occur in the wilderness but rather in rural, suburban, or even urban areas. A classic example is the intoxicated man who was kissing his pet rattlesnake when he was bitten on the lips or tongue. Bites to other areas of the bodies, especially extremities, are also common (**Figure 21-23**).

Snakebites are not as rare as one might think. In the United States, almost 10,000 patients are treated each year for snakebites, and approximately 5 die.[131] It is estimated that worldwide there are approximately 421,000 envenomations annually, resulting in 20,000 deaths, although this number could be much higher because of poor death records in many countries.[129]

Historically, a variety of prehospital treatments have been attempted by patients, bystanders, or sometimes

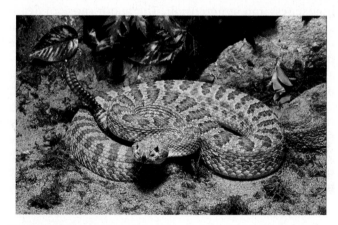
Figure 21-20 Rattlesnake.
© Photos.com/Getty Images.

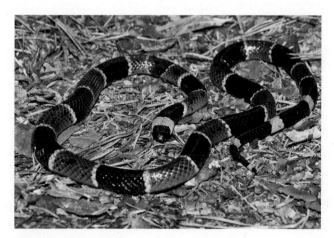
Figure 21-19 Coral snake.
© JasonOndreicka/iStock/Getty Images.

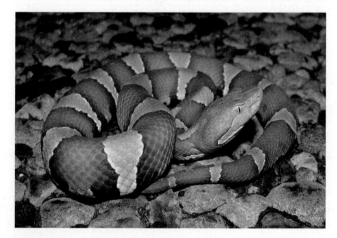
Figure 21-21 Copperhead snake.
© Matt Jeppson/Shutterstock.

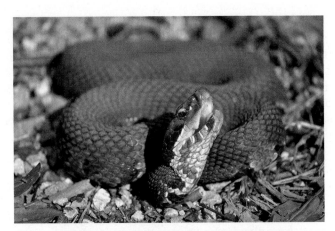

Figure 21-22 Water moccasin (cottonmouth) snake.
© James DeBoer/Shutterstock.

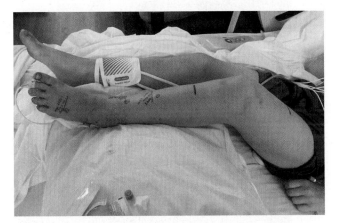

Figure 21-23 Lower left extremity bite from a water moccasin (cottonmouth) snake. Note progressive swelling and ecchymosis.
Courtesy of Ben Abo.

EMS personnel. The only treatment shown to be effective for envenomated pit viper bites is antivenin (antivenom), which is extremely expensive (thousands of U.S. dollars for a single treatment) and thus not routinely carried in first-aid kits. The only street EMS care proven to be helpful is supportive care and transport to the hospital.[132]

The first step in treating snakebite is to *watch for signs of envenomation* (i.e., determine that venom was injected). Only a fraction of bites by pit vipers actually result in envenomation (20% to 25% are dry bites), and the signs of envenomation are fairly distinct. Although signs and symptoms of envenomation usually develop in a few minutes, it is not uncommon for them to be delayed by 6 to 8 hours or perhaps even longer, so transporting to the hospital after a suspected poisonous snakebite is appropriate.[130] Signs of envenomation include the following:

- Severe local redness, swelling, bruising, and pain
- Severe pain and/or tenderness away from bite site (e.g., a bite on the foot with pain or tenderness up in the groin or knee)

- Continued nonsignificant bleeding from the bite
- Paresthesias in the fingers and toes (Paresthesia is unusual sensation, usually caused by damage to nerves or biochemical abnormalities; a feeling of "pins and needles" is a common paresthesia.)
- Metallic taste in the mouth
- Feeling of severe anxiety
- Nausea, vomiting, and abdominal pain

Prehospital Treatment of Suspected Pit Viper Envenomation[130-135]

When managing a patient with a suspected envenomation, the initial care is similar to any other seriously ill or injured patient: Support the ABCs (airway, breathing, circulation), provide oxygen to maintain an adequate oxygen saturation, apply a cardiac monitor, start intravenous therapy (to keep vein open), and monitor the patient's vital signs.

Assess the bite site for signs of envenomation, including erythema, swelling, ecchymosis, tenderness, and the development of blisters or soft-tissue necrosis, and how far pain and/or tenderness travels. Any jewelry or tight clothing should be removed anywhere on the body.

The leading edge of the swelling should be marked with a black pen every 15 minutes to determine the severity of the swelling and rate of progression. Similarly, the leading edge of pain and tenderness should be marked. The involved extremity should be immobilized and positioned at approximately heart level (not elevated or held dependent). Major joints such as the elbow should be maintained in relative extension (less than 45 degrees of flexion). As swelling occurs, constant consideration should be made to ensure any splinting or clothing is not causing circulatory compromise.

If the patient requires pain relief, opiates are preferred for pain relief over NSAIDs because of the risk of bleeding associated with some envenomations and platelet effects with NSAID use.

Do not attempt to kill the snake. A killed or decapitated snake still offers a risk of envenomation to EMS personnel. If circumstances permit, take a photo of the snake from a safe distance. Safety in this scenario cannot be stressed enough.[130]

While a litter rescue is preferred, if necessary, the patient can be slowly walked for evacuation, with frequent rest stops and reassurance to help keep the patient calm. Transport the patient rapidly to an appropriate destination. Notify the receiving facility of the situation while en route so that they can make preparations to receive and treat the patient.

Extremity Immobilization

Pressure immobilization has been used effectively in Australia for field management of *elapid* (cobra, mamba, North American coral) snakebites (**Figure 21-24**).[133] This technique involves immediately wrapping the entire bitten

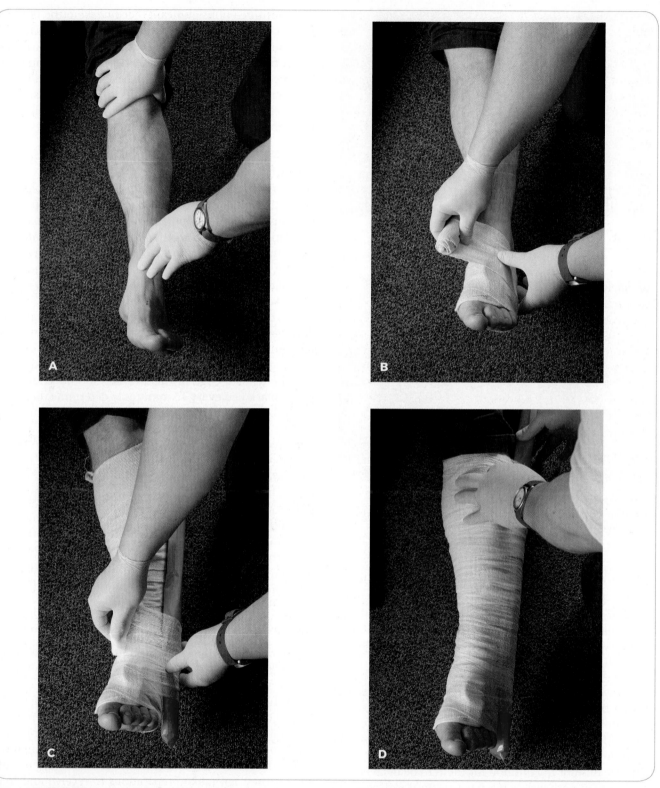

Figure 21-24 Pressure immobilization technique.

extremity with an elastic wrap or bandage as tightly as would be done for a sprain and then splinting and immobilizing the extremity.

If the patient is more than 2 hours from medical attention in an area outside of North America, and the bite is on an arm or leg, it might be reasonable to use the pressure immobilization technique. Place a 2- by 2-inch (5- by 5-centimeter [cm]) cloth pad over the bite site. Next, apply an elastic wrap firmly around the involved limb directly over the padded bite site with a margin of at least 4 to 6 inches (10 to 15 cm) on either side of the wound. Take care to check for adequate circulation in the fingers and toes (normal pulses, feeling, and color). An alternative method is to simply wrap the entire limb as tightly as for a sprain with an elastic bandage. The wrap is meant to impede absorption of venom into the general circulation by containing it within the compressed tissue and microscopic blood and lymphatic vessels near the limb surface. Finally, splint the limb to prevent motion. If the bite is on a hand or arm, also apply a sling. It should be noted that this recommendation is controversial, in that some experts believe that localizing venom in a single area might lead to an increased chance for local tissue damage.

Historically, the following treatments have been recommended; however, they are not supported by the literature and should not be employed:

1. *Rest.* Some recommendations insist that those who have been bitten should always avoid exertion. Deaths from North American snakebite are very rare,[130,136] and it is very unlikely that the exertion of hiking out from a wilderness area will make a victim of a snakebite significantly more ill. If the victim can be carried out, that is ideal. However, if waiting for a carryout will delay the victim's arrival at a hospital, the victim should walk out with whatever assistance can be given.

2. *Catching the snake and bringing it to the hospital.* There are numerous reports of bystanders who tried to catch a suspected poisonous snake and were bitten during the attempt. A single antivenin is used for all pit viper venoms in the United States, and treatment is based on clinical degree of envenomation, relying on the previous signs and symptoms. Therefore, identifying a domestic snake is of minor importance compared with the dangers of attempting to catch the snake.

A digital photograph of the snake might be useful, but identification is not worth the risk of an additional bite.

3. *Suction or incision.* Suction, with or without cutting, has been shown to be useless for venomous snakebite. Snakebite kits consisting of suction devices should be left out of all first-aid kits and should not be used.[137,138]

4. *Electric shock.* Electric shock applied to the snakebite has been shown to be totally ineffective and should never be used.[139,140]

5. *Cold packs.* Cold packs have been shown to increase tissue damage from North American pit viper bites and should not be used.[141]

6. *Splinting, arterial or venous tourniquets, lymph constrictors, or elastic bandages.* Although widely recommended, none of these treatments has been shown to be effective and may worsen local damage to the bite area.[142]

The Wilderness EMS Context Revisited

At the beginning of this chapter, we asked: "When should we think about wilderness EMS; that is, when should we think and work differently from what we do on the street?" The short answer: "It depends."

Time, distance, weather, and terrain all enter into the decision. The decision that a particular patient, in a particular situation, with a particular set of injuries, needs wilderness care rather than street care is a medical decision—one best made by the prehospital care provider directly attending to the patient. If the prehospital care provider at the scene can contact the medical oversight provider, especially in an area where medical control is likely to be familiar with wilderness EMS, the advice is definitely worth seeking. Ultimately, the decision is up to the prehospital care provider at the scene based on scope of practice, local protocols regarding autonomy, and medical oversight.

PHTLS believes that, given a good fund of knowledge, key principles, and training by medical oversight providers in autonomous medical decision making and wilderness medicine, prehospital care providers are capable of making the most appropriate decisions regarding patient care in wilderness settings.

SUMMARY

- While many of the principles of *wilderness* EMS are the same as *street* EMS, preferences and practices may change because of the unique circumstances. Balancing these factors becomes the specialty of wilderness EMS providers.
- Oversight direction by a knowledgeable physician and specialized training for providers who are likely to encounter wilderness EMS situations are integral components of wilderness EMS.
- The acronym LATE—*l*ocate, *a*ccess, *t*reat, *e*xtricate—represents simplified principles in SAR and other wilderness EMS operations.
- Wilderness EMS presents a wide variety of environments and situations requiring unique patient packaging and transport considerations, specialized equipment, modification of standard procedures and protocols, and context-specific safety considerations for both the patient and the responders.
- Initial patient assessment is the same regardless of the environment. The priority of attention is based on the major life threats that can be mitigated immediately at the point of injury.
- In many wilderness situations, responders may have to improvise the tools and methods they use to provide care. They must be skilled in tourniquet use, including improvisational methods, and they must understand how best to adapt standard care practices, such as antibiotic administration, pain management, and cardiopulmonary resuscitation and defibrillation, to the wilderness environment.
- When managing patients in the wilderness, the wilderness EMS providers must also consider food and water requirements and elimination needs.
- A basic principle of wilderness care is that all patients are hypothermic, hypoglycemic, and hypovolemic until proven otherwise.
- Bites and stings are common wilderness problems. Local knowledge and resources are important to help guide the care of these patients, but routine patient care guidelines are still necessary.

SCENARIO RECAP

As first on the scene, you turn on your headlamp and rapidly assess the area and ensure the safety of yourself, the casualty, and his companion. Your communication relay at the top of the canyon relays the progress of the rescue back to the incident commander. The weather seems to be holding with minimal clouds and no thunderstorms developing, and you decide that you will have to remain at this location through the night. No helicopters are available in the area to perform night operations, and you are not able to safely and efficiently move the patient out of this position tonight. You request the rescue helicopter that had been placed on standby to return at first light to hoist the patient from an opening in the canyon about 328 ft (100 m) from your current location.

There is limited room at the patient's location, but you are able to move him off to the side, so you are no longer under the direct path of other rescuers as they descend to your location, and you are able to carefully move the patient to a dry spot and onto an insulating pad.

Your assessment proceeds along the MARCH PAWS algorithm. You have already remotely identified and controlled the *massive hemorrhage* and now evaluate the tourniquet placed by the friend using tubular webbing. It appears to be moderately effective, so you apply a second tourniquet (C-A-T) from your kit adjacent to the first and mark the time it was placed. The second tourniquet completely stopped further bleeding, and you confirm that there is no longer a distal pulse. You perform a blood sweep and detect no other signs of massive hemorrhage. However, when you assess his pelvis, it feels unstable and there is significant pain; therefore you apply a pelvic binder from your medical kit.

He is awake and talking to you with no signs of *airway* compromise. You place your hands on his chest wall and note equal and symmetric chest rise and fall with no signs of *respiratory* distress or chest wall trauma. You check *circulation* by assessing distal pulses and note his heart rate to be rapid with bounding radial pulse

SCENARIO RECAP (CONTINUED)

of 120 beats per minute. His skin is cool and slightly diaphoretic. You treat his *hypothermia* by removing him from the cold water, exposing his skin, and putting dry warm clothes on him. You direct a teammate to prepare a sleeping pad and bag for a hypothermia wrap with additional heating pads. You assess his *head* and see no overt signs of head or back injury; however, he has had a significant fall and possibly a distracting injury, so you consider the possibility of spinal injury and immobilize his spine using a whole-body vacuum splint. He is conscious and alert with an otherwise normal gross neurologic examination. He has some mild nausea but has not vomited, and you give him a 4-mg dose of ondansetron with an orally disintegrating tablet. You treat his *pain* with a 1-gram dose of oral acetaminophen (Tylenol) and give a 100-mg subdissociative dose of intranasal ketamine. This brings his pain from 10 out of 10 down to 2 out of 10 and facilitates the completion of your examination and splinting/treatment.

Based on your standing *antibiotic* order protocol for open fractures, you establish an IV now that all other life threats are addressed and administer 2 grams of IV cefazolin after confirming no allergies. You reassess his body (head to toe) for any other *wounds* or injuries and find the only location requiring attention is the open femur fracture. You grossly irrigate the open fracture site with potable water and bandage. Now you know that you have a prolonged extrication and attempt to convert the tourniquet to another form of bleeding control. You are safely able to transition from a tourniquet to a pressure dressing to control the bleeding. You reassess it frequently and confirm that it maintains control. Distal pulses and sensation are regained.

Last, you complete your patient packaging with appropriate *splints*. For the open femur fracture, you use manual traction and bring the leg to anatomic position and provide *physiologic* splinting, with padding and the vacuum mattress to maintain position. The vacuum mattress now is able to splint the entire body, including neck/back, pelvis, and femur fracture without undue pressure spots. You attend to the suspected right wrist fracture, which was not the most significant injury, once higher priority injuries have been addressed. You allow the patient to sip on fluids through the night and to urinate using an adult diaper that you exchange when needed.

SCENARIO SOLUTION

The team spends the night out with the patient and his companions, and with the preplanning you are well prepared. Your medical training, along with the prolonged field care guidelines, helps you manage the patient through the night. With your stabilization and treatment, the patient does well overnight, and vital signs remain stable. Once immobilized, he has very little pain. As morning arrives, the helicopter is able to hoist the patient out of the canyon. A waiting ambulance assumes care of the patient and transports him to the closest appropriate facility 45 minutes away. Because the patient has been stable overnight, it was determined that a medical helicopter transport was not needed after conferring with medical control. Your field documentation is passed on with the patient to ensure a continuity of patient care. Once out of the field, you complete a final patient care report. You follow up with the hospital and find that the patient is expected to make a full recovery.

References

1. *Merriam-Webster's Collegiate Dictionary*. 11th ed. Springfield, MA: Merriam-Webster; 2014:1432.
2. McGinnis KK. *Rural and Frontier Emergency Medical Services*. Kansas City, MO; National Rural Health Association; 2004.
3. Liffrig JR, Tarter SL, Schimelpfenig T, et al. Wilderness medicine education. In: Auerbach PS, ed. *Auerbach's Wilderness Medicine*. 7th ed. Philadelphia, PA: Elsevier; 2017:2440-2471.
4. Winstead C, Hawkins SC. Wilderness EMS education. In: Hawkins SC, ed. *Wilderness EMS*. Philadelphia, PA: Wolters Kluwer; 2018:61-81.
5. Bennett BL. A time has come for wilderness emergency medical service: a new direction. *Wilderness Environ Med*. 2012;23(1):5-6.

6. Warden CR, Millin MG, Hawkins SC, et al. Medical direction of wilderness and other operational emergency services programs. *Wilderness Environ Med.* 2012;23(1):37-43.

7. Millin M. Wilderness EMS medical oversight. In: Hawkins SC, ed. *Wilderness EMS.* Philadelphia, PA: Wolters Kluwer; 2018:101-110.

8. Russell K, Weber D, Scheele B, et al. Search and rescue in the intermountain west states. *Wilderness Environ Med.* 2013;24:429-433.

9. National Highway Traffic Safety Administration. *The National EMS Scope of Practice Model.* Washington, DC: Department of Transportation/National Highway Traffic Safety Administration; 2005.

10. Millin MG, Johnson DE, Schimelpfenig T, et al. Medical oversight, educational core content, and proposed scopes of practice of wilderness EMS providers: a joint project developed by wilderness EMS educators, medical directors, and regulators using a Delphi approach. *Prehosp Emerg Care.* 2017;21(6):673-681.

11. Smith W. Medical professionals role in search and rescue. In: Rodway G, Weber DC, McIntosh SE, eds. *Mountain Medicine and Technical Rescue.* Herefordshire, UK: Carreg; 2016:207-223.

12. Hawkins SC, Millin MC, Smith W. Wilderness emergency medical services and response systems. In: Auerbach P, ed. *Auerbach's Wilderness Medicine.* 7th ed. Philadelphia, PA: Elsevier; 2017:1200-1213.

13. Johnson DE, Schimelpfenig T, Hubbel F. Minimum guidelines and scope of practice for wilderness first aid. *Wilderness Environ Med.* 2013;24(4):456-462.

14. Tilton B. *Wilderness First Responder.* Guilford, CT: Falcon Guides (Globe Pequot Press); 2010.

15. American Society for Testing and Materials. *Standard Guide for Training First Responders Who Practice in Wilderness, Delayed, or Prolonged Transport Settings.* West Conshohocken, PA: American Society for Testing and Materials; 1995:F1616-F1695.

16. Wilderness Medical Society Curriculum Committee. Wilderness first responder: recommended minimum course topics. *Wilderness Environ Med.* 1999;10:13-19.

17. McNamara EC, Johe DH, Endly DA, eds. *Outdoor Emergency Care.* 5th ed. Lakewood, CO: National Ski Patrol. Brady (Pearson); 2012.

18. Hawkins SC. The relationship between ski patrols and emergency medical services systems. *Wilderness Environ Med.* 2012;23:106-111.

19. Constance BB, Auerbach PS, Johe DH. Prehospital medical care and the National Ski Patrol: how does outdoor emergency care compare to traditional EMS training? *Wilderness Environ Med.* 2012;23:177-189.

20. Spano SJ. National Park Service medicine. In: Auerbach P, ed. *Auerbach's Wilderness Medicine.* 7th ed. Philadelphia, PA: Elsevier; 2017:2487-2497.

21. Smith WR. Integration of tactical EMS in the National Park Service. *Wilderness Environ Med.* 2017;28(2S):S146-S153.

22. Lipman GS, Weichenthal L, Harris NS, et al. Core content for Wilderness Medicine fellowship training of emergency medicine graduates. *Acad Emerg Med.* 2014;21(2):204-207.

23. Hawkins S, Millin M, Smith W. Care in the wilderness. In: Cone D, Brice JH, Delbridge TR, Myers JB, eds. *Emergency Medical Services: Clinical Practice and System Oversight*, Vol 2. 2nd ed. Medical Oversight of EMS. West Sussex, UK: John Wiley & Sons; 2015:377-391.

24. Vines T, Hudson S. Medical considerations in technical rescue. In: *High-Angle Rope Rescue Techniques: Levels I and II.* 4th ed. Burlington, MA: Jones & Bartlett Learning; 2016:224-245.

25. Smith WR. Principles of basic technical rescue, packaging, and patient care integration. In: Hawkins SC, ed. *Wilderness EMS.* Philadelphia, PA: Wolters Kluwer; 2018:101-110.

26. Hawkins SC. WEMS systems. In: Hawkins SC, ed. *Wilderness EMS.* Philadelphia, PA: Wolters Kluwer; 2018:21-59.

27. Zafren K, McCurley L, Shimanski C, et al. Technical rescue. In: Auerbach PS, ed. *Auerbach's Wilderness Medicine.* 7th ed. Philadelphia: Elsevier; 2017:1242-1280.

28. Goodman T, Iserson KV, Strich H. Wilderness mortalities: a 13-year experience. *Ann Emerg Med.* 2001;37:279-283.

29. Gentile DA, Morris JA, Schimelpfenig T, Bass SM, Auerbach PS. Wilderness injuries and illnesses. *Ann Emerg Med.* 1992;21:853-861.

30. Singletary EM, Markenson DS. Injury prevention: decision making, safety, and accident avoidance. In: Auerbach PS, ed. *Auerbach's Wilderness Medicine.* 7th ed. Philadelphia: Elsevier; 2017:593-616.

31. Isaac JE, Johnson DE. *Wilderness and Rescue Medicine.* 6th ed. Burlington, MA: Jones & Bartlett Learning; 2013.

32. Hawkins SC. Setting the record straight to reduce fatalities in sinking vehicles. *Emerg Med News.* 2015;37(8):28-29.

33. Butler FK, Blackbourne LH. Battlefield trauma care then and now: a decade of tactical combat casualty care. *J Trauma Acute Care Surg.* 2012;73:S395-S402.

34. Holcomb JB, Stansbury LG, Champion HR, Wade C, Bellamy RF. Understanding combat casualty care statistics. *J Trauma Acute Care Surg.* 2006;60:397-401.

35. Kelly J, Ritenour AE, McLaughlin DF, et al. Injury severity and causes of death from Operation Iraqi Freedom and Operation Enduring Freedom: 2003-2004 versus 2006. *J Trauma.* 2008;6:S21-S27.

36. Eastridge BJ, Mabry RL, Seguin P, et al. Death on the battlefield (2001-2011): implications for the future of combat casualty care. *J Trauma Acute Care Surg.* 2012;73:S431-S437.

37. Kotwal RS, Montgomery HR, Mabry RL, et al. Eliminating preventable death on the battlefield. *Arch Surg.* 2011;146:1350-1358.

38. Bennett BL, Butler FK, Wedmore I, eds. Tactical combat casualty care: transitioning battlefield lessons learned to other austere environments. *Wilderness Environ Med.* 2017;28(2S):S1-S154.

39. Smith B, Bledsoe BE, Nicolazzo P. General management of trauma in the wilderness. In: Hawkins SC, ed. *Wilderness EMS.* Philadelphia, PA: Wolters Kluwer; 2018:371-392.

40. Smith W. Episode 3: medical direction with Will Smith, MD [podcast]. RAW Medicine website. http://rawmedicine.libsyn.com/episode-3-medical-direction-with-will-smith-md. Published February 1, 2018. Accessed February 20, 2018.

41. Overview. Committee for Tactical Emergency Casualty Care website. http://www.c-tecc.org/about/overview. Accessed February 20, 2018.

42. Smith W, Grange K. Mission success: how a rural EMS agency implemented a tactical EMS program. *JEMS.* 2018;43(1):24-30.

43. Hoffman JR, Mower WR, Wolfson AB, Todd KH, Zucker MI. Validity of a set of clinical criteria to rule out injury to the cervical spine in patients with blunt trauma. National Emergency X-radiography Utilization Study group. *N Engl J Med.* 2000;343:94-99.

44. Vaillancourt C, Stiell IG, Beaudoin T, et al. The out-of-hospital validation of the Canadian c-spine rule by paramedics. *Annals of Emer Med.* 2010;55(1):22.

45. Chan D, Goldberg R, Tascone A, et al. The effect of spinal immobilization on healthy volunteers. *Ann Emerg Med.* 1994;23(1):48.

46. Kwan I, Bunn F, Roberts IG. Spinal immobilisation for trauma patients. *Cochrane Database Syst Rev.* 2001(2):CD002803.

47. Ben-Galim P, Dreiangel N, Mattox KL, et al. Extrication collars can result in abnormal separation between vertebrae in the presence of dissociative injury. *J Trauma.* 2010;69:447-450.

48. Hauswald M, Ong G, Tandeberg D, et al. Out-of-hospital spinal immobilization: its effect on neurologic injury. *Acad Emerg Med.* 1998;5:214-219.

49. Oto B, Corey DJ II, Oswald J, Sifford D, Walsh B. Early secondary neurological deterioration after blunt spinal trauma: a review of the literature. *Acad Emerg Med.* 2015;22:1200-1212.

50. Senz K. New Hampshire rescue squad denies fault in woman's drowning. EMS World website. http://www.emsworld.com/news/10408685/new-hampshire-rescue-squad-denies-fault-in-womans-drowning. Published September 10, 2007. Accessed February 20, 2018.

51. Scheele BM. Technical rescue interface: off-road vehicle and helicopter WEMS response. In: Hawkins SC, ed. *Wilderness EMS.* Philadelphia, PA: Wolters Kluwer; 2018:503-518.

52. Kosequat J, Rush SC, Simonsen I, et al. Efficacy of the mnemonic device "MARCH PAWS" as a checklist for pararescuemen during tactical field care and tactical evacuation. *J Spec Operations Med.* 2017;4:80-84.

53. Hawkins SC, Simon RB, Beissinger JP, Simon D. *Vertical Aid: Essential Wilderness Medicine for Climbers, Trekkers, and Mountaineers.* New York, NY: The Countryman Press; 2017.

54. Davis C. Part 2: management of infectious diseases: general infectious diseases in the wilderness environment. In: Hawkins SC, ed. *Wilderness EMS.* Philadelphia, PA: Wolters Kluwer; 2018:355-370.

55. Keenan S, Riesberg JC. Prolonged field care: beyond the "Golden Hour." *Wilderness Environ Med.* 2017;28(2S):S135-S139.

56. Gomi T. *Everyone Poops.* Brooklyn, NY: Kane/Miller Book Publishers; 1993.

57. Wing-Gaia SL, Askew W. Nutrition, malnutrition and starvation. In: Auerbach PS, ed. *Auerbach's Wilderness Medicine.* 7th ed. Philadelphia, PA: Elsevier; 2017:1964-1985.

58. Kenefick RW, Cheuvront SN, Leon LR, Obrien K. Dehydration and rehydration. In: Auerbach PS, ed. *Wilderness Medicine.* 7th ed. Philadelphia, PA: Elsevier; 2017:2031-2044.

59. Madsen P, Svendsen LB, Jorgenesen LG, et al. Tolerance to head-up tilt and suspension with elevated legs. *Aviat Space Environ Med.* 1998;69:781-784.

60. Mortimer RB. Risks and management of prolonged suspension in an Alpine harness. *Wilderness Environ Med.* 2011;22:77-86.

61. Seddon P. *Harness Suspension: Review and Evaluation on Existing Information.* Colegate, Norwich, UK: Health Safety Executive Books; 2002:CRR 451/2002.

62. Kolb JJ, Smith EL. Redefining the diagnosis and treatment of suspension trauma. *JEMS* website. http://www.jems.com/articles/print/volume-40/issue-6/features/redefining-the-diagnosis-and-treatment-of-suspension-trauma.html. Published June 9, 2015. Accessed February 20, 2018.

63. Prevention and treatment of sunburn. *Med Lett Drugs Ther.* 2004;46:45.

64. Krakowski AC, Goldenberg A. Exposure to radiation from the sun. In: Auerbach PS, ed. *Auerbach's Wilderness Medicine.* 7th ed. Philadelphia, PA: Elsevier; 2017:335-353.

65. Stern RS. Clinical practice. Treatment of photoaging. *N Engl J Med.* 2004;350:1526.

66. Richardson SD. Environmental mass spectrometry: emerging contaminants and current issues. *Anal Chem.* 2012;84:747.

67. Gies P. Photoprotection by clothing. *Photodermal Photimmunol Photomed.* 2007;23:264.

68. Singletary EM, Charlton NP, Epstein JL, et al. Part 15: first aid: 2015 American Heart Association and American Red Cross guidelines update for first aid. *Circulation.* 2015;132(suppl 2): S574-S589.

69. Kragh JF, Walters TJ, Baer DG, et al. Practical use of emergency tourniquets to stop bleeding in major limb trauma. *J Trauma.* 2008;64(2 suppl):38-50.

70. Drew B, Bird D, Matteucci M, Keenan S. Tourniquet conversion: a recommended approach in the prolonged field care setting. *J Spec Operations Med.* 2015;15(3):81-85.

71. Kragh JF, Dubick MA. Bleeding control with limb tourniquet use in the wilderness setting: review of science. *Wilderness Environ Med.* 2017;28(2S):S25-S32.

72. Edlich RF, Rodeheaver GT, Morgan RF, et al. Principles of emergency wound management. *Ann Emerg Med.* 1988; 17(12):1284.

73. Edlich RF, Thacker JG, Buchanan L, Rodeheaver GT. Modern concepts of treatment of traumatic wounds. *Adv Surg.* 1979;13:169.

74. Bhandari M, Thompson K, Adili A, Shaughnessy SG. High and low pressure irrigation in contaminated wounds with exposed bone. *Int J Surg Invest.* 2000;2(3):179.

75. Bhandari M, Adili A, Lachowski RJ. High pressure pulsatile lavage of contaminated human tibiae: an in vitro study. *J Orthop Trauma.* 1998;12(7):479.

76. Bhandari M, Schemitsch EH, Adili A, et al. High and low pressure pulsatile lavage of contaminated tibial fractures: an in vitro study of bacterial adherence and bone damage. *J Orthop Trauma.* 1999;13(8):526.

77. Anglen JO. Wound irrigation in musculoskeletal injury. *J Am Acad Orthop Surg.* 2001;9(4):219.

78. Valente JH, Forti RJ, Freundlich LF, et al. Wound irrigation in children: saline solution or tap water? *Ann Emerg Med.* 2003;41(5):609.

79. Backer HD. Field water disinfection. In: Auerbach PS, ed. *Auerbach's Wilderness Medicine.* 7th ed. Philadelphia, PA: Elsevier; 2017:1985-2030.

80. Griffiths RD, Fernandez RS, Ussia CA. Is tap water a safe alternative to normal saline for wound irrigation in the community setting? *J Wound Care.* 2001;10(10):407.

81. Moscati R, Mayrose J, Fincher L, Jehle D. Comparison of normal saline with tap water for wound irrigation. *Am J Emerg Med.* 1998;16(4):379.

82. Moscati RM, Reardon RF, Lerner EB, Mayrose J. Wound irrigation with tap water. *Acad Emerg Med.* 1998;5(11):1076.

83. Rodeheaver GT, Pettry D, Thacker JG, et al. Wound cleansing by high pressure irrigation. *Surg Gynecol Obstet.* 1975;141(3):357.

84. Edlich RF, Reddy VR. Revolutionary advances in wound repair in emergency medicine during the last three decades: a view toward the new millennium. 5th Annual David R. Boyd, MD, Lecture. *J Emerg Med.* 2001;20(2):167.

85. Singer AJ, Hollander JE, Subramanian S, et al. Pressure dynamics of various irrigation techniques commonly used in the emergency department. *Ann Emerg Med.* 1994;24(1):36.

86. Luck JB, Campagne D, Falcon Bachs R, et al. Pressures of wilderness improvised wound irrigation techniques: how do they compare? *Wilderness Environ Med.* 2016;27(4):476-481.

87. Mellor SG, Cooper GJ, Bowyer GW. Efficacy of delayed administration of benzylpenicillin in the control of infection in penetrating soft tissue injuries in war. *J Trauma.* 1996;40(3 suppl):S128-S134.

88. Hospenthal DR, Murray CK, Andersen RC, et al. Guidelines for the prevention of infection after combat-related injuries. *J Trauma.* 2008;64(3 suppl):S211-S220.

89. Jamshidi R. Wound management. In: Auerbach PS, ed. *Wilderness Medicine.* 7th ed. Philadelphia, PA: Elsevier; 2017: 440-450.

90. Russell KW, Scaife CL, Weber DC, et al. Wilderness Medical Society practice guidelines for the treatment of acute pain in remote environments: 2014 update. *Wilderness Environ Med.* 2014;25:S96-S104.

91. McGladrey L. Psychological first aid and stress injuries. In: Hawkins SC, ed. *Wilderness EMS.* Philadelphia, PA: Wolters Kluwer; 2018:189-202.

92. Switzer JA, Bovard RS, Quinn RH. Wilderness orthopedics. In: Auerbach PS, ed. *Auerbach's Wilderness Medicine.* 7th ed. Philadelphia, PA: Elsevier; 2017:450-492.

93. Kranc DA, Jones AW, Nackenson J, et al. Use of ultrasound for joint dislocation reduction in an austere wilderness setting: a case report. *Prehosp Emerg Care.* 2018[in press].

94. Fulton RL, Voigt WJ, Hilakos AS. Confusion surrounding the treatment of traumatic cardiac arrest. *J Am Coll Surg.* 1995;181:209.

95. Pasquale MD, Rhodes M, Cipolle MD, et al. Defining "dead on arrival": impact on a level I trauma center. *J Trauma.* 1996;41:726.

96. Mattox KL, Feliciano DV. Role of external cardiac compression in truncal trauma. *J Trauma.* 1982;22:934.

97. Shimazu S, Shatney CH. Outcomes of trauma patients with no vital signs on admission. *J Trauma.* 1983;23(3):213.

98. Forgey WW, Wilderness Medical Society. *Practice Guidelines for Wilderness Emergency Care.* 5th ed. Guilford, CT: Globe Pequot Press; 2006.

99. Goth P, Garnett G, Rural Affairs Committee, National Association of EMS Physicians. Clinical guidelines for delayed/prolonged transport. I. Cardiorespiratory arrest. *Prehosp Disaster Med.* 1991;6(3):335.

100. Eisenberg MS, Bergner L, Hallstrom AP. Cardiac resuscitation in the community: importance of rapid provision and implications of program planning. *JAMA.* 1979;241:1905.

101. Kellermann AL, Hackman BB, Somes G. Predicting the outcome of unsuccessful prehospital advanced cardiac life support. *JAMA.* 1993;270(12):1433.

102. Bonnin MJ, Pepe PE, Kimball KT, Clark PS. Distinct criteria for termination of resuscitation in the out-of-hospital setting. *JAMA.* 1993;270(12):1457.

103. Millin MG, Khandker SR, Malki A. Termination of resuscitation of nontraumatic cardiopulmonary arrest: resource document for the National Association of EMS Physicians position statement. *Prehosp Emerg Care.* 2011;15(4):547-554.

104. Leavitt M, Podgorny G. Prehospital CPR and the pulseless hypothermic patient. *Ann Emerg Med.* 1984;13:492.

105. Zafren K, Giesbrecht G, Danzl D, et al. Wilderness Medical Society practice guidelines for the out-of-hospital evaluation and treatment of accidental hypothermia: 2014 update. *Wilderness Environ Med.* 2014;25:S66-S85.

106. Keatinge WR. Accidental immersion hypothermia and drowning. *Practitioner.* 1977;219:183.

107. Olshaker JS. Near drowning. *Emerg Med Clin North Am.* 1992;10(2):339.

108. Bolte RG, Black PG, Bowers RS, et al. The use of extracorporeal rewarming in a child submerged for 66 minutes. *JAMA.* 1988;260(3):377.

109. Orlowski JP. Drowning, near-drowning, and ice-water drowning. *JAMA.* 1988;260(3):390.

110. Cooper MA, Andrews CJ, Holle RL, et al. Lightning-related injuries and safety. In: Auerbach PS, ed. *Auerbach's Wilderness Medicine.* 7th ed. Philadelphia, PA: Elsevier; 2017: 71-117.

111. Davis C, Engeln A, Johnson E, McIntosh S, et al. Wilderness Medical Society practice guidelines for the prevention and treatment of lightning injuries: 2014 update. *Wilderness Environ Med.* 2014;25:S86-S95.

112. Durrer B, Brugger H. Recent advances in avalanche survival. Presented at the Second World Congress on Wilderness Medicine. Aspen, CO; 1995.

113. Van Tilburg C, Grissom CK, Zafren K, et al. Wilderness Medical Society practice guidelines for prevention and management of avalanche and nonavalanche snow burial accidents. *Wilderness Environ Med.* 2017;25(28):23-42.

114. Steinman AM. Cardiopulmonary resuscitation and hypothermia. *Circulation.* 1986;74(6, pt 2):29.

115. Zell SC. Epidemiology of wilderness-acquired diarrhea: implications for prevention and treatment. *J Wild Med.* 1992;3(3):241.

116. Lloyd EL. *Hypothermia and Cold Stress.* Rockville, MD: Aspen Systems; 1986.

117. Maningas PA, DeGuzman LR, Hollenbach SJ, et al. Regional blood flow during hypothermic arrest. *Ann Emerg Med.* 1986;15(4):390.

118. Groves LJ, Cushing TA. General management of medical conditions in the wilderness. In: Hawkins SC, ed. *Wilderness EMS.* Philadelphia, PA: Wolters Kluwer; 2018:393-412.

119. Sampson HA, Muñoz-Furlong A, Campbell RL, et al. Second symposium on the definition and management of anaphylaxis: summary report—Second National Institute of Allergy and Infectious Disease/Food Allergy and Anaphylaxis Network symposium. *J Allergy Clin Immunol.* 2006;117:391.

120. Graif Y, Romano-Zelekha O, Livne I, et al. Allergic reactions to insect stings: results from a national survey of 10,000 junior high school children in Israel. *J Allergy Clin Immunol.* 2006;117:1435.

121. Golden DB. Insect sting anaphylaxis. *Immunol Allergy Clin North Am.* 2007;27:261.

122. Bilò BM, Bonifazi F. Epidemiology of insect-venom ana-phylaxis. *Curr Opin Allergy Clin Immunol.* 2008;8:330.

123. Graft DF. Insect sting allergy. *Med Clin North Am.* 2006;90:211.

124. Valentine MD, Schuberth KC, Kagey-Sobotka A, et al. The value of immunotherapy with venom in children with allergy to insect stings. *N Engl J Med.* 1990;323:1601.

125. Barnard JH. Studies of 400 *Hymenoptera* sting deaths in the United States. *J Allergy Clin Immunol.* 1973;52:259.

126. Gaudio F, Lemery J, Johnson D. Wilderness Medical Society practice guidelines for the use of epinephrine in outdoor education and wilderness settings: 2014 update. *Wilderness Environ Med.* 2014;25:S15-S18.

127. Hawkins S, Weil C, Fitzpatrick D. Letter to the editor: epinephrine autoinjector warning. *Wilderness Environ Med.* 2012;23:371-378.

128. Miller S. Snake bite death statistics worldwide. Paw Nation website. http://animals.pawnation.com/snake-bite-death-statistics-worldwide-2431.html. Accessed January 2018.

129. Kasturiratne A, Wickremasinghe AR, de Silva N, et al. The global burden of snakebite: a literature analysis and modelling based on regional estimates of envenoming and deaths. *PLoS Med.* 2008;5(11):e218.

130. Abo B. Management of animal bites and envenomation. Hawkins SC, ed. *Wilderness EMS.* Philadelphia, PA: Wolters Kluwer; 2018:333-346.

131. O'Neil ME, Mack KA, Gilchrist J, Wozniak EJ. Snakebite injuries treated in United States emergency departments, 2001-2004. *Wilderness Environ Med.* 2007;18(4):281-287.

132. Lavonas EJ, Ruha AM, Banner W, et al. Unified treatment algorithm for the management of crotaline snakebite in the United States: results of an evidence-informed consensus workshop. *BMC Emerg Med.* 2011;11:2.

133. Norris RL, Bush SP, Cardwell MD. Bites by venomous reptiles in Canada, the United States, and Mexico. In: Auerbach PS, ed. *Auerbach's Wilderness Medicine.* 7th ed. Philadelphia, PA: Elsevier; 2017:729-760.

134. Warrell DA. Bites by venomous and nonvenomous reptiles worldwide. In: Auerbach PS, ed. *Auerbach's Wilderness Medicine.* 7th ed. Philadelphia, PA: Elsevier; 2017:760-828.

135. Kanaan NC, Ray J, Stewart M, et al. Wilderness Medical Society practice guidelines for the treatment of pit viper envenomations in the United States and Canada. *Wilderness Environ Med.* 2015;26:472-487.

136. Curry SC, Kunkel DB. Death from a rattlesnake bite. *Am J Emerg Med.* 1985;3(3):227.

137. Bush SP. Snakebite suction devices don't remove venom: they just suck. *Ann Emerg Med.* 2004;43(2):187.

138. Alberts MB, Shalit M, LoGalbo F. Suction for venomous snakebite: a study of "mock venom" extraction in a human model. *Ann Emerg Med.* 2004;43(2):181.

139. Davis D, Branch K, Egen NB, et al. The effect of an electrical current on snake venom toxicity. *J Wild Med.* 1992;3(1):48.

140. Howe NR, Meisenheimer JL Jr. Electric shock does not save snakebitten rats. *Ann Emerg Med.* 1988;17(3):254.

141. Gill KA Jr. The evaluation of cryotherapy in the treatment of snake envenomation. *South Med J.* 1968;63:552.

142. Norris RL. A call for snakebite research. *Wilderness Environ Med.* 2000;11(3):149.

Suggested Reading

Auerbach PS, ed. *Auerbach's Wilderness Medicine.* 7th ed. Philadelphia, PA: Elsevier; 2017.

Hawkins SC, ed. *Wilderness EMS.* Philadelphia, PA: Wolters Kluwer; 2018.

Rodway G, McIntosh S, Weber D, eds. *Mountain Medicine and Technical Rescue: A Manual of the Diploma in Mountain Medicine.* Herefordshire, UK: Carreg; 2016.

CHAPTER 22

Civilian Tactical Emergency Medical Support (TEMS)

Lead Editors:
Alexander L. Eastman, MD, MPH, FACS
Faroukh Mehkri, DO

CHAPTER OBJECTIVES

At the completion of this chapter, you will be able to do the following:

- Describe the components of tactical emergency medical support (TEMS).
- Understand the operational and support functions of TEMS.
- Explain the benefits of a TEMS program.

- Discuss how emergency medical care differs in each of the three phases of care in TEMS.
- Relate how remote assessment methodology may be used on a tactical mission.
- Describe the role of medical support for counterterrorism operations.

SCENARIO

Your emergency medical services (EMS) agency provides coverage for the local special weapons and tactics (SWAT) team and has a rigorous, integrated training program with local law enforcement. Your tactical emergency medical support (TEMS) team is called out for a barricaded gunman holed up in an old mobile home just after sunset. As you are preparing for entry, two SWAT officers cross the suspect's yard and approach the house to prepare for a door pull. Shots ring out from the front window, wounding the SWAT officers. One SWAT officer falls in the doorway of the suspect's home. The second falls near an old pickup truck. A patrol officer standing near you yells, "We need to go get them. Come on!" You grab the patrol officer by the arm and look to the SWAT commander.

- What should your actions be?
- How will you assess and treat the fallen SWAT officers given the danger of the scene?

INTRODUCTION

Tactical emergency medical support (TEMS) is an out-of-hospital system of care dedicated to enhancing the success of special operations law enforcement missions, reducing mission medical liability and risk, and promoting public safety.[1] TEMS builds on the principles of military medicine, wilderness medicine, disaster response, urban search and rescue, and conventional EMS to create a system of care that supports law enforcement missions and maximizes the clinical outcome for casualties in what is often a resource-poor, prolonged-transport environment while minimizing the threat to the prehospital care provider.

This chapter provides a brief overview of TEMS. Participation in TEMS and the provision of **tactical casualty care (TCC)** requires specific training and expertise, just as for any other special operations situation. For a detailed overview of TEMS, the National Association of Emergency Medical Technicians offers a 16-hour course devoted to TEMS: Tactical Emergency Casualty Care (TECC).

History and Evolution of Tactical Emergency Medical Support

The first SWAT team was developed in Los Angeles in 1968. Shortly thereafter, the concept of having a "medic" attached to the SWAT team was advanced, similar to the military model of having a combat medic assigned to the squad. Today, TEMS encompasses a broad spectrum of medical services modified in structure and function to operate within the high-risk, high-speed tactical environment. Broad support for TEMS now exists within both the law enforcement and the medical communities.

Over 20 years ago, the Counter Narcotics and Terrorism Operational Medical Support (CONTOMS) course was developed. This program was developed as an evidence-based TEMS curriculum that selected seasoned emergency medical providers and immersed them in providing medical care in the tactical environment over the course of 56 hours. Through CONTOMS, an injury database was developed to provide the research data needed to support the efficacy of tactical medicine.

Since then, many courses similar to CONTOMS have been developed. The Tactical Combat Casualty Care (TCCC) course, developed by the Committee on Tactical Combat Casualty Care, part of the Defense Health Board of the U.S. Department of Defense, teaches the essential medical interventions needed in the tactical environment, dependent on the specific tactical situation. However, the 16-hour course does not teach the operational components of a tactical incident. Knowledge of tactical movement and planning

are needed for a complete, well-developed TEMS program. The TCCC program and its medical objectives should be included within any TEMS educational program to address emergency medical care issues in the tactical environment.

In 2016, 66 law enforcement officers died from injuries incurred in the line of duty during felonious incidents. In 2013 that number was 27, which represents an increase of over 240% in the number of law enforcement officers killed in the line of duty between 2013 and 2016. This increase, in conjunction with an ever-increasing incidence of active shooter incidents nationwide, has reinforced the need for TEMS.[2] The National Tactical Officers Association (NTOA) has endorsed TEMS, beginning with its original position statement in 1994, and continues to view it as "an important element of tactical law enforcement" for tactical medics.[3] After the September 11, 2001, attacks, both the National Association of EMS Physicians (NAEMSP) and the American College of Emergency Physicians (ACEP) formally endorsed integrating EMS capabilities into law enforcement special operations.[4,5]

The Committee on TCCC (CoTCCC) has established guidelines currently considered to be the standard of care for military prehospital medicine. Both the American College of Surgeons Committee on Trauma (ACS-COT) and the National Association of Emergency Medical Technicians (NAEMT) endorse the TCCC guidelines and offer TCCC training.[6] Though military and law enforcement special operations are unique, similarities exist in the tactical medical care aspects. The NTOA-endorsed TCCC guidelines have provided a strong foundation for the standardization of TEMS protocols.

With the growing recognition that tactical medical care has become an important issue and the work of the CoTCCC to develop the military TCCC educational program, efforts have been under way to adapt the military information to a civilian setting. A civilian CoTCCC counterpart, the Committee on Tactical Emergency Casualty Care (C-TECC), has developed a set of TECC guidelines that closely resemble the CoTCCC guidelines. These guidelines are tailored to address the prehospital high-threat needs of civilian law enforcement.[7] The TECC guidelines have since been incorporated into the National Joint Counterterrorism Awareness Workshop used by the FBI, the Federal Emergency Management Agency, and the National Counterterrorism Center.[8] NAEMT has developed a TECC course for civilian prehospital care providers. This text will primarily use the standard TCCC nomenclature.

TEMS Practice Components

Tactical emergency medical support has several distinctions from conventional EMS. Unlike conventional EMS, comprehensive TEMS programs include health maintenance, preventive medicine (e.g., immunizations, proper sleep practices, and physical fitness), medical threat assessments, and coordination of care with a variety of local medical assets. From an operational perspective, TEMS providers are frequently faced with treat-and-release decisions. These situations will vary from the TEMS operator who has become dehydrated to the angry prisoner who may have been injured in the tactical operation.

Many states include specific addendums to their EMS protocols that address TEMS practice.[9] TEMS providers and their medical directors must be familiar with their local protocols when operating in the tactical environment.

The TEMS medical skill set is consistent with, and often expanded from, conventional EMS. Although skill sets may be similar, in TEMS, the application of these skills is often heavily influenced by the tactical situation and mission profile. For example, the use of a laryngeal mask airway (LMA) may be clinically indicated for a casualty under normal operational conditions, but, if the casualty will need to be dragged across a linear danger zone or carried over rough terrain, the LMA is not a secure airway and, therefore, may not be appropriate.

Barriers to Traditional EMS Access

The scene of a law enforcement special operation presents numerous barriers to traditional EMS access. A geographic perimeter is usually secured. Within that perimeter, it is rarely obvious which, if any, areas are safe for EMS passage or for performance of medical activities. It is imperative that the medical components not become a liability to the SWAT team's mission. Already scarce law enforcement resources should not need to be diverted to the medical support mission.

The time interval from EMS arrival on scene to patient contact has been identified as a significant source of delay in the initiation of prehospital care in conventional EMS operations. In one study, the police action required to secure the scene caused delay in 12% of all observed EMS runs and was the source of the longest delay (39 minutes) from time of EMS arrival to patient contact.[10] This type of delay can be much longer during tactical missions. Integrated TEMS programs minimize delays because the TEMS providers routinely function inside the perimeter as a vital part of the tactical team and can begin treatment of wounds within the first moments of an officer being injured.[11,12]

Some fire and rescue chiefs and EMS administrators may object to their personnel practicing tactical medicine because they perceive it to be too dangerous. When asked why fire fighters under their command enter burning buildings—a clearly dangerous situation—they often respond that firefighting is different from law enforcement

---

Box 22-1 Prehospital Care Provider Safety

Just as an emergency medical technician (EMT) or paramedic should not enter the hot zone of a hazardous materials incident or a fire scene without appropriate personal protective equipment and training, the EMT or paramedic must apply proper equipment and training when entering the tactical setting.

---

operations because firefighting personnel are well trained and appropriately equipped against the fire threat. The same argument is true for TEMS (**Box 22-1**).

It is a violation of basic scene safety principles to utilize EMS personnel who are inadequately trained or equipped for the assignment to enter a secure police perimeter that has not been made safe. However, simply waiting for the patient to be delivered outside the perimeter will result in the unnecessary loss of life or function, whereas far-forward (as close to the point of wounding as possible) medical care in the military has been shown to reduce both mortality and morbidity.[13,14] The duration of the Golden Period is different for each injury and each person, and as such every effort must be made to treat casualties as soon as feasible. The obvious solution is for the medical support of law enforcement special operations to be performed by well-trained and properly equipped TEMS providers who can operate safely within the secured operational perimeter. There are many models for forward operating TEMS personnel. Some include TEMS personnel within the "stack" of the entry team. Others place the TEMS providers within the secured perimeter but not in the direct line of fire, usually near the transport vehicles.

Zones of Operation

During tactical missions, the tactical law enforcement team concept of operation divides the target area into zones of operation. The teams establish an **inner perimeter** and **outer perimeter** as geographic boundaries that define the *safe zone* (outside the outer perimeter where no threat should exist), the *warm zone* (between the outer and inner perimeter where the danger of threat could exist), and the **kill zone** (the area that poses an immediate hazard or in which a responder can become a clear target).[15] In many ways, this structure is analogous to the zones of operation at a hazardous materials incident. It is prudent to recognize that the geographic boundaries of the various zones may change as the situation changes, and, as such, TEMS providers must maintain situational awareness to minimize risk to themselves and their patients.

Phases of Care

The TCC guidelines, whether from TCCC or TECC, divide the delivery of emergency medical care into *phases of care*, based on the tactical situation and the associated threat at the time care is being provided (**Table 22-1**).[7]

Whether using the TCCC or TECC guidelines, the care that is provided in each phase is essentially the same. The phases of care are more dynamic, influenced by minute-to-minute threat assessments, and need not be concentric or contiguous; threat levels change rapidly in the tactical environment. Accordingly, the phases of care may not always coincide with the zones of operation. TEMS personnel must understand the relationship of the two paradigms in order to function effectively in a tactical environment (**Box 22-2**).

Care Under Fire (Direct Threat Care)

During **care under fire (CUF)**, the threat is direct and immediate. Limited protection exists for the casualty and the responder. Operations inside this area are extremely dangerous and should be limited to reconnaissance and tactical team operators. Safe operation within the kill zone during CUF requires the use of appropriate personal protective equipment (e.g., ballistic helmets, goggles, vests, shields, boots) and tactical movements (e.g., light/noise discipline, use of cover/concealment). An officer down in the front yard of a home with a barricaded gunman shooting from a window exemplifies a typical CUF.

Casualty care during this phase entails enormous risk and deviates significantly from the principles of conventional EMS. Immediate actions include threat suppression and evacuation of the casualty to cover/concealment. The sooner the threat can be neutralized, the sooner full medical care resources can be brought to bear to treat the casualty. Until that occurs, trying to have the casualty get to cover is appropriate. If the casualty is responsive and able to move, he or she is directed to

Table 22-1 Phases of Care

Tactical Situation	TCCC	TECC
Immediate or active threat	Care under fire	Direct threat care
Threat contained but could resume	Tactical field care	Indirect threat care
No threat	Tactical evacuation care	Evacuation care

Box 22-2 Tactical Combat Casualty Care Guidelines (Tactical Emergency Casualty Care)

Care Under Fire (Direct Threat Care)

1. Maintain tactical supremacy: Neutralize the threat as soon as possible (e.g., directed fire, smoke, threatening posture, fire suppression, hazardous material mitigation).
2. Ensure cover and concealment: Prevent further injury to casualty or rescuer.
3. Use tourniquet for life-threatening extremity hemorrhage.
4. *Do not:*
   a. Perform invasive airway management.
   b. Perform cardiopulmonary resuscitation.
   c. Employ strict spinal precautions.

Tactical Field Care (Indirect Threat Care)

1. Initial care of the patient should follow MARCH criteria:
   a. **M**assive bleeding: Control bleeding (tourniquet, hemostatic dressing, conventional pressure dressing) for life-threatening hemorrhage.
   b. **A**irway: Assess for obstruction and secure airway with body positioning, nasopharyngeal airway, advanced airways, or surgical airway. (This decision will be based on unit training and protocols.)
   c. **R**espirations: Assess and treat for penetrating chest wounds, sucking chest wounds, and tension pneumothoraces.
   d. **C**irculation: Assess for shock. Establish intravenous or intraosseous access, and initiate fluid resuscitation if medically indicated. (This decision will be based on unit training and protocols.)
   e. **H**ead/**H**ypothermia: Protect the casualty from hypothermia. Heat, chemical, or toxic exposures may also be risk factors. Splint any major fracture, and provide cervical spine immobilization for high-risk mechanism of injury.

Tactical Evacuation Care (Evacuation Care)

1. Provide conventional EMS and transport.
2. Ensure clear routes of egress for prehospital care providers and ambulance.
3. Attend to staging considerations.
4. Stay alert for secondary devices and unconventional threats (e.g., flood, crowds, fire).

move to cover. If the casualty cannot move, a plan for possible rescue may be considered. Medical care in this phase of the operation is directed toward reducing further injury to the casualty, avoiding responder injury, subduing the threat, and controlling life-threatening extremity hemorrhage. Time is not spent on cervical spine immobilization for penetrating neck trauma, airway management, or other "heroic" measures such as cardiopulmonary resuscitation (CPR).

Self-aid and buddy aid are critical components of CUF. Most nonlethal penetrating injuries sustained by officers are usually not fully incapacitating and will not necessarily remove the officer from the operation entirely.[16] Data from military operations in Vietnam, Iraq, and Afghanistan indicate that training soldiers in self-aid and buddy aid significantly decreased mortality, a 67% decrease in fatalities from extremity hemorrhage was appreciated after the initiation of early tourniquet use.[14,17] For example, self-application of a tourniquet to a life-threatening ballistic injury to an extremity could save the victim as well as prevent the TEMS providers from unnecessarily exposing themselves to hostile fire.

Direct pressure and pressure dressings are difficult to perform in a CUF tactical setting and may result in unnecessary blood loss and delay in the evacuation of the casualty to cover. *Tourniquet use for control of extremity hemorrhage is the gold standard during the CUF phase*, with the benefits of stopping the bleeding clearly outweighing the low risk of nerve or vascular damage.[18] The tourniquet should be placed over the clothing as "high and tight" on the extremity as possible. It is vital to ensure that arterial blood flow has been stopped. Nonextremity and junctional wounds are difficult to treat in this phase. An attempt should be made to provide direct pressure to these wounds as the casualty is rapidly moved to a covered position and treatment transitions into the tactical field care phase.

Tactical Field Care (Indirect Threat Care)

During the **tactical field care** phase, threats may continue to exist but are not direct or immediate. For example, in the case of the tactical officer down in the front yard, tactical field care principles would apply once the casualty has been moved behind adequate cover (e.g., a thick brick wall out of the gunman's line of sight) or the threat has been suppressed (**Figure 22-1**). Threat levels vary significantly in this phase of the operation, mandating a flexible and fluid medical response. The TEMS provider must be capable of analyzing dynamic factors, rapidly acquiring data, and quickly weighing all medical decisions in terms of the risks to self and the casualty. In a TEMS scenario, the relatively secure environment may return to a CUF situation at any point.

During tactical field care, if tactically appropriate, care should include a rapid trauma assessment by exposing and

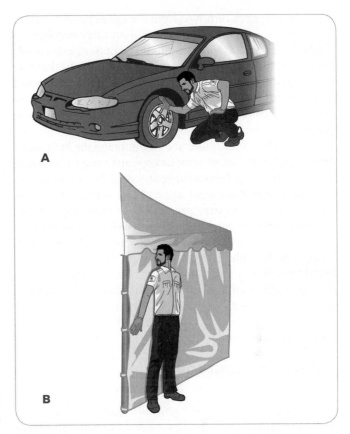

Figure 22-1 A. An example of cover. **B.** An example of concealment.

Courtesy CPL Matt Cain, Ventura Police Department.

assessing all injuries. Interventions should focus on quickly stabilizing the major causes of preventable traumatic death in the tactical environment: compressible hemorrhage, tension pneumothorax, simple airway compromise, and hypothermia.[16,17] The MARCH algorithm should be applied rapidly and initially during tactical field care to address immediate TEMS concerns and stratify the casualty's injuries in order of importance.

Hemorrhage Control

Control of compressible external hemorrhage during tactical field care is critical. Compressible severe external hemorrhage can usually be quickly controlled and should be the first priority. Tourniquets are the first-line treatment of choice for potentially life-threatening extremity hemorrhage when and where application is possible. Any tourniquet placed on an extremity during the CUF phase should be reevaluated to determine the need for its continued use. If bleeding from the injury is determined to not be life threatening, transitioning from a tourniquet to an appropriate pressure dressing may be performed. If the bleeding is life threatening, a tourniquet should be placed "high and tight" in the groin or armpit above the injury, directly on the skin and free of any clothing. It should be placed as snugly as possible, with as much slack removed from the tail as possible before the windlass is tightened. No more than three revolutions (540 degrees) of the windlass should be performed to avoid deforming the chassis of the device.[19] In the event that one tourniquet does not stop the bleeding, it is acceptable and highly recommended to use additional tourniquets side by side until bleeding is controlled, as this provides compression of the artery over a wider area.[17,19]

The current TCCC guidelines recommend the hemostatic dressing Combat Gauze with Celox Gauze and ChitoGauze as alternatives for hemorrhage in areas not amenable to tourniquet use. After application of any of these dressings, 3 minutes of direct firm pressure should be applied.[20-26] Providers should not use older powder- or granule-type agents, as they have been shown to cause thermal burns, foreign body emboli, and *endothelial* (internal lining of blood vessels) toxicity.[27] As a result, it is recommended to use a packable hemostatic-impregnated gauze for wounds to transition zones (i.e., neck, axilla, and groin). The use of hemostatic agents must be approved in advance by the unit's medical director.

Airway Management

Airway management during this phase of care is appropriate if the casualty shows signs of impending airway obstruction or cardiovascular collapse. In conscious casualties with an intact gag reflex, it is recommended that they be allowed to sit up and forward to preserve their own airway. In unconscious casualties, with or without signs of airway compromise, a trauma jaw thrust followed shortly after by a nasopharyngeal airway (NPA) is recommended as a first-line option. After inserting the NPA, place the casualty into the recovery position to maintain the open airway and prevent aspiration of secretions (**Figure 22-2**). If airway

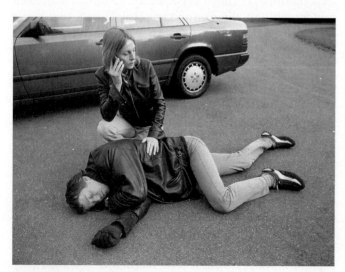

Figure 22-2 A patient who has been placed in the recovery position.
© Cordelia Molloy/Science Photo Library/Science Source.

obstruction develops or persists despite the use of an NPA, a properly trained TEMS provider may consider inserting an endotracheal tube or supraglottic airway device as the tactical situation allows. These devices are not well tolerated unless the casualty is **obtunded**.

In some cases, a surgical cricothyroidotomy may be indicated. Casualties with airway compromise due to maxillofacial trauma or inhalation burns often warrant a cricothyroidotomy as the first-line airway procedure of choice.[6,17,28] TCCC recommends the CricKey device for emergency cricothyrotomy, and recent data have shown 100% success rates in cadaver models with combat medics trained to perform this procedure.[29-31] A cricothyroidotomy is a highly advanced and rarely performed procedure, and training is absolutely crucial to its success. It is up to the TEMS medical director to perform, train, and authorize this intervention, and only a select group of providers—often only physicians—will perform this procedure. In no U.S. region or state is a cricothyroidotomy within the normal scope of paramedic or EMT practice at this time.

Breathing Management

The management of blunt and penetrating chest trauma is especially important for TEMS providers. In particular, the TEMS provider must be comfortable treating penetrating chest wounds and tension pneumothoraces. Cover all open or sucking penetrating wounds on the torso from the lower neck to the umbilicus with an occlusive dressing; numerous different materials are available for improvised use as well as commercially fabricated chest seals, many with excellent adhesive properties. Vented chest seals are preferred and are the recommended option to minimize the risk of developing tension pneumothoraces in sucking chest wounds.

In a casualty with penetrating chest trauma and progressive respiratory distress, it is reasonable to presume the presence of a tension pneumothorax and perform a needle decompression (NDC) on the side of the penetrating trauma to stabilize the patient.[32] Do not rely on findings such as tracheal shift or jugular vein distension, as these signs are late findings and not always present in an early tension pneumothorax or may be difficult to detect in a tactical setting. Even the gold standard of determining absent breath sounds may not be possible in many tactical environments; increasing respiratory distress in the presence of penetrating thoracic trauma is enough to justify performing NDC (**Box 22-3**).

Treat a tension pneumothorax by inserting a 14-gauge (or larger), 3.25-inch (8-centimeter [cm])-long needle with catheter into the casualty's fourth or fifth intercostal space at the anterior axillary line, or alternatively, the second intercostal space at the midclavicular line lateral to the nipple and pointed away from the heart.[33,34] A casualty with penetrating chest trauma, even if a tension pneumothorax is not present, will generally have some degree of hemothorax or pneumothorax as a result of the primary wound. The additional trauma caused by an NDC will not worsen the casualty's condition in the absence of a tension pneumothorax. Successful NDC is confirmed by improvement in the casualty's respiratory status and, if conditions allow, by hearing a rush of air through the decompression needle as the pressure within the chest is relieved.

It is the TCCC recommendation to use a 14-gauge, 8-cm needle and leave the catheter buried to the hub in the casualty.[33-35] The TEMS provider must monitor the casualty after the procedure to ensure the catheter has not become dislodged or clotted with blood and that respiratory distress symptoms have not returned. If respiratory distress symptoms return or the catheter becomes obstructed or dislodged, flush the catheter or perform a second NDC adjacent to the first.[17] After an NDC is performed, proper documentation of the indications for the procedure is important, as the casualty will require a subsequent chest tube or further interventions. One last recommendation is that bilateral NDC should be performed prior to discontinuing resuscitation when a casualty with torso trauma or polytrauma suffers prehospital cardiopulmonary arrest.[20]

Hypothermia

Hypothermia in trauma patients is an independent predictor of mortality.[36] Trauma patients are at high risk for hypothermia, which can occur regardless of the ambient temperature. The longer a patient is exposed to the environment during treatment and evacuation, especially in wet conditions, the more likely the development of hypothermia.[37,38] The TEMS provider must minimize the casualty's exposure to the elements. Whenever possible, replace or remove any wet or bloody clothing. Use any methods available to keep the casualty warm, such as dry blankets, jackets, and sleeping bags. If practical, keep all protective gear on the casualty after ensuring that all injuries have been treated, as this gear will afford protection to the casualty should hostile fire erupt again. TCCC guidelines recommend a Hypothermia Prevention and Management Kit (HPMK) to combat heat loss in TEMS casualties; the HPMK has been shown to help mitigate heat loss effectively.[38]

Vascular Access and Prehospital Fluid Management

Many studies show the benefit of hypotensive ("balanced") resuscitation in trauma patients (see the Shock: Pathophysiology of Life and Death chapter for a detailed discussion).[39,40] Accordingly, delayed intravenous (IV) access is acceptable in certain tactical scenarios. Obtain IV access during the tactical field care phase if medically indicated. While traditional trauma training teaches starting IV lines, the use of a single 18-gauge catheter is adequate in the tactical setting; providers must first strive to do no harm and to minimize delays, especially in the tactical setting. The 18-gauge catheter is adequate for rapid delivery of resuscitation fluids, medication is easier to insert, and supplies available in a medic aid bag are conserved. An IV should not be attempted on an extremity that may have a significant wound proximal to the IV insertion site. The use of a "ruggedized" IV securing system is advisable if the casualty has to be transported a distance before the hand-off to conventional EMS.

If the casualty requires fluid resuscitation or IV medications and IV access cannot be obtained, intraosseous (IO) access is an alternative, as permitted by the TEMS medical director. IO devices are available for use on the sternum and extremities in the absence of a significant injury to the selected site. As with most advanced medical interventions, this procedure requires a strict training program to instill confidence and competence in the TEMS provider. Civilian TEMS injury patterns allow for IO access in both upper and lower extremities with more frequency than military injury patterns. Therefore, it may be appropriate to use the tibial approach for the establishment of the IO line.[41,42] While the proximal humerus can be used, it has been noted that during movement of the casualty in the tactical environment, the location of the IO device at the widest part of the body can easily lead to inadvertent dislodgment.[41-43]

Based on currently accepted hypotensive resuscitation protocols and damage control resuscitation, fluid administration should be reserved for casualties experiencing hemorrhagic shock, as indicated by altered mental status in the absence of a head injury and a weak or absent radial pulse (**Box 22-4**). These findings are indicative of significant blood loss and advanced stages of shock and, coupled with the absence of blood product availability, warrant the administration of fluid.[17,28]

Tactical field care and TEMS have seen much change in the past several years in the realm of fluid management. The choice of resuscitation fluid depends in large part on local protocol and preference. With the advent of whole blood and blood products into the prehospital area, previous recommendations to provide extensive crystalloid fluid administration have been removed. When possible, whole blood is the recommended transfusion strategy in

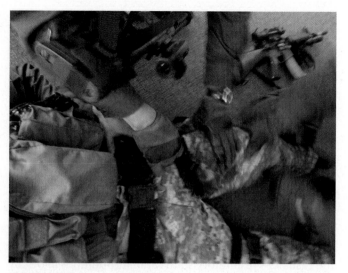

Figure 22-3 Care under fire and extraction.
Courtesy Commander Al Davis, Ventura Police Department.

hemorrhage management.[44-47] Second to this is the transfusion of red blood cells, platelets, and plasma in a 1:1:1 ratio.[48,49] Indeed, large volumes of crystalloid fluid have been shown to worsen outcomes in casualties with large volumes of blood loss.[50,51] Hence, the recommendation is to avoid extensive fluid resuscitation in the field and, along the lines of TCCC recommendations, begin with whole blood as the preferred option and end with crystalloids as a last resort.

Extraction and Evacuation of Casualties

Extraction is the removal of the casualty from the hot to the warm zone (from within the inner perimeter), while evacuation is from the area within the outer perimeter (warm zone) to the cold zone. Casualty extraction is a physically demanding process that interrupts mission flow and potentially places the tactical team in jeopardy during the extraction process from exposure to hostile fire while in a vulnerable situation dealing with a casualty.

Prior to extracting any casualty, the TEMS provider should analyze the transit risk and likelihood of casualty survival. This is a joint decision made with the team leader and ultimately is the decision of the team leader in charge of the overall mission and is influenced by location of injury, weapon of injury, and time of injury.[52] The time required to move a casualty to the safe zone is influenced by the ability of the casualty to assist, the distance involved, the casualty's gear load, relative threat levels of the area, and physical fitness of the team. In some situations, the perpetrator may have a commanding field of fire, creating large unsafe areas, as is the case with the opening scenario. In many civilian tactical operations, the target of the mission may only be one or two perpetrators in a relatively confined location. Missions of these types include high-threat warrant service, narcotics interdiction, and dignitary protection details. These missions tend to be accomplished quickly, with the perpetrator(s) taken into custody or subdued. In these cases, once the area is secured, quick advancement to tactical field care and then to "normal, everyday" EMS care takes place.

The second component of transit risk is the route of travel. Zones of fire are irregularly shaped, noncontiguous geographic areas with dynamic risk levels. Extraction may require crossing linear danger zones, in which case the value of treating in place must be weighed against the need for immediate advanced lifesaving interventions. Commanders must consider their resources prior to initiating a rescue mission. Multiple factors play a role in these high-threat rescues and have historically involved ineffective and unrealistic methods that ultimately increase the risk of unnecessary injury and death. Asymmetric rescues require multiple personnel, potentially specialized equipment (e.g., poleless litter, harnesses, drag straps), and aggressive protective posture prior to implementing egress options (**Figure 22-3**).[53]

Finally, TEMS providers must consider their ability to deliver care during transit; for example, during rapid litter movements across a substantial zone of fire, TEMS providers may not be able to maintain a manual trauma jaw thrust. In this case, inserting an airway adjunct prior to movement may be prudent. The transit risk, or risk of moving a casualty through a potential zone of fire, is related to the time it takes to traverse the zone and the risks associated with both the route of travel and those risks incurred from providing essential care during transit. As with most decisions in the tactical environment, experience and judgment are critical.

Rapid and Remote Assessment Methodology (RAM)

The **Rapid and Remote Assessment Methodology (RAM)** was developed by the CONTOMS Program at the Uniformed Services University of the Health Sciences, the U.S. Department of Defense's medical school.[53] The principal purpose of this assessment algorithm is to maximize the opportunity to extract and treat a salvageable casualty while minimizing risk to TEMS providers from attempting an unnecessary rescue, and the algorithm is most applicable during the CUF phase of TCC (**Figure 22-4**). Unnecessary rescues fall into two categories: those in which the casualty can extract himself or herself and those in which the casualty is already dead (more appropriately termed a "body recovery"). The RAM provides an organized approach to evaluate the totality of circumstances from a protected position before recommending a rescue attempt to the commander.

The first step in conducting a RAM is to determine if the area is secure. If it is, standard EMS care is appropriate after ensuring that the casualty cannot harm TEMS providers. If the area is not secure, use available intelligence to determine whether the casualty is a perpetrator or otherwise represents a threat. Under such circumstances, *no further medical intervention is indicated until the threat has been controlled.* To do otherwise might jeopardize the safety of tactical officers, TEMS providers, and innocent parties. If the casualty is not deemed a perpetrator, a **remote assessment** should be initiated to attempt to evaluate the nature of the injury and the stability of the casualty's condition.

Remote observation is the first technique to be employed during the remote assessment because it allows TEMS providers to gather information without revealing their position or intent to the hostile force. Technology available to SWAT teams can improve the reliability of this assessment. For example, a good pair of binoculars or night-vision goggles can often help to ascertain if the casualty is breathing, the rate and quality of respiration, the presence of life-threatening hemorrhage, and the presence of obvious wounds incompatible with life. In cold weather, a respiratory condensation plume can often be seen from the casualty's mouth if the casualty is breathing. Acoustic surveillance equipment, if available, can be deployed to detect speech, moans, groans, and even respiratory sounds. Thermal imaging technology has improved in recent years and may be considered for application in the RAM.

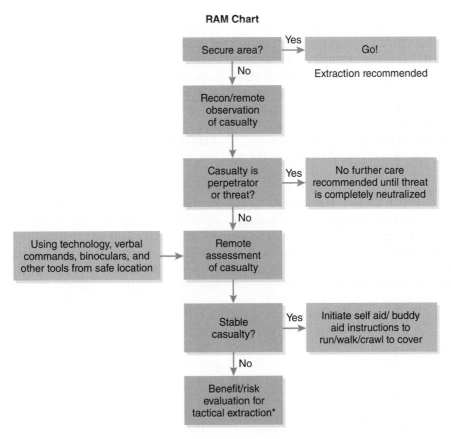

*The benefit/risk evaluation of tactical extraction will depend on the likelihood of survival of casualty. The decision will ultimately be made by the swat commander with significant medical input from the TEMS provider.

Figure 22-4 Rapid and Remote Assessment Methodology (RAM) flow chart.

If the casualty appears stable, self-care instructions and reassurance should be communicated to the casualty, if possible, and medical extraction should await an improvement in the tactical situation. A tactical extraction of the casualty may be determined to be optimal by the commander at any time, but the situation and not the casualty's medical stability should primarily inform this decision. If the casualty is unstable, the risk of extraction must be weighed against the benefits of immediate access to medical care. Although this is a command decision, the commander will rely heavily on the TEMS provider's assessment of the patient's condition and the need for immediate extraction. If the benefit–risk ratio is sufficiently high, the extraction may proceed.

Although the algorithm seems logical it is crucial to have a decision structure that fosters good assessment before emotion overtakes reason and a needless rescue is risked. The military experience is filled with examples of numerous casualties incurred to recover a body or attempt to rescue a casualty who eventually stood up and ran to cover without assistance.[54]

Additional Considerations

Common conventional EMS interventions may be inappropriate in the tactical situation—in particular, cervical spine immobilization and CPR. Cervical spine immobilization is a time-consuming intervention with relatively little value in penetrating trauma.[55,56] An experienced two-person paramedic team requires on average 5.5 minutes to properly perform cervical spine immobilization. This time delay and exposure may be deadly, not only for the casualty but also for the TEMS providers. Accordingly, if the threat of further injury outweighs the risk of spinal injury, cervical spine immobilization should be deferred. However, blunt injury from falls or motor vehicle collisions, in the context of an unreliable physical examination, is a high-risk exception and warrants consideration for cervical spine immobilization if the tactical situation allows.

CPR provides little benefit in traumatic arrest and increases responder exposure.[56] Accordingly, CPR has a very limited role in tactical medical response, and its consideration should be reserved for victims of near-drowning, electrocution, hypothermia, and some toxic exposures.

The diminished emphasis on cervical spine immobilization, CPR, IV access, and fluid management in both phases of care under fire and tactical field care illustrates some of the distinctions between TEMS and conventional EMS. These examples are not meant to substitute for the clinical judgment of the TEMS provider.

Analgesia Considerations

One area of brief consideration is that of TEMS pain management. Early TEMS providers initially used morphine and titrated, as needed, the frequency and dosage during prehospital missions. However, after discovering the potential use for oral transmucosal fentanyl, this medication was added to the TCCC guidelines for mild to moderate pain in casualties with no compromise in airway or mental status.[57,58] Ketamine is another exceptional medication with a wide scope of use and limited contraindications and was added to TCCC guidelines in 2012. Ketamine is not known to cause drops in blood pressure or in respiration rate or effort, nor is it contraindicated in unconscious or obtunded individuals.[57,59] Most operators and casualties requiring analgesia, dissociative amnesia, and procedural sedation can benefit greatly from ketamine use. In 2014 TCCC developed a triple option analgesia approach that can be recommended in the civilian realm as well.[59] Initially, oral medications (e.g., NSAIDs, acetaminophen) are recommended for mild pain with a continually functional member of the team. With moderate pain but without risk of shock or deterioration, oral transmucosal fentanyl is recommended. Finally, if severe pain is suffered by the casualty, and he or she is at risk for or is experiencing shock or pulmonary compromise, ketamine is the agent of choice.[57-59] Recommendations are dependent on local area availability, preference, and the discretion of the TEMS medical director.

Tactical Evacuation Care (Evacuation Care)

Tactical evacuation care takes place in the operational safe zone, beyond the outer perimeter, and is an area of relatively low risk. The outer perimeter isolates the incident and is typically manned by conventional law enforcement patrol personnel with the primary mission of scene control, event isolation, and general public safety. During the tactical evacuation care phase, medical care continues during transport to the receiving trauma center. Akin to conventional EMS care of the trauma patient, it may include the transfer of the casualty to an ambulance or the use of alternative emergency vehicles such as an armored vehicle (**Figure 22-5**). Care during this phase is situation-dependent and based on team standard operating procedures and incident commander decisions. At the incident commander's discretion and as necessary, medical control may be established out of reach of the weapons being used by the perpetrator(s), and additional EMS medical resources may stage in this area.

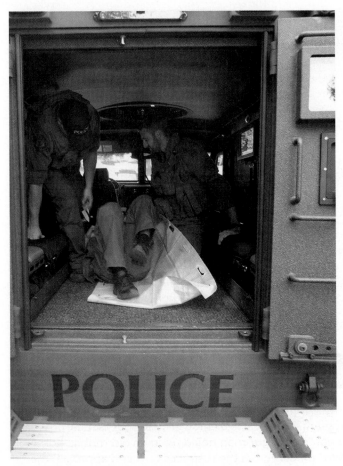

Figure 22-5 Nonstandard tactical evacuation care vehicle.
Courtesy Commander Al Davis, Ventura Police Department.

In the event alternative emergency vehicles are used in transporting the casualty, standard operating procedures should be rehearsed in depth to include the roles of team members who have no medical training. Additional medical equipment should be staged in these vehicles, and all team members should be cross-trained in treating the four preventable causes of death (hemorrhage, airway obstruction, pneumothoraces, and hypothermia) by administering lifesaving interventions such as using tourniquets, NPAs, and chest seals and preventing hypothermia.

Even in an area deemed secure, all emergency responders must remain vigilant. Tactical operations are complex and dynamic. During the 1999 Columbine High School shootings, the assailants targeted emergency responders by placing pipe bombs and improvised explosive devices. Fortunately, due to technical failures, these devices did not detonate. Similarly, the perpetrator of the 2012 Aurora, Colorado, movie theater shooting prepared and placed explosives in his apartment. These devices included trip wires and booby traps with flammable material capable

of killing officers responding to the scene and destroying the building. All of these devices were handled by astute law enforcement personnel without injury.

The FBI has reported several incidents of intentional ambushes of law enforcement personnel, which continue to be on the rise. In addition, terrorist training manuals have been found that explicitly detail operations that use a barricaded suspect to lure law enforcement personnel to a scene in order to ambush them. Diligence and situational awareness are the cornerstones to safe operations by responding law enforcement officers and TEMS providers.

Mass-Casualty Incidents

Mass-casualty incidents (MCIs) involving active shooters are increasingly common and dangerous, and they present a complex interagency collaboration challenge. The Pulse nightclub shooting in Orlando, Florida, represents one tragic example. TEMS providers have a unique role to play in these MCI events. First, TEMS teams tend to bridge law enforcement with fire departments and/or EMS systems. Second, TEMS providers are trained to work in chaotic, dangerous, and resource-poor environments. Third, TEMS providers have broad experience in utilization of various communication mediums, immediate action drills, and mission planning. TEMS providers must be the medical linchpins in a coordinated MCI response system.[34]

Medical Intelligence

Part of the role of the TEMS provider is preplanning, gathering, and maintaining medical intelligence. On local and regional teams, the TEMS provider should have an in-depth knowledge of the local EMS and trauma systems. This knowledge will allow the TEMS provider to make appropriate decisions regarding evacuation care and patient destination if a casualty should occur on the mission. TEMS teams that function remotely in unknown areas, such as wilderness locations, will have to conduct much more in-depth medical planning to develop an operable evacuation plan and extended care plan.

The role of aeromedical evacuation platforms in TEMS may be of great use; however, the TEMS provider must constantly monitor the availability of dedicated aeromedical assets. In addition, the response of an aeromedical evacuation platform to a tactical situation must include appropriate safety precautions to prevent the aeromedical unit from coming under hostile fire.

SUMMARY

- In general, the principles of medical care in the tactical environment are the same as those to which prehospital care providers are accustomed.
- The austerity and danger of the operational environment require that the benefit of every medical intervention be weighed against the risks inherent in delivering that intervention. This determination requires a unique set of decision-making skills.
- The TEMS provider constantly needs to balance the benefit of a particular intervention against the special risks inherent in performing the intervention in this environment.
- The three phases of care in the tactical situation are:

  - Care under fire (direct threat care)—the medical care that is provided while under hostile fire or in an actively hazardous situation
  - Tactical field care (indirect threat care)—the medical care that is provided once the immediate hazard has been suppressed or controlled, knowing that the situation could revert to care under fire
  - Tactical evacuation care (evacuation care)—the medical care that is provided once the situation has been deemed safe, very similar to a standard civilian EMS call
- Medical intelligence gathering allows the TEMS provider to know the environment, geography, and available resources of the area in which the tactical operation will be undertaken.

SCENARIO RECAP

Your emergency medical services (EMS) agency provides coverage for the local special weapons and tactics (SWAT) team and has a rigorous, integrated training program with local law enforcement. Your tactical emergency medical support (TEMS) team is called out for a barricaded gunman holed up in an old mobile home just after sunset. As you are preparing for entry, two SWAT officers cross the suspect's yard and approach the house to prepare for a door pull. Shots ring out from the front window, wounding the SWAT officers. One SWAT officer falls in the doorway of the suspect's home. The second falls near an old pickup truck. A patrol officer standing near you yells, "We need to go get them. Come on!" You grab the patrol officer by the arm and look to the SWAT commander.

- What should your actions be?
- How will you assess and treat the fallen SWAT officers given the danger of the scene?

SCENARIO SOLUTION

The SWAT commander orders you to use your Rapid and Remote Assessment Methodology (RAM) to determine the utility of a rescue effort. You use your binoculars and the SWAT team acoustic device to examine the two fallen officers. The first officer, lying in the doorway of the gunman's mobile home, shows no chest wall movement or signs of respiration around his mouth. Despite calls from his fellow officers, you are unable to detect any audible response on the acoustic device.

The second officer has moved behind the engine block of the old pickup truck. You can visualize bleeding from his lower thigh. Fortunately, you have conducted extensive tactical medical training for your officers. You communicate with him via the secure team radio and instruct him to apply a tourniquet high and tight around his groin region. He secures the device and communicates that he has no further injuries.

Based on your recommendation and the threat assessment, the SWAT commander chooses not to undertake a high-risk rescue of the officer showing no signs of life. You remain in contact with the second injured officer while the negotiators work to convince the suspect to surrender. You contact the local trauma center and inform them of a potential incoming casualty. Thirty minutes later, the suspect surrenders and is taken into custody. Your team evacuates the casualty to the local hospital where he undergoes a vascular repair, saving both his leg and his life.

References

1. Rinnert KJ, Hall WL. Tactical emergency medical support. *Emerg Med Clin N Am*. 2002;20:929-952.
2. Federal Bureau of Investigation. Uniform crime reports. https://ucr.fbi.gov/leoka. Accessed February 16, 2018.
3. National Tactical Officers Association. Position statement on the inclusion of physicians in tactical law enforcement operations. https://www.ntoa.org/sections/tems/tems-position-statement/. Accessed February 16, 2018.
4. Heck JJ, Pierluisi G. Law enforcement special operations and medical support. *Prehosp Emerg Care*. 2001;5:403-406.
5. American College of Emergency Physicians. Policy statement on tactical emergency medical support. *Ann Emerg Med*. 2005;45:108.
6. McSwain NE, Salomone JP, Pons PT, eds. *Prehospital Trauma Life Support Manual*. 7th ed. St. Louis, MO: Mosby; 2011.
7. Callaway DW, Reed S, Shapiro G, et al. The Committee for Tactical Emergency Care (C-TECC): evolution and application of TCCC guidelines to civilian high threat medicine. *J Special Operations Med*. 2011;11:2.
8. Callaway DW. Personal communication; 2012.
9. Massachusetts Department of Public Health. *Emergency Medical Services Pre-hospital Treatment Protocols*. Version 7.02, Appendix U. https://www.mypatrioteducation.com/classes/protocols_702/treatment_protocols_702.pdf. Published February 1, 2008. Accessed November 6, 2017.
10. Campbell JP, Gratton MC, Salomone JA III, et al. Ambulance arrival to patient contact: the hidden component of prehospital response time intervals. *Ann Emerg Med*. 1993;22:1254.
11. Kanable R. Peak performance: well-trained tactical medics can help the team perform at its best. *Law Enforcement Tech*. August 1999.
12. Cooke, MC. How much to do at the accident scene? *BMJ*. 1999;319:1150.
13. Jagoda A, Pietrzek M, Hazen S, et al. Prehospital care and the military. *Mil Med*. 1992;157:11.
14. Bellamy RF. The causes of death in conventional land warfare: implications for combat casualty care research. *Mil Med*. 1984;149:55.
15. Callaway DW. Tactical emergency services. In: Hogan DE, Burstein JL, eds. *Disaster Medicine*. 2nd ed. Philadelphia, PA: Lippincott, Williams and Wilkins; 2007.
16. Gerold KB, Gibbons M, McKay S. The relevance of Tactical Combat Casualty Care (TCCC) guidelines to civilian law enforcement operations. National Tactical Officers TEMS Overview. https://www.east.org/content/documents/MilitaryResources/TCCC/TCCC.pdf. Updated November 1, 2009. Accessed November 6, 2017.
17. Parsons, DL, Mott JC. *Tactical Combat Casualty Care Handbook: Observations, Insights, and Lessons*. Fort Leavenworth, KS: Center for Army Lessons Learned; 2012.
18. Kragh JF, Walters TJ, Baer DG, et al. Survival with emergency tourniquet use to stop bleeding in major limb trauma. *Ann Surg*. 2009;249(1):1-7.
19. Kragh JF, O'Neill ML, Walters TJ, et al. The military emergency tourniquet program's lessons learned with devices and designs. *Mil Med*. 2011;176:10, 1144.
20. Butler FK, Giebner SD, McSwain N, et al., eds. *Prehospital Trauma Life Support*. Military 8th ed. Burlington, MA: Jones & Bartlett Learning; 2014.
21. Bennett BL, Littlejohn LF, Kheirabadi BS, et al. Management of external hemorrhage in Tactical Combat Casualty Care: chitosan-based hemostatic gauze dressings. *J Spec Oper Med*. 2014;14:12-29.
22. Bennett BL, Littlejohn L. Review of new topical hemostatic dressings for combat casualty care. *Mil Med*. 2014;179:497-514.
23. Littlejohn L, Bennett B, Drew B. Application of current hemorrhage control techniques for backcountry care: part 2: hemostatic dressings and other adjuncts. *Wilderness Environ Med*. 2015;26:246-254.
24. Drew B, Bennett B, Littlejohn L. Application of current hemorrhage control techniques for backcountry care. Part 1: tourniquets and hemorrhage control adjuncts. *Wilderness Environ Med*. 2015;26:236-245.
25. Kheirabadi BS, Edens JW, Terrazas IB, et al. Comparison of new hemostatic granules/powders with currently deployed hemostatic products in a lethal model of extremity arterial hemorrhage in swine. *J Trauma*. 2009;66:316-326.
26. Kheirabadi B, Mace J, Terrazas I, et al. Safety evaluation of new hemostatic agents, smectite granules, and kaolin-coated gauze in a vascular injury wound model in swine. *J Trauma*. 2010;68:269-278.
27. Kheirabadi BS, Edens JW, Terrazas IB, et al. Comparison of new hemostatic granules/powders with currently deployed hemostatic products in a lethal model of extremity arterial hemorrhage in swine. *J Trauma*. 2009;66(2):316-326; discussion 327-328.
28. Butler FK Jr, Hagmann J, Butler EG. Tactical combat casualty care in special operations. *Mil Med*. 1996;161(suppl):3-16.
29. Mabry R, Frankfurt A, Kharod C, et al. Emergency cricothyroidotomy in Tactical Combat Casualty Care. *J Spec Oper Med*. 2015;15:11-9.
30. Hessert MJ, Bennett BL. Optimizing emergent surgical cricothyrotomy for use in austere environments. *Wilderness Environ Med*. 2013;24:53-66.
31. Mabry R, Nichols M, Shiner D, et al. A comparison of two open surgical cricothyroidotomy techniques by military medics using a cadaver model. *Ann Emerge Med*. 2014;63:1-5.
32. Tien HC, Jung V, Riool SB, et al. An evaluation of tactical combat casualty care interventions in a combat environment. *J Am Coll Surg*. 2008;207(2):174-178.
33. Hacked HT, Parse LA, Levy AD, et al. Chest wall thickness in military personnel: implications for needle thoracentesis in tension pneumothorax. *Mil Med*. 2008;172:1260-1263.
34. Zengerink I, Brink PR, Laupland KB, et al. Needle thoracostomy in the treatment of tension pneumothorax in trauma patients: what size needle? *J Trauma*. 2008;64:111-114.
35. Givens ML, Ayotte K, Manifold C. Needle thoracostomy: implications of computed tomography chest wall thickness. *Acad Emerg Med*. 2004;11:211-213.
36. Zafren K, Giesbrecht GG, Danzl DF, et al. Wilderness Medical Society practice guidelines for the out-of-hospital evaluation and treatment of accidental hypothermia: 2014 update. *Wilderness Environ Med*. 2014;25(suppl):S66-S85.

37. McKeague AL. Evaluation of patient active warming systems. Military Health System Research Symposium, Tactical Combat Casualty Care breakout session. Ft. Lauderdale, FL. August 2012.

38. Allen PB, Salyer SW, Dubick MA, et al. Preventing hypothermia: comparison of current devices used by the U.S. Army in an in vitro warmed fluid model. *J Trauma*. 2010;69(suppl 1):S154-S161.

39. Revell M, Greaves I, Porter K. Endpoints for fluid resuscitation in hemorrhagic shock. *J Trauma*. 2003;54(suppl 5): S63-S67.

40. Morrison CA, Carrick MM, Norman MA, et al. Hypotensive resuscitation strategy reduces transfusion requirements and severe postoperative coagulopathy in trauma patients with hemorrhagic shock: preliminary results of a randomized controlled trial. *J Trauma*. 2011;70(3):652-663.

41. Benson G. Intraosseous access to the circulatory system: an under-appreciated option for rapid access. *J Perioper Pract*. 2015;25:140-143.

42. Byars DV, Tsuchitani SN, Erwin E, et al. Evaluation of success rate and access time for an adult sternal intraosseous device deployed in the prehospital setting. *Prehosp Disaster Med*. 2011;26:127-129.

43. Lewis P, Wright C. Saving the critically injured trauma patient: a retrospective analysis of 1000 uses of intraosseous access. *Emerg Med J*. 2015;32:463-467.

44. Spinella P, Pidcoke H, Strandenes G, et al. Whole blood transfusion for hemostatic resuscitation of major bleeding. *Transfusion*. 2016;56:S190-S202.

45. Cap A, Pidcoke H, DePasquale M, et al. Blood far forward: time to get moving! *J Trauma*. 2015;78:S2-S6.

46. Stubbs J, Zielinski M, Jenkins D. The state of the science of whole blood: lessons learned at Mayo Clinic. *Transfusion*. 2016;56:S173-S881.

47. Spinella PC, Perkins JG, Grathwohl KW, et al. Warm fresh whole blood is independently associated with improved survival for patients with combat-related traumatic injuries. *J Trauma*. 2009;66:S69-S76.

48. Holcomb J, Spinella P. Optimal use of blood in trauma patients. *Biologicals*. 2010;38:72-77.

49. Borgman MA, Spinella PC, Perkins JG, et al. The ratio of blood products transfused in patients receiving massive transfusions at a combat support hospital. *J Trauma*. 2007;63: 805-813.

50. Ley E, Clond M, Srour M, et al. Emergency department crystalloid resuscitation of 1.5 L or more is associated with increased mortality in elderly and non-elderly trauma patients. *J Trauma*. 2011;70:398-400.

51. Duke MD, Guidry C, Guice J, et al. Restrictive fluid resuscitation in combination with damage control resuscitation: time for adaptation. *J Trauma*. 2012;73:674-678.

52. McKay S, Hoyne S. High threat immediate extraction: the Immediate Reaction Team (IRT) model. *Tactical Edge*. Spring 2007:50-54.

53. Callaway DW. Emergency medical services in disasters. Hogan DE, Burstein JL, eds. *Disaster Medicine*. 2nd ed. Philadelphia, PA: Lippincott, Williams and Wilkins; 2016:127-139.

54. Cloonan C. *Proceedings of the Third International Conference on Tactical Emergency Medical Support*. Bethesda, MD: Uniformed Services University of the Health Sciences; 1999.

55. Arishita GI, Vayer JS, Bellamy RF. Cervical spine immobilization of penetrating neck wounds in a hostile environment. *J Trauma*. 1989;29:332-337.

56. Rosemary AS, Norris PA, Olson SM, et al. Prehospital traumatic cardiac arrest: the cost of futility. *J Trauma*. 1998;38:468-474.

57. Butler FK, Kotwal RS, Buckenmaier CC III, et al. A triple-option analgesia plan for Tactical Combat Casualty Care. *J Spec Oper Med*. 2014;14:13-25.

58. Kotwal R, O'Connor K, Johnson T, et al. A novel pain management strategy for combat casualty care. *Ann Emerg Med*. 2004;44:121-127.

59. Dickey N, Jenkins D, Butler F. Prehospital use of ketamine in battlefield analgesia. Defense Health Board Memorandum. http://www.specialoperationsmedicine.org/documents /TCCC/06%20TCCC%20Reference%20Documents/DHB%20 Memo%20120308%20Ketamine.pdf. Published March 8, 2012. Accessed November 6, 2017.

Suggested Reading

National Association of Emergency Medical Technicians. *PHTLS: Prehospital Trauma Life Support*. Military 9th ed. Burlington, MA: Jones & Bartlett Learning; 2019.

SPECIFIC SKILLS

Ruggedized Intravenous Line

Principle: To insert and secure an intravenous (IV) line when a trauma patient has to be moved, carried, or transported manually over a distance.

When a trauma patient has to be moved, carried, or manually transported over a distance, IV lines placed in the patient often become dislodged in the effort. The U.S. military has developed a method for initiating and securing IV lines that allows for this kind of movement without loss of the IV access. The skill demonstrated has been modified from the military for civilian application.

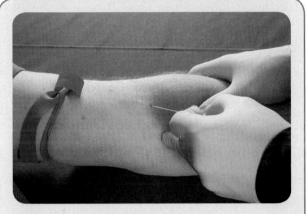

1 The TEMS operator obtains IV access according to the usual procedure, using an 18- or 16-gauge IV catheter.

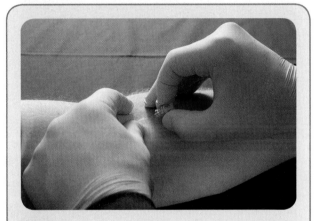

2 The TEMS operator attaches a saline lock to the IV catheter.

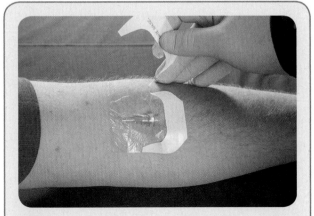

3 The TEMS operator covers the IV catheter and saline lock completely with a transparent wound dressing film (e.g., Tegaderm).

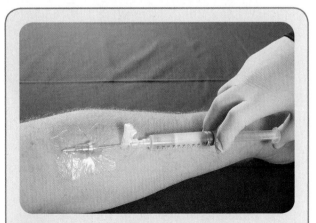

4 The TEMS operator flushes the saline lock with 5 milliliters (ml) of normal saline by puncturing directly through the dressing film and rubber stopper of the saline lock.

(continued)

Ruggedized Intravenous Line *(continued)*

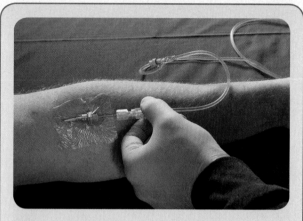

5 The TEMS operator inserts a second IV catheter (18 gauge) directly through the dressing film and rubber stopper of the saline lock and administers fluids and medications through this catheter.

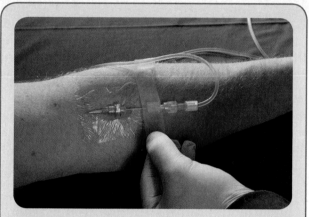

6 The TEMS operator secures the second catheter and attaches the IV line to the arm with circumferential application of a Velcro securing device or tape.

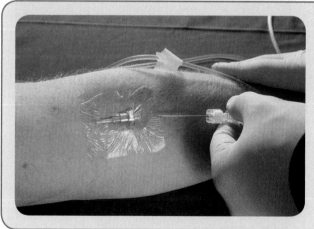

7 If and when the trauma patient must be moved, the securing device or tape, IV line, and second catheter are removed. The primary catheter and saline lock remain in place, thus ensuring rapid IV access once the patient move has been accomplished.

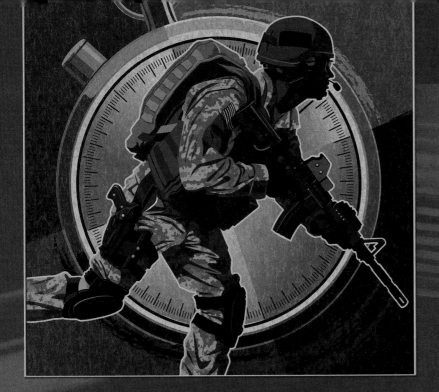

DIVISION **7**

Military Medicine

CHAPTER 23

Introduction to Tactical Combat Casualty Care (TCCC)

Author:
Capt. (Ret) Frank Butler, MD

CHAPTER OBJECTIVES

At the completion of this chapter, you will be able to do the following:

- Describe the transformation in battlefield prehospital trauma care that Tactical Combat Casualty Care (TCCC) has helped to achieve.
- Discuss that the lowest incidence of preventable combat deaths in history has been reported by military units that have trained all unit members in TCCC.
- State the three goals of TCCC.
- List the three phases of TCCC and describe the tactical situation that defines each.
- Describe the membership of the Committee on Tactical Combat Casualty Care (CoTCCC).

- Describe the evidence base for the success of TCCC in helping to avoid preventable deaths.
- Describe how the CoTCCC and the TCCC Working Group succeeded in changing the culture in battlefield trauma care.
- List the U.S. civilian medical organizations that endorse the TCCC Guidelines.
- Describe the transition of TCCC to use in other federal agencies, civilian law enforcement, and civilian EMS settings.

SCENARIO

You are the only medic traveling in a 10-person, four-vehicle convoy through a small village in eastern Iraq. As you pull out on an open road at the end of the village, an improvised explosive device (IED) explodes under the second vehicle. There is no follow-up hostile fire, so the unit sets up a secure perimeter. You proceed to assess the three major casualties at the scene.

Casualty 1 is a soldier with femoral arterial bleeding from a large wound to his right thigh, as well as a right hand amputation with blood oozing from the stump. He is conscious and has a good radial pulse.

Casualty 2 is a soldier with a large open head wound in which mangled gray matter is clearly visible. He is unresponsive, and his breathing is agonal.

Casualty 3 is a civilian bystander with a penetrating injury to his right lower abdomen. He is conscious and in great pain.

(continued)

SCENARIO (CONTINUED)

Evacuation by helicopter is available in 20 minutes, and the flight to the nearest medical treatment facility will take approximately 30 minutes.

· What are some of the considerations in managing these casualties that are not present in most civilian settings?

INTRODUCTION

For U.S. military service members wounded on the battlefield, the most critical phase of care is the period from the time they are injured until they arrive at a medical treatment facility (MTF) capable of providing the surgical care they need. If a casualty survives long enough to reach the care of a combat trauma surgeon, the likelihood is very high that he or she will survive. Almost 90% of our service men and women who die from combat wounds do so before they arrive at an MTF. This fact highlights the importance of the battlefield trauma care provided by combat medics, corpsmen, and pararescuemen (PJs) as well as nonmedical unit members in improving the survival of our country's combat wounded.

Prehospital trauma care on the battlefield varies in many respects from prehospital trauma care as practiced in the civilian sector. The types and severity of the injuries are different from those encountered in civilian settings, and combat medical personnel face multiple additional challenges in caring for their wounded teammates in tactical settings. They must provide care while under hostile fire, often working in the dark, with multiple casualties and limited equipment. In addition, they must often contend with prolonged evacuation times as well as the need for tactical maneuvers superimposed on their efforts to render care. Treatment guidelines developed for the civilian setting do not necessarily translate well to the battlefield. Preventable deaths and unnecessary additional casualties may result if the tactical environment is not considered when developing battlefield trauma care strategies (**Figure 23-1**).

These considerations notwithstanding, at the onset of hostilities in Afghanistan, most U.S. combat medical personnel were being trained using the following civilian-based principles of trauma care:[1]

- Rendering care with no structured consideration of the evolving tactical situation
- No use of tourniquets to control extremity hemorrhage
- Managing external hemorrhage with prolonged direct pressure, precluding the medic from attending to other injuries or rendering care to other casualties
- No use of hemostatic dressings

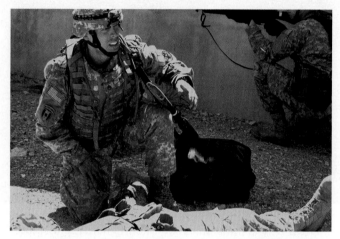

Figure 23-1 Prehospital medicine in the civilian setting differs from the battlefield due to the nature of the environment.
Courtesy of Mr. Jerry Harben/U.S. Army.

- Two large-bore intravenous lines (IVs) started on all patients with significant trauma
- Treatment of hypovolemic shock with large-volume crystalloid fluid resuscitation
- No special considerations for traumatic brain injury (TBI) with respect to avoiding hypotension or hypoxia
- Management of the airway in facial trauma or unconscious casualties with endotracheal intubation
- No specific techniques or equipment to prevent hypothermia and secondary coagulopathy in combat casualties
- Management of pain in combat casualties with intramuscular (IM) morphine—a battlefield analgesic that dates to the Civil War
- No intraosseous (IO) access
- No prehospital electronic monitoring
- No effective nonparenteral analgesic medications
- No prehospital antibiotics
- No delineation of which casualties might benefit most from supplemental oxygen during tactical evacuation
- Spinal precautions applied broadly to casualties with significant trauma, without consideration of tactical concerns or mechanism of injury

Reconsideration of trauma care guidelines for tactical settings had not been accomplished as of 1992, even though the need had long been recognized.[2-4] Tactical Combat Casualty Care (TCCC) is a set of evidence-based, best-practice prehospital trauma care guidelines developed for use on the battlefield. Following the publication of TCCC in 1996,[5] prehospital trauma care in the U.S. military has undergone an unprecedented transformation.

Tourniquets Reconsidered and the Need for TCCC

TCCC began as the result of a Naval Special Warfare biomedical research effort that was undertaken after a striking paradox in battlefield trauma care was identified. Extremity hemorrhage had been reported to be a leading cause of preventable death on the battlefield during the Vietnam conflict.[3,6] Despite this fact, in 1992, U.S. military combat medics, corpsmen, and PJs were not being taught to use a readily available and highly effective treatment for extremity bleeding—a tourniquet.[7-9] This realization led to a systematic review of all aspects of battlefield trauma care. This project was conducted from 1993 to 1996 as a joint effort of Special Operations medical personnel and the Uniformed Services University. This 4-year research effort culminated with the publication of the original TCCC paper in 1996.[5,8,9]

The original TCCC Guidelines provided combat medics and corpsmen with trauma management strategies that combined good medicine with good small-unit tactics. TCCC recognized three goals for trauma care in the tactical environment: (1) *treat the casualty*; (2) *prevent additional casualties*; and (3) *complete the mission*. The original TCCC paper proposed the following:

- A three-phase approach to tactical trauma care to ensure that the care being rendered is tailored to the evolving tactical environment
- Aggressive use of tourniquets to control life-threatening extremity bleeding
- Battlefield antibiotics
- Tactically appropriate fluid resuscitation
- Improved battlefield analgesia (IV vs. IM morphine)
- Nasopharyngeal airways as first-line airway devices
- Surgical airways for maxillofacial trauma with airway obstruction
- Aggressive diagnosis and treatment of tension pneumothorax
- Combat medic input into the TCCC Guidelines
- Scenario-based TCCC training

As the name implies, TCCC is used when casualties are sustained during combat missions. Prehospital trauma care in the military is most commonly provided by enlisted combat medical personnel: medics in the Army, corpsmen in the Navy and Marine Corps, and both medics and pararescuemen (PJs) in the Air Force. TCCC is divided into three phases: Care Under Fire, Tactical Field Care, and Tactical Evacuation Care. In the Care Under Fire phase, combat medical personnel and their units are under effective hostile fire, and the care they can provide to the wounded is very limited. In the Tactical Field Care phase, medical personnel and their casualties are no longer under effective hostile fire, and more extensive care can be provided. Finally, in the Tactical Evacuation Care phase, casualties are transported to a medical facility by an aircraft, ground vehicle, or boat, and there is an opportunity to provide additional medical personnel and equipment to elevate the level of care rendered.

The first TCCC course was taught in 1996 in the Undersea Medical Officer course sponsored by the Navy Bureau of Medicine and Surgery (BUMED). Shortly thereafter, this training was mandated for all SEAL corpsmen.[10] After this introduction, TCCC gradually gained acceptance in U.S.[11-17] and foreign[18] military forces as well as in the civilian law enforcement medical community.[19]

The incorporation of the TCCC Guidelines into the Prehospital Trauma Life Support (PHTLS) course manual was an important milestone in the evolution of TCCC transition. The fourth edition of this manual, published in 1999, contained a chapter on military medicine for the first time, and TCCC was included as part of this chapter.[20] The recommendations contained in the PHTLS textbook carry the endorsement of the American College of Surgeons Committee on Trauma (ACS-COT) and the National Association of Emergency Medical Technicians (NAEMT). TCCC is the only set of battlefield trauma care guidelines ever to have received the endorsements of these internationally respected trauma care organizations and the U.S. Department of Defense (DoD).

The Committee on Tactical Combat Casualty Care and the TCCC Working Group

The need for periodic updates to the TCCC Guidelines was recognized early in the development of TCCC. The original TCCC paper recommended that the TCCC Guidelines be updated as needed by a DoD-sponsored committee established for this purpose.[5] This concept was endorsed by the U.S. Special Operations Command (USSOCOM), and the Committee on Tactical Combat Casualty Care (CoTCCC) was subsequently funded in 2001 as a USSOCOM Biomedical Research Program. The command chosen to execute this project, the Naval Operational Medicine Institute, subsequently conducted the necessary coordination with Navy medicine leaders to ensure that there would be long-term support of this effort. BUMED programmed for financial and personnel support of the CoTCCC beginning in fiscal year 2004. In fiscal years 2007 through 2009, the Office of the Surgeon General of the Army, the U.S. Army Institute of Surgical Research, and the Defense Health Board (DHB) also provided substantial support for the CoTCCC.

CoTCCC Membership

Because the goal of TCCC is to provide the best possible medical care consistent with good small-unit tactics, it is essential that the membership of the CoTCCC include combat medical personnel as well as physicians. It is also critical to have tri-service representation to ensure that differences in doctrine and experience between the Army, Navy, and Air Force medical departments are identified and best practices from each are incorporated into TCCC. The combat medics selected include Navy SEAL corpsmen, Navy corpsmen assigned to Marine units, Ranger medics, Special Forces 18-D medics, Air Force pararescuemen, Air Force aviation medics, and Coast Guard health specialists. Physician membership includes representatives from the trauma surgery, emergency medicine, critical care, and operational medicine communities. Physician assistants, medical planners, and medical educators are also represented.

CoTCCC Alignment

In 2007, due to the increasing visibility of TCCC in the Global War on Terrorism (GWOT), the Navy Medical Support Command proposed that the CoTCCC be moved to a more senior joint command. This proposal was briefed to the offices of the Assistant Secretary of Defense for Health Affairs and the Surgeon for the Joint Chiefs of Staff.

In March 2008, the CoTCCC was relocated to function as a working group of the Trauma and Injury Subcommittee of the Defense Health Board (DHB). The DHB is chartered to provide independent advice and recommendations to the Secretary of Defense through the Under Secretary of Defense for Personnel and Readiness and the Assistant Secretary of Defense for Health Affairs on medical issues, including the care of U.S. service members wounded in combat operations.

Later, on 21 February 2013, by Direction of the Acting Under Secretary of Defense for Personnel and Readiness, the CoTCCC was moved once more, this time to the Joint Trauma System (JTS) to have it co-located with the DoD's combat trauma management system. In 2017, Congress made the JTS the DoD's lead agency for trauma, and the CoTCCC is the prehospital component of the JTS.

TCCC Guideline Updates

Since 2001, and throughout these organizational changes, the CoTCCC has continued to monitor developments in prehospital trauma care. The TCCC Guidelines are updated based on: (1) ongoing review of the published civilian and military prehospital trauma literature; (2) ongoing interaction with military combat casualty care research laboratories; (3) direct input from experienced combat corpsmen, medics, and PJs; (4) input from the service Medical Lessons Learned Centers; (5) case reports discussed at the weekly Joint Theater Trauma System (JTTS) process improvement video teleconferences; (6) observations on the causes of death in combat fatalities gleaned from JTS-Armed Forces Medical Examiner System (AFMES) conferences; and (7) expert opinion from both military and civilian trauma experts.

Each change to the TCCC Guidelines is now supported by a change paper published in the *Journal of Special Operations Medicine*. Guideline changes are also included in revisions of the PHTLS textbook.[21,22]

As the use of TCCC spread from the U.S. military to other agencies within the federal government, allied nations, and the civilian sector, it became important to include representatives from these groups in the TCCC update process, both to secure the benefit of their input and to facilitate communication between them and the CoTCCC. Accordingly, the CoTCCC began to invite liaison members from these groups to participate in its combat trauma care performance improvement process. The CoTCCC voting members and CoTCCC liaison members collectively comprise the TCCC Working Group, and it is through the untiring efforts of this group that the TCCC Guidelines and other TCCC knowledge products have remained state of the art through 16 years of conflict.[8,21]

Although the TCCC Guidelines are best-practice trauma care guidelines customized for use on the battlefield, they are only guidelines. There are no rigid protocols in combat, including TCCC. If the recommended TCCC combat trauma management plan does not work for the specific tactical situation that a combat medic, corpsman, or PJ encounters, then care must be modified to best fit the tactical situation. Scenario-based planning, then, is critical for success in TCCC.[5,13]

Battlefield Trauma Care in 2018

Published evidence and battlefield experience accumulated over the 21 years since TCCC was first published have led all services in the U.S. military and many allied nations to use TCCC concepts to care for their combat wounded. All U.S. combat medics, corpsmen, and PJs are now taught battlefield trauma care techniques based on the TCCC Guidelines. Military units that have trained all their members, medical and nonmedical personnel, in TCCC have documented the lowest incidence of preventable deaths among their casualties in the history of modern warfare.[8] TCCC-based prehospital trauma training is now widespread in the U.S. civilian sector as well.

TCCC Guidelines are reviewed quarterly and updated as needed by the CoTCCC.[23] Proposed changes to the Guidelines must be approved by a two-thirds majority of the CoTCCC to be accepted. Changes recommended by the CoTCCC are then forwarded to the Director of the JTS for final approval.[22] Once approved, updated versions of the TCCC Guidelines are posted on the JTS website as well as the websites of the Military Health System, the DHA (Deployed Medicine), the NAEMT, the *Journal of Special Operations Medicine*, and the Special Operations Medical Association. TCCC-based training now provided to all U.S. combat medical personnel includes the following:

- Phased care in the tactical environment to ensure that good medicine is combined with good small-unit tactics. The three defined phases of care are as follows:
  - Care Under Fire
  - Tactical Field Care
  - Tactical Evacuation (TACEVAC) Care
- Casualty and medic actions during the Care Under Fire phase focus on gaining and maintaining the tactical advantage, with limb tourniquets recommended as the only medical care undertaken in this phase.
- The most thorough guidelines available to optimize the use of limb tourniquets including the use of a second tourniquet when needed to control bleeding; elimination of the distal pulse as a secondary goal for application; and the recommendation to attempt conversion from a tourniquet to other methods of bleeding control if the casualty has not arrived at a definitive care facility after 2 hours of tourniquet time.
- Use of hemostatic dressings to control life-threatening hemorrhage from external bleeding at sites that are not amenable to tourniquet use.
- Use of nasopharyngeal airways to maintain a patent airway when there is no airway obstruction from direct maxillofacial or neck trauma.
- Initial management of the airway in maxillofacial trauma by having the casualty sit up and lean forward, if possible, thus allowing blood to simply drain out of the oropharynx, clearing the airway.
- Surgical airways for maxillofacial or neck trauma when airway compromise is present, and the sit-up-and-lean-forward position is not feasible or not successful.
- Aggressive needle thoracostomy with a 14-gauge, 3.25-inch (8.25-cm) needle for suspected tension pneumothorax.
- A different approach to spinal precautions—they are not emphasized for casualties with penetrating trauma only, but are still recommended, if tactically feasible, when blunt trauma is present.

- IV or IO access only when required for medications or fluid resuscitation.
- The preferential use of a saline lock for IV access as opposed to an IV catheter running fluids at keep vein open (KVO).
- The use of IO devices when vascular access is needed but difficult to obtain.
- Resuscitation of casualties in shock with whole blood or balanced blood components as soon as this becomes logistically feasible in the continuum of care.
- More aggressive fluid resuscitation and supplemental oxygen as needed to avoid hypotension and hypoxia in casualties with TBI.
- The TCCC "Triple-Option Analgesia" plan to provide titrated, faster, safer, and more efficacious battlefield analgesia using oral analgesics when feasible.
- Prevention of hypothermia and secondary coagulopathy with improved technology to prevent heat loss.
- Use of fluoroquinolones and ertapenem on the battlefield to reduce preventable deaths and morbidity from wound infections.
- Combat scenario-based trauma training emphasizing that trauma care on the battlefield must be consistent with good small-unit tactics.
- Better identification of casualties likely to derive the most benefit from supplemental oxygen during TACEVAC.[24]
- The use of tranexamic acid to help prevent death from noncompressible and junctional hemorrhage.
- The use of junctional tourniquets to help prevent death from junctional hemorrhage.
- The hemostatic adjunct XStat as another option for controlling junctional hemorrhage in narrow wound tracts.
- Pelvic binders to help reduce the life-threatening internal bleeding that may accompany pelvic fractures.
- Strategies for management of wounded hostile combatants. Rules of Thumb and the use of specific injury patterns to help determine evacuation priorities.[8,25,26]

Battlefield Experience with TCCC in Iraq and Afghanistan

At the start of the war in Afghanistan, TCCC was used only by Navy SEALs, the 75th Ranger Regiment, the Army Special Missions Unit, Air Force pararescuemen, and a few other innovative units in the U.S. military. The impact of this limited use of TCCC was not well appreciated until the first preventable death analysis was conducted by the U.S. military in Afghanistan as a combined effort of the U.S. Special Operations Command, the U.S. Army Institute of Surgical Research, and the Armed Forces

Medical Examiner System. That study by Holcomb and others examined the first 82 Special Operations fatalities in Iraq and Afghanistan.[27] They found that 8 of the 12 individuals who died from injuries that were potentially survivable might have been saved simply by the proper application of TCCC principles.

In large part, it was the experience with limb tourniquets that was responsible for the adoption of TCCC throughout the U.S. military. Tourniquets were a high-visibility issue for two reasons: the first is that tourniquet use was a radical departure from prehospital trauma care practice—both military and civilian—as it existed 20 years ago. The second is that ubiquitous tourniquet use has clearly been the single most important lifesaving battlefield trauma care advance achieved during the wars in Iraq and Afghanistan.[7,21] U.S. military personnel deployed initially to Afghanistan and Iraq without commercially manufactured tourniquets, but they now routinely carry well-made, effective tourniquets into combat. Limb tourniquets have proven remarkably effective at saving lives in casualties with extremity hemorrhage, with very few complications.[28-33] The strategic messaging regarding tourniquets that drove the spread of TCCC from the Special Operations community to the conventional forces included reports of preventable death from extremity hemorrhage[27,34,35] and documentation of improved survival as the use of extremity tourniquets became more prevalent.[28-33,36-39] These reports were not enough in themselves to effect change; strong leadership by combat unit commanders acting on the advice of well-informed operational medical leaders was needed.

A landmark study published in 2012 by Col. Brian Eastridge and his coauthors examined the causes of death for all 4,596 U.S. military combat deaths that occurred between October 2001 and June 2011. They used autopsy data to judge whether deaths were potentially preventable had optimal treatment been provided.[32] Their findings included: (1) 87% of combat-related deaths occurred in the prehospital setting, (2) 24% of prehospital deaths were potentially preventable, and (3) hemorrhage was the cause of 91% of the preventable deaths on the battlefield.

Additionally, the Eastridge study enabled a comparison of the incidence of death from extremity hemorrhage between the early years of the wars in Iraq and Afghanistan—when tourniquets were not issued to or used by most of the U.S. military and the later years of the war when the TCCC-led use of tourniquets had become widespread throughout U.S. forces. In 2003 to 2006, the preventable death review done by Kelly found a 7.8% incidence of death either solely or significantly due to extremity hemorrhage.[34] Compare this to the 7.4% incidence of death from extremity hemorrhage that was seen in Vietnam.[6] After the use of tourniquets became widespread, beginning in 2005 in Special

Operations and then spreading to conventional forces in the ensuing years, deaths from extremity hemorrhage dropped dramatically.[7] In 2018, based on ongoing surveillance by the JTS weekly trauma teleconferences and the monthly JTS/AFMES teleconferences, deaths from isolated extremity hemorrhage are very rare, and, when they do occur, they are usually the result of the tactical exigencies of the battlefield. All of this was done with no loss of limbs among U.S. casualties in Iraq or Afghanistan due to tourniquet use.[7,29,30]

Other TCCC recommendations, such as moving away from large-volume crystalloid fluid resuscitation, using nasopharyngeal airways instead of endotracheal tubes in tactical field care, and using needle decompression instead of chest tubes for the initial treatment of suspected tension pneumothorax have proven effective, too. These interventions have also helped to reduce both the medical equipment load carried by combat medical personnel as well as their training requirements.[40] Numerous reports published in the medical literature and collected from combat first responders have documented that TCCC is saving lives on the battlefield and is improving the tactical flow of missions on which casualties have been sustained. Tarpey[36] described the use of TCCC by elements of the Third Infantry Division in the initial phase of the war in Iraq. He reported: "The adoption and implementation of the principles of TCCC by the medical platoon of Task Force 1-15 in OIF 1 resulted in overwhelming success. In over 25 days of continuous combat with 32 friendly casualties, many of them serious, we had 0 Killed in Action and 0 Died of Wounds, while simultaneously caring for a significant number of Iraqi civilian and military casualties." Gresham[41] noted that the 101st Airborne Division, "by teaching and using (TCCC) ideas, has achieved one of the highest casualty survival rates in combat of any unit in the Army." In an article in *Tip of the Spear*, the official publication of the U.S. Special Operations Command, Bottoms[42] stated that: "Multiple reports from SOF First Responders have credited TCCC techniques and equipment with saving lives on the battlefield." General Doug Brown, Commander of USSOCOM, sent a letter of appreciation[43] to the Army Surgeon General for the outstanding work done by the U.S. Army Institute of Surgical Research (USAISR) in establishing a pilot program called the TCCC Transition Initiative (described by Butler and Holcomb[37]). This program was established to fast-track new TCCC training and equipment to deploying special operations forces (SOF) units and to collect data about the success of these measures. General Brown stated in his letter[26] that the USAISR's TCCC program had: ". . . produced remarkable advances in our force's ability to successfully manage battlefield trauma."

A team from Madigan Army Medical Center used TCCC-based training to prepare 1,317 combat medics for deployment to Iraq or Afghanistan. Their 2007 study[44]

reported that of the 140 medics who subsequently deployed to Iraq for 1-year periods, "99% indicated that the principles taught in the TCCC course helped with the management of injured casualties during their deployment."

MSG Ted Westmoreland, one of the senior enlisted medics in the Army Special Missions Unit, accumulated extensive experience using TCCC to treat combat casualties in the first few months of the conflict in Afghanistan. In a presentation to the Special Operations Medical Association in December 2005, he made the following recommendation: "Implement TCCC into all service medical training now."[40]

In a paper entitled "Understanding Combat Casualty Care Statistics," Holcomb and his coauthors[45] documented that combat casualties of American forces in Iraq and Afghanistan were experiencing the highest casualty survival rate in U.S. history. They identified TCCC as one of the major factors responsible for this landmark achievement.

In their discussion of the newly developed JTTS, Eastridge et al[46] stated: "Other courses such as Tactical Combat Casualty Care, Emergency War Surgery, and the Joint Forces Combat Trauma Management Course, have revolutionized the way medical providers are trained for wartime deployment."

Beekley, Starnes, and Sebesta[47] reviewed major surgical lessons learned from the conflicts in Iraq and Afghanistan through 2006. Nine of the 19 advances that they highlighted were battlefield trauma management strategies pioneered primarily by TCCC.

Mabry and McManus[33] noted that "the new concept of Tactical Combat Casualty Care has revolutionized the management of combat casualties in the prehospital tactical setting."

In 2008, the Prehospital Trauma Chair for the ACS-COT wrote to the Assistant Secretary of Defense for Health Affairs, stating: "I am writing to offer my congratulations for the recent dramatic advances in prehospital trauma care delivered by the U.S. military. Multiple recent publications have shown that Tactical Combat Casualty Care is saving lives on the battlefield."[48]

Hetzler and Ball, two combat-experienced Special Forces medics, confirmed that "TCCC's identification of causes of combat mortality and essential procedures for their treatment (i.e., tourniquets, needle decompression, etc.) has greatly assisted the medic in focusing the cube space of his gear to the most relevant life threats."[49]

Col. Andy Pennardt reported no potentially preventable deaths among the 201 casualties (including 12 fatalities) sustained by the Army Special Missions Unit during the conflicts in Afghanistan and Iraq through 2009.[50] All combatants in this command had been trained in TCCC prior to 2001.

Based on this experience, accumulated as the course of hostilities in Afghanistan and Iraq progressed, TCCC went from being used by only a few USSOCOM and 18th Airborne Corps units to being used throughout the battle space.[32]

Changing the Culture in Battlefield Trauma Care

Several events that occurred prior to the onset of hostilities in Afghanistan were central to this transformation of battlefield trauma care. The Navy SEAL teams and the 75th Ranger Regiment began training *all* combatants in TCCC prior to the start of the current conflicts. The Army Special Missions Unit and the Air Force pararescue community also implemented TCCC from 1997 to 1998 and quickly adopted the practice of teaching TCCC to *every combatant* so that the most critical lifesaving interventions, like tourniquets, can be accomplished by every one of their unit members.[9,50,51]

After 10 years of intense combat operations in Iraq and Afghanistan by the Ranger Regiment, Kotwal and colleagues reported only one potentially preventable death among 32 combat fatalities (out of 419 casualties) sustained by the 75th Rangers,[51] and the death that was deemed preventable occurred in the hospital, not the prehospital, setting. This finding stands in stark contrast to the 15% to 28% of preventable deaths reported in other studies among U.S. casualties in these conflicts.[27,32,34] Considering the prehospital phase only, potentially preventable deaths among fatalities in the 75th Rangers was zero as compared to 24% in the study by Eastridge et al.[32] The remarkable disparity in potentially preventable deaths between early adopters of TCCC and the rest of the U.S. military was not widely known until the Kotwal study was published in 2011, followed by the Eastridge study in 2012. Observed differences in potentially preventable deaths may be due to differences in the methodology of determining which deaths are considered potentially preventable or differences between the casualty cohorts reported. Nevertheless, in 2017 little disagreement that the interventions pioneered by TCCC reduce preventable deaths during the phase of care when they are most likely to occur has been offered.

As noted earlier, the transition from previous prehospital trauma care regimens to TCCC was well under way in the U.S. military by 2011. This happened because of a very specific sequence of events that has been well documented but is not widely known. When U.S. forces invaded Afghanistan in 2001, there was no JTS in place and thus no mechanism for the systematic review of combat casualty care outcomes in the U.S. military to seek opportunities to improve care.[52] Specifically, from 2001 to 2004, there was no DoD focus on the causes of preventable deaths among U.S. fatalities and how they could have been prevented, and TCCC was primarily used only by those units that had adopted these new concepts before 2001. Adoption of TCCC required a move away from long-standing and firmly entrenched approaches to battlefield trauma care. How did this widespread change of culture finally come about?

The first and most fundamental requirement for changing the culture in battlefield trauma care was to provide a much higher-quality set of recommendations. As recounted in recent publications,[8,9,21] there were three aspects of the TCCC development process that enabled these improved recommendations. First, during the research effort that led to the development of TCCC, existing recommendations for prehospital combat trauma care were held to the same standards of evidence as those applied to proposed changes to that care. Second, the actual conditions that combat medical personnel were likely to encounter on the battlefield were considered in developing the new recommendations. Finally, input from combat medics, corpsmen, and PJs, our country's primary battlefield trauma care providers, was sought and incorporated throughout the TCCC development process.

The second step in changing the culture in battlefield trauma care, and the one that first led to the spread of TCCC beyond the few early adopters, was the first preventable death review of U.S. fatalities from Iraq and Afghanistan. In 2004, the USSOCOM had two critically important questions that needed to be answered: (1) what specifically were our Special Operations combat casualties dying from, and (2) what, if anything, could have been done to prevent those deaths? One might reasonably assume that the DoD had always performed preventable death reviews on its combat fatalities, but, as of 2004, there was no formal process to review combat deaths and to use that information to save the lives of future casualties. USSOCOM called upon Col. John Holcomb, who was then the Commander of the USAISR, to help answer these questions. Col. Holcomb's team found that in Special Operations forces, 15% of combat deaths resulted from injuries that were potentially survivable, and a number of those deaths might have been prevented with simple TCCC measures like a tourniquet.[27] This study sent a clear signal that TCCC training and equipment were needed throughout the Special Operations community, as was methodology for an ongoing evaluation of the impact of these new battlefield trauma care techniques on morbidity and mortality.

The third step in changing the culture also resulted from a collaboration between USSOCOM and USAISR. After the documentation of preventable deaths in the Holcomb study, the leadership of USSOCOM supported the TCCC Transition Initiative, which expedited TCCC equipping and training of deploying USSOCOM units. The project was led by an 18-D Special Forces medic, SFC Dominic Greydanus, and not only provided TCCC training and equipment to deploying Special Operations units,

but also collected feedback from medics, corpsmen, and PJs when these units returned from combat operations. It also provided early documentation of the success of TCCC interventions.[8,21,37]

The fourth event that led to the widespread adoption of TCCC concepts was a U.S. Central Command (CENTCOM) message that required that all combatants deploying to that theater be equipped with a tourniquet and a hemostatic dressing. This requirement was driven by the CENTCOM Surgeon at the time, Lt. Gen. Doug Robb. Although the services have the primary responsibility for training and equipping combatants, this mandate from CENTCOM forced supervising medical officers throughout the services to rethink their many years of medical training that had consistently taught them that the use of extremity tourniquets was a very bad idea.

The fifth key element that helped to change the culture of battlefield trauma care in the military was the excellent documentation of the impact of tourniquet use. It is often difficult to identify with precision which elements of TCCC are responsible for saved lives, but tourniquets are an exception to this rule. The work of Col. John Kragh, an orthopedic surgeon working at the Ibn Sina Hospital in Baghdad, reported that 31 lives were saved with tourniquets at his facility in one 6-month period.[8,28-30] This finding, when extrapolated to all U.S. casualties sustained in Iraq and Afghanistan up to that point in time, indicated that, as early as 2008, well over 1,000 U.S. service members' lives had possibly been saved with tourniquets in those conflicts. Again, these successes with tourniquet use were obtained without loss of limbs to tourniquet ischemia. Col. Kragh's work irrefutably confirmed the lifesaving benefits of what was perhaps the single most controversial aspect of TCCC.[8]

The sixth essential step in changing the culture of the U.S. military to accept TCCC was effective strategic messaging. The success of the TCCC Transition Initiative, Col. Kragh's work, and the decreased incidence of preventable deaths in units that were early TCCC adopters were presented frequently at military medical conferences and in the published medical literature.[29,30,33,36,37,42,44,45,47] The dramatically lower proportion of preventable deaths in the 75th Ranger Regiment compared to that in the broader U.S. military in which TCCC was adopted later was widely acclaimed in the medical literature. This acclamation increased awareness among combat medical personnel and their physician and physician assistant supervisors of the success of TCCC in reducing preventable deaths. These reports also provided TCCC innovators with published evidence that they could present to their unit commanders.[32,51]

Finally, evidence alone is often not effective in driving advances in trauma care,[21] and this and other difficulties inherent in making changes in battlefield trauma care have been identified.[52,53] Divided lines of authority and distributed responsibilities in the military structure make it exceedingly difficult to optimize battlefield trauma care throughout the DoD. Butler, Smith, and Carmona described the problem this way:[52]

> "Just as the United States has hundreds of trauma centers and thousands of autonomous prehospital care systems, which can potentially slow the transition of advances in military prehospital trauma care into use in the civilian sector, the U.S. Military has four armed services, six Geographic Combatant Commands, the U.S. Special Operations Command and the U.S. Transportation Command, all of which play a role in the care of combat casualties. Each of these organizations is authorized to operate autonomously with respect to combat casualty care unless directives are issued at the highest level of the military chain of command, which is the Secretary of Defense (SecDef) acting on the advice of his or her chief medical advisor, the Assistant Secretary of Defense for Health Affairs. Lacking direction in the form of SecDef rule and Joint Staff doctrine, there is no assurance that advances in trauma care will be implemented consistently throughout the various components of the US Military."

Unfortunately, at the Secretary of Defense, Chairman of the Joint Chiefs of Staff, and Service leadership levels, the span of responsibilities is immense. The ability of leaders at this level to focus on and mandate aspects of trauma care that are vigorously debated even among trauma subject matter experts is very limited. Therefore, when change is effected in battlefield trauma care, it typically occurs at a significantly lower level in the military chain of command and benefits only those individuals in that part of the organization.

When TCCC was first proposed in 1996, the recommendations contained in the TCCC Guidelines were presented to a great many people in both civilian and military medical audiences. Even so, very little happened until Rear Admiral Tom Richards, then the Commander of the Naval Special Warfare Command, examined the evidence presented to him and mandated the use of TCCC throughout the Navy SEAL community. Admiral Richards was not a doctor, but his decision paved the way for saving hundreds of lives among U.S. combat casualties.[8,9,21]

A similar occurrence took place in the 75th Ranger Regiment. In 1997, the regiment's commander, Col. Stanley McChrystal, acting on the advice of his Ranger medical personnel, made caring for Rangers wounded in combat one of his "Big Four" priorities by directive in 1997. The Big Four were marksmanship, physical training, small unit tactics, and . . . *medical readiness*.[51] Col. McChrystal understood that on the field of battle, everyone has the potential to be a casualty, and everyone—not just medics—may be the first to encounter a casualty and to render lifesaving care. He expected that *every* Ranger

was going to be engaged in casualty care, and so *every* Ranger received training in TCCC.[21,54]

Likewise, Gen. Doug Brown and VADM Eric Olson at the U.S. Special Operations Command mandated TCCC at a time when it was not the standard of care for prehospital trauma care, either in the U.S. military or in the civilian sector. General John Abizaid at the CENTCOM did much the same thing in requiring the use of tourniquets in Iraq and Afghanistan at a time when conventional wisdom dictated otherwise.

The first takeaway from this discussion of the importance of leadership in advancing battlefield trauma care is that new evidence alone does not drive advances in trauma care—in either the civilian sector or the military—*people* do that.

The second takeaway is that it is often not trauma subject matter experts who are the final decision makers in introducing new standards of trauma care. Both in the military and in the civilian sector, decision makers at senior levels are often not the subject matter experts. As former U.S. Surgeon General Rich Carmona pointed out during the Hartford Consensus IV meeting,[55] it is the responsibility of innovative trauma care experts to inform and inspire senior leaders so that advances in trauma care can be resourced and implemented. It was the senior leaders noted here—all combat commanders, not physicians—who mandated that TCCC be implemented in the military. Effecting positive change in trauma care therefore takes strong senior leaders—acting on the advice of well-informed trauma subject matter experts—with a dedication to continuously improving trauma care and a willingness to invest both their professional reputations and resources to do so.[21,54]

TCCC in the U.S. Department of Defense—2019

As of this writing, due to the successes of TCCC in minimizing preventable combat fatalities and the actions of a great many resolute innovators, TCCC is now used extensively throughout the U.S. military.[8,21,52] USSOCOM mandated TCCC training for its forces[56] in 2005 and, in partnership with the USAISR, established the TCCC Transition Initiative to fast track TCCC training and equipment to its units.[37] The BUMED-directed review of TCCC[57] conducted in 2006/2007 found that TCCC was used not only by Special Operations forces but also by all of the conventional forces in the U.S. military. This has been confirmed by other sources.[1,11,32,58-63] In February 2009, the Army directed that all medical department members receive TCCC training as part of their predeployment trauma preparation.[64]

The DHB, the civilian medical advisory board to the Secretary of Defense, recommended that TCCC be taught to all deploying combatants and to all combatant unit medical providers in August 2009.[65] **Table 23-1** contains the recommended skill sets for combat medical personnel, Combat Lifesavers (nonmedical personnel with extra training in TCCC), and all combatants. In March 2009, Dr. Ward Cascells, the Assistant Secretary of Defense for Health Affairs, recommended to the military services that TCCC be used as the standard for training combat medical personnel to manage combat trauma in the tactical prehospital environment.[66] In 2011 and again in 2014, this recommendation was repeated by Dr. Cascells' successor, Dr. Jonathan Woodson.[67,68]

In 2015, Vice Admiral Matt Nathan, the Navy Surgeon General, addressed a major disconnect in TCCC

Table 23-1 Tactical Combat Casualty Care (TCCC) Skill Sets by Provider Level—1 August 2018				
Skill	**All**	**CLS**	**CM**	**CPM**
Overview of tactical medicine	X	X	X	X
Hemostasis				
Apply tourniquet	X	X	X	X
Apply direct pressure	X	X	X	X
Apply bandage	X	X	X	X
Apply Combat Gauze	X	X	X	X
Apply pressure dressing	X	X	X	X
Apply junctional tourniquets use XStat			X	X
Apply pelvic compression devices			X	X
Casualty movement techniques	X	X	X	X
Airway				
Chin lift/jaw thrust maneuver	X	X	X	X
Nasopharyngeal airway	X	X	X	X
Recovery position	X	X	X	X
Sit-up-and-lean-forward position	X	X	X	X
Extraglottic airway			X	X
Surgical airway			X	X
Endotracheal intubation				X
Breathing				
Treat sucking chest wound	X	X	X	X
Needle thoracostomy		X	X	X
Pulse oximetry monitoring			X	X
Administer oxygen			X	X
Chest tube				X

Skill	All	CLS	CM	CPM
Intravenous Access and IV Therapy				
Assess for shock	X	X	X	X
Start IV line/saline lock			X	X
Obtain IO access			X	X
IV/IO fluid resuscitation			X	X
IV/IO analgesics (morphine, ketamine)			X	X
IV/IO antibiotics			X	X
IV/IO ondansetron			X	X
IV/IO tranexamic acid			X	X
Administer blood products				X
Prevent hypothermia	X	X	X	X
Penetrating Eye Injuries				
Cover eye with rigid shield	X	X	X	X
Field test of visual acuity			X	X
Administer oral moxifloxacin	X	X	X	X
Oral and Intramuscular Medications				
Oral antibiotics	X	X	X	X
Oral analgesia (nonnarcotic)	X	X	X	X
Fentanyl lozenges			X	X
IM antibiotics			X	X
IM ketamine			X	X
IM ondansetron			X	X
Fracture Management				
Splinting	X	X	X	X
Traction splinting			X	X
Management of Burns				
Stop the burning process	X	X	X	X
Cover the burned areas	X	X	X	X
Burn fluid resuscitation			X	X
Electronic Vital Sign Monitoring				
Electronic vital sign monitoring			X	X

Key: All, all deploying combatants; CLS, Combat Lifesaver; CM, Combat Medic (Army 68-Ws, Navy 8404 Corpsmen); CPM, Combat Paramedic (includes SOF Advanced Tactical Practitionerl8-Ds, Expeditionary Combat Medics, PJs, etc.)

Modified from Dr. Frank Butler.

readiness training that had been identified in both JTS/CENTCOM surveys of prehospital trauma care in Afghanistan[69,70]—the need to ensure that medical department officers who supervise combat medical personnel understand TCCC concepts. VADM Nathan's 2015 directive mandated TCCC training for all active duty and reserve physicians, physician assistants, advanced nurse practitioners, nurse generalists, and hospital corpsmen assigned to the Navy BUMED.[71] This directive also sought to address another major issue in TCCC training—the lack of a standardized TCCC curriculum. VADM Nathan's guidance was that all BUMED TCCC training courses will use the curriculum developed by the CoTCCC. The need to use the JTS/CoTCCC curriculum as the standard in training TCCC has been identified in a number of recent reports and is discussed further later in this chapter.[21,72,73]

From the Battlefields of Iraq and Afghanistan to Worldwide Use

Historically, many lessons learned from military combat casualty care have found application in civilian trauma care. This has also been true of TCCC. The United States has just had the longest period of continuous armed conflict in its history, and this has created a unique opportunity to understand and improve battlefield trauma care. Over the past 16 years of caring for combat casualties, many advances have been incorporated into TCCC as new evidence, new technology, and ongoing battlefield experience have accumulated. Many published reports from this period have highlighted the success of TCCC, and it is now used well beyond the U.S. military.

TCCC in Allied Militaries

TCCC has now been implemented by many coalition partner nations[1] and has been recommended as the standard of care for combat first-aid training in member nations by the ABCANZ Armies (formerly America, Britain, Canada, Australia, New Zealand Armies' Program).[74] Canada was one of the earliest international adopters of TCCC. Savage and colleagues noted that, "although the Canadian military experienced increasingly severe injuries during the current conflicts, the Canadian Forces have experienced the highest casualty survival rate in history."[38] They further reported, "Though this success is multifactorial, the determination and resolve of CF leadership to develop and deliver comprehensive, multileveled TCCC packages to soldiers and medics is a significant reason for that and has unquestionably saved the lives of Canadian, Coalition, and Afghan Security Forces." TCCC was also recommended as the battlefield trauma care standard for NATO partner nations by the NATO Special Operations–convened Human Factor and Medicine Expert Panel 224 in 2011.[75] Thanks in large part to allied participation in the TCCC Working Group and to the NAEMT's worldwide educational infrastructure and its leadership in offering TCCC training to countries all around the world,[21,73] TCCC has indeed spread "all around the globe."[76]

PHTLS and the American College of Surgeons Committee on Trauma

In 1996, the nascent TCCC effort benefitted from an interaction between Rear Admiral Mike Cowan, Commander of the Defense Medical Readiness Training Institute, and Dr. Norman McSwain, founder and medical director of the PHTLS program. These two leaders agreed that there should be a military medicine section in the fourth edition of the PHTLS textbook. TCCC concepts were included in that edition[77] and in every subsequent edition. This has been exceptionally helpful in that the PHTLS textbook carries the endorsement of the ACS and the NAEMT; this was the first step toward the mainstreaming of TCCC.[8,9] Beginning with this initial interaction, a robust and ongoing dialogue developed between TCCC, PHTLS, and NAEMT. The strong partnership between NAEMT, PHTLS, the ACS-COT, and TCCC has endured, and these groups have adopted a number of the recommendations made by the CoTCCC regarding prehospital trauma care.[78,79] TCCC, in turn, has benefitted greatly from many aspects of the PHTLS program and the NAEMT educational infrastructure.[21,73]

Hartford Consensus and Stop the Bleed

In recent years, civilian law enforcement officers and EMS responders have been called to bombing incidents, school and mall shootings, and other terror attacks that present tactical situations similar in some respects to those encountered on battlefields. The threat of ongoing hostile fire, treating multiple casualties under cover, and prolonged evacuation times have all come into play. Even in urban settings, getting to, treating, and transporting casualties can require tactics and training outside the parameters of many standard EMS protocols. The mass casualty incidents at Columbine High School, Virginia Tech, Sandy Hook Elementary School, Stoneman Douglas High School in Parkland, Pulse Nightclub in Orlando, and the Las Vegas concert shooting are examples in point. More widespread adoption of applicable TCCC Guidelines into tactical EMS training programs, and application of these principles to tactical law enforcement operations may result in better tactical flow and additional lives saved.[80]

The dramatic increase in terrorist attacks and so-called active-shooter incidents creates the potential for a great many additional lives to be saved by using TCCC concepts. Public awareness of such events has caused tremendous acceleration in the usual interchange of information between military and civilian trauma care experts via initiatives like the Hartford Consensus,[55,81,82] the White House Stop the Bleed campaign,[83] TCCC-based courses offered by NAEMT, and the development of the civilian Tactical Emergency Casualty Care (TECC) program. These initiatives and many other local, state, and regional efforts have ensured that the advances in prehospital trauma care pioneered by TCCC, the JTS, and military medicine are being used to save lives in civilian trauma care practice with increasing frequency.[84,86]

TCCC and Wilderness Medicine

Another of the earliest and most productive of the partnerships formed by TCCC with civilian medical organizations was that between TCCC and the Wilderness Medical Society (WMS). The wilderness environment is similar in some respects to the battlefield. In both settings, the patient and the care provider are often in remote locations where evacuation may be delayed and complicated, significant and ongoing hazard may be present during the time that care is being provided, the equipment available for treatment is very limited, the environments may be extreme, and those providing care are often not paramedics, emergency physicians, or trauma surgeons.[87,88] The overlap in the austerities of the combat and the wilderness settings has resulted in collaboration between military and wilderness medicine experts in many areas. TCCC emphasizes the need to consider the specific tactical scenario in formulating a treatment plan for a casualty, and many combat trauma scenarios occur in wilderness areas. TCCC and the WMS conducted a workshop in which they developed guidelines for combat casualty care in wilderness settings.[89] Fentanyl lozenges recommended for analgesia in TCCC[90] were previously recommended for use in wilderness trauma care in 1999.[91] Hemostatic dressings and tourniquets used in TCCC are the mainstays for controlling life-threatening external hemorrhage in the wilderness.[92,93] TCCC-based techniques are now used to train medical personnel who provide care to trauma victims in our country's national parks.[94] A 2-day TCCC preconference held at the 2016 annual meeting of the WMS resulted in a supplement to the WMS-sponsored journal *Wilderness and Environmental Medicine* dedicated to topics in TCCC.[88]

The American College of Emergency Physicians (ACEP)

The endorsement of the ACS-COT of the TCCC-led use of prehospital tourniquets and hemostatic dressings has been discussed previously.[55,78,81,82] The ACEP likewise endorsed tourniquets and hemostatic dressings for the control of life-threatening external hemorrhage in the prehospital setting.[95]

Additionally, the ACEP has endorsed some of the TCCC-led advances in prehospital analgesia. The survey of prehospital trauma care in Afghanistan in November 2012 led by Col. (retired) Russ Kotwal, Col. Stacy Shackelford, and Col. Erin Edgar, produced very valuable feedback from combat medical providers about the state of battlefield analgesia in U.S. forces.[69] There was a clear and consistent message from medics, corpsmen, and PJs all over Afghanistan that they were happy with the analgesia options recommended by TCCC at the time, but that these options needed to be forged into a structured and coherent approach to battlefield analgesia. The JTS and the CoTCCC subsequently developed "Triple Option Analgesia." This plan for battlefield analgesia provides faster, safer, and more effective relief of pain from combat injuries than the IM morphine that has been used by the U.S. Military since the Civil War.[90] The Triple Option Analgesia plan incorporates the use of fentanyl lozenges pioneered by the 75th Ranger Regiment and the Army Special Missions Unit and ketamine pioneered by our colleagues in the United Kingdom and the U.S. Air Force PJ community. This plan customizes the analgesia choice to best suit the casualty's level of pain and his or her physiologic status. The ACEP's policy on out-of-hospital analgesia and sedation[96] mirrors the Triple Option Analgesia plan. The agreement between these guidelines is compelling evidence that the Triple Option Analgesia plan is sound and that the lack of an FDA indication for fentanyl lozenges and ketamine as analgesics for acute pain does not preclude them from being best practice options based on available clinical evidence. This will be discussed more in the following section.

Lessons Learned Are Not Really Lessons Learned—Unless We Actually Learn Them

Despite 16 years of continuous warfare, we have not incorporated all the prehospital trauma care lessons learned from Iraq and Afghanistan into our country's battlefield trauma care plan for future conflicts. Specifically, the items below are needed to translate lessons learned into improvements in combat casualty care going forward.[21,52]

1. The command structure of the U.S. military requires definitive action at senior levels for effective change to be enacted. For TCCC to save as many lives as possible, commanders at every level must mandate that TCCC will be the standard for battlefield trauma care. They must also ensure that all combatants and medical personnel are trained in the current version of

TCCC as developed by the DoD's lead agency, the JTS, and taught through a standardized, high-quality curriculum. These measures will ensure that combat units are fully prepared to use TCCC concepts to treat casualties on the battlefield. The recent DoD Instruction makes TCCC the U.S. military standard for battlefield trauma care and mandates TCCC training for all members of the U.S. Armed Services.[97] This is an excellent first step and requires definitive follow-up action by both line and medical senior leadership.

2. The parent organization for the CoTCCC, the JTS, should be made a permanent entity within the Military Health System and should be recognized as the DoD's lead organization for trauma care. The JTS should be a direct resource for the battlefield trauma care provider, senior military medical leaders, the military services, and the Combatant Commands. This step has presently been mandated by law but has not yet been fully implemented by the DoD.

3. To support continuous performance improvement in combat casualty care, all trauma care data in the U.S. military should be entered into the DoD Trauma Registry maintained by the JTS. Prehospital care documentation has been historically very difficult to capture and should be a point of emphasis for the combat unit command structure.

4. Multiple factors can affect the mortality rate during combat operations: the maturity of the theater, the presence or absence of air superiority, the theater geography, the casualty transport times involved, the lethality of the hostile forces, innovations in personal protection equipment, and the protection afforded from advances in aircraft and armored vehicles. Consequently, historically used metrics such as Killed in Action and Died of Wounds rates do not provide a completely accurate assessment of the quality of care provided to casualties. In assessing the effectiveness of combat casualty care, a robust performance improvement process must include reviews of the injuries sustained by and the care provided to both surviving casualties and all combat fatalities with a focus on preventing death. This information should be assessed on an ongoing basis by the JTS and the Armed Forces Medical Examiner System at established intervals as dictated by the number of U.S. combat casualties sustained.[52] These assessments should be forwarded to senior medical and combat leaders who have the authority to implement any remedial action that may be indicated.

5. There is no DoD-wide program to ensure that newly recommended technology, techniques, and medications in combat casualty care, with regard to both TCCC and in-hospital care, are quickly and reliably made available to those who care for casualties.[21,52] A medical Rapid Fielding Initiative program should be established to expedite delivery of newly recommended combat casualty care equipment and associated training to deployed and deploying forces and to gather feedback on the initial experience with the newly fielded equipment. The importance of this lack is especially high in TCCC because the prehospital phase of care is where the greatest numbers of preventable deaths occur. The 2005–2006 TCCC Transition Initiative conducted as a joint effort of USSO-COM and the USAISR is an excellent model.[37]

6. Combat casualty care research should be focused on prevention of fatalities that result from potentially survivable injuries. Research should be preferentially directed toward interventions that are most likely to reduce preventable combat deaths.

7. Even during peace intervals, training on TCCC Guidelines and JTS Clinical Practice Guidelines should be provided for all medical department personnel who may be called on to treat combat casualties. For trauma surgical teams and those who provide TACEVAC care, this training should be coupled with on ongoing trauma care experience in civilian trauma centers to sustain essential trauma skills. TCCC training and trauma practicums should be conducted continuously so that the military's combat trauma care capability does not languish in times of peace. Service and Geographic Combatant Commanders should work in partnership to ensure that this training is reliably accomplished.

8. A high-quality, standardized TCCC training course should be used to train medical personnel in TCCC.[21,73] Many combat trauma courses represented as TCCC courses have been found to contain material substantially different from the TCCC recommendations developed by the CoTCCC. These variations have been directly associated with documented adverse casualty care events.[97] In the absence of a standard TCCC course with a professionally developed curriculum, "TCCC Training" in the DoD can include anything from an hour of PowerPoint slides to 11 days of inappropriate training. As

of this writing there is no DoD-wide oversight over the quality of TCCC instruction or the accuracy of the messaging. The TCCC course offered through the educational infrastructure of the NAEMT provides TCCC training that uses the standard curriculum developed by the CoTCCC. This training option has been used by both U.S. and allied military units since 2009 at a minimal cost. NAEMT courses also provide a TCCC certification card endorsed by the JTS, the CoTCCC, the NAEMT, and the ACS-COT.[72] No other training course offers this level of endorsement by nationally recognized trauma organizations. This course has been identified by both the JTS and medical personnel supporting the Marine Corp as the best option available at the time of this writing.[72,73] To increase its availability to military users, NAEMT TCCC training could be added to course offerings under the auspices of the Uniformed Services University of the Health Sciences (USUHS) Military Training Network.[21,72]

9. The TCCC for Medical Personnel course should be prerequisite training for any physician, physician assistant, nurse, or Medical Service Corps officer in the DoD who may lead, supervise, or support any aspect of battlefield trauma care. This requirement should be strongly and consistently enforced. The 2012 and 2013 surveys of prehospital trauma care in Afghanistan[69,70] found a major disconnect between the battlefield trauma care knowledge fund of medics, corpsmen, and PJs and those who supervise them. The U.S. military in the past has variably taught physicians and other medical supervisors the Advanced Trauma Life Support course and then assigned them to combat units with the expectation that they will be able to effectively supervise medics who have been taught battlefield trauma care based on TCCC concepts.[52] A 2017 survey of Army physicians and physician assistants found that only about half had had TCCC training.[98] This puts both combat medical personnel and the casualties that they will be expected to care for at a significant disadvantage. Physicians, physician assistants, nurses, and Medical Service Corps officers should be proficient in TCCC so they can effectively oversee the training and equipping of their medics and/or supervise the delivery of battlefield trauma care.

10. A Battlefield Trauma Care Medical Panel should be established as a joint effort of the DoD and the FDA.[21,25,52] Care of our nation's combat wounded is not well served by the current FDA regulatory structure. For example, ketamine, which does not have an analgesic indication from the FDA, can be and is extensively used off-label by physicians for analgesia. Ketamine is especially useful for battlefield analgesia in casualties with hemodynamic or pulmonary compromise for whom opioids are contraindicated.[90,96,99] Ketamine cannot, however, be marketed or produced in delivery systems designed for battlefield analgesia despite its proven success in combat because of regulatory constraints. Ketamine supplied in 50-milligram (mg) or 100-mg manufactured unit-dose delivery systems (that could be designed for IM, intranasal, or IV use) would be a very useful addition to medical kits on the battlefield. However, unit-dose packaging for analgesic use is not allowed by the FDA, because there is no approved indication for that use. Unit medical personnel are therefore forced to either draw up the medication into syringes before combat actions (leading to wastage and an increased potential for diversion) or to draw up the medication from multidose vials in the middle of a combat engagement (increasing the risk of medication error and slowing the medic down as he or she attempts to treat multiple casualties).[21,22]

Another example is dried plasma. The available evidence shows that colloids and crystalloids are the *least* desirable options for fluid resuscitation of casualties in hemorrhagic shock.[22,52,100] Dried plasma is a much better option and is used by most of our coalition partner nations. It is not available to most medics in the U.S. military because of the FDA regulatory structure.[22,52,100]

Medical devices, many of which are intended for battlefield use, and medications used to treat victims of weapons of mass destruction are already handled by the FDA using processes distinct from the typical regulatory approach for new medications. Appropriate special treatment should be extended to medications and blood components that have been identified as the best-practice options for battlefield trauma care.[22,52]

11. Documentation of prehospital care in combat casualties must be improved if the U.S. military is to optimize combat casualty care and to continue to advance battlefield trauma care. Consistent documentation of the critical aspects of TCCC (e.g., time of tourniquet application, tranexamic acid dose and time, analgesic doses/times, and antibiotics given) is essential to optimal care. Documentation of

TCCC is also essential to efforts to improve battlefield trauma care through the JTS performance improvement process. Despite the importance of this aspect of combat casualty care, prehospital care documentation is often not accomplished.[21,69,101] Medical personnel from the 75th Ranger Regiment developed a simple and well-designed TCCC card and a more detailed electronic after-action report, and they demonstrated that reliable documentation of prehospital care is possible if the appropriate command emphasis is present.[101] Building on the regiment's success with these dual formats, the CoTCCC has consistently advocated for the use of these two documentation tools throughout the DoD and has updated them recently to include new treatment recommendations in the TCCC Guidelines. Nevertheless, it will take strong and sustained command emphasis in combat units to replicate the Rangers' success in this aspect of care throughout the U.S. military.[21,54,101]

SUMMARY

- Combat medical personnel often face multiple challenges in caring for the wounded on the battlefield. These include the threat of hostile fire, working in the dark, multiple casualties, limited medical equipment, and prolonged evacuation times.
- Ignoring the tactical environment when developing battlefield trauma care strategies may increase the number of preventable deaths.
- There are three goals in TCCC: (1) treat the casualty, (2) prevent additional casualties, and (3) complete the mission.
- TCCC is divided into three phases: Care Under Fire, Tactical Field Care, and Tactical Evacuation Care.
- In Care Under Fire, combat medical personnel and casualties are under effective hostile fire, and tactical considerations predominate. In this phase, medical care should be limited to controlling extremity hemorrhage with tourniquets.
- In Tactical Field Care, medical personnel and casualties are not under effective hostile fire. More extensive care can be provided.
- In Tactical Evacuation Care, casualties are transported to a medical treatment facility by aircraft, ground vehicle, or boat. An opportunity exists here to provide additional medical personnel and equipment, raising the level of care that can be delivered.
- The TCCC Guidelines are published in the military version of the PHTLS course manual. They are the only set of battlefield trauma care guidelines to

- receive the dual endorsement of the ACS-COT and the NAEMT.
- The CoTCCC updates TCCC Guidelines based on ongoing review of the published civilian and military prehospital trauma literature, ongoing interaction with military combat casualty care research laboratories, direct input from experienced combat medical personnel, input from the service Medical Lessons Learned Centers, case reports discussed at the weekly JTS process improvement teleconferences, and expert opinion from both military and civilian trauma specialists.
- The single most successful TCCC intervention reported to date is the reintroduction of tourniquet use on the battlefield.
- TCCC is now used throughout the U.S. military and the militaries of numerous allied nations to train combat medical personnel to manage trauma in the tactical prehospital environment. Adoption of TCCC Guidelines into civilian tactical EMS systems is under way, and TCCC principles are now saving lives in those settings as well.
- For TCCC to save as many lives as possible, commanders at every level in the U.S. military need to mandate that TCCC will be the standard for battlefield trauma care.
- These senior leaders also need to ensure that all combatants and medical personnel are trained in the current version of TCCC as developed by the DoD's lead agency for trauma, the JTS, and taught through a standardized, high-quality curriculum.

SCENARIO RECAP

You are the only combat medic traveling in a 10-person, four-vehicle convoy through a small village in eastern Iraq. As you pull out on an open road at the end of the village, an IED explodes under the second vehicle. There is no follow-up hostile fire, so the unit sets up a secure perimeter. You proceed to assess the three major casualties at the scene.

Casualty 1 is a soldier with femoral arterial bleeding from a large wound on the right thigh, as well as a right hand amputation with blood oozing from the stump. He is conscious and has a good radial pulse.

Casualty 2 is a soldier with a large open head wound in which mangled gray matter is clearly visible. He is unresponsive, and his breathing is agonal.

Casualty 3 is a civilian bystander with a penetrating injury to his right lower abdomen. He is conscious and in great pain.

Evacuation by helicopter is available in 20 minutes, and the flight to the nearest medical treatment facility will take approximately 30 minutes.

SCENARIO SOLUTION

- **What are some of the considerations in managing these casualties that are not present in most civilian settings?**
  Factors that the medic must take into consideration in this scenario include the following:
  - What is the threat of hostile fire?
  - What is the best way to move the casualties to cover?
  - Should the medic attend to the casualties immediately or assist the unit in suppressing hostile fire?
  - Which of the injuries noted are immediately life threatening?
  - What are the most effective interventions for addressing these injuries in this combat setting?
  - What is the threat to evacuation platforms from hostile fire?
  - How long will evacuation take?
  - What type of evacuation platform is best for this situation?

References

1. Butler FK, Blackbourne LH. Battlefield trauma care then and now: a decade of tactical combat casualty care. *J Trauma Acute Care Surg.* 2012;73(6)(Suppl 5):S395-402. doi:10.1097/TA.0b013e3182754850.
2. Heiskell LE, Carmona RH. Tactical emergency medical services: an emerging subspecialty in emergency medicine. *Ann Emerg Med.* 1994;23:778-785.
3. Bellamy RF. How shall we train for combat casualty care? *Mil Med.* 1987;152(12):617-621.
4. Baker MS. Advanced trauma life support: is it acceptable stand-alone training for military medicine? *Mil Med.* 1994;159(9):581-590.
5. Butler FK, Hagmann J, Butler EG. Tactical combat casualty care in special operations. *Mil Med.* 1996;161(Suppl):1-16.
6. Maughon JS. An inquiry into the nature of wounds resulting in killed in action in Vietnam. *Mil Med.* 1970;135:8-13.
7. Butler FK. Military history of increasing survival: the US military experience with tourniquets and hemostatic dressings in the Afghanistan and Iraq conflicts. *Bull Am Coll Surg.* 2015 Sep;100(1 Suppl):60-64.
8. Butler FK. Two decades of saving lives on the battlefield: tactical combat casualty care turns 20. *Mil Med.* 2017;182(3):e1563-e1568.
9. Butler FK. Tactical Combat Casualty Care: beginnings. *Wilderness Environ Med.* 2017 Jun;28(Suppl 2):S12-S17.
10. Richards TR. Commander, Naval Special Warfare Command letter. 1500 Ser 04/0341; 9 April 1997.
11. Butler FK, Holcomb JB, Giebner SD, McSwain NE, Bagian J. Tactical Combat Casualty Care 2007: evolving concepts and battlefield experience. *Mil Med.* 2007;172(Suppl):1-19.

12. Holcomb, JB. The 2004 Fitts lecture: current perspective on combat casualty care. *J Trauma.* 2005;59(4):990-1002.

13. Butler FK. Tactical medicine training for SEAL mission commanders. *Mil Med.* 2001;166(7):625-631.

14. DeLorenzo, RA. Medic for the millennium: the US Army 91W healthcare specialist. *Mil Med.* 2001;166(8):685-688.

15. Pappas CG. The Ranger medic. *Mil Med.* 2001;166(5):394-400.

16. Allen RC, McAtee JM. *Pararescue Medications and Procedures Manual.* Hurlburt Field, FL: Air Force Special Operations Command; 1999.

17. Malish RG. The medical preparation of a special forces company for pilot recovery. *Mil Med.* 1999;164(12):881-884.

18. Krausz MM. Resuscitation strategies in the Israeli Army. Presentation to the Institute of Medicine Committee on Fluid Resuscitation for Combat Casualties, 17 September 1998.

19. McDevitt I. *Tactical Medicine.* Boulder, CO: Paladin Press; 2001.

20. McSwain NE, Frame S, Paturas JL, eds. *Prehospital Trauma Life Support Manual.* 4th ed. Akron, OH: Mosby; 1999.

21. Butler FK. Leadership lessons learned in tactical combat casualty care. *J Trauma Acute Care Surg.* 2017 Jun;82(6 Suppl 1):S16-S25.

22. Butler FK, Blackbourne LH, Gross KR. The combat medic aid bag: 2025. CoTCCC top ten recommended battlefield trauma care research, development, and evaluation priorities for 2015. *J Spec Oper Med.* 2015;15(4):7-19.

23. Butler FK. Tactical combat casualty care: update 2009. *J Trauma.* 2010;69(Suppl):S10-S13.

24. Grissom CK, Weaver LK, Clemmer TP, Morris AH. Theoretical advantage of oxygen treatment for combat casualties during medical evacuation at high altitude. *J Trauma.* 2006;61(2):461-467.

25. McSwain NE, Frame S, Salomone JP, eds. *Prehospital Trauma Life Support Manual.* 5th ed. Akron, OH: Mosby; 2003.

26. McSwain NE, Salomone JP, eds. *Prehospital Trauma Life Support Manual,* 6th ed. Akron, OH: Mosby; 2006.

27. Holcomb JB, McMullen NR, Pearse L, et al. Causes of death in special operations forces in the global war on terrorism: 2001-2004. *Ann Surg.* 2007;245(6):986-991.

28. Kragh J, Walters T, Westmoreland T, et al. Tragedy into drama: an American history of tourniquet use in the current war. *J Spec Oper Med.* 2013;13:5-25.

29. Kragh JF, Walters TJ, Baer, DJ, et al. Survival with emergency tourniquet use to stop bleeding in major limb trauma. *Ann Surg.* 2009;249(1):1-7. doi:10.1097/SLA.0b013e31818842ba.

30. Kragh JF, Walters TJ, Baer DG, et al. Practical use of emergency tourniquets to stop bleeding in major limb trauma. *J Trauma.* 2008;64(2)(Suppl):S38-S49. doi:10.1097/TA.0b013e31816086b1.

31. Caravalho J. OTSG Dismounted Complex Blast Injury Task Force: final report. 18 June 2011:44-47.

32. Eastridge BJ, Mabry RL, Seguin P, et al. Death on the battlefield (2001-2011): implications for the future of combat casualty care. *J Trauma Acute Care Surg.* 2012;73(6)(Suppl 5):S431-S437.

33. Mabry R, McManus JG. Prehospital advances in the management of severe penetrating trauma. *Crit Care Med.* 2008;36(7)(Suppl):S258-266.

34. Kelly JF, Ritenhour AE, McLaughlin DF, et al. Injury severity and causes of death from Operation Iraqi Freedom and Operation Enduring Freedom: 2003–2004 versus 2006. *J Trauma.* 2008; 64(2)(Suppl):S21-S27. doi:10.1097/TA.0b013e318160b9fb.

35. Beekley AC, Sebesta JA, Blackbourne LH, Herbert GS, Kauvar DS, Baer DG, Walters TJ, Mullenix PS, Holcomb JB. Prehospital tourniquet use in Operation Iraqi Freedom: effect on hemorrhage control and outcomes. *J Trauma.* 2008;64:S28-S37.

36. Tarpey M. Tactical combat casualty care in Operation Iraqi Freedom. *US Army Med Dept J.* 2005;April-June:38-41.

37. Butler FK, Holcomb JB. The tactical combat casualty care transition initiative. *US Army Med Dept J.* 2005; April-June:33-37.

38. Savage E, Forestier C, Withers N, Tien H, Pannel D. Tactical combat casualty care in the Canadian forces: lessons learned from the Afghan War. *Can J Surg.* 2011;59:S118-S123.

39. Tien HC, Jung V, Rizoli SB, Acharya SV, MacDonald JC. An evaluation of tactical combat casualty care interventions in a combat environment. *J Am Coll Surg.* 2008;207:174-178.

40. Butler FK, Holcomb JB, Giebner SD, McSwain NE, Bagian J. Tactical combat casualty care 2007: evolving concepts and battlefield experience. *Mil Med.* 2007;172(Suppl):1-19.

41. Gresham J. Giving back, again: Master Sgt. Luis Rodriguez and the tactical combat casualty care course. *Faircount's The Year in Veterans Affairs and Military Medicine.* 2006;2005-2006:136-139.

42. Bottoms M. Tactical combat casualty care: saving lives on the battlefield. *Tip of the Spear* (Command Publication of the US Special Operations Command). 2006;June:34-35.

43. Brown BD. Letter of Commendation to Army Medical Command. Commander, US Special Operations Command, 17 August 2005.

44. Sohn VY, Miller JP, Koeller CA, et al. From the combat medic to the forward surgical team: the Madigan model for improving trauma readiness of brigade combat teams fighting the global war on terror. *J Surg Res.* 2007;138(1):25-31.

45. Holcomb JB, Stansbury LG, Champion HR, Wade C, Bellamy RF. Understanding combat casualty care statistics. *J Trauma.* 2006;60(2):397-401.

46. Eastridge BJ, Jenkins D, Flaherty S, Schiller H, Holcomb JB. Trauma system development in a theater of war: experiences from Operation Iraqi Freedom and Operation Enduring Freedom. *J Trauma.* 2006;61(6):1366-1372.

47. Beekley AC, Starnes BW, Sebesta JA. Lessons learned from modern military surgery. *Surg Clin N Am.* 2007;87(1):157-184.

48. Salomone JP. Letter to Assistant Secretary of Defense for Health Affairs, 10 June 2008.

49. Hetzler MR, Ball JA. Thoughts on aid bags: part one. *J Spec Oper Med.* 2008;8(3):47-53.

50. Pennardt A. TCCC in one special operations unit. Presentation at CoTCCC Meeting, 3 February 2009.

51. Kotwal RS, Montgomery HR, Kotwal BM, et al. Eliminating preventable death on the battlefield. *Arch Surg.* 2011;146(12):1350-1358. doi:10.1001/archsurg.2011.213.

52. Butler FK, Smith DJ, Carmona RH. Implementing and preserving advances in combat casualty care from Iraq and Afghanistan throughout the US military. *J Trauma Acute Care Surg.* 2015 Aug;79(2):321-326.

53. Mabry RL, DeLorenzo R. Challenges to improving combat casualty survival on the battlefield. *Mil Med.* 2014 May;179(5):477-482.

54. Kotwal R, Montgomery H, Conklin C, et al. Leadership and a casualty response system for eliminating preventable death. *J Trauma Acute Care Surg.* 2017 Jun;82(6 Suppl 1):S9-S15.

55. Jacobs LM and the Joint Committee to Create a National Policy to Enhance Survivability from Intentional Mass Shooting Events. The Hartford Consensus IV: a call for increased national resilience. *Conn Med J.* 2016;80:239-244.

56. Brown BD. Special operations combat medic critical task list. Commander, US Special Operations Command letter, 9 March 2005.

57. Bureau of Medicine and Surgery (Navy Surgeon General) Message 111622Z: Tactical combat casualty care training, December 2006.

58. Holcomb, JB. The 2004 Fitts lecture: current perspective on combat casualty care. *J Trauma.* 2005;59(4):990-1002.

59. US Marine Corps Message 02004Z: Tactical Combat Casualty Care (TCCC) and Combat Lifesaver (CLS) fundamentals, philosophies, and guidance, August 2006.

60. US Coast Guard Message 221752Z: Tactical medical response program, November 2006.

61. Hostage GM. USSOCOM visit to the pararescue medical course at Kirtland AFB September 2005. Air Force Education and Training Command letter, 8 September 2005.

62. Kiley KC. Operational needs statement for medical simulation training centers for combat lifesavers and tactical combat casualty care training. Army Surgeon General letter DASG-ZA, 1 September 2005.

63. Blackbourne LH, Baer DG, Eastridge BJ, et al. Military medical revolution: military trauma system. *J Trauma Acute Care Surg.* 2012;73(6)(Suppl 5):S388-S394. doi:10.1097/TA.0b013e31827548df.

64. All Army Activities Message 0902031521Z: Mandatory predeployment trauma training for Army medical department personnel, 3 February 2009.

65. Holcomb JB, Wilensky G. Tactical combat casualty care and minimizing preventable fatalities in combat. Defense Health Board memorandum, 6 August 2009. Military Health System website. https://health.mil/About-MHS/OASDHA/Defense-Health-Agency/Defense-Health-Board/Reports. Accessed March 21, 2018.

66. Casscells W. Tactical combat casualty care. Assistant Secretary of Defense for Health Affairs memorandum, 4 March 2009.

67. Woodson J. Tactical combat casualty care. Assistant Secretary of Defense for Health Affairs Memorandum. 23 August 2011.

68. Woodson J. Tactical combat casualty care for deploying personnel. Assistant Secretary of Defense for Health Affairs Memorandum. 14 February 2014.

69. Kotwal RS, Butler FK, Edgar EP, Shackelford SA, Bennett DR, Bailey JA. Saving lives on the battlefield: a joint trauma system review of prehospital trauma care in combined joint operating area Y Afghanistan (CJOA-A) executive summary. *J Spec Oper Med.* 2013;13(1):77-80.

70. Sauer SW, Robinson JB, Smith MP, et al. Saving lives on the battlefield (part II): one year later: a joint theater trauma system & joint trauma system review of pre-hospital trauma care in combined joint operating area Y Afghanistan (CJOA-A). USCENTCOM Report. 2014.

71. Nathan ML. BUMEDINST 1510.25A Navy medicine tactical combat casualty care program. http://www.med.navy.mil/directives/ExternalDirectives/1510.25A.pdf. Accessed March 21, 2018.

72. Gross KR. Establishing a DoD standard for TCCC training: joint trauma system. White paper to the US Military Services Surgeons General. 11 September 2015. https://www.naemt.org/docs/default-source/education-documents/tccc/tccc-updates_092017/tccc-reference-materials/06-tccc-reference-documents/jts-white-paper-tccc-training-150910-v12.pdf?sfvrsn=884cd92_2. Accessed March 23, 2018.

73. Goforth C, Antico D. TCCC Standardization: the time is now. *J Spec Oper Med.* 2016;16:53-56.

74. Amor SP. ABCA Armies' Program Chief of Staff letter. February 22, 2011.

75. Irizzary D. Training NATO special forces medical personnel: opportunities in technology-enabled training systems for skill acquisition and maintenance. *J Special Ops Med.* 2013 Nov;(Suppl). doi:10.14339/STO-MP-HFM-224.

76. Holcomb J. Major scientific lessons learned in the trauma field over the last two decades. *PLoS Med.* 2017;14:e1002339.

77. McSwain NE, Frame S, Paturas JL, eds. *Prehospital Trauma Life Support Manual.* 4th ed. Akron, OH: Mosby; 1999.

78. Bulger E, Snyder D, Schoelles K, et al. An evidence-based prehospital guideline for external hemorrhage control: American College of Surgeons Committee on Trauma. *Prehosp Emerg Care.* 2014;18:163-173.

79. Stuke L, Pons P. Guy J, et al. Prehospital spine immobilization for penetrating trauma-review and recommendations from the prehospital trauma life support executive committee. *J Trauma.* 2011;71(3):763-769.

80. Butler FK, Carmona R. Tactical combat casualty care: from the battlefields of Afghanistan and Iraq to the streets of America. *The Tactical Edge.* 2012;86-91. http://public.ntoa.org/default.asp?action=issue&year=2012&season=1%20-%20Winter&pub=Tactical%20Edge. Accessed March 22, 2018.

81. Jacobs LM, Wade DS, McSwain NE, et al. The Hartford consensus: THREAT, a medical disaster preparedness concept. *J Am Coll Surg.* 2013;217(5):947-953.

82. Jacobs LM, McSwain NE Jr, Rotondo MF, et al. Improving survival from active shooter events: the Hartford Consensus. *J Trauma Acute Care Surg.* 2013 Jun;74(6):1399-1400.

83. Levy M, Jacobs L. A call to action to develop programs for bystanders to control severe bleeding. *JAMA Surg.* 2016;151(12):1103-1104.

84. Callaway D, Robertson J, Sztajnkrycer M. Law enforcement-applied tourniquets: a case series of life-saving interventions. *Prehosp Emerg Care.* 2015;19:320-327.

85. Pons P, Jerome J, McMullen J, et al. The Hartford Consensus on active shooters: implementing the continuum of prehospital trauma response. *J Emerg Med.* 2015;49:878-885.

86. Callaway DW. Translating tactical combat casualty care lessons learned to the high-threat civilian setting: tactical emergency casualty care and the Hartford consensus. *Wilderness Environ Med.* 2017 Jun;28(2 Suppl):S140-S145.

87. Butler FK, Bennett B, Wedmore CI. Tactical combat casualty care and wilderness medicine: advancing trauma

care in austere environments. *Emerg Med Clin North Am.* 2017;35:391-407.

88. Bennett BL, Butler FK Jr, Wedmore IS. Tactical combat casualty care: transitioning battlefield lessons learned to other austere environments. *Wilderness Environ Med.* 2017;28(2 Suppl):S3-S4.

89. Butler FK, Zafren K, eds. Tactical management of wilderness casualties in special operations. *Wilderness Environ Med.* 1998;9(2);62-117.

90. Butler FK, Kotwal RS, Buckenmaier CC III, et al. A triple-option analgesia plan for tactical combat casualty care. *J Spec Operations Med.* 2014;14:13-25.

91. Weiss E. Medical considerations for wilderness and adventure travelers. *Med Clin North Am.* 1999;83(4):885-902.

92. Drew B, Bennett B, Littlejohn L. Application of current hemorrhage control techniques for backcountry care: part one, tourniquets and hemorrhage control adjuncts. *Wilderness Environ Med.* 2015;26:236-245.

93. Littlejohn L, Bennett B, Drew B. Application of current hemorrhage control techniques for backcountry care: part two, hemostatic dressings and other adjuncts. *Wilderness Environ Med.* 2015;26:246-254.

94. Smith WWR. Integration of tactical EMS in the National Park Service. *Wilderness Environ Med.* 2017;28(2 Suppl):S146-S153.

95. American College of Emergency Physicians. Out-of-hospital severe hemorrhage control: policy statement. *Ann Emerg Med.* 2015 Dec;66(6):693.

96. American College of Emergency Physicians. Out-of-hospital use of analgesia and sedation. *Ann Emerg Med.* 2016 Feb;67(2):305-306.

97. Department of Defense Instruction 1322.24: Military readiness training. Washington, DC: The Pentagon; 16 March 2018.

98. Gross K. Establishing a DoD standard for TCCC training. US Army Institute of Surgical Research letter to the service Surgeons General and the Medical Officer of the Marine Corps, 11 September 2015. https://www.naemt.org/docs/default-source/education-documents/tccc/tccc-updates_092017/tccc-reference-materials/06-tccc-reference-documents/jts-white-paper-tccc-training---cover-ltradb7ab32fe31667a9799ff0000a338da.pdf?sfvrsn=ac86cd92_2. Accessed March 23, 2018.

99. Gurney J, Turner C, Burelison D, et al. Tactical combat casualty care training, knowledge and utilization in the Army. *J Trauma.* (publication pending).

100. Cousins R, Anderson S, Dehnisch F, et al. It's time for EMS to administer ketamine analgesia. *Prehosp Emerg Care.* 2017;21:408-410.

101. Butler FK, Holcomb JB, Kotwal RS, et al. Fluid resuscitation for hemorrhagic shock in tactical combat casualty care: TCCC guidelines proposed change 14-01. *J Spec Oper Med.* 2014;14:13-38.

102. Kotwal RS, Butler FK, Montgomery HR, et al. The tactical combat casualty care casualty card. *J Spec Oper Med.* 2013;13:82-86.

CHAPTER 24

© Ralf Hiemisch/Getty Images.

Care Under Fire

Authors:
Capt. (Ret) Frank Butler, MD
Master Sgt. (Ret) Harold Montgomery
Command Master Chief Petty Officer (Ret) Eric Sine

CHAPTER OBJECTIVES

At the completion of this chapter, you will be able to do the following:

- Discuss the impact of the tactical environment on the management of combat trauma.
- Describe techniques that can be used to quickly move casualties to cover while the unit is engaged in a firefight.
- Discuss the rationale for early use of a tourniquet to control life-threatening extremity bleeding during Care Under Fire.
- Explain why spinal immobilization is not a critical need in combat casualties with only penetrating trauma.

SCENARIO

Your unit is in a five-vehicle convoy moving through a small Iraqi village when a command-detonated improvised explosive device (IED) explodes under the second vehicle. Moderate sniper fire follows, and the rest of the convoy is busily engaged in suppressing it. You are a medic in the disabled vehicle, which is not on fire and is right side up. You are not injured and are able to assist. The person next to you has bilateral mid-thigh traumatic amputations. There is heavy arterial bleeding from the left stump and only mild oozing of blood from the right stump. The casualty is conscious and in moderate pain. What do you do?

- What phase of care are you in?
- What is your immediate concern?
- Should you treat the casualty or return fire? Why?
- What is your next action?
- Should you put a tourniquet on the right stump? Why?
- What are your next actions?

INTRODUCTION

As reflected in the Tactical Combat Casualty Care (TCCC) guidelines for Care Under Fire shown in **Table 24-1** and **Figure 24-1**, very limited medical care should be attempted while the casualty and the unit are under effective hostile fire. Suppression of hostile fire and moving the casualty to a safe position are major considerations at this point. Significant delays for a detailed examination and thorough treatment of all injuries are not advisable while under effective enemy fire.

Casualties who have sustained injuries that are not life threatening and that do not preclude further participation in the fight should continue to assist the unit in suppressing hostile fire. It may also be critical for the combat medic, corpsman, or pararescueman (PJ) to help suppress hostile fire before attempting to provide care. This can be especially true in small-unit operations in which friendly firepower is limited and every weapon in the unit may be needed to prevail.

Moving Casualties in Tactical Settings

In Care Under Fire, the best first step in saving a casualty is usually to control the tactical situation. An axiom of TCCC is that "The best medicine on the battlefield is fire superiority." If hostile fire cannot be effectively suppressed or the unit is unable to break contact with the enemy, it may be necessary to move the casualty to cover. Casualties whose wounds do not prevent them from moving themselves to cover should do so to avoid exposing the medic or other aid providers to unnecessary hazard. If unable to move and unresponsive, the casualty is likely beyond help, and risking the lives of rescuers by subjecting them to enemy fire in an unprotected area at this point in the engagement is usually not warranted. If a casualty *is* responsive but unable to move, a rescue plan should be developed, as follows:

1. Determine the potential risk to the rescuers, keeping in mind that *rescuers should not move into a zeroed-in position* (i.e., where there is effective concentration of enemy fire). Did the casualty trip a booby trap or mine? Where is fire coming from? Is it direct or indirect (e.g., rifle, machine gun, grenade, mortar)? Are there electrical, fire, chemical, water, mechanical, or other environmental hazards?

2. Consider your assets. What can rescuers provide in the way of covering fire, screening, shielding, and rescue-applicable equipment?

3. Make sure all personnel understand their role in the rescue and which movement technique

Table 24-1 Basic Management Plan for Care Under Fire

1. Return fire and take cover.
2. Direct or expect casualty to remain engaged as a combatant, if appropriate.
3. Direct casualty to move to cover and apply self-aid if able.
4. Try to keep the casualty from sustaining additional wounds.
5. Casualties should be extricated from burning vehicles or buildings and moved to places of relative safety. Do what is necessary to stop the burning process.
6. Stop life-threatening external hemorrhage if tactically feasible:
   - Direct casualty to control hemorrhage by self-aid if able.
   - Use aCoTCCC-recommended limb tourniquet for hemorrhage that is anatomically amenable to tourniquet use.
   - Apply the limb tourniquet over the uniform clearly proximal to the bleeding site(s). If the site of the life-threatening bleeding is not readily apparent, place the tourniquet "high and tight" (as proximal as possible) on the injured limb, and move the casualty to cover.
7. Airway management is generally best deferred until the Tactical Field Care phase.

is to be used (e.g., drag, carry, rope, stretcher, etc.). If possible, let the casualty know what the plan is so that he or she can assist as much as possible by rolling to a certain position, attaching a dragline to his or her web gear, and identifying hazards.

4. Management of the airway is temporarily deferred until the casualty is safe from hostile fire or other hazard. This minimizes the risk to the rescuer and avoids the difficulty of attempting to manage the airway while dragging the casualty.

Usually, the fastest method for moving a casualty is dragging him or her along the long axis of the body by two rescuers (**Figure 24-2**). This drag can be used in buildings, shallow water, and snow and down stairs. It can be accomplished with the rescuers standing or crawling. The use of the casualty's web gear, tactical vest, a dragline, poncho, clothing, or improvised harness makes this method easier. However, holding the casualty under the arms is all that is necessary. A one-rescuer drag can be used for short distances, but it is more difficult for the rescuer, is slower, and is less controlled (**Figure 24-3**).

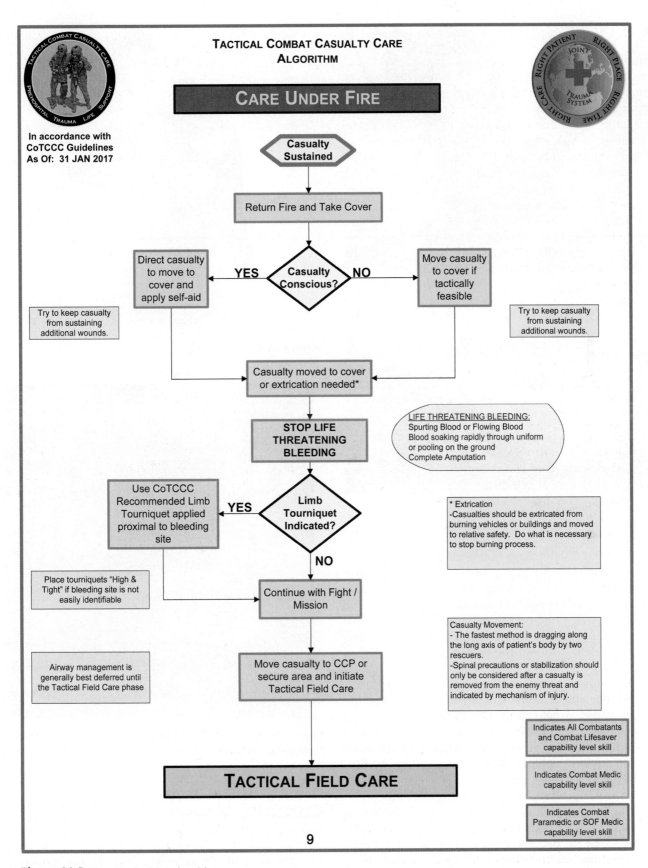

Figure 24-1 Care Under Fire algorithm.

Courtesy of Harold Montgomery. Retrieved from https://deployedmedicine.com/market/11/content/87.

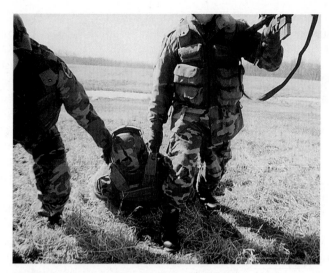

Figure 24-2 Two-person drag.

Courtesy of Dr. Mel Otten.

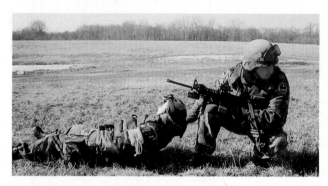

Figure 24-3 One-person drag.

Courtesy of Dr. Mel Otten.

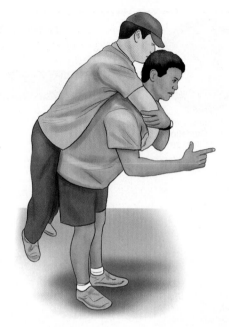

Figure 24-4 Hawes carry.

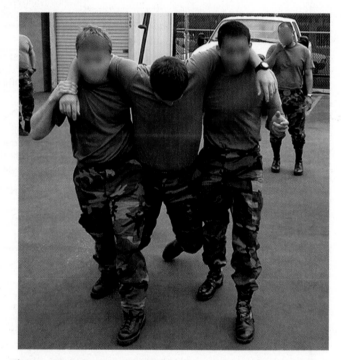

Figure 24-5 SEAL Team THREE carry: Both rescuers hold the casualty by the belt in the rear.

Courtesy of Dr. Frank Butler.

The great disadvantage of dragging is that the casualty is in contact with the ground, and this can cause additional injury in rough terrain. Carrying the casualty may be a better option when tactically feasible. The Hawes carry is a one-person technique that allows for rapid movement (**Figure 24-4**). If the casualty can maintain an upright position, the rescuer stands in front of the casualty and squats down. The casualty's arms are moved around the neck of the rescuer and held in place. The rescuer stands and leans forward, assuming the weight of the casualty, and then moves to the desired location. This carry avoids the greater lifting effort and difficulty of carrying a very heavy load in an awkward position entailed by older carry techniques like the fireman's carry. Members of SEAL Team THREE devised and use a two-person carry based on having one of the casualty's arms draped over each of the rescuers' shoulders. The rescuers use the hand closest to the casualty to lift him or her by the belt at the waist. If the casualty is conscious and can hold on to each of the two rescuers with his or her arms, then the rescuers' free arms may be used to employ their weapons if necessary (**Figure 24-5**).

Casualty Movement and Spinal Immobilization

Movement of the casualty will often be the most problematic aspect of providing TCCC.[1] Performing spinal immobilization prior to moving a trauma patient with a potential spinal injury is a long-standing principle of care; however, this practice should be reevaluated in the combat setting. Arishita, Vayer, and Bellamy examined the value of cervical spine immobilization in penetrating neck injuries in Vietnam and found that in only 1.4% of casualties with penetrating neck injuries would immobilization of the cervical spine have been of possible benefit.[2] Because the time required to accomplish cervical spine immobilization was found to be 5.5 minutes, even when applied by experienced emergency medical technicians (EMTs), the authors concluded that the potential hazards to both casualty and providers outweighed the potential benefit of immobilization. Kennedy and his coauthors reported similar findings of no cervical spine injuries in 105 victims of gunshot wounds to the head.[3] Other papers examining the value of cervical spine immobilization in civilian trauma cases also found few data to support this practice in trauma victims with a mechanism of injury limited to penetrating trauma.[4,5]

In casualty scenarios in which the casualty has suffered blunt trauma and is under effective hostile fire (e.g., an ambush in which an IED causes a vehicle to be overturned and the explosion is followed by small arms fire) stabilization of the cervical spine may be medically indicated but tactically contraindicated. The combat medic, corpsman, or PJ must weigh the risk of injury from hostile fire against the risk of worsening any potential spinal cord injury when making decisions about how and when to move the casualty to cover.

The wounding pattern seen in IED injuries depends on whether the explosion occurred when the casualty was riding in a vehicle (mounted IED attack) or as the casualty stepped on the IED (dismounted IED attack). The latter mechanism of injury was seen in increasing numbers in Afghanistan during the 2010–2012 time period and resulted in an injury pattern referred to as Dismounted Complex Blast Injury (DCBI).[6] Spinal injuries may result from either type of IED attack, and this must be considered when treating IED casualties.[7] Appropriate spinal precautions should be taken as tactically feasible.

Hemorrhage Control

In combat casualties, early control of significant external hemorrhage is *the* most important intervention. Hemorrhage remains the predominant cause of preventable death in combat fatalities.[8] The renewed focus on prehospital tourniquet use is one example of the lifesaving potential of the TCCC guidelines. Before the onset of hostilities of Afghanistan in 2001, most military medics were taught that a tourniquet should be used only as a last resort to control extremity hemorrhage.[9] A study of 2,600 combat fatalities incurred during the Vietnam conflict[10] noted that the incidence of death from extremity

hemorrhage was 7.4%. In 2003 to 2006, the preventable death review of 982 combat fatalities done by Kelly found a 7.8% incidence of death either solely or significantly due to extremity hemorrhage.[11] After the widespread implementation of the tourniquet recommendations from the TCCC guidelines, a 2012 comprehensive study of 4,596 U.S. combat fatalities from 2001 to 2011 noted that only 2.6% of total combat fatalities resulted from extremity hemorrhage.[12] This dramatic decrease in deaths from extremity hemorrhage resulted from the now ubiquitous fielding of modern tourniquets and aggressive training of all potential first responders on tourniquet application.[9]

Control of significant bleeding from injuries like scalp lacerations and external torso injuries is also a high priority, but the tactical imperative to maintain fire superiority and move the casualty to cover dictates that *only life-threatening extremity bleeding should warrant any intervention during Care Under Fire*. Both the casualty and the other unit members should disregard minor wounds insofar as possible during Care Under Fire to maximize the unit's firepower. If a tourniquet is required during Care Under Fire, the casualty should apply it to himself or herself, if at all possible. Tourniquet application should take place under the best cover immediately available to the casualty.

Tourniquets

Background

Tourniquet use was widely disparaged by prehospital trauma care courses used by the military in the recent past, despite extremity hemorrhage having been the leading cause of preventable death in combat fatalities during the Vietnam conflict.[10,13-16] The reluctance to employ tourniquets to control life-threatening extremity hemorrhage on the battlefield was even more difficult to understand in light of the fact that tourniquets are routinely used for short periods of time during orthopedic surgical procedures without causing adverse effects due to tourniquet ischemia.[1,13] Recognition of this lethal paradox was the primary driver for the combined U.S. Special Operations Command and Uniformed Services University of the Health Sciences research effort that resulted in the development of TCCC.[13] The opportunity to effectively address a leading cause of preventable death on the battlefield with prehospital tourniquets compelled a reexamination of this aspect of battlefield trauma care. The continuation of that effort into other aspects of prehospital combat casualty care led to the publication of the first set of TCCC guidelines in 1996.[1,13]

Despite the publication of the original TCCC guidelines in *Military Medicine*, the vast majority of the U.S. military was not using extremity tourniquets at the start of the conflicts in Afghanistan and Iraq, which allowed preventable deaths from extremity hemorrhage to continue.

Then, in 2004, at the request of the U.S. Special Operations Command, Holcomb and his colleagues examined all deaths in Special Operations forces from the start of the Global War on Terrorism in 2001 until November 2004. They found that bleeding from extremity wounds was either the sole cause of death or a significant factor in 3 of the 12 potentially preventable deaths among the 82 combat fatalities reviewed.[17] Beekley noted that 4 of the 7 deaths that occurred in a series of 165 casualties with severe extremity injuries could have been saved by the timely use of properly placed and functional tourniquets.[18] Kelly documented 77 deaths in which extremity hemorrhage was the sole cause of a potentially preventable death or a significant contributing factor in his study of 982 combat fatalities occurring between 2003 and 2006.[11] Eastridge found 120 deaths from extremity hemorrhage in his comprehensive study of 4,596 combat fatalities from Afghanistan and Iraq between 2001 and 2011.[8]

There was a paucity of reporting on prehospital emergency tourniquet use on the battlefield prior to the conflicts in Iraq and Afghanistan. Colonel John Kragh's work has now confirmed the lifesaving benefit and low incidence of complications from prehospital tourniquet use in combat casualties.[19,20] Although tourniquets have been in use on the battlefield for centuries,[21] only recently have Colonel Kragh and other authors clearly shown that tourniquets save lives in combat without causing harm.[22-26] By June 2011, Colonel Brian Eastridge's landmark study "Death on the Battlefield"[8] found that potentially preventable deaths from extremity hemorrhage had dropped from the 7.8% of deaths due solely or significantly to extremity hemorrhage noted in the Kelly study[11] to 2.6% (as calculated over the entire study period), a decrease of 67%. Because of their proven lifesaving value, tourniquets are now ubiquitous on the modern battlefield.

Several papers have called for a reevaluation of tourniquet use in the civilian prehospital environment as well.[27-31] Both the American College of Surgeons Hartford Consensus program, led by Dr. Lenworth Jacobs, and the Stop the Bleed campaign, led by White House medical staffers Doctors David Marcozzi, Kathryn Brinsfield, and Richard Hunt, have advocated for the aggressive TCCC approach to the use of extremity tourniquets to control life-threatening extremity hemorrhage in civilian settings, especially in mass-casualty events resulting from active shooter incidents and terrorist bombings.[32,33] Recent studies have documented the lifesaving benefit of extremity tourniquets in civilian settings.[34-36] The Scerbo paper[36] clearly documents the importance of applying tourniquets as quickly as possible when they are indicated, even in civilian settings.

Which Tourniquets?

There are currently a variety of tourniquets available on the market, and some are more effective at controlling

extremity haemorrhage than others.[37,38] In a comparative evaluation of tourniquets available at the time, the 2005 U.S. Army Institute of Surgical Research identified three that were 100% effective in stopping arterial blood flow.[37] These were the Combat Application Tourniquet (C-A-T), the SOF™ Tactical Tourniquet (SOFTT), and the Emergency and Military Tourniquet (EMT™), a pneumatic device. The C-A-T and SOFTT are both windlass devices that are lightweight and relatively inexpensive. These tourniquets can be readily applied to one's own or another's extremity, and are rugged, reliable, and small enough to be easily carried. The C-A-T has been designated as an item of individual issue to ground combatants in all services and has proven effective and reliable in the current conflicts (**Figure 24-6**).[19,20] The SOFTT has also performed well in combat, although it is not as widely used as the C-A-T at present. Combat medic experience has found that the SOFTT may be a better choice if the casualty has a stocky, muscular build with large thighs and needs a tourniquet in that location (**Figure 24-7**). The EMT has been found to perform

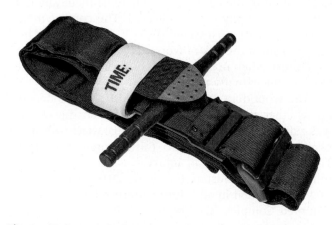

Figure 24-6 Combat Application Tourniquet (C-A-T).
© Looka/Shutterstock

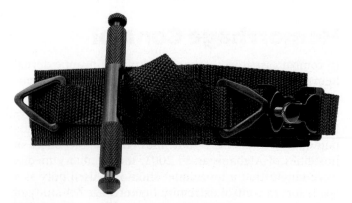

Figure 24-7 SOF Tactical Tourniquet (SOFTT).
Courtesy of Tactical Medical Solutions, LLC.

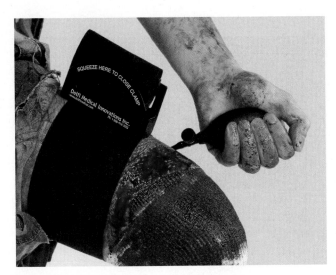

Figure 24-8 Emergency and Military Tourniquet.
Courtesy of Delfi Medical. Retrieved from http://www.delfimedical.com/emergency-military-tourniquet/.

very well in emergency departments,[19] but it is considerably more expensive than the C-A-T (**Figure 24-8**). Furthermore, its inflatable cuff may develop leaks if it has had prolonged time in the field with heat and cold stress as well as incidental trauma to the cuff.

More recent laboratory studies have found that some newer tourniquets, such as the Tactical Mechanical Tourniquet, may perform as well as the currently fielded devices.[39] At this point in time, however, the U.S. military has more experience with combat tourniquets than any military force in history,[38] and the accumulated positive evidence on the use of the C-A-T and the SOFTT in combat settings must be considered in making future decisions about tourniquet acquisition and fielding. That said, there has not been a comprehensive comparative study of commercially available tourniquets performed since the 2005 Walters study.[37] The CoTCCC is currently undertaking a review of the tourniquet literature to determine if the evidence base is strong enough to recommend additional tourniquets in TCCC.

Tourniquet Application

Death from extremity hemorrhage can be prevented by aggressive use of tourniquets unless the site of bleeding is too proximal on the extremity to apply a tourniquet. Because of their effectiveness at hemorrhage control, the speed with which they can be applied, and the lack of a requirement to hold sustained direct pressure on the bleeding site, tourniquets are the best option for temporary control of life-threatening extremity hemorrhage in the tactical environment.

Tourniquets are far more effective at saving lives when applied before the casualty has gone into hemorrhagic shock.[19] As noted previously, past concerns about ischemic damage to extremities from brief periods of tourniquet use

have proven to be unfounded when tourniquets are used appropriately and for short periods of time.[20,40,41] Tourniquets have been found to be safe if left on for less than 2 hours.[42] Prolonged (> 6 hours) use of a tourniquet can potentially result in the loss of a limb, but there were no reports of limb loss in U.S. casualties due to tourniquet ischemia in a large review of tourniquet use in Iraq and Afghanistan.[15]

The first decision to be made in caring for a casualty who has been wounded in one or more extremities is whether the extremity bleeding is severe enough to necessitate tourniquet use. The following are examples of the various ways in which life-threatening bleeding may present; they depict clinical situations in which tourniquet use is indicated[32] (**Figure 24-9**).

- Pulsatile or steady bleeding is noted.
- Blood is seen pooling on the ground.
- The overlying uniform or clothes are soaked with blood.
- Dressings applied to the bleeding site are ineffective and become soaked with blood.
- There is a traumatic amputation of the arm or leg.
- There has been prior bleeding and the victim is now in shock (unconscious or confused).

Every combatant on the battlefield should be able to apply a tourniquet to his or her own bleeding extremity and to the arm or leg of any other unit member who requires it. Hemorrhage control by nonmedical personnel has been a key element in reducing preventable deaths on the battlefield.[43] When applied, tourniquets should be placed over the uniform just proximal to the site of the severe bleeding. If the bleeding site cannot be precisely located due to darkness or the need for expedited application during an engagement with hostile forces, the tourniquet should be applied as proximally on the extremity as feasible.[42] If bleeding does not stop after the first tourniquet has been tightened, a second tourniquet should be applied adjacent to the first.

Tourniquets should never be placed directly over a joint. They should also never be placed over a holster or a pocket containing bulky objects that would make tightening the tourniquet more difficult or make tourniquet application more painful for the casualty. During Care Under Fire, tourniquets should be tightened as necessary to stop the bleeding from the distal injury. Having the tourniquet placed over the uniform is not ideal, but Care Under Fire is not the right time to expose the wound for a thorough examination. Rather, the bleeding should be stopped, and both the casualty and the care provider should move to cover as quickly as possible. Once time permits in the Tactical Field Care phase, the wound should be exposed and reevaluated, and a replacement tourniquet should be applied directly to the casualty's skin.

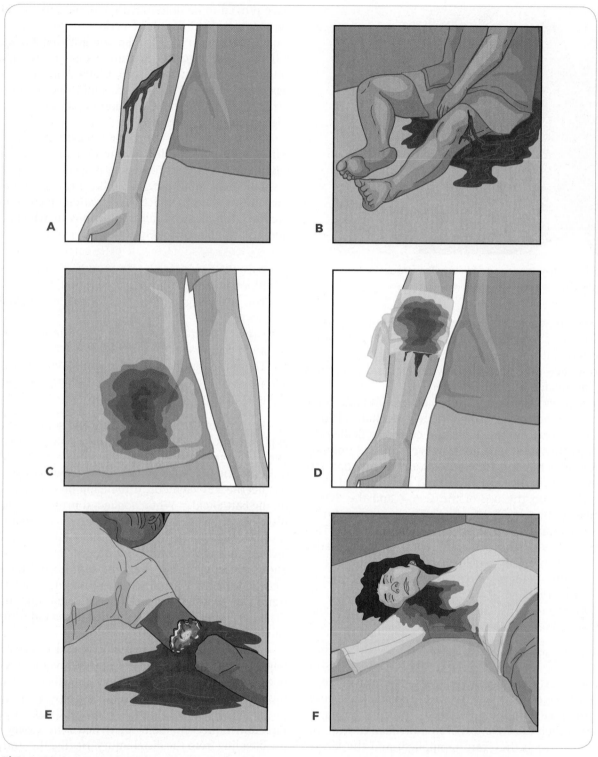

Figure 24-9 Life-threatening bleeding. **A.** Pulsatile or steadily flowing bleeding from the wound. **B.** Blood seen pooling on the ground. **C.** Overlying clothes are soaked with blood. **D.** Bandages covering wound are soaked with blood. **E.** Bleeding from a traumatic amputation. **F.** Prior bleeding with victim now in shock (unconscious or confused).

The U.S. military experience with tourniquets during the conflicts in Iraq and Afghanistan has provided some additional teaching points about these devices:

- Waiting too long to apply a needed tourniquet is a mistake, and it may prove fatal.
- Casualties who have had tourniquets applied should be rechecked periodically to ensure that hemorrhage is still controlled. If bleeding has recurred, the tourniquet should be tightened, or a second tourniquet applied.
- Tourniquets cause significant pain when tightened. This pain does not mean that the tourniquet has been applied incorrectly or that it should be removed. Tourniquet pain should be managed with analgesics as recommended in the TCCC Triple Option Analgesia plan in Tactical Field Care.[44,45]

Tourniquet mistakes to avoid include:

- Not having an effective commercial tourniquet available for use
- Not using a tourniquet when one is indicated
- Waiting too long to put a tourniquet on when one is needed
- Not using a second tourniquet when one is needed
- Using a tourniquet for minor bleeding
- Applying the tourniquet more proximally than is required to stop bleeding (except when a tourniquet is applied during Care Under Fire above a bleeding site that is not readily locatable. In this instance, the tourniquet should be applied "high and tight"—as proximal as feasible on the injured extremity)
- Not tightening the tourniquet enough to effectively control the bleeding
- Periodically loosening the tourniquet to allow blood flow to the injured extremity

The time of tourniquet application should always be documented. This has customarily been accomplished by writing the letter "T" on the casualty's forehead along with the time. This should be done with an indelible ink marker to ensure that this important information does not wash or wipe off. Either on the involved extremity or a piece of tape applied to the casualty's chest is an alternative location for noting tourniquet application time. The information should also be recorded on the individual's TCCC Casualty Card. If the casualty has multiple tourniquets with significantly different times of application, this should be noted clearly in the first responder care documentation.

All manufactured tourniquets are designed for a single use. A separate group of tourniquets should be used for training, and training tourniquets should not subsequently be issued to individuals for use in combat. Many military units have evolved to a single-tour, single-use policy for tourniquets.

Direct pressure and compression dressings are less desirable than tourniquets during Care Under Fire because the need for direct pressure may result in lethal delays in getting the casualty and the rescuer to cover. Furthermore, these interventions provide less definitive control of life-threatening extremity hemorrhage, especially while the casualty is being moved.[38,46]

A final note about tourniquets: They should be protected from exposure to the elements during combat deployments. In 2013, Weppner and colleagues studied tourniquets that were carried by Marine Corps personnel on their plate carriers during a deployment, comparing them to tourniquets that were carried inside individual first aid kits (IFAKs).[47] Of the plate carrier-exposed tourniquets, 46 (12%) broke when tested as opposed to none among those carried in IFAKs.

Hemostatic Agents

The requirement to hold direct pressure on the bleeding site for 3 minutes after the application of a hemostatic agent is tactically infeasible when the casualty and the responder are under effective hostile fire. Therefore, the use of hemostatic agents in the Care Under Fire phase is not recommended. When its application can be achieved in a safer setting, however, a hemostatic dressing can be a highly effective option for controlling life-threatening hemorrhage when a tourniquet cannot be applied to the bleeding site. This subject is discussed more fully in the Tactical Field Care chapter.

Airway

No immediate management of the airway should be anticipated at this point because of the need to move the casualty to cover as quickly as possible.[1] Because most preventable deaths on the battlefield are caused by hemorrhage, addressing any significant external hemorrhage (either with a tourniquet during Care Under Fire or with other hemorrhage control options during Tactical Field Care) will help to prevent the casualty from going into hypovolemic shock and thereby requiring airway management. A penetrating injury that is severe enough to result in immediate loss of consciousness such as penetrating head trauma will have a high probability of proving fatal during the Care Under Fire phase. Airway control should be deferred until Tactical Field Care and until after major external hemorrhage has been addressed.

SUMMARY

- In Care Under Fire, the need for medical care must be weighed against the need to move to cover and to suppress hostile fire rapidly.
- During Care Under Fire, very limited medical care should be attempted while under effective hostile fire. Suppression of hostile fire and moving the casualty to cover are priorities.
- Casualties who can maintain their combat effectiveness should remain engaged as combatants during Care Under Fire.
- The combat medic or corpsman may have to help suppress hostile fire before providing care to casualties.
- If the casualty has sustained a gunshot wound, is unable to move, and is unresponsive, he or she is likely beyond help. Risking additional lives by exposure to fire in the open to move the casualty to cover during Care Under Fire may not be warranted.
- If the casualty is responsive and able to move to cover, he or she should do so immediately.
- If the casualty is responsive but unable to move to cover, a rescue plan should be implemented as outlined in this chapter.
- The fastest method for moving a casualty is dragging along the long axis of the body by two rescuers.
- One-person drags are slower than two-person drags but have the advantage of exposing only one rescuer to additional risk.
- The Hawes carry can be used by one rescuer and may be useful in some situations.
- A two-person carry used by SEAL Team THREE requires one of the casualty's arms over each of the rescuers' shoulders and is a useful option for a two-rescuer carry.
- With penetrating injury to the head or neck, in the absence of significant blunt force trauma, immobilization of the cervical spine during Care Under Fire is not warranted.
- During Care Under Fire, when treating combat casualties with known or suspected blunt spinal trauma, the first responder must weigh the risk of injury from hostile fire to the casualty and the responder while immobilizing the spine against the risk of causing or worsening a spinal cord injury.
- The wounding pattern of mounted IED injuries is characterized by both penetrating injury and blast injury from the explosion and possibly blunt injury from motor vehicle trauma. In these settings, injury to the spine is more common, and appropriate precautions should be taken.
- Immediate control of extremity hemorrhage with a tourniquet is the most important lifesaving intervention in Care Under Fire and is the only medical care that should be considered before the casualty is moved to cover.
- Tourniquets save lives in combat when used appropriately. They are most effective when applied before the casualty has gone into shock from blood loss.
- Tourniquets are safe when applied for less than 2 hours.
- Three tourniquets have been shown to be 100% effective in stopping arterial blood flow and are recommended for use in TCCC: the Combat Application Tourniquet (C-A-T), the SOF Tactical Tourniquet (SOFTT), and the Emergency and Military Tourniquet (EMT).
- Tourniquets should be placed just proximal to the site of the hemorrhage.
- Tourniquets should never be placed directly over a joint or over pockets containing bulky items.
- The time of tourniquet application should be noted both somewhere on the casualty and on the TCCC Casualty Card.
- The use of hemostatic agents in the Care Under Fire phase is not recommended because of the requirement to hold direct pressure on the bleeding site for 3 minutes after application. This is an unacceptably long period of time during Care Under Fire.
- Airway management is usually best deferred until the Tactical Field Care phase and until after major external hemorrhage has been addressed.

SCENARIO RECAP

Your unit is in a five-vehicle convoy moving through a small Iraqi village when a command-detonated IED explodes under the second vehicle. Moderate sniper fire follows, and the rest of the convoy is busily engaged in suppressing it. You are a medic in the disabled vehicle, which is not on fire and is right side up. You are not injured and are able to assist. The person next to you has bilateral mid-thigh traumatic amputations. There is heavy arterial bleeding from the left stump and only mild oozing of blood from the right stump. The casualty is conscious and in moderate pain. What do you do?

SCENARIO SOLUTION

- **What phase of care are you in?**
  You are in the Care Under Fire phase.
- **What is your immediate concern?**
  The casualty may exsanguinate quickly from arterial bleeding.
- **Should you treat the casualty or return fire? Why?**
  You should treat the casualty's extremity hemorrhage. The rest of the convoy is providing suppressive fire, and applying a tourniquet is a fast and easy lifesaving intervention.
- **What is your next action?**
  Place a tourniquet on the stump of the casualty's left thigh.
- **Should you put a tourniquet on the right stump? Why?**
  No. The bleeding from the right stump is minimal at this point. Wait until the Tactical Field Care phase, but recheck often.
- **What are your next actions?**
  Drag the casualty out of the vehicle and move to the best cover. Return fire if needed. Communicate the casualty's status to the team leader.

References

1. Butler FK, Hagmann J, Butler EG. Tactical combat casualty care in special operations. *Mil Med.* 1996;161(Suppl):3-16.

2. Arishita GI, Vayer JS, Bellamy RF. Cervical spine immobilization of penetrating neck wounds in a hostile environment. *J Trauma.* 1989;29(3):332-337.

3. Kennedy FR, Gonzalez P, Beitler A, Sterling-Scott R, Fleming AW. Incidence of cervical spine injury in patients with gunshot wounds to the head. *South Med J.* 1994;87(6):621-623.

4. Stuke L, Pons P, Guy J, et al. Prehospital spine immobilization for penetrating trauma - review and recommendations from the Prehospital Trauma Life Support Executive Committee. *J Trauma.* 2011;71(3):763-769. doi:10.1097/TA.0b013e3182255cb9.

5. Lustenberger T, Talving P, Lam L, et al. Unstable cervical spine fracture after penetrating neck injury: a rare entity in an analysis of 1,069 patients. *J Trauma.* 2011;70(4):870–872. doi:10.1097/TA.0b013e3181e7576e.

6. Caravalho J. Report of the Army Dismounted Complex Blast Injury Task Force. 2011, June 18. Breakaway Media, LLC. https://www.jsomonline.org/TCCCEsp/06%20TCCC%20Documentos%20de%20Referencia/DCBI%20Task%20Force%20Report%20Final%20(Redacted)%20110921.pdf. Accessed April 9, 2018.

7. Comstock S, Pannell D, Talbot M, et al. Spinal injuries after improvised explosive device incidents: implications for Tactical Combat Casualty Care. *J Trauma.* 2011;71(5)(Suppl 1):S413-S417. doi:10.1097/TA.0b013e318232e575.

8. Eastridge BJ, Mabry R, Seguin P, et al. Death on the battlefield (2001-2011): implications for the future of combat casualty care. *J Trauma Acute Care Surg.* 2012;73(6)(Suppl 5):S431-S437. doi:10.1097/TA.0b013e3182755dcc.

9. Butler FK, Blackbourne LH. Battlefield trauma care then and now: a decade of tactical combat casualty care. *J Trauma Acute Care Surg.* 2012;73(6)(Suppl 5):S395-S402. doi:10.1097/TA.0b013e3182754850.

10. Maughon JS. An inquiry into the nature of wounds resulting in killed in action in Vietnam. *Mil Med.* 1970;135(1):8-13.

11. Kelly JF, Ritenhour AE, McLaughlin DF, et al. Injury severity and causes of death from Operation Iraqi Freedom and Operation Enduring Freedom: 2003-2004 versus 2006. *J Trauma.* 2008;64(Suppl 2):S21-S27. doi:10.1097/TA.0b013e318160b9fb.

12. Kotwal RS, Butler FK, Edgar EP, Shackelford SA, Bennett DR, Bailey JA. Saving lives on the battlefield: a joint trauma system review of pre-hospital trauma care in combined joint operating area—Afghanistan (CJOA-A). 2013, January 30. http://www.jsomonline.org/TCCC/CENTCOM%20Prehospital%20Final%20Report%2020130130.pdf. Accessed September 6, 2013.

13. Butler FK. Tactical combat casualty care—beginnings. *Wilderness Env Med.* 2017;28:S12-S17.

14. Butler F, Smith D, Carmona R. Implementing and preserving the advances in combat casualty care from Iraq and Afghanistan throughout the US military. *J Trauma Acute Care Surg.* 2015;79:321-326.

15. Kragh J, Walters T, Westmoreland T, et al. Tragedy into drama: an American history of tourniquet use in the current war. *J Spec Oper Med.* 2013;13:5-25.

16. Bellamy RF. The causes of death in conventional land warfare: implications for combat casualty care research. *Mil Med.* 1984;149:55-62.

17. Holcomb JB, McMullen NR, Pearse L, et al. Causes of death in Special Operations Forces in the Global War on Terror. *Ann Surg.* 2007;245(6):986-991.

18. Beekley AC, Sebesta JA, Blackbourne LH, et al. Prehospital tourniquet use in Operation Iraqi Freedom:

effect on hemorrhage control and outcomes. *J Trauma.* 2008;64(Suppl 2):S28-S37.

19. Kragh JF, Walters TJ, Baer DG, et al. Practical use of emergency tourniquets to stop bleeding in major limb trauma. *J Trauma.* 2008;64(Suppl 2):S38-S50. doi:10.1097/TA.0b013e31816086b1.

20. Kragh JF, Walters TJ, Baer DG, et al. Survival with emergency tourniquet use to stop bleeding in major limb trauma. *Ann Surg.* 2009;249(1):1-7. doi:10.1097/SLA.0b013e31818842ba.

21. Mabry RL. Tourniquet use on the battlefield. *Mil Med.* 2006;171(5):352-356.

22. Mabry RL, Holcomb JB, Baker A, et al. US Army Rangers in Somalia: an analysis of combat casualties on an urban battlefield. *J Trauma.* 2000;49(3):515.

23. Tarpey MJ. Tactical combat casualty care in Operation Iraqi Freedom. *U.S. Army Med Dept J.* 2005;April-June:38-41.

24. Mucciarone JJ, Llewellyn CH, Wightman JM. Tactical Combat Casualty Care in the assault on Punta Paitilla Airfield. *Mil Med.* 2006;171(8):687-690.

25. Beekley AC, Starnes BW, Sebesta JA. Lessons learned from modern military surgery. *Surg Clin N Am.* 2007;87(1):157-184.

26. Tien HC, Jung V, Rizoli SB, Acharya SV, MacDonald JC. An evaluation of Tactical Combat Casualty Care interventions in a combat environment. *J Am Coll Surg.* 2008;207(2):174-178. doi:10.1016/j.jamcollsurg.2008.01.065.

27. Dorlac WC, Debakey ME, Holcomb JB, et al. Mortality from isolated civilian penetrating extremity injury. *J Trauma.* 2005;59(1):217-222.

28. Kalish J, Burke P, Feldman J, et al. The return of tourniquets: original research evaluates the effectiveness of prehospital tourniquets for civilian penetrating extremity injuries. *J Em Med Serv.* 2008;33(8):44-54. doi:10.1016/S0197-2510(08)70289-4.

29. Doyle GS, Taillac PP. Tourniquets: a review of current use with proposals for expanded prehospital use. *Prehosp Emerg Care.* 2008;12(2):241-256. doi:10.1080/10903120801907570.

30. Markov N, Dubose J, Scott D, et al. Anatomic distribution and mortality of arterial injury in the wars in Afghanistan and Iraq with comparison to a civilian benchmark. *J Vasc Surg.* 2012;56(3):728-736. doi:10.1016/j.jvs.2012.02.048.

31. Butler F, Carmona R. Tactical combat casualty care: from the battlefields of Afghanistan to the streets of America. *The Tactical Edge,* Winter 2012. National Tactical Officers Association. http://public.ntoa.org/AppResources/publications/Articles/2167.pdf. Accessed April 17, 2018.

32. Jacobs LM, Wade DS, McSwain NE, et al. The Hartford Consensus: THREAT, a medical disaster preparedness concept. *J Am Coll Surg.* 2013;217:947-953.

33. Levy MJ, Jacobs LM. A call to action to develop programs for bystanders to control severe bleeding. *JAMA Surg.* 2016;151(12):1103-1104. doi:10.1001/jamasurg.2016.2789.

34. Pons O, Jerome J, McMullen J, et al. The Hartford Consensus on active shooters: implementing the continuum of prehospital trauma response. *J Emerg Med.* 2015;49:878-885.

35. Zietlow J, Zietlow S, Morris D, et al. Prehospital use of hemostatic bandages and tourniquets: translation from military experience to implementation in civilian trauma center. *J Spec Oper Med.* 2015;15:48-53.

36. Scerbo M, Holcomb J, Taub E, et al. The trauma center is too late: major limb trauma without a pre-hospital tourniquet has increased death from hemorrhagic shock. *J Trauma Acute Care Surg.* 2017;83:1165-1172.

37. Walters TJ, Wenke JC, Greydanus DJ, Kauvar DS, Baer DG. Laboratory evaluation of battlefield tourniquets on human volunteers. US Army Institute of Surgical Research Technical Report 2005-05, September 2005. Defense Technical Information Center. http://www.dtic.mil/cgi-bin/GetTRDoc?AD=ADA441140. Accessed April 17, 2018.

38. Butler FK. The US military experience with tourniquets and hemostatic dressings in the Afghanistan and Iraq conflicts. *Bull Am College Surg.* 2015;100(Sept Suppl):60-65.

39. Gibson R, Aden J, Dubick M, Kragh J. Preliminary comparison of pneumatic models of tourniquet for prehospital control of limb bleeding in a manikin model. *J Spec Oper Med.* 2016;16:21-27.

40. Lakstein D, Blumenfeld A, Sokolov T, et al. Tourniquets for hemorrhage control on the battlefield: a 4-year accumulated experience. *J Trauma.* 2003;54(Suppl 5):S221-225.

41. Butler FK, Holcomb JB, Giebner SG, McSwain NE, Bagian J. Tactical Combat Casualty Care 2007: evolving concepts and battlefield experience. *Mil Med.* 2007;172(Suppl 11):1-19.

42. Shackelford SA, Butler FK Jr, Kragh JF Jr, et al. Optimizing the use of limb tourniquets in Tactical Combat Casualty Care: TCCC guidelines change 14-02. *J Spec Oper Med.* 2015;15:17-31.

43. Kotwal RS, Montgomery HR, Kotwal BM, et al. Eliminating preventable death on the battlefield. *Arch Surgery.* 2011;146(12):1350-1358. doi:10.1001/archsurg.2011.213.

44. Holcomb JB, Butler FK, Rhee P. Hemorrhage control devices: tourniquets and hemostatic dressings. *Bull Am College Surg.* 2015;100(Sept Suppl):66-71.

45. Butler FK, Kotwal RS, Buckenmaier CC III, et al. A triple-option analgesia plan for Tactical Combat Casualty Care. *J Spec Oper Med.* 2014;14:13-25.

46. Carey ME. Analysis of wounds incurred by US Army Seventh Corps personnel treated in corps hospitals during Operation Desert Storm, February 20 to March 10, 1991. *J Trauma.* 1996;40(Suppl 3):S165-S169.

47. Weppner J, Lang M, Sunday R, Debiasse N. Efficacy of tourniquets exposed to the Afghanistan combat environment stored in Individual First Aid Kits versus on the exterior of plate carriers. *Mil Med.* 2013;178:334-337.

SPECIFIC SKILLS

Combat Application Tourniquet (C-A-T)

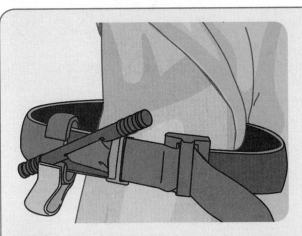

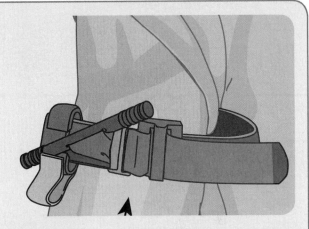

1 **A. Two-handed application**. Route the band around the injured limb, pass the tip through the slit of the buckle, and position the C-A-T above the bleeding site. **B. One-handed application**. Insert the injured limb through the loop in the band, and position the C-A-T above the bleeding site. If, based on the situation, you cannot be sure or cannot take the additional time to determine where the bleeding is coming from, the C-A-T can be effectively applied over clothing as high on the arm or leg as possible. The C-A-T must not be applied over solid objects within the clothing.

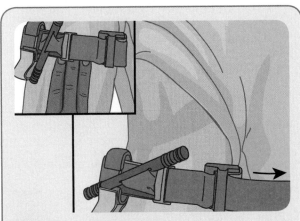

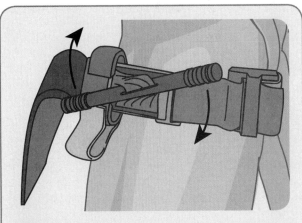

2 Pull the self-adhering band *tightly*, and fasten it back on itself all the way around the limb but not over the rod clips. The band should be tight enough that the tips of three fingers cannot be slid between the band and the limb. If the tips of three fingers slide under the band, retighten and resecure.

3 Twist the windlass rod until the bleeding stops.

(continued)

Combat Application Tourniquet (C-A-T) *(continued)*

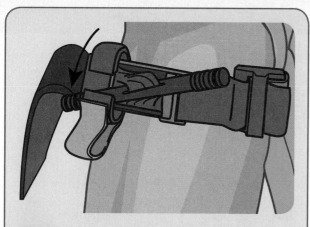

4 Snap one end of the windlass rod inside one of the rod clips to lock it in place. If the bleeding resumes, consider additional tightening or applying a second C-A-T side-by-side with the first.

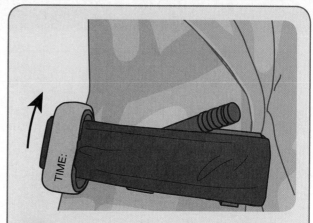

5 Route the self adhering band between the rod clips over the windlass rod. Continue to adhere the band around the extremity. Secure with the gray TIME strap. Record the time of application.

CHAPTER **25**

Tactical Field Care

Authors:
Capt. (Ret) Frank Butler, MD
Capt. (Ret) Stephen Giebner, MD
Master Sgt. (Ret) Harold Montgomery

CHAPTER OBJECTIVES
At the completion of this chapter, you will be able to do the following:

- Discuss the need to establish a security perimeter at the onset of Tactical Field Care.
- List the common causes of altered mental status on the battlefield.
- Explain the implications of altered mental status in a combat casualty regarding his or her arms and communications gear.
- Describe the relative urgency of life-threatening conditions listed in the MARCH algorithm.
- List the progressive strategies for controlling massive external hemorrhage in Tactical Field Care and the indications for each.
- Discuss the difficulties inherent in using direct pressure alone for controlling external hemorrhage.
- Describe airway control techniques and devices appropriate to the Tactical Field Care phase.
- State the preferred surgical airway option in Tactical Combat Casualty Care (TCCC), and explain its preference.
- List the criteria for the diagnosis of tension pneumothorax on the battlefield.
- Describe the appropriate use of pulse oximetry in prehospital combat casualty care.
- Describe the initial treatment of tension pneumothorax on the battlefield.
- Demonstrate the appropriate procedure for needle decompression (NDC) of a suspected tension pneumothorax in both of the recommended sites.
- Describe the subsequent management of a tension pneumothorax when the initial treatment is not successful.

- Describe the management of a tension pneumothorax when the initial treatment is successful, but the symptoms later recur.
- Discuss the appropriate use of pulse oximetry in prehospital combat casualty care.
- Discuss the pitfalls associated with interpretation of pulse oximeter readings.
- Describe the TCCC management for open pneumothorax.
- Discuss the treatment with supplemental oxygen of casualties who have known or suspected smoke inhalation.
- Describe the progressive strategy for controlling external hemorrhage in Tactical Field Care.
- Discuss the indications for applying a circumferential pelvic compression device in TCCC.
- List the preferred circumferential pelvic compression devices.
- Demonstrate the application of a circumferential pelvic compression device.
- Discuss the indications for removing or converting a tourniquet in Tactical Field Care.
- Demonstrate the conversion of an extremity tourniquet to another means of extremity hemorrhage control.
- Discuss the reevaluation of limb tourniquets that were placed during Care Under Fire including reinforcement with a second tourniquet, replacement with another tourniquet, replacement with another means of hemorrhage control, and removal.

- Discuss the options for hemorrhage control when an injection of XStat proves insufficient.
- Describe the most useful indicators of shock during Tactical Field Care.
- List the indications for establishing intravenous (IV) or intraosseous (IO) access in Tactical Field Care.
- Discuss the options for establishing access to the circulatory system for administration of medications and/or resuscitation.
- Demonstrate the appropriate procedure for constructing a field-ruggedized saline lock.
- Discuss the indications, contraindications, and hazards of using sternal IO devices.
- Demonstrate the correct procedure for inserting a sternal IO device.
- Describe the expected survival benefit resulting from tranexamic acid (TXA) use in casualties who are in or at risk of hemorrhagic shock.
- Discuss the need for early administration of TXA in casualties at risk of death from hemorrhage.
- Demonstrate the preparation and administration of a TXA infusion.
- Describe per oral fluid resuscitation in Tactical Field Care including indications and patient selection.
- List acceptable resuscitation fluids for casualties in hemorrhagic shock in order of preference.
- Describe the advantages of blood products over colloids or crystalloids for fluid resuscitation of casualties in hemorrhagic shock during TCCC.
- Discuss the dangers of administering large quantities of crystalloid fluids to a casualty who has noncompressible bleeding sites.
- Describe the factors that can worsen traumatic brain injury (TBI) by causing secondary injury to the brain.
- Recite the target blood pressures for resuscitation of a casualty in hemorrhagic shock with and without a concurrent TBI.
- Demonstrate the calculation of the total body surface area (TBSA) of burns using the rule of nines.
- Discuss the impact of known or suspected inhalation injury on a casualty's airway management.
- Demonstrate the calculation of fluid resuscitation requirements for a casualty with burns greater than 20% TBSA using the United States Army Institute of Surgical Research (USAISR) rule of tens.
- Explain the relative urgency of burn injury compared to concurrent penetrating and/or blunt trauma.
- Explain the need of burn victims for protection against hypothermia.
- Discuss the importance of hypothermia prevention in any seriously injured combat casualty.

- List the preferred methods to accomplish hypothermia prevention in TCCC.
- Explain the benefit of providing hypothermia prevention concurrently with fluid resuscitation.
- Describe the management of obvious or suspected penetrating eye trauma in a tactical setting.
- Describe the TCCC Triple-Option Analgesia plan for managing the pain of combat wounds.
- Explain the choice of ondansetron as the preferred antiemetic in TCCC.
- Recite the correct dosage and administration of ondansetron.
- Demonstrate the proper technique for preparing and administering an IV ketamine infusion.
- Discuss the rationale for early antibiotic intervention in combat casualties.
- List the factors involved in selecting antibiotics for use on the battlefield.
- Discuss the identification of casualties who should receive antibiotics in TCCC.
- List the antibiotics recommended for use in TCCC.
- Discuss the most advantageous timing of antibiotic administration in combat casualties.
- Explain the benefit of an indications for advanced electronic monitoring in Tactical Field Care.
- Describe the signs and symptoms that indicate the presence of a closed extremity fracture.
- Describe the proper splinting of a fractured extremity.
- Discuss the role of cardiopulmonary resuscitation (CPR) in combat casualties during Tactical Field Care.
- Discuss the diagnostic and therapeutic utility of bilateral NDC in a casualty with significant torso trauma and cardiac arrest.
- Describe the proper documentation of casualty care in TCCC.
- Discuss the selection of a location for a casualty collection point.
- Describe the Joint Trauma System (JTS) recommended evacuation priorities for casualties with various wounding patterns and physiologic statuses.
- Discuss the management of wounded hostile combatants during Tactical Field Care.
- Explain the importance of communicating with the casualty, tactical leadership, and the evacuation system.
- Describe the actions required to prepare the casualty for evacuation.
- Describe the proper transition of the care of the casualty to medical personnel on the tactical evacuation (TACEVAC) platform.

SCENARIO

While on patrol in the city of Mosul, an infantry platoon comes under small arms fire. The point man is hit and falls to the ground. The platoon reacts to the contact, rapidly eliminating the ambushing force. The point man is the only casualty in your unit. The platoon leader tells you to take care of the wounded man while the other unit members establish a security perimeter. In your rapid initial assessment for life-threatening conditions, you find a gunshot entry wound on the casualty's right upper back. The exit wound is in the right axilla, and there is heavy pulsatile bleeding from it. The casualty is breathing slightly fast but is awake, alert, and responding appropriately. There are no other wounds.

- What phase of tactical combat casualty care (TCCC) are you in?
- What is your immediate concern and how do you address it?
- While addressing your immediate concern, what should you be doing simultaneously?
- What should you do after you finish your first intervention?
- What do you evaluate next?
- Should you treat for a tension pneumothorax? Why?
- What do you want to do after that?
- What interventions come next if the casualty is in shock?
- What should this casualty's evacuation priority be?

INTRODUCTION

In a casualty scenario, you enter the Tactical Field Care phase of TCCC once the unit is no longer receiving effective hostile fire. Tactical Field Care also includes tactical situations where a casualty is sustained in the absence of hostile fire, such as a serious injury from a parachute accident, a motor vehicle crash, or a fall.

The casualty should be moved to the best available cover and concealment. Although light discipline is a necessity in conditions of reduced ambient light, a white or red light can be used under cover of a poncho or other cover if this is essential to the care of the casualty and the tactical conditions permit. Equipment limitations and environmental extremes are still factors that will affect the care that can be delivered.

Box 25-1 lists the TCCC Guidelines for Tactical Field Care.

Establishing a Security Perimeter

As the medic or another unit member begins to address the casualty's injuries, the mission leadership should ensure that a security perimeter is established. Mission personnel should constantly maintain their situational awareness with respect to the potential threat from hostile forces.

Box 25-1 Basic Management Plan for Tactical Field Care—August 1, 2018

1. Establish a security perimeter in accordance with unit tactical standard operating procedures and/or battle drills. Maintain tactical situational awareness.
2. Triage casualties as required. Casualties with an altered mental status should have weapons and communications equipment taken away immediately.
3. Massive Hemorrhage
   a. Assess for unrecognized hemorrhage and control all sources of bleeding. If not already done, use a CoTCCC-recommended limb tourniquet to control life-threatening external hemorrhage that is anatomically amenable to tourniquet use or for any traumatic amputation. Apply directly to the skin 2–3 inches above the bleeding site. If bleeding is not controlled with the first tourniquet, apply a second tourniquet side-by-side with the first.
   b. For compressible (external) hemorrhage not amenable to limb tourniquet use or as an adjunct to tourniquet removal, use Combat Gauze as the CoTCCC hemostatic dressing of choice.

(continued)

Box 25-1 Basic Management Plan for Tactical Field Care—August 1, 2018 (*continued*)

- Alternative hemostatic adjuncts:
  - Celox Gauze or
  - ChitoGauze or
  - XStat (best for deep, narrow-tract junctional wounds)
- Hemostatic dressings should be applied with at least 3 minutes of direct pressure (optional for XStat). Each dressing works differently, so if one fails to control bleeding, it may be removed and a fresh dressing of the same type or a different type applied. (Note: XStat is not to be removed in the field, but additional XStat, other hemostatic adjuncts, or trauma dressings may be applied over it.)
- If the bleeding site is amenable to use of a junctional tourniquet, immediately apply a CoTCCC-recommended junctional tourniquet. Do not delay in the application of the junctional tourniquet once it is ready for use. Apply hemostatic dressings with direct pressure if a junctional tourniquet is not available or while the junctional tourniquet is being readied for use.

4. Airway Management
   a. Conscious casualty with no airway problem identified:
      - No airway intervention required
   b. Unconscious casualty without airway obstruction:
      - Place casualty in the recovery position
      - Chin lift or jaw thrust maneuver or
      - Nasopharyngeal airway or
      - Extraglottic airway
   c. Casualty with airway obstruction or impending airway obstruction:
      - Allow a conscious casualty to assume any position that best protects the airway, to include sitting up.
      - Use a chin lift or jaw thrust maneuver.
      - Use suction if available and appropriate.
      - Nasopharyngeal airway or
      - Extraglottic airway (if the casualty is unconscious)
      - Place an unconscious casualty in the recovery position.
   d. If the previous measures are unsuccessful, perform a surgical cricothyroidotomy using one of the following:
      - Cric-Key technique (preferred option)
      - Bougie-aided open surgical technique using a flanged and cuffed airway cannula of less than 10 mm outer diameter,

6–7 mm internal diameter, and 5–8 cm of intratracheal length
      - Standard open surgical technique using a flanged and cuffed airway cannula of less than 10 mm outer diameter, 6–7 mm internal diameter, and 5–8 cm of intratracheal length (least desirable option)
      - Use lidocaine if the casualty is conscious.
   e. Cervical spine stabilization is not necessary for casualties who have sustained only penetrating trauma.
   f. Monitor the hemoglobin oxygen saturation in casualties to help assess airway patency.
   g. Always remember that the casualty's airway status may change over time and requires frequent reassessment.

Notes:

- *The i-gel is the preferred extraglottic airway because its gel-filled cuff makes it simpler to use and avoids the need for cuff inflation and monitoring. If an extraglottic airway with an air-filled cuff is used, the cuff pressure must be monitored to avoid overpressurization, especially during TACEVAC on an aircraft with the accompanying pressure changes.*
- *Extraglottic airways will not be tolerated by a casualty who is not deeply unconscious. If an unconscious casualty without direct airway trauma needs an airway intervention, but does not tolerate an extraglottic airway, consider the use of a nasopharyngeal airway.*
- *For casualties with trauma to the face and mouth, or facial burns with suspected inhalation injury, nasopharyngeal airways and extraglottic airways may not suffice and a surgical cricothyroidotomy may be required.*
- *Surgical cricothyroidotomies should not be performed on unconscious casualties who have no direct airway trauma unless use of a nasopharyngeal airway and/or an extraglottic airway has been unsuccessful in opening the airway.*

5. Respiration/Breathing
   a. Assess for tension pneumothorax and treat as necessary.
      1. Suspect a tension pneumothorax and treat when a casualty has significant torso trauma or primary blast injury and one or more of the following:
         - Severe or progressive respiratory distress
         - Severe or progressive tachypnea
         - Absent or markedly decreased breath sounds on one side of the chest

Box 25-1 Basic Management Plan for Tactical Field Care—August 1, 2018 (*continued*)

- Hemoglobin oxygen saturation <90% on pulse oximetry
- Shock
- Traumatic cardiac arrest without obviously fatal wounds

2. Initial treatment of suspected tension pneumothorax:
   - If the casualty has a chest seal in place, burp or remove the chest seal.
   - Establish pulse oximetry monitoring.
   - Place the casualty in the supine or recovery position unless he or she is conscious and needs to sit up to help keep the airway clear as a result of maxillofacial trauma.
   - Decompress the chest on the side of the injury with a 14-gauge or a 10-gauge, 3.25-inch needle/catheter unit.
   - If a casualty has significant torso trauma or primary blast injury and is in traumatic cardiac arrest (no pulse, no respirations, no response to painful stimuli, no other signs of life), decompress both sides of the chest before discontinuing treatment.

3. The NDC should be considered successful if:
   - Respiratory distress improves, or
   - There is an obvious hissing sound as air escapes from the chest when NDC is performed (this may be difficult to appreciate in high-noise environments), or
   - Hemoglobin oxygen saturation increases to 90% or greater (note that this may take several minutes and may not happen at altitude), or
   - A casualty with no vital signs has return of consciousness and/or radial pulse.

4. If the initial NDC fails to improve the casualty's signs/symptoms from the suspected tension pneumothorax:
   - Perform a second NDC on the same side of the chest at whichever of the two recommended sites was not previously used. Use a new needle/catheter unit for the second attempt.
   - Consider, based on the mechanism of injury and physical findings, whether decompression of the opposite side of the chest may be needed.

5. If the initial NDC was successful, but symptoms later recur:

- Perform another NDC at the same site that was used previously. Use a new needle/catheter unit for the repeat NDC.
- Continue to re-assess!

6. If the second NDC is also not successful:
   - Continue on to the Circulation section of the TCCC Guidelines.

b. All open and/or sucking chest wounds should be treated by immediately applying a vented chest seal to cover the defect. If a vented chest seal is not available, use a non-vented chest seal. Monitor the casualty for the potential development of a subsequent tension pneumothorax. If the casualty develops increasing hypoxia, respiratory distress, or hypotension and a tension pneumothorax is suspected, treat by burping or removing the dressing or by needle decompression.

c. Initiate pulse oximetry. All individuals with moderate/severe TBI should be monitored with pulse oximetry. Readings may be misleading in the settings of shock or marked hypothermia.

d. Casualties with moderate/severe TBI should be given supplemental oxygen when available to maintain an oxygen saturation >90%.

Notes:

- *If not treated promptly, tension pneumothorax may progress from respiratory distress to shock and traumatic cardiac arrest.*
- *Either the 5th intercostal space (ICS) in the anterior axillary line (AAL) or the 2nd ICS in the mid-clavicular line (MCL) may be used for needle decompression (NDC). If the anterior (MCL) site is used, do not insert the needle medial to the nipple line.*
- *The needle/catheter unit should be inserted at an angle perpendicular to the chest wall and just over the top of the lower rib at the insertion site. Insert the needle/catheter unit all the way to the hub and hold it in place for 5–10 seconds to allow decompression to occur.*
- *After the NDC has been performed, remove the needle and leave the catheter in place.*

6. Circulation
   a. Bleeding
      - A pelvic binder should be applied for cases of suspected pelvic fracture:
        - Severe blunt force or blast injury with one or more of the following indications:
          - Pelvic pain

(*continued*)

Box 25-1 Basic Management Plan for Tactical Field Care—August 1, 2018 (*continued*)

- Any major lower limb amputation or near amputation
- Physical exam findings suggestive of a pelvic fracture
- Unconsciousness
- Shock

– Reassess prior tourniquet application. Expose the wound and determine if a tourniquet is needed. If it is needed, replace any limb tourniquet placed over the uniform with one applied directly to the skin 2–3 inches above the bleeding site. Ensure that bleeding is stopped. If there is no traumatic amputation, a distal pulse should be checked. If bleeding persists or a distal pulse is still present, consider additional tightening of the tourniquet or the use of a second tourniquet side-by-side with the first to eliminate both bleeding and the distal pulse. If the reassessment determines that the prior tourniquet was not needed, then remove the tourniquet and note time of removal on the TCCC Casualty Card.

– Limb tourniquets and junctional tourniquets should be converted to hemostatic or pressure dressings as soon as possible if three criteria are met: the casualty is not in shock; it is possible to monitor the wound closely for bleeding; and the tourniquet is not being used to control bleeding from an amputated extremity. Every effort should be made to convert tourniquets in less than 2 hours if bleeding can be controlled with other means. Do not remove a tourniquet that has been in place more than 6 hours unless close monitoring and lab capability are available.

– Expose and clearly mark all tourniquets with the time of tourniquet application. Note tourniquets applied and time of application; time of re-application; time of conversion; and time of removal on the TCCC Casualty Card. Use a permanent marker to mark on the tourniquet and the casualty card.

b. IV Access

– Intravenous (IV) or intraosseous (IO) access is indicated if the casualty is in hemorrhagic shock or at significant risk of shock (and may therefore need fluid resuscitation), or if the casualty needs medications, but cannot take them by mouth.

- An 18-gauge IV or saline lock is preferred.
- If vascular access is needed but not quickly obtainable via the IV route, use the IO route.

c. Tranexamic Acid (TXA)

– If a casualty is anticipated to need significant blood transfusion (for example, presents with hemorrhagic shock, one or more major amputations, penetrating torso trauma, or evidence of severe bleeding):

- Administer 1 g of tranexamic acid in 100 ml normal saline or lactated Ringer as soon as possible but NOT later than 3 hours after injury. When given, TXA should be administered over 10 minutes by IV infusion.
- Begin the second infusion of 1 g TXA after initial fluid resuscitation has been completed.

d. Fluid Resuscitation

– Assess for hemorrhagic shock (altered mental status in the absence of brain injury and/or weak or absent radial pulse).

– The resuscitation fluids of choice for casualties in hemorrhagic shock, listed from most to least preferred, are whole blood*; plasma, red blood cells (RBCs) and platelets in a 1:1:1 ratio*; plasma and RBCs in a 1:1 ratio; plasma or RBCs alone; Hextend; and crystalloid (lactated Ringer or Plasma-Lyte A). (NOTE: Hypothermia prevention measures [Section 7] should be initiated while fluid resuscitation is being accomplished.)

- If not in shock:
  - No IV fluids are immediately necessary.
  - Fluids by mouth are permissible if the casualty is conscious and can swallow.
- If in shock and blood products are available under an approved command or theater blood product administration protocol:
  - Resuscitate with whole blood,* or, if not available
  - Plasma, RBCs, and platelets in a 1:1:1 ratio,* or, if not available
  - Plasma and RBCs in a 1:1 ratio, or, if not available
  - Reconstituted dried plasma, liquid plasma or thawed plasma alone or RBCs alone
  - Reassess the casualty after each unit. Continue resuscitation until a palpable

Box 25-1 Basic Management Plan for Tactical Field Care—August 1, 2018 (*continued*)

radial pulse, improved mental status or systolic BP of 80–90 is present.

- If in shock and blood products are not available under an approved command or theater blood product administration protocol due to tactical or logistical constraints:
  - Resuscitate with Hextend, or if not available
  - Lactated Ringer or Plasma-Lyte A
  - Reassess the casualty after each 500-ml IV bolus.
  - Continue resuscitation until a palpable radial pulse, improved mental status, or systolic BP of 80–90 mm Hg is present.
  - Discontinue fluid administration when one or more of the above end points has been achieved.
  - If a casualty with an altered mental status due to suspected TBI has a weak or absent radial pulse, resuscitate as necessary to restore and maintain a normal radial pulse. If BP monitoring is available, maintain a target systolic BP of at least 90 mm Hg.
  - Reassess the casualty frequently to check for recurrence of shock. If shock recurs, re-check all external hemorrhage control measures to ensure that they are still effective and repeat the fluid resuscitation as outlined above.

  e. Refractory Shock
  - If a casualty in shock is not responding to fluid resuscitation, consider untreated tension pneumothorax as a possible cause of refractory shock. Thoracic trauma, persistent respiratory distress, absent breath sounds, and hemoglobin oxygen saturation <90% support this diagnosis. Treat as indicated with repeated NDC or finger thoracostomy/chest tube insertion at the 5th ICS in the AAL, according to the skills, experience, and authorizations of the treating medical provider. Note that if finger thoracostomy is used, it may not remain patent and finger decompression through the incision may have to be repeated. Consider decompressing the opposite side of the chest if indicated based on the mechanism of injury and physical findings.

Note:

- *Currently, neither whole blood nor apheresis platelets collected in theater are FDA compliant*

because of the way they are collected. Consequently, whole blood and 1:1:1 resuscitation using apheresis platelets should be used only if all of the FDA-compliant blood products needed to support 1:1:1 resuscitation are not available, or if 1:1:1 resuscitation is not producing the desired clinical effect.

7. Hypothermia Prevention
   a. Minimize casualty's exposure to the elements. Keep protective gear on or with the casualty if feasible.
   b. Replace wet clothing with dry if possible. Get the casualty onto an insulated surface as soon as possible.
   c. Apply the Ready-Heat Blanket from the Hypothermia Prevention and Management Kit (HPMK) to the casualty's torso (not directly on the skin) and cover the casualty with the Heat-Reflective Shell (HRS).
   d. If an HRS is not available, the previously recommended combination of the Blizzard Survival Blanket and the Ready-Heat Blanket may also be used.
   e. If the items mentioned above are not available, use dry blankets, poncho liners, sleeping bags, or anything that will retain heat and keep the casualty dry.
   f. Warm fluids are preferred if IV fluids are required.
8. Penetrating Eye Trauma
   a. If a penetrating eye injury is noted or suspected:
      - Perform a rapid field test of visual acuity and document findings.
      - Cover the eye with a rigid eye shield (NOT a pressure patch.)
      - Ensure that the 400 mg moxifloxacin tablet in the Combat Wound Medication Pack (CWMP) is taken if possible and that IV/IM antibiotics are given as outlined below if oral moxifloxacin cannot be taken.
9. Monitoring
   a. Initiate advanced electronic monitoring if indicated and if monitoring equipment is available.
10. Analgesia
    a. Analgesia on the battlefield should generally be achieved using one of three options:
       - Option 1
         • Mild to moderate pain
         • Casualty is still able to fight
           - TCCC Combat Wound Medication Pack (CWMP)

(*continued*)

Box 25-1 Basic Management Plan for Tactical Field Care—August 1, 2018 (*continued*)

- Tylenol—650 mg bilayer caplet, 2 PO every 8 hours
- Meloxicam—15 mg PO once a day
  - Option 2
    - Moderate to severe pain
    - Casualty IS NOT in shock or respiratory distress AND
    - Casualty IS NOT at significant risk of developing either condition
      - Oral transmucosal fentanyl citrate (OTFC) 800 µg
    - Place lozenge between the cheek and the gum
    - Do not chew the lozenge
  - Option 3
    - Moderate to severe pain
    - Casualty IS in hemorrhagic shock or respiratory distress OR
    - Casualty IS at significant risk of developing either condition
      - Ketamine 50 mg IM or IN

Or

      - Ketamine 20 mg slow IV or IO
        - Repeat doses q30min prn for IM or IN
        - Repeat doses q20min prn for IV or IO
        - End points: Control of pain or development of nystagmus (rhythmic back-and-forth movement of the eyes)

Notes:

- *Casualties may need to be disarmed after being given OTFC or ketamine.*
- *Document a mental status exam using the AVPU method prior to administering opioids or ketamine.*
- *For all casualties given opioids or ketamine— monitor airway, breathing, and circulation closely.*
- *Directions for administering OTFC:*
  - *Recommend taping lozenge-on-a-stick to casualty's finger as an added safety measure OR utilizing a safety pin and rubber band to attach the lozenge (under tension) to the patient's uniform or plate carrier.*
  - *Reassess in 15 minutes.*
  - *Add second lozenge, in other cheek, as necessary to control severe pain.*
  - *Monitor for respiratory depression.*
- *IV Morphine is an alternative to OTFC if IV access has been obtained.*
  - *5 mg IV/IO*
  - *Reassess in 10 minutes.*

- *Repeat dose every 10 minutes as necessary to control severe pain.*
- *Monitor for respiratory depression.*
- *Naloxone (0.4 mg IV or IM) should be available when using opioid analgesics.*
- *Both ketamine and OTFC have the potential to worsen severe TBI. The combat medic, corpsman, or PJ must consider this fact in his or her analgesic decision, but if the casualty is able to complain of pain, then the TBI is likely not severe enough to preclude the use of ketamine or OTFC.*
- *Eye injury does not preclude the use of ketamine. The risk of additional damage to the eye from using ketamine is low and maximizing the casualty's chance for survival takes precedence if the casualty is in shock or respiratory distress or at significant risk for either.*
- *Ketamine may be a useful adjunct to reduce the amount of opioids required to provide effective pain relief. It is safe to give ketamine to a casualty who has previously received morphine or OTFC. IV Ketamine should be given over 1 minute.*
- *If respirations are noted to be reduced after using opioids or ketamine, provide ventilatory support with a bag-valve-mask or mouth-to-mask ventilations.*
- *Ondansetron, 4 mg orally dissolving tablet (ODT)/ IV/IO/IM, every 8 hours as needed for nausea or vomiting. Each 8-hour dose can be repeated once at 15 minutes if nausea and vomiting are not improved. Do not give more than 8 mg in any 8-hour interval. Oral ondansetron is NOT an acceptable alternative to the ODT formulation.*
- *Reassess—reassess—reassess!*

11. Antibiotics: recommended for all open combat wounds
    a. If able to take PO meds:
       - Moxifloxacin (from the CWMP), 400 mg PO once a day
    b. If unable to take PO meds (shock, unconsciousness):
       - Ertapenem, 1 g IV/IM once a day
12. Inspect and dress known wounds.
13. Check for additional wounds.
14. Burns*
    a. Facial burns, especially those that occur in closed spaces, may be associated with inhalation injury. Aggressively monitor airway status and oxygen saturation in such patients and consider early surgical airway for respiratory distress or oxygen desaturation.

Box 25-1 Basic Management Plan for Tactical Field Care—August 1, 2018 (*continued*)

b. Estimate total body surface area (TBSA) burned to the nearest 10% using the Rule of Nines.

c. Cover the burn area with dry, sterile dressings. For extensive burns (>20%), consider placing the casualty in the Heat-Reflective Shell or Blizzard Survival Blanket from the Hypothermia Prevention Kit in order to both cover the burned areas and prevent hypothermia.

d. Fluid resuscitation (USAISR Rule of Ten)
   - If burns are greater than 20% of TBSA, fluid resuscitation should be initiated as soon as IV/IO access is established. Resuscitation should be initiated with lactated Ringer, normal saline, or Hextend. If Hextend is used, no more than 1000 ml should be given, followed by lactated Ringer or normal saline as needed.
   - Initial IV/IO fluid rate is calculated as %TBSA x 10 ml/hr for adults weighing 40–80 kg.
   - For every 10 kg ABOVE 80 kg, increase initial rate by 100 ml/hr.
   - If hemorrhagic shock is also present, resuscitation for hemorrhagic shock takes precedence over resuscitation for burn shock. Administer IV/IO fluids per the TCCC Guidelines in Section (6).

e. Analgesia in accordance with the TCCC Guidelines in Section (10) may be administered to treat burn pain.

f. Prehospital antibiotic therapy is not indicated solely for burns, but antibiotics should be given per the TCCC Guidelines in Section (11) if indicated to prevent infection in penetrating wounds.

g. All TCCC interventions can be performed on or through burned skin in a burn casualty.

h. Burn patients are particularly susceptible to hypothermia. Extra emphasis should be placed on barrier heat loss prevention methods.

15. Splint fractures and re-check pulses.

16. Communication
   a. Communicate with the casualty if possible. Encourage, reassure, and explain care.
   b. Communicate with tactical leadership as soon as possible and throughout casualty

treatment as needed. Provide leadership with casualty status and evacuation requirements to assist with coordination of evacuation assets.

   c. Communicate with the evacuation system (the Patient Evacuation Coordination Cell) to arrange for TACEVAC. Communicate with medical providers on the evacuation asset if possible and relay mechanism of injury, injuries sustained, signs/symptoms, and treatments rendered. Provide additional information as appropriate.

17. Cardiopulmonary resuscitation (CPR)
   a. Resuscitation on the battlefield for victims of blast or penetrating trauma who have no pulse, no ventilations, and no other signs of life will not be successful and should not be attempted. However, casualties with torso trauma or polytrauma who have no pulse or respirations during TFC should have bilateral needle decompression performed to ensure they do not have a tension pneumothorax prior to discontinuation of care. The procedure is the same as described in section 5.a above.

18. Documentation of Care
   a. Document clinical assessments, treatments rendered, and changes in the casualty's status on a TCCC Card (DD Form 1380). Forward this information with the casualty to the next level of care.

19. Prepare for evacuation.
   a. Complete and secure the TCCC Card (DD 1380) to the casualty.
   b. Secure all loose ends of bandages and wraps.
   c. Secure hypothermia prevention wraps/blankets/straps.
   d. Secure litter straps as required. Consider additional padding for long evacuations.
   e. Provide instructions to ambulatory patients as needed.
   f. Stage casualties for evacuation in accordance with unit standard operating procedures.
   g. Maintain security at the evacuation point in accordance with unit standard operating procedures.

*See Chapter 32, *Treatment of Burn Casualties in Tactical Combat Casualty Care*, for discussion of this guideline.

Source: Courtesy of the Committee on Tactical Combat Casualty Care.

Disarming Casualties With Altered Mental Status and Securing Their Communications Equipment

Armed combatants with altered mental status pose a serious threat of injury or death to others in their unit if they happen to employ their weapons accidentally or inappropriately. In the combat setting, altered mental status may be due to traumatic brain injury (TBI), shock, and/or analgesic medications. Anyone noted to have an altered mental status should be disarmed immediately, including secondary weapons and explosive devices.[1] If the casualty is carrying communications equipment, it should likewise be removed to prevent inappropriate and/or compromising radio transmissions.

The MARCH Mnemonic

With other mission personnel ensuring that a security perimeter has been established, and weapons and communications gear having been secured if necessary, the medical evaluation and treatment of the casualty (or casualties) begins. If life-threatening compressible hemorrhage (e.g., external hemorrhage from extremities or the neck, groin, shoulder, or axillary areas) is present, this bleeding should be addressed immediately with an extremity tourniquet, a hemostatic agent, a junctional tourniquet, or XStat as outlined in the following section.

The acronym MARCH helps the provider recall the key initial steps in caring for a combat casualty. The letters refer to the following elements of care:

M—Massive bleeding: Establish immediate control of massive external bleeding with a combat application tourniquet (C-A-T) or SOF™ Tactical Tourniquet (SOFTT), a Committee on Tactical Combat Casualty Care (CoTCCC)-recommended hemostatic dressing, a CoTCCC-recommended junctional tourniquet, or XStat.

A—Airway: Check the airway and open it as needed.

R—Respirations/breathing: Treat tension pneumothorax with needle decompression (NDC) and treat open pneumothorax with a vented chest seal as needed.

C—Circulation: Assess hemodynamic status and take action as appropriate. Initiate intravenous (IV) or intraosseous (IO) access, administer tranexamic acid (TXA), and begin fluid resuscitation with blood products (if possible) as indicated.

H—Head/hypothermia: If moderate to severe head injury is present, perform the additional elements of care outlined in this chapter to manage TBI. Prevent hypothermia to help the casualty maintain a normal coagulation profile.

Massive Hemorrhage

Caring for a casualty during Tactical Field Care begins by assessing for any massive external hemorrhage (**Box 25-2** and **Figure 25-1**). If ongoing massive external hemorrhage

---

Box 25-2 Tactical Field Care Guideline 3: Massive Hemorrhage

3. Massive Hemorrhage
   a. Assess for unrecognized hemorrhage and control all sources of bleeding. If not already done, use a CoTCCC-recommended limb tourniquet to control life-threatening external hemorrhage that is anatomically amenable to tourniquet use or for any traumatic amputation. Apply directly to the skin 2–3 inches above the bleeding site. If bleeding is not controlled with the first tourniquet, apply a second tourniquet side-by-side with the first.
   b. For compressible (external) hemorrhage not amenable to limb tourniquet use or as an adjunct to tourniquet removal, use Combat Gauze as the CoTCCC hemostatic dressing of choice.
      – Alternative hemostatic adjuncts:
        · Celox Gauze or
        · ChitoGauze or

   · XStat (best for deep, narrow-tract junctional wounds)
   – Hemostatic dressings should be applied with at least 3 minutes of direct pressure (optional for XStat). Each dressing works differently, so if one fails to control bleeding, it may be removed and a fresh dressing of the same type or a different type applied. (Note: XStat is not to be removed in the field, but additional XStat, other hemostatic adjuncts, or trauma dressings may be applied over it.)
   – If the bleeding site is amenable to use of a junctional tourniquet, immediately apply a CoTCCC-recommended junctional tourniquet. Do not delay in the application of the junctional tourniquet once it is ready for use. Apply hemostatic dressings with direct pressure if a junctional tourniquet is not available or while the junctional tourniquet is being readied for use.

Source: Courtesy of the Committee on Tactical Combat Casualty Care.

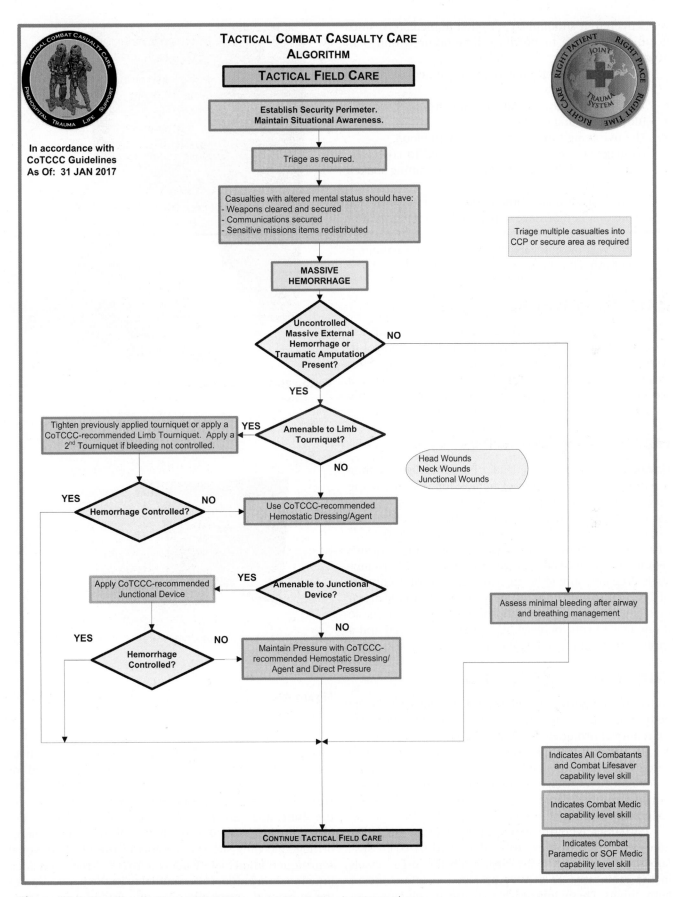

Figure 25-1 Algorithm for Tactical Field Care Guideline 3: Massive Hemorrhage.

is discovered, it should be controlled immediately, since death from severe hemorrhage may occur within 5 to 10 minutes.

Life-threatening bleeding can be identified as follows[2]:

- There is pulsatile or steady bleeding from the wound.
- Blood is pooling on the ground.
- The overlying clothes are soaked with blood.
- Bandages or makeshift bandages used to cover the wound are ineffective and steadily becoming soaked with blood.
- There is a traumatic amputation of the arm or leg. (Note that hemorrhage may be delayed in onset after the amputation has occurred.
- There was prior severe bleeding, and the patient is now in shock (unconscious, confused, pale).

Extremity Hemorrhage

If life-threatening extremity bleeding is still present, use a CoTCCC-recommended limb tourniquet to control it. Apply the tourniquet directly to the skin 2 to 3 inches (5 to 7.6 centimeters [cm]) above the bleeding site. If bleeding is not controlled with the first tourniquet, apply a second tourniquet side-by-side with the first.[2-7]

Hemostatic Dressings

Having moved out of Care Under Fire, there is now time to employ a wider variety of hemostatic options. If the external hemorrhage is occurring at a site not amenable to limb tourniquet use, use Combat Gauze™ as the CoTCCC hemostatic dressing of choice (**Figure 25-2**).[3,6,8-12] Alternative hemostatic dressings include Celox Gauze™ (**Figure 25-3**) and ChitoGauze (**Figure 25-4**).[13,14] Hemostatic dressings should be applied with at least 3 minutes of direct pressure. The different types of hemostatic dressings have somewhat different mechanisms of action, so if one fails to control bleeding, it may be removed and a fresh dressing of the same type or a different type applied.

Junctional Hemorrhage

Junctional hemorrhage is bleeding from the areas of the body where the extremities or the head join the torso. Extremity tourniquets are not suitable for use in these areas so other interventions to stop the bleeding must be employed.[15] Also implicit in this definition is the fact that junctional hemorrhage is compressible hemorrhage—it can be controlled with methods that do not involve open abdominal or thoracic surgery.

Casualties who are wounded by stepping on a dismounted improvised explosive device (IED) often sustain severe external hemorrhage from the large vessels in the groin area or at very proximal sites on one or both thighs These injuries led to the development of

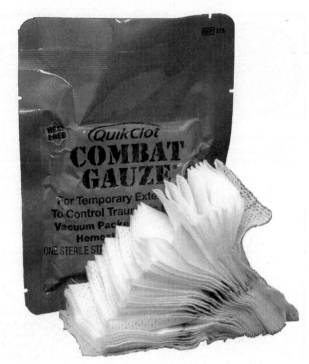

Figure 25-2 Combat Gauze®.
Courtesy of Z-Medica.

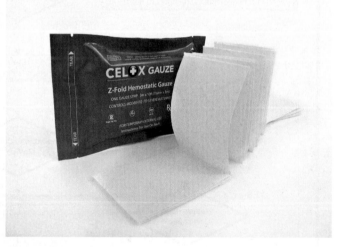

Figure 25-3 Celox Gauze®.
Courtesy of Medtrade Products Ltd.

junctional tourniquets designed to stop bleeding at these sites. The three junctional tourniquets recommended for use by the CoTCCC[9,15-17] are the Combat Ready Clamp (the CRoC), the SAM Junctional Tourniquet (SJT), and the Junctional Emergency Treatment Tool (JETT) depicted in **Figures 25-5** through **25-7**. If the external hemorrhage bleeding site is amenable to use of a junctional tourniquet, immediately apply a CoTCCC-recommended junctional tourniquet. Do not delay in the application of the junctional tourniquet once it is ready for use. Apply

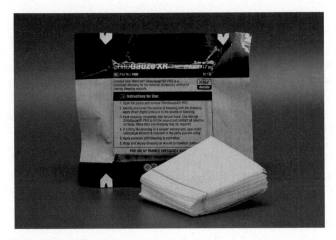

Figure 25-4 ChitoGauze.

Courtesy of Tricol Biomedical, Inc.

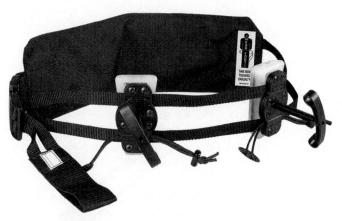

Figure 25-6 Junctional Emergency Treatment Tool (JETT).

Courtesy of North American Rescue.

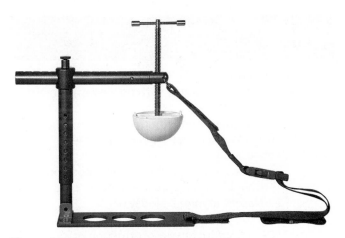

Figure 25-5 Combat Ready Clamp (CRoC).

Courtesy of Combat Medical Systems.

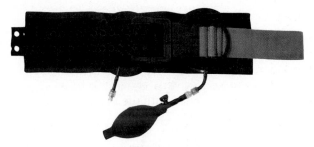

Figure 25-7 SAM Junctional Tourniquet (SJT).

Courtesy of SAM Medical Products.

hemostatic dressings with direct pressure if a junctional tourniquet is not available or while the junctional tourniquet is being readied for use.[15]

XStat

XStat was cleared for use by the Food and Drug Administration (FDA) in April 2014; it offers another option for controlling external hemorrhage. The XStat applicator syringe contains approximately 90 small, compressed foam sponges that expand when they come into contact with blood. The FDA clearance letter[18] states that XStat should be used:

"... as a hemostatic device for the control of bleeding from junctional wounds in the groin or axilla not amenable to tourniquet application in adults and adolescents. XStat™ is a temporary device for use up to four (4) hours until surgical care is acquired. XStat is intended for use in the battlefield. XStat is not indicated for use in: the thorax; the pleural cavity; the

mediastinum; the abdomen; the retroperitoneal space; the sacral space above the inguinal ligament; or tissues above the clavicle."

Recent innovations with the XStat device include a smaller diameter application device and a newer version of the compressed sponges that are not coated with chitosan.

XStat is best for deep, narrow-tract junctional wounds, especially those involving the hard-to-compress subclavian vessels.[19-21] The application of direct pressure over the site of application is optional for XStat. The expansion of the sponges within the wound cavity is designed to create an internal source of pressure at the bleeding site, but external pressure may be applied as well if bleeding is not well controlled. Note that XStat is not to be removed in the field, but additional XStat, other hemostatic adjuncts, or trauma dressings may be applied over it. The battlefield experience with this relatively new hemostatic adjunct has been limited to date, but in animal studies, XStat was successful in stopping hemorrhage in a highly lethal bleeding model that included injury to both the subclavian artery and the subclavian vein.[20,21]

Injuries to the subclavian vessels as in these studies have a high mortality rate due to the large diameter

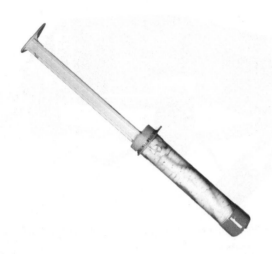

Figure 25-8 XStat 30.
Courtesy of RevMedx.

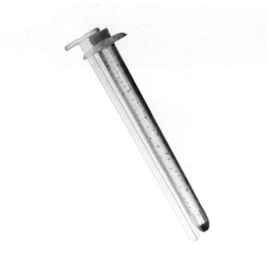

Figure 25-9 XStat 12.
Courtesy of RevMedx.

of these vessels resulting in a high rate of bleeding and the difficulty in applying direct external pressure to the bleeding site due to the overlying clavicle. In one case series, 61% of patients who sustained penetrating trauma to the subclavian vessels died before arriving at a hospital.[22] The original XStat 30 device and the newer XStat 12 device for smaller wounds are shown in **Figure 25-8** and **Figure 25-9**.

Airway

Overview

Airway obstruction on the battlefield is most often due to maxillofacial trauma, which may result in disrupted airway anatomy and the intrusion of blood, teeth, or other tissues into the airway.

Kelly's autopsy study of the causes of death in 982 combat fatalities in Afghanistan and Iraq found that 232 individuals in this cohort died from potentially survivable injuries.[23] Mabry reviewed these findings and determined that 18 (1.8%) of the fatalities with potentially survivable injuries died from airway obstruction. Of note, all 18 of these fatalities had sustained penetrating trauma to the face or neck.[24] Nine of these fatalities had injuries to major vascular structures as well; eight had significant airway hemorrhage. Surgical airways were attempted in five cases, but none of these procedures were successful. No cases were identified in which the casualties had been rendered unconscious by TBI or hemorrhagic shock and subsequently died of airway obstruction with no direct maxillofacial trauma. **Box 25-3** and **Figure 25-10** present the Tactical Field Care guideline for airway management.

Box 25-3 Tactical Field Care Guideline 4: Airway Management

4. Airway Management
   a. Conscious casualty with no airway problem identified:
      - No airway intervention required
   b. Unconscious casualty without airway obstruction:
      - Place casualty in the recovery position
      - Chin lift or jaw thrust maneuver or
      - Nasopharyngeal airway or
      - Extraglottic airway
   c. Casualty with airway obstruction or impending airway obstruction:
      - Allow a conscious casualty to assume any position that best protects the airway, to include sitting up
      - Use a chin lift or jaw thrust maneuver
      - Use suction if available and appropriate
      - Nasopharyngeal airway or
      - Extraglottic airway (if the casualty is unconscious)
      - Place an unconscious casualty in the recovery position.
   d. If the previous measures are unsuccessful, perform a surgical cricothyroidotomy using one of the following:
      - Cric-Key technique (preferred option)
      - Bougie-aided open surgical technique using a flanged and cuffed airway cannula of less than 10 mm outer diameter, 6–7 mm internal diameter, and 5–8 cm of intratracheal length

Source: Courtesy of the Committee on Tactical Combat Casualty Care.

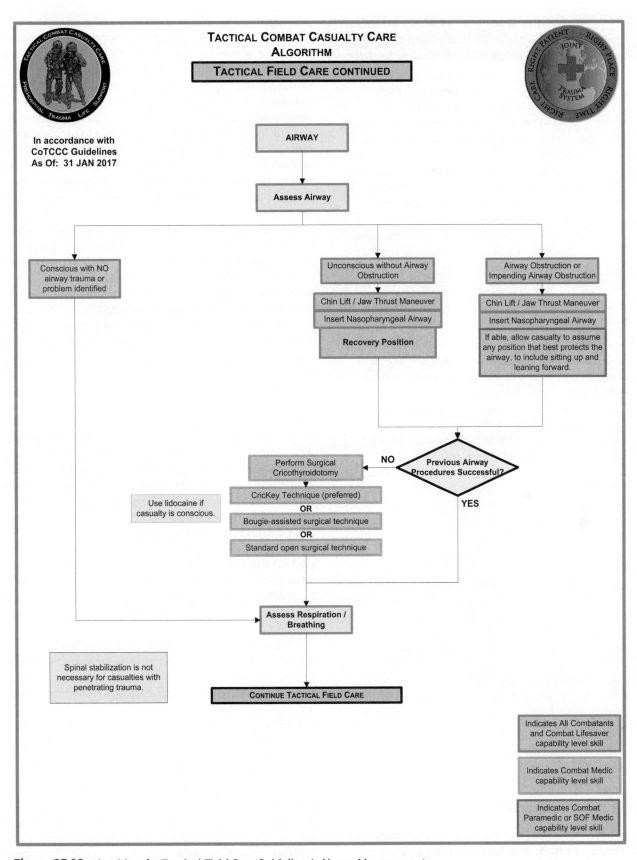

Figure 25-10 Algorithm for Tactical Field Care Guideline 4: Airway Management.

Courtesy of Mr. Harold Montgomery. Retrieved from https://deployedmedicine.com/market/11/content/87

Box 25-3 Tactical Field Care Guideline 4: Airway Management (*continued*)

- Standard open surgical technique using a flanged and cuffed airway cannula of less than 10 mm outer diameter, 6–7 mm internal diameter, and 5–8 cm of intra-tracheal length (least desirable option)
- Use lidocaine if the casualty is conscious.

e. Cervical spine stabilization is not necessary for casualties who have sustained only penetrating trauma.

f. Monitor the hemoglobin oxygen saturation in casualties to help assess airway patency.

g. Always remember that the casualty's airway status may change over time and requires frequent reassessment.

Notes:

- *The i-gel is the preferred extraglottic airway because its gel-filled cuff makes it simpler to use and avoids the need for cuff inflation and monitoring. If an extraglottic airway with an air-filled cuff is used, the cuff pressure must be monitored to avoid overpressurization, especially during TACEVAC on an aircraft with the accompanying pressure changes.*

- *Extraglottic airways will not be tolerated by a casualty who is not deeply unconscious. If an unconscious casualty without direct airway trauma needs an airway intervention, but does not tolerate an extraglottic airway, consider the use of a nasopharyngeal airway.*

- *For casualties with trauma to the face and mouth, or facial burns with suspected inhalation injury, nasopharyngeal airways and extraglottic airways may not suffice and a surgical cricothyroidotomy may be required.*

- *Surgical cricothyroidotomies should not be performed on unconscious casualties who have no direct airway trauma unless use of a nasopharyngeal airway and/or an extraglottic airway have been unsuccessful in opening the airway.*

Source: Courtesy of the Committee on Tactical Combat Casualty Care.

Airway Procedures

Unconscious casualties should have their airways opened with the head tilt–chin lift or jaw-thrust maneuver.

If spontaneous ventilations are present and there is no airway obstruction, further airway management is best achieved with a nasopharyngeal airway (NPA). An NPA is better tolerated than an oropharyngeal airway if the casualty regains consciousness,[25] and an NPA is less likely to be dislodged during transport.[26] Also, trismus (a strong contraction of the jaw muscles) is commonly encountered in head-injured patients, making an oral airway difficult to place. A review of NPA use on the battlefield found no reported instances of vomiting and aspiration complicating the use of this device in a combat setting.[27] Since the time of that review, one casualty with severe TBI who had vomiting and aspiration with an NPA in place was discussed during one of the Joint Trauma System weekly trauma teleconferences. Although intracranial insertion of NPAs is rare, it has been reported in the literature.[28-32] This complication has not been reported in any U.S. casualties from Iraq and Afghanistan.

Unconscious casualties should be placed in the semiprone recovery position to prevent aspiration of blood, mucus, or vomitus (**Figure 25-11**).

Another option for managing the airway in an unconscious patient is an extraglottic airway (EGA), commonly referred to as supraglottic airway.[33] EGAs have been used widely and with excellent success in the civilian sector over the past two decades—in the prehospital setting, in the emergency department (ED), and in the operating room (OR).[34-48]

The original TCCC Guidelines published in 1996 recommended the laryngeal mask airway (LMA) as an option for airway management during tactical evacuation (TACEVAC) care. In 2012, the CoTCCC and the Defense Health Board revisited this issue and expanded the recommendation to supraglottic airways generically, rather than singling out the LMA as the preferred option.[49]

Successful insertion of an EGA is more easily accomplished than endotracheal intubation for care providers who do not have extensive and current experience with intubation. Accordingly, the CoTCCC now recommends the use of EGAs in Tactical Field Care as well as during TACEVAC.[33]

Excess cuff pressure may be a contributing factor to the small incidence of compression neuropraxias involving nerves that travel through the pharynx after EGA use.[50-53] Overpressurization may occur with a change in ambient pressure (as with ascent to altitude) or as a result of overinflation of the cuff.[50] One case series of patients who developed this complication found that the lingual nerve was the most commonly affected (22 patients). Also affected were the recurrent laryngeal nerve (17 patients), the hypoglossal nerve (11 patients), the glossopharyngeal nerve (3 patients), the inferior alveolar nerve (2 patients), and the infraorbital nerve (1 patient).[50] Additional factors that may predispose to such injuries include an inappropriately sized EGA, misplacement of the device, patient positioning, and poor insertion technique.[33,50] If an EGA with a cuff that must be

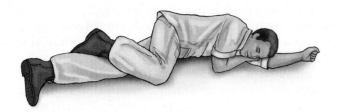

Figure 25-11 Semi-prone recovery position.
Courtesy of Mr. Harold Montgomery.

inflated with air after insertion is used, the cuff pressure must be monitored, especially during and after changes in altitude during casualty transport.[33,54-57]

The evidence available at the time of this writing suggests that the i-gel EGA (**Figure 25-12**) performs as well or better than other EGAs.[37,38,45,58-66] It is easy to train and simple to use. In addition, the gel-filled cuff on the i-gel eliminates the need to inflate the cuff with air after insertion as required with other EGAs. There is also no need to monitor cuff pressure during casualty evacuation flights. The i-gel thus simplifies EGA use and eliminates the need for the medic to carry a cuff manometer as part of his or her medical kit.[33]

No matter what EGA option is chosen, EGAs will not be tolerated by a casualty unless he or she is deeply unconscious. If the casualty's ability to tolerate an EGA is in doubt, an NPA may be a better option.[33]

As noted previously, life-threatening airway obstruction in the combat setting typically results from trauma to the face or neck. In such casualties, blood in the airway and/or disrupted airway anatomy may preclude good visualization of the vocal cords. Conscious casualties with maxillofacial trauma are often able to protect their own airways by the simple act of sitting up and leaning forward, so that blood drains out of the mouth through gravity and as the result of a protective cough reflex, rather than entering the trachea. This point is reflected in the TCCC airway management guideline that calls for the casualty to be allowed to assume whatever position allows him or her to breathe most easily, including sitting upright if required (**Figure 25-13**). Conscious casualties with maxillofacial trauma should not be forced into the supine position if they are able to breathe more comfortably in the sitting position.

If an airway obstruction develops or persists despite efforts to manage the airway with the sit-up and lean-forward position, an NPA, or an EGA, a more definitive airway will be required. In the civilian sector, this has often meant endotracheal intubation (ETI). The ability of experienced paramedical personnel to perform ETI in civilian prehospital settings has been well documented.[67-76] Many studies, however, report ETI success as the procedure is performed on nontraumatic cardiac arrest patients. Most studies also reported use of training methodologies

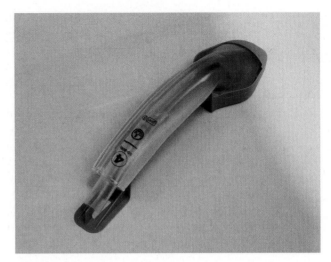

Figure 25-12 The i-gel extraglottic airway.
Science History Images/Alamy Stock Photo.

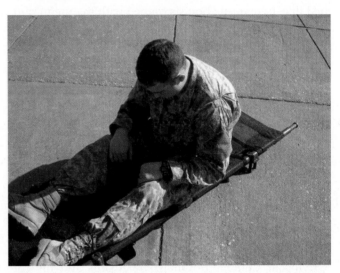

Figure 25-13 Simulated casualty sitting in the tripod position.
Courtesy of Mr. Harold Montgomery.

beyond just mannequin training—cadaver training, OR intubations, supervised initial intubations, or a combination of these methods in teaching the skill. They also stressed the importance of continued experience with ETI to maintain proficiency. Considerations for ETI in the battlefield trauma setting are somewhat different, however, and outlined as follows[26]:

1. No studies have examined the ability of well-trained but relatively inexperienced military medics to perform ETI on the battlefield.
2. Most corpsmen and medics have never performed an intubation on a live casualty or even a cadaver.
3. Standard ETI techniques entail the use of a tactically compromising white light in the

laryngoscope. There was a fatality from the use of a white light on the battlefield during an attempted intubation on an Israeli Special Operations mission.[27]

4. ETI may be extremely challenging in casualties with maxillofacial injuries.[77-78]

5. Esophageal intubation may go unrecognized more easily in the tactical setting, with potentially fatal results for the casualty.[78] In a recent study that included combat medic/corpsman intubations as well as physician and physician-assistant intubations done in prehospital Battalion Aid Station settings, only 22.5% had end-tidal CO_2 monitoring confirmation of the correct position for the ET tube.[79]

ETI may be difficult to accomplish even in the hands of more experienced paramedical personnel and even under less austere conditions.[80,81] One study that examined first-time intubationists trained with mannequin intubations alone noted an initial success rate of only 42% in the ideal setting of the OR with paralyzed patients.[75] Another study examined intubations performed by emergency medical technicians (EMTs) who had been trained in intubation and found that only 53 of 103 patients were successfully intubated.[59] A third paper documented that, even in civilian settings with experienced paramedical personnel, the tube was found misplaced in 27 of 108 prehospital intubations upon arrival in the ED.[82] One report of successful mastery of intubation skills by military combat medical personnel used mannequin intubation by just-trained corpsmen as an outcome measure.[83] This may not be an accurate indicator of success under actual battlefield conditions.

The REACH study (Registry of Emergency Airways Arriving at Combat Hospitals) by Adams and his colleagues found a relatively higher success rate in prehospital intubations.[79] However, most of these casualties (81%) were received from Battalion Aid Stations or Forward Surgical Teams where a nurse anesthetist or physician could perform the intubation in somewhat more favorable settings.

ETI in civilian trauma patients is more successful and has fewer complications when it is done with rapid-sequence intubation (RSI). Most combat medical personnel, however, are not trained and sustained in this procedure, and without RSI, intubation attempts in a casualty who is not deeply unconscious (a predictor of poor outcomes in combat casualties) will be vigorously resisted by the casualty and should not be attempted.

If the less invasive measures outlined previously do not provide an acceptable airway, then a surgical airway (cricothyrotomy) is preferable to intubation, and combat corpsmen and medics should be trained to do this procedure.[26,77] Cricothyroidotomy has been reported to

be safe and effective in trauma patients,[84] but it is not without complications.[85,86] Even so, cricothyroidotomy is believed to provide the best chance for successful airway management in the setting of airway compromise from maxillofacial trauma in tactical settings. One of the 12 potentially preventable deaths noted by Holcomb and his colleagues[78] was an individual with maxillofacial trauma who was managed with attempted ETI instead of a surgical airway. The casualty died from airway obstruction, and the tube was found at autopsy to be in a false passage instead of the trachea. MacDonald and Tien described a 19-year-old Afghan man with extensive maxillofacial injuries from an IED blast.[87] His respiratory rate was elevated, and his oxygen saturation was unsatisfactory even on supplemental oxygen. The medic attending him performed a successful surgical airway with subsequent improvement of the casualty's condition. The medic also performed an NDC of a suspected tension pneumothorax, and the casualty survived his injuries. Surgical airways have been performed successfully and with good results in Special Operations units that practice this skill frequently and use live tissue as part of their training.[49] Developing and sustaining the ability to reliably perform surgical airways is one of the most compelling reasons for combat medical personnel to obtain live tissue training. Note that a surgical airway is *not* indicated simply for unconsciousness when there is no maxillofacial trauma. An NPA or an EGA should suffice for these casualties. Surgical airways can be performed under local anesthesia with lidocaine in a casualty who is awake.

In his analysis of 72 prehospital surgical airways, Mabry found that (1) 66% of the patients died (not necessarily from airway obstruction), (2) those patients injured by gunshot wounds to the head or thorax all died, (3) the largest group of survivors had gunshot or blast-related wounds to the face and/or neck, and (4) the failure rate for the procedure performed by combat medics was 33% compared to 15% for physicians and physician assistants.[88] The latter finding should be evaluated in light of a possible difference in the tactical situations in which combat medics and the more advanced providers would likely have performed the procedure (point of injury versus battalion aid station). Mabry also noted that while the failure rate for surgical airways in the combat setting is three to five times higher than reported in civilian settings, surgical airways in civilian prehospital settings are performed by paramedic-level providers, whereas most military medics are typically trained to the EMT-Basic level.

Mabry and colleagues studied the ability of combat medics to perform cricothyroidotomies using the Cric-Key as opposed to the standard surgical technique without using this device. In this crossover study, 15 U.S. Army 68 Whiskey medics, were found to perform the surgical airway in less time with the Cric-Key than with the standard surgical procedure (34 seconds vs. 65 seconds).[89] There were also no first-attempt failures with the Cric-Key (15 of 15 successful insertions) as compared to a 66% success rate (10 of 15 attempts) when using the standard procedure. Two of the individuals who experienced a failed surgical airway procedure on their first attempt were successful on subsequent attempts, while three of the study participants did not succeed in achieving airway cannulation despite multiple attempts.

Based on this comparison, the CoTCCC identified the Cric-Key as the preferred device for the performance of surgical airways in the prehospital combat environment.[90] If this device is not available, the procedure should be performed with the assistance of a bougie. In addition, a purposed cricothyroidotomy tube should be used to secure the airway rather than using an endotracheal tube that has been modified and repurposed as a cricothyroidotomy tube. Endotracheal tubes are too long to be suitable for this purpose without being shortened, and the lack of flanges on these tubes allows them to be dislodged from the surgical site and slip down into the tracheobronchial tree.

The steps involved in performing a surgical airway in the tactical prehospital environment are:

1. Identify the cricothyroid membrane between the thyroid cartilage and the cricoid cartilage.
2. Grasp and hold the trachea with the nondominant hand to stabilize the airway.
3. Make a vertical skin incision from the inferior edge of the thyroid cartilage to the top of the cricoid cartilage using a #10 scalpel. Incise down to the cricothyroid membrane.
4. Dissect the tissues to expose the membrane.
5. Make a horizontal incision through the cricothyroid membrane.
6. Insert the Cric-Key with the Melker airway.
7. Confirm placement by feeling the tracheal rings and looking for skin tenting.
8. Remove the Cric-Key, leaving the airway in place.
9. Inflate the cuff with 10 milliliters (ml) of air.
10. Connect a bag and valve and ventilate the casualty if he or she is not breathing. Check for breath sounds bilaterally. Secure the airway.

The following clinical points (John B. Holcomb, MD, oral communication, June 2017) should be kept in mind while performing the surgical airway:

- The three most common mistakes in performing this procedure are:
  - making the initial incision too small;
  - making the initial incision too small; and
  - making the initial incision too small.
- I always use my left hand to stabilize the soft tissue of the neck and do all the operating with my right. I never move my left, as it keeps my exposure intact.

- I always start the vertical skin incision at the inferior border of the thyroid cartilage.
- In my opinion, I make a vertical skin incision and then a transverse incision in the cricothyroid membrane. The CT membrane is much wider than it is tall, so incising it transversely works with the anatomy rather than against it.
- I would avoid "stab" maneuvers. . . . In the excitement of this technical exercise, it's easy to go through the back wall of the trachea and injure the esophagus. That's bad.
- After incising the CT membrane, put a finger through it and feel the tracheal rings. It confirms placement and properly dilates the membrane to accept the tube.
- One of the more common errors I have seen from interns and medics is to place the trach tube into the trachea above the thyroid cartilage, so that is also a teaching point.

Bennett and others performed a review of cricothyroidotomy training at a U.S. Naval Hospital and found five specific gaps in the training[91]: (1) limited anatomic instruction, (2) lack of "hands-on" familiarization with laryngeal anatomy, (3) nonstandardized step-by-step training in the surgical technique involved, (4) anatomically incorrect training mannequins, and (5) lack of standardized refresher training frequency. The authors recommended incorporating a preliminary step into cricothyroidotomy training in which students use a skin marking device to illustrate on a fellow student exactly where they would make the incision for the cricothyroidotomy. This excellent recommendation adds a measure of adrenalin to the student's learning experience in that it is immediately obvious to the instructor if the student identifies the site for the incision incorrectly, and that realization, combined with the simulated casualty's awareness of the results, will immediately reinforce either that knowledge of the anatomy has been mastered or that further instruction is needed.

Thermal or toxic gas injuries are important considerations in certain tactical situations. These injuries may result in airway edema that can be aggravated by aggressive fluid administration leading to acute upper airway obstruction. Inhalation injury should be suspected if fire occurs in the casualty's presence in a confined space or if the casualty has facial burns, singeing of the nasal hairs, or carbonaceous sputum. Sore throat, hoarseness, and wheezing may also be noted. For these casualties, NPAs and EGAs will likely not suffice, and cricothyroidotomy is the airway intervention of choice.

Final points of emphasis regarding management of the airway in Tactical Field Care[33]:

- Surgical airways should not be performed simply because a casualty is unconscious. This option should

- be used only when less invasive measures have not been adequate to secure an open airway.
- Stabilization of the cervical spine with a C-collar is not needed for casualties who have sustained only penetrating trauma (without blunt force trauma).
- Pulse oximetry monitoring is a useful adjunct in assessing airway patency, and capnography should be used when it becomes available to ensure correct positioning of EGAs and the Cric-Key.
- Suctioning should be used as an adjunct to airway management when needed to remove blood and vomitus from the oropharynx. When required, suctioning should be accomplished quickly (less than 10 seconds in duration) to avoid hypoxia and gently to avoid mucosal damage.
- The casualty's airway status may change quickly; he or she should be frequently reassessed.

Respiration/Breathing

Tension Pneumothorax

Physiology

Tension pneumothorax has been defined in varying terms,[91-95] but these definitions have a common element—an injury to the lung that results in air leaking out of the lung parenchyma into the pleural space where it is trapped and produces a resulting rise in the intrapleural pressure.[96] The definition of tension pneumothorax also varies in animal studies of this disorder.[97-101] Even though a tension pneumothorax is developing and a shift in the position of intrathoracic organs has occurred, the patient may not immediately decompensate. Innocencio reported a patient found to have tension pneumothorax by ultrasound who was still clinically stable without exhibiting significant dyspnea or hypotension.[102]

Combat casualties on the battlefield who develop a tension pneumothorax are typically breathing spontaneously in the period shortly after wounding.[103] In contrast, many of the published papers on tension pneumothorax discuss patients who are being mechanically ventilated when they develop their tension pneumothoraces.[91,94,95,104] Tension pneumothorax in this setting may have a more rapidly progressive course than is seen in spontaneously breathing patients.[96] Lehigh-Smith and Harris observe that: "In ventilated patients, [tension pneumothorax] presents rapidly with consistent signs of respiratory and cardiac compromise. In contrast, awake patients show greater variation in their presentations, which are generally more progressive, with slower decompensation."[95] Roberts reported that, in 183 tension pneumothorax patients, 86 were breathing without assistance and 97 were receiving assisted ventilation. Of the spontaneously breathing patients, 50% were hypoxic

whereas 92% of the assisted ventilation patients were hypoxic.[91] When examining the course of tension pneumothorax in the two different groups, patients who were receiving assisted ventilation had a much higher incidence of hypotension (12.6 times as frequent) and cardiac arrest (17.7 times as frequent) as patients who were breathing spontaneously.[91]

Hypoxemia has been noted to occur reliably before the onset of shock in animal models of tension pneumothorax.[92,101] If tension pneumothorax is not treated quickly enough, however, the rise in intrapleural pressure may progress enough to cause hypotension by compressing the heart and great vessels. At this point, the combat medical provider may be unable to tell whether shock is due to noncompressible hemorrhage or to tension pneumothorax. NDC will be successful in treating hypotension only when the hypotension has been caused by a tension pneumothorax.

As air continues to accumulate in the pleural space, if the elevated intrapleural pressure is not relieved, the hypoxemia and shock may cause traumatic cardiac arrest. NDC of the chest is an effective intervention in this circumstance. The late Dr. Norman McSwain, the father of PHTLS, pioneered the use of NDC to relieve tension pneumothorax.[105] NDC of tension pneumothorax is one of only a few interventions that has been shown to improve survival in patients who have suffered a traumatic cardiac arrest.[106-109]

Tension Pneumothorax in Combat Casualties

Tension pneumothorax was reported as a significant cause of preventable combat fatalities during the Vietnam conflict.[103,110-112] NDC was not routinely used as a prehospital intervention to treat tension pneumothorax in Vietnam.[103] The incidence of preventable death resulting from tension pneumothorax has been reduced in the recent Middle Eastern conflicts. One reason for the decrease is that U.S. combatants now use personal protective equipment that provides significant protection for the chest and back, although it should be noted that chest wounds may still result from bullets or shrapnel impacting near the edge of the body armor and traveling into the chest.[112] Also, since 1997 U.S. combat medics, corpsmen, and pararescuemen (PJs) trained in TCCC have been taught to treat suspected tension pneumothorax with NDC. These two innovations have combined to produce a marked reduction in preventable deaths from tension pneumothorax. Eastridge's 2012 study found tension pneumothorax to have caused only 0.2% of deaths among U.S. combat fatalities in the Afghanistan and Iraq conflicts.[113] This represents a decrease of over 90% in preventable deaths caused by tension pneumothorax when compared to the estimated 3% to 4% reported by McPherson in Vietnam.[103]

Management of Suspected Tension Pneumothorax in TCCC: A Chronology

The original 1996 TCCC Guidelines recommended NDC (rather than a chest tube as used by Special Operations medics at the time) as the initial treatment for suspected tension pneumothorax.[114] No specific recommendations were made in that paper about what length needle should be used for NDC. The most frequently used needle length for NDC prior to 2007 was 2 inches (5 cm).[115]

Harcke reported in 2007 that there had been two U.S. combat-related fatalities from tension pneumothorax in which the 2-inch (5-cm) needles used for NDC had not penetrated into the pleural space.[115] His subsequent review of thoracic computed tomography (CT) scans in 100 U.S. military fatalities was done to determine the mean chest wall thickness. In this series the mean chest wall thickness was 2.11 inches (5.36 cm).[116] Harcke and his co-authors recommended that a 3.25-inch (8-cm) needle/catheter unit be used for NDC. A needle of that length would produce a 99% assurance of reaching the pleural space. Both the U.S. Army and the CoTCCC quickly responded to this new information by adopting the recommendation for a 3.25-inch (8-cm) needle NDC.[117,118] Other studies have also recommended that needles longer than 2 inches (5 cm) be used for NDC.[119-121]

There have been no published reports of preventable U.S. combat fatalities due to tension pneumothorax as a result of failed NDC since the 2007 Harcke paper was published, and use of a 3.25-inch (8-cm) needle for NDC became the standard in the U.S. military.[96]

A successful reversal of traumatic cardiac arrest was presented during a Joint Trauma System (JTS) weekly trauma teleconference in 2010. This casualty had sustained multiple injuries and had no vital signs upon arrival at the medical treatment facility (MTF) with CPR under way. No NDC had been attempted during prehospital care. The ED physician immediately performed bilateral NDC with subsequent return of vital signs. This was clearly an opportunity for improvement, and the TCCC Guidelines were soon modified to recommend bilateral NDC in casualties with torso trauma or polytrauma who suffer a prehospital traumatic cardiac arrest.[122] In 2012, the TCCC Guidelines were modified again to make the fourth or fifth intercostal space (ICS) at the midaxillary line a recommended alternate site for NDC in addition to the previously recommended second ICS at the midclavicular line (MCL).[123]

A recent review of tension pneumothorax by the CoTCCC addressed the following questions regarding the management of this disorder[96]:

- When should a tension pneumothorax be suspected in a combat casualty?

- What should be the initial treatment of a suspected tension pneumothorax?
- How should the casualty be positioned for NDC?
- What device should be used for NDC?
- What anatomic site should be used for NDC?
- What is the best NDC technique?
- What findings indicate that NDC has been successful?
- What should be done if the initial NDC is not successful?
- What should be done if the initial NDC is successful, but signs/symptoms subsequently recur?
- What should be done if the second NDC is also not successful?
- What should be the prehospital treatment of refractory shock?

When Should a Tension Pneumothorax Be Suspected in a Combat Casualty?

The original TCCC paper in 1996 contained this statement recommending an aggressive approach to the treatment of suspected tension pneumothorax:

> Progressive, severe respiratory distress on the battlefield resulting from unilateral penetrating or blunt chest trauma should be considered to represent a tension pneumothorax and that hemithorax decompressed with a 14-gauge catheter. The diagnosis in this setting should not rely on such typical clinical signs such as absence of breath sounds, tracheal shift, and hyperresonance on percussion because these signs may not always be present and, even if they are, they may be exceedingly difficult to appreciate on the battlefield. . . it is technically easy to perform, and may be lifesaving if the patient does in fact have a tension pneumothorax.[114]

In its most recent review of this topic, the CoTCCC considered the issue of whether treatment for suspected tension pneumothorax should be initiated based on respiratory symptoms even in the absence of shock if the casualty has an injury that is severe enough and in the appropriate anatomic location to produce a tension pneumothorax.[96] A number of papers addressing this topic were included in the review.[92,94,95,124-130] Consideration was given to the fact that if tension pneumothorax is not treated promptly with NDC or thoracostomy, traumatic cardiac arrest may ensue. There were two deaths noted during the monthly JTS/Armed Forces Medical Examiner System (AFMES) Mortality Conferences in which postmortem CT scans were found to show blood and air in one hemithorax and a resulting mediastinal shift, but with no definite evidence of attempted NDC. The quantity of blood noted in the hemithoraces was not of sufficient magnitude to produce lethal hemorrhagic shock and no other lethal injuries were found (E.L. Mazuchowski, written communication, June 2017).[96]

Similarly, a paper by Tien and colleagues from the Canadian military reported seven casualties who had arrived at medical treatment facilities with no vital signs and with no evidence of prehospital NDC.[131] A study from the civilian sector noted that failure to treat for a possible tension pneumothorax is the most common error in the management of prehospital cardiac arrest; the incidence of tension pneumothorax in 144 patients with traumatic cardiac arrest was 9.7%.[132] Combat medical providers must be cognizant of the fact that tension pneumothorax is a reversible cause of traumatic cardiac arrest.

Box 25-4 and **Figure 25-14** present the updated 2018 TCCC recommendations for when to treat a suspected tension pneumothorax.

Box 25-4 Tactical Field Care Guideline 5a: Respiration/Breathing: Tension Pneumothorax

5. Respiration/Breathing
  a. Assess for tension pneumothorax and treat as necessary.
  1. Suspect a tension pneumothorax and treat when a casualty has significant torso trauma or primary blast injury and one or more of the following:
    · Severe or progressive respiratory distress
    · Severe or progressive tachypnea
    · Absent or markedly decreased breath sounds on one side of the chest
    · Hemoglobin oxygen saturation <90% on pulse oximetry
    · Shock
    · Traumatic cardiac arrest without obviously fatal wounds
  2. Initial treatment of suspected tension pneumothorax:
    · If the casualty has a chest seal in place, burp or remove the chest seal.
    · Establish pulse oximetry monitoring.
    · Place the casualty in the supine or recovery position unless he or she is conscious and needs to sit up to help keep the airway clear as a result of maxillofacial trauma.
    · Decompress the chest on the side of the injury with a 14-gauge or a 10-gauge, 3.25-inch needle/catheter unit.
    · If a casualty has significant torso trauma or primary blast injury and is in traumatic cardiac arrest (no pulse, no respirations, no response to painful stimuli, no other signs of life), decompress both sides of the chest before discontinuing treatment.
  3. The NDC should be considered successful if:
    · Respiratory distress improves, or
    · There is an obvious hissing sound as air escapes from the chest when NDC is performed (this may be difficult to appreciate in high-noise environments), or
    · Hemoglobin oxygen saturation increases to 90% or greater (note that this

may take several minutes and may not happen at altitude), or
    · A casualty with no vital signs has return of consciousness and/or radial pulse.
  4. If the initial NDC fails to improve the casualty's signs/symptoms from the suspected tension pneumothorax:
    · Perform a second NDC on the same side of the chest at whichever of the two recommended sites was not previously used. Use a new needle/catheter unit for the second attempt.
    · Consider, based on the mechanism of injury and physical findings, whether decompression of the opposite side of the chest may be needed.
  5. If the initial NDC was successful, but symptoms later recur:
    · Perform another NDC at the same site that was used previously. Use a new needle/catheter unit for the repeat NDC.
    · Continue to reassess!
  6. If the second NDC is also not successful:
    · Continue on to the Circulation section of the TCCC Guidelines.

Notes:

■ *If not treated promptly, tension pneumothorax may progress from respiratory distress to shock and traumatic cardiac arrest.*

■ *Either the 5th intercostal space (ICS) in the anterior axillary line (AAL) or the 2nd ICS in the mid-clavicular line (MCL) may be used for needle decompression (NDC). If the anterior (MCL) site is used, do not insert the needle medial to the nipple line.*

■ *The needle/catheter unit should be inserted at an angle perpendicular to the chest wall and just over the top of the lower rib at the insertion site. Insert the needle/catheter unit all the way to the hub and hold it in place for 5–10 seconds to allow decompression to occur.*

■ *After the NDC has been performed, remove the needle and leave the catheter in place.*

Source: Courtesy of the Committee on Tactical Combat Casualty Care.

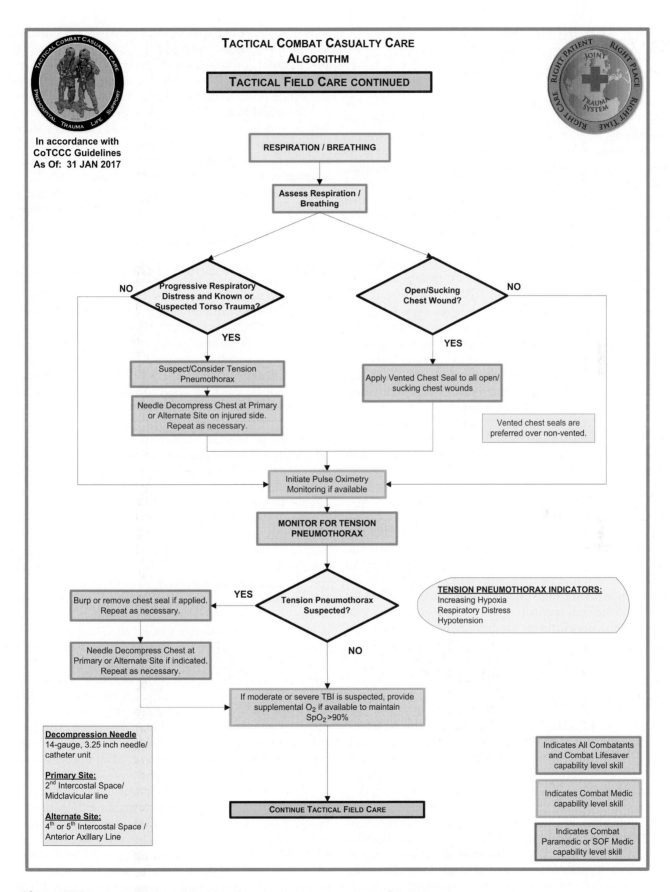

Figure 25-14 Algorithm for Tactical Field Care Guideline 5: Respiration/Breathing.

What Should Be the Initial Treatment of a Suspected Tension Pneumothorax?

If a Chest Seal Is Present

The TCCC Guidelines now state that if the casualty was previously treated for an open pneumothorax with a chest seal and that seal is still in place, if he or she is subsequently suspected of having a tension pneumothorax, then the first step in treatment is to "burp" the chest seal—that is, lift up the edge of the seal. The seal can also be completely removed if needed. These maneuvers allow the accumulated air under pressure in the pleural space to escape.[105]

Based on recent studies by Kheirabadi and Kotora and their colleagues,[133,134] the CoTCCC recommended in 2013 that vented chest seals be used to treat open pneumothoraces in order to prevent the potential subsequent development of a tension pneumothorax.[135] Recent reports from the battlefield, however, have found that most of the chest seals being used by U.S. combat forces in 2017 are still the older, nonvented type.[136] Furthermore, even if the chest seals are vented, they may on occasion become obstructed with clotted blood and not function effectively to relieve increased intrapleural pressure.[137]

Recommendation: "If the casualty is suspected of having a tension pneumothorax and has a chest seal in place, burp or remove the chest seal."[96]

Pulse Oximetry Monitoring

Next, pulse oximetry monitoring should be established to monitor hemoglobin oxygen saturation (Spo_2). This will allow the combat medical provider to obtain a baseline for SpO_2, which will be important for two reasons: (1) to determine whether hypoxia is present and (2) to provide a reference point from which to judge the success or failure of further treatment.

Recommendation: "Establish pulse oximetry monitoring."[96]

How Should the Casualty Be Positioned for NDC?

Attempts at NDC may not be successful if the tip of the needle rests in a blood-filled region of the pleural space rather than an air-filled space. Because tension pneumothorax may be accompanied by hemothorax, optimal positioning of the patient is a consideration in ensuring that NDC has the best chance to be successful.

There may be a theoretical advantage to performing NDC with the casualty in the sitting position because this maneuver would allow blood in the chest cavity to move to a dependent position and cause air to rise to the most superior location in the pleural space. This maneuver, however, may be difficult to accomplish in a severely

injured casualty and may be ill-advised in other situations, as when there is still an active threat of hostile fire. A sitting position is also contraindicated in casualties who may have a spinal cord injury. Finally, moving a casualty into the sitting position may result in decreased blood flow to the brain and heart, which may be detrimental to a casualty in shock. For these reasons, most casualties should be maintained in the supine position (for NDC at either the anterior or lateral site) or in the recovery position (an alternative for NDC at the lateral site) prior to NDC.

Recommendation: "Place the casualty in the supine or recovery position unless he or she is conscious and needs to sit up and lean forward to help keep the airway clear as a result of maxillofacial trauma."[96]

What Device Should Be Used for NDC?

Needle length is an important consideration in NDC,[138] and the needle/catheter length recommended prior to 2008 was 2 inches (5 cm).[115] However, both CT studies and clinical reports have noted that 2-inch (5-cm) needles are too short to reliably penetrate the chest wall and enter the pleural space[115,120,121,124,125,139-143] and therefore should not be used for NDC. As noted previously, two U.S. combat-related fatalities in the recent Middle Eastern conflicts were identified in which 2-inch (5-cm) needles failed to penetrate the chest wall and the casualties died with an unrelieved tension pneumothorax.[115] Both the U.S. Army[117] and the CoTCCC[144] modified their recommendations for NDC to call for a 3.25-inch (8-cm) needle shortly after the findings of Harcke and his coauthors became known. The 3.25-inch (8-cm), 14-gauge needle was also recommended for use in the wilderness setting.[145] Since this change was made and the longer needles began to be used for NDC in the U.S. military, no further deaths from tension pneumothorax in U.S. combat casualties due to failed NDC have been identified.[96] A 2013 autopsy study reported 7 failures in 13 attempts at NDC when the anterior site for NDC was used.[116] The authors stated: "While the literature has noted catheter length to be an important element in failure of NDC, it was not a factor in our cases. The change to 8-cm angiocatheters from 5-cm angiocatheters based on published chest wall thickness data appears to have eliminated this cause for an unsuccessful (NDC)." This report also found that none of the 16 combat fatalities in the case series died solely (or primarily) as a result of an unrelieved tension pneumothorax.

A study from the Mayo Clinic retrospectively reviewed 91 NDC procedures performed on 70 patients.[124] When 2-inch (5-cm) needles were used for NDC, as was the practice prior to March 2011, the success rate was 41%. After March 2011, 3.25-inch (8-cm) NDC needles were used, and the success rate rose to 83%. There were no complications reported with either length needle. The NDC site that was used in this study was the second ICS at the MCL. The recent CoTCCC review of this topic identified no evidence that suggested that NDC needles longer than 3.25 inches (8 cm) were needed to perform this procedure with reliable success.[96]

With 3.25 inches (8 cm) thus considered to be the suitable length for needles that will be used to perform NDC, the next consideration is the preferred needle gauge. Holcomb found that a 14-gauge needle was as effective as tube thoracostomy for treating tension pneumothorax in an animal study with an observation period of 4 hours,[100] but subsequent animal studies have questioned whether a 14-gauge needle has the flow capacity required to decompress a tension pneumothorax.[97-99,146] These seemingly contradictory findings may be due to variations in the animal models used, especially with respect to the amount of blood in the chest cavity, the severity of the initial pleural overpressure, and the amount of air introduced into the pleural space throughout the study to simulate an ongoing air leak.[96] The reasons for failure of 14-gauge needles noted in these studies included migration of the catheter out of the thoracic cavity, kinking of the catheter after the needle was withdrawn, inadequate flow rate, and immersion of the needle tip in blood.[97-99,146] The study by Leatherman in 2017 recommended using a 10-gauge needle for NDC rather than the currently used 14-gauge needle.[97] That paper identified no clinical studies in which the safety and efficacy of 10-gauge and 14-gauge needles were compared.

Although the animal model studies discussed above merit consideration, clinical experience with 3.25-inch (8-cm) 14-gauge needles has been generally favorable.[96,116] As noted previously, the Mayo Clinic reported a success rate of 83% using 14-gauge, 3.25-inch needles for NDC.[124]

Other commercially available needles that have been proposed for the treatment of suspected tension pneumothorax include the Russell PneumoFix (a 12-gauge, 4-inch [11-cm] device) and the Enhanced Pneumothorax Needle (a 14-gauge, 3-inch [8.6-cm] device).[5] These both have a Veress-type configuration that deploys a blunt-tipped cannula to cover the point of the needle after entering the pleural space. A PUBMED search conducted on these two devices in 2017 found no published studies of their clinical use. Furthermore, no animal or clinical data were found in the 2017 CoTCCC review of NDC to document that a 4-inch (11-cm) needle length is needed (in preference to a 3.25-inch/8-cm needle) to reliably decompress a tension pneumothorax.[96]

Additional devices that have been proposed for NDC based on animal models of tension pneumothorax include[96]:

- Vygon Catheter[142]
- ThoraQuik device[147]
- 5-mm laparoscopic trocar[146]
- Modified Veress needle[98,148]
- Reactor-bladed trochar device[149,150]

The primary concern regarding the use of larger and/or longer needles and other devices is that the incidence of iatrogenic complications may increase. Potentially lethal complications may be caused by NDC, including injury to the heart, pulmonary vessels, subclavian artery, and lungs.[150-152] Serious injuries could also occur to structures outside the thoracic cavity such as the liver or spleen. No published reports or JTS documentation of major complications from NDC in U.S. combat casualties during the Afghanistan and Iraq conflicts were identified in the 2017 CoTCCC review of this topic, but this observation was made while the military was using 14-gauge needles, initially 2 inches (5 cm) in length and now 3.25 inches (8 cm) in length.[96]

Recommendation: "Decompress the chest on the side of the injury with a 14-gauge or a 10-gauge, 3.25-inch (8-cm) needle/catheter unit."[96e]

What Site Should Be Used for NDC?

Most of the complications noted earlier have resulted from NDC performed at the second ICS at the MCL, but that observation must be considered in light of the fact that, until recently, the anterior site for NDC was the site recommended and most frequently used.[96] The CoTCCC review identified no prospective trials or retrospective case series that compared the complication rate from NDC at the anterior site (second ICS at the MCL) to that at the lateral site (fifth ICS at the anterior axillary line [AAL]). Papers were found in this review that suggested that the proximity of the heart and great vessels increase the risk associated with use of the anterior site for NDC.[96,153] Additionally, at least two studies found that prehospital personnel often perform NDC intended for the second ICS in the MCL more medially than recommended, thereby putting the heart and great vessels at increased risk,[151,154] although no major complications resulting from these NDCs were identified.[131] Inaba found that Navy corpsmen using a cadaver model were able to locate the anterior NDC site correctly only 18% of the time but located the lateral NDC site with 78% accuracy.[155] **Figure 25-15** and **Figure 25-16** show NDCs intended to be done at the second ICS in the MCL being performed more medially than intended.

The lateral site for NDC (the fifth ICS at the AAL) has been proposed by multiple authors as safer and/or associated with a higher success rate than the anterior site.[95,103,116,119,143,150,153,155-159] The lateral site is now recommended as the primary site for NDC in the 10th edition of *Advanced Trauma Life Support* (ATLS).[160] Other studies, however, still recommend or describe the use of the second ICS at the MCL for NDC.[106,124,128,142,161]

Harcke and colleagues reported that 6 of the 13 NDC attempts at the anterior site actually entered the pleural space in the 16 combat fatalities studied, whereas 4 of 4 of the NDC procedures attempted at the

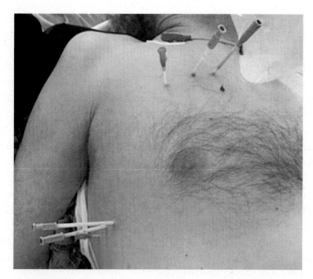

Figure 25-15 This clinical photo from a civilian trauma center shows multiple needle decompressions in both the anterior and the lateral locations. Note that two of the needles in the anterior site have been inserted at locations medial to the midclavicular line.

Courtesy of Dr. Warren Dorlac.

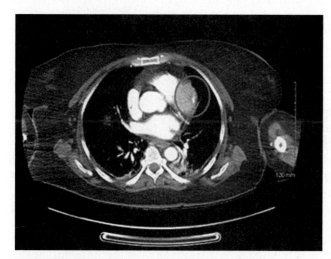

Figure 25-16 This CT image from a civilian trauma center shows a catheter that was used to perform needle decompression located in the myocardium.

Courtesy of Dr. Jay Johannigman.

lateral site entered the pleural space.[116] Leatherman and his colleagues found in a cadaver model that NDC devices inserted at the lateral position were dislodged less frequently than those placed at the anterior site during combat casualty transport.[162] In another study, Beckett and colleagues found that the 14-gauge, 1.5-inch angiocatheters used for NDC were more likely to become occluded at the lateral site than when placed at the anterior site.[163]

The topic of preferred site for NDC was discussed during a CoTCCC Working Group teleconference held on

December 14, 2017. Although the papers cited previously might seem to favor the lateral site for NDC, further considerations were highlighted during the teleconference[96]:

1. The anterior site has been widely used for NDC during combat operations in Iraq and Afghanistan and there have been no reports of major procedural complications in U.S. casualties as a result.
2. Contingencies encountered on the battlefield may make it more advantageous to use either the anterior site or the lateral site, depending on the particular circumstances of a given casualty scenario, and medics should be able to use either site as required for a specific casualty.
3. No clinical studies comparing the safety and success rates of NDC at the lateral site to the anterior site had been reported.

The latter point was congruent with a 2012 Defense Health Board report on management of suspected tension pneumothorax in TCCC that stated: "No definitive literature was found that establishes the superiority of the second ICS at the MCL over the fourth or fifth intercostal site at the AAL as the preferred site for NDC of a presumed tension pneumothorax."[123] Following the teleconference, the majority of participants favored including both of the NDC sites without specifying a preferred site.

Recommendation: "Either the fifth ICS in the AAL or the second ICS in the MCL may be used for NDC. If the anterior (MCL) site is used, do not insert the needle medial to the nipple line."[96]

Figure 25-17 and **Figure 25-18** illustrate NDC being performed at the second ICS in the MCL in a cadaver model. **Figure 25-19** and **Figure 25-20** illustrate NDC being performed at the fifth ICS at the AAL in a cadaver model.

What Is the Best NDC Technique?

Following its review, the CoTCCC made the following recommendations about the technique that should be used for NDC:

1. Insert the needle/catheter unit at a 90-degree angle (perpendicular) to the chest wall. If the device is inserted at an angle, the distance the needle will have to travel through the chest wall will be increased and the likelihood of entering into the pleural space will be decreased. Also, if the needle is inserted at a cephalad angle, the risk of injury to the intercostal vessels that travel along the inferior aspect of the rib above the intercostal space will be increased.
2. Insert the needle at the superior aspect of the lower rib at whichever insertion site is used. Again, this is done to avoid the intercostal vessels located at the inferior aspect of the rib above.

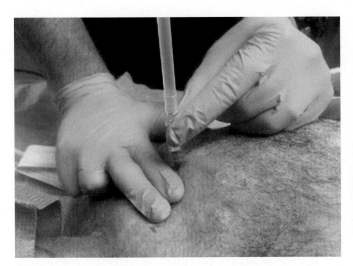

Figure 25-17 Needle decompression performed at the second ICS at the MCL in a cadaver model.

Courtesy of Lt. Col. Mark Buzzelli.

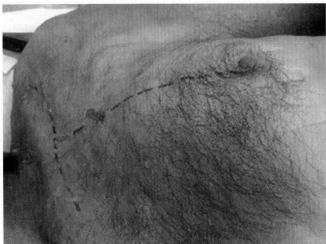

Figure 25-18 Needle decompression performed at the second ICS at the MCL with the needle removed and the catheter left in place in a cadaver model.

Courtesy of Lt. Col. Mark Buzzelli.

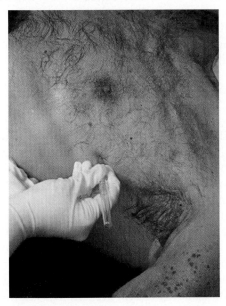

Figure 25-19 Needle decompression being performed at the fifth ICS at the AAL in a cadaver model.

Courtesy of Maj. Andrew Hall.

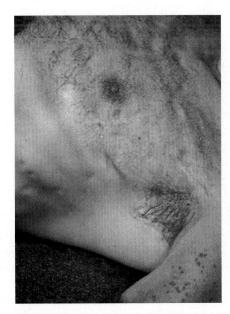

Figure 25-20 Needle decompression at the fifth ICS at the AAL with the needle removed and the catheter left in place in a cadaver model.

Courtesy of Maj. Andrew Hall.

3. Insert the needle and catheter together all the way to the hub. The 2013 Harcke paper reported a number of instances in which the catheter was found to be kinked within the chest wall and did not enter the pleural space.[116] This may have occurred because the individual performing the NDC was hesitant to insert the needle all the way for fear of causing iatrogenic injury. Alternatively, the NDCs may have been attempted using a misapplied carryover technique from IV access wherein the needle is inserted only part way initially, and then the catheter is inserted all the way as it is threaded into the vein (Dr. Ted Harcke, oral communication, April 2017).

4. Hold the needle/catheter unit—with the needle still in place—in place for 5 to 10 seconds after insertion. This allows for full decompression of the pleural space. The rigid structure of the needle helps to ensure adequate flow of pressurized air from the pleural space and eliminates the possibility of the catheter kinking after the initial decompression, as has been suggested.[164] This aspect of the technique is already

commonly performed by combat medical personnel (Mr. Harold Montgomery, oral communication, December 2017).

5. After the initial 5- to 10-second decompression, remove the needle in order to decrease the likelihood of iatrogenic injury. Leave the catheter in place so that it can provide ongoing decompression in the event of a continuing leak of air from the lung into the pleural space. The presence of the catheter also alerts subsequent care providers that NDC has been performed. Regardless of this visual indicator, the treating medic should note the NDC and the time that it was performed on the TCCC Casualty Card (DD 1380). Even though the catheter has been left in place, it cannot be assumed that the catheter will continue to decompress the pleural space—it may kink or become occluded with clotted blood.

6. Should a casualty with thoracic trauma or polytrauma sustain a traumatic cardiac arrest, both sides of the chest should be decompressed to ensure that the arrest is not due to an unrecognized tension pneumothorax on either side of the chest.[96]

Recommendation: "Use the technique described here to perform NDC.

If a casualty has significant torso trauma or primary blast injury and is in traumatic cardiac arrest (no pulse, no respirations, no response to painful stimuli, no other signs of life), decompress both sides of the chest before discontinuing treatment."[96]

What Findings Indicate That NDC Has Been Successful?

It may be difficult for a prehospital provider to determine that NDC has been successful at relieving the suspected tension pneumothorax.[75,165] In his study, Aho defined success as ". . . documented improvement in respiratory status (increased oxygenation, decreased respiratory rate, or an improvement in ventilator requirements) or cardiovascular status (normalized heart rate and/or blood pressure or a return of pulses), or a documented general improvement in the patient's condition as per the provider after needle thoracostomy was performed."[33]

In combat settings, multiple NDC procedures are commonly performed on a casualty during prehospital care.[96,166] One explanation for this is a lack of perceived improvement following NDC that may be due to the presence of respiratory distress caused by conditions other than tension pneumothorax (e.g., pulmonary contusion, hemothorax, or bronchial injury).[166] In its review of tension pneumothorax, the CoTCCC found no clearly

defined metrics of success for NDC in the medical literature, and offered the items below as indicators that tension pneumothorax has been effectively treated.

Recommendation: "An NDC procedure should be considered successful if:

- Respiratory distress improves, or
- There is an obvious hissing sound as air escapes from the chest when NDC is performed (this may be difficult to appreciate in high-noise environments), or
- Hemoglobin oxygen saturation increases to 90% or greater (note that this may take several minutes and may not happen at altitude), or
- A casualty with no vital signs has return of consciousness and/or radial pulse."[96]

If there is no improvement in signs/symptoms after NDC is performed, other causes must be considered. In casualties with penetrating thoracic trauma, respiratory distress and hemodynamic instability may be caused by hemothorax. In casualties with blunt trauma, pulmonary contusions, flail chest, or pain from rib fractures may produce respiratory distress in the absence of tension pneumothorax.[96]

What Should Be Done If the Initial NDC Is Not Successful?

There will be some casualties with suspected tension pneumothorax in whom the symptoms of respiratory distress, hypoxia, and/or shock are not relieved by NDC, leading to repeated attempts at NDC.[166] Animal studies have found that, in some cases, the tip of the needle is immersed in a coexistent hemothorax, which prevents the air in the pleural space from escaping. If the initial NDC was performed with the casualty in the supine position, blood would be expected to be pooled at the posterior aspect of the chest. Therefore, if the initial NDC was attempted at the lateral site, another attempt should be made at the anterior site, where the needle would be less likely to be occluded by blood. Another possible cause of failed NDC is failure of the needle to penetrate into the pleural space, possibly because of an unusually thick chest wall or a technical error in performing the NDC.[96]

Recommendation: "If the initial NDC fails to improve the casualty's signs/symptoms from the suspected tension pneumothorax:

- Perform a second NDC—on the same side of the chest—at whichever of the two recommended sites was not previously used. Use a new needle/catheter unit for the second attempt.
- Consider—based on the mechanism of injury and physical findings—whether decompression of the opposite side of the chest may be needed."[96]

What Should Be Done If the Initial NDC Is Successful but Signs/Symptoms Subsequently Recur?

If there is a positive response to the first NDC, that is clinical evidence that a tension pneumothorax was present and that it was effectively decompressed. Following the initial NDC, however, when the needle is removed, the catheter may kink, become occluded, or migrate out of the pleural space. Any of these events would allow the reaccumulation of air in the pleural space and a recurrence of the tension pneumothorax.[96]

Should this occur, NDC should be repeated on the same side of the chest using a new needle/catheter unit.

In a review of the casualties from the battle of Mogadishu in 1993, Dr. Ken Zafren noted: "I did find research that showed that needle thoracostomies were likely to remain patent. If a needle thoracostomy becomes obstructed, it is simpler to put in a second one rather than attempt a chest tube in the field. The second needle thoracostomy should be just as effective as the first one. Continuous monitoring and reassessment of patients is necessary whether a needle or chest tube is in place."[167,168]

Recommendation: "If the initial NDC was successful, but symptoms later recur:

- Perform another NDC at the same site that was used previously. Use a new needle/catheter unit for the repeat NDC.
- Continue to reassess!"[96]

What Should Be Done If the Second NDC Is Also Not Successful?

If the second NDC also does not improve the casualty's condition, the observed signs and symptoms may be caused by hemorrhagic shock. The combat medical provider should therefore proceed to the next step in the sequence of care outlined in the TCCC Guidelines—Circulation.

Recommendation: "If the second NDC is also not successful:

- Continue on to the Circulation section of the TCCC Guidelines."[96]

What Is the Prehospital Treatment of Refractory Shock?

Untreated tension pneumothorax may cause shock and preventable death in a combat casualty, but shock from noncompressible torso hemorrhage is a much more frequent cause of preventable death on the battlefield than tension pneumothorax.[113] If the treating combat medical provider has performed two NDCs without improvement, he or she should proceed to the measures outlined in the Refractory Shock portion of the Circulation section of the TCCC Guidelines.

Once all of the hemostatic and fluid resuscitation interventions recommended for hemorrhagic shock have been performed (if indicated), if shock persists, unrelieved tension pneumothorax should be reconsidered as a possible cause of the refractory shock.[96,104] Findings of significant thoracic trauma, continuing respiratory distress, unilateral absence of breath sounds, and hemoglobin oxygen saturation <90% would all support this diagnosis.[96] Since the casualty will have had two failed NDCs by this point, more definitive measures may be needed to treat the suspected tension pneumothorax.[73] Performing a simple finger thoracostomy will ensure that the pleural cavity has been successfully entered and decompressed.[96,130] No evidence was identified in the CoTCCC review, however, that a finger thoracostomy (without chest tube insertion) will continue to remain patent and thus continue to prevent tension pneumothorax in the presence of an ongoing air leak from the lung injury.[96] A tube thoracostomy will drain blood from the chest as well as definitively decompress any tension pneumothorax that may be present. The use of chest tubes in the prehospital setting, especially on the battlefield, is a topic that has been discussed at length in the literature.[95,104,114,126,128,130,145,169-171] These two more-invasive procedures should be performed only by combat medical personnel who have the appropriate skills, experience, equipment, and authorization. If they are to be part of the battlefield trauma care plan, training is paramount. The importance of experience in chest tube insertion was emphasized in a 2017 study that found the complication rate for this procedure was significantly higher when the procedure was performed by interns (17%) than when performed by resident physicians (7%).[172]

In the case of refractory shock, consideration should also be given to decompressing the contralateral side of the chest if that is deemed appropriate based on the injury pattern. Other interventions that may alleviate shortness of breath include ketamine administration for pain control and supplemental oxygen.[96]

Recommendation: "If a casualty in shock is not responding to fluid resuscitation, consider untreated tension pneumothorax as a possible cause of refractory shock. Thoracic trauma, persistent respiratory distress, absent breath sounds, and hemoglobin oxygen saturation <90% support this diagnosis. Treat as indicated with repeated NDC or finger thoracostomy/chest tube insertion at the fifth ICS in the AAL, according to the skills, experience, and authorizations of the treating combat medical provider. Note that if finger thoracostomy is used, it may not remain patent and finger decompression through the incision may have to be repeated.

Consider decompressing the opposite side of the chest if indicated based on the mechanism of injury and physical findings."[96]

Open Pneumothorax

An open pneumothorax results from an injury that penetrates the chest wall and may or may not include injuries to the underlying lung and pulmonary blood vessels. On the battlefield, these injuries are usually caused by bullets or fragments from blasts. The pathophysiology of open pneumothorax was well described by Dolley and Brewer during World War II[173]:

> When a chest wall injury extends through the parietal pleura into the pleural cavity (normally only a potential space), two openings are present to admit air into the thorax. While on inspiration air enters the chest through both of these openings, it is only by way of the trachea and bronchi that air, with its necessary oxygen, can reach the pulmonary alveoli. It is evident that the percentage of air that reaches the lungs through the trachea is in inverse proportion to the size of the chest wall opening. When this differential is sufficiently great, not enough oxygen is available to sustain life even with the deepest inspiratory effort. The prompt application of a reasonably air-tight dressing to close the chest wall opening averts this disaster.

When the chest wall opening is large enough (usually two-thirds or more of the diameter of the trachea),

air preferentially flows into the chest cavity via the defect in the chest wall instead of into the lung via the trachea, as the casualty inhales. (Note: The adult trachea is 2.0 to 2.5 cm in diameter; a nickel is 2 cm in diameter.) Air entering through the defect in the chest wall allows the lung on the affected side to collapse (**Figure 25-21**). This prevents normal gas exchange in that lung, causing dyspnea and (potentially) hypoxia and hypercarbia. The risk of death associated with isolated open pneumothorax is not well described, but no fatalities during Operation Enduring Freedom (OEF) and Operation Iraqi Freedom (OIF) have been attributed specifically to this injury alone.[174] Even if an open pneumothorax is not fatal in itself, the resultant impediment to pulmonary gas exchange could contribute to secondary brain injury in casualties with trauma to the brain.

The immediate treatment for an open pneumothorax is to seal the opening with an occlusive dressing (**Box 25-5** and Figure 25-14) to prevent air from entering the pleural space through the defect in the chest wall. This helps to restore air flow into the lung during inspiration, but it could lead to the development of a tension pneumothorax, because there is typically an underlying lung injury. A dressing secured on only three sides was used in the past to prevent tension pneumothorax.[175-177] The intent of the three-sided dressing was to have the open side act as a flutter valve to release any air pressure that may build up in the pleural space. There is, however, little evidence to document the efficacy of this type of dressing in practice, and it takes longer to construct

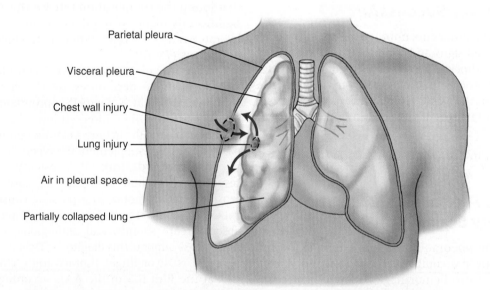

Figure 25-21 Because of the proximity of the chest wall to the lung, it would be extremely difficult for the chest wall to be injured by penetrating trauma and the lung not to be injured. Sealing the hole in the chest wall does not stop any air leakage that may be occurring from the injured lung.

than simply using a commercially available vented chest seal.[178]

Commercially available vented and unvented chest seals have been evaluated in an animal study for the treatment of open pneumothorax and prevention of tension pneumothorax.[179] In that study, 200-ml increments of air were injected into the pleural cavity of thoracotomized swine every 5 minutes to simulate an ongoing air leak from the lung into the pleural space until either tension pneumothorax developed or the volume of air injected equaled 100% of the animal's estimated total lung capacity. The authors reported no tension pneumothoraces in animals treated with vented chest seals (incorporating a one-way valve that allowed air to leave but not to enter the pleural space). Tension pneumothoraces did occur in the animals treated with chest seals without valves.

A vented chest seal, then, is the preferred treatment, but no matter what dressing or seal is used to close an open chest wound, it is crucial to monitor the casualty for signs of a developing tension pneumothorax.[178] When time, provider skills, and circumstances allow, a thoracostomy tube should be placed in the same side of the chest as the open pneumothorax. This is typically accomplished in an MTF.

Despite the 2013 recommendation by the CoTCCC that chest seals be vented, a recent study by Schauer and colleagues found that the majority of chest seals placed for 62 combat casualties with penetrating chest trauma were not vented.[180] This was attributed to both lack of predeployment TCCC training for deploying combat units and to the slow response time of the military medical logistical system in incorporating newly recommended TCCC equipment items. The need for both improved TCCC training for U.S. combat forces and a TCCC Equipment Rapid Fielding Initiative has been previously noted in multiple papers.[181-183]

A recent study by Kheirabadi and colleagues found that there were significant differences in performance between various types of vented chest seals when studied in an animal model of hemo/pneumothorax.[184] The laminar valves used in the Russell and the Sentinel chest seals were found to perform more reliably. The other types of chest seals tested in this model were either detached by blood and increasing intrapleural pressure, or blood clogged the valve and led to recurrence of tension physiology. As of this writing, however, the CoTCCC has made no recommendation regarding preferred types of vented chest seals.

Pulse Oximetry

Pulse oximeters are now commonly included in the medical kits carried by medics, corpsmen, and PJs. Although this device has no role during Care Under Fire, a pulse oximeter is a useful tool in Tactical Field Care (**Box 25-6**) and Tactical Evacuation Care. Oxygen saturation monitoring should be used in conjunction with other findings from the physical examination to assess for a patent airway and adequate ventilation. Physical examination is poor at detecting hypoxemia. Central cyanosis (a blue coloration of the tongue and mucous membranes) requires 5 grams per deciliter (g/dl) of desaturated hemoglobin and is an unreliable indicator of hypoxemia, particularly in the presence of hemorrhagic shock. The ability to detect cyanosis is reduced in typical field conditions and is effectively eliminated during

---

Box 25-5 Tactical Field Care Guideline 5b: Respiration/Breathing: Open/Sucking Chest Wounds

5. Respiration/Breathing
    b. All open and/or sucking chest wounds should be treated by immediately by applying a vented chest seal to cover the defect. If a vented chest seal is not available, use a non-vented chest seal. Monitor the casualty for the potential development of a subsequent tension pneumothorax. If the casualty develops increasing hypoxia, respiratory distress, or hypotension and a tension pneumothorax is suspected, treat by burping or removing the dressing or by needle decompression.

Source: Courtesy of the Committee on Tactical Combat Casualty Care.

Box 25-6 Tactical Field Care Guideline 5c and 5d: Respiration/Breathing: Pulse Oximetry

5. Respiration/Breathing
    c. Initiate pulse oximetry. All individuals with moderate/severe TBI should be monitored with pulse oximetry. Readings may be misleading in the settings of shock or marked hypothermia.
    d. Casualties with moderate/severe TBI should be given supplemental oxygen when available to maintain an oxygen saturation >90%.

Source: Courtesy of the Committee on Tactical Combat Casualty Care.

night combat operations in which the use of white lights is discouraged.

An understanding of the functional basis of pulse oximetry is helpful in interpreting the information provided by pulse oximeters. The purpose of pulse oximetry is to measure the percent of total hemoglobin in peripheral arterial blood that is saturated with oxygen (SpO_2).[185-195] The light absorption spectra of oxygenated hemoglobin differs from the spectra of reduced (nonoxygenated) hemoglobin. When two compounds with differing absorption spectra are together in solution, the ratio of their concentrations can be determined from the ratio of the light absorbed at two different wavelengths. From these measurements, the oxygen saturation of arterial blood can be calculated.

An arterial oxygen hemoglobin saturation of 95% or higher indicates that there is an adequate airway and that oxygen is being adequately exchanged in the lungs. Decreases in oxygen saturation may indicate an inadequate airway or pulmonary problems such as tension pneumothorax, hemothorax, sucking chest wound, or pulmonary contusion. Low hemoglobin oxygen saturations should trigger reassessment of the casualty to determine if a lifesaving intervention is indicated. Low oxygen saturation levels also help to determine which casualties need urgent evacuation as well as providing an indication of which casualties will benefit the most from supplemental oxygen if it is available in Tactical Field Care or Tactical Evacuation Care. It is important to note that good hemoglobin oxygen saturations may be seen in casualties shortly before they go into hypovolemic shock. Pulse oximetry is *not* useful as an indicator of impending hypovolemic shock.

Pulse oximetry is easily performed, but care must be taken in interpreting the results displayed by the device. Although pulse oximetry can give accurate estimations of oxygenation, it cannot measure the adequacy of ventilation since it does not measure carbon dioxide in the blood.[192] The absence of an adequate pulse waveform in a casualty in shock makes the readings obtained inaccurate. Poor perfusion is the main cause of failure to obtain a satisfactory signal. **Box 25-7** lists factors that may affect the readings obtained by pulse oximetry.

In combat settings, transport of casualties by helicopter may contribute to decreased hemoglobin oxygen saturation depending on the cabin altitude during transport. This decrease is a normal result of the lower partial pressure of oxygen at altitude. Gross movement results in loss of signal, but vibration at frequencies that fall within the possible range of heart rate may lead to erroneous values. A small (1%–2%) difference may be seen between a reading taken from a finger and the ear, particularly if the finger is dependent. Compounds that absorb light at the same wavelengths as oxygenated hemoglobin will result in falsely high readings.[192] The

---

Box 25-7 Factors Affecting Readings or Limiting Performance of Pulse Oximeters

Factors affecting readings
- Artificially low reading
- Shock
- Methemoglobin
- Cold extremity

Factors limiting performance
- Inability to obtain or interference with reading
  - Shock
  - Vascular injury
  - Motion artifact
  - Excessive ambient light
  - Skin pigmentation
  - Nail polish or nail coverings
- Pulse oximetry cannot assess:
  - Ventilatory status
  - Oxygen saturations below 83% with same degree of accuracy
- Altitude lowers oxygen saturation in normal individuals as well as casualties unless supplemental oxygen is used.
- Carboxyhemoglobin may cause a falsely high oxygen saturation reading.

---

most common and potentially most dangerous of these is carboxyhemoglobin, which may give falsely normal or high saturation readings in a casualty with smoke inhalation or exposure to other sources of carbon dioxide. Methemoglobin also interferes with light absorption. Methemoglobinemia may occur in casualties treated with dapsone, primaquine, or other related antimalarials.[194,195] Excessive ambient light may saturate the detector and give erroneous readings.[8] Xenon and infrared lamps are the sources most likely to give problems, but intense daylight as well as fluorescent and incandescent light may also interfere.

Pulse oximetry should be used in casualties who are unconscious or who have injuries associated with impaired oxygenation (e.g., blast injuries, chest contusion, and penetrating injuries of the chest). It should also be used to monitor casualties who have TBI to help ensure that hemoglobin oxygen saturation is maintained at greater than 90%. Hemoglobin oxygen saturation is increasingly considered the "fifth vital sign" in trauma care. Combat medics, corpsmen, and PJs have reported pulse oximetry to be very useful during mass-casualty events.[196] Casualties exhibiting obvious clinical signs of airway obstruction, tension pneumothorax, or hemorrhage should be managed accordingly, without undue delay to attempt pulse oximetry. When a casualty does have an abnormal pulse oximetry reading, the combat medic should reassess the casualty immediately to determine why the reading is abnormal.

Hypoxemia may worsen outcomes in casualties with moderate to severe TBI. The Brain Trauma Foundation emphasizes the need for all patients with moderate to severe TBI to be monitored with pulse oximetry and for the arterial hemoglobin oxygen saturation to be maintained at 90% or higher. This recommendation is included in the TCCC Guidelines.[193,197]

Pulse oximetry should not be considered a portable "all-in-one" monitor of oxygenation, pulse rate, rhythm regularity, and overall cardiopulmonary well-being. Overreliance on pulse oximetry may lead to delays in therapy or inappropriate decision making in the field environment. Pulse oximeters, like tourniquets and hemostatic agents, require adequate training to ensure their appropriate use.

Oxygen Administration

Combat medics do not typically carry oxygen cylinders into the field as part of their medical loadouts due to their weight and the potential for explosions secondary to ballistic damage to the cylinders. There are now, however, relatively small (11-pound [lb]; 5-kilogram [kg]), low-pressure oxygen concentrators that could be carried on convoys and used at casualty collection points. These devices would allow supplemental oxygen (at flows of up to 3 liters/minute) to be used during Tactical Field Care.[198]

Because of its potential benefit, supplemental oxygen should be provided whenever possible to casualties in shock[199] or with TBI as noted previously. If oxygen is available during Tactical Field Care, the guidelines for supplemental oxygen in Tactical Evacuation Care should be followed.

Although the current recommendations for administering oxygen in TCCC reflect the indications for oxygen mentioned earlier, a 2004 study by Stockinger and McSwain challenged the ubiquitous use of prehospital oxygen in trauma patients in the civilian sector.[200] This study reviewed 5,090 trauma patients not requiring assisted ventilation who were transported to the level I trauma center at Charity Hospital in New Orleans. Of these patients, 2,203 (43.3%) received (prehospital) oxygen and 2,887 (56.7%) did not receive oxygen. The authors noted that patients who received (prehospital) oxygen had a higher mortality than those who did not (2.3% vs. 1.1%, $p = 0.011$). After the results above were corrected for injury severity score (ISS), mechanism of injury, and age, the study found that those who received (prehospital) oxygen fared worse or no better than those who did not receive it. The authors concluded that "supplemental oxygen does not improve survival in traumatized patients who are not in respiratory distress."[200] This reinforces the TCCC recommendation that oxygen be given selectively to casualties with a particular need for it as a result of pulmonary compromise. This study neither supports nor refutes the TCCC recommendation that supplemental oxygen be provided to casualties in hemorrhagic shock, since no subgroup analysis was done for that condition.

Hypoxia in casualties with TBI is associated with unfavorable outcomes,[201] so casualties with moderate to severe TBI should receive supplemental oxygen when needed to maintain their oxygen saturation above 90%. Furthermore, hyperoxia causes cerebral vasoconstriction independently of the effects of hypocapnia and may help to reduce intracranial pressure.[202,203] Hyperoxia also increases cerebral tissue oxygenation[199] and improves cerebral metabolism in casualties with severe head injury.[204] For casualties with moderate to severe TBI, then, supplemental oxygen should be given at the highest inspired fraction of oxygen achievable as early in the continuum of care as possible.[197]

Oxygen should also be administered as soon as available for casualties with known or suspected smoke inhalation since carbon monoxide is a common product of combustion and may cause tissue hypoxia even in the present of normal hemoglobin oxygen saturation readings.[205] As noted previously, carboxyhemoglobin is mistaken for oxyhemoglobin by pulse oximetry, thereby masking the presence of hypoxemia.

Circulation

Bleeding

Improved control of external hemorrhage has been the signature advance in battlefield trauma care during the conflicts in Iraq and Afghanistan, with extremity tourniquets in particular responsible for saving many hundreds of lives in those conflicts.[206-210] Having previously controlled any massive *external* hemorrhage earlier in Tactical Field Care (Guideline 3: Massive Hemorrhage), attention should now be directed toward a more comprehensive evaluation of all hemorrhage. Potential sources of life-threatening *internal* hemorrhage must be addressed and prior interventions in external hemorrhage reassessed (**Box 25-8** and **Figure 25-22**).

Pelvic Fractures

Pelvic fractures have been seen with increasing frequency in the recent conflicts in Iraq and Afghanistan as a result of the increased use of convoy operations in the open terrain of the Middle East and the prevalence of IED attacks. Vehicular IED attacks result in both blast and blunt force trauma capable of causing pelvic fractures in

---

Box 25-8 Tactical Field Care Guideline 6a: Circulation: Bleeding

6. Circulation
   a. Bleeding
      - A pelvic binder should be applied for cases of suspected pelvic fracture:
         • Severe blunt force or blast injury with one or more of the following indications:
            - Pelvic pain
            - Any major lower limb amputation or near amputation
            - Physical exam findings suggestive of a pelvic fracture
            - Unconsciousness
            - Shock
      - Reassess prior tourniquet application. Expose the wound and determine if a tourniquet is needed. If it is needed, replace any limb tourniquet placed over the uniform with one applied directly to the skin 2 to 3 inches above the bleeding site. Ensure that bleeding is stopped. If there is no traumatic amputation, a distal pulse should be checked. If bleeding persists or a distal pulse is still present, consider additional tightening of the tourniquet or the use of a second tourniquet side-by-side with the first to eliminate both bleeding

and the distal pulse. If the reassessment determines that the prior tourniquet was not needed, then remove the tourniquet and note time of removal on the TCCC Casualty Card.
      - Limb tourniquets and junctional tourniquets should be converted to hemostatic or pressure dressings as soon as possible if three criteria are met: the casualty is not in shock; it is possible to monitor the wound closely for bleeding; and the tourniquet is not being used to control bleeding from an amputated extremity. Every effort should be made to convert tourniquets in less than 2 hours if bleeding can be controlled with other means. Do not remove a tourniquet that has been in place more than 6 hours unless close monitoring and lab capability are available.
      - Expose and clearly mark all tourniquets with the time of tourniquet application. Note tourniquets applied and time of application; time of re-application; time of conversion; and time of removal on the TCCC Casualty Card. Use a permanent marker to mark on the tourniquet and the casualty card.

Source: Courtesy of the Committee on Tactical Combat Casualty Care.

---

the occupants while antipersonnel IEDs often cause pelvic fractures in association with lower extremity amputations and penetrating trauma to the pelvis and abdomen.

Pelvic fracture should be suspected in any casualty who suffers severe blunt force or blast injury and has one or more of the following indications[211]:

• Pelvic pain
• Any major lower limb amputation or near amputation
• Physical exam findings suggestive of a pelvic fracture
• Unconsciousness
• Shock

A circumferential pelvic binding device (CPBD) should be applied for cases of suspected pelvic fracture. The CoTCCC recommends three CPBDs based on research published by Shackelford and colleagues: the T-POD, the SAM Pelvic Sling, and the PelvicBinder.[211] As of this writing there is insufficient evidence to determine which of these devices is most successful at reducing bleeding from a pelvic fracture. Another option for stabilizing and compressing a suspected pelvic fracture is to use one of the two circumferential junctional tourniquets

recommended by the CoTCCC: the Sam Junctional Tourniquet (SJT) or the Junctional Emergency Treatment Tool (JETT).[211]

Limb Tourniquets

Life-threatening extremity hemorrhage should have been previously addressed with a limb tourniquet in the Care Under Fire phase and again when checking for massive hemorrhage at the beginning of Tactical Field Care.

Prior limb tourniquet application should be reassessed at this point to ensure that all significant extremity bleeding has been controlled. A limb tourniquet is still the first step to gain control of any life-threatening extremity hemorrhage in locations amenable to tourniquet placement if this has not already been accomplished. Hemorrhage control in combat casualties takes precedence over infusing fluids or providing oxygen. Even when treating a casualty who is in shock from his or her wounds, fluid resuscitation does not take priority over controlling external hemorrhage.

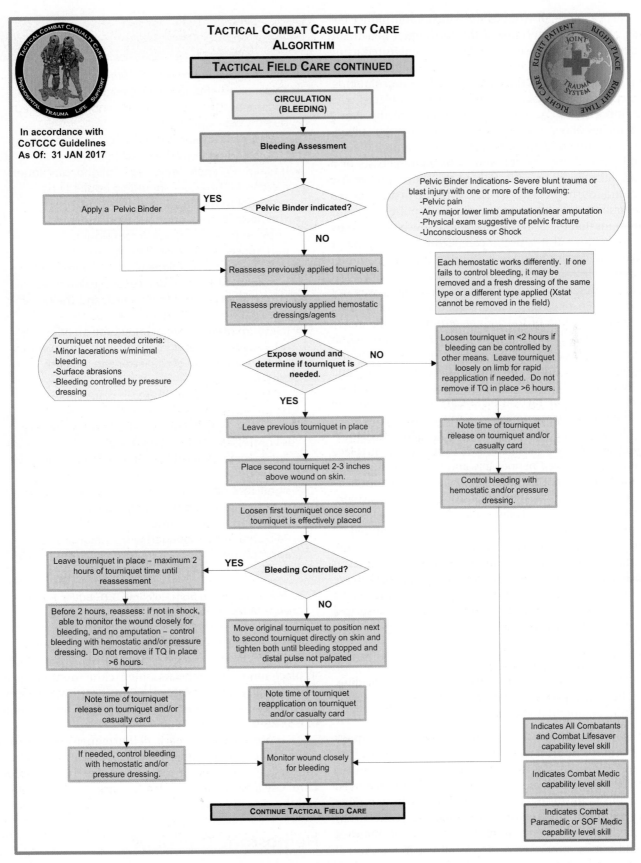

Figure 25-22 Algorithm for Tactical Field Care Guideline 6a: Bleeding.

Courtesy of Mr. Harold Montgomery. Retrieved from https://deployedmedicine.com/market/11/content/87

Next, expose all wounds for which a tourniquet has been applied to determine if the tourniquet is actually needed. Wound exposure should be accomplished using trauma shears rather than an unguarded blade to prevent further injury to the extremity. If the tourniquet is, in fact, needed, replace any limb tourniquet placed over the uniform with another applied directly to the skin 2 to 3 inches above the bleeding site. Ensure that bleeding is controlled. If there is no traumatic amputation, a distal pulse should be checked. If bleeding persists or a distal pulse is still present, tighten the tourniquet or use a second tourniquet side-by-side with the first as needed to eliminate both bleeding and the distal pulse.[212,213] It is important that the distal arterial blood flow be stopped by the tourniquet. If it is not, a compartment syndrome or expanding hematoma may develop in the limb, creating an avoidable complication for the casualty.[213] If the reassessment determines that the prior tourniquet was not needed, then remove the tourniquet, dress the wound, and note the time of tourniquet removal on the TCCC Casualty Card.[212,213] This step is needed because when tourniquets are applied during Care Under Fire, both the decision and the application are carried out rapidly due to the urgency of the tactical situation. A careful reassessment is needed in Tactical Field Care to assure that the bleeding was severe enough to warrant the tourniquet.

Hemorrhage control does not stop with the initial tourniquet application. Casualties with tourniquets in place should be rechecked periodically and each time he or she is moved to ensure that the hemorrhage is still controlled.

Tourniquet application typically causes the casualty significant pain, but this does not signify incorrect application or that the tourniquet should be discontinued.[214] Pain should be managed with analgesics as appropriate, taking care not to give narcotic analgesics to casualties in shock. For casualties with severe tourniquet pain who are in shock, ketamine is the preferred analgesic option.[215]

Limb tourniquets and junctional tourniquets should be converted to hemostatic or pressure dressings as soon as feasible if three criteria are met[212]:

- The casualty is not in shock.
- It is possible to monitor the wound closely for bleeding.
- The tourniquet is not being used to control bleeding from an amputated extremity.

Every effort should be made to convert tourniquets in less than 2 hours if bleeding can be controlled by other means, such as hemostatic dressings. It is important to note that the tourniquet should not actually be removed from the limb during this process but slowly loosened after an alternative method of hemorrhage control has been applied. Most importantly, tourniquet removal should not be attempted if the casualty is in shock or if the evacuation time to a medical facility is expected to be 2 hours or less. Do not remove a tourniquet that has been

---

Box 25-9 Key Points Regarding the Use of Tourniquets

- Waiting too long to place a tourniquet is a mistake.
- Tourniquets should be applied just proximal to the site of the severe bleeding and never placed directly over a joint.
- Tourniquets should be tightened as necessary to stop bleeding from the distal injury.
- If bleeding is not controlled with one tourniquet, a second tourniquet should be applied just proximal to the first.
- The need for a second tourniquet is especially applicable when applying tourniquets to generously sized lower extremities.
- If a distal pulse is still present, the tourniquet should be tightened, or a second tourniquet applied just proximal to the first, and the pulse should be checked again.
- If a tourniquet is used, it should be an effective arterial tourniquet and not an ineffective venous tourniquet, as use of the latter can increase bleeding.
- Casualties with tourniquets in place should be rechecked periodically to ensure that the tourniquet is still working, and that hemorrhage is controlled.
- Pulses distal to every tourniquet should checked.
- Correctly applied tourniquets can cause significant pain, but this pain does not signify that the tourniquet has been applied incorrectly or that it should be removed.
- Pain should be managed with analgesics as appropriate, but don't use opioids for patients in shock.

Source: Reproduced from Holcomb, J. B., Butler, F. K., & Rhee, P. M. (2015). Hemorrhage control devices: Tourniquets and hemostatic dressings. Bulletin of the American College of Surgeons, 100(1), 66-70. Used with permission.

---

in place more than 6 hours unless close monitoring and lab capability are available.[212] Considerations regarding tourniquet use and tourniquet conversion are presented in **Box 25-9** and **Box 25-10**.

Expose and clearly mark all tourniquets with the time of tourniquet application, time of reapplication, time of conversion, and time of removal on the TCCC Casualty Card. Use a permanent marker to mark on the tourniquet and the casualty card.[212,216]

Hemostatic Dressings

The HemCon® dressing and the granular agent QuikClot® were the hemostatic agents previously recommended by the CoTCCC based on their success in controlling severe bleeding in animal models.[217,218] These agents worked effectively,[219-221] although some cutaneous burns were reported with granular QuikClot use.[219,222]

A number of newer hemostatic agents subsequently became available after HemCon and QuikClot were introduced. These newer agents also underwent testing at the USAISR.[223] The USAISR studies found the newer agents, Combat Gauze and WoundStat™, to be consistently more effective than HemCon and QuikClot. No significant exothermic reaction was noted with either Combat Gauze or

---

Box 25-10 Considerations Regarding Tourniquet Removal

Do not convert the tourniquet if:

- The casualty is in shock.
- You cannot closely monitor the wound for re-bleeding.
- The extremity distal to the tourniquet has been traumatically amputated.
- The tourniquet has been on for more than 6 hours.
- The casualty will arrive at a medical treatment facility within 2 hours after time of application.
- Tactical or medical considerations make transition to other hemorrhage control methods inadvisable.

Source: Committee on Tactical Combat Casualty Care. Key Points. In: TFC Hemorrhage Control Pocket Guide. https://deployedmedicine.com/market/11. Published January 19, 2018. Accessed November 26, 2018.

WoundStat. Celox was also found to outperform HemCon and QuikClot, although it performed less effectively than WoundStat in the USAISR model of severe femoral bleeding (**Figure 25-23**). A summary of the relative characteristics of the various hemostatic agents is shown in **Figure 25-24**.

Based on these results, the TCCC Guidelines were changed to recommend Combat Gauze (Figure 25-2) as the first-line treatment for life-threatening hemorrhage that is not amenable to tourniquet placement. Although WoundStat was more effective, subsequent studies at USAISR demonstrated that WoundStat use resulted in the formation of occlusive thrombi in the injured vessels as well as evidence of toxicity to the endothelial cells.[224] Concern over the implications of these findings for casualties halted its distribution to the U.S. military.

In addition, combat medics involved in evaluating the options for hemostatic agents voiced a strong preference for a gauze-type agent rather than a powder or granule. This was based on their combat experience that powder or granular agents do not work well in wounds in which the bleeding vessel is at the bottom of a narrow wound tract. A gauze-based hemostatic agent is more easily applied in the depth of such wounds. Powder or granular agents also present an ocular hazard when used in windy situations like evacuation by helicopter. They can also be difficult to remove from wounds when the casualty reaches definitive care.

To assure effectiveness, Combat Gauze should be applied over the bleeding site with 3 minutes of sustained direct pressure. Simply applying the agents without maintaining pressure is not adequate to achieve the best

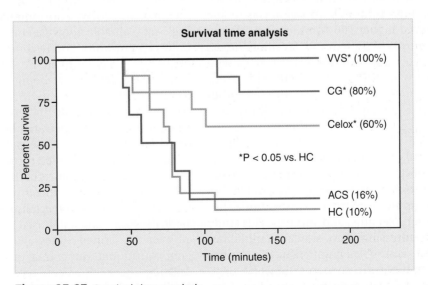

Figure 25-23 Survival time analysis.
Courtesy of Dr. Bijan Kheirabadi.

Hemostatic agent comparison

	QC ACS*	Hem Con	Celox	Woundstat	Combat gauze
Hemostatic efficacy	+	+	+++	++++	++++
Side effect	None	None	Unknown	Yes	None
Ready to use	√	√	√	√	√
Training requirement	+	+	+	+++	++
Lightweight and durable	++	+++	+++	++	+++
2 years' shelf life	√	√	√	√	√
Stable in extreme condition	√	√	√	√	√
FDA approved	√	√	√	√	√
Biodegradable	No	No	Yes	No	No
Cost ($)	~ 30	~ 75	~ 25	30–35	~ 25

Figure 25-24 Hemostatic agent comparison.
Courtesy of Dr. Bijan Kheirabadi.

possible hemostatic effect.[225] Afterward, a pressure dressing can be applied to cover both the wound and the Combat Gauze and to maintain some degree of pressure.

Combat Gauze is now the most widely used hemostatic dressing on the battlefield.[226,227] The first report of Combat Gauze use in combat noted a 79% success rate in 14 applications among Israeli Defense Force (IDF) personnel.[228] A later, larger case series from the IDF published in 2015 documented 122 uses of Combat Gauze with 88.6% success.[229] Combat Gauze was also found to be effective (93% first attempt, 100% second attempt) in one animal study using a femoral bleeding model—even when the animals were acidotic and coagulopathic.[227] Combat Gauze has also proven safe and effective when used in civilian EMS systems.[230,231]

Hemostatic dressing technology continues to evolve. A 2012 study from the Naval Medical Research Unit in San Antonio found that both Celox Gauze and Chito Gauze produced higher 150-minute survival rates in the standardized USAISR femoral bleeding model than Combat Gauze.[232] Survival was 9/10 animals with Celox Gauze, 7/10 with ChitoGauze, 7/10 with Combat Gauze XL, and 6/10 with Combat Gauze. Another study that compared Combat Gauze, Celox Gauze, and ChitoGauze using a consensus swine groin injury model found that all three products were similar in efficacy when used by a test group of 24 Navy corpsmen who had had little or no personal experience applying hemostatic dressings. Animals were then resuscitated and monitored for 150 minutes in order to assess initial hemostasis, blood loss, rebleeding, and survival. This study found that the three dressings were similar in initial hemostasis, blood loss, and rebleeding.[233] ChitoGauze has also been used with success in civilian settings.[234]

Celox Gauze and ChitoGauze have now been recommended by the CoTCCC as alternates to Combat Gauze.[235,236] To date, however, neither of these two alternate choices has been tested in the hemostatic safety model described by Kheirabadi.[224]

Use of Tourniquets and Hemostatic Dressings in the Civilian Sector

The American College of Surgeons–sponsored Hartford Consensus advocated for the use of tourniquets and hemostatic dressings by first responders in the civilian sector.[32] Of special importance is the use of these devices by law enforcement officers, because they are often the first responders to an accident or crime scene. Mass shootings at schools, malls, concerts, and transportation hubs present tactical situations that are in some respects similar to those encountered on battlefields. The threat of ongoing hostile fire, treating multiple casualties under cover, and prolonged evacuation times have all come into play. Tourniquets and hemostatic dressings are valuable tools in this setting that enable law enforcement officers to become lifesaving first responders.[206,237-240] Lives saved by law enforcement officers using these devices are being reported with increasing frequency.[241,242]

The tragic increase in terrorist attacks and active-shooter incidents perpetrated by disturbed and disgruntled individuals creates the potential for a great many additional lives to be saved through the use of TCCC concepts. Thanks to the efforts of the Hartford Consensus, the White House Stop the Bleed program, and the initiative of innovative trauma specialists, tourniquets and hemostatic dressings are being used with increasing frequency all over the United States and the world.[206,237-240,243-245] Limb tourniquets, junctional tourniquets, and hemostatic dressings have also been recommended by Wilderness Medical Society authors for use in austere environments in nonmilitary settings.[246,247]

Dismounted Complex Blast Injury and Junctional Tourniquets

Pressure-activated IEDs were used with increasing frequency by insurgent forces in Afghanistan starting in 2010. These devices produce an injury complex that has been designated dismounted complex blast injury (DCBI) and is characterized by severe injuries to one or both lower extremities, usually accompanied by upper extremity, urogenital, pelvic, and/or abdominal trauma. Multiple amputations are common.[248] Lower extremity amputations can be quite high, soft-tissue damage is often massive, and control of hemorrhage may be difficult to achieve with tourniquets and Combat Gauze. The prevalence of DCBI in casualties from Afghanistan led to the development of devices designed to apply sustained pressure to the large arteries in the groin.

As discussed previously in the Massive Hemorrhage section, if a lower extremity wound is not amenable to tourniquet application and bleeding from it cannot be controlled by hemostatic agents or pressure dressings, the treating combat medic should consider immediate application of mechanical direct pressure using one of the three CoTCCC-recommended junctional tourniquets: the CRoC, the JETT, or the SAM Junctional Tourniquet.[249-251]

XStat

XStat was discussed previously in the Massive Hemorrhage section. At this point in Tactical Field Care, any sites that have had XStat used to control bleeding should be reevaluated, and more Xstat may be applied if needed to control residual bleeding. XStat, unlike other hemostatic dressings, should not be removed by combat medical personnel in the field after it has been applied, but more XStat may be added and/or a different hemostatic dressing applied with direct pressure may be used in conjunction with the XStat.[216,252]

Hemorrhage Control—Direct Pressure

In most cases, control of external hemorrhage can be accomplished by simply applying direct pressure on the bleeding vessel. This is true even for major vessels like the carotid or femoral arteries. However, casualties with life-threatening hemorrhage often bleed to death when direct pressure is the only treatment available to achieve hemostasis.

Why does this happen? For direct pressure to be effective, it must be applied, preferably with both hands, using significant force, and with the casualty on a surface firm enough to provide effective counterpressure. Consequently, direct pressure is typically ineffectively applied while the casualty is being moved. Additionally, discontinuation of pressure to check the status of the bleeding site during transport must be avoided. The pressure must be applied without interruption until the casualty reaches a location at which surgical repair of the vessel can be accomplished or hemostatic adjuncts applied. For these reasons, tourniquets and hemostatic dressings are the favored methods for controlling life-threatening external hemorrhage on the battlefield.

Wounds with minimal external bleeding that do not involve injury to major blood vessels may be dressed with a gauze bandage or simply ignored until the casualty reaches definitive care.

Noncompressible Torso Hemorrhage (NCTH)

For internal hemorrhage from wounds to the chest, abdomen, or pelvis, the most crucial lifesaving measures are administration of TXA (discussed in a later section), resuscitation with whole blood (instead of crystalloid or asanguinous colloids), and rapid transportation to a facility where definitive surgical control of the hemorrhage can be achieved. NCTH may cause shock and death despite relatively unimpressive entrance wounds. Transport of a casualty with suspected NCTH should be accomplished on an emergent basis. Avoiding platelet-impairing nonsteroidal anti-inflammatory drugs (NSAIDs), overly aggressive prehospital crystalloid-based fluid resuscitation, and the clotting dysfunction caused by hypothermia can improve survival in casualties with NCTH.

Emerging Hemostatic Technologies

Several promising new technologies to assist with hemorrhage control are being evaluated at the time of this writing. These include resuscitative endovascular occlusion of the aorta (REBOA) and ResQFoam™, an intraperitoneally injected polyurethane self-expanding foam.[226]

Resuscitative Endovascular Occlusion of the Aorta

In REBOA, after femoral artery access has been gained, a catheter with a balloon is introduced and passed retrograde up to the desired site of occlusion.[253,254] When the balloon is inflated, distal flow—and NCTH below the site of occlusion—is stopped. This procedure has to date been done mostly in MTFs under fluoroscopic guidance. With modifications, however, the device has been used in austere environments[255] and might be feasible for use by prehospital medical providers.[256] The CoTCCC is presently exploring how REBOA could be developed as a far-forward capability as part of what has been designated as Advanced Resuscitative Care (ARC).[257-259]

One concern about performing REBOA in the prehospital environment is that, if there is a bleeding site above the balloon occlusion, the rate of bleeding from that site may actually be increased. Another major limitation of REBOA is the relatively short period of time that the balloon can remain inflated without causing distal ischemic damage. REBOA in aortic Zone 1 (from the origin of the left subclavian artery to the celiac artery) can only be used to occlude flow for 30 minutes without incurring distal ischemic damage. Zone 2 is not used. Zone 3 (from the lower of the two renal arteries to the aortic bifurcation) can be occluded for 60 minutes. Therefore, the patient will need to be in the OR within a very short time after REBOA has been accomplished. There are two factors that may allow this interval to be extended. The first is the emerging technique of partial REBOA, where the balloon is inflated sufficiently to slow the rate of blood flow in the aorta but not completely stop it.[260,261] The second factor is intermittent REBOA wherein periods of occlusion are alternated with periods of balloon deflation to allow distal flow. Laboratory study of the optimal use of this technique is currently underway at the Naval Medical Research Unit San Antonio (J. Glaser, oral communication, May 2018). Both partial and intermittent REBOA are designed to reduce the burden of ischemia distal to the occlusion site and extend the time that this intervention may be used to control NCTH. At the time of this writing, the combination of whole blood resuscitation and a customized plan for intermittent Zone 1 REBOA has been designated Advanced Resuscitative Care and approved as the newest addition to TCCC.

ResQFoam

ResQFoam is a product that has been developed with funding from the Defense Advanced Research Projects Agency (DARPA) as a collaborative effort of Harvard Medical School and the Massachusetts General Hospital. This technology entails the mixing and percutaneous injection of two liquid precursors—a polyol phase and an isocyanate phase—into the peritoneal cavity.[262] Once the precursor materials have been mixed, the resulting compound rapidly expands approximately 35-fold inside the abdomen. It then transitions into a solid foam that conforms to the anatomy of the abdominal organs in a process that takes approximately 1 minute. The resulting compound creates a local tamponading effect that reduces the rate of intra-abdominal hemorrhage and prolongs survival.[262] ResQFoam is designed not to adhere to the abdominal organs and tissues, allowing for easier removal at surgery.[262] This product has been extensively tested in animal models and found to increase survival in lethal models of liver and iliac artery hemorrhage.[263-267] ResQFoam is currently undergoing clinical trials and may

be cleared for use by the FDA in the near future. If and when ResQFoam is approved by the FDA, along with REBOA and whole blood transfusion, it could be a third pillar of ARC.[259]

ResQFoam may offer two advantages over REBOA for use in austere environments. It may prove to be more feasible technically for far-forward medical personnel who do not have a great deal of experience with obtaining arterial access. It may also safely control bleeding for a longer period of time in the prehospital phase than does REBOA, although the extended safe times for Zone 1 REBOA currently being evaluated using partial or intermittent REBOA may negate this relative advantage in the future. Lastly, because ResQFoam induces a diffuse increase in intraperitoneal pressure, it may provide a benefit in casualties who have solid organ or vascular injury proximal to the aortic bifurcation.

Intravenous Access

In civilian trauma care, it is common practice to establish IV access in the prehospital setting for all individuals who have suffered significant trauma. In tactical military settings, this practice has a number of disadvantages. Starting IVs entails costs in both time and equipment. On the battlefield, it is important not to burden the medic with carrying extra equipment and not to burden the mission commander with a delay in tactical flow in order to perform a procedure if it is not really needed. Intravenous supplies and fluids should be conserved for those casualties who truly need them. Therefore, only individuals requiring fluid resuscitation for shock and those who need intravenous medications should have an IV started (**Box 25-11** and **Figure 25-25**). The option of using

---

Box 25-11 Tactical Field Care Guideline 6b: Circulation: IV Access

6. Circulation
   b. IV Access
      - Intravenous (IV) or intraosseous (IO) access is indicated if the casualty is in hemorrhagic shock or at significant risk of shock (and may therefore need fluid resuscitation), or if the casualty needs medications, but cannot take them by mouth.
        · An 18-gauge IV or saline lock is preferred.
        · If vascular access is needed but not quickly obtainable via the IV route, use the IO route.

Source: Courtesy of the Committee on Tactical Combat Casualty Care.

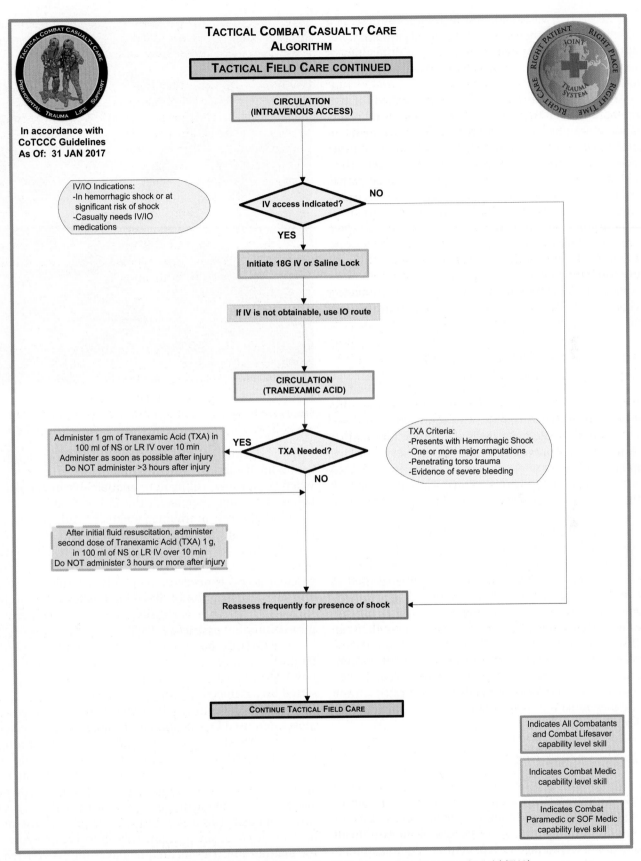

Figure 25-25 Algorithm for Tactical Field Care Guideline 6b: IV Access and 6c: Tranexamic Acid (TXA).

Courtesy of Mr. Harold Montgomery. Retrieved from https://deployedmedicine.com/market/11/content/87

intraosseous (IO) vascular access techniques as described later eliminates the need to start IVs on all casualties preemptively in order to avoid the potential difficulties of establishing IV access in a casualty who may later go into shock.

Although civilian practice in the past called for two large-bore (14- or 16-gauge) IV catheters for fluid resuscitation in trauma victims,[268] a recent review in the *American Journal of Nursing* found that an 18-gauge catheter is adequate for transfusion of blood products even when rapid transfusion is required.[269] Eighteen-gauge catheters are easier to insert than the larger 14- or 16-gauge catheters, an important consideration for combat medical personnel, many of whom do not have extensive or recent experience establishing IV access.[270] Because the battlefield environment must be considered inherently contaminated, it is good practice to replace IV lines started in the field with new ones that are inserted using accepted sterile techniques once time allows in the hospital setting.[271,272]

Securing Intravenous Lines for Casualty Movement

Intravenous lines started in the field often become dislodged during casualty transport. To address this problem, the 75th Ranger Regiment devised a system for securing IV lines that has proved successful in the field. The first step in their system is insertion of an 18-gauge, 1.25-inch (3-cm) catheter along with a saline lock. The saline lock is then secured by applying a sheet of transparent wound dressing film over the site. Fluids and medications are then given by inserting a second 18-gauge, 1.25-inch (3-cm) needle and catheter through the film dressing and saline lock, then withdrawing the needle. The second catheter is left in place, and the IV line secured to the arm with a device that has a circumferential Velcro® strap. The combination of transparent film dressing and the line-locking device provides for IV access that can withstand rugged handling (**Figure 25-26**). If the IV line must be discontinued temporarily to facilitate movement on the field, the locking strap, IV line, and second catheter can be quickly disconnected. The first catheter and saline lock remain in place under the film, providing for quick IV access later.

Intraosseous Access

It may be difficult to establish IV access in casualties in shock. An intraosseous (IO) device offers an alternative route for administering fluids and medications in this situation.[273,274] This allows the medic to avoid more difficult and invasive techniques such as central venous cannulation or saphenous cutdown.[271] Intraosseous access is also far easier to obtain than IV access when casualty care is

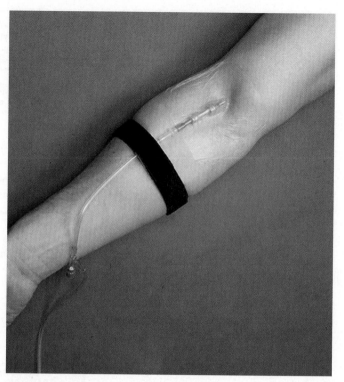

Figure 25-26 Ranger ruggedized field IV.
Courtesy of North American Rescue.

being performed in the dark. The CoTCCC began advocating for IO access as an alternative for vascular access when IV access was difficult or unattainable in 2003, long before it became popular in the U.S. civilian sector for prehospital access in trauma patients.[271] Although IO access can typically be obtained reliably and rapidly, serious complications, including osteomyelitis, can result from IO devices. This option should therefore be used only when vascular access is needed emergently for fluid resuscitation or administration of lifesaving medications and peripheral IV access is not easily obtained.[275] IO access is now commonly practiced in civilian EMS systems.[276]

The CoTCCC has not to date recommended a specific IO device as a preferred option. One option is the Teleflex FAST-1®. This device can be quickly and easily inserted by paramedics.[277] In a 2011 survey,[277] the FAST-1 (**Figure 25-27**) was the IO device most favorably rated and most often used by U.S. military combat medical personnel. The FAST-1 delivers fluid and medications through the bone marrow of the sternal manubrium. Using the sternal notch as a reference point, an adhesive patch is applied that provides a target area for insertion. The device is then aligned with the target, and firm, steady pressure is applied. This action inserts a small, stainless steel tip connected to an infusion tube into the marrow of the manubrium. This technique makes the FAST-1 readily applicable in low-light environments. A clear plastic dome attaches via a Velcro ring, keeping the site clean

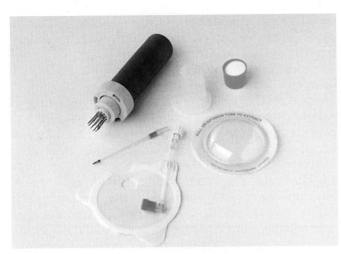

Figure 25-27 Teleflex FAST-1.
Courtesy of Teleflex, Inc.

and visible. The FAST-1 device is not spring-loaded, and its configuration renders accidental autoinjection into the medic's hand (a possibility with some devices) unlikely. A disadvantage of the FAST-1 (and other devices that use the sternum for IO access) is that the casualty's body armor must be removed to insert the device. Doing so makes the casualty more vulnerable to further injury from hostile fire.

The EZ-IO® intraosseous infusion system has also been widely used by coalition forces in Iraq and Afghanistan. The original EZ-IO device was not approved for sternal IO access. This was a problem in that its tibial plateau insertion site may be injured or missing in combat casualties. However, the EZ-IO system subsequently included needles of various lengths, allowing IO access at the sternum and at six other sites on the proximal humerus, proximal tibia, and distal tibia. The EZ-IO is small, lightweight, and easy to use. The EZ-IO tibial device (drill type) was the second most used device in the 2011 Navy Operational Medical Lessons Learned Survey and was very close to the FAST-1 in user preference ratings. Both manual and battery-powered versions are available. Combat medical personnel have noted several disadvantages of the EZ-IO system: the need to construct protection for the infusion needle during transport, significant pain when fluids are administered at tibial sites, and loss of potential insertion sites due to extremity trauma. Furthermore, care must be taken not to use a tibial needle at a sternal infusion site. The AFMES noted that use of the wrong needle for a sternal IO resulted in inadvertent passage of the longer tibial needle through the interior aspect of the sternum, with subsequent infusion of resuscitation fluid into the mediastinum.[278,279]

A key aspect of IO devices is the flow rate that can be achieved with each device and at the various potential insertion sites. In a 2015 study, Pasley and others[280] used a fresh human cadaver model to study the respective flow rates of the three most commonly used IO sites: sternum (FAST-1), humeral head (EZ-IO), and proximal tibia (EZ-IO). The volume of 0.9% saline solution infused into each site using 300 mm Hg pressure over a period of 5 minutes was measured. Sixteen cadavers were used, and the mean volumes of fluid infused at each site were 469 ml for the sternum, 286 ml for the humerus, and 154 ml for the tibia. The tibial site was noted to have the greatest number of insertion difficulties. Also of note, Burgert found in an animal model that it took twice as long to transfuse 900 ml of whole blood through a humeral IO compared with an 18-gauge IV.[281] However, since IO devices can be used simultaneously at sternal, tibial, and humeral (IO) sites, rapid infusion can be achieved intraosseously by using multiple IO infusions. Multiple IO infusions have been routinely used by the British Medical Emergency Response Team caring for casualties during TACEVAC.[282] Due to physical configuration, specific evacuation platforms may make some potential IO sites easier to access than others during TACEVAC.[283]

Intraosseous infusion has been used widely in Iraq and Afghanistan and has proven a valuable option for the combat medic, corpsman, and PJ.[271,283] Although one report has questioned the use of IO devices when rapid transfusion of blood products is required,[284] a 2013 study by Lewis and colleagues[285] reported 1,014 uses of IO devices in caring for combat casualties in Afghanistan between 2006 and 2013 with 5,124 separate infusions of blood products. The authors concluded that "IO access can be used to administer a wide variety of life-saving medications quickly, easily and with low-complication rates. This highlights its valuable role as an alternative method of obtaining vascular access, vital when resuscitating the critically injured trauma patient."

Tranexamic Acid

Hemorrhage is the leading cause of preventable death in combat casualties.[286-288] The widespread use of commercially manufactured limb tourniquets in the U.S. military has almost eliminated death from isolated extremity hemorrhage.[289] Junctional hemorrhage can now be effectively addressed with CoTCCC-recommended hemostatic dressings or junctional tourniquets.[290,291] Noncompressible hemorrhage is now the cause of 67% of hemorrhagic deaths on the battlefield.[288]

TXA is a lysine analog that binds to the lysine receptor sites in plasminogen, preventing its transformation into plasmin and thereby inhibiting the breakdown of clots in the fibrinolytic process. TXA does not promote the formation of new clots: it stabilizes clots that have already formed, which may be of benefit in establishing hemostasis in bleeding casualties. TXA has other properties in addition to its antifibrinolytic activity. It has been shown to reduce inflammation and to stabilize the vascular endothelium.[292] Both of these properties may be of benefit in bleeding trauma patients. TXA is not approved by the FDA for use in trauma despite the findings outlined here, so use of TXA in this setting is off-label.[293]

The CRASH-2 study examined the effect of TXA as an intervention to reduce death from hemorrhage in 20,211 trauma patients.[294] In that study, a small but statistically significant benefit from TXA use was found. There was no difference in the rate of vascular occlusive events between the two arms of the study, and no unexpected adverse events from TXA use were reported. Subgroup analysis of the CRASH-2 data that examined the impact of the timing of TXA administration on the 1,063 deaths from bleeding in the CRASH-2 study found that the risk of death due to bleeding was significantly reduced (5.3% vs. 7.7%) if TXA was given within 1 hour of injury.[293] When TXA was given 1 to 3 hours after injury, the decrease in mortality remained significant (4.8% vs. 6.1%), but when TXA was administered more than 3 hours after injury, mortality was increased compared to controls.

The findings of the CRASH-2 study were compelling, but their applicability to the care of combat casualties was uncertain. Different mechanisms of wounding, differences in injury patterns, longer delays to evacuation, and differences in trauma systems made it less than obvious that TXA would provide similar benefits to individuals wounded in combat. The Military Application of Tranexamic Acid in Trauma Emergency Resuscitation Study (MATTERs) was carried out at a Role 3 facility in Afghanistan to examine this question.[295] In this case series of 896 combat casualties who received blood, mortality in casualties who received TXA was reduced compared to those who did not (17.4% vs. 23.9%; *p* = 0.03), despite the fact that those receiving TXA were more seriously injured (ISS 25.2 vs. 22.5). In the subgroup of casualties who received *massive* transfusions, however, mortality was markedly lower in the TXA group (14.4%) as compared to the no-TXA group (28.1%; *p* = 0.004.)

In the MATTERs study, both deep venous thrombosis (DVT) and pulmonary embolism (PE) were increased in the TXA group (PE in the massive transfusion TXA group was 3.2% vs. 0% in the no-TXA massive transfusion group), but no fatalities from PE were reported in this study. The CRASH-2 and MATTERs findings support the use of TXA in combat casualties who are in hemorrhagic shock or at significant risk for that condition. Accordingly, TXA was added to the TCCC Guidelines in 2011.[296,297]

In his 2011 review of the literature on TXA[298] Col. Andre Cap concluded that: "This inexpensive and safe drug should be incorporated into trauma clinical practice guidelines and treatment protocols. . . . TXA should be adopted for use in bleeding trauma patients because it is the only drug with prospective clinical evidence to support this application." A later study using a swine model found that TXA is also effective when administered by the intraosseous route.[298]

In the years following the CRASH-2 study, a number of studies examining the use of TXA in elective surgery appeared in the medical literature. A 2013 meta-analysis reviewed 46 randomized controlled trials involving 2,925 patients and found that the use of TXA in elective major orthopedic surgery reduced total blood loss by a mean of 408 ml.[299] In his 2017 study Sabbag[300] noted that "IV TXA has gained substantial popularity in primary total hip arthroplasty (THA) and total knee arthroplasty (TKA) and is now commonly used for revision hip and knee arthroplasties as well." This paper addressed the question of whether or not TXA was safe to use in patients who had a previous history of DVT. Their retrospective study of 1,262 patients who had undergone either THA or TKA found that patients who had a history of venous thromboembolism (VTE) did not have an increased risk of recurrent VTE when TXA was used as an adjunct to their surgery. Ramirez and colleagues state that "Currently, TXA may be the best pharmacologic option for prehospital hemostatic interventions, and its administration in the field has been shown to be feasible in both civilian and military settings."[301]

The finding of the CRASH-2 timing subgroup analysis that TXA given more than 3 hours after injury increased mortality[293] has unfortunately led to the misperception that giving TXA at any time before the 3-hour point is equally acceptable when using this drug in trauma patients. A best-practice summary published in *Annals of Emergency Medicine* states: "According to the available evidence, tranexamic acid has been shown to significantly decrease mortality in bleeding trauma patients, with no significant increase in serious prothrombotic complications if administered within 3 hours of injury" and recommends its use in patients who require resuscitation with blood products, especially massive transfusion patients.[302] This approach does not reflect the fact that CRASH-2 showed that the greatest benefit from TXA use in trauma was seen when it was given within 1 hour of injury. Furthermore, the studies of TXA given before elective surgery produced Level A evidence that TXA reduces blood loss and does not increase the risk of thromboembolic complications when given *before the bleeding starts* in elective surgery. The best way to prevent death from hemorrhage is to prevent the causative hemorrhage. Col. John Kragh found in his 2009 tourniquet study that when tourniquets were applied before the onset of shock, survival was 90%. When shock was already present at the time of tourniquet application, survival dropped to 10%.[303] The implication for TCCC is that to obtain the maximal survival benefit from the hemostatic effect of TXA, TXA should be given as soon as possible after injury (see Figure 25-23). This is reflected in the wording of the August 1, 2018, TCCC Guidelines[304] (see Box 25-11).

The second dose of TXA is typically given after the casualty arrives at a Role 2 or Role 3 medical facility. This dose may be given in the field if evacuation is delayed and fluid resuscitation is completed before arrival at the medical facility. If the second dose of TXA is administered during Tactical Field Care or Tactical Evacuation Care, it should be given just as directed for the first dose.

Additional information on intravenous administration of TXA obtained from *Physician's Desk Reference*[305] includes:

- To avoid hypotension, administer at a rate not to exceed 100 milligram (mg; 1 ml) per minute.
- May be administered together with replacement therapy.
- Prepare the same day the solution is to be used; discard any remaining solution after single use.
- May be mixed with most solutions for infusion, such as electrolyte, carbohydrate, amino acid, and dextran solutions.
- Do not add heparin to injection or mix with blood; do not mix with solutions containing penicillin.

The question of whether or not TXA can be safely mixed with Hextend™ has been raised. A 2016 study was performed to address that issue.[306] The authors found that mixing TXA with Hextend caused no evidence of incompatibility on visual inspection or by digital turbidimeter. To date, this study has resulted in no change in the *Physician's Desk Reference* recommendations[305] nor a change in the TCCC recommendation to mix TXA in normal saline (NS) or lactated Ringer (LR) solution.

In October 2013, the assistant secretary of defense expanded prehospital use of TXA from Special Operations forces to all forces in the U.S. military. The approval letter noted that TXA is not FDA approved for trauma and is therefore considered an off-label use subject to a provider's clinical judgment. The letter required the military services to establish service-specific policies regarding TXA administration, develop training and education plans, accumulate outcome data and monitor adverse events associated with TXA use, and assume all costs for implementation.[307]

The JTS recently examined the data in the Department of Defense (DoD) Trauma Registry to further evaluate the impact of TXA in combat casualties. Howard's 2017 study is the largest study to date of TXA use in combat casualties (3,773).[308] All of these casualties received at least one unit of red blood cells (RBCs). The authors did not find a significant impact of TXA use on mortality, but they did note that TXA use was associated with a higher rate of DVT. Caveats in this study included a note that physicians and combat medical providers have been cautious about the use of this new medication and have received training that suggests that TXA should only be given to the most seriously injured patients.[308] If TXA administration is delayed until the casualty is in shock, the time for maximal benefit has likely passed.[303,309] Additionally, Howard's study did not include a subgroup analysis based on elapsed time from injury until TXA administration, as the CRASH-2 timing subgroup analysis did.[308] Finally, the preponderance of undocumented prehospital care makes it difficult to determine what was or was not done in the prehospital phase of care, when TXA administration would be expected to have had the most benefit.[290,310]

A civilian TXA study examining the prehospital use of TXA found a benefit from using this medication early in the continuum of care for trauma patients.[311] In this study, early (24-hour) mortality was found to be significantly lower in the TXA group (5.8%) than the control group (12.4%). The most pronounced mortality difference was observed in patients who were more severely injured.

A review of TXA use in austere environments[312] produced the following recommendation: "Our recommendation based on the current literature advocates the use of early bolus TXA in the prehospital setting in those patients at risk of significant uncontrolled bleeding. The benefit is most pronounced when given early after injury (less than 1 hour) and, combined with the extensive literature on prophylactic administration in elective surgery, may be most beneficial when given before the development of hemorrhagic shock. We recommend withholding repeat dosing until coagulation status has been determined and redosing at that time for a LY30 greater than 43% on TEG."

A large meta-analysis of trauma and postpartum hemorrhage patients treated with TXA[309] found that "*Immediate* treatment improved survival by more than 70% (OR 1.72, 95% confidence interval [CI] 1.42–2.10; $p < 0.0001$). Thereafter, the survival benefit decreased by 10% for every 15 min of treatment delay until 3 h, after which there was no benefit." There was no increase in vascular occlusive events with TXA use.

Despite the power of the amassed evidence as discussed, the novelty of TXA in prehospital trauma care has resulted in its continued underuse or delayed use in battlefield trauma care, as recently noted by Schauer and his coauthors.[313]

Fluid Resuscitation

A Historical Perspective on Fluid Resuscitation in TCCC

Despite its widespread use at the initiation of the TCCC effort in 1992, the benefit of large-volume prehospital fluid resuscitation with crystalloid solutions in trauma patients had not been well established.[314-325] Civilian trauma courses of that time generally recommended initial fluid resuscitation with 2 liters of a crystalloid solution—either LR or NS.

The beneficial effect from crystalloid and colloid fluid resuscitation in hemorrhagic shock had been demonstrated largely in animal models in which the volume of hemorrhage was controlled experimentally and resuscitation was initiated after the hemorrhage had been stopped—these were referred to as "controlled hemorrhage" models.[326,327] In contrast, multiple studies using "uncontrolled hemorrhagic" shock models found that aggressive fluid resuscitation performed before definitive control of bleeding had been accomplished was associated with either no improvement in survival or increased mortality when compared to no resuscitation or hypotensive resuscitation.[328-334] The vasodilation, increased hydrostatic pressure, and dilution of clotting factors that accompany crystalloid fluid resuscitation may interfere with the clotting process at the bleeding site and paradoxically worsen the chance for survival. Aggressive fluid resuscitation did, however, improve outcomes for rats with uncontrolled hemorrhagic shock in two studies.[327,335] Both studies used rat tail amputation models that may not correlate well with uncontrolled hemorrhage on the battlefield from intrathoracic or intra-abdominal injuries. Other studies noted that fluid resuscitation proved beneficial only after previously uncontrolled hemorrhage had been stopped.[336-338]

Among studies that addressed this issue in trauma patients, one large study of 6,855 trauma casualties found that, although hypotension was associated with a significantly higher mortality rate, the administration of prehospital IV fluids did not reduce this mortality.[332] A retrospective analysis of individuals with ruptured abdominal aortic aneurysms showed a survival rate of 30% for those who were treated with aggressive preoperative colloid fluid replacement, in contrast to a 77% survival rate for those in whom fluid resuscitation was delayed until the time of operative repair.[339] The author of that study strongly recommended that aggressive fluid resuscitation be withheld until the time of surgery in patients with this disorder. Bickell and colleagues published a large, prospective, randomized trial that addressed fluid resuscitation in the setting of uncontrolled hemorrhage.[340] The authors studied 598 patients with penetrating torso trauma. They found that aggressive prehospital fluid resuscitation of hypotensive patients with penetrating wounds of the chest and abdomen was associated with a higher mortality than was seen in those in whom aggressive volume replacement was withheld until the time of surgical repair. Further analysis of these data found that this difference was most significant in those casualties with wounds of the chest. Abdominal wounds showed little difference in survival between early and delayed fluid resuscitation.[341] Although confirmation of these findings in other similarly designed trials was not available, there were no human studies found that demonstrated any definite benefit from large-volume prehospital fluid replacement with crystalloids in casualties with ongoing hemorrhage. This impacts battlefield care because continuing hemorrhage must be suspected in battlefield casualties with penetrating abdominal or thoracic wounds until surgical repair of their injuries has been accomplished.

In light of the studies mentioned previously, the recommendation in the original TCCC paper was to withhold aggressive fluid resuscitation from individuals with penetrating torso trauma and uncontrolled hemorrhage.[342] At a Special Operations workshop on urban warfare casualties in 1998, however, there was a clear consensus among the panelists that should a casualty with uncontrolled hemorrhage have mental status changes or become unconscious (correlating to systolic blood pressure [SBP] of 50 mm Hg or less), the casualty should be given enough fluid to resuscitate him or her to the point that mentation improves (correlating to SBP of 70 mm Hg or above). Panel members also stressed the importance of not administering IV fluids in large volumes with the goal of achieving "normal" blood pressure in casualties with penetrating torso wounds, because that could result in disruption of any clot forming at the site of the vascular injury in these casualties.[343]

Hespan® (6% hetastarch) was recommended in the 1996 TCCC paper as a better choice for fluid resuscitation in the Tactical Field Care phase than LR solution or NS.[342] Both LR and NS are crystalloids in which the primary osmotically active particle is sodium. Because the sodium ion distributes throughout the entire extracellular fluid compartment, crystalloids move rapidly from the intravascular space to the extravascular space. This shift has significant implications for fluid resuscitation. If a trauma casualty is infused with 1,000 ml of LR, only 200 ml of that volume will remain in the intravascular space 1 hour later.[344-346] This presents little problem in urban civilian settings because the typical time for transport of the casualty to the hospital in urban trauma systems is less than 15 minutes,[332,347] after which surgical control of hemorrhage can be rapidly achieved and resuscitation with blood products can be accomplished. In military settings, however, where several hours or more may pass before a casualty arrives at an MTF, effective volume resuscitation may be difficult to sustain with crystalloids. The large hetastarch molecule, on the other hand, is retained in the intravascular space, and there is no osmotic loss of fluid into the interstitium. To the contrary, hetastarch osmotically promotes fluid influx *into* the vascular space *from* the interstitium so that an infusion of hetastarch results in an intravascular volume expansion somewhat larger than the volume of fluid infused.[346] This effect is sustained for 8 hours or longer.[348] Although concerns existed about coagulopathies and changes in immune function associated with the use of hetastarch,[349,350] these effects were not seen with infusions of less than 1,500 ml.[351] Hetastarch was found a safe and effective alternative to LR in resuscitating casualties with controlled hemorrhagic shock.[352,353] Hetastarch had also been reported to be an acceptable alternative to LR for intraoperative fluid replacement.[354]

There were other reasons to prefer hetastarch over crystalloids in tactical settings. Infusion of crystalloids to maintain intravascular volume when surgical control of noncompressible hemorrhage is delayed may result in the need for combat medical personnel to carry large volumes of crystalloid in their rucksacks.[355] This significant weight burden is tactically undesirable. The extravascular fluid shift caused by crystalloids may also cause edema and dysfunction in the lungs, the abdomen, the brain, or the muscle compartments of the extremities.[342,355]

Combat fluid resuscitation conferences[356] were held in 2001 under the sponsorship of the Office of Naval Research and the U.S. Army Medical Research and Materiel Command. Conferees endorsed the concepts of (1) limited (hypotensive) fluid resuscitation in the setting of uncontrolled hemorrhage and (2) the use of the synthetic colloid Hextend to provide the advantages of lighter weight and smaller volume in the rucksack. Hespan (hetastarch in saline solution) had been found to result in increased blood loss compared to the same hetastarch molecule in a balanced electrolyte solution with a lactate buffer and physiologic levels of glucose (Hextend).[357]

Col. John Holcomb recommended a technique of hypotensive fluid resuscitation in the field in casualties with uncontrolled hemorrhage.[358] Whereas the 1996 TCCC Guidelines called for Special Operations medics to give 1,000 ml of Hespan to all casualties meeting the requirements for resuscitation, Holcomb proposed that all casualties in shock (defined by weak or absent peripheral pulses or altered mental status in the absence of TBI) be given a 500-ml bolus of Hextend. This was to be administered as rapidly as possible using manual pressure on the IV bag or inflatable IV bag cuffs. If no improvement was noted in 30 minutes, the bolus was to be repeated once. This approach had the following advantages:

1. Better logistics. Not all casualties would require 1,000 ml of Hextend, thus saving fluid and time for other casualties.
2. Decreased rebleeding. Basing the titration of fluids upon a monitored physiologic response could avoid the problem of excessive blood pressure elevation and fatal rebleeding from previously clotted injury sites. The potential for aggressive resuscitation to cause rebleeding at a mean systolic pressure of 94 mm Hg had been demonstrated in animal models of uncontrolled

hemorrhage.[359] Interestingly, this recommendation for "hypotensive" resuscitation was reminiscent of similar principles employed in World War II by Beecher.[360]
3. Simplified training. Basing the fluid therapy on the premise of responders versus nonresponders followed the lead of the American College of Surgeons (ACS) Committee on Trauma in the ATLS course and allowed for a single approach to casualties with both controlled and uncontrolled hemorrhage.

Col. Holcomb's recommendation was included in TCCC Guidelines in 2003 (Military Medicine section in *Prehospital Trauma Life Support–Military*, revised fifth edition), and Hextend was widely used for a time as a front-line resuscitation fluid. Combat medics reported good and sustained results when they used it for hypotensive resuscitation in shock victims.[361]

Fluid Resuscitation in TCCC–2019

At the time of this writing there has been an increasing awareness that when a casualty is in shock from blood loss, the best fluid with which to treat that condition is whole blood.[362-373] Whole blood has the optimal mix of red blood cells, plasma, and platelets to restore intravascular volume, increase oxygen-carrying capacity, and promote hemostasis. In situations where it is not logistically feasible to provide whole blood for fluid resuscitation, studies have shown that outcomes are improved with earlier and increased use of plasma, platelets, and red blood cells.[374,375]

As noted earlier, the fluid of choice for the resuscitation of casualties in hemorrhagic shock in TCCC in the past was Hextend. There have been, however, been reports of adverse effects from large-volume resuscitation with both crystalloids and colloids.[376-381] In his review of hemorrhagic shock, Cannon noted that "Isotonic crystalloid resuscitation has been used for decades in the early management of bleeding. However, these solutions have no intrinsic therapeutic benefit except to transiently expand the intravascular volume. When isotonic crystalloid is administered in large volumes, the risk of complications, including respiratory failure, compartment syndromes (both abdominal and extremity), and coagulopathy, increases."[382] Col. Andre Cap summed it up this way: "The historic role of crystalloid and colloid solutions in trauma resuscitation represents the triumph of hope and wishful thinking over physiology and experience."[365]

As the conflict in Afghanistan progressed, the U.S. and its coalition partners increased their use of blood products during TACEVAC and even in Tactical Field Care.[366,383,384] In the Afghanistan theater, resuscitation with red blood cells and plasma in a 1:1 ratio during TA-CEVAC was pioneered by the British Medical Emergency Response Team (MERT). The practice was associated with improved casualty survival even with relatively short evacuation times.[385,386] Improvements in survival resulting from the use of prehospital blood products could well become even more significant in immature theaters with longer evacuation times.[366] Shackelford's review of prehospital blood product administration in 502 casualties from the Afghanistan conflict found that 3 (5%) of 55 casualties who received early blood transfusion—either in the prehospital phase of care or within minutes of injury—died within 24 hours as compared to 85 (19%) of 447 who received delayed or no transfusion (unadjusted $p = 0.013$).[383] In the U.S. civilian sector, the Mayo Clinic in Rochester, Minnesota, and Memorial Hermann Hospital in Houston, Texas, now provide prehospital administration of blood component therapy (1:1 plasma and RBCs) for trauma patients in shock.[387-389] Many civilian deaths from severe NCTH occur well within 60 minutes following injury, underscoring the need for aggressive early hemostasis and hemostatic fluid resuscitation.[390] Spinella and Cap noted that in order for the U.S. military to achieve the desired goal of zero preventable deaths in its combat casualties, increased emphasis must be placed on prehospital resuscitation using whole blood.[391]

The standards committee of the American Association of Blood Banks (AABB) recently reviewed the issue of using group O low titer blood for patients of unknown blood type who are in hemorrhagic shock. Standard 5.15.1 in the 31st edition of the *Standards for Blood Banks and Transfusion Services* that came into effect on April 1, 2018, now endorses the use of group O low-titer whole blood for recipients of known or unknown ABO group in patients with hemorrhagic shock. Standard 5.27.1 provides that the definition of "low titer" shall be made locally by each transfusion service and that the transfusion service must have a policy specifying which patients are eligible to receive whole blood (WB), the maximum quantity of WB per patient, and how to monitor for potential adverse events post transfusion. Regarding these changes, Yazer and colleagues proclaimed, "With the regulatory impediments removed, the determination of the efficacy of cold-stored, low titer WB in civilian patients with massive hemorrhage will now begin in earnest."[392]

Although WB offers the most physiologic benefit for resuscitating casualties in shock, this option may be precluded by the challenges of combat medical logistics. In this setting, dried plasma may be the best option available to combat medical personnel.[366] Plasma provides fibrinogen as well as other hemostatic factors. It also restores lost intravascular volume, whereas crystalloids and colloids restore only fluid volume with no hemostatic factors, thus producing an iatrogenic addition to trauma-associated coagulopathy.[366,393,394] Dried plasma can be stored without refrigeration and may be carried and used by combat medical personnel when other blood components are not logistically feasible. Although dried plasma has been used for some time by the militaries of several nations (e.g., United Kingdom, France, Germany, Netherlands, and Israel),[393,395,396] until 2018 there was no FDA-approved dried plasma product available to U.S. forces, although some U.S. Special Operations units carried and used the French dried plasma product under a treatment protocol.[366] While there is general acceptance of the premise that plasma is a better fluid to use in resuscitating casualties in hemorrhagic shock than either crystalloids or colloids, there is currently a lack of clinical studies that document a survival advantage from the use of dried plasma alone in prehospital fluid resuscitation. Also lacking are studies that provide good evidence regarding optimal treatment regimens for prehospital fluid resuscitation using plasma alone. Despite these gaps in evidence, it remains that "combat casualties often have a coagulopathy, coagulopathy increases mortality, and plasma administration reduces the coagulopathy."[366] (Author's note: At the time of this writing, the DoD-FDA panel established by congressional mandate to make recommendations on medical products with special applicability to battlefield trauma care has approved the French freeze-dried product FLyP™ for use in treating casualties with hemorrhagic shock. The U.S. military is working with the manufacturer of FLyP™ to explore ways to increase the production to meet the demand created by the FDA approval.)

In consideration of the items discussed previously, the CoTCCC revised its fluid resuscitation guidelines in 2014. The updated TCCC fluid resuscitation guideline emphasizes the importance of resuscitation with whole blood when practical and with other blood products in a balanced 1:1:1 ratio when whole blood is not available. The synthetic hetastarch Hextend and the crystalloid solutions LR and PlasmaLyte-A® are recommended for use only when no blood products are available. **Box 25-12** and **Figure 25-28** show the current CoTCCC recommendations for fluid resuscitation, in order of their physiologic benefit to casualties in hemorrhagic shock.[366]

Providers should always recognize the importance of hypotensive resuscitation in the setting of uncontrolled hemorrhage and avoid over-resuscitation. Fluid resuscitation in Tactical Field Care may be directed toward clinical improvement as evidenced by an improved state of consciousness or restoration of a normal radial pulse. If blood pressure monitoring is available, resuscitation should be titrated to a target systolic blood pressure of 80 to 90 mm Hg.[366]

Box 25-12 Tactical Field Care Guideline 6d: Circulation: Fluid Resuscitation

d. Fluid Resuscitation
- Assess for hemorrhagic shock (altered mental status in the absence of brain injury and/or weak or absent radial pulse).
- The resuscitation fluids of choice for casualties in hemorrhagic shock, listed from most to least preferred, are whole blood plasma, red blood cells (RBCs), and platelets in a 1:1:1 ratio*; plasma and RBCs in a 1:1 ratio; plasma or RBCs alone; Hextend; and crystalloid (lactated Ringer or Plasma-Lyte A). (NOTE: Hypothermia prevention measures [Section 7] should be initiated while fluid resuscitation is being accomplished.)
  - If not in shock:
    - No IV fluids are immediately necessary.
    - Fluids by mouth are permissible if the casualty is conscious and can swallow.
  - If in shock and blood products are available under an approved command or theater blood product administration protocol:
    - Resuscitate with whole blood,* or, if not available
    - Plasma, RBCs, and platelets in a 1:1:1 ratio,* or, if not available
    - Plasma and RBCs in a 1:1 ratio, or, if not available
    - Reconstituted dried plasma, liquid plasma, or thawed plasma alone or RBCs alone
    - Reassess the casualty after each unit. Continue resuscitation until a palpable

radial pulse, improved mental status or systolic BP of 80–90 is present.
  - If in shock and blood products are not available under an approved command or theater blood product administration protocol due to tactical or logistical constraints:
    - Resuscitate with Hextend, or if not available
    - Lactated Ringer or Plasma-Lyte A
    - Reassess the casualty after each 500 ml IV bolus.
    - Continue resuscitation until a palpable radial pulse, improved mental status, or systolic BP of 80–90 mm Hg is present.
    - Discontinue fluid administration when one or more of the above end points has been achieved.
- If a casualty with an altered mental status due to suspected TBI has a weak or absent radial pulse, resuscitate as necessary to restore and maintain a normal radial pulse. If BP monitoring is available, maintain a target systolic BP of at least 90 mm Hg.
- Reassess the casualty frequently to check for recurrence of shock. If shock recurs, re-check all external hemorrhage control measures to ensure that they are still effective and repeat the fluid resuscitation as outlined above.

Source: Courtesy of the Committee on Tactical Combat Casualty Care.

Resuscitation of Casualties with Traumatic Brain Injury

The TCCC Guidelines call for a modified fluid resuscitation approach to casualties suffering from both hemorrhagic shock and TBI. In these casualties, unconsciousness or altered mental status may be caused by either the head injury or the hypovolemic shock. Additionally, there are fluid resuscitation considerations particular to optimizing survival in casualties who have both hemorrhagic shock and TBI. Hypotension in the presence of TBI is associated with a significant increase in mortality.[397] Both the magnitude and the duration of the prehospital hypotensive episode have been found to contribute to increased mortality.[398] If the hypotension occurs in a casualty who is

also hypoxic, the odds of death for that casualty are more than twice as great as for casualties with hypotension or hypoxia alone.[399] If a casualty with an altered mental status and suspected TBI has a weak or absent peripheral pulse, he or she should be resuscitated as necessary to maintain a palpable radial pulse, thus ensuring adequate cerebral perfusion pressure.[400] If blood pressure monitoring is available in Tactical Field Care, a systolic pressure of at least 90 mm Hg should be maintained.[366]

Oral Rehydration in Combat Casualties

Trauma surgeons attached to forward-deployed MTFs have noted that many casualties are kept on nothing-by-mouth

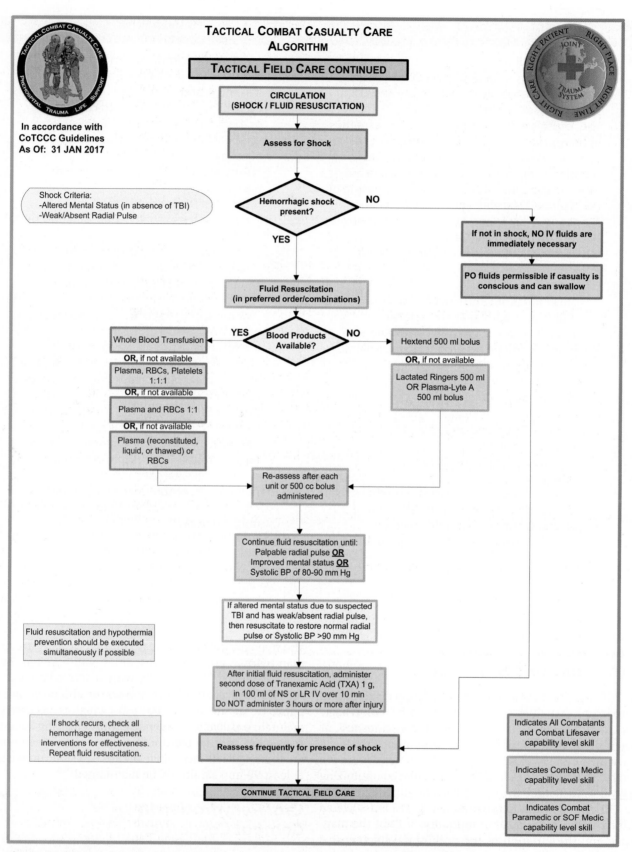

Figure 25-28 Algorithm for Tactical Combat Casualty Care Guideline 6.d: Fluid Resuscitation.

Courtesy of Mr. Harold Montgomery. Retrieved from https://deployedmedicine.com/market/11/content/87

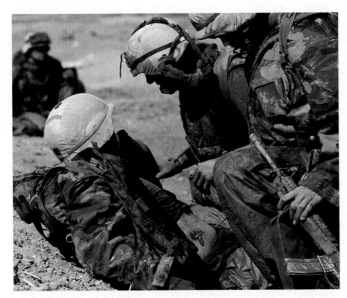

Figure 25-29 Marine with abdominal wound drinking water.
Courtesy of Dr. David Callaway.

(NPO) status for prolonged periods in anticipation of eventual surgery to repair their wounds. With transportation delays superimposed on the dehydration often present in combat operations before wounding, these casualties often come to surgery significantly dehydrated. Dehydration adversely affects survival in hypovolemic shock,[343] and the risk of emesis and aspiration is judged to be very low in casualties given only oral fluids for rehydration.[342] Therefore, oral fluids are recommended for all casualties with a normal state of consciousness and the ability to swallow, including those with penetrating torso trauma (**Figure 25-29**).

Refractory Shock

Some casualties may not have a favorable response to fluid resuscitation, even when blood products are used. Should this occur, a thorough reassessment of the casualty must be performed. The combat medical provider should review hemorrhage control measures, to include the following:

- Ensure that all external hemorrhage is controlled.[401]
- Apply a pelvic binder if indicated.[383]
- Administer TXA if hemorrhagic shock is present or likely to occur.[402]
- Perform or continue fluid resuscitation with blood products if possible.[366]

Should the shock persist after all of these interventions have been performed (if indicated), the combat medical provider should consider the possibility of untreated tension pneumothorax as a possible cause of refractory shock.[401,403] This potential diagnosis is supported by findings of thoracic trauma, persistent respiratory distress, absent breath sounds on one side of the chest, and hemoglobin oxygen saturation <90%. If a casualty in shock has already had at least two failed NDCs and has not responded to fluid resuscitation efforts, additional measures should be considered.[404] These measures may include either simple (finger) thoracostomy or tube thoracostomy. Both of these measures, correctly performed, will provide definitive decompression of the hemithorax. Tube thoracostomy will also drain the blood from the chest and help the lung to reexpand. Only combat medical providers with the appropriate skills, equipment, and authorizations should perform these invasive procedures.

Why not insert a chest tube as the initial treatment for tension pneumothorax? Although chest trauma that results in pneumothorax or hemothorax will be treated with prompt tube thoracostomy when the casualty reaches an MTF, placing chest tubes in the prehospital *combat* setting has not been shown to improve outcomes. In a 1985 Israeli Defense Force (IDF) study Rosenblatt found that only 8 of 16 chest tubes placed by physicians in the prehospital combat setting were inserted correctly and for the appropriate indications.[405] A 2015 study, also from the IDF, reported on 35 chest tubes that had been placed in the prehospital setting after failed NDC, but the difference in outcomes associated with the use of this more invasive intervention as used prehospital were not well described.[406] There are more recent reports from *civilian* EMS systems that finger thoracostomy or tube thoracostomy can be safely and effectively performed by prehospital personnel if NDC is not successful in relieving a suspected tension pneumothorax.[403,407-412] If the injury pattern sustained by a casualty in refractory shock suggests that both sides of the chest might be at risk for tension pneumothorax, the combat medical provider should consider bilateral chest decompression.[401]

Future Research in Fluid Resuscitation for Hemorrhagic Shock

The optimal resuscitation strategy for combat casualties in shock remains a research topic of great importance in military medicine. Because combat missions do not lend themselves well to the conduct of prospective, randomized, blinded studies on fluid resuscitation, optimal resuscitation strategies will have to be based on the best available evidence from animal studies, evidence found in the civilian prehospital trauma literature, and retrospective studies from combat theaters. Animal models used in studies addressing battlefield fluid resuscitation issues should include a significant delay to surgical repair, simulating the prolonged evacuation times that combat operations often entail. Care should be taken in extrapolation of the results of resuscitation fluid studies in the civilian sector to the battlefield, because transport times to the hospital in urban areas are typically shorter than those seen in combat. Additionally, resuscitation studies must address shock in the settings of both controlled and uncontrolled hemorrhage because of the different physiologic considerations in these two clinical conditions.

Two publications outlined a number of promising research areas that may pave the way for further advances in fluid resuscitation in battlefield trauma care.[366,393] Among the most important of these are the following:

1. Develop new methodologies to make type O low titer (universal donor) whole blood available throughout the continuum of care for combat casualties. Better blood storage methods and improved technology for cold storage in far-forward military environments may help make FDA-compliant universal donor whole blood available at the point of injury and during TACEVAC.[393]

2. Unit-based programs allowing combat units to identify individuals with type O low anti-A, low anti-B titer (universal donor) blood have been demonstrated. These individuals serve as donors enabling whole blood transfusions in tactical situations where casualties require emergent treatment for hemorrhagic shock but cold-stored universal donor whole blood is not available. Methods for whole blood transfusion when cold-stored type O low titer whole blood is not available need further development.[364,365,371-373,391]

3. In battlefield trauma care scenarios, there may be no way to make whole blood or other blood components available. In such settings, reconstituted dried plasma is preferred over crystalloids or colloids. The pressing need for an FDA-approved dried plasma product to be carried and used by combat medics was identified by the CoTCCC as the number one research priority in battlefield trauma care in 2015.[393,413]

4. The impact of all battlefield fluid resuscitation strategies on outcomes must be determined, especially with respect to patient selection for fluid resuscitation, types and quantities of blood products used, the timing of fluid resuscitation after injury, and end points of resuscitation. In the U.S. military, this will require better documentation of TCCC care and careful study of the casualty information contained in the DoD Trauma Registry.[393]

Hypothermia Prevention

Hypothermia and Coagulopathy on the Battlefield

Hypothermia poses a far greater risk to a trauma victim than to an otherwise healthy person. Hypothermia-induced coagulopathy is well described and may occur in a casualty with even mild hypothermia. It results from decreases in platelet function, decreased coagulation cascade enzyme activity, and alterations of the fibrinolytic system.[414-416]

Risk factors for prehospital hypothermia include a Glasgow Coma Scale (GCS) score of 8 or less, low ambient temperatures, a wet patient,[4] female gender, nighttime, winter season, motorcycle/bicycle accidents, ISS of 9 or greater, shock, preclinical volume replacement, and prehospital transport time.[418] Hypothermia in trauma victims is not limited to cold environments, however; it can also occur in warm ambient temperatures. Hemorrhagic shock results in a decreased ability to produce heat and to maintain normal body temperature. This predisposes shock victims to hypothermia, which can contribute to coagulopathy that, in turn, increases blood loss, worsening the hemorrhagic shock.[419-421] Patients with severe burn injury are also at increased risk of hypothermia.[422]

As many as 66% of civilian trauma patients arrive in emergency departments with core temperatures of less than 36°C (96.8°F), and hypothermia is associated with increased mortality.[423] In 2006, hypothermia was found to be more prevalent in combat trauma victims than was previously realized, and this was found to contribute independently to increased mortality.[424] Evacuation of a casualty to a medical facility may be delayed for many hours in military settings, increasing the likelihood that hypothermia will complicate trauma management. This problem is exacerbated in helicopter evacuation, where the casualty is exposed to cooler temperatures at altitude and significant wind chill in an open cabin. The importance of preventing hypothermia in combat casualties was emphasized in a memo from the office of the Assistant Secretary of Defense for Health Affairs, which recommends that body temperature in combat casualties be maintained as close to 98.6°F (37°C) as possible.[425]

Aggressive prevention of hypothermia in casualties is an essential element of care, and simple interventions have proven effective in decreasing the incidence of hypothermia during prolonged evacuations.[426] Because of the physics of heat transfer, it is much easier to prevent hypothermia than to correct it. Therefore, prevention of heat loss should start as soon after wounding as the tactical situation permits. **Box 25-13** and **Figure 25-30** present the Tactical Field Care guideline for hypothermia

7. Hypothermia Prevention
   a. Minimize casualty's exposure to the elements. Keep protective gear on or with the casualty if feasible.
   b. Replace wet clothing with dry if possible. Get the casualty onto an insulated surface as soon as possible.
   c. Apply the Ready-Heat Blanket from the Hypothermia Prevention and Management Kit (HPMK) to the casualty's torso (not directly on the skin) and cover the casualty with the Heat-Reflective Shell (HRS).
   d. If an HRS is not available, the previously recommended combination of the Blizzard Survival Blanket and the Ready-Heat Blanket may also be used.
   e. If the items mentioned above are not available, use dry blankets, poncho liners, sleeping bags, or anything that will retain heat and keep the casualty dry.
   f. Warm fluids are preferred if IV fluids are required.

Source: Courtesy of the Committee on Tactical Combat Casualty Care.

prevention. Exposure to the elements should be minimized, and the casualty should be placed on an insulated surface as soon as possible. Protective gear should be kept on or with the casualty, if feasible. After immediately life-threatening issues are addressed, wet clothing should be replaced with dry clothes, if possible.

The Ready-Heat™ Blanket can provide heating up to 104°F (40°C) for up to 8 hours. It should be placed on the casualty's chest to provide active warming (**Figure 25-31**), with care taken not to place it directly on bare skin to prevent possible burns. The casualty should then be wrapped in the Heat-Reflective Shell (HRS™). The HRS allows easy access to the casualty for reassessment and possible interventions (e.g., IVs or tourniquets) by means of the Velcro strips down each side. The HRS also utilizes a mummy-like sleeping bag configuration that covers the head, reducing heat loss from the scalp (**Figure 25-32**). Both the Ready-Heat Blanket and the HRS are found in the current version of the hypothermia prevention and management kit (HPMK®), which is a commercially available item (**Figure 25-33**). This protective ensemble was shown in U.S. Army Institute of Surgical Research (USAISR) studies to be effective in preventing heat loss.[427]

If the HPMK is not available, the previously recommended Blizzard™ survival blanket/Ready-Heat Blanket/Thermo-Lite™ cap combination can be used, with care taken to prevent helicopter rotor wash from blowing off the cap.[428] If none of these items is available, then blankets, ponchos, sleeping bags, or other field expedient materials should be used to keep the casualty warm and dry.

If IV fluid warmers are available in Tactical Field Care, they should be used to reduce cooling caused by cool fluids or blood products. Fluid warming should be considered for any casualty who has hypotension (SBP <90 mm Hg), has received more than 1,000 ml of fluid, or who requires a blood transfusion. Intravenous tubing should be insulated if possible, because fluids may cool significantly while traversing the tubing.[429]

The Wilderness Medical Society practice guidelines for hypothermia prevention and treatment recommend that hypothermic individuals who have been immersed in water be maintained in a horizontal position to minimize the risk of postural hypotension from standing and that movement should be minimized during transport to reduce the risk of ventricular fibrillation that may result from a sudden increase in the volume of cooled blood returning to the heart.[430]

The measures outlined earlier can be accomplished concurrently with fluid resuscitation if the casualty requires that intervention.[431] Removal of wet clothing and the use of active warming blankets have also been recommended for use in preventing hypothermia in the civilian sector.[432] The HPMK used by the U.S. military (with good success in Iraq and Afghanistan) has also been proposed as the preferred method of preventing hypothermia in wilderness settings.[433]

Effective hemorrhage control and fluid resuscitation will help maintain the casualty's ability to generate heat. Additional measures should be applied as needed throughout Tactical Field Care and Tactical Evacuation Care and should be used as far forward in the field as possible (**Box 25-14**). Items 1 to 5 on this list do not require a power source. Items 6 and 7 are devices that require power and can deliver heat to the casualty via warmed fluids.

Penetrating Eye Trauma

The single most important item to remember about combat eye trauma is that, for the most part, it can be prevented (**Figure 25-34**). Unit-issued protective eyewear is very successful at stopping the fragments of metal from explosions that cause the vast majority of eye injuries.[434]

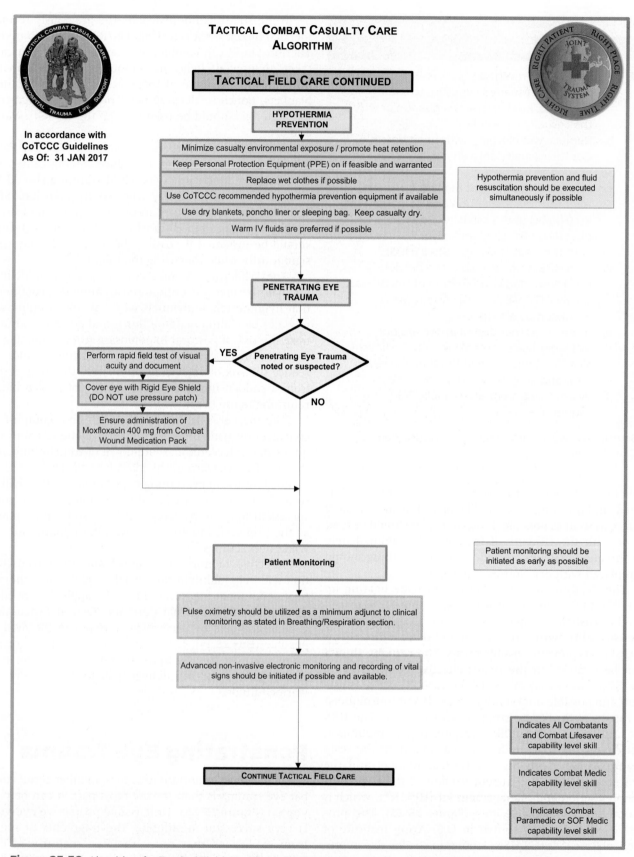

Figure 25-30 Algorithm for Tactical Field Care Guideline 7: Hypothermia Prevention, 8: Penetrating Eye Trauma, and 9: Monitoring.

Courtesy of Mr. Harold Montgomery. Retrieved from https://deployedmedicine.com/market/11/content/87

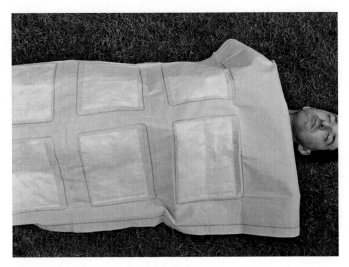

Figure 25-31 Ready-Heat Blanket.

© Jones and Bartlett Learning. Ready-Heat Blankets provided courtesy of TechTrade, L.L.C.

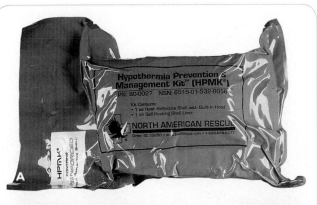

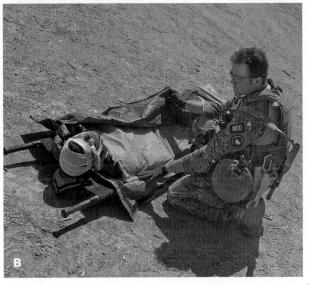

Figure 25-33 Hypothermia prevention and management kit (HPMK).

(**A**) and (**B**) Courtesy of North American Rescue.

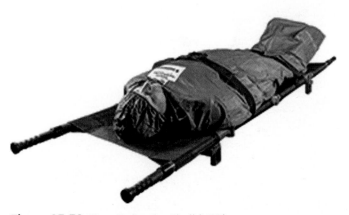

Figure 25-32 Heat-Reflective Shell (HRS).

Courtesy of North American Rescue.

Box 25-14 Additional Hypothermia Prevention Measures

- TechStyles Thermo-Lite Hypothermia Prevention System Cap
- Blizzard Survival Blanket, NSN 6532-01-524-6932
- TechTrade Ready-Heat Blanket, NSN 6532-01-525-4063
- North American Rescue Heat Reflective Shell
- North American Rescue Hypothermia Prevention and Management Kit (HPMK), NSN 6515-01-532-8056
- Thermal Angel, NSN 6515-01-500-3521
- Belmont FMS 2000, NSN 6515-01-370-5019
- Bair Hugger, NSN 6530-01-463-6823

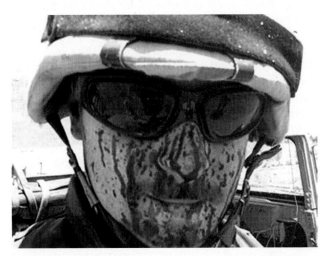

Figure 25-34 Soldier with facial fragment injuries whose eyes are protected by eye armor.

Courtesy of Tom Mader.

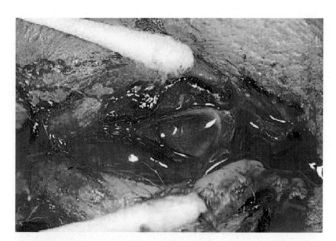

Figure 25-35 Obvious open globe injury.
Courtesy of Dr. Paul Auerbach.

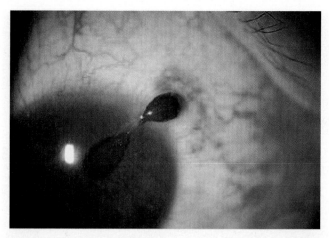

Figure 25-36 Open globe eye injury with peaked pupil and iris protrusion.
Courtesy of Dr. Paul Auerbach.

When penetrating eye trauma due to shrapnel or any other foreign body is suspected (**Figure 25-35, Figure 25-36,** and **Figure 25-37**), the paramount concerns when caring for the casualty in the prehospital setting are to do nothing that will exert pressure on the injured globe and to protect the eye from further injury. Any manipulation or additional pressure on the eye will raise intraocular pressure and potentially result in the expulsion of intraocular contents through the corneal or scleral defect. Manipulation of the globe or the eyelids to obtain a better view of the injured globe should be avoided. Ultrasound should not be used to identify foreign bodies in the globe since the probe will likely increase intraocular pressure.

The appropriate management for obvious or suspected penetrating eye trauma during Tactical Field Care (**Box 25-15** and Figure 25-27) is to tape a rigid shield (**Figure 25-38**) over the eye to protect it from any inadvertent contact that might increase intraocular pressure. If no rigid eye shield is available, an intact set of protective eyewear may be taped in place over the casualty's eyes (**Figure 25-39**). No dressings or bandages should be placed between the rigid shield and the eye to avoid placing pressure on a potentially open globe. Pressure dressings may result in an avoidable permanent loss of vision, and so are *not* part of the care of an injured eye (**Figure 25-40**).

When an open globe injury is observed or suspected, a rapid check of visual acuity should be performed (if the tactical situation permits) before covering the eye with a shield. A useful approach to quantifying visual acuity is (from best to worst acuity levels) (1) able to read print, (2) can count the number of fingers held up, (3) can see hand motion, and (4) can see light. Vision should be checked with the other eye closed or covered. The results of the rapid field test of visual acuity should be documented on the TCCC Casualty Card and in the TCCC After-Action Report.

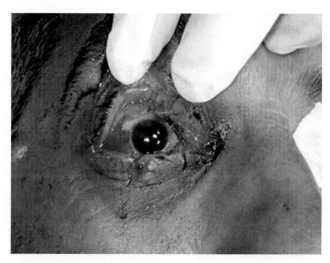

Figure 25-37 This soldier suffered a blast injury. The treating medic, seeing the eyelid lacerations, placed an eye shield and evacuated the patient without examining the eye further. On closer examination, the attending ophthalmologist discovered a full-thickness scleral wound. Because the combat medic placed a shield and not a patch, no ocular contents were expulsed. The laceration was closed, and the eye was saved.
Courtesy of Dr. Robb Mazzoli.

The final important element of care is to administer an antibiotic that will help to prevent the development of posttraumatic endophthalmitis, an infection of the anterior and posterior chambers inside the eye. This type of intraocular infection typically has devastating visual results, with only 30% of victims in one study retaining visual acuity greater than or equal to 20/400.[435] *Staphylococcus epidermidis* is the most common pathogen implicated, but *Bacillus cereus* is another

Box 25-15 Tactical Field Care Guideline 8:
Penetrating Eye Trauma

8. Penetrating Eye Trauma
   a. If a penetrating eye injury is noted or
      suspected:
      – Perform a rapid field test of visual acuity
        and document findings.
      – Cover the eye with a rigid eye shield (NOT
        a pressure patch).
      – Ensure that the 400 mg moxifloxacin
        tablet in the Combat Wound Medication
        Pack (CWMP) is taken if possible and that
        IV/IM antibiotics are given as outlined
        below if oral moxifloxacin cannot be
        taken.

Source: Courtesy of the Committee on Tactical Combat
Casualty Care.

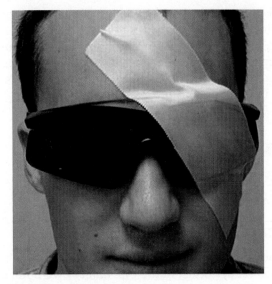

Figure 25-39 Protecting a suspected eye injury with
protective eyewear taped in place.
Courtesy of Dr. Robb Mazzoli.

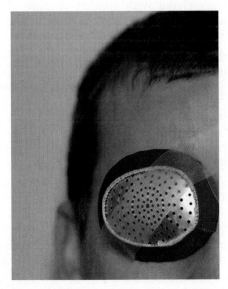

Figure 25-38 Protecting a suspected eye injury with a rigid
eye shield taped in place.
Courtesy of Stephen Giebner.

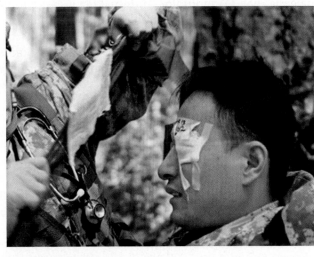

Figure 25-40 Incorrect treatment of a suspected eye injury
with a pressure patch.
Courtesy of Dr. Robb Mazzoli.

aggressive pathogen often isolated in intraocular infections. The casualty with a penetrating eye injury needs
broad spectrum coverage with an antibiotic that has
good penetration into the eye. Moxifloxacin 400 mg
once per day, given as soon as possible after wounding, is the treatment of choice in the prehospital environment if the casualty is able to take medications by
mouth. If the casualty is unable to take oral medications, ertapenem, 1 g IV, IO, or IM, should be administered. No topical antibiotics (ointments or eye drops)
should be used on an unrepaired penetrating injury of

the eye. The casualty should be evacuated as soon as
feasible.

These elements of care are consistent with the recommendations in the *Emergency War Surgery Manual* and
with the recommendations for managing eye trauma in
austere environments found in Auerbach's textbook,
Wilderness Medicine.[436] In Iraq and Afghanistan, casualties with eye trauma due to intraocular shrapnel or other
foreign bodies who had removal of the foreign body delayed for several days had no worse visual outcomes as
long as aggressive antibiotic therapy was provided and

the penetrating injury to the eye was repaired as soon as possible after the injury was sustained.[437]

As simple as these guidelines for managing combat eye injuries might seem to be, Col. Robb Mazzoli and colleagues reported a noncompliance rate of approximately 95% in Afghanistan from 2010 to 2012.[438]

Analgesia

The TCCC Triple-Option Analgesia Plan

Background

At the start of the war in Afghanistan, most prehospital medical personnel in the U.S. military were still using IM morphine—a legacy analgesic option that was used at the Battle of Bull Run in the U.S. Civil War, almost 150 years ago.[439-442] The original TCCC paper had recommended that this method of treating pain on the battlefield be discontinued and that morphine be used IV. Intravenous morphine has a much more rapid onset of analgesia than IM morphine, thus making it easier to titrate the required dose of pain medication and reducing the risk of an opioid overdose.[443] Unfortunately, TCCC had not been widely implemented in U.S. military units prior to 2001, and IM morphine was still the prevailing standard in many combat units for relieving pain on the battlefield at that time.

The conflicts in Iraq and Afghanistan saw a steady increase in the use of TCCC recommendations throughout the U.S. military. Furthermore, TCCC itself changed throughout the war years as new technologies became available and battlefield trauma care experience was gained. These changes included updated recommendations for battlefield analgesia. In 2004, a breakthrough paper by Kotwal, O'Connor, and colleagues described the initial combat use of oral transmucosal fentanyl citrate (OTFC), an analgesic option that provides pain relief that is nearly as rapid and as potent as that obtained with IV morphine.[442] The use of OTFC lozenges eliminated the need to start an IV to provide effective analgesia and was quickly adopted by TCCC. Ketamine was also identified by TCCC as a safe and effective analgesic option for battlefield use in 2012.[439] The last major advance in battlefield analgesia occurred as a result of the combined JTS/U.S. Central Command assessment of prehospital care in Afghanistan that resulted in the first "Saving Lives on the Battlefield" report.[444] During that assessment, a number of the combat medics, corpsmen, and PJs interviewed noted that, although they liked the analgesic options

recommended by TCCC at that point in time, the recommendations needed to be simplified and shaped into a more definitive plan. They did not believe that the TCCC Guidelines at that time provided enough clear and specific guidance on which analgesic option to use in specific casualty situations.[445] The TCCC Triple-Option Analgesia strategy was subsequently developed as a direct result of this request from combat medical personnel and is shown in **Box 25-16** and **Figure 25-41**.

As with all medications that are recommended by TCCC for use in treating combat casualties, an appropriate program of instruction should be conducted for combat units, and unit personnel should have been screened for medication allergies before these medications are used on the battlefield.

TCCC Analgesic Option 1: The TCCC Combat Wound Medication Pack

The pain associated with combat wounds is variable, depending on the location and severity of the wounds. Beecher[446] noted in his World War II survey that many men were not in severe pain despite having sustained serious wounds in battle. Obviously, if a casualty's wounds are not significantly painful, potent analgesia is not required.

To treat mild to moderate pain, the preferential COX-2 inhibitor, meloxicam (Mobic®), is the recommended analgesic.[445] Many analgesics prescribed for mild to moderate pain belong to the nonsteroidal anti-inflammatory drug (NSAID) class of medications. Most drugs in this class inhibit platelet function and prolong bleeding time due to their inhibition of cyclooxygenase-1 production.[443,447-449] Analgesic medications that adversely affect platelet function should not be used in a combat setting because normal platelet function is essential to the body's ability to establish hemostasis. This is critical when an individual sustains a vascular or solid organ injury that produces severe bleeding.[443] Meloxicam (one 15-mg tablet once a day) was chosen because it is a preferential COX-2 inhibitor that spares platelet function.[450,451] It also has a mild side effect profile, has proven effective in relieving postoperative pain, and has a 24-hour duration of action.[445]

To augment analgesia and to shorten the time to onset of effect, two 650-mg bilayer acetaminophen (Tylenol®) tablets are recommended along with meloxicam. This medication provides 8 hours of analgesia due to its extended-release formulation. Acetaminophen, like meloxicam, has no adverse effect on platelet function and does not interfere with hemostasis.

Box 25-16   Tactical Field Care Guideline 10: Analgesia

10. Analgesia

  a. Analgesia on the battlefield should generally be achieved using one of three options:

    – Option 1
- Mild to moderate pain
- Casualty is still able to fight.
  - TCCC Combat Wound Medication Pack (CWMP)
    - Tylenol—650 mg bilayer caplet, 2 PO every 8 hours
    - Meloxicam—15 mg PO once a day

    – Option 2
- Moderate to severe pain
- Casualty IS NOT in shock or respiratory distress AND
- Casualty IS NOT at significant risk of developing either condition.
  - Oral transmucosal fentanyl citrate (OTFC) 800 µg
    - Place lozenge between the cheek and the gum.
    - Do not chew the lozenge.

    – Option 3
- Moderate to severe pain
- Casualty IS in hemorrhagic shock or respiratory distress OR
- Casualty IS at significant risk of developing either condition.
  - Ketamine 50 mg IM or IN

    Or

  - Ketamine 20 mg slow IV or IO
    - Repeat doses q30min prn for IM or IN
    - Repeat doses q20min prn for IV or IO
    - End points: Control of pain or development of nystagmus (rhythmic back-and-forth movement of the eyes)

Notes:

- *Casualties may need to be disarmed after being given OTFC or ketamine.*
- *Document a mental status exam using the AVPU method prior to administering opioids or ketamine.*
- *For all casualties given opioids or ketamine— monitor airway, breathing, and circulation closely*
- *Directions for administering OTFC:*
  - *Recommend taping lozenge-on-a-stick to casualty's finger as an added safety measure OR*

utilizing a safety pin and rubber band to attach the lozenge (under tension) to the patient's uniform or plate carrier.
- *Reassess in 15 minutes.*
- *Add second lozenge, in other cheek, as necessary to control severe pain.*
- *Monitor for respiratory depression.*

- *IV Morphine is an alternative to OTFC if IV access has been obtained.*
  - *5 mg IV/IO*
  - *Reassess in 10 minutes.*
  - *Repeat dose every 10 minutes as necessary to control severe pain.*
  - *Monitor for respiratory depression.*

- *Naloxone (0.4 mg IV or IM) should be available when using opioid analgesics.*

- *Both ketamine and OTFC have the potential to worsen severe TBI. The combat medic, corpsman, or PJ must consider this fact in his or her analgesic decision, but if the casualty is able to complain of pain, then the TBI is likely not severe enough to preclude the use of ketamine or OTFC.*

- *Eye injury does not preclude the use of ketamine. The risk of additional damage to the eye from using ketamine is low and maximizing the casualty's chance for survival takes precedence if the casualty is in shock or respiratory distress or at significant risk for either.*

- *Ketamine may be a useful adjunct to reduce the amount of opioids required to provide effective pain relief. It is safe to give ketamine to a casualty who has previously received morphine or OTFC. IV Ketamine should be given over 1 minute.*

- *If respirations are noted to be reduced after using opioids or ketamine, provide ventilatory support with a bag-valve-mask or mouth-to-mask ventilations.*

- *Ondansetron, 4 mg orally dissolving tablet (ODT)/IV/IO/IM, every 8 hours as needed for nausea or vomiting. Each 8-hour dose can be repeated once at 15 minutes if nausea and vomiting are not improved. Do not give more than 8 mg in any 8-hour interval. Oral ondansetron is NOT an acceptable alternative to the ODT formulation.*

- *Reassess—reassess—reassess!*

Source: Courtesy of the Committee on Tactical Combat Casualty Care.

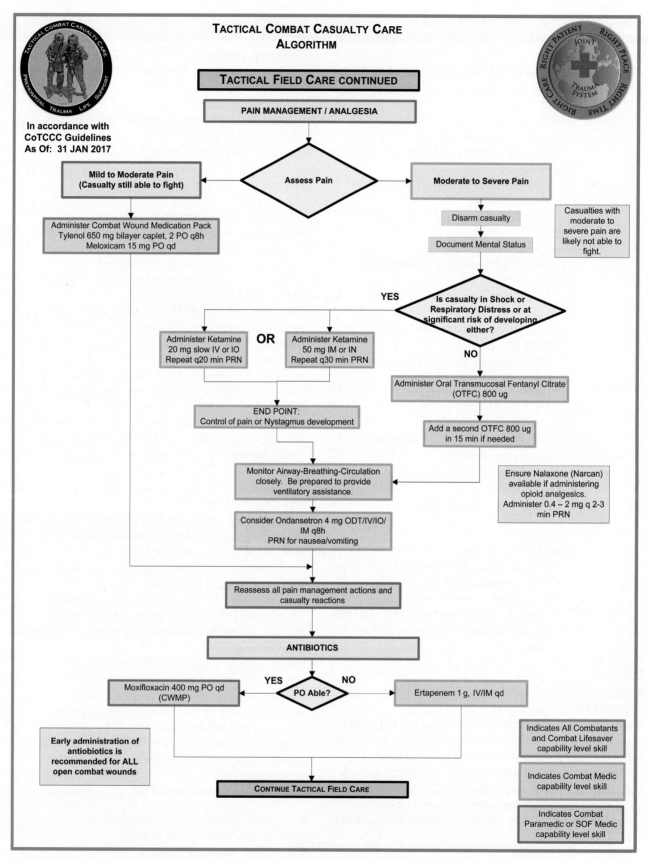

Figure 25-41 Algorithm for Tactical Field Care Guideline 10: Analgesia and 11: Antibiotics

Courtesy of Mr. Harold Montgomery. Retrieved from https://deployedmedicine.com/market/11/content/87

In addition to their platelet-sparing qualities, meloxicam and extended-release acetaminophen have the distinct advantage of not producing sedation or an altered state of consciousness, as many analgesics do. This means that they are able to achieve some measure of analgesia without reducing combat effectiveness. They also avoid the logistical difficulties of controlled medications. Anecdotal experience from casualties in Iraq shows this combination to be very effective in treating pain from minor penetrating soft-tissue injuries.[442,452]

These two oral pain medications should be carried by individual combatants as part of the combat wound medication pack (CWMP) and should be self-administered by the casualty as soon as feasible after an injury is sustained, if the pain from the wound is significant enough to require analgesia, if the casualty is able, and if the casualty has no allergies to either medication.

TCCC Analgesic Option 2: Oral Transmucosal Fentanyl Citrate (OTFC) Lozenges

If the casualty requires more potent pain relief (bony injuries are often the most painful combat wounds), then the more potent analgesic options recommended in TCCC should be employed. The use of OTFC was introduced and recommended for battlefield application independently by Kotwal and O'Connor in 2004. They and others published a retrospective case series documenting that OTFC is an alternative for safe, effective, rapid-onset, noninvasive pain management in a prehospital combat or austere environment.[442]

OTFC is recommended when a casualty has severe pain but is hemodynamically stable and not at risk for pulmonary dysfunction. OTFC is a valuable option for the combat medic because it provides potent, rapid analgesia without requiring intravenous access. Starting an IV for the sole purpose of providing analgesia is not an optimal plan in that (1) it requires significant time, which is always an important consideration in time-intensive tactical settings; (2) IV access is a perishable skill that may be difficult to perform for combat medics who do not do it routinely; and (3) starting an IV at night is difficult even when night vision devices are used.[453]

Management of the pain of acute combat trauma with OTFC is an off-label use of this medication. An FDA safety warning states that the medication is intended only for cancer patients who are narcotic tolerant and have breakthrough pain. OTFC has, however, been reported to be safe and effective for a variety of indications other than breakthrough cancer pain.[454-460] It has also been recommended as a good choice for analgesia in wilderness environments.[461]

Fentanyl provides effects ranging from analgesia at blood levels of 1 to 2 nanograms per milliliter (ng/ml), to surgical anesthesia and profound respiratory depression at levels of 10 to 20 ng/ml. The maximum serum concentration achieved following a 1,600-microgram (mcg) dose of OTFC was 2.51 ng/ml in clinical efficacy trials.[462] Respiratory depression is reported to occur at serum levels above 2 ng/ml, corresponding to doses greater than 800 mcg. An 800-mcg dose of OTFC, however, was found to produce no respiratory depression even in volunteers with no pain stimulus.[463] Additionally, casualties suffering from combat trauma with severe pain have been noted to tolerate large doses of narcotics without respiratory depression because of the powerful stimulant effect of their pain, as long as there is no associated shock.[464]

In a review of the analgesic options available to combat medical personnel in the prehospital battlefield setting, Wedmore and colleagues noted that OTFC "appears to be ideal for administering safe, rapid-onset, oral opiate analgesia in the prehospital austere setting."[452] Kacprowicz and colleagues found that OTFC was ". . . uniquely suited for the management of pain in the combat setting."[465] Over 280 uses of this medication by U.S. combat forces in Iraq and Afghanistan have been documented, and results to date indicate that this medication is safe and effective for use in relieving the pain of combat trauma when used appropriately.[466]

Given the documented safety and efficacy of OTFC in combat trauma, the CoTCCC recommends OTFC for use in casualties who are not in shock or experiencing respiratory distress or at risk for either condition. The initial dose is 800 mcg transbuccally for a casualty who does not otherwise require IV access. As an added safety measure, the simple act of taping the lozenge-on-a-stick preparation to the casualty's finger is recommended. Should the casualty inadvertently absorb a dose significant enough to exceed the desired analgesic effect, the resulting somnolence will cause relaxation of the supporting arm. As the arm relaxes, the fentanyl lozenge will be pulled from the casualty's mouth, preventing further absorption. Naloxone, however, must be readily available whenever any narcotic is administered.

Most of the experience to date with OTFC on the battlefield has been with the Actiq® brand. Other formulations of this medication may have different clinical effects for similar dosages based on variations in bioavailability.

The presence of hemorrhagic shock is a contraindication to opioid analgesics—including both morphine and fentanyl—because of their cardiorespiratory depressant effect. When there is severe pain, but the casualty is not in or at significant risk for shock, OTFC is the analgesic of choice. If there is moderate to severe pain and the casualty is in shock or at risk of shock or pulmonary compromise, ketamine is the agent of choice.[445]

TCCC Analgesic Option 3: Ketamine

Ketamine is another option for battlefield analgesia.[439] This agent may be useful in two specific battlefield settings. The first is when the analgesia provided by morphine and/or fentanyl is not adequate and additional analgesic effect is desired without increasing the opioid dose. The second is when the casualty is in respiratory distress or hemorrhagic shock and opioids are contraindicated. Opioids should also be administered with caution in casualties who have a high risk of going into shock (e.g., casualties with severe DCBI, penetrating wounds of the chest and/or abdomen, or pelvic fractures). NCTH has been the most common cause of preventable death in the Iraq and Afghanistan conflicts,[467,468] and OTFC or morphine may cause hypotension, which could increase the risk of death in casualties with severe hemorrhage.[439] The hypoxia and hypotension that may be associated with opiate use may also worsen outcomes in TBI.[439] Acute respiratory depression, excessive sedation, and nausea are all known side effects of opioids with profound operational implications.[469] Ketamine offers prehospital providers the ability to relieve pain without the potential adverse effects of opioids.

Because ketamine is highly lipid soluble, its clinical effects appear within 1 minute of administration when given intravenously and within 5 minutes when given intramuscularly.[470] It has been used extensively in acute care medicine and has a low frequency of serious adverse effects in doses used for analgesia.[470-474] Ketamine is known for its advantageous effects on hemodynamic stability, airway maintenance, and respiration in comparison to opioids, as well as for its low cost, broad range of clinical applications, ease of storage, and excellent therapeutic index.[475,476] When administered to combat casualties in smaller (analgesic) doses, ketamine does not usually impair airway patency or respiration, and it does not worsen hemorrhagic shock, the leading cause of potentially preventable death on the battlefield.[467,477-479] As the dose-related effect of ketamine transitions from analgesia to anesthesia, nystagmus (a rhythmic back-and-forth movement of the eyes) emerges as a side effect of ketamine. The appearance of nystagmus, then, should be an end point indicator for ketamine dosage.[439] Published reports support the concept that low-dose ketamine may serve as an effective adjuvant to opioids and other analgesic agents.[478,480-482]

Ketamine may be administered via intranasal, IM, IO, and IV routes. Intramuscularly, ketamine may be given at a dose of 50 to 100 mg and the dose may be repeated every 30 minutes to 1 hour as necessary to control severe pain or until the casualty develops nystagmus. Ketamine may also be given intranasally at a dose of 50 mg using a nasal atomizer. This dose, too, may be repeated every 30 minutes to 1 hour as necessary to control severe pain or until the casualty develops nystagmus. If IV or IO access has been obtained, ketamine may be given as a 20-mg slow IV/IO push over 1 minute. The casualty should be reassessed in 5 to 10 minutes and repeat doses given every 5 to 10 minutes as necessary to control severe pain or, again, until nystagmus appears. Any casualty receiving ketamine should be monitored for signs of respiratory difficulty or agitation. In the past, ketamine was believed to be contraindicated in the presence of head injury or possible eye injury.[439] More recent evidence indicates that neither of these two injuries should preclude the use of ketamine in a combat casualty who is experiencing severe pain but has or is at risk for hemodynamic or pulmonary compromise.[445] The two remaining conditions that are considered absolute contraindications to ketamine use are age less than 3 years and a history of schizophrenia. Neither is a significant problem in deployed combat forces.[445]

At higher doses, the utility of ketamine is limited by undesirable psychomimetic effects (e.g., excessive sedation, cognitive dysfunction, hallucinations, and nightmares), but lower doses, like those recommended earlier, have rarely been associated with adverse effects.[482] In a review of analgesic options for relief of pain on the battlefield, Black and McManus[483] noted that "ketamine in subanesthetic doses is an almost ideal analgesic because of its profound pain relief, its potentiation of opioids, its role in preventing opioid hyperalgesia, and its large margin of safety." In a case series of 13 patients given prehospital ketamine for chemical restraint, Burnett[484] reported a significant incidence of adverse effects, but the mean dose of ketamine administered in that study was much larger than the doses recommended for analgesia in TCCC (8 of 13 patients received 500 mg), and all side effects were successfully managed. The authors pointed out that, in their EMS system, ketamine is the prehospital drug of choice for chemical restraint in patients with excited delirium syndrome. Laryngospasm is an infrequently reported side effect of ketamine. If this problem occurs, a brief period of ventilation with a bag-mask device will typically resolve it.[484] The frequency of respiratory compromise following procedural sedation and analgesia with ketamine was lower in pediatric patients than that seen in other analgesics, including fentanyl.[485] Anecdotal reports suggest that given the larger diameter of the adult airway, simple airway repositioning is typically sufficient to relieve airway compromise following ketamine administration.[439]

While the desirable clinical features of ketamine administration (e.g., preservation of spontaneous respiration) are numerous, providers must be prepared to deal with its potential side effects.[439] Among the best-known side effects following ketamine administration are emergence reactions—patients may make spontaneous utterances and purposeless motions or exhibit agitation. The FDA-approved package insert includes a special note stating that emergence reactions occur in approximately 12% of patients.[486] Although emergence reactions generally occur when higher doses of ketamine than those recommended earlier are used (i.e., anesthetic doses rather than analgesic doses), management of this condition may require restraint of the casualty.[487]

Benzodiazepines in Triple-Option Analgesia

Midazolam and other benzodiazepines are commonly used in EDs to reduce the dysphoric side effects that may result from larger doses of ketamine. The lower subdissociative doses of ketamine recommended by the CoTCCC, however, will minimize the incidence of dysphoric symptoms and generally eliminate the need for the concomitant use of a benzodiazepine medication that may cause respiratory compromise. Of special note, benzodiazepines should not be administered after opioids have been given. Case reports in the weekly JTS teleconferences have included instances of respiratory arrest associated with the use of opioids followed by administration of benzodiazepines.

Management of Nausea and Vomiting in TCCC

Trauma victims who have received opiates often experience nausea and vomiting. Ondansetron should be given as needed to manage these symptoms,[488] and it replaces the previously recommended promethazine as the medication of choice for nausea and vomiting in TCCC. Ondansetron has a favorable safety profile and has been documented to be effective in treating nausea and vomiting in both the ED and prehospital settings. It does not carry the potential for central and autonomic nervous system side effects that promethazine does. Ondansetron may be administered either in parenteral form (IV, IM, or IO) or as an orally disintegrating tablet. The use of ondansetron to treat the nausea and vomiting associated with combat wounds or analgesic opioids is an off-label use. This fact notwithstanding, ondansetron is increasingly being used in the U.S. military and in civilian sectors to treat acute nausea and vomiting from multiple etiologies.[488] The current TCCC Guidelines include the following recommendation:

Ondansetron, 4 mg orally dissolving tablet (ODT)/IV/ IO/IM, every 8 hours as needed for nausea or vomiting. Each 8-hour dose can be repeated once at 15 minutes if nausea and vomiting are not improved. Do not give more than 8 mg in any 8-hour interval. Oral ondansetron is *not* an acceptable alternative to the ODT formulation.

IV Morphine

Morphine sulfate remains an excellent choice for analgesia if IV access has been obtained and the casualty is stable with respect to pulmonary and hemodynamic status.[443] The IV route is preferred over the IM route because of the much more rapid onset of analgesia—several minutes when given IV contrasted to 30 to 60 minutes when given IM.[443] The delayed onset of pain relief makes it difficult to effectively titrate analgesic effect using IM therapy. The risk of an unintentional overdose of morphine increases if repeated IM injections are given during the time it takes for the initial dose to work.

Emerging Evidence Related to TCCC Triple-Option Analgesia

As noted previously, IM morphine was the predominant medication used for battlefield analgesia at the start of the war in Afghanistan. This was an excellent example of battlefield trauma care based on tradition rather than the available evidence. Respondents in a survey of combat medical personnel conducted by the Naval Operational Medical Lessons Center[489] indicated that IM morphine was the most commonly used battlefield analgesic but rated it less effective than either IV morphine or ketamine.

Anecdotal reports from operational settings have described individuals with severe pain refractory to morphine who responded quickly to ketamine.[452] The authors of "Saving Lives on the Battlefield" reported that, although ketamine had been used less frequently than morphine and OTFC, combat medical personnel rated it more effective than IM morphine at providing rapid relief of pain.[439,444]

One of the challenges in ascertaining the efficacy of the TCCC Triple-Option Analgesia plan in combat casualties is the poor rate of documentation regarding the severity of the casualty's pain, the medication administered to treat the pain, and the effectiveness of the treatment rendered. In a retrospective study of 8,913 casualties abstracted from DoD Trauma Registry records from September 1, 2007, through June 30, 2011, prehospital analgesic administration was documented for only 1,313 cases (15%), and prehospital pain assessment was documented for only 581 cases (7%).[490] Many of the casualties were not severely injured, with the median ISS score being 5 with a 98.7% survival rate. The authors concluded that "Prehospital pain assessment, management, and documentation remain primary targets for performance improvement and optimization on the battlefield."

Shackelford and others examined records on 309 combat casualties from October 2012 to March 2013 and reported that at the point of injury 200 of the 309 casualties received no analgesic medication, 33 casualties received OTFC, 30 received IV morphine, 24 received IM morphine, and 15 received IV or IM ketamine. During TACEVAC care, 116 received IV or IM ketamine, 87 received IV fentanyl, 35 received IV morphine, and only 5 received IM morphine.[491] In their 2015 survey of prehospital analgesia practice in tactical settings Schauer and his colleagues found that the most common analgesic medication administered at that point in time was OTFC, that Special Operations units had higher adherence rates to TCCC analgesia recommendations than conventional forces, and that less than half of all combat casualties in the study received pain medication at the point of injury.[492]

Given the poor rate of documentation of prehospital care in combat casualties, evidence from the civilian sector has been valuable in evaluating the efficacy of TCCC analgesic recommendations. A small prospective, randomized, double-blind trial evaluating ED patients with moderate to severe acute abdominal, flank, or musculoskeletal pain examined the efficacy of IV ketamine and IV morphine. The primary outcome measure was reduction in pain 30 minutes after administration of analgesia. Forty-five patients were enrolled in each arm of the study. Ketamine at a nondissociative dose provided analgesia and safety comparable to that of IV morphine for acute pain.[493] A small prospective, randomized, double-blind, placebo-controlled trial (30 patients in each group) published in 2017 found that ketamine at 0.3 mg/kg IV piggyback over 15 minutes administered as an adjunct to IV morphine resulted in more effective analgesia than morphine alone without an increase in adverse events related to analgesia. Patients who received ketamine in addition to IV morphine reported a significantly higher satisfaction score with their pain management.[494]

At the time of this writing, the TCCC Triple-Option Analgesia strategy for relieving the pain of combat wounds on the battlefield has gained wide acceptance in the U.S. military.[441,495] The American College of Emergency Physicians recommends an approach that mirrors the TCCC Triple-Option Analgesia plan in its policy statement on out-of-hospital analgesia and sedation.[480] The Wilderness Medicine Society practice guidelines for management of pain in austere environments also include an oral combination of an NSAID and acetaminophen, OTFC, and ketamine.[496]

Nonsteroidal Anti-inflammatory Drugs in Combat Forces

As noted previously, platelet dysfunction increases the risk of death from hemorrhage in a casualty with significant trauma and bleeding. A 2008 study noted an increase in mortality in trauma patients taking aspirin.[497] Harris reported that NSAID use by soldiers at a forward operating base in Afghanistan was prevalent enough to place 75% of the individuals at that base at risk for a self-induced coagulopathy.[498] In EDs, Toradol® is a medication frequently used for indications like migraine headaches and severe back pain. Toradol is an NSAID that can inhibit platelet function for 7 to 10 days.[499,500] It is important to note that adverse effects on clotting due to NSAIDs may persist for a week or more after the last dose of a medication like aspirin or ibuprofen is taken. Therefore, medications that decrease platelet function should *not be used at all* by troops deployed in support of combat operations, because these individuals may be called upon to conduct missions on short notice.[445] Because NCTH is still the leading cause of potentially preventable death on the battlefield, this is a clear opportunity to improve. It is also important to recognize that platelet dysfunction is an important consideration, even for casualties with relatively minor wounds until they have been evacuated to an MTF or their operating base. The first wounds sustained by a casualty in combat may, unfortunately, not be the last.

Antibiotics

Despite historically low case-fatality rates in OIF and OEF, infections still cause significant late morbidity and mortality in combat casualties.[501] The factors contributing to wound infection on the battlefield, like mechanism and pattern of injury and ISS, are variable.[502] Furthermore, the bacteriology of combat wound infections may change from conflict to conflict based on the microbial environment in the theater and evolving patterns of antibiotic resistance.[503]

The need for early administration of antibiotics was recognized over 50 years ago, when Poole[504] observed that ". . . the greatest lesson learned from World War II may have been the benefit of the use of penicillin prophylactically in the surgical units closest to the front." Scott[505] commented after the Korean War that, "In any tactical situation where the casualty cannot reach the aid station until 4 or 5 hours or longer after wounding, antibiotic therapy by the aidman in the field is most desirable."

Early antibiotics are commonly used upon arrival at the ED in the treatment of patients with significant trauma.[506] Antibiotics are not used in most civilian prehospital emergency medical systems because of the relatively short transport times typically encountered in the urban environment. However, definitive care for casualties may be significantly delayed in combat settings due to the longer distances to be covered and tactical constraints on evacuation helicopters and ground vehicles.[507]

Battlefield antibiotics for combat casualties were proposed in the original TCCC Guidelines.[508] Antibiotics must be given as soon as possible after injury to maximize their ability to prevent wound infections. Intramuscular benzyl penicillin started within 1 hour of wounding was found to be effective in preventing streptococcal infections in a swine model of wound infection. If administration was delayed until 6 hours after wounding, however, the medication was not effective.[509] In another animal model, delaying antibiotic administration from 2 hours to either 6 or 24 hours had a "profoundly detrimental effect on the infection rate regardless of the timing of surgery."[510] A review of antibiotic use on the battlefield recommended that antibiotics be used if arrival at an MTF was anticipated to be 3 hours or more.[511] However, no evidence was cited in this review to document the efficacy of antibiotics administered beyond the 1-hour period in preventing wound infections. The importance of early antibiotics has been noted in several reports discussing the battlefield management of combat casualties. Mabry and his colleagues[512] noted a 15-hour delay before treatment at a forward surgical facility for most of the casualties wounded in the battle of Mogadishu in 1993. The wound infection rate in those casualties was approximately 30%. In contrast, Tarpey[513] reported no infections in the 32 casualties from Task Force 1-15 (Third Infantry Division), which was involved in the drive to Baghdad at the start of the war in Iraq. Early antibiotics were administered on the battlefield, and the reported negligible rate of infections was achieved despite casualty evacuation often being delayed on this operation. There were no reports of adverse effects from the use of battlefield antibiotics documented in a 2007 review of TCCC as used on the battlefields of the Global War on Terrorism.[514] Extremity injuries have been prevalent in the recent conflicts,[502] and infections have been a cause of significant morbidity. Osteomyelitis has been reported to occur in 9% of type III tibia fractures.[515] Extremity infections have been associated with decreased success in limb salvage, an increase in additional surgical procedures and late amputations, and a decrease in the likelihood of the casualty being able to return to duty.[515] Infection prevention measures, including antibiotics, should begin as soon as possible after wounding.[515-517]

Tactical Field Care Guideline 11: Antibiotics is shown in **Box 25-17** and Figure 25-43.

> **Box 25-17** Tactical Field Care Guideline 11: Antibiotics
>
> 11. Antibiotics: recommended for all open combat wounds
>   a. If able to take PO meds:
>   - Moxifloxacin (from the CWMP), 400 mg PO once a day
>   b. If unable to take PO meds (shock, unconsciousness):
>   - Ertapenem, 1 g IV/IM once a day
>
> *Source:* Courtesy of the Committee on Tactical Combat Casualty Care.

Parenteral (IV or IM) administration of antibiotics is required in casualties who are unconscious or who cannot take medications by mouth due to maxillofacial injuries. It is also required for casualties in shock, in whom the gastrointestinal tract blood flow may be inadequate for absorption of oral medications. Ertapenem (Invanz®) was recommended by Hospenthal as a better choice for a parenteral antibiotic in TCCC than cefotetan because of ertapenem's once-a-day dosing, excellent coverage, and good safety profile.[511] This recommendation was also endorsed in a more recent review of this topic.[516] Ertapenem should not be mixed or co-infused with other medications to prevent crystallization, and it should not be mixed with diluents containing dextrose (alpha-D-glucose). It may be administered IM if needed. Cefotetan was subsequently removed from the TCCC Guidelines because ertapenem had become the prevalent choice for a TCCC antibiotic by 2017.[518]

The logistical burden of carrying, reconstituting, and injecting parenteral medications makes the use of oral antibiotics an attractive alternative when oral administration is possible.[519] In choosing antibiotic agents as part of the medic's loadout, characteristics like effectiveness across a broad range of potential bacterial pathogens, minimal side effects, environmental stability, simple and infrequent dosage regimens, and comparatively low cost are all highly desirable. In 2002, O'Connor and Butler proposed the fourth-generation fluoroquinolones gatifloxacin and moxifloxacin as good choices for oral battlefield antibiotics.[507] Gatifloxacin was selected initially based on its lower cost to the military compared to moxifloxacin. Gatifloxacin was later reported to cause disorders of glucose metabolism,[520] so the CoTCCC recommended moxifloxacin as the best replacement oral antibiotic. This choice was endorsed by Hospenthal and his colleagues in 2011.[516] Moxifloxacin has the additional advantage of excellent intraocular penetration when taken systemically (as opposed to some antibiotics that

---

Box 25-18 Combat Wound Medication Pack

The CWMP is a small blister package included in the individual first aid kits of deployed service members. It contains a 400 mg tablet of moxifloxacin, a single 15 mg tablet of meloxicam, and two 650 mg caplets of extended-release acetaminophen.

Box 25-19 Tactical Field Care Guideline 16: Communication

16. Communication
    a. Communicate with the casualty if possible. Encourage, reassure, and explain care.
    b. Communicate with tactical leadership as soon as possible and throughout casualty treatment as needed. Provide leadership with casualty status and evacuation requirements to assist with coordination of evacuation assets.
    c. Communicate with the evacuation system (the Patient Evacuation Coordination Cell) to arrange for TACEVAC. Communicate with medical providers on the evacuation asset if possible and relay mechanism of injury, injuries sustained, signs/symptoms, and treatments rendered. Provide additional information as appropriate.

Source: Courtesy of the Committee on Tactical Combat Casualty Care.

---

require intravitreal injection) and is effective for most gram-positive and gram-negative bacteria that are potential etiologic agents for postinjury endophthalmitis.[521] A 400-mg tablet of moxifloxacin is part of the CWMP (**Box 25-18**) carried by deployed service members.[518]

Ideally, the choice of antibiotics should be based on a careful consideration of the anatomic location of the wounds sustained as well as any information that may be available about the local microbiology and antibiotic susceptibility. Prophylactic antibiotic therapy should be accompanied by wound irrigation, surgical debridement of the wound, immunization for tetanus, and appropriate postsurgical care of the wound in order to minimize the risk of wound infections.[522] Ertapenem and moxifloxacin are not ideal prophylaxis for every type of wound, but they are safe and effective broad-spectrum antibiotics. They are also recommended for prehospital care of penetrating wounds of the chest or abdomen in the current JTS Infection Prevention Clinical Practice Guideline.[523] A recent review of the use of antibiotics for combat wounds by Murray recommended that levofloxacin be considered as a replacement for moxifloxacin because the former agent is more effective against gram-negative bacteria, including *Pseudomonas aeruginosa*. Moxifloxacin was noted to have more activity against anaerobes than levofloxacin, but this agent has recently been associated with increasing rates of resistant intra-abdominal bacteria, especially *Bacteroides* species.[522]

It is important that unit medics screen their troops for medication allergies when providing the units with CWMPs. For individuals who should not take moxifloxacin or ertapenem, consultation with the unit physician regarding appropriate substitute antibiotics for that individual is indicated. The unit corpsman, medic, or PJ should likewise be aware of any allergies that unit members may have to other medications recommended in the TCCC Guidelines.

Communication

Being physically wounded may generate significant anxiety and fear above and beyond the usual psychological

trauma of combat. Talking frankly with casualties about their injuries and describing the treatments being rendered will help to reduce their anxiety. Offering reassurance by emphasizing that everything possible is being done on their behalf and that they will be well cared for will also help. This type of communication is just as important on the battlefield as it is in the MTF and should be a part of the treatment regimen (**Box 25-19** and **Figure 25-42**). Be honest about the injuries sustained, but maintain a positive attitude about treatment and outcome.

Other aspects of communication are also important. The individual providing care to the casualty should ensure that a request for casualty evacuation is being submitted if warranted by the casualty's injuries. The evacuation request must include the information required by the standardized 9-Line MEDEVAC request and, depending on the requirements of the specific theater in which the casualty occurs, may also require reporting of MIST information (mechanism/injuries/symptoms/treatments) to the patient evacuation coordination cell.[524]

The individual providing care to the casualty or other designated unit members should likewise ensure that tactical leadership is kept informed of the casualty's status. If time and communications capabilities allow, it is also helpful to provide casualty information to both the medical personnel on the evacuation platform and to providers at the MTF to which the casualty will be transported.[524]

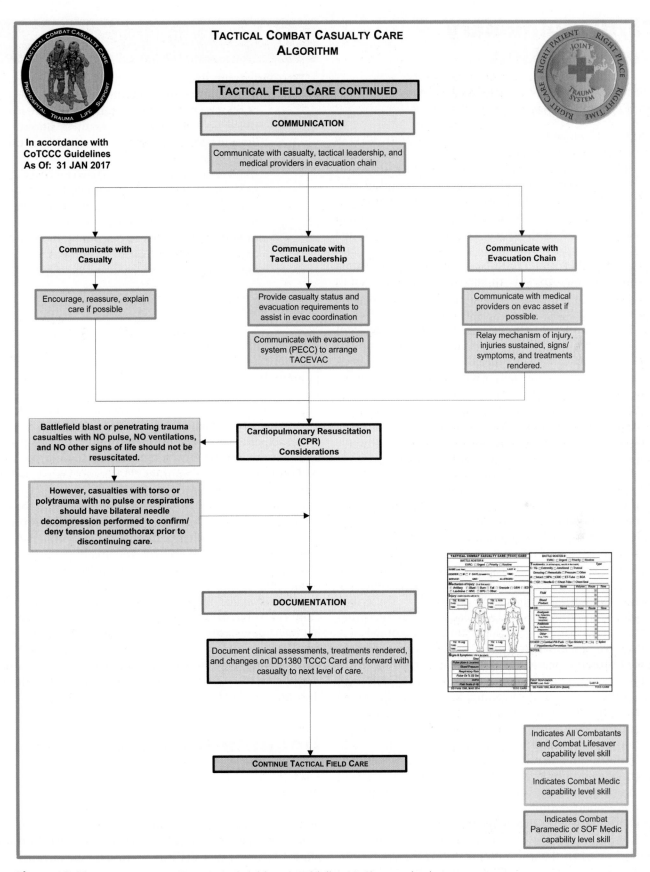

Figure 25-42 Algorithm including Tactical Field Care Guideline 16: Communication.

Courtesy of Mr. Harold Montgomery. Retrieved from https://deployedmedicine.com/market/11/content/87

Cardiopulmonary Resuscitation

Cardiopulmonary Resuscitation in Tactical Settings

CPR was developed to attempt to maintain some level of perfusion and oxygenation in cardiac arrest victims until defibrillation and advanced cardiac life support measures can be employed. Although CPR may be useful in normovolemic cardiac patients who have intact anatomy, it will not be successful and is not appropriate for combat casualties on the battlefield who have sustained trauma severe enough to cause loss of pulse, respirations, and other signs of life.[525,526] Prehospital resuscitation of trauma victims in cardiac arrest is an exercise in futility, even in urban settings where the casualty is close to a trauma center. Branney and colleagues reported only a 2% survival rate (14 of 708) among casualties who underwent thoracostomy after arriving at a hospital ED with absent vital signs.[527] Rosemurgy and others reported no survivors in 138 trauma casualties who sustained a prehospital cardiac arrest and for whom CPR was attempted.[528] The authors recommended that CPR not be attempted for patients who suffer a prehospital *traumatic* cardiac arrest, even in the civilian setting, because of the large economic costs and the uniformly unsuccessful results.

Even in individuals with nontraumatic cardiac arrest (i.e., those who have had a sudden cardiac death with no injuries) survival declines rapidly if spontaneous circulation is not promptly restored. Only 2% to 10% of patients with out-of-hospital cardiopulmonary arrest survive to hospital discharge. The chance of survival declines by 10% for every minute that defibrillation is delayed and there is no spontaneous circulation.[529] Even an 8-minute delay until defibrillation may be too long.[530] These data are bleak for individuals with cardiac arrest on the battlefield, where early defibrillation cannot be accomplished, and where blood loss and severe injuries to vital organs make restoration of spontaneous circulation far more difficult to achieve than in nontraumatic cardiac arrest.

In the tactical combat setting, the cost of attempting CPR on the battlefield on casualties with inevitably fatal wounds will be measured in additional lives lost as combat medical personnel are exposed to hostile fire while performing CPR and care is withheld from casualties with potentially survivable wounds. Successful completion of the unit's mission may also be unnecessarily jeopardized by these efforts. Although some studies have shown a small incidence of survival when casualties with traumatic cardiac arrest undergo immediate resuscitative thoracostomy[531] or when the arrest occurs during transport or in the ED,[532] point-of-injury CPR should be considered in the combat prehospital setting only in the case of selected disorders such as hypothermia, near drowning, or electrocution where there is a higher likelihood of responding to

---

Box 25-20 Tactical Field Care Guideline 17: Cardiopulmonary Resuscitation

17. Cardiopulmonary Resuscitation (CPR)
    a. Resuscitation on the battlefield for victims of blast or penetrating trauma who have no pulse, no ventilations, and no other signs of life will not be successful and should not be attempted. However, casualties with torso trauma or polytrauma who have no pulse or respirations during TFC should have bilateral needle decompression performed to ensure they do not have a tension pneumothorax prior to discontinuation of care. The procedure is the same as described in section 5.a.

Source: Courtesy of the Committee on Tactical Combat Casualty Care.

CPR than in combat injuries such as hemorrhagic shock or severe head trauma that result in prehospital cardiopulmonary arrest.[525] Guidance regarding CPR in Tactical Field Care is presented in **Box 25-20** and Figure 25-42.

A 2011 study of 52 military casualties who suffered a prehospital traumatic cardiac arrest found that all survivors experienced arrest during transport to the hospital and that the longest duration of cardiac arrest associated with survival was 24 minutes.[533] Hemorrhagic shock is the leading cause of preventable death in combat casualties, and in animal models of arrest from this disorder, chest compressions have not been shown to improve survival.[534] This highlights the importance of achieving definitive hemorrhage control and treating shock with blood products as soon as possible in order to prevent the occurrence of traumatic cardiac arrest.[535]

Unrecognized tension pneumothorax is one potentially reversible cause of cardiopulmonary arrest in combat casualties. Casualties with torso trauma or polytrauma who have no pulse or respirations during Tactical Field Care should have bilateral NDC performed to ensure that they do not have an occult tension pneumothorax prior to discontinuation of care.[536,537]

Documentation of Care

Documenting Care on the Battlefield

Eastridge and colleagues found that 87% of combat fatalities in Iraq and Afghanistan occurred in the prehospital phase of combat casualty care.[538] Despite the obvious importance of recording the care provided in the prehospital phase, Eastridge noted that less than 10% of combat casualties had documentation of prehospital care.[538] The continuing lack of adequate documentation of battlefield trauma care rendered to U.S. casualties is a clear obstacle to ongoing CoTCCC and JTS efforts to improve that care. This requirement continues to be poorly fulfilled across the services.[539-542]

Documentation of care rendered on the battlefield is not simply an administrative requirement. It directly impacts the further care rendered to the casualty. When a tourniquet was applied and if and when the first dose of TXA was administered are examples of information crucial to other providers in the casualty's continuum of care. Furthermore, review of prehospital care rendered and outcomes achieved helps shape battlefield trauma care in the future.

In 2007, a CoTCCC working group was convened to address the lack of prehospital care documentation in the conflicts in Iraq and Afghanistan. At that point in time, there were over 30,000 casualties from these conflicts, but fewer than 10% of those casualties' records had any documentation of the care that was provided before the casualty reached an MTF. Unit-level reporting formats were used in almost all cases of successful documentation. In many instances, the first responders providing care were not medical personnel. Documentation of care provided by nonmedical first responders requires a format that these providers can understand and use effectively. Three possible choices for battlefield trauma care documentation were reviewed at the conference. One was the DoD paper form 1380 most commonly used at the time. Another was the Battlefield Medical Information System–Tactical (BMIS-T), a personal digital assistant-based software program. Neither of these two options was felt to sufficiently meet the needs of the prehospital providers in the tactical environment. The third option was a casualty card used by the 75th Ranger Regiment. This card was recognized by the working group as an immediate, cost-effective, and easily fielded interim solution. It was developed largely by Ranger medics, had proven easy to use, and was very well accepted by the Rangers and by other Special Operations groups. Using this card, the regiment had effectively documented the prehospital care provided to almost all of the approximately 450 battle injury and nonbattle injury casualties they had sustained in Iraq and Afghanistan by the time of the conference. The data collected were used to create the Ranger Prehospital Trauma Registry, the single best unit-based trauma registry to emerge from these conflicts. This registry, in turn, eventually enabled the most comprehensive study on prehospital care rendered by a combat unit in these two theaters.[543,544] The card was recommended by conference attendees and endorsed by the CoTCCC as the preferred method for documenting TCCC on the battlefield. This "TCCC Casualty Card" was endorsed by the Defense Health Board[545] and adopted as the standard format for documenting prehospital care by the Department of the Army. The governing Army regulation (AR 40-66 Medical Record Administration and Healthcare Documentation) was amended to permit the TCCC Casualty Card (DA Form 7656) to become a part of a health record

without a medical officer's signature as required for the old DD 1380 Field Medical Card. The other services, however, did not follow the Army's lead in adopting the TCCC Casualty Card. Consequently, there remained a need for a form that would be acceptable to and used by all of the services. The Defense Medical Materiel Program Office (DMMPO) noted this need and initiated an effort to develop a single form approved for use across the DoD. That initiative resulted in an updated version of the TCCC Casualty Card developed in 2013 as a joint effort of the CoTCCC, the DMMPO, and the JTS.[542]

The new card (**Figure 25-43**) maintains the simple format of the previous TCCC Casualty Card, but incorporates a number of modifications that allow for better documentation of prehospital care:

- The casualty battle roster number (to link to the DoD Trauma Registry)
- Better definition of the mechanism of injury
- Improved documentation of tourniquet use
- A section to record the use of junctional tourniquets
- A section to document the use of prehospital plasma and blood
- A section to document the hemoglobin oxygen saturation level
- A section for documentation of pain level
- A section for supraglottic airway use
- A space for the type of supraglottic airway
- A space to document the type of chest seal used
- Adds ketamine in the analgesic section
- A section to document the use of TXA
- Provides a space for documentation of an eye shield
- A space for documentation of CWMP usage
- A space for documentation of hypothermia prevention equipment

The TCCC Casualty Card should be completed by the first responder caring for each casualty and by all subsequent prehospital medical providers (**Box 25-21** and Figure 25-42). It should be attached to the casualty during the evacuation process. Once the casualty reaches a Level III care facility, the TCCC card should be transcribed by the hospital's patient administration department into the prescribed format to initiate the casualty's longitudinal electronic medical record.

The TCCC Casualty Card should also be supplemented by a more complete TCCC casualty After-Action Report (AAR) once the unit has returned to base.

The challenges entailed in documenting battlefield trauma care are well recognized, but this is a key element not only in assuring optimal care for the individual casualty but also in the JTS performance improvement process. The new TCCC Casualty Card and the TCCC AAR are excellent tools to help accomplish this, but success will ultimately depend on unit line and medical leadership making documentation of care a priority for unit combat medical personnel. The 75th Ranger Regiment has proven that with strong leadership, this can be done well.[541,543,544]

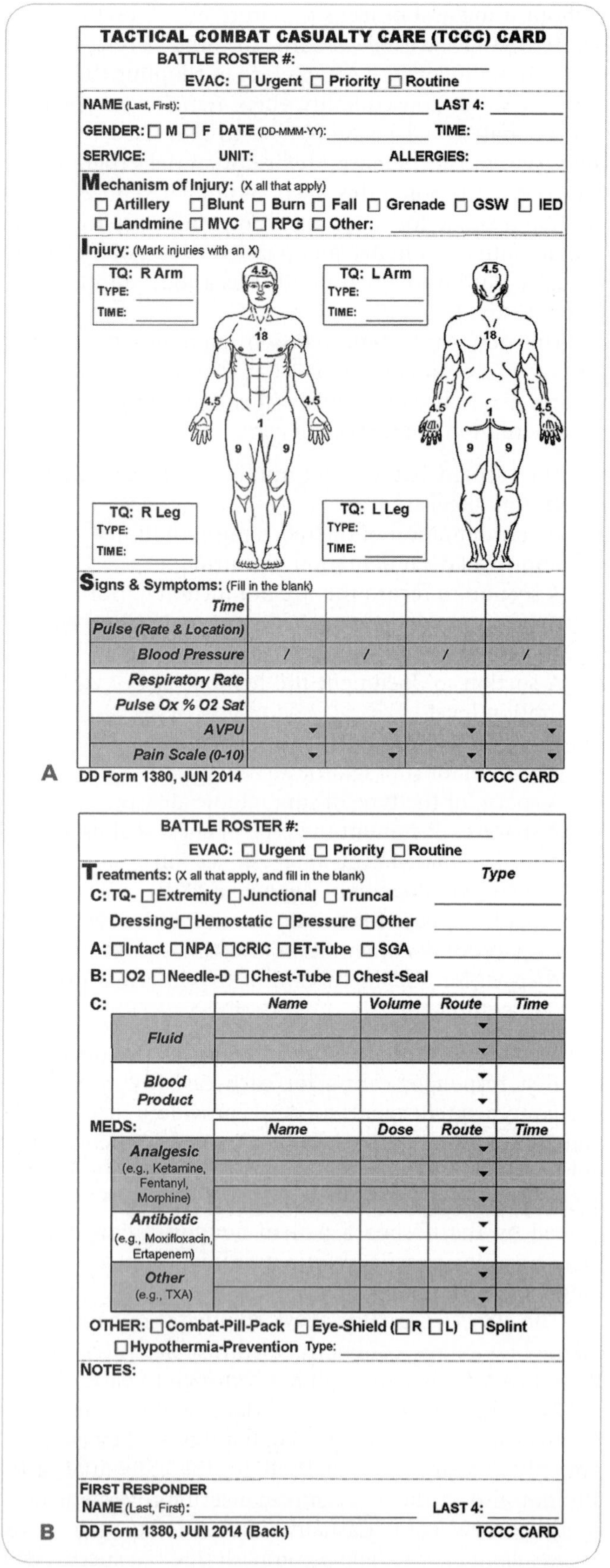

TACTICAL COMBAT CASUALTY CARE (TCCC) CARD

BATTLE ROSTER #: ________

EVAC: ☐ Urgent ☐ Priority ☐ Routine

NAME (Last, First): ________ LAST 4: ________

GENDER: ☐ M ☐ F DATE (DD-MMM-YY): ________ TIME: ________

SERVICE: ________ UNIT: ________ ALLERGIES: ________

Mechanism of Injury: (X all that apply)

☐ Artillery ☐ Blunt ☐ Burn ☐ Fall ☐ Grenade ☐ GSW ☐ IED

☐ Landmine ☐ MVC ☐ RPG ☐ Other: ________

Injury: (Mark injuries with an X)

Signs & Symptoms: (Fill in the blank)

Time				
Pulse (Rate & Location)				
Blood Pressure	/	/	/	/
Respiratory Rate				
Pulse Ox % O2 Sat				
AVPU				
Pain Scale (0-10)				

A DD Form 1380, JUN 2014 TCCC CARD

BATTLE ROSTER #: ________

EVAC: ☐ Urgent ☐ Priority ☐ Routine

Treatments: (X all that apply, and fill in the blank) *Type*

C: TQ- ☐ Extremity ☐ Junctional ☐ Truncal ________

Dressing- ☐ Hemostatic ☐ Pressure ☐ Other ________

A: ☐ Intact ☐ NPA ☐ CRIC ☐ ET-Tube ☐ SGA ________

B: ☐ O2 ☐ Needle-D ☐ Chest-Tube ☐ Chest-Seal ________

C:

	Name	Volume	Route	Time
Fluid				
Blood Product				

MEDS:

	Name	Dose	Route	Time
Analgesic (e.g., Ketamine, Fentanyl, Morphine)				
Antibiotic (e.g., Moxifloxacin, Ertapenem)				
Other (e.g., TXA)				

OTHER: ☐ Combat-Pill-Pack ☐ Eye-Shield (☐ R ☐ L) ☐ Splint

☐ Hypothermia-Prevention Type: ________

NOTES:

FIRST RESPONDER

NAME (Last, First): ________ LAST 4: ________

B DD Form 1380, JUN 2014 (Back) TCCC CARD

Figure 25-43 TCCC Casualty Card.

Courtesy of U.S.AISR.

Box 25-21 Tactical Field Care Guideline 18: Documentation of Care

18. Documentation of Care

a. Document clinical assessments, treatments rendered, and changes in the casualty's status on a TCCC Card (DD Form 1380). Forward this information with the casualty to the next level of care.

Source: Courtesy of the Committee on Tactical Combat Casualty Care.

Box 25-22 Tactical Field Care Guideline 19: Prepare for Evacuation

19. Prepare for evacuation.

a. Complete and secure the TCCC Card (DD 1380) to the casualty.

b. Secure all loose ends of bandages and wraps.

c. Secure hypothermia prevention wraps/blankets/straps.

d. Secure litter straps as required. Consider additional padding for long evacuations.

e. Provide instructions to ambulatory patients as needed.

f. Stage casualties for evacuation in accordance with unit standard operating procedures.

g. Maintain security at the evacuation point in accordance with unit standard operating procedures.

Source: Courtesy of the Committee on Tactical Combat Casualty Care.

Preparing the Casualty for Evacuation

Transitioning from Tactical Field Care to TACEVAC is a critical point in the casualty's continuum of care. This transition includes preparing the casualty for transport on one of a number of possible evacuation platforms—aircraft, ground vehicles, or water craft. Some of the essential elements in this preparation are securing loose dressings and straps, casualty marking, and completion of the TCCC Casualty Card (**Box 25-22** and **Figure 25-44**). These actions will help to ensure a smooth handover of the casualty to TACEVAC personnel.[524]

These actions are made more challenging by the tactical environment and may occur in loud noise conditions, such as under spinning helicopter rotor blades

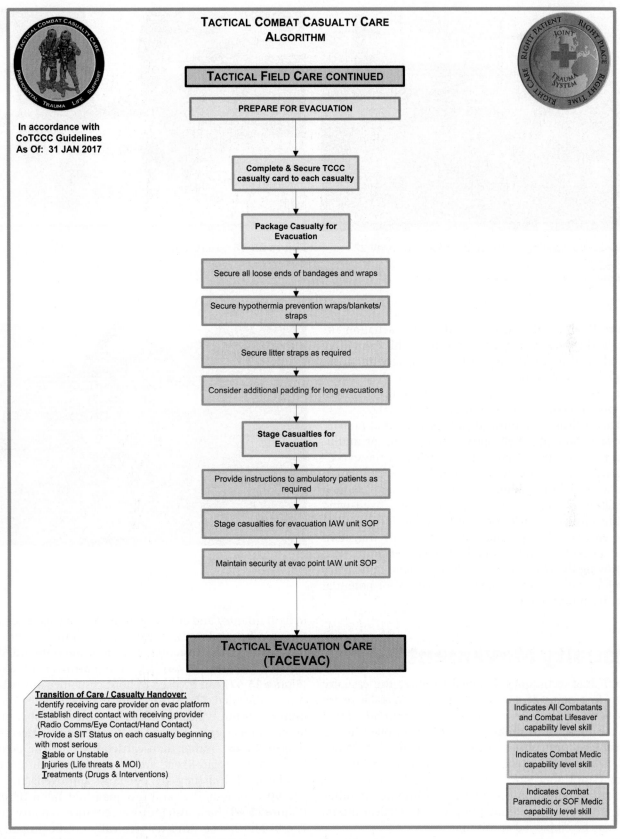

Figure 25-44 Algorithm for Tactical Field Care Guideline 19: Prepare for Evacuation.

Courtesy of Mr. Harold Montgomery. Retrieved from https://deployedmedicine.com/market/11/content/87

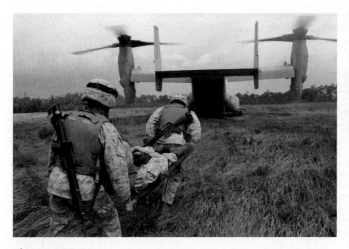

Figure 25-45 Loading a simulated casualty on an MV-22 Osprey.
Courtesy of 2nd Marine Division, Marine Corps Base Camp Lejeune, N.C.

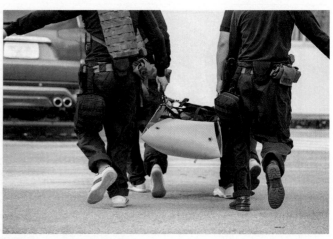

Figure 25-46 Sked SK-200.
© Prath/Shutterstock.

(**Figure 25-45**), at the tail of a fixed-wing evacuation aircraft, in the back of a truck with other vehicles moving around nearby, or on small boats rocking back and forth in rough seas. A smooth transfer of care in these hectic environments is facilitated by preplanned procedures, rehearsals, and effective communication.[524]

The tactical force must identify, secure, and prepare the evacuation site (helicopter landing zone or ambulance exchange point) prior to the arrival of the evacuation platform. Casualties are moved to the evacuation site and staged for loading as required for the particular evacuation platform to be used (helicopter, fixed-wing aircraft, ground vehicle, or boat.) Tactical force leaders must ensure full accountability during this transition phase for both casualties and the tactical personnel who are moving the casualties onto the evacuation platforms as well as continuing to maintain alertness for potential threat from hostile forces.[524]

Casualty Movement

Tactical drag techniques designed to move the casualty to the first point of cover as quickly as possible were described previously. (See Chapter 24, *Care Under Fire*.) Because the tactical situation is more controlled in the Tactical Field Care phase, further movement of casualties on the battlefield may be accomplished more easily than during Care Under Fire. The casualty can be disarmed, if indicated, and mission-essential gear distributed to other team members. If the unit has access to tactical litters, they may be employed at this time.

The type of litter used on missions is largely dependent on the type of unit and the mission profile. Skedco™ litters are some of the most commonly used tactical litters

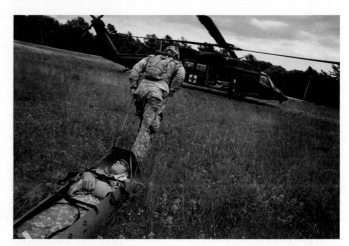

Figure 25-47 PJ Sked.
© Boston Globe/Contributor/Getty Images.

in light infantry and airborne units. As drag/slide devices, they can be used to carry gear and ammunition into the mission and carry casualties out. Both the standard Sked SK-200® (**Figure 25-46**) and the narrower PJ Sked® (**Figure 25-47**) can be used to hoist casualties into a helicopter if needed. The Stokes litter may be used by rescue units but is not typically carried by ground combat units. Stokes litters can be dragged by two rescuers, if necessary (**Figure 25-48**), rather than carried by four. The Foxtrot Litter® and Ranger Sked® are other drag/slide litters that can be used, but they are not hoist approved. The Raven 90C® bi-fold litter and the quad-fold Talon II® litter (**Figure 25-49**) have also found acceptance in many units. The bi-fold Raven litter will typically not fit properly in standard H-60 MEDEVAC/TAEVAC platforms, whereas the Talon II litter has collapsible handles and will fit into those aircraft.

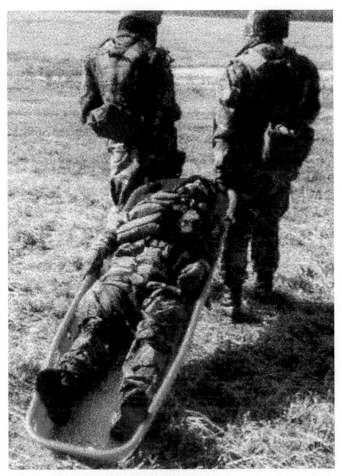

Figure 25-48 Stokes basket drag.
Courtesy of Dr. Mel Otten.

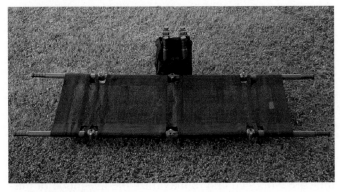

Figure 25-49 Talon II litter.
Courtesy of Mr. Dom Greydanus.

The Talon II is probably the most popular litter across the services. It is a component of the warrior aid and litter kit, which was a standard item in the Stryker and mine-resistant ambush-protected (MRAP) brigades. The grips on the Talon help make this litter advantageous for transporting a casualty in rough terrain. The "Army standard litter" is another option for a tactical litter. It does not have preinstalled litter straps, so these will need to be carried on the mission as well. Moving a casualty by litter in rough terrain is difficult, no matter which litter option is used.

An improvised litter can be made from a poncho, poncho liner, blanket, field jacket, door, or other field-expedient materials. If the casualty is a victim of blunt trauma and spinal injury is suspected, a rigid litter that provides adequate support to help protect the spinal cord from sustaining secondary injury should be used, if at all possible. A cervical collar can be improvised from a SAM® splint or other material and applied to the casualty before moving if needed to provide cervical stabilization. As noted previously, spinal precautions are not needed when the mechanism of wounding is penetrating trauma only. The meta-analysis on spine immobilization by Velopoulos and colleagues found that this intervention, when performed for patients with only penetrating trauma, is "associated with increased mortality and has not been shown to have a beneficial effect on mitigating neurologic deficits."[546] The Eastern Association of Surgical Trauma practice management guideline on spinal immobilization contained in that paper is in agreement with the preceding TCCC recommendation that spinal immobilization is not needed for trauma patients who have suffered only penetrating trauma.

When moving casualties over long distances, tourniquets, dressings, splints, and IV lines should be checked periodically to ensure they are intact and functioning. Casualties should be protected as much as possible from environmental hazards (e.g., sun, rain, wind, cold, snow, blowing sand, insects) prior to and during transport, and observed for signs of hypothermia, dehydration, and heat illness.

If no litter is available, the tactical drags and carries may be used in Tactical Field Care.

Wounded Hostile Combatants

Military medics may be called upon to render initial care for wounded hostile combatants. Medically speaking, the tenets of trauma care do not change. Tactical considerations, however, add an extra dimension to the care of these casualties. Even though wounded, enemy personnel may still act as hostile combatants and employ any weapons, ordnance, or communications devices (such as cellphones) they may be carrying to inflict harm on the individual rendering care and other unit members. Therefore, enemy casualties remain hostile combatants until they indicate surrender, are separated from all of their weapons and communications gear, and are proven to no longer pose a threat. For obvious reasons, then, no medical care for wounded hostile combatants should be attempted during Care Under Fire. In Tactical Field Care, combat medical personnel should not attempt to provide medical care for wounded hostile combatants until the tactical situation permits and these individuals have been rendered safe by other members of the unit. Rendering hostiles safe includes restraining them with flex cuffs or other such devices, searching them for hidden weapons and ordnance, and segregating them from other captured hostiles.

Once the medic is sure that wounded hostile combatants have been rendered safe, medical care should be provided in accordance with Tactical Field Care guidelines for U.S. forces. Thereafter, the wounded hostiles should be safeguarded from further injury and sped to the rear as medically and tactically feasible.

Calling for Tactical Evacuation (TACEVAC)

A medic caring for a casualty in Tactical Field Care must consider the degree of urgency for the casualty to reach an MTF. During the conflicts in Afghanistan and Iraq, the practice for requesting evacuation has been to prioritize casualties using the NATO doctrinal system. In this classification system, there are three categories:

A—Urgent evacuation within 2 hours
B—Priority evacuation within 4 hours
C—Routine evacuation within 24 hours

The following are offered as suggestions for how different injury patterns should be classified under this system. Note that these are examples only and the evacuation category may need modification based upon the findings in and condition of a particular casualty.

CAT A—Urgent (Denotes a Critical, Life-Threatening Injury)

- Significant injuries from a dismounted IED attack
- Gunshot wound or penetrating shrapnel to chest, abdomen, or pelvis
- Blunt chest, abdominal, or pelvic trauma with suspected noncompressible hemorrhage
- Ongoing airway difficulty
- Ongoing respiratory difficulty
- Unconscious casualty
- Known or suspected spinal injury
- Hemorrhagic shock
- External bleeding that is difficult to control
- Extremity injury with absent distal pulses
- Moderate/severe TBI
- Burns greater than 20% TBSA

Note that by Secretary of Defense directive, all casualties categorized as CAT A in the Afghanistan theater

of operations should be able to be evacuated to an MTF with a surgical capability within 60 minutes from the time that the evacuation mission is approved.[547]

CAT B—Priority (Serious Injury)

- Isolated, open extremity fracture with bleeding controlled
- Extremity injury with a tourniquet in place
- Penetrating or other serious eye injury
- Significant soft-tissue injury without major bleeding
- Burns of 10% to 20% TBSA

CAT C—Routine (Mild to Moderate Injury)

- Concussion (mild TBI)
- Gunshot wound to extremity—bleeding controlled without tourniquet
- Minor soft-tissue shrapnel injury
- Closed fracture with intact distal pulses
- Burns of <10% TBSA

Opportunities to Improve in TCCC

Reports have emerged from the wars in Afghanistan and Iraq that document potentially preventable deaths among U.S. combat casualties.[548-550] These reports reinforce the need to focus on improved battlefield trauma care interventions, technology, and training to avoid preventable death. Aspects of care that need to be modified or reinforced to ensure optimal combat casualty care are also identified during weekly trauma teleconferences conducted by the JTS. Finally, as noted in the 2017 Journal of Trauma TCCC Leadership Lessons paper, it does not matter how good the plan is if it is not adopted and well executed.[551] Leadership from the line combat community is an essential factor in the training and use of TCCC by combat units.[552,553] Battlefield trauma care is an essential component of a combat unit leader's responsibility and must be addressed as such in order to optimize the survival of unit members when they are wounded and to maximize the likelihood of mission success when casualties are sustained.[551]

The following have been identified as potential problems in the performance of TCCC that should be emphasized during training:

- Failure to control extremity bleeding with a tourniquet:
  - Initial tourniquet not adequately tightened
  - No second tourniquet used when needed to help control bleeding
  - No reassessment of the casualty to ensure that hemorrhage remains controlled

- Failure to use Combat Gauze when there is external hemorrhage that is not amenable to tourniquet use
- Failure to attempt to convert a tourniquet to other means of hemorrhage control after 2 hours of tourniquet time
- Failure to control junctional hemorrhage with Combat Gauze or junctional tourniquets
- Not administering TXA as early as possible when indicated[554]
- Administering morphine or OTFC to casualties in or at significant risk of shock
- Inability to perform an adequate surgical airway[555]
- Failure to document prehospital care[556-558]
- Failure to use whole blood as soon as feasible to resuscitate casualties in hemorrhagic shock[556]

- Failure to administer prehospital antibiotics[559]
- Use of platelet-impairing NSAIDs by combatants in theater, resulting in self-induced coagulopathies[560]
- Failure to treat suspected tension pneumothorax with NDC[561]
- Failure to provide adequate analgesia (or any analgesia) on the battlefield[562]
- Administering midazolam to casualties who have previously been given opioid analgesics
- Failure to use a rigid eye shield and administer an antibiotic for casualties with known or suspected penetrating eye injury[563]
- Use of ocular pressure dressings in casualties with known or suspected penetrating eye injury[563]

SCENARIO RECAP

While on patrol in the city of Mosul, an infantry platoon comes under small arms fire. The point man is hit and falls to the ground. The platoon reacts to the contact, rapidly eliminating the ambushing force. The point man is the only casualty in your unit. The platoon leader tells you to care for the wounded man while the other unit members establish a secure perimeter. In your rapid initial assessment for life-threatening conditions, you find a gunshot entry wound on the casualty's right upper back. The exit wound is in the right axilla, and there is heavy pulsatile bleeding from this site. The casualty is breathing slightly fast but is awake, alert, and responding appropriately. There are no other wounds.

SCENARIO SOLUTION

- **What phase of TCCC are you in?**
  You are in Tactical Field Care.

- **What is your immediate concern, and how do you address it?**
  Your immediate concern is the life-threatening external hemorrhage from the axillary wound. Expose the wound and push a Combat Gauze dressing directly onto the site of maximal bleeding. Hold firm, direct pressure with both hands for a minimum of 3 minutes.

- **While addressing your immediate concern, what should you be doing simultaneously?**
  While holding direct pressure, you talk to the casualty, checking both airway and mental status. While you are doing this, you note that the casualty is becoming increasingly drowsy.

- **What should you do after you finish your first intervention?**
  You check for other sources of external bleeding. You find none.

- **What do you evaluate next?**
  After confirming that there is no other significant external bleeding, you check his airway and breathing. You notice that his airway is clear, but his breathing is deep, rapid, and appears labored.

(continued)

SCENARIO SOLUTION (CONTINUED)

- **Should you treat for a tension pneumothorax? Why?**
  Yes—the casualty has a chest wound, labored breathing, and is in shock. You perform an NDC of the right chest and note the hiss of escaping air. His breathing becomes slower and easier.

- **What do you want to do after that?**
  After treating the tension pneumothorax, check the left radial pulse (not the right because of his wound.) It is not palpable. You consider that although external hemorrhage has been controlled, there may also be noncompressible torso hemorrhage at internal bleeding sites.

- **What interventions come next since the casualty is in shock?**
  Start an IV or IO and administer TXA. After that has been done, initiate fluid resuscitation with cold-stored type O low-titer blood if that is available or, alternatively, with type O low-titer or type O untitered fresh whole blood from a unit-based walking blood bank program. If whole blood is not available, use red blood cells and plasma in a 1:1 ratio or reconstituted dried plasma if these products are available. If no blood products are available, begin fluid resuscitation with 500 ml of Hextend.

- **What should this casualty's evacuation priority be?**
  Urgent surgical.

References

1. Butler FK, Hagmann JH, Richards DT. Tactical management of urban warfare casualties in special operations. *Mil Med*. 2000;165(4)(Suppl):1–48.

2. Holcomb JB, Butler FK, Rhee P. Hemorrhage control devices: tourniquets and hemostatic dressings. *Bull Am Coll Surg*. 2015 Sep;100(1 Suppl):66-70.

3. Butler F. Military history of increasing survival: the U.S. Military experience with tourniquets and hemostatic dressings in the Afghanistan and Iraq conflicts. *J Spec Oper Med*. 2015 Winter;15(4):149-152.

4. Kragh J, Dubick M. Bleeding control with limb tourniquet use in the wilderness setting: review of science. *Wilderness Environ Med*. 2017;28:S25-S32.

5. Shackelford SA, Butler FK, Kragh JF, et al. Optimizing the use of limb tourniquets in Tactical Combat Casualty Care: TCCC guidelines change 14-02. *J Spec Oper Med*. 2015;15: 17-31.

6. Drew B, Bennett B, Littlejohn L. Application of current hemorrhage control techniques for backcountry care: part one, tourniquets and hemorrhage control adjuncts. *Wilderness Environ Med*. 2015 Jun;26(2):236-245.

7. Kragh J, Walters T, Westmoreland T, et al. Tragedy into drama: an American history of tourniquet use in the current war. *J Spec Oper Med*. 2013;13:5-25.

8. Schauer S, April M, Naylor J, et al. QuikClot® use by ground forces in Afghanistan the prehospital trauma registry experience. *J Spec Oper Med*. 2017;17:101-106.

9. Littlejohn L, Bennett B, Drew B. Application of current hemorrhage control techniques for backcountry care: part two, hemostatic dressing and other adjuncts. *Wilderness Environ Med*. 2015 Jun;26(2):246-254.

10. Shina A, Lipsky A, Nadler R, et al. Prehospital use of hemostatic dressings by the Israel Defense Forces Medical Corps: a case series of 122 patients. *J Trauma Acute Care Surg*. 2015 Oct;79(4 Suppl 2):S204-S209.

11. Johnson D, Bates S, Nukalo S, et al. The effects of QuickClot Combat Gauze on hemorrhage control in the presence of hemodilution and hypothermia. *Ann Med Surg*. 2014;3:21-25.

12. Kheirabadi B. Evaluation of topical hemostatic agents for combat wound treatment. *U.S. Army Med Dep J*. 2011 Apr-Jun:25-37.

13. Bennett BL, Littlejohn LF, Kheirabadi BS, et al. Management of external hemorrhage in Tactical Combat Casualty Care: chitosan-based hemostatic gauze dressings. *J Spec Oper Med*. 2014;14:12-29.

14. Bennett BL. Bleeding control using hemostatic dressings: lessons learned. *Wilderness Environ Med*. 2017;28:S39-S49.

15. Kotwal RS, Butler FK, Gross KR, et al. Management of junctional hemorrhage in Tactical Combat Casualty Care: TCCC guidelines proposed change 13-03. *J Spec Oper Med*. 2013 Winter;13(4):85-93.

16. Dickey NW, Jenkins DH. Combat Ready Clamp addition to the Tactical Combat Casualty Care Guidelines 2011-07. Defense Health Board memorandum dated 23 September 2011. https://health.mil/About-MHS/OASDHA/Defense -Health-Agency/Defense-Health-Board/Reports. Accessed December 12, 2018.

17. Conley S, Littlejohn L, Henao J, et al. Control of junctional hemorrhage in a consensus swine model with hemostatic gauze products following minimal training. *Mil Med*. 2015;180:1189-1195.

18. Food and Drug Administration. De novo classification request for XStat. January 28, 2013. http://www.accessdata.fda.gov/cdrh_docs/reviews/k130218.pdf. Accessed December 12, 2018.

19. Sims K, Montgomery H, Dituro P, et al. Management of external hemorrhage in Tactical Combat Casualty Care: the adjunctive use of XStat™ compressed hemostatic sponges: TCCC guidelines change 15-03. *J Spec Oper Med.* 2016;16:19-28.

20. Cestero RF, Song BK. The effect of hemostatic dressings in a subclavian artery and vein transection porcine model. Naval Medical Research Unit San Antonio Technical Report TR-2013-012. 2013.

21. Mueller G, Pineda T, Xie H, et al. A novel sponge-based wound stasis dressing to treat lethal noncompressible hemorrhage. *J Trauma Acute Care Surg.* 2012;73:S134-139.

22. Demetriades D, Rabinowitz B, Pezikis A, et al. Subclavian vascular injuries. *Br J Surg.* 1987;74:1001-1003.

23. Kelly JF, Ritenour AE, McLaughlin DF, et al. Injury severity and causes of death from Operation Iraqi Freedom and Operation Enduring Freedom: 2003-2004 versus 2006. *J Trauma.* 2008 Feb;64(2)(Suppl):S21-S26.

24. Mabry RL, Edens JW, Pearse L, Kelly JF, Harcke H. Fatal airway injuries during Operation Enduring Freedom and Operation Iraqi Freedom. *Prehosp Emerg Care.* 2010;14(2):272-277. doi:10.3109/10903120903537205.

25. Alexander RH, Proctor HJ, eds. *ATLS® for Doctors Student Manual.* Chicago, IL: American College of Surgeons; 1993.

26. Butler FK, Hagmann J, Butler EG. Tactical combat casualty care in special operations. *Mil Med.* 1996;161(Suppl):3-16.

27. Butler FK, Holcomb JB, Giebner SD, McSwain NE, Bagian J. Tactical combat casualty care 2007: evolving concepts and battlefield experience. *Mil Med.* 2007;172(11)(Suppl):1-19.

28. Muzzi DA, Losasso TJ, Cucchiara RF. Complication from a nasopharyngeal airway in a patient with a basilar skull fracture. *Anesthesiology.* 1991;74:366-368.

29. Schade K, Borzotta A, Michaels A. Intracranial malposition of nasopharyngeal airway. *J Trauma.* 2000;49:967-968.

30. Martin JE, Mehta R, Aarabi B, Ecklund JE, Martin AH, Ling GSF. Intracranial insertion of a nasopharyngeal airway in a patient with craniofacial trauma. *Mil Med.* 2004;169:496-497.

31. Ellis DY, Lambert C, Shirley P. Intracranial placement of nasopharyngeal airways: is it all that rare? *Emerg Med J.* 2006;23:661-663.

32. Steinbruner D, Mazur R, Mahoney PF. Intracranial placement of a nasopharyngeal airway in a gunshot victim. *Emerg Med J.* 2007;24:311.

33. Otten M, Montgomery H, Butler F. Extraglottic airways in Tactical Combat Casualty Care. *J Spec Oper Med.* 2017;17:19-28.

34. Shavit I, Aviram E, Hoffmann Y, Biton O, Glassberg E. Laryngeal mask airway as a rescue device for failed endotracheal intubation during scene-to-hospital air transport of combat casualties. *Eur J Emerg Med.* 2017; Epub ahead of print June 27, 2017.

35. Gill RK, Tarat A, Pathak D, Dutta S. Comparative study of two laryngeal mask airways: proseal laryngeal mask airway and supreme laryngeal mask airway in anesthetized paralyzed adults undergoing elective surgery. *Anesth Essay and Res.* 2017;11:23-27.

36. van Tulder R, Schriefl C, Roth D, et al. Laryngeal tube practice in a metropolitan ambulance service: a five-year retrospective observational study (2009-2013). *Prehosp Emerg Care.* 2016 Apr;26:1-7.

37. Das A, Majumdar S, Mukherjee A, et al. i-gel™ in ambulatory surgery: a comparison with LMA-Proseal™ in paralyzed anaesthetized patients. *J Clin Diagn Res.* 2014;8:80-84.

38. Ekinci O, Abitagaoglu S, Turan G, Sivrikaya Z, Bosna G. The comparison of ProSeal and I-gel laryngeal mask airways in anesthetized adult patients under controlled ventilation. *Saudi Med J.* 2014;35:432-436.

39. Jaoua H, Djaziri L, Bousselmi J, et al. Evaluation of a new supraglottic airway device in ambulatory surgery: the i-gel. *Tunis Med.* 2014;92:239-244.

40. Duckett J, Fell P, Han K, Kimber C, Taylor C. Introduction of the i-gel supraglottic airway device for prehospital airway management in a UK ambulance service. *Emerg Med J.* 2014;31:505-507.

41. Ostermayer D, Gausche-Hill M. Supraglottic airways: the history and current state of prehospital airway adjuncts. *Prehosp Emerg Care.* 2014;18:106-115.

42. Goliash G, Ruetzler A, Fischer H, et al. Evaluation of advanced airway management in absolutely inexperienced hands: a randomized manikin trial. *Eur J Emerg Med.* 2013;20:310-314.

43. Barreira SR, Souza CM, Fabrizia F, Azevedo AB, Lelis TG, Lutke C. Prospective, randomized clinical trial of laryngeal mask airway Supreme(®) used in patients undergoing general anesthesia. *Braz J Anesthesiol.* 2013;63:456-460.

44. Studer NM, Horn GT, Studer LL, Armstrong JH, Danielson PD. Feasibility of supraglottic airway use by combat lifesavers on the modern battlefield. *Mil Med.* 2013;178:1202-1207.

45. Jeon W, Cho S, Baek S, Kim K. Comparison of the Proseal LMA and intersurgical i-gel during gynecological laparoscopy. *Korean J Anesthesiol.* 2012 Dec;63(6):510-514.

46. Mayglothling J, Duane T, Gibbs M, et al. Emergency tracheal intubation immediately following traumatic brain injury: an Eastern Association for the Surgery of Trauma practice management guideline. *J Trauma Acute Care Surg.* 2012;73:S333-S340.

47. Theiler L, Gutzmann M, Kleine-Brueggeney M, et al. i-gel™ supraglottic airway in clinical practice: a prospective observational multicenter study. *Brit J Anaesthesia.* 2012;109:990-995.

48. Timmerman A. Supraglottic airways in difficult airway management: successes, failures, use and misuse. *Anaesthesia.* 2011;66:45-56.

49. Dickey NW. Supraglottic airway use in tactical evacuation care 2012-06. Defense Health Board Memorandum dated September 17, 2012. https://health.mil/About-MHS/OASDHA/Defense-Health-Agency/Defense-Health-Board/Reports. Accessed July 6, 2018.

50. Thiruvenkatarajan V, Van Wijk RM, Rajbhoj A. Cranial nerve injuries with supraglottic airway devices: a systematic review of published case reports and series. *Anaesthesia.* 2015;70:344-359.

51. Endo K, Okabe Y, Maruyama Y, Tsukatani T, Furukawa M. Bilateral vocal cord paralysis caused by laryngeal mask airway. *Am J Otolarnygol.* 2007 Mar-Apr;28(2):126-129.

52. Brimacombe J, Clarke G, Keller C. Lingual nerve injury associated with the ProSeal laryngeal mask airway: a case report and review of the literature. *Br J Anaesthesia*. 2005;95:420-423.

53. Bruce IA, Ellis R, Kay NJ. Nerve injury and the laryngeal mask airway. *J Laryngol Otol*. 2004;18:899-901.

54. Miyashiro RM, Yamamoto LG. Endotracheal tube and laryngeal mask airway cuff pressures can exceed critical values during ascent to higher altitude. *Pediatr Emerg Care*. 2011;27:367-370.

55. Wilson GD, Sittig SE, Schears GJ. The laryngeal mask at altitude. *J Emerg Med*. 2008 Feb;34(2):171-174.

56. U. S. Air Force. *Air Force Instruction* 48-307, Vol 1. 9 January 2017; 76.

57. Britton T, Blakeman TC, Eggert J, Rodriquez D, Ortiz H, Branson RD. Managing endotracheal tube cuff pressure at altitude: a comparison of four methods. *J Trauma Acute Care Surg*. 2014;77:S240-S244.

58. Radhika KS, Sripriya R, Ravishankar M, et al. Assessment of suitability of i-gel and laryngeal mask airway-supreme for controlled ventilation in anesthetized paralyzed patients: a prospective randomized trial. *Anesth Essays Res*. 2016;10(1):88-93.

59. Ohchi F, Komasawa N, Imagawa K, et al. Evaluation of the efficacy of six supraglottic devices for airway management in devices airway management in dark conditions: a crossover randomized simulation trial. *J Anesth*. 2015 Dec;29(6):887-892.

60. Taxak S, Gopinath A, Saini S, et al. A prospective study to evaluate and compare laryngeal mask airway ProSeal and i-gel airway in the prone position. *Saudi J Anaesth*. 2015;9:446-450.

61. Gupta B, Gupta S, Hilam B, et al. Comparison of three supraglottic airway devices for airway rescue in the prone position: a manikin-based study. *J Emerg Trauma Shock*. 2015;8:188-192.

62. Middleton PM, Simpson PM, Thomas RE, Bendall JC. Higher insertion success with the i-gel supraglottic airway in out-of-hospital cardiac arrest: a randomized controlled trial. *Resuscitation*. 2014;85:893-897.

63. Haske D, Schempf B, Gaier G, Neiderberger C. Performance of the i-gel during pre-hospital cardiopulmonary resuscitation. *Resuscitation*. 2013;564:72-77.

64. Russo S, Cremer S, Galli T, et al. Randomized comparison of the i-gel™, the LMA Supreme™, and the Laryngeal Tube Suction-D using clinical and fiberoptic assessments in the elective patients. *BMC Anesthesiol*. 2012;18:1-9.

65. Henlin T, Sotak M, Kovaricek P, et al. Comparison of five 2nd-generation supraglottic airway devices for airway management performed by novice military operators. *BioMed Res Internat*. 2015;ID 201898:1-8.

66. Wharton NM, Gibbison B, Haslam GM, Muchatua N, Cook TM. I-gel insertion by novices in manikins and patients. *Anaesthesia*. 2008;63:991-995.

67. Smith JP, Bodai BI. The urban paramedic's scope of practice. *JAMA*. 1985;253(4):544-548.

68. Sladen A. Emergency endotracheal intubation: who can—who should? *Chest*. 1979;75(5):535-536.

69. Stewart RD, Paris PM, Winter PM, Pelton GH, Cannon GM. Field endotracheal intubation by paramedical personnel:

success rates and complications. *Chest*. 1984;85(3): 341-345.

70. Jacobs LM, Berrizbeitia LD, Bennet B, Madigan C. Endotracheal intubation in the prehospital phase of emergency medical care. *JAMA*. 1983;250(16):2175-2177.

71. Pointer JE. Clinical characteristics of paramedics' performance of endotracheal intubation. *J Emerg Med*. 1988;6(6): 505-509.

72. Lavery RF, Doran J, Tortella BJ, Cody RP. A survey of advanced life support practices in the United States. *Prehosp Disaster Med*. 1992;7(2):144-150.

73. DeLeo BC. Endotracheal intubation by rescue squad personnel. *Heart Lung*. 1977;65:851-854.

74. Trooskin SZ, Rabinowitz S, Eldridge C, McGowan D, Flancbaum L. Teaching endotracheal intubation using animals and cadavers. *Prehosp Disaster Med*. 1992;7(2):179-182.

75. Stewart RD, Paris PM, Pelton GH, Garretson D. Effect of varied training techniques on field endotracheal intubation success rates. *Ann Emerg Med*. 1984;13(11):1032-1036.

76. Cameron PA, Flett K, Kaan E, Atkin C, Dziukas L. Helicopter retrieval of primary trauma patients by a paramedic helicopter service. *Aust N Z J Surg*. 1993;63(10):790-797.

77. Zajtchuk R, Jenkins DP, Bellamy RF, Quick CM, Moore CC. Combat casualty care guidelines for Operation Desert Storm. Washington, DC: Office of the Army Surgeon General; 1991.

78. Holcomb JB, McMullin NR, Pearse L, et al. Causes of death in Special Operations Forces in the global war on terrorism. *Ann Surg*. 2007;245(6):986-991.

79. Adams BD, Cuniowski PA, Muck A, DeLorenzo RA. Registry of emergency airways arriving at combat hospitals. *J Trauma*. 2008;64(6):1548-1554. doi:10.1097/TA.0b013e3181728c41.

80. Reinhart DJ, Simmons G. Comparison of placement of the laryngeal mask airway with endotracheal tube by paramedics and respiratory therapists. *Ann Emerg Med*. 1994;24(2):260-263.

81. Stratton SJ, Kane G, Gunter CS, et al. Prospective study of manikin-only versus manikin and human subject endotracheal intubation training of paramedics. *Ann Emerg Med*. 1991;20(12):1314-1318.

82. Katz SH, Falk JL. Misplaced endotracheal tubes by paramedics in an urban emergency medical services system. *Ann Emerg Med*. 2001;37(1):32-37.

83. Calkins MD, Robinson TD. Combat trauma airway management: endotracheal intubation versus laryngeal mask airway versus Combitube use by Navy SEAL and reconnaissance combat corpsmen. *J Trauma*. 1999;46(5): 927-932.

84. Salvino CK, Dries D, Gamelli R, Murphy-Macabobby M, Mashall W. Emergency cricothyroidotomy in trauma victims. *J Trauma*. 1993;34(4):503-505.

85. McGill J, Clinton JE, Ruiz E. Cricothyrotomy in the emergency department. *Ann Emerg Med*. 1982;11(7):361-364.

86. Erlandson MJ, Clinton JE, Ruiz E, Cohen J. Cricothyrotomy in the emergency department revisited. *J Emerg Med*. 1989;7(2):115-118.

87. MacDonald JC, Tien HC. Emergency battlefield cricothyrotomy. *CMAJ*. 2008;178(9):1133–1135.

88. Mabry R. An analysis of battlefield cricothyrotomy in Iraq and Afghanistan. *J Spec Oper Med*. 2012;12(1):17-23.

89. Mabry R, Nichols M, Shiner D, et al. A comparison of two open surgical cricothyroidotomy techniques by military medics using a cadaver model. *Ann Emerg Med.* 2014;63:1-5.

90. Mabry R, Frankfurt A, Kharod C, Butler F. Emergency cricothyroidotomy in Tactical Combat Casualty Care. *J Spec Oper Med.* 2015;15:11-19.

91. Bennett B, Cailteux-Zevallos B, Kotora J. Cricothyroidotomy bottom-up training review: battlefield lessons learned. *Mil Med.* 2011;176(11):1311-1319.

92. Roberts DJ, Leigh-Smith S, Faris PD, et al. Clinical presentation of patients with tension pneumothorax: a systematic review. *Ann Surg.* 2015;261:1068-1078.

93. Simpson G. Tension pneumothorax case report is misleading. *Thorax.* 2011;67:355(ltr).

94. Waydhas C, Sauerland S. Pre-hospital pleural decompression and chest tube placement after blunt trauma: a systematic review. *Resuscitation.* 2007;72:11-25.

95. Leigh-Smith S, Harris T. Tension pneumothorax: time for a re-think? *Emerg Med J.* 2005;22:8-16.

96. Butler FK, Holcomb JB, Shackelford S, et al. Management of suspected tension pneumothorax in Tactical Combat Casualty Care: TCCC guidelines change 17-02. *J Spec Oper Med.* 2018;18(2):19-35.

97. Leatherman M, Fluke L, McEvoy C, et al. Bigger is better: comparison of alternative devices for tension hemopneumothorax and pulseless electrical activity in a Yorkshire swine model. *J Trauma Acute Care Surg.* 2017 Dec;83(6):1187-1194.

98. Lubin D, Tang A, Friese R, et al. Modified Veres needle compression of tension pneumothorax: a randomized crossover animal study. *J Trauma Acute Care Surg.* 2013;75: 1071-1075.

99. Martin M, Satterly S, Inaba K, Blair K. Does needle thoracostomy provide adequate and effective decompression of tension pneumothorax? *J Trauma Acute Care Surg.* 2012;73(6):1412-1417.

100. Holcomb JB, McManus JB, Kerr ST, Pusateri AE. Needle versus tube thoracostomy in a swine model of traumatic tension hemopneumothorax. *Prehosp Emerg Care.* 2009;13(1):18–27.

101. Barton ED, Rhee P, Hutton KC, Rosen P. The pathophysiology of tension pneumothorax in ventilated swine. *J Emerg Med.* 1997;15:147-153.

102. Inocencio M, Childs J, Chilstrom M, Berona K. Ultrasound findings in tension pneumothorax: a case report. *J Emerg Med.* 2017;52:e217-e220.

103. McPherson JJ, Feigin DS, Bellamy RF. Prevalence of tension pneumothorax in fatally wounded combat casualties. *J Trauma.* 2006;60(3):573-578.

104. Lee C, Revell M, Steyn R. The prehospital management of chest injuries: a consensus statement. Faculty of pre-hospital care, Royal College of Surgeons of Edinburgh. *Emerg Med J.* 2007;24:220-224.

105. McSwain NE. The McSwain Dart: device for relief of tension pneumothorax. *Med Instrum.* 1982;16(5):249-250.

106. Weichenthal L, Crane D, Rond L. Needle thoracostomy in the prehospital setting: a retrospective observational study. *Prehosp Emerg Care.* 2016;20:399-403.

107. Leis CC, Hernandez CC, Blanoc MJ, Paterna PC, Hernandez RE, Torres EC. Traumatic cardiac arrest: should advanced life support be initiated? *J Trauma Acute Care Surg.* 2013;74(2):634-638.

108. Mistry N, Bleetman A, Roberts KJ. Chest decompression during the resuscitation of patients in prehospital traumatic cardiac arrest. *Emerg Med J.* 2009;26(10):738-740.

109. Warner KJ, Copass MK, Bulger EM. Paramedic use of needle thoracostomy in the prehospital environment. *Prehosp Emerg Care.* 2008;12(2):162-168.

110. Lockey D, Crewdson K, Davies G. Traumatic cardiac arrest: who are the survivors? *Ann Emerg Med.* 2006;48(3):240-244.

111. Bellamy RF. The causes of death in conventional land warfare: implications for combat casualty care research. *Milit Med.* 1984;149:55-62.

112. Mabry RL, Holcomb JB, Baker AM, et al. United States Army Rangers in Somalia: an analysis of combat casualties on an urban battlefield. *J Trauma.* 2000;49(3):515-528.

113. Eastridge BJ, Mabry RL, Seguin P, et al. Death on the battlefield (2001-2011): implications for the future of combat casualty care. *J Trauma Acute Care Surg.* 2012;73(6)(Suppl 5): S431-S437.

114. Butler FK, Hagmann J, Butler EG. Tactical combat casualty care in special operations. *Milit Med.* 1996;161(Suppl):3-16.

115. Harcke HT, Pearse LA, Levy AD, Getz JM, Robinson SR. Chest wall thickness in military personnel: implications for needle thoracentesis in tension pneumothorax. *Milit Med.* 2007;172(12):1260-1263.

116. Harcke HT, Mabry RL, Mazuchowski EL. Needle thoracentesis decompression: observations from post-mortem computer tomography and autopsy. *J Spec Oper Med.* 2013;13:53-58.

117. Kiley KC. Management of soldiers with tension pneumothorax. U.S. Army Surgeon General memorandum dated 25 Aug 2006.

118. Butler FK, Giebner SD, McSwain N, Pons P, eds. *Prehospital Trauma Life Support Manual.* 8th ed—Military Version. Burlington, MA: Jones and Bartlett Learning; 2014.

119. Goh S, Xu WR, Teo LT. Decompression of tension pneumothoraces in Asian trauma patients: greater success with lateral approach and longer catheter lengths based on computed tomography chest wall measurements. *Eur J Trauma Emerg Surg.* 2018 Oct;44(5):767-771.

120. Zengerink I, Brink PR, Laupland KB, et al. Needle thoracostomy in the treatment of tension pneumothorax in trauma patients: what size needle? *J Trauma.* 2008;64(1):111–114.

121. Givens ML, Ayotte K, Manifold C. Needle thoracostomy: implications of computed tomography chest wall thickness. *Acad Emerg Med.* 2004;11(2):211-213.

122. Dickey NW, Jenkins D. Needle decompression of tension pneumothorax and cardiopulmonary resuscitation Tactical Combat Casualty Care Guideline Recommendations 2011-8. Defense Health Board Memorandum dated October. 11, 2011. https://health.mil/About-MHS/OASDHA/Defense -Health-Agency/Defense-Health-Board/Reports. Accessed October 29, 2018.

123. Dickey N. Needle decompression of tension pneumothorax: Tactical Combat Casualty Care Recommendations 2012-5. Defense Health Board Memorandum dated July 6, 2012. https://health.mil/About-MHS/OASDHA/Defense -Health-Agency/Defense-Health-Board/Reports. Accessed October 29, 2018.

124. Aho J, Thiels C, El Khatin M, et al. Needle thoracostomy: clinical effectiveness is improved using a longer angiocatheter. *J Trauma.* 2016;80:272-277.

125. Cantwell K, Burgess S, Patrick I, et al. Improvement in the prehospital recognition of tension pneumothorax: the effect of a change to paramedic guidelines and education. *Injury.* 2013;45:71-76.

126. Davis DP, Pettit K, Rom CD, et al. The safety and efficacy of prehospital needle and tube thoracostomy by aeromedical personnel. *Prehosp Emerg Care.* 2005;9:191-197.

127. Eckstein M, Suyehara D. Needle thoracostomy in the prehospital setting. *Prehosp Emerg Care.* 1998;2:132-135.

128. Chen J, Nadler R, Schwartz D, et al. Needle thoracostomy for tension pneumothorax: the Israeli Defense Forces experience. *Can J Surg.* 2015;58:S118-S124.

129. Kong V, Sartorius B, Clarke D. Traumatic tension pneumothorax: experience from 115 consecutive patients in a trauma service in South Africa. *Eur J Trauma Emerg Surg.* 2016;42:55-59.

130. High K, Brywczynski J, Guillamondegui O. Safety and efficacy of thoracostomy in the air medical environment. *Air Med J.* 2016;35:227-230.

131. Tien HC, Jung V, Rizoli SB, Acharya SV, MacDonald JC. An evaluation of Tactical Combat Casualty Care interventions in a combat environment. *J Am Coll Surg.* 2008;207(2):174-178.

132. Peters J, Ketelaars R, van Wageningen B, et al. Prehospital thoracostomy in patients with traumatic circulatory arrest: results from a physician-staffed helicopter emergency medical service. *Eur J Emerg Med.* 2017;24:96-100.

133. Kheirabadi BS, Terrazas IB, Koller A, et al. Vented versus unvented chest seals for treatment of pneumothorax and prevention of tension pneumothorax in a swine model. *J Trauma Acute Care Surg.* 2013;75(1):150-156.

134. Kotora JG, Henao J, Littlejohn LF, Kirchner S. Vented chest seals for the prevention of tension pneumothorax in a communicating pneumothorax. *J Emerg Med.* 2013;45:686-694.

135. Butler FK, Dubose JJ, Otten EJ, et al. Management of open pneumothorax in the tactical environment: TCCC guidelines change 13-02. *J Spec Oper Med.* 2013;13:81-86.

136. Schauer SG, April MD, Naylor JF, et al. Chest seal placement for penetrating chest wounds by prehospital ground forces in Afghanistan. *J Spec Oper Med.* 2017;17:85-89.

137. Kheirabadi B, Terrazas I, Miranda N, et al. Do vented chest seals differ in efficacy? An experimental evaluation using a swine hemopneumothorax model. *J Trauma Acute Care Surg.* 2017;83:182-189.

138. Britten S, Palmer SH, Snow TM. Needle thoracocentesis in tension pneumothorax: insufficient cannula length and potential failure. *Injury.* 1996;27(5):321-322.

139. Lamblin A, Turc J, Bylicki O, et al. Measure of chest wall thickness in French soldiers: which technique to use for needle decompression of tension pneumothorax at the front? *Milit Med.* 2014;179:783-786.

140. Schroeder E, Valdez C, Krauthamer A, et al. Average chest wall thickness at two anatomic locations in trauma patients. *Injury.* 2013;44:1183-1185.

141. Kaserer A, Stein P, Simmen H, et al. Failure rate of prehospital chest decompression after severe thoracic trauma. *Am J Emerg Med.* 2017 Mar;35(3):469-474.

142. Rottenstreich M, Fay S, Gendler S, et al. Needle thoracotomy in trauma. *Milit Med.* 2015;180:1211-1213.

143. Bach PT, Solling C. Failed needle decompression of bilateral spontaneous tension pneumothorax. *Acta Anesthesiol Scand.* 2015 Jul;59(6):807-810.

144. Butler FK, Bennett B, Wedmore I. Tactical Combat Casualty Care and wilderness medicine: advancing trauma care in austere environments. *Emerg Med Clin N America.* 2017;35:391-407.

145. Littlejohn LF. Treatment of thoracic trauma: lessons from the battlefield adapted to all austere environments. *Wilderness Environ Med.* 2017 Jun;28(2S):S69-S73.

146. Hatch Q, Debarros M, Johnson E, et al. Standard laparoscopic trocars for the treatment of tension pneumothorax: a superior alternative to needle decompression. *J Trauma Acute Care Surg.* 2014;77:170-175.

147. Rathinam S, Quinn DW, Bleetman A, Wall P, Steyn RS. Evaluation of ThoraQuik: a new device for the treatment of pneumothorax and pleural effusion. *Emerg Med J.* 2010;28:750-753.

148. Fluke L, Fitch J, Restrepo R, Gamble C, Polk TM. Novel modified Veress needle is superior to angiocatheter for decompression of tension pneumothorax in a Yorkshire swine model. Poster presented at 29th Annual Scientific Assembly of the Eastern Association for the Surgery of Trauma; January 2016; San Antonio, TX.

149. Kuckelman J, Derickson M, Phillips C, et al. Evaluation of a novel thoracic entry device versus needle decompression in a tension pneumothorax swine model. *Am J Surgery.* 2018 May;215(5):832-835.

150. Riwoe D, Poncia H. Subclavian artery laceration: a serious complication of needle decompression. *Emerg Med Australas.* 2011;23(5):651-653.

151. Butler KL, Best IM, Weaver L, Bumpers HL. Pulmonary artery injury and cardiac tamponade after needle decompression of a suspected tension pneumothorax. *J Trauma.* 2003;54(3):610-611.

152. Rawlins R, Brown KM, Carr CS, Cameron CR. Life-threatening haemorrhage after anterior needle aspiration of pneumothoraces: a role for lateral needle aspiration in emergency decompression of spontaneous pneumothorax. *Emerg Med J.* 2003;20(4):383-384.

153. Wernick B, Hon H, Mubang R, et al. Complications of needle thoracostomy: a comprehensive clinical review. *Int J Crit Illn Inj Sci.* 2015 Jul-Sep;5(3):160-169.

154. Netto F, Shulman H, Rizoli S, et al. Are needle decompressions for tension pneumothoraces being performed appropriately for appropriate indications? *Am J Emerg Med.* 2008;26(5):597-602.

155. Inaba K, Karamanos E, Skiada D, et al. Cadaveric comparison of the optimal site for needle decompression of tension pneumothorax by prehospital care providers. *J Trauma Acute Care Surg.* 2015;79:1044-1048.

156. Chang S, Ross S, Kiefer D, et al. Evaluation of 8.0-cm needle at the fourth anterior axillary line for needle chest decompression of tension pneumothorax. *J Trauma Acute Care Surg.* 2014;76:1029-1034.

157. Schreiber M. The death of another sacred cow. *Arch Surg.* 2012;147:818-819.

158. Inaba K, Branco BC, Eckstein M, et al. Optimal positioning for emergent needle thoracostomy: a cadaver-based study. *J Trauma*. 2011;71:1099-1103.

159. Heng K, Bystrzycki A, Fitzgerald M, et al. Complications of intercostal catheter insertion using EMST techniques for chest trauma. *ANZ J Surg*. 2004;74:420-423.

160. American College of Surgeons. Advanced Trauma Life Support—10th edition changes. American College of Surgeons emDocs website. http://www.emdocs.net/ready-atls-10th-edition-updates/. Accessed 30 October 2018.

161. Sanchez LD, Straszewski S, Saghir A, et al. Anterior versus lateral needle decompression of tension pneumothorax: comparison by computed tomography chest wall measurement. *Acad Emerg Med*. 2011 Oct;18(10):1022-1026.

162. Leatherman ML, Held JM, Fluke LM, et al. Relative device stability of anterior versus axillary needle decompression for tension pneumothorax during casualty movement: preliminary analysis of a human cadaver model. *J Trauma Acute Care Surg*. 2017 Jul;83(1 Suppl 1):S136-S141.

163. Beckett A, Savage E, Pannell D, Acharya S, Kirkpatrick A, Tien H. Needle decompression for tension pneumothorax in Tactical Combat Casualty Care: do catheters placed in the midaxillary line kink more often than those in the midclavicular line? *J Trauma*. 2011;71:S408-S412.

164. Jones R, Hollingsworth J. Tension pneumothoraces not responding to needle thoracentesis. *J Emerg Med*. 2002;19(2):176-177.

165. Naik ND, Hernandez MC, Anderson JR, Ross EK, Zielinski MD, Aho JM. Needle decompression of tension pneumothorax with colorimetric capnography. *Chest*. 2017;152:1015-1020.

166. McKenzie M, Parrish E, Miles E, et al. A case of prehospital traumatic arrest in a U.S. Special Operations soldier. *J Spec Oper Med*. 2016;16:93-96.

167. Gupta A, Rattan A, Kumar S, Rathi V. Delayed tension pneumothorax: identification and treatment in traumatic bronchial injury. *J Clin Diagn Res*. 2017;11:12-13.

168. Butler FK, Hagmann J, eds. Tactical management of urban warfare casualties in special operations. *Milit Med*. 2000;165:1-48.

169. Pritchard J, Hogg K. Pre-hospital finger thoracostomy in patients with traumatic cardiac arrest. *Emerg Med J*. 2017;34:417-418.

170. Massarutti D, Trillo G, Berlot G, et al. Simple thoracostomy in prehospital management is safe and effective: a 2-year experience by helicopter emergency crews. *Eur J Emerg Med*. 2006;13(5):276-280.

171. Rosenblatt M, Lemer J, Best LA, Peleg H. Thoracic wounds in Israeli battle casualties. *J Trauma*. 1985;25:350-354.

172. Sritharen Y, Hernandez MC, Haddad NN, et al. External validation of a tube thoracostomy complication classification system. *World J Surg*. 2018 Mar;42(3):736-741.

173. Dolley F, Brewer L. Chest injuries. *Ann Surg*. 1942;116(5):668-686.

174. Eastridge BJ, Mabry RL, Seguin P, et al. Death on the battlefield (2001-2011): implications for the future of combat casualty care. *J Trauma Acute Care Surg*. 2012;73(6)(Suppl 5):S431-S437.

175. Szul AC, Davis LB, Maston BG, Wise D, Sparacino LR, eds. *Emergency War Surgery*. 3rd U.S. revision. Washington, DC: The Borden Institute; 2004.

176. McSwain NE, Salome JP, Pons PT, eds. *Prehospital Trauma Life Support*. 6th ed. St. Louis, MO: Mosby; 2006:280.

177. Hodgetts TJ, Hanian CG, Newey CG. Battlefield first aid: a simple, systematic approach for every soldier. *J R Army Med Corps*. 1999;145(2):55-59.

178. Butler F, Dubose J, Otten E, et al: Management of open pneumothorax in Tactical Combat Casualty Care: TCCC guidelines change 13-02. *J Spec Oper Med*. 2013;13:81-86.

179. Kheirabadi BS, Terrazas IB, Koller A, et al. Vented versus unvented chest seals for treatment of pneumothorax and prevention of tension pneumothorax in a swine model. *J Trauma Acute Care Surg*. 2013;75(1):150-156.

180. Schauer SG, April MD, Naylor JF, et al. Chest seal placement for penetrating chest wounds by prehospital ground forces in Afghanistan. *J Spec Oper Med*. 2017;17:85-89.

181. Butler FK. Leadership lessons learned in Tactical Combat Casualty Care. *J Trauma Acute Care Surg*. 2017 Jun;82(6 Suppl 1):S16-S25.

182. Butler F. Two decades of saving lives on the battlefield: Tactical Combat Casualty Care turns 20. *Mil Med*. 2017;182:e1563-e1568.

183. Butler FK, Smith DJ, Carmona RC. Implementing and preserving advances in combat casualty care from Iraq and Afghanistan throughout the U.S. military. *J Trauma Acute Care Surg*. 2015 Aug;79(2):321-326.

184. Kheirabadi B, Terrazas I, Miranda N, et al. Do vented chest seals differ in efficacy? An experimental evaluation using a swine hemopneumothorax model. *J Trauma Acute Care Surg*. 2017;83:182-189.

185. Schnapp LM, Cohen NH. Pulse oximetry: uses and abuses. *Chest*. 1990;98:1244-1250.

186. Hanning CD, Alexander-Williams JM. Pulse oximetry: a practical review. *BMJ*. 1995;311(7001):367-370.

187. Moran RF, Clausen JL, Ehrmeyer SS, Feil M, Van Kessel Al, Eichhorn JH. Oxygen content, hemoglobin oxygen, "saturation," and related quantities in blood: terminology, measurement, and reporting. National Committee for Clinical Laboratory Standards 1990; C25-P:10:1-49.

188. Huch A, Huch R, Konig V, et al. Limitations of pulse oximetry. *Lancet*. 1988;1(8581):357-358.

189. Hansen JE, Casaburi R. Validity of ear oximetry in clinical exercise testing. *Chest*. 1987;91(3):333-337.

190. Ries AL, Prewitt LM, Johnson JJ. Skin color and ear oximetry. *Chest*. 1989;96(2):287-290.

191. Shapiro BA, Crane RD. Blood gas monitoring: yesterday, today, and tomorrow. *Crit Care Med*. 1989;17(6):573-581.

192. Davidson JA, Hosie HE. Limitations of pulse oximetry: respiratory insufficiency—a failure of detection. *BMJ*. 1993;307(6900):372-373.

193. Badjatia N, Carney N, Crocco TJ, et al. Brain Trauma Foundation; BTF Center for Guidelines Management. Guidelines for the prehospital management of traumatic brain injury. 2nd ed. *Prehosp Emerg Care*. 2008;12(Suppl 1):S1-S52.

194. Trillo RA Jr, Aukburg S. Dapsone-induced methemoglobinemia and pulse oximetry. *Anesthesiology*. 1992;77(3):594-596.

195. Sin DD, Shafran SD. Dapsone- and primaquine-induced methemoglobinemia in HIV-infected individuals. *J Acquir Immune Defic Syndr Hum Retrovirol*. 1996;12(5):477-481.

196. Butler FK, Holcomb JB, Giebner SD, McSwain NE, Bagian J. Tactical combat casualty care 2007: evolving concepts and battlefield experience. *Mil Med*. 2007;172(11)(Suppl):1-19.

197. Dickey NW. Management of traumatic brain injury in Tactical Combat Casualty Care 2012-04. Defense Health Board memorandum dated 26 July 2012. https://health.mil/About-MHS/OASDHA/Defense-Health-Agency/Defense-Health-Board/Reports. Accessed November 14, 2018.

198. Rybak M, Huffman L, Nahourali R, et al. Ultraportable oxygen concentrator use in U.S. Army Special Operations forward area surgery: a proof of concept in multiple environments. *Mil Med*. 2017;182:e1649-e1652.

199. Grissom CK, Weaver LK, Clemmer TP, Morris AH. Theoretical advantage of oxygen treatment for combat casualties during medical evacuation at high altitude. *J Trauma*. 2006;61(2):461-467.

200. Stockinger ZT, McSwain NE. Prehospital supplemental oxygen in trauma patients: its efficacy and implications for military medical care. *Mil Med*. 2004;169(8):609-612.

201. Chi JH, Knudson MM, Vassar MJ, et al. Prehospital hypoxia affects outcome in patients with traumatic brain injury: a prospective multicenter study. *J Trauma*. 2006;61(5):1134-1141.

202. Floyd TF, Clark JM, Gelfand R, et al. Independent cerebral vasoconstrictive effects of hyperoxia and accompanying arterial hypocapnia at 1 ATA. *J Appl Physiol*. 2003;95(6):2453-2461.

203. Tisdall MM, Taylor C, Tachtsidis I, Leung TS, Elwell CE, Smith M. The effect of cerebral tissue oxygenation index of changes in the concentrations of inspired oxygen and end-tidal carbon dioxide in healthy adult volunteers. *Anesth Analg*. 2009;109(3):906-913.

204. Tolias C, Reinert M, Seiler R, Gilman C, Scharf A, Bullock MR. Normobaric hyperoxia-induced improvement in cerebral metabolism and reduction in intracranial pressure in patients with severe head injury: a prospective historical cohort-matched study. *J Neurosurg*. 2004;101(3):435-444.

205. Montgomery H, Butler F, Kerr W, et al. TCCC guidelines comprehensive review and update: TCCC guidelines change 16-03. *J Spec Oper Med*. 2017;17:21-38.

206. Butler F. Military history of increasing survival: the U.S. military experience with tourniquets and hemostatic dressings in the Afghanistan and Iraq conflicts. *J Spec Oper Med*. 2015;15:149-152.

207. Kragh J, Walters T, Westmoreland T, et al. Tragedy into drama: an American history of tourniquet use in the current war. *J Spec Oper Med*. 2013;13:5-25.

208. Kragh JF, Walters TJ, Baer, DJ, et al. Survival with emergency tourniquet use to stop bleeding in major limb trauma. *Ann Surg*. 2009;249:1-7.

209. Kragh JF, Walters TJ, Baer DG, et al. Practical use of emergency tourniquets to stop bleeding in major limb trauma. *J Trauma*. 2008;64(Suppl 2):S38-S50.

210. Eastridge BJ, Mabry RL, Seguin P, et al. Prehospital death on the battlefield (2001-2011): implications for the future of combat casualty care. *J Trauma Acute Care Surg*. 2012;73(6 Suppl 5):S431-S437.

211. Shackelford S, Hammesfahr R, Morissette D, et al. The use of pelvic binders in Tactical Combat Casualty Care: TCCC guidelines change 16-02. *J Spec Oper Med*. 2017;17:135-147.

212. Shackelford SA, Butler FK, Kragh JF, et al. Optimizing the use of limb tourniquets in Tactical Combat Casualty Care: TCCC Guidelines Change 14-02. *J Spec Oper Med*. 2015;15:17-31.

213. Kragh JF, Walters TJ, Baer DG, et al. Practical use of emergency tourniquets to stop bleeding in major limb trauma. *J Trauma*. 2008;64(2)(Suppl):S38-S49.

214. Holcomb JB, Butler FK, Rhee P. Hemorrhage control devices: tourniquets and hemostatic dressings. *J Spec Oper Med*. 2015 Winter;15(4):153-156.

215. Butler FK, Kotwal RS, Buckenmaier CC III, et al. A Triple-Option Analgesia plan for Tactical Combat Casualty Care. *J Spec Oper Med*. 2014;14:13-25.

216. Montgomery H, Butler F, Kerr W, et al. TCCC guidelines comprehensive review and update: TCCC guidelines change 16-03. *J Spec Oper Med*. 2017;17:21-38.

217. Pusateri AE, Modrow HE, Harris RA, et al. Advanced hemostatic dressing development program: animal model selection criteria and results of a study of nine hemostatic dressings in a model of severe large venous hemorrhage and hepatic injury in swine. *J Trauma*. 2003;55(3):518-526.

218. Alam HB, Uy GB, Miller D, et al. Comparative analysis of hemostatic agents in a swine model of lethal groin injury. *J Trauma*. 2003;54(6):1077-1082.

219. Butler FK, Holcomb JB, Giebner SD, McSwain NE, Bagian J. Tactical combat casualty care 2007: evolving concepts and battlefield experience. *Mil Med*. 2007;172(11)(Suppl):1-19.

220. Rhee P, Brown C, Martin M, et al. QuikClot® use in trauma for hemorrhage control: case series of 103 documented uses. *J Trauma*. 2008;64(4):1093-1099.

221. Wedmore I, McManus JG, Pusateri AE, Holcomb JB. A special report on the chitosan-based hemostatic dressing: experience in current combat operations. *J Trauma*. 2006;60(3):655-658.

222. McManus J, Hurtado T, Pusateri A, Knoop KJ. A case series describing thermal injury resulting from zeolite use for hemorrhage control in combat operations. *Prehosp Emerg Care*. 2007;11(1):67-71.

223. Kheirabadi BS, Edens JW, Terrazas IB, et al. Comparison of new hemostatic granules/powders with currently deployed hemostatic products in a lethal model of extremity arterial hemorrhage in swine. *J Trauma*. 2009;66(2):316-326.

224. Kheirabadi B, Mace J, Terrazas I, et al. Safety evaluation of new hemostatic agents, smectite granules, and kaolin-coated gauze in a vascular injury wound model in swine. *J Trauma*. 2010;68(2):269-278.

225. Watters JM, Van PY, Hamilton GJ, Sambasivan C, Differding JA, Schreiber M. Advanced hemostatic dressings are not superior to gauze for care under fire scenarios. *J Trauma*. 2011;70(6):1413-1419.

226. Butler F, Blackbourne L, Gross KL. The Combat Medic Aid Bag: 2025—CoTCCC Top 10 recommended battlefield

trauma care research, development, and evaluation priorities for 2015. *J Spec Oper Med.* 2015;15:7-19.

227. Causey MW, McVay DP, Miller S, Beekley A, Martin M. The efficacy of Combat Gauze in extreme physiologic conditions. *J Surg Res.* 2012;177(2):301-305.

228. Ran Y, Hadad E, Daher S, et al. QuikClot Combat Gauze for hemorrhage control in military trauma: January 2009 Israel Defense Force experience in the Gaza Strip: a preliminary report of 14 cases. *Prehosp Disaster Med.* 2010;25(6):584-588.

229. Shina A, Lipsky A, Nadler R, et al. Prehospital use of hemostatic dressings by the Israel Defense Forces Medical Corps: a case series of 122 patients. *J Trauma Acute Care Surg.* 2015;79:s204-s209.

230. Leonard J, Zietlow H, Morris D, et al. A multi-institutional study of hemostatic gauze and tourniquets in rural civilian trauma. *J Trauma Acute Care Surg.* 2016;81:441-444.

231. Zietlow J, Zietlow S, Morris D, et al. Prehospital use of hemostatic bandages and tourniquets: translation from military experience to implementation in civilian trauma center. *J Spec Oper Med.* 2015;15:48-53.

232. Rall JM, Cox JM, Songer A, et al. Naval Medical Research Unit San Antonio. Comparison of novel hemostatic gauzes to QuikClot Combat Gauze in a standardized swine model of uncontrolled hemorrhage. Technical Report 2012-22 dated March 23, 2012. https://docplayer.net/14834086-Naval-medical-research-unit-san-antonio-technical-report-tr-2012-22.html. Accessed December 3, 2018.

233. Conley S, Littlejohn L, Henao J, et al. Control of junctional hemorrhage in a consensus swine model with hemostatic gauze products following minimal training. *Mil Med.* 2015;180:1189-1195.

234. te Grotenhuis T, van Grunsven P, Heutz W, Tan E. Prehospital use of hemostatic dressings in emergency medical services in the Netherlands: a prospective study of 66 cases. *Injury.* 2016;47:1007-1011.

235. Bennett BL, Littlejohn LF, Kheirabadi BS, et al. Management of external hemorrhage in Tactical Combat Casualty Care: chitosan-based hemostatic gauze dressings. *J Spec Oper Med.* 2014;14:12-29.

236. Bennett BL. Bleeding control using hemostatic dressings: lessons learned. *Wilderness Environ Med.* 2017;28:S39-S49.

237. Jacobs LM, Wade DS, McSwain NE, et al. The Hartford consensus: THREAT, a medical disaster preparedness concept. *J Am Coll Surg.* 2013;217:947-953.

238. Levy MJ, Jacobs LM. A call to action to develop programs for bystanders to control severe bleeding. *JAMA Surg.* 2016 Dec 1;151(12):1103-1104.

239. Jacobs LM, Joint Committee to Create a National Policy to Enhance Survivability from Intentional Mass Shooting Events. The Hartford consensus IV: a call for increased national resilience. *Conn Med J.* 2016;80:239-244.

240. Jacobs LM, McSwain NE Jr, Rotondo MF, et al. Improving survival from active shooter events: the Hartford consensus. *J Trauma Acute Care Surg.* 2013 Jun;74(6):1399-1400.

241. Callaway D, Robertson J, Sztajnkrycer M. Law enforcement-applied tourniquets: a case series of life-saving interventions. *Prehosp Emerg Care.* 2015;19:320-327.

242. Pons P, Jerome J, McMullen J, et al. The Hartford consensus on active shooters: implementing the continuum

of prehospital trauma response. *J Emerg Med.* 2015; 49:878-885.

243. Holcomb J. Major scientific lessons learned in the trauma field over the last two decades. *PLoS Med.* 2017;14: e1002339.

244. Butler FK. Leadership lessons learned in Tactical Combat Casualty Care. *J Trauma Acute Care Surg.* 2017 Jun;82(6 Suppl 1):S16-S25.

245. Butler FK. TCCC updates: two decades of saving lives on the battlefield: Tactical Combat Casualty Care turns 20. *J Spec Oper Med.* 2017 Summer;17(2):166-172.

246. Drew B, Bennett B, Littlejohn L. Application of current hemorrhage control techniques for backcountry care: part one, tourniquets and hemorrhage control adjuncts. *Wilderness Environ Med.* 2015 Jun;26(2):236-245.

247. Littlejohn L, Bennett BL, Drew B. Application of current hemorrhage control techniques for backcountry care: part two, hemostatic dressing and other adjuncts. *Wilderness Environ Med.* 2015 Jun;26(2):246-254.

248. Caravalho J, Dismounted Complex Injury Task Force. *Report of the Army Dismounted Complex Injury Task Force.* https://armymedicine.health.mil/reports/. Published June 18, 2011. Accessed December 3, 2018.

249. Kotwal RS, Butler FK Jr. Junctional hemorrhage control for Tactical Combat Casualty Care. *Wilderness Environ Med.* 2017 Jun;28(2S):S33-S38.

250. Kotwal RS, Butler FK, Gross KR, et al. Management of junctional hemorrhage in Tactical Combat Casualty Care. *J Spec Oper Med.* 2013 Winter;13:85-93.

251. Dickey NW, Jenkins DH. Combat Ready Clamp addition to the Tactical Combat Casualty Care guidelines 2011-07. Defense Health Board memorandum dated September 23, 2011. https://health.mil/About-MHS/OASDHA/Defense-Health-Agency/Defense-Health-Board/Reports. Accessed December 3, 2018.

252. Sims K, Montgomery H, Dituro P, et al. Management of external hemorrhage in Tactical Combat Casualty Care: the adjunctive use of XStat™ compressed hemostatic sponges: TCCC Guidelines change 15-03. *J Spec Oper Med.* 2016;16:19-28.

253. Rasmussen T, Eliason J. Military-civilian partnership in device innovation: development, commercial and application of resuscitative endovascular balloon occlusion of the aorta. *J Trauma Acute Care Surg.* 2017 Oct;83(4):732-735.

254. DuBose J, Scalea T, Brenner M, et al. The AAST prospective aortic occlusion for resuscitation in trauma and acute care surgery (AORTA) registry: data on contemporary utilization and outcomes of aortic occlusion and resuscitative balloon occlusion of the aorta (REBOA). *J Trauma Acute Care Surg.* 2016;81:409-419.

255. Manley J, Mitchell B, DuBose J, Rasmussen T. A modern case series of resuscitative endovascular balloon occlusion of the aorta (REBOA) in an out-of-hospital, combat casualty care setting. *J Spec Oper Med.* 2017;17:1-8.

256. Reva V, Hörer T, Makhnovskiy A, et al. Field and en route resuscitative endovascular balloon occlusion of the aorta: a feasible military reality? *J Trauma Acute Care Surg.* 2017 Jul;83(1 Suppl 1):S170-S176.

257. Holcomb JB. Transport time and preoperating room hemostatic interventions are important: improving

outcomes after severe truncal injury. *Crit Care Med.* 2018 Mar;46(3):447-453.

258. Butler F, Giebner S. CoTCCC Meeting 4-6 August 2015 Meeting Minutes. http://www.naemt.org/docs/default-source/education-documents/tccc/tccc-updates_092017/tccc-reference-materials/03-cotccc-meeting-minutes/cotccc-meeting-minutes-1508.pdf?sfvrsn=1783cd92_2. Published September 20, 2017. Accessed December 10, 2018.

259. Butler F, Giebner S. CoTCCC Meeting 31 January—01 February 2017 Meeting Minutes. http://www.naemt.org/docs/default-source/education-documents/tccc/tccc-updates_092017/tccc-reference-materials/03-cotccc-meeting-minutes/cotccc-meeting-minutes-1702.pdf?sfvrsn=2283cd92_2. Published September 20, 2017. Accessed December 10, 2018.

260. Dubose J. How I do it: partial resuscitative endovascular balloon occlusion of the aorta (P-REBOA). *J Trauma Acute Care Surg.* 2017;83:197-199.

261. Johnson M, Neff L, Williams T, et al. Partial resuscitative balloon occlusion of the aorta (P-REBOA): clinical techniques and rationale. *J Trauma Acute Care Surg.* 2016;81:S133-S137.

262. Chang J, Holloway B, Zamisch M, Hepburn MJ, Ling GS. ResQFoam for the treatment on non-compressible hemorrhage on the front line. *Mil Med.* 2015;180(9):932-933.

263. Rago A, Sharma U, Sims K, King D. Conceptualized use of self-expanding foam to rescue special operators from abdominal exsanguination. *J Spec Oper Med.* 2015;15:39-45.

264. Rago A, Duggan M, Hannett P, et al. Chronic safety assessment of hemostatic self-expanding foam: 90-day survival study and intramuscular biocompatibility. *J Trauma Acute Care Surg.* 2015;79:s78-s84.

265. Rago A, Marini J, Duggan M, et al. Diagnosis and deployment of a self-expanding foam for abdominal exsanguination: translation questions for human use. *J Trauma Acute Care Surg.* 2015;78:607-613.

266. Rago A, Duggan M, Beagle J, et al. Self-expanding foam for prehospital treatment of intra-abdominal hemorrhage: 28-day survival and safety. *J Trauma Acute Care Surg.* 2014;77:S127-S133.

267. Rago A, Duggan M, Marini J, et al. Self-expanding foam improves survival following a lethal, exsanguinating iliac artery injury. *J Trauma Acute Care Surg.* 2014;77:73-77.

268. Alexander RH, Proctor HJ, eds. *ATLS® for Doctors Student Manual.* Chicago, IL: American College of Surgeons; 1993.

269. Stupnyckyj C, Smolarek S, Reeves C, McKeith J. Changing blood transfusion policy and practice. *Am J Nursing.* 2014;114:50-59.

270. Butler FK, Hagmann J, Butler EG. Tactical combat casualty care in special operations. *Mil Med.* 1996;161(Suppl):3-16.

271. Butler FK, Holcomb JB, Giebner SD, McSwain NE, Bagian J. Tactical combat casualty care 2007: evolving concepts and battlefield experience. *Mil Med.* 2007;172(11)(Suppl):1-19.

272. Lawrence DW, Lauro AJ. Complications from I.V. therapy: results from field-started and emergency department-started I.V.'s compared. *Ann Emerg Med.* 1988;17(4):314-317.

273. Dubick MA, Holcomb JB. A review of intraosseous vascular access: current status and military application. *Mil Med.* 2000;165(7):552-559.

274. Calkins MD, Fitzgerald G, Bentley TB, Burris D. Intraosseous infusion devices: a comparison for potential use in special operations. *J Trauma.* 2000;48(6):1068-1074.

275. Luck R, Haines C, Mull C. Intraosseous access. *J Emerg Med.* 2010;39:468-475.

276. Santos D, Carron PN, Yersin B, Pasquier M. EZ-IO(®) intraosseous device implementation in a pre-hospital emergency service: a prospective study and review of the literature. *Resuscitation.* 2013;84:440-445.

277. Findlay J, Johnson DL, Macnab AJ, MacDonald D, Shellborn R, Susak L. Paramedic evaluation of adult intraosseous infusion system. *Prehosp Disaster Med.* 2006;21:329-334.

278. Naval Operational Medical Lessons Learned Center Report: Combat Medical Personnel Evaluation of Battlefield Trauma Care Equipment. November 19, 2011 (For official use only—available to DoD personnel through official request to the Joint Trauma System.)

279. Harcke HT, Mazuchowski E. Feedback to the field: perforation of the sternum by an intraosseous infusion device. National Association of Emergency Medical Technicians website. https://www.naemt.org/docs/default-source/education-documents/tccc/tccc-updates_092017/tccc-reference-materials/10-feedback-to-the-field/ft2f-6-perforation-of-the-sternum-by-an-io-infusion.pdf?sfvrsn=c18bcd92_2. Accessed December 14, 2018.

280. Pasley J, Miller C, DuBose J, et al. Intraosseous infusion rate under high pressure: a cadaveric comparison of anatomic sites. *J Trauma Acute Care Surg.* 2015;78:295-299.

281. Burgert J, Mozer J, Williams T, et al. Effects of intraosseous transfusion of whole blood on hemolysis and transfusion time in a swine model of hemorrhagic shock: a pilot study. *AANA J.* 2014;82(3):198-202.

282. Kehoe A, Jones A, Marcus S, et al. Current controversies in military prehospital care. *J R Army Med Corps.* 2011;157(3 Suppl 1):S305-S309.

283. Rush S, D'Amore J, Boccio E. A review of the evolution of intraosseous access in tactical setting and a feasibility study of a human cadaver model for a humeral head approach. *Mil Med.* 2014;179:24-28.

284. Harris M, Balog R, Devries G. What is the evidence of utility for intraosseous blood transfusion in damage-control resuscitation? *J Trauma Acute Care Surg.* 2013;75:904-906.

285. Lewis P, Wright C. Saving the critically injured trauma patient: a retrospective analysis of 1000 uses of intraosseous access. *Emerg Med J.* 2015 Jun;32:463-467.

286. Kelly JF, Ritenour AE, McLaughlin DF, et al. Injury severity and causes of death from Operation Iraqi Freedom and Operation Enduring Freedom: 2003-2004 versus 2006. *J Trauma.* 2008 Feb;64(2)(Suppl):S21-S26.

287. Holcomb JB, McMullin NR, Pearse L, et al. Causes of death in special operations forces in the global war on terrorism. *Ann Surg.* 2007;245(6):986-991.

288. Eastridge BJ, Mabry RL, Seguin P, et al. Death on the battlefield (2001-2011): implications for the future of combat casualty care. *J Trauma Acute Care Surg.* 2012;73(6)(Suppl 5):S431-S437.

289. Butler FK. Military history of increasing survival: the U.S. military experience with tourniquets and hemostatic dressings in the Afghanistan and Iraq conflicts. *Bull Am College Surg.* 2015 Sep;100(1 Suppl):60-64.

290. Kotwal RS, Butler FK, Gross KR, et al. Management of junctional hemorrhage in Tactical Combat Casualty Care: TCCC guidelines proposed change 13-03. *J Spec Oper Med.* 2013 Winter;13(4):85-93.

291. Kotwal RS, Butler FK Jr. Junctional hemorrhage control for Tactical Combat Casualty Care. *Wilderness Environ Med.* 2017 Jun;28(2S):S33-S38.

292. Diebel LN, Martin JV, Liberati DM. Early tranexamic acid administration ameliorates the endotheliopathy of trauma and shock in an in vitro model. *J Trauma Acute Care Surg.* 2017 Jun;82(6):1080-1086.

293. CRASH-2 collaborators, Roberts I, Shakur H, et al. The importance of early treatment with tranexamic acid in bleeding trauma patients: an exploratory analysis of the CRASH-2 randomized controlled trial. *Lancet.* 2011;377 (9771):1096-1110.

294. CRASH-2 trial collaborators, Shakur H, Roberts I, et al. Effects of tranexamic acid on death, vascular occlusive events, and blood transfusion in trauma patients with significant haemorrhage (CRASH-2): a randomised, placebo-controlled trial. *Lancet.* 2010;376:23-32.

295. Morrison JJ, Dubose JJ, Rasmussen TE, Midwinter MJ. Military Application of Tranexamic Acid in Trauma Emergency Resuscitation (MATTERs) study. *Arch Surg.* 2012;147(2):113-119.

296. Dickey NW, Jenkins D. Defense Health Board Recommendation for the Addition of Tranexamic Acid to the Tactical Combat Casualty Care Guidelines. Defense Health Board memorandum dated September 23, 2011. https://health.mil /About-MHS/OASDHA/Defense-Health-Agency/Defense -Health Board/Reports. Accessed December 18, 2018.

297. Cap AP, Baer DG, Orman JA, Aden J, Ryan K, Blackbourne LH. Tranexamic acid for trauma patients: a critical review of the literature. *J Trauma.* 2011;71(1 Suppl):S9-S14.

298. Boysen S, Pang J, Mikler J, et al. Comparison of tranexamic acid plasma concentrations when administered via intraosseous and intravenous routes. *Am J Emerg Med.* 2017;35: 227-233.

299. Huang F, Wu D, Ma G, Yin Z, Wang Q. The use of tranexamic acid to reduce blood loss and transfusion in major orthopedic surgery: a meta-analysis. *J Surg Res.* 2014 Jan;186(1): 318-327.

300. Sabbag OD, Abdel MP, Amundson AW, Larson DR, Pagnano MW. Tranexamic acid was safe in arthroplasty patients with a history of venous thromboembolism: a matched outcome study. *J Arthroplasty.* 2017 Sep;32(9S):S246-S250.

301. Ramirez R, Spinella P, Bochichio G. Tranexamic acid update in trauma. *Crit Care Clin.* 2017;33:85-99.

302. Harvey V, Perrone J, Kim P. Does the use of tranexamic acid improve trauma mortality? *Ann Emerg Med.* 2014;63: 460-462.

303. Kragh JF Jr, Walters TJ, Baer DG, et al. Survival with emergency tourniquet use to stop bleeding in major limb trauma. *Ann Surg.* 2009;249:1-7.

304. Montgomery HR, Butler FK, Kerr W, et al. TCCC guidelines comprehensive review and update: TCCC guidelines change 16-03. *J Spec Oper Med.* 2017;17:21-38.

305. Tranexamic Acid. Physician's Desk Reference website. http:// www.pdr.net/drug-summary/Cyklokapron-tranexamic -acid-1885.8271. Accessed December 18, 2018.

306. Studer N, Yassin A, Keen D. Compatibility of hydroxyethyl starch and tranexamic acid for battlefield co-administration. *Mil Med.* 2016;181:1305-1307.

307. Woodson J. Use of TXA in Combat Casualty Care. Assistant Secretary of Defense for Health Affairs memo. October 9, 2013. National Association of Emergency Medical Technicians website. http://www.naemt.org/docs/default-source /education-documents/tccc/tccc-updates_092017/tccc -reference-materials/06-tccc-reference-documents/asdha -memo-131009-expanded-use-of-txa.pdf?sfvrsn=8584cd92 _2. Accessed December 18, 2018.

308. Howard JT, Stockinger ZT, Cap AP, Bailey JA, Gross KR. Military use of TXA in combat trauma: does it matter? *J Trauma Acute Care Surg.* 2017 Oct;83(4):579-588.

309. Gayet-Ageron A, Prieto-Merino D, Ker K, et al. Effect of treatment delay on the effectiveness and safety of antifibrinolytics in acute severe haemorrhage: a meta-analysis of individual patient-level data from 40138 bleeding patients. *Lancet.* 2018 Jan 13;391(10116):125-132.

310. Butler FK, Bennett B, Wedmore I. Tactical Combat Casualty Care and wilderness medicine: advancing trauma care in austere environments. *Emerg Med Clin North Am.* 2017 May;35(2):391-407.

311. Wafaisade A, Lefering R, Bouillon B, et al. Prehospital administration of tranexamic acid in trauma patients. *Crit Care.* 2016 May 12;20(1):143.

312. Huebner BR, Dorlac WC, Cribari C. Tranexamic acid use in prehospital uncontrolled hemorrhage. *Wilderness Environ Med.* 2017 Jun;28(2S):S50-S60.

313. Schauer SG, April MD, Naylor JF, et al. Prehospital administration of tranexamic acid by ground forces in Afghanistan: the prehospital trauma registry experience. *J Spec Oper Med.* 2017;17:55-58.

314. Smith JP, Bodai BI. The urban paramedic's scope of practice. *JAMA.* 1985;253(4):544-548.

315. Krausz MM. Controversies in shock research: hypertonic resuscitation—pros and cons. *Shock.*1995;3(1):69-72.

316. Smith JP, Bodai BI, Hill AS, Frey CF. Prehospital stabilization of critically injured patients: a failed concept. *J Trauma.* 1985;25(1):65-70.

317. Dronen SC, Stern S, Baldursson J, Irvin C, Syverud S. Improved outcome with early blood administration in a near-fatal model of porcine hemorrhagic shock. *Am J Emerg Med.* 1992;10(6):533-537.

318. Chudnofsky CR, Dronen SC, Syverud SA, Hedges JR, Zink BJ. Early versus late fluid resuscitation: lack of effect in porcine hemorrhagic shock. *Ann Emerg Med.* 1989;18(2):122-126.

319. Bickell WH. Are victims of injury sometimes victimized by attempts at fluid resuscitation? *Ann Emerg Med.* 1993;22(2): 225-226.

320. Chudnofsky CR, Dronen SC, Syverud SA, Zink BJ, Hedges JR. Intravenous fluid therapy in the prehospital management of hemorrhagic shock: improved outcome with hypertonic saline/6% Dextran 70 in a swine model. *Am J Emerg Med.* 1989;7(4):357-363.

321. Kaweski SM, Sise MJ, Virgilio RW. The effect of prehospital fluids on survival in trauma patients. *J Trauma.* 1990;30(10): 1215-1218.

322. Deakin CD, Hicks IR. AB or ABC: prehospital fluid management in major trauma. *J Accid Emerg Med.* 1994;11(3):154-157.

323. Krausz MM, Bar-Ziv M, Rabinovici R, Gross D. "Scoop and run" or stabilize hemorrhagic shock with normal saline or small-volume hypertonic saline? *J Trauma*. 1992;33(1):6-10.

324. Kowalenko J, Stern S, Dronen S, Wang X. Improved outcome with hypotensive resuscitation of uncontrolled hemorrhagic shock in a swine model. *J Trauma*. 1992;33(3):349-353.

325. Kramer GC, Perron PR, Lindsey DC, et al. Small-volume resuscitation with hypertonic saline dextran solution. *Surgery*. 1986;100(2):239-247.

326. Krausz MM, Klemm O, Amstislavsky T, Horovitz M. The effect of heat load and dehydration on hypertonic saline solution treatment on uncontrolled hemorrhagic shock. *J Trauma*. 1995;38(5):747-752.

327. Krausz MM, Horn Y, Gross D. The combined effect of small volume hypertonic saline and normal saline solutions in uncontrolled hemorrhagic shock. *Surg Gynecol Obstet*. 174(5):363-368.

328. Gross D, Landau EH, Klin B, Krausz MM. Treatment of uncontrolled hemorrhagic shock with hypertonic saline solution. *Surg Gynecal Obstet*. 1990;170(2):106-112.

329. Stern SA, Dronen SC, Birrer P, Wang X. Effect of blood pressure on hemorrhage volume and survival in a near-fatal hemorrhage model incorporating a vascular injury. *Ann Emerg Med*. 1993;22(2):155-163.

330. Bickell WH, Bruttig SP, Millnamow GA, O'Benar J, Wade CE. Use of hypertonic saline/dextran versus lactated Ringer's solution as a resuscitation fluid after uncontrolled aortic hemorrhage in anesthetized swine. *Ann Emerg Med*. 1992;21(9):1077-1085.

331. Dontigny L. Small-volume resuscitation. *Can J Surg*. 1992; 35(1):31-33.

332. Gross D, Landau EH, Assalia A, Krausz MM. Is hypertonic saline resuscitation safe in "uncontrolled" hemorrhagic shock? *J Trauma*. 1988;28(6):751-756.

333. Shaftan GW, Chiu CJ, Dennis C, Harris B. Fundamentals of physiological control of arterial hemorrhage. *Surgery*. 1965;58(5):851-856.

334. Milles G, Koucky CJ, Zacheis HG. Experimental uncontrolled arterial hemorrhage. *Surgery*. 1966;60(2):434-442.

335. Sindlinger JF, Soucy DM, Greene SP, Barber AE, Illner H, Shires GT. The effects of isotonic saline volume resuscitation in uncontrolled hemorrhage. *Surg Gynecol Obstet*. 1993;177(6):545-550.

336. Landau EH, Gross D, Assalia A, Krausz MM. Treatment of uncontrolled hemorrhagic shock by hypertonic saline and external counterpressure. *Ann Emerg Med*. 1989;18(10): 1039-1043.

337. Rabinovici R, Krausz MM, Feurstein G. Control of bleeding is essential for a successful treatment of hemorrhagic shock with 7.5 per cent sodium chloride solution. *Surg Gynecol Obstet*. 1991;173(2):98-106.

338. Landau EH, Gross D, Assalia A, Feigin E, Krausz MM. Hypertonic saline infusion in hemorrhagic shock treated by military antishock trousers (MAST) in awake sheep. *Crit Care Med*. 21(10):1554-1562.

339. Crawford ES. Ruptured abdominal aortic aneurysm. *J Vasc Surg*. 1991;13(2):348-350.

340. Bickell WH, Wall MJ, Pepe PE, et al. Immediate versus delayed fluid resuscitation for hypotensive patients with penetrating torso injuries. *N Engl J Med*. 1994;331(17): 1105-1109.

341. Wall MJ. Audiovisual presentation at the 53rd annual meeting of the American Association for the Surgery of Trauma. 1994.

342. Butler FK, Hagmann J, Butler EG. Tactical combat casualty care in special operations. *Mil Med*. 1996;161(Suppl): 3-16.

343. Butler FK, Hagmann JH, Richards DT. Tactical management of urban warfare casualties in special operations. *Mil Med*. 2000;165(4)(Suppl):1-48.

344. Rainey TG, Read CA. The pharmacology of colloids and crystalloids. In: Chernow B, ed. *The Pharmacologic Approach to the Critically Ill Patient*. 2nd ed. Baltimore, MD: Williams & Wilkins; 1988:219-240.

345. Carey JS, Scharschmidt BF, Culliford AT, Greenlee JE, Scott CR. Hemodynamic effectiveness of colloid and electrolyte solutions for replacement of simulated operative blood loss. *Surg Gynecol Obstet*. 1970;131(4):679-686.

346. Marino PL. Colloid and crystalloid resuscitation. In: Marino PL. *The ICU Book*. Malvern, PA: Williams & Wilkins; 1991:205–216.

347. Strauss RG. Review of the effects of hydroxyethyl starch on the blood coagulation system. *Transfusion*. 1981;21(3): 299-302.

348. Mortelmans Y, Merckx E, van Nerom C, et al: Effect of an equal volume replacement with 500cc 6% hydroxyethyl starch on the blood and plasma volume of healthy volunteers. *Eur J Anesthesiol*. 1995;12(3):259-264.

349. Napolitano LM. Resuscitation following trauma and hemorrhagic shock: is hydroxyethyl starch safe? *Crit Care Med*. 1995;23(5):795-797.

350. Dalrymple-Hay MB, Aitchison R, Collins P, Sekhar M, Colvin B. Hydroxyethyl starch induced acquired von Willebrand's disease. *Clin Lab Haematol*. 1992;14(3):209-211.

351. Via D, Kaufman C, Anderson D, Stanton K, Rhee P. Effect of hydroxyethyl starch on coagulopathy in a swine model of hemorrhagic shock resuscitation. *J Trauma*. 2001;50(6):1076-1082.

352. Shatney CH, Deepika K, Militello PR, Majerus TC, Dawson RB. Efficacy of hetastarch in the resuscitation of patients with multisystem trauma and shock. *Arch Surg*. 1983;118(7):804-809.

353. Falk JL, O'Brien JF, Kerr R. Fluid resuscitation in traumatic hemorrhagic shock. *Crit Care Clin*. 1992;8(2):323-340.

354. Ratner LE, Smith GW. Intraoperative fluid management. *Surg Clin North Am*. 1993;73(2):229-241.

355. Pearce FJ, Lyons WS. Logistics of parenteral fluids in battlefield resuscitation. *Mil Med*. 1999;164(9):653-655.

356. Champion HR. Combat fluid resuscitation: introduction and overview of conferences. *J Trauma*. 2003;54(5)(Suppl):S7-S12.

357. Gan TJ, Bennett-Guerrero E, Phillips-Bute B, et al. Hextend®, a physiologically balanced plasma expander for large volume use in major surgery: a randomized phase III clinical trial. Hextend® Study Group. *Anesth Analg*. 1999;88(5): 992-998.

358. Holcomb JB. Fluid resuscitation in modern combat casualty care: lessons learned from Somalia. *J Trauma*. 2003; 54(Suppl 5):S46-S51.

359. Sondeen J, Coppes VG, Holcomb JB. Blood pressure at which rebleeding occurs after resuscitation in swine with aortic injury. *J Trauma*. 2003;54(Suppl 5):S110–S117.

360. Beecher HK. *Resuscitation and Anesthesia for Wounded Men: The Management of Traumatic Shock*. Springfield, IL: Charles C Thomas; 1949.

361. Butler FK, Holcomb JB, Giebner SD, McSwain NE, Bagian J. Tactical combat casualty care 2007: evolving concepts and battlefield experience. *Mil Med*. 2007;172(11)(Suppl):1-19.

362. Butler FK. Fluid resuscitation in Tactical Combat Casualty Care—yesterday and today. *Wilderness Environ Med*. 2017 Jun;28(2S):S74-S81.

363. Butler FK, Bennett B, Wedmore I. Tactical Combat Casualty Care and wilderness medicine: advancing trauma care in austere environments. *Emerg Med Clin North Am*. 2017 May;35(2):391-407.

364. Fisher A, Miles E, Cap A, et al. Tactical damage control resuscitation. *Mil Med*. 2015;180:869-875.

365. Cap A, Pidcoke H, DePasquale M, et al. Blood far forward: time to get moving! *J Trauma Acute Care Surg*. 2015;78:S2-S6.

366. Butler FK, Holcomb JB, Kotwal RS, et al. Fluid resuscitation for hemorrhagic shock in Tactical Combat Casualty Care: TCCC guidelines change 14-01. *J Spec Oper Med*. 2014;14: 13-38.

367. Jenkins D, Rappold J, Badloe J, et al. THOR position paper on remote damage control resuscitation: definitions, current practice, and knowledge gaps. *Shock*. 2014;41:3-12.

368. Joint Trauma System Clinical Practice Guideline: Damage Control Resuscitation. February 1, 2013. Joint Trauma System website. https://jts.amedd.army.mil/assets/docs/cpgs/JTS _Clinical_Practice_Guidelines_(CPGs)/Damage_Control _Resuscitation_03_Feb_2017_ID18.pdf. Accessed December 27, 2018.

369. Kauvar DS, Holcomb JB, Norris GC, Hess JR. Fresh whole blood transfusion: a controversial military practice. *J Trauma*. 2006 Jul;61(1):181-184.

370. Spinella PC, Perkins JG, Grathwohl KW, et al. Warm fresh whole blood is independently associated with improved survival for patients with combat-related traumatic injuries. *J Trauma*. 2009;66:S69-S76.

371. Strandenes G, Hervig T, Bjerkvig C, et al. The lost art of whole blood transfusions in austere environments. *Curr Sports Med Rep*. 2015;15:11-15.

372. Strandenes G, De Pasquale M, Cap A, et al. Emergency whole-blood use in the field: a simplified protocol for collection and transfusion. *Shock*. 2014;41(Suppl 1):76-83.

373. Strandenes G, Skogrand H, Spinella P, Hervig T, Rein EB. Donor performance of combat readiness skills of special forces soldiers are maintained immediately after whole blood donation: a study to support the development of a prehospital fresh whole blood transfusion program. *Transfusion*. 2013 Mar;53(3):526-530.

374. Holcomb, JB. Optimal use of blood products in severely injured trauma patients. *Hematology Am Soc Hematol Educ Program*. 2010;2010:465-469.

375. Holcomb J, Spinella P. Optimal use of blood in trauma patients. *Biologicals*. 2010;38:72-77.

376. Bickell WH, Wall MJ, Pepe PE, et al. Immediate versus delayed fluid resuscitation for hypotensive patients with penetrating torso injuries. *N Engl J Med*. 1994;331(17): 1105-1109.

377. Kasotakis G, Sideris A, Yang Y, et al. Aggressive early crystalloid resuscitation adversely affects outcomes in adult blunt trauma patients: an analysis of the Glue Grant database. *J Trauma Acute Care Surg*. 2013;74:1215-1221.

378. Zarychanski R, Abou-Setta A, Turgeon A, et al. Association of hydroxyethyl starch admission with mortality and acute kidney injury in critically ill patients requiring volume resuscitation. *JAMA*. 2013;309:678-688.

379. Ley E, Clond M, Srour M, et al. Emergency department crystalloid resuscitation of 1.5 L or more is associated with increased mortality in elderly and non-elderly trauma patients. *J Trauma*. 2011;70:398-400.

380. Duke MD, Guidry C, Guice J, et al. Restrictive fluid resuscitation in combination with damage control resuscitation: time for adaptation. *J Trauma Acute Care Surg*. 2012;73:674-678.

381. Lissauer ME, Chi A, Kramer ME, Scalea TM, Johnson SB. Association of 6% Hetastarch resuscitation with adverse outcomes in critically ill trauma patients. *Am J Surg*. 2011;202(1):501.

382. Cannon J. Hemorrhagic shock. *N Engl J Med*. 2018;378: 370-379.

383. Shackelford S, Del Junco D, Powell-Dunford N, et al. Association of prehospital blood product transfusion during medical evacuation of combat casualties in Afghanistan with acute and 30-day survival. *JAMA*. 2017;318:1581-1591.

384. Wild G, Anderson D, Lund P. Round Afghanistan with a fridge. *J R Army Med Corps*. 2013;159:24-29.

385. Morrison JJ, Oh J, Dubose JJ, et al. En-route care capability from point of injury impacts mortality after severe wartime injury. *Ann Surg*. 2013;257:330-334.

386. Apodaca A, Olson C, Bailey J, et al. Performance improvement evaluation of forward aeromedical evacuation platforms in Operation Enduring Freedom. *J Trauma Acute Care Surg*. 2013;75:S157-S163.

387. Holcomb J, Donathan D, Cotton B, et al. Prehospital transfusion of plasma and red blood cells in trauma patients. *Prehosp Emerg Care*. 2015 January-March;19(1):1-9.

388. Stubbs J, Zielinski M, Jenkins D. The state of the science of whole blood: lessons learned at Mayo Clinic. *Transfusion*. 2016;56:S173-S181.

389. Holcomb JB, Swartz MD, DeSantis SM, et al. Multicenter observational prehospital resuscitation on helicopter study. *J Trauma Acute Care Surg*. 2017;83:S83-S91.

390. Holcomb J. Transport time and pre-operating room hemostatic interventions are important: improving outcomes after severe truncal injury. *Crit Care Med*. 2018 Mar;46: 447-453.

391. Spinella P, Pidcoke H, Strandenes G, et al. Whole blood transfusion for hemostatic resuscitation of major bleeding. *Transfusion*. 2016;56:S190-S202.

392. Yazer M, Cap A, Spinella P. Raising the standards on whole blood. *J Trauma Acute Care Surg*. 2018 Jun;84(6 Suppl 1): S14-S17.

393. Butler FK, Blackbourne LH, Gross KR. The combat medic aid gag—2025: CoTCCC top ten recommended battlefield trauma care research, development, and evaluation priorities for 2015. *J Spec Oper Med*. 2015;15:7-19.

394. Holcomb JB, Pati S. Optimal trauma resuscitation with plasma as the primary resuscitative fluid: the surgeon's perspective. *Hematology*. 2013;2013:656-659.

395. Glassberg E, Nadler R, Rasmussen T, et al. Point-of-injury use of reconstituted freeze-dried plasma as a resuscitative fluid: a special report for prehospital trauma care. *J Trauma Acute Care Surg*. 2013;75:S111-S114.

396. Martinaud C, Ausset S, Deshayes A, et al. Use of freeze-dried plasma in French intensive care unit Afghanistan. *J Trauma*. 2011;71:1761-1765.

397. Manley G, Knudson MM, Morabito D, et al. Hypotension, hypoxia, and head injury: frequency, duration, and consequences. *Arch Surg*. 2001;136(10):1118-1123.

398. Spaite DW, Hu C, Bobrow BJ, et al. Association of out-of-hospital hypotension depth and duration with traumatic brain injury mortality. *Ann Emerg Med*. 2017 Oct;70(4):522-530.

399. Spaite D, Hu C, Bobrow B, et al. The effect of combined out-of-hospital hypotension and hypoxia on mortality in major traumatic brain injury. *Ann Emerg Med*. 2017;69:62-72.

400. Lednar WM, Poland GA, Holcomb JB, Butler FK. Recommendations Regarding the Tactical Combat Casualty Care Guidelines on Fluid Resuscitation. Defense Health Board memorandum. December 10, 2010. Defense Health Agency website. https://health.mil/About-MHS/OASDHA/Defense-Health-Agency/Defense-Health-Board/Reports. Accessed December 31, 2018.

401. Butler F, Holcomb J, Shackelford S, et al. Management of suspected tension pneumothorax in Tactical Combat Casualty Care. TCCC guidelines change 17-02. *J Spec Oper Med*. 2018 Summer;18(2):19-35.

402. Dickey NW, Jenkins D. Addition of Tranexamic Acid to the Tactical Combat Casualty Care Guidelines. Defense Health Board memorandum. September 23, 2011. Defense Health Agency website. https://health.mil/About-MHS/OASDHA/Defense-Health-Agency/Defense-Health-Board/Reports. Accessed December 31, 2018.

403. Lee C, Revell M, Porter K, Steyn R. The prehospital management of chest injuries: a consensus statement. Faculty of Pre-hospital Care, Royal College of Surgeons of Edinburgh. *Emerg Med J*. 2007 Mar;24(3):220-224.

404. Jones R, Hollingsworth J. Tension pneumothoraces not responding to needle thoracocentesis. *Emerg Med J*. 2002 Mar;19(2):176-177.

405. Rosenblatt M, Lemer J, Best LA, Peleg H. Thoracic wounds in Israeli battle casualties during the 1982 evacuation of wounded from Lebanon. *J Trauma*. 1985 Apr;25(4):350-354.

406. Chen J, Nadler R, Schwartz D, et al. Needle thoracostomy for tension pneumothorax: the Israeli Defense Forces experience. *Can J Surg*. 2015;58:S118-S124.

407. Pritchard J, Hogg K. Pre-hospital finger thoracostomy in patients with traumatic cardiac arrest. *Emerg Med J*. 2017;34:417-418.

408. Littlejohn LF. Treatment of thoracic trauma: lessons from the battlefield adapted to all austere environments. *Wilderness Environ Med*. 2017;28:S69-S73.

409. High K, Brywczynski J, Guillamondegui O. Safety and efficacy of thoracostomy in the air medical environment. *Air Med J*. 2016;35:227-230.

410. Massarutti D, Trillo G, Berlot G, et al. Simple thoracostomy in prehospital management is safe and effective: a 2-year experience by helicopter emergency crews. *Eur J Emerg Med*. 2006;13:276-280.

411. Davis DP, Pettit K, Rom CD, et al. The safety and efficacy of prehospital needle and tube thoracostomy by aeromedical personnel. *Prehosp Emerg Care*. 2005;9:191-197.

412. Leigh-Smith S, Harris T. Tension pneumothorax—time for a rethink? *Emerg Med J*. 2005;22:8-16.

413. Dickey NW, Jenkins D, Butler FK. Use of Dried Plasma in Prehospital Battlefield Resuscitation 2011-04. Defense Health Board memorandum. August 8, 2011. Defense Health Agency website. https://health.mil/About-MHS/OASDHA/Defense-Health-Agency/Defense-Health-Board/Reports. Accessed January 1, 2019.

414. Wolberg AS, Meng ZH, Monroe DM III, Hoffman M. A systematic evaluation of the effect of temperature on coagulation enzyme activity and platelet function. *J Trauma*. 2004;56(6):1221-1228.

415. Watts DD, Trask A, Soeken K, Perdue P, Dols S, Kaufmann C. Hypothermic coagulopathy in trauma: effect of varying levels of hypothermia on enzyme speed, platelet function, and fibrinolytic activity. *J Trauma*. 1998;44(5):846-854.

416. Vardon F, Mrozek S, Geeraerts T, Fourcade O. Accidental hypothermia in severe trauma. *Anaesth Crit Care Pain Med*. 2016;35:355-361.

417. Lapostolle F, Couvreur J, Koch F, et al. Hypothermia in trauma victims at first arrival of ambulance personnel: an observational study with assessment of risk factors. *Scand J Trauma Resusc Emerg Med*. 2017;25:43.

418. Wesuter M, Brück A, Lippross S, et al. Epidemiology of accidental hypothermia in polytrauma patients: an analysis of 15,230 patients on the TraumaRegister DGU®. *J Trauma Acute Care Surg*. 2016;81:905-912.

419. Peng RY, Bongard FS. Hypothermia in trauma patients. *J Am Coll Surg*. 1999;188(6):685-696.

420. Fries D, Innerhofer P, Schobersberger W. Coagulation management in trauma patients. *Curr Opin Anaesthesiol*. 2002;15(2):217-223.

421. Carr ME Jr. Monitoring of hemostasis in combat trauma patients. *Mil Med*. 2004;169(Suppl 12):11-15.

422. Steele J, Atkins J, Vizcaychipi M. Factors at scene and in transfer related to the development of hypothermia in major burns. *Ann Burns Fire Disasters*. 2016;29:103-107.

423. Joint Theater Trauma System Clinical Practice Guideline. Hypothermia prevention, monitoring, and management. Joint Trauma System website. https://jts.amedd.army.mil/assets/docs/cpgs/JTS_Clinical_Practice_Guidelines_(CPGs)/Hypothermia_Prevention_Monitoring_Management_20_Sep_2012_ID23.pdf. Published September 18, 2012. Accessed January 2, 2019.

424. Arthurs Z, Cuadrado D, Beekley, et al. The impact of hypothermia on trauma care at the 31st combat support hospital. *Am J Surg*. 2006;191(5):610-614.

425. Winkenwerder W. Defense-wide Policy on Combat Trauma Casualty Hypothermia Prevention and Treatment. Assistant Secretary of Defense for Health Affairs memorandum. February 16, 2006. https://www.health.mil/Reference-Center. Accessed January 2, 2019.

426. Husum H, Olsen T, Murad M, Wisborg T, Gilbert M. Preventing post-injury hypothermia during prolonged prehospital evacuation. *Prehosp Disaster Med*. 2002;17(1):23-26.

427. Allen PB, Salyer SW, Dubick MA, Holcomb JB, Blackbourne LH. Preventing hypothermia: comparison of current devices used by the U.S. Army with an in vitro warmed fluid model. *J Trauma*. 2010;69(Suppl):S154-S161.

428. Lednar WM, Poland GA, Holcomb JB, Butler FK. Tactical Combat Casualty Care Guidelines on the Prevention of Hypothermia. Defense Health Board memorandum. December 10, 2010. https://health.mil/About-MHS/OASDHA/Defense-Health-Agency/Defense-Health-Board/Reports. Accessed January 2, 2019.

429. Singleton W, McLean M, Smale M, et al. An analysis of the temperature change in warmed intravenous fluids during administration in cold environments. *Air Med J*. 2017;36:127-130.

430. Zafren K, Giesbrecht G, Danzl D, et al. Wilderness Medical Society practice guidelines for the out-of-hospital evaluation and treatment of accidental hypothermia. *Wilderness Environ Med*. 2014;25:425-445.

431. Montgomery H, Butler F, Kerr W, et al. TCCC guidelines comprehensive review and update: TCCC guidelines change 16-03. *J Spec Oper Med*. 2017;17:21-38.

432. Perlman R, Callum J, Laflamme C, et al. A recommended early goal-directed management guideline for the prevention of hypothermia-related transfusion, morbidity, and mortality in severely injured trauma patients. *Crit Care*. 2016;20:107.

433. Bennett BL, Holcomb JB. Battlefield trauma-induced hypothermia: transitioning the preferred method of casualty rewarming. *Wilderness Environ Med*. 2017;28:S82-S89.

434. Calvano C. Rigid eye shields: a crucial gap in the individual first aid kit commentary. *J Spec Oper Med*. 2013;13(3):29-30.

435. Kressloff MS, Castellarin AA, Zarbin MA. Endophthalmitis. *Surv Ophthalmol*. 1998;43(3):193-224.

436. Butler FK, Chalfin S. The eye in the wilderness. In: Auerbach PS, ed. *Wilderness Medicine*. 7th ed. St. Louis, MO: Mosby; 2016.

437. Lyer MH, Weber ED, Weichel ED, et al. Delayed intraocular foreign body removal without endophthalmitis during Operations Iraqi Freedom and Enduring Freedom. *Ophthalmology*. 2007;114:1439-1447.

438. Mazzoli RA, Gross KR, Butler FK. The use of rigid eye shields (Fox shields) at the point of injury for ocular trauma in Afghanistan. *J Trauma Acute Care Surg*. 2014;17:56-62.

439. Dickey N. Prehospital use of ketamine in battlefield analgesia 2012-03. Defense Health Board memorandum. March 8, 2012. https://health.mil/About-MHS/OASDHA/Defense-Health-Agency/Defense-Health-Board/Reports. Accessed March 29, 2019.

440. Butler FK. Tactical Combat Casualty Care—beginnings. *Wilderness Environ Med*. 2017 Jun;28(2S):S12-S17.

441. Butler FK, Bennett B, Wedmore CI. Tactical Combat Casualty Care and wilderness medicine: advancing trauma care in austere environments. *Emerg Med Clin North Am*. 2017 May;35(2):391-407.

442. Kotwal RS, O'Connor KC, Johnson TR, Mosely DS, Meyer DE, Holcomb JB. A novel pain management strategy for combat casualty care. *Ann Emerg Med*. 2004;44(2):121-127.

443. Butler FK, Hagmann J, Butler EG. Tactical Combat Casualty Care in special operations. *Mil Med*. 1996 Aug;161 Suppl:3-16.

444. Kotwal RS, Butler FK, Edgar EP, Shackelford SA, Bennett DR, Bailey JA. Saving lives on the battlefield: a joint trauma system review of pre-hospital trauma care in combined joint operating area Afghanistan (CJOA-A) executive summary. *J Spec Oper Med*. 2013 Spring;13(1):77-85.

445. Butler FK, Kotwal RS, Buckenmaier CC III, et al. A Triple-Option Analgesia plan for Tactical Combat Casualty Care: TCCC guidelines change 13-04. *J Spec Oper Med*. 2014 Spring;14(1):13-25.

446. Beecher HK. Pain in men wounded in battle. *Bull US Army Med Dep*. 1946;5:445-454.

447. Vonkeman HE, van de Laar MA. Nonsteroidal anti-inflammatory drugs: adverse effects and their prevention. *Semin Arthritis Rheum*. 2010;39(4):294-312.

448. Van Ryn J, Kink-Eiband M, Kuritsch I, et al. Meloxicam does not affect the antiplatelet effect of aspirin in healthy male and female volunteers. *J Clin Pharmacol*. 2004;44(7):777-784.

449. Knijff-Dutmer EA, Kalsbeek-Batenburg EM, Koerts J, van de Laar MA. Platelet function is inhibited by non-selective non-steroidal anti-inflammatory drugs but not by cyclooxygenase-2-selective inhibitors in patients with rheumatoid arthritis. *Rheumatology (Oxford)*. 2002;41(4):458-461.

450. Rinder HM, Tracey JB, Souhrada M, Wang C, Gagnier RP, Wood CC. Effects of meloxicam on platelet function in healthy adults: a randomized, double-blind, placebo-controlled trial. *J Clin Pharmacol*. 2002;42(8):881-886.

451. de Meijer A, Vollaard H, de Metz M, Verbruggen B, Thomas C, Novakova I. Meloxicam, 15 mg/day, spares platelet function in healthy volunteers. *Clin Pharmacol Ther*. 1999;66(4):425-430.

452. Wedmore IS, Johnson T, Czarnik J, Hendrix S. Pain management in the wilderness and operational setting. *Emerg Med Clin North Am*. 2005;23(2):585-601, xi-xii.

453. Schwartz RB, Charity BM. Use of night vision goggles and low-level light source in obtaining intravenous access in tactical conditions of darkness. *Mil Med*. 2001;166(11):982-983.

454. Lind GH, Marcus MA, Mears SL, et al. Oral transmucosal fentanyl citrate for analgesia and sedation in the emergency department. *Ann Emerg Med*. 1991;20(10):1117-1120.

455. Gauna AA, Kang SK, Triano ML, Swatko ER, Vanston VJ. Oral transmucosal fentanyl citrate for dyspnea in terminally ill patients: an observational case series. *J Palliat Med*. 2008;11(4):643-648.

456. Collado F, Torres LM. Association of transdermal fentanyl and oral transmucosal fentanyl citrate in the treatment of opioid naive patients with severe chronic noncancer pain. *J Opioid Manag*. 2008;4(2):111-115.

457. Mahar PJ, Rana JA, Kennedy CS, Christopher NC. A randomized clinical trial of oral transmucosal fentanyl citrate versus intravenous morphine sulphate for initial control of pain in children with extremity injuries. *Pediatric Emerg Care*. 2007;23(8):544-548.

458. MacIntyre PA, Margetts L, Larsen D, Barker L. Oral transmucosal fentanyl citrate versus placebo for painful dressing changes: a crossover trial. *J Wound Care.* 2007;16(3):118-121.

459. Aronoff GM, Brennan MJ, Pritchard DD, Ginsberg B. Evidence-based oral transmucosal fentanyl citrate (OTFC) dosing guidelines. *Pain Med.* 2005;6(4):305-314.

460. Landy SH. Oral transmucosal fentanyl citrate for the treatment of migraine headache pain in outpatients: a case series. *Headache.* 2004;44(8):762-766.

461. Weiss EA. Medical considerations for the wilderness and adventure travelers. *Med Clin North Am.* 1999;83(4):885-902, v-vi.

462. U.S. Food and Drug Administration Center for Drug Evaluation and Research. *NDA 20–747: Clinical Pharmacology and Biopharmaceutics Review of Actiq® (Oral Transmucosal Fentanyl Citrate).* Rockville, MD: U.S. Food and Drug Administration; 1997.http://www.accessdata.fda.gov/drugsatfda_docs/label/2011/20747orig1s029rems.pdf. Accessed April 2, 2019.

463. Lee M, Kern SE, Kisicki JC, Egan TD. A pharmacokinetic study to compare two simultaneous 400 microg doses with a single 800 microg dose of oral transmucosal fentanyl citrate. *J Pain Symptom Manage.* 2003;26(2):743-747.

464. Butler FK, Hagmann JH, Richards DT. Tactical management of urban warfare casualties in special operations. *Mil Med.* 2000;165(4)(Suppl):1-48.

465. Kacprowicz R, Johnson T, Mosely D. Fentanyl for pain control in special operations. *J Spec Oper Med.* 2008;8(1):48-53.

466. Wedmore IS, Kotwal RS. McManus JG, et al. Safety and efficacy of oral transmucosal fentanyl citrate for prehospital pain control on the battlefield. *J Trauma Acute Care Surg.* 2012; 73(6)(Suppl 5):S490-S495.

467. Eastridge BJ, Mabry RL, Seguin P, et al. Death on the battlefield (2001-2011): implications for the future of combat casualty care. *J Trauma Acute Care Surg.* 2012;73(6)(Suppl 5):S431-S437.

468. Kelly JF, Ritenour AE, McLaughlin DF, et al. Injury severity and causes of death from Operation Iraqi Freedom and Operation Enduring Freedom: 2003-2004 versus 2006. *J Trauma.* 2008;64(2)(Suppl):S21-S26.

469. Jennings PA, Cameron P, Bernard S, et al. Morphine and ketamine is superior to morphine alone for out-of-hospital trauma analgesia: a randomized controlled trial. *Ann Emerg Med.* 2012;59(6):497-503.

470. Alonso-Serra HM, Weslet K. National Association of EMS Physicians Standards and Clinical Practices Committee. Prehospital Pain Management. *Prehosp Emerg Care.* 2003;7(4):482-488.

471. Cherry DA, Plummer JL, Gourlay GK, Coates KR, Odgers CL. Ketamine as an adjunct to morphine in the treatment of pain. *Pain.* 1995;62(1):119-121.

472. Howes MC. Ketamine for paediatric sedation/analgesia in the emergency department. *Emerg Med J.* 2004;21(3):275-280.

473. Porter K. Ketamine in prehospital care. *Emerg Med J.* 2004;21(3):351-354.

474. Jennings PA, Cameron P, Bernard S. Ketamine as an analgesic in the pre-hospital setting: a systematic review. *Acta Anaesthiol Scand.* 2011;55(6):638-643.

475. Gaydos SJ, Webb CM, Walters PL, King MR, Wildzunas RM. Comparison of the effects of ketamine and morphine on the performance of representative military tasks. U.S. Army Aeromedical Research Laboratory Report No. 2010-17. August 2010. http://www.dtic.mil/cgi-bin/GetTRDoc?AD=ADA528747. Accessed April 2, 2019.

476. Craven R. Ketamine. *Anaesthesia.* 2007; 62(Suppl 1):48-53.

477. White PF, Way WL, Trevor AJ. Ketamine-its pharmacology and therapeutic uses. *Anesthesiology.* 1982;56(2):119-136.

478. Subramaniam K, Subramaniam B, Steinbrook RA. Ketamine as adjuvant analgesic to opioids: a quantitative and qualitative systematic review. *Anesth Analg.* 2004;99(2):482–495.

479. Porter K. Ketamine in prehospital care. *Emerg Med J.* 2004;21(3):351-354.

480. American College of Emergency Physicians Policy Statement. Out of hospital use of analgesia and sedation. *Ann Emerg Med.* 2016;67:305-306.

481. Schmid RL, Sandler AN, Katz J. Use and efficacy of low-dose ketamine in the management of acute postoperative pain: a review of current techniques and outcomes. *Pain.* 1999;82(2):111-125.

482. Buvanendran A, Kroin J. Multimodal analgesia for controlling acute postoperative pain. *Curr Opin Anesthesiol.* 2009;22(5):588-593.

483. Black IH, McManus J. Pain management in current combat operations. *Prehosp Emerg Care.* 2009;13(2):223-227.

484. Burnett AM, Salzmann JG, Griffith KR, Kroeger B, Frascone RJ. The emergency department experience with prehospital ketamine: a case series of 13 patients. *Prehosp Emerg Care.* 2012;16(4):553-559.

485. Roback MG, Wathen JE, Bajaj L, Bothner JP. Adverse events associated with procedural sedation in a pediatric emergency department: a comparison of common parenteral drugs. *Acad Emerg Med.* 2005;12(6):508-513.

486. Ketamine Hydrochloride Injection, U.S.P. [package insert]. Lake Forest, IL: Bioniche Pharma USA, LLC; 2008.

487. Guldner GT, Petinaux B, Clemens P, Foster S, Antoine S. Ketamine for procedural sedation and analgesia by nonanesthesiologists in the field: a review for military health care providers. *Mil Med.* 2006;171(6):484-490.

488. Onifer D, Butler F, Gross K, et al. Replacement of promethazine with ondansetron for treatment of opioid and trauma-related nausea and vomiting in tactical combat casualty care. *J Spec Oper Med.* 2015;15:17-24.

489. Naval Medical Lessons Learned Center. Combat Medical Personnel Evaluation of Battlefield Trauma Care Equipment Initial Report. November 2011.

490. Gerhardt R, Reeves P, Kotwal R, et al. Analysis of prehospital documentation of injury-related pain assessment and analgesic administration on the contemporary battlefield. *Prehosp Emerg Care.* 2016;20:37-44.

491. Shackelford SA, Fowler M, Schultz K, Summers A, et al. Prehospital pain medication use by U.S. Forces in Afghanistan. *Mil Med.* 2015;180:304-309.

492. Schauer S, Robinson J, Mabry R, Howard J. Battlefield analgesia: TCCC guidelines are not being followed. *J Spec Oper Med.* 2015;15:85-89.

493. Motov S, Rockoff B, Cohen V, et al. Intravenous subdissociative-dose ketamine versus morphine for

analgesia in the emergency department: a randomized controlled trial. *Ann Emerg Med*. 2015;66:222-229.

494. Sin B. The use of ketamine for acute treatment of pain: a randomized, double-blind, placebo-controlled trial. *J Emerg Med*. 2017;52:601-608.

495. Wedmore I, Butler F. Battlefield analgesia in Tactical Combat Casualty Care. *Wilderness Environ Med*. 2017;28: S109-S116.

496. Russell KW, Scaife CL, Weber DC, et al. Wilderness Medical Society practice guidelines for the treatment of acute pain in remote environments: 2014 update. *Wilderness Environ Med*. 2014;25(Suppl):S96-S104.

497. Ivascu FA, Howells GA, Junn FS, Bair HA, Bendick PJ, Janczyk RJ. Predictors of mortality in trauma patients with intracranial hemorrhage on preinjury aspirin or clopidogrel. *J Trauma*. 2008;65(4):785-788.

498. Harris M, Baba R, Nahouraii R, Gould P. Self-induced bleeding diathesis in soldiers at a FOB in south eastern Afghanistan. *Mil Med*. 2012;177(8):928-929.

499. Singer AJ, Mynster CJ, McMahon BJ. The effect of IM ketorolac on bleeding time: a prospective, interventional, controlled study. *Am J Emerg Med*. 2003;21(5):441-443.

500. Greer IA. Effect of ketorolac tromethamine on hemostasis. *Pharmacotherapy*. 1990;10(6 pt 2):71S-76S.

501. Blyth D, Yun H, Tribble D, Murray C. Lessons of war: combat-related injury infections during the Vietnam War and Operation Iraqi and Enduring Freedom. *J Trauma Acute Care Surg*. 2015 Oct;79(4 Suppl 2):S227-S235.

502. Murray CK, Hsu JR, Solomkin JS, et al. Prevention and management of infections associated with combat-related extremity injuries. *J Trauma*. 2008 Mar;64(3 Suppl): S239-251.

503. Murray CK. Epidemiology of infections associated with combat-related injuries in Iraq and Afghanistan. *J Trauma*. 2008 Mar;64(3 Suppl):S232-S238.

504. Poole LT. Army progress with penicillin. *Br J Surg*. 1944;32(125):110–111.

505. Scott R Jr. Care of the battle casualty in advance of the aid station. Medical Science Publication No. 4, Volume 1. U.S. Army Medical Department Office of Medical History website. http://history.amedd.army.mil/booksdocs/korea /recad1/ch1-4.html. Accessed March 14, 2019.

506. Hopkins T, Daley M, Rose D, et al. Presumptive antibiotic therapy for civilian trauma injuries. *J Trauma Acute Care Surg*. 2016 Oct;81(4):765-774.

507. O'Connor K, Butler F. Antibiotics in tactical combat casualty care 2002. *Mil Med*. 2003;168(11):911-914.

508. Butler FK, Hagmann J, Butler EG. Tactical combat casualty care in special operations. *Mil Med*. 1996;161(Suppl):3-16.

509. Mellor SG, Cooper GJ, Bowyer GW. Efficacy of delayed administration of benzylpenicillin in the control of infection in penetrating soft tissue injuries in war. *J Trauma*. 1996;40(Suppl 3):S128-S134.

510. Penn-Barwell J, Murray C, Wenke J. Early antibiotics and debridement independently reduce infection in an open fracture model. *J Bone Joint Surg Br*. 2012 Jan;94(1): 107-112.

511. Hospenthal DR, Murray CK, Anderson RC, et al. Guidelines for prevention of infection after combat-related injuries. *J Trauma*. 2008;64(3)(Suppl):S211-S220.

512. Mabry RL, Holcomb JB, Baker AM, et al. United States Army Rangers in Somalia: an analysis of combat casualties on an urban battlefield. *J Trauma*. 2000;49(3):515-528.

513. Tarpey MJ. Tactical Combat Casualty Care in Operation Iraqi Freedom. *U.S. Army Med Dep J*. April-June 2005;38-41.

514. Butler FK, Holcomb JB, Giebner SD, McSwain NE, Bagian J. Tactical combat casualty care 2007: evolving concepts and battlefield experience. *Mil Med*. 2007;172(11) (Suppl):1-19.

515. Yun H, Murray C, Nelson K, Bosse M. Infection after orthopaedic trauma: prevention and treatment. *J Orthop Trauma*. 2016 Oct;30 Suppl 3:S21-S26.

516. Hospenthal DR, Murray CK, Andersen RC, et al. Guidelines for the prevention of infections associated with combat-related injuries: 2011 update: endorsed by the Infectious Diseases Society of America and the Surgical Infection Society. *J Trauma*. 2011 Aug;71(2 Suppl 2):S210-234.

517. Lack W, Karunakar M, Angerame M, et al. Type III open tiba fractures: immediate antibiotic prophylaxis minimizes infection. *J Orthop Trauma*. 2016;29(1):1-6.

518. Montgomery H, Butler F, Kerr W, et al. TCCC guidelines comprehensive review and update: TCCC guidelines change 16-03. *J Spec Oper Med*. 2017;17:21-38.

519. Butler FK, Hagmann JH, Richards DT. Tactical management of urban warfare casualties in special operations. *Mil Med*. 2000 Apr;165(4 Suppl):1-48.

520. Yamada C, Nagashima K, Takahashi A, et al. Gatifloxacin acutely stimulates insulin secretion and chronically suppresses insulin biosynthesis. *Eur J Pharmacol*. 2006;553(1-3):67-72.

521. Ahmed S, Kuruvilla O, Chin Yee D, et al. Intraocular penetration of systemic antibiotics in eyes with penetrating ocular injury. *J Ocul Pharmacol Ther*. 2014 Dec;30(10):823-830.

522. Murray CK. Field wound care: prophylactic antibiotics. *Wilderness Environ Med*. 2017 Jun;28(2S):S90-S102.

523. Saeed O, Tribble D, Biever K, Kavanaugh M, Crouch H. Joint Trauma System Clinical Practice guideline: infection prevention in combat-related injuries. https://jts.amedd .army.mil/assets/docs/cpgs/JTS_Clinical_Practice_Guidelines _(CPGs)/Infection_Prevention_in_Combat-Related_Injuries _08_Aug_2016_ID24.pdf. Updated August 8, 2016. Accessed March 14, 2019.

524. Montgomery H, Butler F, Kerr W, et al. TCCC guidelines comprehensive review and update: TCCC guidelines change 16-03. *J Spec Oper Med*. 2017;17:21-38.

525. Butler FK, Hagmann J, Butler EG. Tactical combat casualty care in special operations. *Mil Med*. 1996;161(Suppl):3-16.

526. Battistella FD, Nugent W, Owings JT, Anderson JT. Field triage of the pulseless trauma patient. *Arch Surg*. 1999;134(7):742-745.

527. Branney SW, Moore EE, Feldhaus KM, Wolfe RE. Critical analysis of two decades of experience with postinjury emergency department thoracotomy in a regional trauma center. *J Trauma*. 1988;45(1):87-94.

528. Rosemurgy AS, Norris PA, Olson SM, Hurst JM, Albrink MH. Prehospital traumatic cardiac arrest: the cost of futility. *J Trauma*. 1993;35(3):468-473.

529. Wieneke H, Konorza T, Breuckmann F, Reinsch N, Erbel R. Automatic external defibrillator—mode of operation and clinical use (in German). *Dtsch Med Wochenschr.* 2008;133(42):2163-2167.

530. De Maio VJ, Stiell IG, Wells GA, Spaite DW; Ontario Prehospital Advanced Life Support Study Group. Optimal defibrillation response intervals for maximum out-of-hospital cardiac arrest survival rates. *Ann Emerg Med.* 2003;42(2):242-250.

531. Mitchell T, Waldrep K, Sams V, et al. An 8-year review of Operation Enduring Freedom and Operation Iraqi Freedom resuscitative thoracotomies. *Mil Med.* 2015;180:33-36.

532. Evans C, Petersen A, Meier E, et al. Prehospital traumatic cardiac arrest: management and outcomes from the resuscitation outcomes consortium epistry-trauma and PROPHET registries. *J Trauma Acute Care Surg.* 2016;81(2):285-293.

533. Tarmey N, Park C, Bartels O, et al. Outcomes following military traumatic cardiorespiratory arrest: a prospective observational study. *Resuscitation.* 2011;82:1194-1197.

534. Jeffcoach D, Gallegos J, Jesty S, et al. Use of CPR in hemorrhagic shock, a dog model. *J Trauma Acute Care Surg.* 2016;81(1):27-33.

535. Smith J, Le Clerc S, Hunt P. Challenging the dogma of traumatic cardiac arrest management: a military perspective. *Emerg Med J.* 2015 Dec;32(12):955-960.

536. Dickey N, Jenkins D. Needle Decompression of Tension Pneumothorax and Cardiopulmonary Resuscitation Tactical Combat Casualty Care guideline recommendations 2011-08. Defense Health Board memo. October 11, 2011. https://health.mil/About-MHS/OASDHA/Defense-Health-Agency/Defense-Health-Board/Reports. Accessed April 5, 2019.

537. Mistry N, Bleetman A, Roberts K. Chest decompression during the resuscitation of patients in prehospital traumatic cardiac arrest. *Emerg Med J.* 2009;26(10):738-740.

538. Eastridge BJ, Mabry RL, Seguin P, et al. Death on the battlefield (2001-2011): implications for the future of combat casualty care. *J Trauma Acute Care Surg.* 2012;73(6)(Suppl 5):S431-S437.

539. Eastridge BJ, Mabry R, Blackbourne LH, Butler FK. We don't know what we don't know: prehospital data in combat casualty care. *U.S. Army Med Dep J.* 2011 Apr-Jun;11-14.

540. Caravalho J. Dismounted Complex Injury Task Force. Report of the Army Dismounted Complex Injury Task Force. https://armymedicine.health.mil/reports. Published June 18, 2011. Accessed April 8, 2019.

541. Butler F. Leadership lessons learned in tactical combat casualty care. *J Trauma Acute Care Surg.* 2017 Jun;82(6 Suppl 1):S16-S25.

542. Kotwal RS, Butler FK, Montgomery HR, et al. The Tactical Combat Casualty Care Casualty Card. *J Spec Oper Med.* 2013;13:82-86.

543. Kotwal RS, Butler FK, Edgar EP, Shackelford SA, Bennett DR, Bailey JA. Saving lives on the battlefield: a joint trauma system review of pre-hospital trauma care in combined joint operating area—Afghanistan (CJOA-A).

January 30, 2013. Defense Technical Information Center website. https://apps.dtic.mil/dtic/tr/fulltext/u2/a573744.pdf. Accessed April 8, 2019.

544. Kotwal RS, Montgomery HR, Kotwal BM, et al. Eliminating preventable death on the battlefield. *Arch Surgery.* 2011;146:1350-1358.

545. Wilensky G, Holcomb J. Tactical Combat Casualty Care and Minimizing Preventable Fatalities in Combat. Defense Health Board memorandum. August 6, 2009. https://health.mil/About-MHS/OASDHA/Defense-Health-Agency/Defense-Health-Board/Reports. Accessed April 8, 2019.

546. Velopulos C, Shihab H, Lottenberg L, et al. Prehospital spine immobilization/spinal motion restriction in penetrating trauma: a practice management guideline from the Eastern Association for the Surgery of Trauma (EAST). *J Trauma Acute Care Surg.* 2018 May;84(5):736-744.

547. Kotwal R, Howard J, Orman J, et al. The effect of a golden hour policy on morbidity and mortality of combat casualties. *JAMA Surg.* 2016;151:15-24.

548. Holcomb JB, McMullin NR, Pearse L, et al. Causes of death in special operations forces in the global war on terrorism. *Ann Surg.* 2007;245(6):986-991.

549. Eastridge BJ, Mabry RL, Seguin P, et al. Death on the battlefield (2001-2011): implications for the future of combat casualty care. *J Trauma Acute Care Surg.* 2012;73(6)(Suppl 5):S431-S437.

550. Kelly JF, Ritenour AE, McLaughlin DF, et al. Injury severity and causes of death from Operation Iraqi Freedom and Operation Enduring Freedom: 2003-2004 versus 2006. *J Trauma.* 2008;64(2)(Suppl):S21-S26.

551. Butler F. Leadership lessons learned in tactical combat casualty care. *J Trauma Acute Care Surg.* 2017;82:S16-S25.

552. Kotwal R, Montgomery H, Miles E, et al. Leadership and a casualty response system for eliminating preventable death. *J Trauma Acute Care Surg.* 2017;82:S9-S15.

553. Butler F, Smith D, Carmona R. Implementing and preserving the advances in combat casualty care from Iraq and Afghanistan throughout the U.S. military. *J Trauma Acute Care Surg.* 2015;79:321-326.

554. Schauer SG, April MD, Naylor JF, et al. Prehospital administration of tranexamic acid by ground forces in Afghanistan: the prehospital trauma registry experience. *J Spec Oper Med.* 2017;17:55-58.

555. Mabry R. An analysis of battlefield cricothyrotomy in Iraq and Afghanistan. *J Spec Oper Med.* 2012;12:17-23.

556. Butler F. Fluid resuscitation in Tactical Combat Casualty Care: yesterday and today. *Wilderness Environ Med.* 2017;28:S74-S81.

557. Kotwal RS, Butler FK, Montgomery HR, et al. The Tactical Combat Casualty Care Casualty Card. *J Spec Oper Med.* 2013;13:82-86.

558. Eastridge BJ, Mabry RL, Blackbourne LH, Butler FK. We don't know what we don't know: prehospital data in combat casualty care. *U.S. Army Med Dep J.* 2011 Apr-Jun;11-14.

559. Murray CK, Hospenthal DR, Kotwal RS, Butler FK. Efficacy of point-of-injury combat antimicrobials. *J Trauma.* 2011 Aug;71(2 Suppl 2):S307-S313.

560. Harris M, Baba R, Nahouraii R, Gould P. Self-induced bleeding diathesis in soldiers at a FOB in South Eastern Afghanistan. *Mil Med.* 2012 Aug;177(8):928-929.

561. Butler FK Jr, Holcomb JB, Shackelford S, et al. Management of suspected tension pneumothorax in Tactical Combat Casualty Care: TCCC guidelines change 17-02. *J Spec Oper Med.* 2018 Summer;18(2):19-35.

562. Gerhardt R, Reeves P, Kotwal R, et al. Analysis of prehospital documentation of injury-related pain assessment and analgesic administration on the contemporary battlefield. *Prehosp Emerg Care.* 2016;20:37-44.

563. Mazzoli R, Gross K, Butler F. The use of rigid eye shields (Fox shields) at the point of injury for ocular trauma in Afghanistan. *J Trauma Acute Care Surg.* 2014 Sep;77(3 Suppl 2):S156-162.

CHAPTER **26**

Tactical Evacuation Care

Authors:
Capt. (Ret) Frank Butler, MD
Senior Master Sgt. Travis Shaw
Col. Jay Johannigman, MD
Lt. Col. (Ret) John Gandy, MD

CHAPTER OBJECTIVES

At the completion of this chapter, you will be able to do the following:

- Delineate the scope of Tactical Evacuation (TACEVAC) Care and its inclusion of both casualty evacuation (CASEVAC) and medical evacuation (MEDEVAC).
- Describe the differences between Tactical Field Care and Tactical Evacuation Care.
- Describe the additional interventions that may be indicated given the increased stability of the circumstances and the additional personnel and equipment that should be available in TACEVAC.
- Describe which casualties are most likely to benefit from supplemental oxygen.
- Discuss the indications for and administration of tranexamic acid during tactical evacuation.

- List the indications for transfusions in the field and discuss the requirement to do so under protocol.
- Discuss the management of moderate to severe traumatic brain injury, including impending cerebral herniation, during TACEVAC.
- Discuss the use of extraglottic airways during TACEVAC.
- Discuss the need to monitor and adjust pressure in air-filled airway cuffs during TACEVAC.
- Describe the importance of and the methods for documenting casualty care.
- Discuss the role of cardiopulmonary resuscitation in combat casualties during TACEVAC.
- Describe the management of wounded hostile combatants during TACEVAC.

SCENARIO

You are a medic aboard a medical evacuation (MEDEVAC) Black Hawk helicopter that has landed in a secure landing zone (LZ) in the mountains of southeastern Afghanistan to extract a Ranger who has multiple shrapnel wounds from a rocket-propelled grenade (RPG) blast. The LZ altitude is 6,000 feet (ft; 1,800 meters [m]), and the ambient temperature is 64°F (18°C). The casualty, who has been stabilized by the platoon medic, is able to converse normally and has a tourniquet over his uniform on his upper right thigh. The trousers are cut open below the tourniquet, and there is a pressure dressing around his lower thigh and another around his middle calf. His right shirtsleeve is missing, and there is a pressure dressing around his right upper arm. There is a saline lock in his left antecubital fossa. The platoon medic tells you the casualty lost a lot of blood from his thigh wound and was drowsy and confused before the tourniquet was applied 30 minutes ago. He received

(continued)

SCENARIO (CONTINUED)

2 units of cold-stored type O low-titer whole blood to which he responded well. He has been stable since. The wounds with pressure dressings were all packed with Combat Gauze underneath. He has taken moxifloxacin 400 milligrams (mg) by mouth and has an 800-microgram (mcg) fentanyl lozenge in his right cheek. He has been drinking water from his canteen.

- What are your considerations for the care of this casualty during the 30-minute helicopter flight back to the Combat Support Hospital?
- What do you do first?
- What do you do next?
- Should you start an intravenous (IV) line through the saline lock in anticipation of the need for a second whole blood transfusion?
- Should you remove the tourniquet?
- Should you remove the fentanyl lozenge?
- What else do you want to do?
- Is there anything else to attend to during the flight to the Combat Support Hospital?

INTRODUCTION

The term *casualty evacuation*, or CASEVAC, is used to describe the unregulated movement of casualties from the point of wounding to the first point of surgical care (Role 2 Forward Surgical Team or Role 3 Combat Support Hospital). CASEVAC platforms are typically armed tactical assets that bear no Red Cross markings. These may be aircraft, vehicles, or maritime vessels of opportunity. During the drive on Baghdad in Operation Iraqi Freedom, some casualties were moved to the rear on tanks because MEDEVAC aircraft and vehicles were not feasible given the tactical circumstances.

The term *medical evacuation*, or MEDEVAC, refers to medically regulated casualty movement using dedicated medical evacuation platforms (typically rotary-wing aircraft or, less commonly, ground vehicles). These are crewed by medical attendants and generally have more medical treatment equipment available than nonmedical platforms. MEDEVAC platforms are predesignated assets that bear Red Cross markings and carry no offensive weaponry such as rockets or missiles. MEDEVAC movements may include both clearing casualties from the battlefield and moving casualties between medical treatment facilities.

Because casualty movement following Tactical Field Care (TFC) may be either CASEVAC or MEDEVAC, the third phase of care in Tactical Combat Casualty Care (TCCC) is designated Tactical Evacuation (TACEVAC) Care to encompass both types of platforms.

In contrast, the term *aeromedical evacuation* is typically used to describe the aeromedical transfer of casualties between medical treatment facilities in theater or to a Role 4 hospital outside the theater of combat. Aeromedical evacuation is beyond the scope of TCCC but will be discussed in a later chapter. En route care is a more general term that includes all of these types of casualty transport.

Tactical Evacuation Care Versus Tactical Field Care

Evacuation of the wounded from the battlefield using ground, air, or maritime platforms presents an opportunity to bring in additional medical equipment and personnel. This allows for more advanced (electronic) monitoring and therapeutic measures as outlined in the TCCC Guidelines for the Tactical Evacuation (TACEVAC) Care phase (**Box 26-1**). For example, the TACEVAC provider may have more options for airway management, fluid resuscitation, and prevention of hypothermia than were available in Care Under Fire or TFC. As noted in the 2012 TCCC update paper:[1]

Recent reviews of this topic have offered the possibility for significant improvements in care through providing evacuation providers trained to at least the critical care flight paramedic level, ensuring that blood and plasma are available for casualties in hemorrhagic shock, using the most capable evacuation platforms available, ensuring TCCC training for all evacuation providers, and having advanced airway options, intravenously administered medications, and other interventions routinely available for critical casualties. The survival advantage has been found to be the greatest, as would be expected, in the subset of casualties with severe but not overwhelming injuries.

Box 26-1 Basic Management Plan for Tactical Evacuation Care—1 August 2018

1. **Transition of Care**
   a. Tactical force personnel should establish evacuation point security and stage casualties for evacuation.
   b. Tactical force personnel or the medic should communicate patient information and status to TACEVAC personnel as clearly as possible. The minimum information communicated should include stable or unstable, injuries identified, and treatments rendered.
   c. TACEVAC personnel should stage casualties on evacuation platforms as required.
   d. Secure casualties in the evacuation platform in accordance with unit policies, platform configurations, and safety requirements.
   e. TACEVAC medical personnel should reassess casualties and reevaluate all injuries and previous interventions.

2. **Massive Hemorrhage**
   a. Assess for unrecognized hemorrhage and control all sources of bleeding. If not already done, use a CoTCCC-recommended limb tourniquet to control life-threatening external hemorrhage that is anatomically amenable to tourniquet use or for any traumatic amputation. Apply directly to the skin 2-3 inches above the bleeding site. If bleeding is not controlled with the first tourniquet, apply a second tourniquet side-by-side with the first.
   b. For compressible (external) hemorrhage not amenable to limb tourniquet use or as an adjunct to tourniquet removal, use Combat Gauze as the CoTCCC hemostatic dressing of choice.
      - Alternative hemostatic adjuncts:
        · Celox Gauze or
        · ChitoGauze or
        · XStat (best for deep, narrow-tract junctional wounds)
      - Hemostatic dressings should be applied with at least 3 minutes of direct pressure (optional for XStat). Each dressing works differently, so if one fails to control bleeding, it may be removed and a fresh dressing of the same type or a different type applied. (Note: XStat is not to be removed in the field, but additional XStat, other hemostatic adjuncts, or trauma dressings may be applied over it.)
      - If the bleeding site is amenable to use of a junctional tourniquet, immediately apply a CoTCCC-recommended junctional tourniquet. Do not delay in the application of the junctional tourniquet once it is ready for use. Apply hemostatic dressings with direct pressure if a junctional tourniquet is not available or while the junctional tourniquet is being readied for use.

3. **Airway Management**
   a. Conscious casualty with no airway problem identified:
      - No airway intervention required
   b. Unconscious casualty without airway obstruction:
      - Place casualty in the recovery position.
      - Chin lift or jaw thrust maneuver or
      - Nasopharyngeal airway or
      - Extraglottic airway
   c. Casualty with airway obstruction or impending airway obstruction:
      - Allow a conscious casualty to assume any position that best protects the airway, to include sitting up.
      - Use a chin lift or jaw thrust maneuver.
      - Use suction if available and appropriate.
      - Nasopharyngeal airway or
      - Extraglottic airway (if the casualty is unconscious)
      - Place an unconscious casualty in the recovery position.
   d. If the previous measures are unsuccessful, assess the tactical and clinical situations, the equipment at hand, and the skills and experience of the person providing care, and then select one of the following airway interventions:
      - Endotracheal intubation or
      - Perform a surgical cricothyrotomy using one of the following:
        · Cric-Key technique (Preferred option)
        · Bougie-aided open surgical technique using a flanged and cuffed airway cannula of less than 10 mm outer diameter, 6-7 mm internal diameter, and 5-8 cm of intratracheal length
        · Standard open surgical technique using a flanged and cuffed airway cannula of less than 10 mm outer diameter, 6-7 mm internal diameter, and 5-8 cm of intratracheal length (Least desirable option)
        · Use lidocaine if the casualty is conscious.

(continued)

Box 26-1 Basic Management Plan for Tactical Evacuation Care—1 August 2018 (*continued*)

e. Cervical spine stabilization is not necessary for casualties who have sustained only penetrating trauma.

f. Monitor the hemoglobin oxygen saturation in casualties to help assess airway patency. Use capnography monitoring in this phase of care if available.

g. Always remember that the casualty's airway status may change over time and requires frequent reassessment.

Notes:

- The i-gel is the preferred extraglottic airway because its gel-filled cuff makes it simpler to use and avoids the need for cuff inflation and monitoring. If an extraglottic airway with an air-filled cuff is used, the cuff pressure must be monitored to avoid overpressurization, especially during TACEVAC on an aircraft with the accompanying pressure changes.

- Extraglottic airways will not be tolerated by a casualty who is not deeply unconscious. If an unconscious casualty without direct airway trauma needs an airway intervention, but does not tolerate an extraglottic airway, consider the use of a nasopharyngeal airway.

- For casualties with trauma to the face and mouth, or facial burns with suspected inhalation injury, nasopharyngeal airways and extraglottic airways may not suffice, and a surgical cricothyroidotomy may be required.

- Surgical cricothyroidotomies should not be performed on unconscious casualties who have no direct airway trauma unless use of a nasopharyngeal airway and/or an extraglottic airway have been unsuccessful in opening the airway.

4. **Respiration/Breathing**

a. Assess for tension pneumothorax and treat as necessary.

- Suspect a tension pneumothorax and treat when a casualty has significant torso trauma or primary blast injury and one or more of the following:
  - Severe or progressive respiratory distress
  - Severe or progressive tachypnea
  - Absent or markedly decreased breath sounds on one side of the chest
  - Hemoglobin oxygen saturation <90% on pulse oximetry
  - Shock
  - Traumatic cardiac arrest without obviously fatal wounds

- Initial treatment of suspected tension pneumothorax:
  - If the casualty has a chest seal in place, burp or remove the chest seal.

- Establish pulse oximetry monitoring.
- Place the casualty in the supine or recovery position unless he or she is conscious and needs to sit up to help keep the airway clear as a result of maxillofacial trauma.
- Decompress the chest on the side of the injury with a 14-gauge or a 10-gauge, 3.25-inch needle/catheter unit.
- If a casualty has significant torso trauma or primary blast injury and is in traumatic cardiac arrest (no pulse, no respirations, no response to painful stimuli, no other signs of life), decompress both sides of the chest before discontinuing treatment.

- The NDC should be considered successful if:
  - Respiratory distress improves, or
  - There is an obvious hissing sound as air escapes from the chest when NDC is performed (this may be difficult to appreciate in high-noise environments), or
  - Hemoglobin oxygen saturation increases to 90% or greater (note that this may take several minutes and may not happen at altitude), or
  - A casualty with no vital signs has return of consciousness and/or radial pulse.

- If the initial NDC fails to improve the casualty's signs/symptoms from the suspected tension pneumothorax:
  - Perform a second NDC on the same side of the chest at whichever of the two recommended sites was not previously used. Use a new needle/catheter unit for the second attempt.
  - Consider, based on the mechanism of injury and physical findings, whether decompression of the opposite side of the chest may be needed.

- If the initial NDC was successful, but symptoms later recur:
  - Perform another NDC at the same site that was used previously. Use a new needle/catheter unit for the repeat NDC.
  - Continue to reassess!

- If the second NDC is also not successful:
  - Continue on to the Circulation section of the TCCC Guidelines.

b. Initiate pulse oximetry if not previously done. All individuals with moderate/severe TBI should be monitored with pulse oximetry. Readings may be misleading in the settings of shock or marked hypothermia.

c. Most combat casualties do not require supplemental oxygen, but administration of oxygen may be of benefit for the following types of casualties:
   - Low oxygen saturation by pulse oximetry
   - Injuries associated with impaired oxygenation
   - Unconscious casualty
   - Casualty with TBI (maintain oxygen saturation >90%)
   - Casualty in shock
   - Casualty at altitude
   - Known or suspected smoke inhalation

d. All open and/or sucking chest wounds should be treated by immediately applying a vented chest seal to cover the defect. If a vented chest seal is not available, use a nonvented chest seal. Monitor the casualty for the potential development of a subsequent tension pneumothorax. If the casualty develops increasing hypoxia, respiratory distress, or hypotension and a tension pneumothorax is suspected, treat by burping or removing the dressing or by needle decompression.

Notes:
- If not treated promptly, tension pneumothorax may progress from respiratory distress to shock and traumatic cardiac arrest.
- Either the 5th intercostal space (ICS) in the anterior axillary line (AAL) or the 2nd ICS in the midclavicular line (MCL) may be used for needle decompression (NDC). If the anterior (MCL) site is used, do not insert the needle medial to the nipple line.
- The needle/catheter unit should be inserted at an angle perpendicular to the chest wall and just over the top of the lower rib at the insertion site. Insert the needle/catheter unit all the way to the hub and hold it in place for 5-10 seconds to allow decompression to occur.
- After the NDC has been performed, remove the needle and leave the catheter in place.

5. **Circulation**
   a. Bleeding
      - A pelvic binder should be applied for cases of suspected pelvic fracture:
        - Severe blunt force or blast injury with one or more of the following indications:
          - Pelvic pain
          - Any major lower limb amputation or near amputation
          - Physical exam findings suggestive of a pelvic fracture
          - Unconsciousness
          - Shock

      - Reassess prior tourniquet application. Expose the wound and determine if a tourniquet is needed. If it is needed, replace any limb tourniquet placed over the uniform with one applied directly to the skin 2-3 inches above the bleeding site. Ensure that bleeding is stopped. If there is no traumatic amputation, a distal pulse should be checked. If bleeding persists or a distal pulse is still present, consider additional tightening of the tourniquet or the use of a second tourniquet side-by-side with the first to eliminate both bleeding and the distal pulse. If the reassessment determines that the prior tourniquet was not needed, then remove the tourniquet and note time of removal on the TCCC Casualty Card.
      - Limb tourniquets and junctional tourniquets should be converted to hemostatic or pressure dressings as soon as possible if three criteria are met: the casualty is not in shock; it is possible to monitor the wound closely for bleeding; and the tourniquet is not being used to control bleeding from an amputated extremity. Every effort should be made to convert tourniquets in less than 2 hours if bleeding can be controlled with other means. Do not remove a tourniquet that has been in place more than 6 hours unless close monitoring and lab capability are available.
      - Expose and clearly mark all tourniquets with the time of tourniquet application. Note tourniquets applied and time of application; time of reapplication, time of conversion, and time of removal on the TCCC Casualty Card. Use a permanent marker to mark on the tourniquet and the casualty card.

   b. IV Access
      - Reassess need for IV access.
      - IV or IO access is indicated if the casualty is in hemorrhagic shock or at significant risk of shock (and may therefore need fluid resuscitation), or if the casualty needs medications, but cannot take them by mouth.
        - An 18-gauge IV or saline lock is preferred.
        - If vascular access is needed but not quickly obtainable via the IV route, use the IO route.

(continued)

Box 26-1 Basic Management Plan for Tactical Evacuation Care—1 August 2018 (*continued*)

c. Tranexamic Acid (TXA)
  – If a casualty is anticipated to need significant blood transfusion (for example: presents with hemorrhagic shock, one or more major amputations, penetrating torso trauma, or evidence of severe bleeding):
    · Administer 1 gm of tranexamic acid in 100 ml Normal Saline or Lactated Ringers as soon as possible but NOT later than 3 hours after injury. When given, TXA should be administered over 10 minutes by IV infusion.
    · Begin second infusion of 1 gm TXA after initial fluid resuscitation has been completed.

d. Fluid Resuscitation
  – Assess for hemorrhagic shock (altered mental status in the absence of brain injury and/or weak or absent radial pulse).
  – The resuscitation fluids of choice for casualties in hemorrhagic shock, listed from most to least preferred, are: whole blood*; plasma, RBCs, and platelets in a 1:1:1 ratio*; plasma and RBCs in a 1:1 ratio; plasma or RBCs alone; Hextend; and crystalloid (Lactated Ringer's or Plasma-Lyte A). (NOTE: Hypothermia prevention measures [Section 7] should be initiated while fluid resuscitation is being accomplished.)
    · If not in shock:
      - No IV fluids are immediately necessary.
      - Fluids by mouth are permissible if the casualty is conscious and can swallow.
    · If in shock and blood products are available under an approved command or theater blood product administration protocol:
      - Resuscitate with whole blood*, or, if not available
      - Plasma, RBCs, and platelets in a 1:1:1 ratio*, or, if not available
      - Plasma and RBCs in a 1:1 ratio, or, if not available
      - Reconstituted dried plasma, liquid plasma, or thawed plasma alone, or RBCs alone
      - Reassess the casualty after each unit. Continue resuscitation until a palpable radial pulse, improved mental status, or systolic BP of 80 to 90 is present.
    · If in shock and blood products are not available under an approved command

or theater blood product administration protocol due to tactical or logistical constraints:
    - Resuscitate with Hextend, or, if not available
    - Lactated Ringer's or Plasma-Lyte A
    - Reassess the casualty after each 500 ml IV bolus.
    - Continue resuscitation until a palpable radial pulse, improved mental status, or systolic BP of 80 to 90 mm Hg is present.
    - Discontinue fluid administration when one or more of the above end points has been achieved.
  – If a casualty with an altered mental status due to suspected TBI has a weak or absent radial pulse, resuscitate as necessary to restore and maintain a normal radial pulse. If BP monitoring is available, maintain a target systolic BP of at least 90 mm Hg.
  – Reassess the casualty frequently to check for recurrence of shock. If shock recurs, recheck all external hemorrhage control measures to ensure that they are still effective, and repeat the fluid resuscitation as outlined above.

e. Refractory Shock
  – If a casualty in shock is not responding to fluid resuscitation, consider untreated tension pneumothorax as a possible cause of refractory shock. Thoracic trauma, persistent respiratory distress, absent breath sounds, and hemoglobin oxygen saturation <90% support this diagnosis. Treat as indicated with repeated NDC or finger thoracostomy/chest tube insertion at the 5th ICS in the AAL, according to the skills, experience, and authorizations of the treating medical provider. Note that if finger thoracostomy is used, it may not remain patent and finger decompression through the incision may have to be repeated. Consider decompressing the opposite side of the chest if indicated based on the mechanism of injury and physical findings.

Note:
· Currently, neither whole blood nor apheresis platelets collected in theater are FDA-compliant because of the way they are collected. Consequently, whole blood and 1:1:1 resuscitation using apheresis platelets should be used only if all the FDA-compliant blood products needed to support 1:1:1 resuscitation are not available, or if 1:1:1 resuscitation is not producing the desired clinical effect.

6. **Traumatic Brain Injury**
   a. Casualties with moderate/severe TBI should be monitored for:
      - Decreases in level of consciousness
      - Pupillary dilation
      - SBP should be >90 mm Hg
      - O_2 sat >90
      - Hypothermia
      - End-tidal CO_2 (If capnography is available, maintain between 35 and 40 mm Hg.)
      - Penetrating head trauma (if present, administer antibiotics.)
      - Assume a spinal (neck) injury until cleared.
   b. Unilateral pupillary dilation accompanied by a decreased level of consciousness may signify impending cerebral herniation; if these signs occur, take the following actions to decrease intracranial pressure:
      - Administer 250 ml of 3 or 5% hypertonic saline bolus.
      - Elevate the casualty's head 30 degrees.
      - Hyperventilate the casualty.
        - Respiratory rate 20
        - Capnography should be used to maintain the end-tidal CO_2 between 30 and 35 mm Hg
        - The highest oxygen concentration (FIO_2) possible should be used for hyperventilation.

   Notes:
   - Do not hyperventilate the casualty unless signs of impending herniation are present.
   - Casualties may be hyperventilated with oxygen using the bag-valve-mask technique.

7. **Hypothermia Prevention**
   a. Minimize casualty's exposure to the elements. Keep protective gear on or with the casualty if feasible.
   b. Replace wet clothing with dry if possible. Get the casualty onto an insulated surface as soon as possible.
   c. Apply the Ready Heat Blanket from the Hypothermia Prevention and Management Kit (HPMK) to the casualty's torso (not directly on the skin) and cover the casualty with the Heat Reflective Shell (HRS).
   d. If an HRS is not available, the previously recommended combination of the blizzard survival blanket and the Ready Heat Blanket may also be used.
   e. If the items mentioned above are not available, use poncho liners, sleeping bags, or anything that will retain heat and keep the casualty dry.

   f. Use a portable fluid warmer capable of warming all IV fluids, including blood products.
   g. Protect the casualty from wind if doors must be kept open.

8. **Penetrating Eye Trauma**
   a. If a penetrating eye injury is noted or suspected:
      - Perform a rapid field test of visual acuity and document findings.
      - Cover the eye with a rigid eye shield (NOT a pressure patch.)
      - Ensure that the 400 mg moxifloxacin tablet in the Combat Wound Medication Pack (CWMP) is taken if possible and that IV/IM antibiotics are given as outlined below if oral moxifloxacin cannot be taken.

9. **Monitoring**
   a. Initiate advanced electronic monitoring if indicated and if monitoring equipment is available.

10. **Analgesia**
    a. Analgesia on the battlefield should generally be achieved using one of three options:
       - Option 1
         - Mild to Moderate Pain
         - Casualty is still able to fight
           - TCCC CWMP
             - Tylenol: 650 mg bilayer caplet, 2 PO every 8 hours
             - Meloxicam: 15 mg PO once a day
       - Option 2
         - Moderate to Severe Pain
         - Casualty IS NOT in shock or respiratory distress AND
         - Casualty IS NOT at significant risk of developing either condition.
           - Oral transmucosal fentanyl citrate (OTFC) 800 mcg
             - Place lozenge between the cheek and the gum.
             - Do not chew the lozenge.
       - Option 3
         - Moderate to Severe Pain
         - Casualty IS in hemorrhagic shock or respiratory distress, OR
         - Casualty IS at significant risk of developing either condition.
           - Ketamine 50 mg IM or IN
           Or
           - Ketamine 20 mg slow IV or IO
             - Repeat doses q30min prn for IM or IN.

(continued)

Box 26-1 Basic Management Plan for Tactical Evacuation Care—1 August 2018 (*continued*)

- · Repeat doses q20min prn for IV or IO.
- · End points: Control of pain or development of nystagmus (rhythmic back-and-forth movement of the eyes)

Notes:
- · Casualties may need to be disarmed after being given OTFC or ketamine.
- · Document a mental status exam using the AVPU method prior to administering opioids or ketamine.
- · For all casualties given opioids or ketamine—monitor airway, breathing, and circulation closely.
- · Directions for administering OTFC:
  - – Recommend taping lozenge-on-a-stick to casualty's finger as an added safety measure OR utilizing a safety pin and rubber band to attach the lozenge (under tension) to the patient's uniform or plate carrier.
  - – Reassess in 15 minutes.
  - – Add second lozenge, in other cheek, as necessary to control severe pain.
  - – Monitor for respiratory depression.
- · IV Morphine is an alternative to OTFC if IV access has been obtained.
  - – 5 mg IV/IO
  - – Reassess in 10 minutes.
  - – Repeat dose every 10 minutes as necessary to control severe pain.
  - – Monitor for respiratory depression.
- · Naloxone (0.4 mg IV or IM) should be available when using opioid analgesics.
- · Both ketamine and OTFC have the potential to worsen severe TBI. The combat medic, corpsman, or PJ must consider this fact in his or her analgesic decision, but if the casualty can complain of pain, then the TBI is likely not severe enough to preclude the use of ketamine or OTFC.
- · Eye injury does not preclude the use of ketamine. The risk of additional damage to the eye from using ketamine is low and maximizing the casualty's chance for survival takes precedence if the casualty is in shock or respiratory distress or at significant risk for either.
- · Ketamine may be a useful adjunct to reduce the amount of opioids required to provide effective pain relief. It is safe to give ketamine to a casualty who has previously received morphine or OTFC. IV Ketamine should be given over 1 minute.
- · If respirations are noted to be reduced after using opioids or ketamine, provide ventilatory support with a bag-valve-mask or mouth-to-mask ventilations.
- · Ondansetron, 4 mg ODT/IV/IO/IM, every 8 hours as needed for nausea or vomiting. Each 8-hour dose can be repeated once at 15 minutes if nausea and vomiting are not improved. Do not give more than 8 mg in any 8-hour interval. Oral ondansetron is NOT an acceptable alternative to the ODT formulation.
- · Reassess—reassess—reassess!

11. **Antibiotics: Recommended for All Open Combat Wounds**
    a. If able to take PO meds:
       – Moxifloxacin (from CWMP) 400 mg PO once a day
    b. If unable to take PO meds (shock, unconsciousness):
       – Ertapenem, 1 gm IV/IM once a day
12. **Inspect and Dress Known Wounds.**
13. **Check for Additional Wounds.**
14. **Burns**
    a. Facial burns, especially those that occur in closed spaces, may be associated with inhalation injury. Aggressively monitor airway status and oxygen saturation in such patients and consider early surgical airway for respiratory distress or oxygen desaturation.
    b. Estimate total body surface area (TBSA) burned to the nearest 10% using the Rule of Nines.
    c. Cover the burn area with dry, sterile dressings. For extensive burns (>20%), consider placing the casualty in the heat-reflective shell or blizzard survival blanket from the hypothermia prevention kit to both cover the burned areas and prevent hypothermia.
    d. Fluid resuscitation (USAISR Rule of Ten)
       – If burns are greater than 20% of TBSA, fluid resuscitation should be initiated as soon as IV/IO access is established. Resuscitation should be initiated with Lactated Ringer's, normal saline, or Hextend. If Hextend is used, no more than 1,000 ml should be given, followed by Lactated Ringer's or normal saline as needed.
       – Initial IV/IO fluid rate is calculated as %TBSA x 10 ml/hr for adults weighing 40-80 kg.
       – For every 10 kg ABOVE 80 kg, increase initial rate by 100 ml/hr.
       – If hemorrhagic shock is also present, resuscitation for hemorrhagic shock takes precedence over resuscitation for burn shock. Administer IV/IO fluids per the TCCC Guidelines in Section (6).
    e. Analgesia in accordance with the TCCC Guidelines in Section (10) may be administered to treat burn pain.
    f. Prehospital antibiotic therapy is not indicated solely for burns, but antibiotics should be given per the TCCC Guidelines in Section (11) if indicated to prevent infection in penetrating wounds.

g. All TCCC interventions can be performed on or through burned skin in a burn casualty.

h. Burn patients are particularly susceptible to hypothermia. Extra emphasis should be placed on barrier heat loss prevention methods and IV fluid warming in this phase.

15. **Reassess Fractures and Recheck Pulses.**

16. **Communication**

a. Communicate with the casualty if possible. Encourage, reassure, and explain care.

b. Communicate with medical providers at the next level of care as feasible and relay mechanism of injury, injuries sustained, signs/symptoms, and treatments rendered. Provide additional information as appropriate.

17. **CPR in TACEVAC Care**

a. Casualties with torso trauma or polytrauma who have no pulse or respirations during TACEVAC should have bilateral needle decompression performed to ensure they do not have a tension pneumothorax. The procedure is the same as described in Section (4a) above.

b. CPR may be attempted during this phase of care if the casualty does not have obviously fatal wounds and will be arriving at a facility with a surgical capability within a short period of time. CPR should not be done at the expense of compromising the mission or denying lifesaving care to other casualties.

18. **Documentation of Care**

a. Document clinical assessments, treatments rendered, and changes in the casualty's status on a TCCC Card (DD Form 1380). Forward this information with the casualty to the next level of care.

* The term "Tactical Evacuation" includes both Casualty Evacuation (CASEVAC) and Medical Evacuation (MEDEVAC) as defined in Joint Publication 4-02.

Source: Courtesy of the Committee on Tactical Combat Casualty Care.

2012 Defense Health Board TACEVAC Care Recommendations

In 2011, the Committee on TCCC (CoTCCC) identified numerous issues pertaining to TACEVAC Care and briefed them to the Department of Defense (DoD) Defense Health Board (DHB). The DHB, in turn, submitted a number of specific recommendations to senior line and medical leaders in the military for improving TACEVAC care in Afghanistan and Iraq:[2]

1. Develop a US Advanced TACEVAC Care Capability

    In the near term and on a limited basis, pilot this capability where tactically feasible and where a high probability of critical casualties exists.

    a. Structure this capability after the successful MERT [United Kingdom's Medical Emergency Response Team] model to the extent possible.

    b. Consider an emergency medicine or critical care physician-led team.

    c. Ensure that capability includes current best practices, as indicated in the Joint Trauma System (JTS) Clinical Practice Guidelines and TCCC TACEVAC Care Guidelines [Box 26-1], including fluid resuscitation, advanced airway capabilities, and intravenous medications.

    d. Use this capability when possible for the most critical casualties.

    e. Ensure that trauma care procedures and outcomes are documented comprehensively.

    f. Utilize the most capable platform available. (CH-47/CH-53/CV-22)

    g. Use the outcomes from this pilot effort to inform further tactical evacuation system-wide changes.

2. Ensure that TACEVAC platforms are staffed with in-flight care providers to meet or exceed the civilian standard. Such platforms should each include at least two of the following providers during critical care casualty transport, and at least one of the following providers per critical casualty:

    a. Critical care-trained flight paramedic

    b. Critical care-trained flight nurse

    c. Critical care-capable, flight-trained physician

    d. Critical care-trained certified nurse practitioner or physician assistant

3. Ensure routine availability of packed red blood cells and plasma on TACEVAC platforms for critical casualties. TCCC Guidelines pertaining to resuscitation should be followed, which include:

    a. Limiting the amount of crystalloid infused

    b. Using hypotensive resuscitation with Hextend® when blood is unavailable. (Note that the updated TCCC Guidelines on fluid resuscitation call for the use of whole blood when feasible.)

4. Provider Skill Level and Oversight
    Staff TACEVAC platforms with providers who are trained and experienced in trauma care.

    a. Recommended training includes:

    • Ongoing intensive care unit/trauma experience

    • Experience at service trauma training centers

- Other trauma rotations that provide ongoing trauma patient contact
- TCCC training

b. Trauma training should be the primary focus of pre-deployment competencies for individuals who provide trauma care on TACEVAC platforms. Supervising physicians in TACEVAC units should have similar training and experience. Commanders' unit status reports should convey provider training level information.

c. In-theater oversight of TACEVAC systems should be provided by a qualified medical officer with EMS experience.

d. Dedicated personnel should be assigned to prehospital care cells as part of both the deployed JTS staff, and within the JTS structure in CONUS [continental United States].

5. Response Time
TACEVAC planning should aim to optimize evacuation time for all likely tactical contingencies.

a. Define hostile fire evacuation options in mission planning as a supplement to dedicated MEDEVAC platforms.

b. Consider the use of armed, armored CASEVAC aircraft to avoid evacuation delays due to ground fire.

c. Consider the use of modular medical packages for deployment on tactical aircraft designated to perform TACEVAC duties.

6. Standardization, Documentation Procedures, and Quality Assurance

a. Standardized TACEVAC care capability should be a *joint* requirement.

b. Standard protocols for TACEVAC care, as outlined in the TACEVAC section of the TCCC Guidelines, should be accepted across the Services as the standard of care during in-theater evacuation.

c. Improve TACEVAC care documentation procedures and implement process improvement measures.

- Collect TCCC cards from grounds medics and analyze data.
- Ensure reliable entry into Joint Theater Trauma Registry (JTTR) and on the casualty's Electronic Medical Record (EMR).
- Enhance prehospital data fields in the Joint Trauma Registry (now the DoD Trauma Registry).
- Integrate data collection between the JTTR, EMR systems, unit-based Pre-hospital Trauma Registry, and the Office of the Armed Forces Medical Examiner.
- Include flight care documentation in commander unit status report.
- Incorporate flight reviews of TACEVAC care in JTTS quality assurance measures.
- Conduct a follow-up when no pre-hospital data is provided for a casualty.

It now lies with the services, the geographic combatant commanders, and the U.S. Special Operations Command to consider these recommendations and decide what actions to take. As of this writing, these organizations have already begun to adapt some of the most important recommendations like Critical Care Flight Paramedics and increased availability of blood products during TACEVAC.

Specific Aspects of Care in TACEVAC

Massive Hemorrhage

The casualty should be reassessed for any unrecognized hemorrhage, and all significant external bleeding should be controlled. Use a CoTCCC-recommended limb tourniquet to control life-threatening external hemorrhage and for any traumatic amputation that is anatomically amenable to limb tourniquet use. Apply the tourniquet directly to the skin 2 to 3 inches (5–8 centimeters [cm]) above the bleeding site. If bleeding is not controlled with the first tourniquet, apply a second tourniquet side-by-side with the first. If the bleeding is not amenable to limb tourniquet application, Combat Gauze, junctional tourniquets, or XStat may be used.

Airway

The opportunity to carry additional equipment and work in a more secure environment allows for an expanded range of airway interventions. Most airway fatalities in combat are related to direct maxillofacial trauma.[3] Even so, airway problems in this setting may still be best managed by allowing the casualty to maintain the sit-up-and-lean-forward position if the casualty is conscious and the maneuver is not proscribed by requirements for spinal precautions.

Endotracheal intubation may be more feasible in this phase of care if the intubationist has the skill and experience to accomplish this procedure in a casualty with airway trauma. Schwartz and colleagues reported success in performing endotracheal intubation with the aid of night-vision goggles.[4] If endotracheal intubation is performed during TACEVAC, waveform capnography should be used.[5]

If a nasopharyngeal airway (NPA) is judged insufficient to manage the airway or a more reliable airway is desired, extraglottic airways (EGAs) are another alternative in this phase of care. The laryngeal mask airway (LMA) was recently reported to be useful as a rescue airway for combat casualties being transported by helicopter when endotracheal intubation had failed.[6] Of the 65 casualties who were reported, 47 were successfully intubated.

Of the 18 casualties in whom intubation failed, 16 of the 18 had an LMA placed successfully. Other EGAs besides the LMA may also be useful, especially in the subset of patients who are unconscious but have no direct maxillofacial trauma causing airway obstruction.[7]

Decreased pressure at altitude will result in an increase in the volume of gas enclosed in spaces with flexible shapes, such as air-filled cuffs in endotracheal (ET) tubes and supraglottic airways. If there is restricted space in which the cuff can expand, the pressure inside the cuff will increase because the volume cannot. Overpressurization of EGA cuffs is associated with barotraumatic palsies of the cranial nerves that pass through the oropharynx.[8-11] Such palsies can occur even without a change in ambient pressure, but the decrease in atmospheric pressure associated with helicopter transport of combat casualties results in increasing pressure inside the volume-limited cuff and an increased risk of barotraumatic neuropraxia. If a device with an air-filled cuff is used, medical personnel must monitor the pressure in the cuff and adjust it as needed, especially during and after changes in altitude during flight.

The CoTCCC has recommended the i-gel® as the preferred EGA in TCCC because the i-gel's gel-filled cuff makes the device simpler to use than EGAs with air-filled cuffs. (See the Tactical Field Care chapter.) The i-gel has a gel-filled cuff that does not increase in volume or cause elevated cuff pressures at altitude and thus does not require venting at altitude. Eliminating the risk of volume expansion at altitude lowers the potential for cuff overpressurization and reduces the risk of cranial nerve palsies.[5] It also eliminates the need to monitor cuff pressure, an important consideration in TACEVAC via aircraft.

EGAs are not well tolerated unless the casualty is deeply unconscious. If there is doubt about whether or not the casualty will tolerate an EGA, an NPA might be a better choice in the absence of direct maxillofacial trauma. As with endotracheal intubation, waveform capnography should be used in the TACEVAC phase of care if an EGA is placed.[5]

Note that EGAs may not be appropriate for those with serious burns affecting the upper airway. Intubation or a surgical airway may be required for these casualties. A surgical airway using the Cric-Key device remains a valuable option if the provider has the requisite skill and the other measures mentioned previously have failed.[12]

Respirations/Breathing

Any gas trapped in the pleural space will also expand at altitude, thus increasing the risk of producing a tension pneumothorax. Casualties with chest trauma should be watched for respiratory distress, hypoxia, and/or hypotension with a high index of suspicion for tension pneumothorax. This is especially true for any casualty who has previously been treated for an open pneumothorax (sucking chest wound) or has already been treated with needle thoracostomy (needle decompression or NDC). If a casualty with a chest seal in place has increasing respiratory difficulty, "burp" (lift up one side) or remove the chest seal. If respiratory distress persists, treat for suspected tension pneumothorax with NDC. (This procedure is outlined in the Tactical Field Care chapter.)

Oxygen is often available on TACEVAC platforms. Many trauma victims do not require supplemental oxygen, but some conditions may warrant its application. Casualties with injuries that impair ventilation (unconsciousness) or gas exchange (inhalation injury from burns or exposure to smoke or toxic fumes), casualties with blunt or penetrating pulmonary injury, casualties in shock, or any casualty with low oxygen saturation on pulse oximetry may benefit from supplemental oxygen.[13] Casualties being transported by air should be monitored for a drop in oxygen saturation due to the lower oxygen partial pressures at altitude. They should receive supplemental oxygen if the Spo_2 drops below 90 mm Hg.

Hypoxia in casualties with traumatic brain injury (TBI) is associated with unfavorable outcomes,[14] so casualties with moderate to severe TBI should be carefully monitored for adequate oxygenation and given supplemental oxygen, when available, to maintain an oxygen saturation of greater than 90%. (This is discussed further in the Tactical Field Care chapter.) Furthermore, hyperoxia causes cerebral vasoconstriction independently of the effects of hypocapnia and may therefore help to reduce intracranial pressure.[15,16] Hyperoxia has also been shown to increase cerebral tissue oxygenation[16] and to improve cerebral metabolism in casualties with severe head injury.[17-19] For casualties with moderate to severe TBI, then, supplemental oxygen should be given at the highest inspired fraction of oxygen achievable as early in the continuum of care as possible.[19]

Circulation—Bleeding

Hemorrhage is the leading cause of preventable death in combat casualties.[20] Early and definitive control of external hemorrhage using the TCCC interventions described previously has been shown to produce dramatic reductions in preventable deaths.[21] The TACEVAC phase usually offers an opportunity to reassess the casualty in a more controlled environment. Assessment of wounds and external hemorrhage control as described previously should continue to be a priority. To the extent possible, all areas of the casualty's body should be examined for additional wounds, and the adequacy of hemorrhage control measures previously employed should be reassessed. The TACEVAC phase may also provide the first opportunity to employ junctional hemorrhage control devices[22] or XStat[23] as discussed in TFC.[24-26] Furthermore, if the casualty meets the criteria for pelvic binder placement and a pelvic binder has not been placed previously, it is appropriate at this time.[27]

It is also appropriate during TACEVAC to reassess the continued need of a tourniquet to achieve or maintain hemorrhage control. The presence of shock or an anticipated time of 2 hours or less from tourniquet placement until arrival at a medical treatment facility are contraindications to tourniquet removal in the field. If the tourniquet has been on for 2 hours and the casualty is not in shock, the previous extremity bleeding sites should be rechecked to see if it is possible to remove the tourniquet and control bleeding with other methods.[28] Tourniquet replacement may be facilitated by the use of Combat Gauze, which should be applied with direct pressure. (This is discussed further in the Tactical Field Care chapter.) If a tourniquet remains necessary, it should be removed from over the uniform *after* replacing it with another tourniquet applied directly to the skin 2 to 3 inches (5–8 cm) above the wound. As time and the tactical situation permit, a distal pulse check should be accomplished. If there is ongoing hemorrhage or a persistent distal pulse, the tourniquet should be tightened, or a second tourniquet applied just proximal to the first.

Circulation—Tranexamic Acid

Administration of tranexamic acid (TXA) has been shown to confer a survival benefit in trauma victims who are in or at risk of hemorrhagic shock. Just as in TFC, TXA should be administered as soon as possible when indicated, but not more than 3 hours after the injury was sustained.[29-31]

Circulation—Fluid Resuscitation

Recent experience in resuscitating severely injured casualties who require massive transfusions (10 or more units of packed red blood cells [RBCs]) has shown that the resuscitation fluid that conveys the most physiologic benefit is whole blood.[32-35] If whole blood is not logistically feasible, studies have shown that infusing plasma and RBCs in a 1:1 ratio increases survival over the previously used crystalloids and colloids.[33,35-40] Administration of blood products as soon as possible after wounding has been shown to convey a survival benefit in critically injured combat casualties.[41] Early administration of plasma (i.e., within the first 6 hours after injury) is critical to maximize casualty survival if whole blood is not used.[42] This practice, known as damage control resuscitation (DCR), helps to restore clotting factors lost due to bleeding, improve coagulation status, and restore oxygen-carrying capability.[36,42-46] Blood component therapy initiated in the TACEVAC phase may be a

factor in the increased survival noted in critically injured casualties in studies of TACEVAC care and survival.[47,48] The use of RBCs and whole blood has a good safety profile in the deployed setting.[40] Decreased use of crystalloids in resuscitation has been associated with improved outcomes.[49,50]

Safe and effective administration of whole blood or blood component therapy requires that: (1) obtaining the blood or blood components for transport into prehospital settings must be logistically feasible in the area of operations or a unit-based walking blood bank must be established, (2) a protocol coordinated with the appropriate blood-banking facilities and approved by both theater and unit medical leadership must be in place, and (3) combat medical personnel must be well trained in the transfusion protocol.

The details of the protocol may vary depending on the maturity of the theater, service guidelines, the specific tactical scenario(s) envisioned, and the blood-banking logistics in the area of operations. In general, though, the following items should be addressed:

- Training of combat medical personnel in the protocol
- Documentation of this training
- Retraining interval
- Which blood products will be used (whole blood, RBCs, plasma)
- Ratio of plasma to RBC units infused
- ABO and Rh compatibility issues
- Transport container to be used
- Transport container handling instructions
- Storage temperature requirements
- Storage temperature documentation requirements
- Disposition of unused units upon return of containers
- Maximum time allowed for transport in a container
- Numbers and types of units to be transported
- Indications for transfusion
- Procedure for transfusion
- Equipment required
- Pretransfusion check of units
- Protective equipment required
- Transfusion rate
- Transfusion pressure
- Warming of units
  - Monitoring during transfusion
  - End points of resuscitation
  - Administration of adjuncts like calcium
  - Management of transfusion reactions
  - Documentation of transfusion

The JTS has published a clinical practice guideline for administering whole blood to casualties in hemorrhagic shock.[51]

If whole blood or plasma and RBCs are not available, hypotensive resuscitation with Hextend should be carried out with an initial 500-milliliter (ml) bolus, followed by a second bolus in 30 minutes if clinically indicated.[33,35,52] If necessary, resuscitation may be continued with crystalloid solutions or additional Hextend in a casualty who has already received two 500-ml boluses of Hextend. Both Hextend and crystalloids replace intravascular volume but do not replace oxygen-carrying capacity or clotting factors. They also contribute to dilutional coagulopathy.

Providers should always recognize the importance of hypotensive resuscitation in the setting of uncontrolled hemorrhage and avoid over-resuscitation to avoid promoting additional hemorrhage in casualties with noncompressible hemorrhage from wounds to the torso. Blood pressure monitoring will typically be present on TACEVAC platforms. Regardless of the fluids used, resuscitation should be titrated to a target systolic blood pressure of 80–90 mm Hg. If the casualty has sustained a TBI, however, the target systolic blood pressure is 90 mm Hg or higher.[52]

Prevention of Hypothermia

Efforts to prevent hypothermia should continue during Tactical Evacuation Care. Given the potential for heat loss due to wind chill and the lower temperatures encountered at altitude, the casualty must be aggressively protected against cold stress during evacuation. Hypothermia may occur rapidly in conditions that expose the casualty to water, wind, and cold surfaces like the floor of a vehicle or aircraft (**Figure 26-1**). Even in warm ambient temperatures, it is possible for the casualty to become significantly hypothermic if appropriate measures to preserve core temperature are not employed. Casualties in shock are at increased risk of hypothermia because they are not able to generate body heat at a normal rate.[53]

Traumatic Brain Injury in TACEVAC Care

Prevention of hypoxia and hypotension is especially important in casualties with TBI because these conditions may result in secondary injury to the traumatized brain. Casualties with moderate to severe TBI should be monitored carefully for the following:

1. Decreases in level of consciousness
2. Pupillary dilation
3. Systolic blood pressure maintained at >90 mm Hg
4. Hemoglobin oxygen saturation maintained at >90%
5. Hypothermia
6. P_{CO_2} maintained within 35–40 mm Hg (if capnography is available)[19]

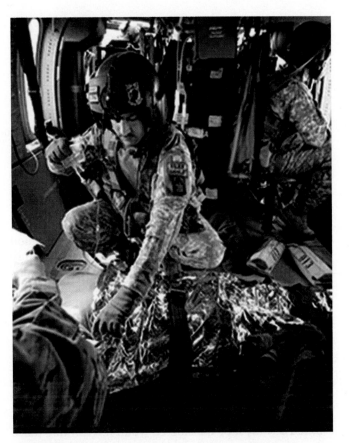

Figure 26-1 If helicopter doors must stay open for the firepower provided by the door gunner, wind could cause casualties to become hypothermic during transport.

U.S. Navy photo by Petty Officer Daniel Gay.

If penetrating head trauma is present, antibiotics should be administered. Providers should assume a cervical spine injury, until cleared, in TBI casualties when the mechanism of injury includes blunt trauma.[19]

Unilateral pupillary dilation accompanied by a decreased level of consciousness may signify impending cerebral herniation; if these signs occur, take the following actions to decrease intracranial pressure:

1. Administer 250 ml of 3% or 5% hypertonic saline IV/intraosseous (IO) bolus.
2. Elevate the casualty's head 30 degrees.
3. Hyperventilate the casualty.
   a. Respiratory rate should be 20 breaths/min.
   b. Capnography should be used to maintain the end-tidal carbon dioxide ($ETCO_2$) between 30 and 35 mm Hg.
   c. The highest oxygen concentration (FIO_2) possible should be used for hyperventilation.

Do not hyperventilate casualties unless signs of impending herniation are present. Hyperventilation with supplemental oxygen may be carried out using a bag-mask device if a definitive airway has not been placed for other indications.[19]

Electronic Monitoring

Casualty assessment is typically difficult inside TACEVAC platforms due to high noise and vibration levels and the need to avoid using lights at night for tactical safety reasons. For instance, helicopter transport impairs or precludes the provider's ability to auscultate the lungs[54,55] and even to palpate the carotid pulse.[56] To provide for continued quality assessment of the casualty's status during transport under such conditions, electronic monitoring should be available during TACEVAC care. Electronic monitoring systems capable of providing blood pressure, heart rate, pulse oximetry, and capnography are commercially available and should be used for seriously injured casualties. As an example of the need for such monitoring, the presence of esophageal intubation will have to be determined by a decrease in oxygen saturation or an absence of expired carbon dioxide because it will be impossible to hear breath sounds inside a noisy aircraft or vehicle. A national sample of 250 air transport agencies reported that more than 75% of these agencies monitored oxygenation and ventilation during transport.[57] The significant effect of altitude on oxygenation (**Table 26-1**) must be considered when interpreting pulse oximetry readings while operating in mountainous regions and during aircraft evacuation in airframes with unpressurized cabins.[58,59]

Analgesia

The use of appropriate analgesics should be continued in the TACEVAC phase. Remember that medications that impair platelet function should not be used in combat casualties. Oral transmucosal fentanyl citrate is a good option when the casualty is not in or at risk of shock or pulmonary compromise.[60-62] Opioids are contraindicated in casualties in hemorrhagic shock or with respiratory difficulty. Ketamine is the preferred option for casualties whose pain is severe but in whom opioids should not be used.[62,63]

Casualty Movement

Casualty evacuation conditions are typically chaotic due to the challenges of patient onloading and offloading, uneven terrain, rotor wash, deafening aircraft noise, hectic turnover, and hazardous tactical situations. Casualties should be thoroughly reassessed after movement; all interventions should be rechecked after a casualty has been moved to or from a CASEVAC platform.

Conventional litters should be available during TACEVAC. The casualty should be made as comfortable as possible on a litter and kept warm and dry. If an improvised litter is used, it should be padded, and any field-expedient materials used to treat the casualty should be replaced with conventional splints, tourniquets, and dressings as soon as feasible.

Cardiopulmonary Resuscitation (CPR) During TACEVAC

The prognosis for trauma patients with prehospital cardiac arrest is very poor. Casualties with torso trauma or polytrauma who lose their pulse or respirations during TACEVAC should have bilateral needle decompression performed to ensure they do not have a tension pneumothorax.[64]

CPR is appropriate during this phase of care if the casualty does not have obviously fatal wounds and will be arriving at a facility with a surgical capability within a short period of time. CPR should not be performed at the expense of compromising the mission or denying lifesaving care to other casualties.

If the evacuation platform has the appropriate personnel and equipment, resuscitative thoracostomy may be indicated if the casualty has a cardiopulmonary arrest during transport. A recent study noted that of 29 patients who arrested en route, 13 (44.8%) had a transient return of spontaneous circulation, and 3 (10.3%) survived to 30 days.[65]

Care for Wounded Hostile Combatants

In the TACEVAC phase, the principles of care are the same for wounded hostile combatants as for coalition forces *after* the prisoner security measures have been accomplished. (These measures are described in the Tactical Field Care chapter.) The Rules of Engagement may dictate the evacuation process for wounded hostile combatants,

Table 26-1 Approximate Pulse Oximetry Values for Healthy Volunteers at Altitude	
Altitude	**Oxygen Saturation**
Sea level	97%
5,000 ft (1,500 m)	96%
8,000 ft (2,400 m)	93%
12,000 ft (3,700 m)	86%

Source: Courtesy of Dr. Frank Butler.

but proper prisoner-handling procedures must be maintained throughout, with particular attention to restraint and security. Remember that each hostile combatant in your custody represents a potential threat not only to the provider but also to the unit and the TACEVAC platform as well. They may be wounded, and you may be providing them with lifesaving care, but wounded hostile combatants still pose a very real threat. Ensure that they are kept away from and are physically blocked from vehicle exits and access to aircraft systems and controls. Additionally, awareness of the medic's and team's weapons is of special importance when working in a confined area

with an enemy combatant. Medics' rifles are often slung in the aircraft when treating coalition casualties. This practice should be avoided when wounded hostile combatants or local nationals are onboard.

In an era in which hostile forces routinely use suicide bomber tactics, the concealment of improvised explosive devices (IEDs) on hostile combatant casualties or even on apparently friendly local national casualties is an additional concern. This has led some evacuation units to require that all noncoalition casualties be searched thoroughly for IEDs before they are loaded onto an evacuation platform.[46]

SUMMARY

- Additional medical equipment and personnel should be provided in the TACEVAC phase of care. This allows for an enhanced level of medical care compared to Care Under Fire and Tactical Field Care.
- Expansion of intrapleural gas due to the lower pressure at altitude may result in a tension pneumothorax. Casualties with torso trauma should be monitored for severe or increasing respiratory distress with a high index of suspicion for tension pneumothorax.
- Oxygen should be administered if available to casualties who: (1) have injuries that interfere with respirations or oxygenation, (2) have a low oxygen saturation on pulse oximetry, (3) are in shock, (4) have TBI and an SpO_2 below 90 mm Hg, or (5) have suspected smoke inhalation injury.
- EGAs and ET tube cuffs that are filled with air must be monitored for pressure changes in the cuff during flights and adjusted as needed. This monitoring is not required if the airway has a cuff filled with gel rather than air, such as the i-gel.
- During the TACEVAC phase, a thorough examination for additional wounds should be performed. The adequacy of hemorrhage control measures previously employed should be reassessed and replaced or enhanced as needed.
- Electronic monitoring systems capable of displaying blood pressure, heart rate, pulse oximetry, and capnography should be used during evacuation.
- Fluid resuscitation should be continued as needed with the goal of maintaining a palpable

peripheral pulse and normal mentation. If electronic blood pressure monitoring is available, resuscitate to a systolic blood pressure of 80-90 mm Hg.
- Whole blood or plasma/RBCs administered in a 1:1 ratio should be used in the tactical evacuation care phase, if logistically feasible.
- Blood products, if used, must be administered by a provider trained in blood transfusion and under a preapproved protocol.
- If a casualty with TBI is unconscious and has a weak or absent peripheral pulse, resuscitate as necessary to maintain a systolic blood pressure of at least 90 mm Hg.
- Altitude affects oxygenation in aircraft with unpressurized cabins, and this should be considered when interpreting pulse oximetry readings.
- Casualties with moderate to severe TBI should be monitored carefully for signs of impending cerebral herniation, and steps should be taken to lower intracranial pressure if decreasing level of consciousness and unilateral pupillary dilation are noted.
- Casualties should be aggressively protected against hypothermia during evacuation.
- Proper prisoner handling procedures should be maintained throughout the treatment and evacuation of wounded hostile combatants and local nationals.
- All noncoalition casualties should be searched thoroughly for IEDs and weapons before being loaded onto an evacuation platform.

SCENARIO RECAP

You are a medic aboard a MEDEVAC Black Hawk helicopter that has landed in a secure LZ in the mountains of southeastern Afghanistan to extract a Ranger who has multiple shrapnel wounds from an RPG blast. The LZ altitude is 6,000 ft (1,800 m), and the ambient temperature is 64°F (18°C). The casualty, who has been stabilized by the platoon medic, is able to converse normally and has a tourniquet over his uniform on his upper right thigh. The trousers are cut open below the tourniquet, and there is a pressure dressing around his lower thigh and another around his middle calf. His right shirtsleeve is missing, and there is a pressure dressing around his right upper arm. There is a saline lock in his left antecubital fossa. The platoon medic tells you the casualty lost a lot of blood from his thigh wound and was drowsy and confused before the tourniquet was applied 30 minutes ago. He received 2 units of cold-stored type O low-titer whole blood to which he responded well. He has been stable since. The wounds with pressure dressings were all packed with Combat Gauze underneath. He has taken moxifloxacin 400 mg by mouth and has an 800-mcg fentanyl lozenge in his right cheek. He has been drinking water from his canteen.

SCENARIO SOLUTION

- **What are your considerations for the care of this casualty during the 30-minute helicopter flight back to the Combat Support Hospital?**
  This casualty is now apparently stable but had been noted to be in hemorrhagic shock earlier.
- **What do you do first?**
  You check all the pressure dressings and see no signs of bleeding from these wounds. You check for a palpable pulse at the right ankle and find none. Right and left radial and left popliteal pulses are palpable. You check for other wounds and find none of significance.
- **What do you do next?**
  You confirm that he is responsive—he answers questions appropriately and has a good radial pulse.
- **Should you start an IV line through the saline lock in anticipation of the need for a second whole blood transfusion?**
  Yes, it is probably a good idea start an IV line through the saline lock. You can run a crystalloid solution at a keep vein open rate to assure the line's readiness.
- **Should you remove the tourniquet?**
  No, you should not remove the tourniquet. Even though pressure dressings over Combat Gauze are present on the distal wounds, you will risk further bleeding by releasing the tourniquet's pressure, and the casualty will be at the emergency department within 2 hours of the tourniquet's application. It is better at this point not to remove the tourniquet. If feasible, you may replace it with another tourniquet applied directly to the skin 2-3 inches (5-8 cm) above the site of the bleeding.
- **Should you remove the fentanyl lozenge?**
  Yes, you should remove the fentanyl lozenge because the casualty was previously in shock. If the casualty's pain level requires analgesia, ketamine is a better analgesic option in casualties who are in or at risk for hemorrhagic shock. Opioids may cause cardiorespiratory depression and must be used with caution in casualties who have recently been hypotensive or who are in danger of going into shock.
- **What else do you want to do?**
  You also want to establish electronic monitoring of the casualty. You place a pulse oximeter from the Propaq aboard the helicopter on a finger of the casualty's left hand. Pulse rate is 100 beats/min, and oxygen saturation is 92%.
- **Is there anything else to attend to during the flight to the Combat Support Hospital?**
  Yes, you should be concerned about the oxygen saturation, but this decrease is likely due to the altitude. You should keep a careful eye on this during the flight. Administer supplemental oxygen as needed to maintain an oxygen saturation of 90% or higher. You should also keep the casualty warm during the flight to the Combat Support Hospital.

References

1. Butler FK, Blackbourne LH. Battlefield trauma care then and now: a decade of tactical combat casualty care. *J Trauma Acute Care Surg.* 2012;73(6)(Suppl 5):S395-S402.

2. Dickey N, Jenkins D, Butler F. *Tactical evacuation care improvements within the Department of Defense.* Defense Health Board Memo dated 8 August 2011. Military Health System website. https://health.mil/About-MHS/OASDHA/Defense-Health-Agency/Defense-Health-Board/Reports. Accessed June 12, 2018.

3. Mabry RL, Edens JW, Pearse L, et al. Fatal airway injuries during Operation Enduring Freedom and Operation Iraqi Freedom. *Prehosp Emerg Care.* 2010;14:272-277.

4. Schwartz RB, Gillis WL, Miles RJ. Orotracheal intubation in darkness using night vision goggles. *Mil Med.* 2001;166(11):984-986.

5. Otten E, Montgomery H, Butler F. Extraglottic airways in tactical combat casualty care: TCCC Guidelines change 17-01 28 August 2017. *J Spec Oper Med.* 2017;17:19-28.

6. Shavit I, Aviram E, Hoffmann Y, Biton O, Glassberg E. Laryngeal mask airway as a rescue device for failed endotracheal intubation during scene-to-hospital air transport of combat casualties. *Eur J Emerg Med.* 2018 Oct;25(5):368-371. doi:10.1097/MEJ.0000000000000480.

7. Dickey N. *Supraglottic airway use in tactical evacuation care.* Defense Health Board Memo dated 17 September 2012. Military Health System website. https://health.mil/About-MHS/OASDHA/Defense-Health-Agency/Defense-Health-Board/Reports. Accessed June 12, 2018.

8. Bruce IA, Ellis R, Kay NJ. Nerve injury and the laryngeal mask airway. *J Laryngol Otol.* 2004;18:899-901.

9. Brimacombe J, Clarke G, Keller C. Lingual nerve injury associated with the ProSeal laryngeal mask airway: a case report and review of the literature. *Br J Anaesthesia.* 2005;95:420-423.

10. Endo K, Okabe Y, Maruyama Y, Tsukatani T, Furukawa M. Bilateral vocal cord paralysis caused by laryngeal mask airway. *Am J Otolaryngol.* 2007 Mar-Apr;28(2):126-129.

11. Thiruvenkatarajan V, Van Wijk RM, Rajbhoj A. Cranial nerve injuries with supraglottic airway devices: a systematic review of published case reports and series. *Anaesthesia.* 2015;70:344-359.

12. Mabry R, Frankfurt A, Kharod C, Butler F. Emergency cricothyroidotomy in tactical combat casualty care. *J Spec Oper Med.* 2015;15:11-19.

13. Grissom CK, Weaver LK, Clemmer TP, Morris AH. Theoretical advantage of oxygen treatment for combat casualties during medical evacuation at high altitude. *J Trauma.* 2006;61(2):461-467.

14. Chi JH, Knudson MM, Vassar MJ, et al. Prehospital hypoxia affects outcome in patients with traumatic brain injury: a prospective multicenter study. *J Trauma.* 2006;61(5):1134-1141.

15. Floyd T, Clark J, Gelfand R, et al. Independent cerebral vasoconstrictive effects of hyperoxia and accompanying arterial hypocapnia at 1 ATA. *J Appl Physiol.* 2003;95(6):2453-2461.

16. Tisdall M, Taylor C, Tachtisidis I, et al. The effect of cerebral tissue oxygenation index of changes in the concentrations of inspired oxygen and end-tidal carbon dioxide in healthy adult volunteers. *Anesth Analg.* 2009;109(3):906-913.

17. Tolias C, Reinert M, Seiler R, et al. Normobaric hyperoxia-induced improvement in cerebral metabolism and reduction in intracranial pressure in patients with severe head injury: a prospective historical cohort-matched study. *J Neurosurg.* 2004;101(3):435-444.

18. Tolias CM, Kumaria A, Bullock MR. Hyperoxia and traumatic brain injury. *J Neurosurg.* 2009;110(3):607-609.

19. Dickey N. *Management of traumatic brain injury in tactical combat casualty care.* Defense Health Board Memo dated 26 July 2012. Military Health System website. https://health.mil/About-MHS/OASDHA/Defense-Health-Agency/Defense-Health-Board/Reports. Accessed June 12, 2018.

20. Eastridge BJ, Mabry R, Seguin P, et al. Pre-hospital death on the battlefield: implications for the future of combat casualty care. *J Trauma Acute Care Surg.* 2012;73(6)(Suppl 5):S431-S437. doi:10.1097/TA.0b013e3182755dcc.

21. Kotwal RS, Montgomery HR, Kotwal BM, et al. Eliminating preventable death on the battlefield. *Arch Surgery.* 2011;146(12):1350-1358. doi:10.1001/archsurg.2011.213.

22. Kotwal RS, Butler FK, Gross KR, et al. Management of junctional hemorrhage in tactical combat casualty care. *J Spec Oper Med.* 2013;13:Winter:85-93.

23. Sims K, Bowling F, Montgomery H, et al. Management of external hemorrhage in tactical combat casualty care: the adjunctive use of XStat™ compressed hemostatic sponges. TCCC Guidelines Change 15-03. *J Spec Oper Med.* 2016;16:19-28.

24. Dickey N, Jenkins D. *Combat ready clamp addition to the tactical combat casualty care guidelines.* Defense Health Board Memo dated 23 September 2011. Military Health System website. https://health.mil/About-MHS/OASDHA/Defense-Health-Agency/Defense-Health-Board/Reports. Accessed June 12, 2018.

25. Tovmassian RV, Kragh JF, Dubick MA, Baer DG, Blackbourne LH. Combat ready clamp medic technique. *J Spec Oper Med.* 2012;12(4):72-78.

26. Dubick M, Kragh JF, eds. Evaluation of the combat ready clamp to control bleeding in human cadavers, manikins, swine femoral artery hemorrhage model and swine carcasses. U.S. Army Institute of Surgical Research Technical Report, June 2012. dtic.mil/cgi-bin/GetTRDoc?AD=ADA569685. Accessed June 12, 2018.

27. Shackelford S, Hammesfahr R, Morissette D, et al. The use of pelvic binders in tactical combat casualty care: TCCC guidelines change 16-02. *J Spec Oper Med.* 2017;17:135-147.

28. Shackelford SA, Butler FK, Kragh JF, et al. Optimizing the use of limb tourniquets in tactical combat casualty care: TCCC guidelines change 14-02. *J Spec Oper Med.* 2015;15:17-31.

29. Dickey N, Jenkins D. *Addition of tranexamic acid to the tactical combat casualty care guidelines.* Defense Health Board Memo dated 23 September 2011. Military Health System website. https://health.mil/About-MHS/OASDHA/Defense-Health-Agency/Defense-Health-Board/Reports. Accessed June 12, 2018.

30. Morrison JJ, Dubose JJ, Rasmussen TE, Midwinter MJ. Military application of tranexamic acid in trauma emergency resuscitation study (MATTERs). *Arch Surg.* 2011;147(2):113-119. doi:10.1001/archsurg.2011.287.

31. CRASH-2 Collaborators, Roberts I, Shakur H, et al. The importance of early treatment with tranexamic acid in bleeding trauma patients: an exploratory analysis of the CRASH-2 randomized controlled trial. *Lancet.* 2011;377(9771):1096-1101. doi:10.1016/S0140-6736(11)60278-X.

32. Spinella PC, Perkins JG, Grathwohl KW, et al. Warm fresh whole blood is independently associated with improved survival for patients with combat-related traumatic injuries. *J Trauma.* 2009;66:S69-S76.

33. Butler FK, Holcomb JB, Kotwal RS, et al. Fluid resuscitation for hemorrhagic shock in tactical combat casualty care: TCCC guidelines proposed change 14-01. *J Spec Oper Med.* 2014;14:13-38.

34. Strandenes G, DePasquale M, Cap A, et al. Emergency whole-blood use in the field: a simplified protocol for collection and transfusion. *Shock.* 2014;41(Suppl 1):76-83.

35. Butler FK. Fluid resuscitation in tactical combat casualty care—yesterday and today. *Wilderness Environ Med.* 2017;28:S74-S81.

36. Holcomb JB, Wade CE, Michalek JE, et al. Improved plasma and platelet to red blood cell ratios improves outcome in 466 massively transfused civilian trauma patients. *Ann Surg.* 2008;248(3):447-458. doi:10.1097/SLA.0b013e318185a9ad.

37. Streets CG. Lessons from the battlefield in the management of major trauma. *Br J Surg.* 2009;96(8):831-832. doi:10.1002/bjs.6617.

38. Hess JR, Holcomb JB. Transfusion practice in military trauma. *Transfusion Med.* 2008;18(3):143-150. doi:10.1111/j.1365-3148.2008.00855.x.

39. Beekley AC, Starnes BW, Sebesta JA. Lessons learned from modern military surgery. *Surg Clin N Am.* 2007;87(1):157-184.

40. Borgman MA, Spinella PC, Perkins JG, et al. The ratio of blood products transfused affects mortality in patients receiving massive transfusions at a combat support hospital. *J Trauma.* 2007;63(4):805-813.

41. Shackelford S, Del Junco D, Powell-Dunford N, et al. Association of prehospital blood product transfusion during medical evacuation of combat casualties in Afghanistan with acute and 30-day survival. *JAMA.* 2017;318:1581-1591.

42. Zink KA, Sambasivan CN, Holcomb JB, Chisholm G, Schreiber MA. A high ratio of plasma and platelets to packed red blood cells in the first 6 hours of massive transfusion improves outcomes in a large multicenter study. *Am J Surg.* 2009;197(5):565-570. doi:10.1016/j.amjsurg.2008.12.014.

43. Holcomb JB, Spinella PC. Optimal use of blood in trauma patients. *Biologicals* 2010;38(1):72-77. doi:10.1016/j.biologicals.2009.10.007.

44. Holcomb JB. Damage control resuscitation. *J Trauma.* 2007;62(6 Suppl):S36-S37.

45. Holcomb JB. Optimal use of blood products in severely injured trauma patients. *Hematology Am Soc Hematol Educ.* 2010;2010:465-469. doi:10.1182/asheducation-2010.1.465.

46. Kotwal RS, Butler FK, Edgar EP, Shackelford SA, Bennett DR, Bailey JA. Saving lives on the battlefield: a joint trauma system review of pre-hospital trauma care in combined joint operations area—Afghanistan (CJOA-A). Final report of the U.S. Central Command Pre-Hospital Trauma Care Assessment Team dated 30 January 2013. *J Spec Oper Med.* 2013 Spring;13(1):77-85.

47. Morrison JJ, Oh J, Dubose JJ, et al. En-route care capability from point of injury impacts mortality after severe wartime injury. *Ann Surg.* 2013;257(2):330-334. doi:10.1097/SLA.0b013e31827eefcf.

48. Apodaca A, Olson CM Jr, Bailey J, Butler FK, Eastridge BJ, Kuncir E. Performance improvement evaluation of forward aeromedical evacuation platforms in Operation Enduring Freedom. *J Trauma Acute Care Surg.* 2013;75(2)(Suppl 2):S157-S163. doi:10.1097/TA.0b013e318299da3e.

49. Duke MD, Guidry C, Guice J, et al. Restrictive fluid resuscitation in combination with damage control resuscitation: time for adaptation. *J Trauma Acute Care Surg.* 2012;73(3):674-678. doi:10.1097/TA.0b013e318265ce1f.

50. Morrison CA, Carrick MM, Norman MA, et al. Hypotensive resuscitation strategy reduces transfusion requirements and severe postoperative coagulopathy in trauma patients with hemorrhagic shock: preliminary results of a randomized controlled trial. *J Trauma.* 2011;70(3):652-663. doi:10.1097/TA.0b013e31820e77ea.

51. Cap AP, Beckett A, Benov A, et al. Joint Trauma System Clinical Practice Guideline 21: whole blood transfusion. Joint Trauma System website. http://jts.amedd.army.mil/assets/docs/cpgs/JTS_Clinical_Practice_Guidelines_(CPGs)/Whole_Blood_Transfusion_15_May_2018_ID21.pdf. Accessed June 13, 2018.

52. Lednar WM, Poland GA, Holcomb JB, Butler FK. *Tactical combat casualty care guidelines on fluid resuscitation.* Defense Health Board Memo dated 2010 December 10. Military Health System website. https://health.mil/About-MHS/OASDHA/Defense-Health-Agency/Defense-Health-Board/Reports. June 13, 2018.

53. Bennett BL, Holcomb JB. Battlefield trauma-induced hypothermia: transitioning the preferred method of casualty rewarming. *Wilderness Environ Med.* 2017;28:S82-S89.

54. Fromm RE Jr, Varon J. Air medical transport. *J Fam Pract.* 1993;36(3):313-318.

55. Fromm RE Jr, Dellinger RP. Transport of critically ill patients. *J Intensive Care Med.* 1992;7(5):223-233.

56. Hunt RC, Carroll RG, Whitley TW, Bryan-Berge DM, Dufresne DA. Adverse effect of helicopter flight on the ability to palpate carotid pulses. *Ann Emerg Med.* 1994;24(2):190-193.

57. Perez L, Klofas E, Wise L. Oxygenation/ventilation of transported intubated adult patients: a national survey of organizational practices. *Air Med J.* 2000;19(2):55-58.

58. Pilmanis AA. Presentation at USSOCOM Biomedical Initiatives Steering Committee. August 2004.

59. Luks AM, Swenson ER. Pulse oximetry at high altitude. *High Alt Med Biol.* 2011;12(2):109-119. doi:10.1089/ham.2011.0013.

60. Kotwal R, O'Connor KC, Johnson TR, Mosely DS, Meyer DE, Holcomb JB. A novel pain management strategy for combat casualty care. *Ann Emerg Med.* 2004;44(2):121-127.

61. Wedmore IS, Kotwal RS, McManus JG, et al. Safety and efficacy of oral transmucosal fentanyl citrate for prehospital pain control on the battlefield. *J Trauma Acute Care Surg.* 2012;73(6)(Suppl 5):S490-S495. doi:10.1097/TA.0b013e3182754674.

62. Butler FK, Kotwal RS, Buckenmaier CC III, et al. A triple-option analgesia plan for tactical combat casualty care. *J Spec Oper Med.* 2014;14:13-25.

63. Dickey N. *Prehospital use of ketamine in battlefield analgesia.* Defense Health Board Memo dated 8 March 2012.

Military Health System website. https://health.mil/About-MHS/OASDHA/Defense-Health-Agency/Defense-Health-Board/Reports. Accessed June 13, 2018.

64. Dickey N. *Needle decompression of tension pneumothorax tactical combat casualty care recommendations.* Defense Health Board Memorandum dated July 6, 2012. Military Health System website. https://health.mil/About-MHS/OASDHA/Defense-Health-Agency/Defense-Health-Board/Reports. Accessed June 13, 2018.

65. Morrison J, Poon H, Rasmussen T, et al. Resuscitative thoracotomy following wartime injury. *J Trauma Acute Care Surg.* 2013;24(3):809-814. doi:10.1097/TA.0b013e31827e1d26.

CHAPTER 27

Scenarios

Authors:
Capt. (Ret) Frank Butler, MD
Master Sgt. (Ret) Harold Montgomery
Col. (Ret) Rob DeLorenzo, MD
Col. Peter Cuenca
Col. (Ret) Robert Gerhardt, MD

CHAPTER OBJECTIVES   At the completion of this chapter, you will be able to do the following:

- Apply and adapt the tenets of Tactical Combat Casualty Care (TCCC) to the care of casualties in the context of realistic combat scenarios.

INTRODUCTION

From the lessons learned in the wars in Vietnam, Iraq, and Afghanistan, we now recognize that the leading causes of preventable combat-related deaths are hemorrhage, airway obstruction, and tension pneumothorax.[1-6] A study of battlefield mortality from Iraq and Afghanistan found that hemorrhage accounted for 90.9% of preventable prehospital deaths (with truncal being the most common site, followed by junctional and extremity hemorrhage); airway obstruction accounted for 7.9% of preventable deaths; and tension pneumothorax was responsible for the remaining 1.1%.[3]

Beyond intervening to prevent imminent death, there are a number of combat casualty care conditions requiring immediate attention to reduce suffering, morbidity, and disability.[7-11] This includes shock management, analgesia, infection prophylaxis, spinal cord protection, traumatic brain injury (TBI) treatment, and hypothermia prevention. Ensuring the best outcome for the casualty requires that life threats and the other conditions listed previously be addressed rapidly, often within the first few minutes after wounding. The battlefield first responder and other far-forward medical providers are critical to this effort.

Combat medical personnel are charged with rapid decision making, immediate action, and competent technical performance under a wide range of challenging, austere, and dangerous conditions. To illustrate the performance of casualty care in the combat environment, several scenarios will be presented in this chapter. Each scenario presents some of the unique features of the combat environment and describes the key medical assessments and interventions performed by combat medical personnel. The scenarios are themed in such a way that the focus is on a defined set of clinical problems. Not every Tactical Combat Casualty Care (TCCC) principle is highlighted in every scenario; rather, the scenarios are intended to illustrate how combat medical personnel must combine good medicine with good small-unit tactics to optimize the care provided to each casualty on the battlefield.

The text in this chapter is not intended to suggest that the answers provided are the only acceptable answers. Other answers may turn out to be just as good or better, depending on the totality of the injuries sustained and evolving tactical circumstances.

Scenario 1: Gunshot Wound on a Night Patrol

You are a medic operating in Afghanistan as part of a combat element on a nighttime direct-action mission. While moving by foot along the edge of a cultivated field, one man in your four-person team is shot and falls into an irrigation ditch. You and your uninjured teammates take immediate cover and begin returning fire. You call to the wounded man, asking how badly he is hit. He responds, telling you that he's been shot in the left leg just above the knee. He is under effective cover but cannot move.

1. **What do you know about the wounded man already?**

   He is alert enough to speak coherently, so he probably has an acceptable blood pressure, at least for the moment, and his airway is open.

2. **What do you want to know next?**

   You need to determine how badly he is bleeding and whether he has other injuries. Fire from four hostiles is keeping you and the other two team members very busy, and you cannot leave your cover without getting shot yourself. While you and your other teammates continue the firefight, you ask the casualty if he can tell how much blood is coming out of the wound. He tells you he cannot tell, but his leg is really messed up and he can feel blood on the trousers of his uniform. You ask him if he has been hit anywhere else. He says he does not think so, but his leg really hurts.

3. **What do you do next?**

   You tell the casualty to put a tourniquet on his leg and then get back in the fight if he can. In the Care Under Fire phase, the best thing a medic can do for the casualty and the rest of his team may be to take cover and return fire (**Figure 27-1**). If a medic gets killed trying to get to a casualty, he has done the casualty, the rest of the team, and himself no good. In a situation like this one, the overriding concern is suppression of enemy fire, and every gun, including the medic's and the casualty's, may be needed. Casualties who are able should remain engaged in the firefight and/or the prosecution of the mission. This casualty was equipped with a tourniquet and trained to use it on himself and others. Because his wound was at a site where a tourniquet could be effectively applied above it, he was able to address potentially life-threatening extremity hemorrhage via self-aid. Both he and the medic were able to remain under cover and involved in the fight. In this way, the risk of further injury to the casualty,

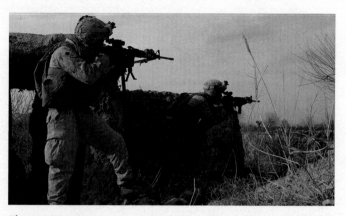

Figure 27-1 Cover and return fire are the priorities in the Care Under Fire phase.
Courtesy of Lance Cpl. James Clark/U.S. Marine Corps.

the medic, and the other members of the team was minimized.

After several minutes of intense fighting, your team eliminates all hostile fire, and you are able to tend to the casualty. You find him lying on his back in 2 inches of muddy water at the bottom of the irrigation ditch with a limb tourniquet in place on the injured leg. He is alert and oriented, but in great pain. He has a strong radial pulse. He tells you again that the gunshot wound to his left leg is his only injury. When you cut open his trousers leg, there is an open fracture of his femur. His pain is so great, he stops you from doing a sweep of his leg.

4. **What is the greatest tactical need at this point?**

   Your team needs to call for extraction. Since it is difficult to move the casualty and the four hostiles are now neutralized, you elect to call for an evacuation at your current location.

5. **What do you need to do for the casualty?**

   Ensure hemorrhage control, rule out other injuries, provide pain relief, administer antibiotics, prepare him to move, and protect him from hypothermia.

6. **How do you do all that?**

   You cannot use a light because the enemy may be nearby, and he will not let you manipulate his injured leg. Since you cannot see or feel well enough to assess for sites of bleeding, amount of blood lost, or to determine if he is still bleeding, you elect to place a second tourniquet higher on his left thigh. You sweep everything other than his left leg and find no other injuries. His clinical status has not changed.

   You give him the moxifloxacin from his Combat Wound Medication Pack (CWMP) and place one 800-microgram (mcg) oral transmucosal fentanyl citrate (OTFC) lozenge in his cheek. You gently place a large dressing over the entire wounded area. You splint the casualty's left leg alongside his right. You check to make sure both tourniquets are still tight and in place. The casualty's clinical status has not changed—he is alert and still in severe pain—so you give him a second OTFC lozenge in his other cheek.

You have elected to leave his body armor on since you may get into another firefight, so you put a Ready-Heat Blanket over him just below the bottom edge of his armor, placing it on top of his t-shirt (to prevent burns that may result from direct contact with the skin), and you cover him up with the Heat Reflective Shell.

7. **What does the casualty need more than anything else at this point?**
He needs continued control of his bleeding and expedited evacuation.

8. **What should you be doing for him until he gets to more advanced care?**
Continue to monitor his clinical status. You notice that he is drowsy.

9. **What is the most significant possible cause of a decline in mental status in this casualty?**
Ongoing blood loss.

10. **What else do you want to know?**
 • Pulse character? His radial pulse is now rapid and weak.
 • Tourniquets OK? They are both still in place, but you suspect that the wound is still bleeding. It is nighttime, so it is hard to be sure if there is ongoing bleeding from his wound.
 • Breathing OK? His breathing is slightly rapid but not labored.

11. **What is most likely happening?**
The casualty is going into hemorrhagic shock.

12. **What makes you think so?**
 • Mental status and radial pulse character have deteriorated.
 • Even though the tourniquets look okay, you suspect continued bleeding.
 • Breathing is slightly rapid.
 • 1,600 mcg of OTFC is not that large a dose for a young, healthy male in acute pain. It is unlikely that this amount could have caused the change in mental status observed in this casualty.
 • Hemorrhage is the number one cause of preventable combat death.

13. **What do you do?**
You tighten both tourniquets.

14. **What else?**
Because this casualty will need significant blood transfusion due to his hemorrhagic shock, you want to infuse 1 gram (g) of tranexamic acid (TXA) in 100 milliliters (ml) of normal saline (NS). It is difficult to start an intravenous line (IV) at night, so you place a sternal intraosseous (IO) device.

15. **What next?**
Next you resuscitate the casualty with a unit of whole blood. If whole blood is not available, use RBCs and plasma or reconstituted dried plasma if those products are available. If they are not, give him 500 ml of Hextend. Ten minutes after the resuscitation fluids are infused, the casualty is a little less drowsy and his radial pulse is stronger. You check the tourniquets, and they are still in place and tight. You can detect no bleeding.

16. **What next?**
You complete the TCCC casualty card while waiting for the evacuation helicopter to arrive.

Scenario 2: Rocket-Propelled Grenade Attack in an Urban Environment

While you are on patrol in an urban environment, your squad comes under small arms fire and rocket-propelled grenade (RPG) attack. The point man and a second man are hit. The squad reacts to the contact, rapidly eliminating the ambushing hostiles. There are no other casualties. A secure perimeter is established, and the squad leader instructs you to take care of the casualties.

You move to Casualty 1 and quickly check for massive external hemorrhage. You discover a gunshot wound with a small hole that is likely the entrance wound on his right upper back, and what appears to be a larger exit wound in his right axilla. You see pulsatile bleeding from the axillary wound. His airway is open, and his breathing is rapid but unlabored. His mental status is normal.

1. **What is your immediate concern?**
The bleeding is life threatening and must be controlled.

2. **How do you handle it?**
You immediately expose the area, pack Combat Gauze into the wound, and hold direct pressure for 3 minutes. While you are performing these actions, you talk to the casualty in order to check both his airway and mental status. After 3 minutes, the external bleeding appears controlled, so you build a pressure dressing over the Combat Gauze. This dressing also covers the entrance wound.

You notice the casualty is more anxious and is growing short of breath. The pressure dressing in okay, so you look for other sources of bleeding but find none. Suddenly, the casualty becomes unresponsive. His left radial pulse is not palpable. His breathing grows more rapid and shallow.

3. **What do you think is going on?**

Given the location of the chest wound and the sudden decompensation, you suspect a tension pneumothorax.

4. **What are you going to do about it?**

You perform a needle decompression (NDC) of the right chest and hear the soft hiss of escaping air. The casualty becomes conscious again and you note that his breathing is less labored.

5. **What next?**

You recheck the casualty's pulse. His radial pulse is now normal.

6. **What next?**

You move to Casualty 2, who reports that he was hit on his right side. He denies loss of consciousness, and his mental status is normal. There is no massive external hemorrhage. He complains of shortness of breath and appears anxious. Upon examination, the only injury you find is a shrapnel wound in the midaxillary line on his right side at nipple level. The wound is approximately 1 inch (2.5 centimeters) in diameter. Sucking and hissing sounds are coming from the wound. His pulse oximetry reading shows an oxygen saturation of 88%.

7. **What is the diagnosis?**

Open pneumothorax (or sucking chest wound)

8. **How can you help this man?**

You apply a vented chest seal over the wound, and the casualty's breathing quickly improves. His pulse oximetry reading improves to 95% over several minutes.

9. **What else do you want to know?**

- Is there an exit wound? You can't find one.
- Are there signs of shock? He is alert and oriented, and his radial pulse is strong.
- Are there other injuries? You find none.

Medical evacuation (MEDEVAC) for the two casualties is requested from headquarters. In anticipation of a helicopter evacuation (**Figure 27-2**), you prepare the casualties for flight including saline lock, TXA, antibiotics, and analgesia.

10. **Which analgesic would you use?**

Casualty 1 is not complaining of severe pain, so you elect to defer analgesic medications. You use ketamine for Casualty 2 because he has an injury that might impair respiration.

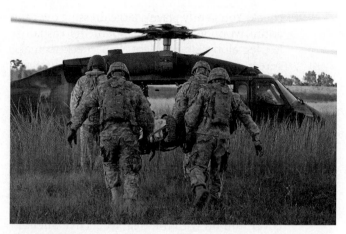

Figure 27-2 Evacuation by air requires special considerations.
Courtesy of Kimberly Lamb, U.S. Army.

You place both casualties in Hypothermia Prevention and Management Kits (HPMKs) to ensure that the cold environment of helicopter flight does not induce hypothermia. You plan to remind the flight paramedic to keep the doors closed during the flight, if possible.

11. **What do you do next?**

You complete the TCCC casualty card while waiting for the evacuation helicopter to arrive.

The casualties are picked up by an Army DUSTOFF helicopter. Immediately after takeoff, the casualty with the back-to-right axilla gunshot wound develops sudden-onset shortness of breath and hypoxemia as measured by pulse oximetry. The flight paramedic recalls Boyle's Law, by which gas expands at altitude, thus potentially causing air trapped in the pleural space to expand and convert a simple pneumothorax to a tension pneumothorax. She responds by performing NDC, and the casualty's condition immediately improves.

12. **What should she do now?**

Continue to monitor both casualties' respiration, blood pressure, and oxygen saturation as well as watch for any signs of external hemorrhage.

The DUSTOFF unit delivers both casualties to the Role 3 medical treatment facility (MTF) and communicates their clinical histories to the emergency medical staff.

Scenario 3: Rocket-Propelled Grenade Attack on a Convoy

You are riding with a squad in the back of a cargo Humvee along a road at the outskirts of a small Afghani village. When you stop at an intersection, a lone attacker located about 160 feet (ft; 50 meters [m]) away takes aim with an RPG and fires the rocket. The warhead explodes near the right front wheel. The vehicle sustains moderate damage to its right side and veers into a concrete barrier. Small flames erupt from the engine compartment.

Everyone in your vehicle is shaken, but they all scramble to exit the vehicle. You grab your rifle and medical kit and hit the ground running. The soldier who was riding in the front passenger seat makes it only a few meters from the Humvee and then falls to the ground. You stop to help the casualty even though there is no cover where he is lying. The rest of the unit takes cover near the side of the road. Hostile small arms fire is incoming from several locations. Rounds from hostile fire are striking the ground near you and the casualty.

1. **What should you do first to help the casualty?**
   You immediately move him to cover.
2. **How do you move him?**
   You use the one-person drag.
3. **Why?**
   - You do not have help since the other squad members are providing security.
   - The ground you have to cross is fairly smooth.
   - You can stabilize the casualty's cervical spine (blunt trauma) by cradling his head and neck with your forearms.

You drop behind cover that gives you a hasty fighting position. The casualty is conscious but has facial wounds and is having difficulty breathing. A quick look reveals that he has no massive external hemorrhage. You start firing back at the enemy. After a 5-minute firefight, hostile fire is eliminated. The squad sets up a security perimeter, and the squad leader gives you the go-ahead to care for the casualty. Because there may still be a risk of sniper fire, you want to relocate the casualty to better cover behind a low stone wall nearby. He is still alert but having trouble breathing and is unable to walk at this point. As you evaluate him for airway status, you find that he has a disfigured right zygomatic arch, a broken jaw, and there is blood in his mouth. There are swelling, bruising, and abrasions over the right side of his neck. He is not talking and does not respond to questions about neck pain. He responds to deep pain with barely audible moaning. His radial pulse is strong. His breathing is labored, and blood is gurgling from his mouth. Opening his body armor and blouse, you observe that the rise and fall of his chest are symmetrical, but there is little excursion.

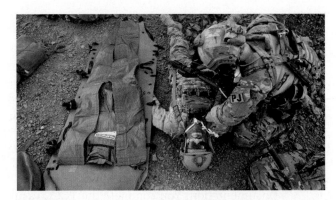

Figure 27-3 Addressing acute breathing problems is usually best deferred until the Tactical Field Care or Tactical Evacuation Care phase.

Paula Bronstein/Getty Images.

4. **What is your primary concern?**
   The casualty is still breathing spontaneously, but he is having airway difficulty. The disrupted anatomy and bleeding from injuries to his lower face and neck could be blocking his airway.
5. **What do you do?**
   The casualty's clinical status and the mechanism of his injuries make it impossible to rule out a spinal injury, so you do not attempt to place him in a sit-up-and-lean-forward position. Taking care to keep his neck stable, you do a chin lift and notice that the casualty's respirations get a little deeper, but his breathing is still labored. His oxygen saturation is 65%.
6. **What next?**
   You judge that the casualty does not yet have an adequate airway and elect to do a cricothyrotomy. As you perform this procedure, you give the squad leader the information he needs for a 9-line MEDEVAC request (**Figure 27-3**). He lets you call over one of the Combat Lifesavers in the squad to help you out. After the procedure is performed and the Cric-Key is in place, the casualty becomes more alert and his oxygen saturation improves to 94%. You secure the cricothyrotomy tube. Your squad leader tells you to prepare for MEDEVAC by helicopter in 30 minutes.
7. **What else do you want to do for this casualty?**
   Stabilize his cervical spine.
8. **How do you do that?**
   You do not have a cervical collar (C-collar) with you, so you use manual in-line stabilization. The MEDEVAC helicopter will have a C-collar and a rigid litter.
9. **What else should you consider?**
   - Reevaluate for massive external hemorrhage. Again, you find none.

- TXA? Not indicated because the radial pulse is normal.
- IV or IO fluids? Not indicated at this point.
- Hypothermia prevention? Yes.
- Analgesia? The casualty cannot speak but appears uncomfortable and indicates "yes" when asked if he is in pain. You give him ketamine 50 mg intramuscularly (IM).
- Antibiotics? Yes, you administer ertapenem 1 g IM.

10. What next?
Documentation. You complete the TCCC casualty card while waiting for the evacuation helicopter to arrive.

When the MEDEVAC helicopter arrives, you, the Combat Lifesaver, and the flight paramedic place the casualty on a rigid litter and apply a C-collar. You brief the flight paramedic on the casualty's course so far and give him the casualty's TCCC card.

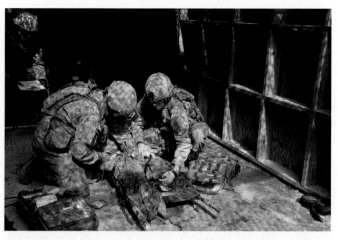

Figure 27-4 Traumatic amputations require the application of a tourniquet.
Courtesy of Lori Newman, JBSA-Fort Sam Houston Public Affairs.

Scenario 4: Dismounted Improvised Explosive Device Attack

You are a medic in a 12-man Marine squad moving into a small village. One patrol member steps on a pressure plate-activated improvised explosive device (IED). Three patrol members are injured. Unhurt members of the patrol form a perimeter around the casualties. There is no follow-on hostile fire, at least for the moment.

1. What phase of care are you in right now?
You are in the Tactical Field Care phase because there is no incoming fire at present, but the patrol is alert for any hostile fire that may ensue.

2. What do you do first?
You do a rapid triage of your casualties. Casualty 1 is obviously dead from a devastating head wound. Casualty 2 has multiple small fragment wounds to the back of his arms and legs and to his buttocks, but there is no obvious major hemorrhage. He is alert and oriented. Casualty 3 has sustained a traumatic amputation of his left leg just below the hip, with additional pelvic and inguinal wounds. He is bleeding heavily from multiple points in and around the amputation site. He is agitated, making loud but incomprehensible sounds, and is thrashing about with his remaining extremities.

3. How do you begin caring for the casualties?
You divide the labor. You direct a squad Combat Lifesaver to evaluate Casualty 2 with the

shrapnel wounds. You take Casualty 3 with the amputation and apply a tourniquet above the amputation site (**Figure 27-4**).

4. Whose Combat Application Tourniquet are you using?
One of your own. You would normally use the casualty's, but you are in a real hurry, and you don't have time to inspect the casualty's tourniquet to make sure it wasn't damaged in the blast.

5. Where do you apply it?
You apply the tourniquet as high on the femoral stump as you can get it. You continue to tighten the tourniquet but cannot get a good purchase on the stump, and there is still significant bleeding, both from the amputation site and the inguinal wounds.

6. What now?
You break out your Combat Gauze and, with help from another patrol member, apply it to the bleeding sites with 3 minutes of firm direct pressure. The bleeding is still not controlled.

7. What next?
You break out your junctional tourniquet and apply it while another unit member maintains direct pressure over the Combat Gauze. The hemorrhage is now controlled.

The squad sends in the 9-line MEDEVAC request along with a warning of the RPG hazard in the nearby village. The squad is then directed to move the casualties on foot to a landing zone (LZ) in an open area 0.6 miles (1 kilometer [km]) away from the village.

Casualty 2 takes his CWMP. He continues to function as a unit member and assists with the mission. Casualty 3, however, although still conscious, is now confused. His radial pulse is not palpable, and his carotid pulse is thready and rapid.

8. **What is the most likely diagnosis for Casualty 3?**
    Hemorrhagic shock.

9. **What treatment do you provide Casualty 3?**
    The unit delays its movement so that care can be rendered. You place a sternal IO device and infuse 1 g of TXA in 100 ml of NS after which you flush the IO line. While the TXA solution infuses, you draw a unit of type O low-titer whole blood from one of the unit's preidentified universal donors. As soon as the unit is drawn, you administer it to the casualty. When the blood is in, the casualty's carotid pulse gets a little stronger, and his radial becomes palpable. He is alert but confused. He is breathing adequately and is not complaining of pain at the moment.

10. **Now that you have IO access, are there other medications you would give Casualty 3?**
    Yes, ertapenem.

11. **What further care is required?**
    You place a pulse oximeter on Casualty 3. His oxygen saturation is 95%. The mission commander gives the order to move out for the designated LZ. The deceased casualty is moved with a two-person drag. Casualty 3 is moved using a three-person carry. The Marines carrying Casualty 3 monitor the site of the previous hemorrhage to ensure that it does not begin to bleed again. The other five patrol members provide security during the movement to the LZ.

    The patrol arrives at the LZ. The helicopter is 10 minutes out. It has been about 45 minutes since Casualty 3 received the first unit of whole blood. His status is the same.

12. **What next?**
    You draw and infuse a second unit of type O low-titer whole blood.

13. **What else do you want to do?**
    You thoroughly reassess both casualties and find no new conditions requiring immediate treatment. You place Casualty 3 in an HPMK after rechecking to ensure that his previous hemorrhage remains controlled.

14. **What next?**
    You complete TCCC casualty cards while waiting for the evacuation helicopter to arrive.

15. **In addition to monitoring for continued hemorrhage control, what is Casualty 3 likely to need during the 20-minute MEDEVAC flight?**
    He may need further fluid resuscitation, preferably with whole blood or plasma and packed red blood cells if available. High-flow supplemental oxygen should be started using a reservoir mask. If his mental status continues to improve and pain becomes an issue, he may need ketamine.

Scenario 5: Fast-Roping Casualty in an Urban Environment

A 14-man Special Operations assault team fast-ropes from a helicopter hovering about 80 ft (25 m) above the ground for a building assault in a high-threat urban environment. On exiting, one of the last members of the team loses his grip and falls to the ground (**Figure 27-5**). The helicopter, unable to loiter at the scene or evacuate the casualty, departs quickly with its escort gunship. You, one of two medics on the team, attend immediately to the casualty. The mission commander instructs the rest of the team to form a defensive perimeter. There are hostiles all around you in the streets, and the unit begins to take sporadic fire from several directions. The casualty is unconscious.

1. **What is the first priority?**
    Provide cover for the team, including the casualty.

2. **Why?**
    There are many armed hostiles in street crowds all around you. It is unlikely that the team can eliminate all hostile fire. The best way to deal with injuries is to prevent them. The team takes cover behind a nearby low wall.

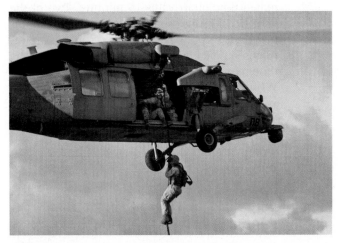

Figure 27-5 Not all combat-related trauma involves weapons. Falls represent an important mechanism of injury on the battlefield.

3. **How do you move the casualty?**

You and another team member move him using a two-man carry, taking care to minimize head and neck movement.

4. **The low wall provides effective cover from incoming fire. What phase of care are you now in?**

You are in the Tactical Field Care phase, but a very high-risk version of it.

5. **What do you do next?**

Safely behind cover, you begin your assessment of the casualty. He is still unresponsive; you find no signs of external hemorrhage. He has a patent airway, adequate breathing, and a strong radial pulse. You note bilateral open femur fractures and are aware of the high incidence of spinal and pelvic fractures in high falls. While maintaining improvised cervical stabilization, you remove his weapons, helmet, and body armor to facilitate your examination. Your further assessment reveals symmetrical and responsive pupils and ecchymosis at the left mastoid area (Battle's sign). The casualty remains unresponsive. You place a pulse oximeter on his finger; his oxygen saturation is 94%.

6. **What is the diagnosis?**

Traumatic brain injury due to blunt trauma and bilateral femur fractures. You cannot rule out spinal injury or pelvic fracture, and he may have noncompressible abdominal or thoracic hemorrhage.

You inform the team leader of the urgency of the casualty's condition. The team leader reports back that the mission has been altered to accommodate the casualty and four armored Humvees have been dispatched for evacuation. Their estimated time of arrival is 15 minutes. Two of the vehicles have litters, but one of the team members finds a door nearby and you use it as an improvised rigid litter so that you can minimize the time required on-scene once the vehicles arrive.

7. **What do you do next?**

While continuing to monitor him, you apply the C-collar that you thought to bring for this type of mission, and you insert an i-gel extraglottic airway. (Note that a field-expedient cervical collar can also be made from a SAM splint.) You then insert a saline lock.

8. **Does the casualty need any medications?**

His radial pulse is strong, but because of the high probability of noncompressible hemorrhage in a fall of this magnitude, you elect to administer TXA. The casualty remains unconscious, so he does not need analgesics. He has open femur fractures, so you administer IV antibiotics after the TXA is infused.

9. **What next?**

The door effectively splints the femur fractures after you have secured his legs to the door with tactical tape. You put a Ready-Heat Blanket over the casualty's t-shirt and place him into a Heat Reflective Shell. You then put his helmet back on and lay his body armor over him.

The vehicles were due to arrive 10 minutes ago but have not yet appeared. The team members continue to maintain security and minimize incoming hostile fire.

10. **What next?**

You reassess the casualty and note his respirations have become very shallow and his left pupil is now dilated. He remains unresponsive.

11. **What's happening clinically with this casualty?**

Cerebral herniation.

12. **What can you do about it?**

You have no oxygen in TFC. You use a bag-mask device to ventilate the casualty. Capnography is not available, so you use a ventilation rate of 20 breaths/min. You elevate the head of the improvised rigid litter 30 degrees. You would give 250 ml of 3% saline IV if you had it, but you do not. You monitor his oxygen saturation with the pulse oximeter, and it remains above 90%.

13. **What next?**

You complete the TCCC casualty card while waiting for the evacuation vehicles to arrive.

The vehicles arrive shortly thereafter. You have unit members help you carefully move the casualty into one of the vehicles and secure the improvised litter as best you can. Everyone else mounts up in the other vehicles, and the convoy moves out.

References

1. Gerhardt RG, Mabry RL, De Lorenzo RA, Butler FK. Fundamentals of combat casualty care. IN: Savitsky E, Eastridge B, eds. *Combat Casualty Care—Lessons Learned from OEF and OIF.* Fort Detrick, MD: Borden Institute; 2011.

2. Butler, FK Jr, Blackbourne LH. Battlefield trauma care then and now: a decade of tactical combat casualty care. *J Trauma Acute Care Surg.* 2012;73(6)(Suppl 5): S395-S402. doi:10.1097/TA.0b013e3182754850.

3. Eastridge BJ, Mabry RL, Seguin P, et al. Death on the battlefield (2001-2011): implications for the future of combat casualty care. *J Trauma Acute Care Surg.* 2012;73(6)(Suppl5):S431-S437.doi:10.1097/TA.0b013e3182755dcc.

4. Kotwal RS, Montgomery HR, Mechler KK. A prehospital trauma registry for tactical combat casualty care. *J Spec Oper Med.* 2011;11(3):127-128.

5. Pannell D, Brisebois R, Talbot M, et al. Causes of death in Canadian Forces members deployed to Afghanistan and implications on tactical combat casualty care provision. *J Trauma.* 2011;71(5)(Suppl 1):S401-S407. doi:10.1097/TA.0b013e318232e53f.

6. Deal VT, McDowell D, Benson P, et al. Tactical combat casualty care February 2010. Direct from the battlefield: TCCC lessons learned in Iraq and Afghanistan. *J Spec Ops Med.* 2010;10(3):77-119.

7. Committee on Tactical Combat Casualty Care. Tactical Combat Casualty Care Guidelines, September 17, 2012. Defense Health System website. http://www.health.mil /Libraries/120917_TCCC_Course_Materials/TCCC-Guidelines-120917.pdf. Accessed June 6, 2013.

8. Gerhardt, RG, Adams BD, De Lorenzo RA, et al. Panel synopsis: pre-hospital combat health support 2010: what should our azimuth be? *J Trauma.* 2007;62(Suppl 6):S15-S16.

9. Adams BD, Cuniowski PA, Muck A, De Lorenzo RA. Registry of emergency airways at combat hospitals. *J Trauma.* 2008;64(6):1548-1554. doi:10.1097/TA.0b013e3181728c41.

10. Bell RS, Vo AH, Neal CJ, et al. Military traumatic brain and spinal column injury: a 5-year study of the impact blast and other military grade weaponry on the central nervous system. *J Trauma.* 2009;66(4)(Suppl 5):S104-111. doi:10.1097/TA.0b013e31819d88c8.

11. Morrison JJ, Dubose JJ, Rasmussen TE, Midwinter MJ. Military Application of Tranexamic Acid in Trauma Emergency Resuscitation (MATTERs) study. *Arch Surg.* 2012;147(2):113-119. doi:10.1001/archsurg.2011.287.

CHAPTER **28**

Aeromedical Evacuation in a Combat Theater

Authors:
Col. Kimberlie Biever
Col. Jay Johannigman, MD

CHAPTER OBJECTIVES

At the completion of this chapter, you will be able to do the following:

- Define the terms *CASEVAC, MEDEVAC, TACEVAC,* and *aeromedical evacuation* (AE).
- State the difference between a casualty and a patient in the AE chain.
- Discuss the limitations on combat casualty care imposed by the environment of a rotary-wing platform.
- Recognize techniques and procedures to ensure safety during rotary-wing evacuation.
- Discuss the concepts and requirements of en route care.
- Specify the common stressors of AE, and discuss the effects and management of each.

SCENARIO

You are the senior flight nurse on an aeromedical evacuation (AE) team aboard a MEDEVAC C-130 transferring a patient from the Role 3 hospital in Kandahar, Afghanistan, to Craig Joint Theater Hospital in Bagram. As the aircraft makes its final approach, it comes under small arms fire. Two of your team members are wounded. Casualty 1 has sustained a gunshot wound to his right inguinal area with heavy bleeding. Casualty 2 has an injury to her left thigh with pulsatile bleeding. The aircraft banks away from the approach, and there is no further incoming fire.

- What phase of tactical combat casualty care (TCCC) are you in?
- You now need to do two things simultaneously. What are they?
- What do you do next?

INTRODUCTION

History of Aeromedical Casualty Movement

The concept of moving combat casualties by air has been recognized since the early days of aviation. The first recorded movement of combat casualties by air is thought to have occurred in 1870 during the Franco-Prussian War. At the siege of Paris, 160 wounded French soldiers were flown out over the Prussian lines in hot-air balloons.[1] Limited attempts at movement of casualties by air occurred during World War I and through the 1920s and 1930s.

Large-scale casualty movement by air did not occur until World War II, during which more than 1.4 million casualties were moved by air, with only 46 deaths occurring in flight.[1] It must be noted that the majority of these flights originated in rear staging areas for hospital-treated casualties who had been transported from the battlefield by the more traditional means of ground evacuation. Aeromedical evacuation (AE) from the battlefield was not readily practiced during World War II because of the limitations of the fixed-wing aircraft of the era.

The development of rotary-wing aircraft in the mid-1940s created dramatic new capabilities for evacuation of the injured combatant. The first movement of a casualty by helicopter occurred in Burma in 1944.[2] During the Korean War, more than 17,700 casualties were flown by the newly introduced rotary-wing aircraft, many directly from the battle zone.[1] The introduction of a helicopter evacuation system in Korea is usually credited as the most important causative factor in the improved survival rate among combat casualties seen in this conflict.

The rotary-wing evacuation system developed even further during the Vietnam War, when by 1967, more than 94,000 casualties had been flown out of combat zones by helicopters like the venerable UH-1.[3] The comparative success of the Vietnam evacuation system led to its widespread adaptation by civilian programs within the continental United States (CONUS), beginning in the mid-1970s. The majority of current civilian "life flight" programs trace their roots to the experience provided by the military AE units of Korea and Vietnam.[1,4]

En Route Care

The introduction of rotary-wing evacuation aircraft sparked the recognition that a variety of missions may be involved in the movement of casualties—from the point of wounding, through the initial resuscitation, to the final point of care. Recent experience gained from AE during Operation Iraqi Freedom and Operation Enduring

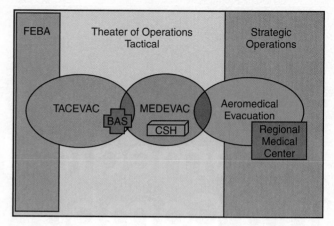

Figure 28-1 Schematic representation of the continuum of evacuation.
Courtesy of Stephen Giebner, MD.

Freedom has significantly increased the understanding and appreciation of the AE process. The most significant of these revisions is the recognition of the role of continuous, high-intensity medical care throughout the continuum of care from the point of wounding to the point of final, definitive care and rehabilitation. AE is a continuum of care, usually associated with some form of transportation or movement (rotary wing, fixed wing, or other) while medical care is ongoing (**Figure 28-1**). The term *en route care* is employed to encompass and characterize this seamless continuum of medical care from point-of-injury providers (field medics, battalion aid station physicians, and physician assistants), through theater facilities (Role 2 and 3 theater hospitals), and onward to Role 4 medical treatment facilities (MTFs), both out of the theater of conflict and in CONUS. From there, they are treated further at rehabilitation centers and Veterans Affairs hospitals. The Committee on Tactical Combat Casualty Care revised the definitions of its third phase of care to reflect operational, doctrinal, and logistical, and medical concerns. The phrase *tactical evacuation care* (TACEVAC) encompasses casualty evacuation (CASEVAC) and medical evacuation (MEDEVAC) operations into a spectrum of continuous en route care from the point of wounding to the first MTF. Although doctrinal differences exist among the service branches regarding terminology and definitions of phases of care, for purposes of the following discussion, casualty movement may be described as follows:

1. **CASEVAC:** Evacuation of a casualty from the battlefield to a Role 2 or Role 3 MTF using available tactical platforms (i.e., vehicles not dedicated to medical missions.) Tactical platforms may include movement aboard ships, land vehicles, or aircraft and in the future, may

include trains.[5] CASEVAC assets are owned by line commanders and are an integral part of combat missions. They are designed accordingly, with armor and offensive weaponry such as crew-served automatic weapons, rockets, and missiles. "CASEVAC is considered unregulated movement of casualties to and between treatment facilities."[6]

2. **MEDEVAC**: Timely evacuation of a casualty from the battlefield to an MTF, or from one MTF to another within the tactical theater using dedicated medical assets, usually marked with a red cross, while performing en route care by medical personnel. These evacuation assets are not part of the offensive forces; they are part of the casualty care plan. MEDEVAC assets may be rotary-wing or fixed-wing aircraft like the C-130 dedicated to medical missions, or they may include ground ambulance-type vehicles.

3. **Tactical Evacuation Care**: En route care from the battlefield to a theater Role 2 or Role 3 MTF, including both CASEVAC and MEDEVAC.

4. **Aeromedical evacuation (AE)**: A term most commonly utilized by the U.S. Air Force to designate the movement of a casualty ("patient") under medical supervision from a point of care within the theater to a more rearward location, such as regional hospital or CONUS. Traditionally, this phase of movement has employed fixed-wing jet aircraft such as the C-17.

In the process of AE, a wounded soldier is considered a *casualty* until he or she reaches the first point of definitive medical care. Once entered into the medical care system, the casualty is considered a "patient" (although this text uniformly uses "casualty").

In practice, the lines separating CASEVAC, MEDEVAC, and AE are blurred at times because doctrine, circumstances, and medical care require flexibility (Figure 28-1). In recent years, prehospital care capabilities across all phases of casualty care and movement have significantly improved, reflecting advancements in medical technology, pharmacology, and casualty management doctrine. In theaters such as Afghanistan, where the evacuation system is well established, the transport distances are relatively short, and there is definitive air superiority, it is common for a U.S. combat casualty to be evacuated by helicopter within 30 minutes of injury, be at a forward surgical facility or a combat support hospital within 30 minutes, and on the way back to CONUS within 48 hours of wounding. In the next 10 or 20 years, this casualty movement may be augmented with a capability for remote monitoring and by medical equipment that automatically intervenes to stabilize the casualty en route.

Tactical Evacuation (TACEVAC) Care

Principles

Although CASEVAC, MEDEVAC, and AE can all involve the transport of casualties by air, they may be functionally very different. In CASEVAC, casualties are moved from the point of injury to a place of initial surgical care or an aid station to stabilize the patient and await onward movement. In most cases, this is a relatively short transport accomplished by rotary-wing aircraft, although it can be conducted using ground vehicles or watercraft. TACEVAC aircraft must frequently fly into the forward edge of the battle area (FEBA) and may come under enemy fire. The aircraft used in this mission may be tactical aircraft that are designated for a single mission (*aircraft of opportunity*) or may have had a secondary CASEVAC role designated during pre-mission planning. When the tactical situation allows, dedicated aircraft designed and equipped for medical missions (e.g., an *air ambulance*) may be used for MEDEVAC (**Figure 28-2**). En route care is the continuation of the provision of care during movement or evacuation between the health service support capabilities in the roles of care, without clinically compromising the patient's condition.[6]

Casualties needing evacuation from the field are, by definition, recently injured and may be quite unstable. Essential care must be focused on lifesaving maneuvers that enhance survival while minimizing additional risk to the casualty, the unit's mission, and the evacuation crew. Tactical imperatives to accomplish the mission or prevent further casualties may impose severe limitations on medical capabilities during TACEVAC. It is desirable to keep ground time in the forward area to a minimum, and therefore, most CASEVAC/MEDEVAC care is delivered during flight in a noisy, turbulent, and crowded environment, very different from a hospital trauma bay.

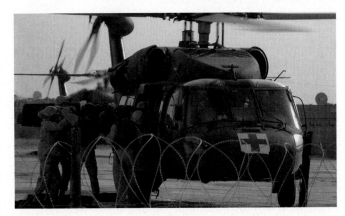

Figure 28-2 UH-60 Black Hawk MEDEVAC helicopter.
Courtesy of SPC Algernon E, Crawley Jr/U.S. Department of Defense.

Excellent tactical flying and pre-mission planning are essential to keep the aircraft, crew, and casualties safe. Consideration must be given to whether the medical needs of the casualty justify the risk and exposure that a TACEVAC mission generates for the casualty's unit and the TACEVAC platform and its crew. (These issues are discussed further in Chapter 26, *Tactical Evacuation Care*.) Alternative modes of evacuation (ground, water) and the impact of delayed transport should be included in the decision-making process.[5]

Medical Care

TACEVAC operations occur after the Care Under Fire and/or Tactical Field Care phases and may allow for increased visibility and opportunities for intervention. Hemorrhage control, airway management, respiratory support as needed, intravenous (IV) access, treatment of shock, and hypothermia prevention are the core of treatment in these phases. Once under way in a TACEVAC platform, the limitations imposed by space, noise, lighting, and combat conditions may continue to impose severe limitations on care.

Equipment used during TACEVAC should be lightweight and robust enough to withstand the rugged environment. In the setting of nighttime tactical conditions, light sources should be minimized and subdued light (e.g., Phantom light, Petzl light) or infrared light sources in conjunction with night-vision devices used. White lights should be avoided because of their adverse impact on the crew's vision and because they may provide a targeting profile for the enemy. TACEVAC providers should be practiced in medical care techniques in darkened conditions while under way in tactical vehicles and aircraft.

Preparation of the Casualty

The principles of casualty preparation for TACEVAC fall under the same guidelines as discussed in Care Under Fire and Tactical Field Care. For TACEVAC by air, a landing zone (LZ) should be prepared in accordance with standard guidance (**Box 28-1**). Helicopter safety is critical in TACEVAC operations. Engine-running onloads and offloads are the norm, and rotors will be turning. It is imperative that everyone who assists in loading patients

---

Box 28-1 Preparation for CASEVAC by Air

1. Determine the number of casualties to be moved, the requirement for movement by helicopter, and the urgency of the movement; evaluate the tactical situation.
   · Note that in some cases it is faster and safer to move casualties by ground than by air.
   · Not all casualties require urgent evacuation.
   · The tactical situation may preclude evacuation by air (e.g., heavy enemy fire).
   · Environmental conditions, such as darkness, bad weather, or lack of a suitable landing zone, may prevent evacuation by air.

2. Locate and mark a suitable helicopter landing zone (HLZ) or pickup site.
   · HLZ should be as flat as possible, with even terrain and no surrounding large trees, wires, or tall structures.
   · HLZ should be a minimum of 100 ft (30 m) in diameter, or larger if a CH-47 or MH-53 will be landing.
   · Mark (or prepare to mark) the zone as per protocol (VS-17 panels, smoke, chemical lights, strobe lights, vehicle lights).
   · If possible, have a wind indicator (wind sock, ribbon on stick) just outside the HLZ, easily visible to the pilot.
   · In a tactical situation, keep the HLZ as inconspicuous as possible to prevent the enemy from zeroing in on it.

3. Prepare the casualties for flight.
   · If possible, perform any urgent medical procedures, such as splinting, applying dressings, or starting IV lines, while still on the ground.
   · Move the casualties near the HLZ, and stage them perpendicular to the line of approach/departure of the aircraft, but well outside the HLZ.
   · Protect the casualties' ears with earplugs. Protect the eyes with goggles or bandages. Litter bearers should have earplugs and goggles in place.

4. Load the casualties.
   · Do not approach the helicopter until the crew has seen you and given you positive clearance to approach the aircraft.
   · Do not approach the rear of the aircraft unless you are specifically directed to go there by the aircraft crew. (The CH-46, CH-47, and CH/MH-53 have rear loading ramps, and you will probably be directed to load casualties there. Do not approach from the rear of an H-60 or any other helicopter with a tail rotor.)
   · Load the casualties as directed by the aircraft crew.
   · Minimize the time that the aircraft is on the ground
   · As soon as loading is complete, exit the rotor disc and clear the HLZ.

on and off helicopters be familiar with rotary-wing operational procedures under all conditions.

Casualties should have eye and ear protection, as should all members of the loading crew. Most helicopters should be approached from the nose or the sides. Personnel should never enter the rotor disc area (area under rotor blades) unless they have been cleared to enter by the helicopter crew. If the helicopter is on a slope, personnel should approach and depart from the downslope side.[1,7]

A standard method of calling for a TACEVAC is the nine-line evacuation request (**Box 28-2**). Other methods are also used, but regardless of the method, it should be specified during pre-mission planning so that everyone involved with the operation is familiar with the chosen format.

MTF to MTF MEDEVAC

The term MEDEVAC also applies to the movement of a patient from one MTF to another MTF within the theater, for example, the movement of a casualty from a Role 2 forward resuscitative surgical team to a Role 3 combat support hospital or field hospital. MEDEVAC also describes the movement of a patient from a combat support hospital (CSH)/Expeditionary Medical Support System (EMEDS) to a regional staging facility, theater air hub, aeromedical staging facility). Both of these movements are components of AE. Patient transport from MTF to MTF may include the capabilities of MEDEVAC units, which include flight paramedics and critical care flight paramedics, but also may include the en route critical

---

Box 28-2 Standard Nine-Line MEDEVAC Request (Unregulated Patient Movement)

Line 1: Location of Casualty/HLZ (Helicopter Landing Zone)
Location can be given in grid coordinates, latitude/longitude, or any other system that is clearly understood by all parties. In hostile areas the HLZ coordinates should be encrypted to prevent enemy forces from ascertaining the location of the HLZ.

Line 2: Radio Frequency and Call Sign
Radio the frequency and call sign of the unit requesting the MEDEVAC. Again, in hostile situations this should be encrypted.

Line 3: Evacuation Precedence
  A Urgent
  B Urgent/surgical
  C Priority
  D Routine
  E Convenience

Each letter is preceded by the number of casualties in each category. For example, "3 ALPHA, 2 BRAVO, 1 CHARLIE" means there are three urgent casualties, two urgent surgical casualties, and 1 priority casualty requiring MEDEVAC.

Line 4: Special Equipment Requests
This line requests specialized extraction or medical equipment.

  A None
  B Hoist required
  C Extraction equipment
  D Ventilator required

Line 5: Numbers of Litter and Ambulatory Patients
  L Litter casualties
  A Ambulatory casualties

Each category is preceded by the number of casualties. For example, "3 LIMA, 2 ALPHA" means three litter casualties and two ambulatory casualties require MEDEVAC.

Line 6: Evacuation Site Security
This indicates the level of hostile threat in the area.

  N No threat
  P Possible enemy troops in the area
  E Enemy troops in the area
  X Hot HLZ, armed escort needed

Line 7: Marking of Evacuation Site
  A Colored panels (VS-17 panel)
  B Pyrotechnic signals
  C Smoke
  D No designation
  E Other means of designation

Line 8: Casualty Nationalities and Combat Status
  A U.S. Military
  B U.S. Civilian
  C Non-U.S. Military
  D Non-U.S. Civilian
  E Enemy prisoner of war

Line 9: NBC/Terrain Specifics
  N Nuclear
  B Biologic
  C Chemical

Describe any terrain features that may help the crew locate the HLZ from the air or that may affect their approach, such as trees, electrical wires, or sloping terrain.

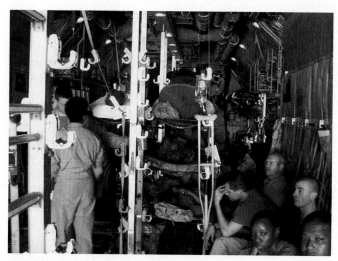

Figure 28-3 En route care during MEDEVAC.
Courtesy of Dr. Jay Johannigman.

care capabilities of nurses from one of the services. Military critical care nurses may be embedded in deployed MEDEVAC units and augment flight paramedics to immediately and aggressively resuscitate casualties as they are evacuated from the battlefield or transported, following lifesaving damage control surgery.

MTF to MTF MEDEVAC operations may involve either rotary-wing or fixed-wing tactical aircraft (**Figure 28-3**). As the duration of medical missions extends sufficiently to require the use of fixed-wing aircraft, the considerations for MEDEVAC missions more closely reflect those discussed next for AE.

Aeromedical Evacuation

Doctrine and Principles

In AE, patients who have received appropriate medical care and are stable (or stabilized) are flown relatively long distances in fixed-wing aircraft. This is considered regulated movement and requested through the TRANSCOM Regulating and Command and Control Evacuation System (TRAC2eS), a patient movement automated information system comprising transportation, logistics, and clinical decision elements. TRAC2eS is used at the global and theater levels, matching medical treatment capabilities to available transport. Some aircraft used for AE, like the C-130, are capable of dirt-strip operations, but in most cases a fixed airfield is necessary. Strategic patient movement via AE aircraft may occasionally be at risk from enemy fire, but usually not to the same extent as TACEVAC aircraft. Duration of flight (and, thus, length of in-flight medical care) is usually longer in AE than in TACEVAC flights. It is not unusual to have AE missions last 10 to 12 hours.

The medical support crew of an AE mission usually consists of persons specifically trained in the requirements and challenges of the flight environment. A typical AE crew consists of two flight nurses and three aeromedical technicians. Physicians are not normally part of an AE crew. Flight nurses and AE technicians are trained regarding altitude physiology, nursing considerations in the AE environment, aircraft power and oxygen systems, emergency procedures, AE aircraft configuration, and survival. The standard AE crew can be pared down or augmented as required.

Role of Critical Care Air Transport Team

The medical experiences garnered from more than a decade of current military operations have challenged portions of conventional AE doctrine. The fluidity of the battle space and the mobility of maneuvering forces have put increasing emphasis on a medical capability that is equally fluid. Traditional AE doctrine provided for the movement of a stable casualty who had received extensive care at an advanced facility (Role 3). It has become increasingly apparent that tactical combat considerations as well as evolving medical support doctrine will emphasize the capability to move casualties who have been "stabilized" at far-forward facilities (Role 2) but are not yet "stable." For the purposes of this discussion, a *stabilized* casualty is defined as a casualty with (1) hemorrhage controlled, (2) shock treated, (3) airway controlled, and (4) fractures splinted.

The development of the critical care air transport team (CCATT) arose from the need to provide en route care for stabilized, but not necessarily stable, casualties from forward locations (**Figure 28-4**). A CCATT is composed of an intensivist-trained physician (anesthesia, surgery, emergency medicine, or pulmonary medicine), a critical care nurse, and a respiratory therapist. The CCATT's equipment is self-contained and self-carried (**Figure 28-5**) and can provide care for three critically ill intubated patients or a total of six critical patients. All of the medical equipment that the CCATT carries has been tested and approved for use in flight.

A CCATT functions to augment a standard AE team and provides extended capability to far-forward locations via the provision of continuous en route intensive care. This concept ensures that the critically ill casualty may be moved rearward without degrading the capabilities of the forward medical units. CCATTs may be co-located at AE hubs, theater hospitals, or at other rearward locations. CCATTs are moved forward with the airframe and aeromedical crew as medical circumstances dictate. A CCATT may be effectively employed to provide continuous critical care from the battlefield rearward to CONUS, thus ensuring seamless en route care.

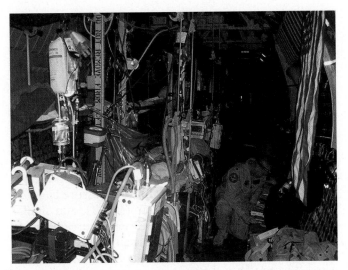

Figure 28-4 Critical care air transport team (CCATT) evacuation.

Courtesy of Dr. Jay Johannigman.

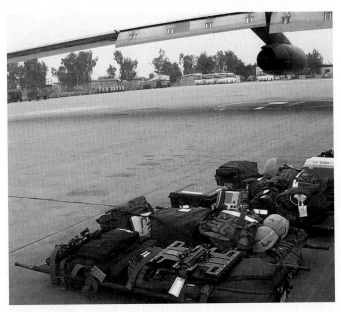

Figure 28-5 CCATT equipment load.

Courtesy of Dr. Jay Johannigman.

Other specialized aeromedical transport teams are available as needed. For example, the U.S. Army Burn SMART (Special Medical Augmentation Response Team) is based out of the Institute of Surgical Research at San Antonio Military Medical Center. Burn SMARTs specialize in transport of critically injured burn casualties, multiple-trauma casualties with burns, and victims of chemical blister agents. During Operation Iraqi Freedom and Operation Enduring Freedom, a specialized pulmonary CCATT team was stationed at Landstuhl Regional Medical Center and was available with advanced pulmonary rescue equipment, including extracorporeal devices to maintain oxygenation.

Stressors of Aeromedical Evacuation

During air transport, casualties may be exposed to a variety of environmental stressors that may adversely affect their medical outcome and complicate the provision of care. These elements are collectively referred to as the "stressors of flight." Stressors common to both rotary-wing and fixed-wing aircraft may include elevated ambient-noise levels, vibration, decreased atmospheric pressure, hypoxia, dehydration, and thermal stress.[1,4,7,8] Patient packaging and meticulous handoff between care teams can help to prevent complications from the stressors of AE.

Ambient Noise

High levels of ambient noise can damage hearing and make situational awareness pertaining to the casualty difficult. It is important that both the casualty and the prehospital care provider have hearing protection, like earplugs, headsets, or flight helmets. It is virtually impossible to hear breath sounds or take a manual blood pressure (BP) reading in a helicopter, and it is difficult in most fixed-wing aircraft, making electronic monitoring technology a requisite for optimal care. Hearing protection makes these tasks even more difficult. Recent advances have introduced wireless headsets to facilitate crew communication and provide hearing protection.

Vibration

Vibration is a recognized stressor that results in physical fatigue and poses challenges to the provision of ongoing medical care. Vibration impairs the evaluation of a casualty in flight by compromising physical examination (e.g., pulse and BP detection), and in some instances by interfering with electronic monitoring equipment. In preparation for long-duration AE flights, it is desirable to establish redundant means of monitoring casualties and their vital signs (e.g., electronic BP monitoring as well as invasive arterial lines to measure BP; pulse oximetry and mechanical spirometers to monitor ventilation).

The combination of vibration, turbulence, low-light conditions, and limited space creates extremely challenging working conditions for the medical crew providing casualty care. It is possible to accomplish most medical procedures in flight; however, it will be more challenging than performing the same procedure on the ground. If possible, medical procedures like starting IV lines, applying splints or dressings, and airway procedures (e.g., endotracheal intubation) should be accomplished before flight.[4,5] If a particular potential problem (e.g., unstable airway) is a concern, it is prudent to address this issue aggressively before transport rather than midway through a flight at altitude and in the dark.[4] With this in mind, it is important for the care provider to err on the side of over-preparation before AE.

Decreased Atmospheric Pressure

Since the inception of aviation, it has been recognized that as an aircraft ascends in altitude, the ambient atmospheric pressure decreases. Boyle's law states that, for a given amount of gas, pressure and volume are inversely proportional. In practical terms, this means that as an aircraft ascends to altitude, any gas trapped in the body or in a closed space will either expand in volume or, if expansion is not possible, will create a pressure differential that may result in pressure-related injury, or barotrauma. Conversely, as the aircraft descends, ambient pressure increases, and gas trapped in a space that is able to change in its dimensions will decrease in volume. For example, if a (theoretically perfectly elastic) balloon contains 1 liter of gas at sea level (ambient pressure = 760 mm Hg), that balloon will expand in volume to 2 liters at 18,000 feet (ft; 5,486 meters [m]) above sea level (ambient pressure = 380 mm Hg).[1,4] Most fixed-wing aircraft are pressurized, meaning that the pressure inside the aircraft cabin (cabin altitude) is maintained at a higher level than the outside ambient pressure. This will decrease pressure-related effects as the aircraft ascends and descends. However, most aircraft cannot maintain sea-level pressure up to their typical cruising altitudes. For example, the C-130 can maintain sea-level cabin pressure only up to an altitude of about 18,000 feet.[9] Even commercial aircraft routinely have cabin altitudes of 6,000 to 8,000 ft (1,829–2,438 m) when at cruising altitude.[1,4] Most helicopters are not pressurized, so the aircraft altitude and the cabin altitude are the same.

Boyle's law can have potentially disastrous consequences for casualties during AE. Care must be taken to provide adequate means of decompression for the medically relevant closed spaces of the human body. Gas trapped in distensible spaces in the body such as the intestines, the middle ear, or the chest will expand as altitude increases and contract as altitude decreases. A casualty with a simple pneumothorax at low altitude may develop a life-threatening tension pneumothorax as the gas in the chest expands on ascent. Therefore, a pneumothorax must be appropriately treated with a decompressive device, such as a chest tube, before flight. The presence of an untreated pneumothorax is one of the few absolute contraindications to AE.[8] MEDEVAC may be possible without a chest tube if the helicopter maintains a low altitude; however, the medic should monitor the casualty carefully and be prepared to perform a needle decompression if signs or symptoms of a tension pneumothorax appear.

Gas in the intestines, ears, and sinuses will usually find a means of decompression during ascent. On descent, however, air must be added to the middle ear and sinuses to prevent ear and sinus "squeeze." If the patient is unconscious, has injury to the maxillofacial area, or has other pathology (e.g., a cold), ventilation of the middle ears and sinuses may be difficult. Comatose or semiconscious patients may become combative as a result of pain from occult ear or sinus squeeze. Appropriate management of patients at risk for these events may include the administration of nasal decongestants (e.g., phenylephrine nasal spray) before flight.[4,7,8]

Gas-filled bladders on medical equipment are also affected by changes in atmospheric pressure. On ascent, gas in endotracheal (ET) tube cuffs, IV pressure bags, air splints, military antishock trousers (MAST), and similar devices will expand. This can increase pressure on tissues enough to cause damage. On descent, volume will decrease. Medics should avoid the use of air splints in flight if possible. MAST and IV pressure bags should be closely monitored, and air added or removed as necessary.[4,7,8] Air-filled cuffs on ET tubes and extraglottic airways must be monitored to ensure that cuff pressure remains within recommended limits during ascent and descent. Even minor volume changes can lead to pressure necrosis of the trachea or air leakage around the cuff.

Altitude Hypoxia

As an aircraft ascends and the ambient pressure decreases, the partial pressure of oxygen in the air decreases. Therefore, as altitude increases, the available oxygen in the atmosphere decreases, and measures must be undertaken to prevent hypoxia.[1,4,7,8] For a healthy individual, altitude hypoxia is usually not significant below altitudes of 10,000 feet (3,048 m). For casualties with respiratory compromise or preexisting anemia, however, altitude hypoxia may pose a significant problem at much lower altitudes.

Altitude hypoxia is readily treated with the provision of supplemental oxygen.[1,4] Not all trauma victims will need oxygen during flight, especially if the cabin altitude is maintained at or below 10,000 feet. Monitoring with pulse oximetry is the preferred way to determine the need for supplemental oxygen, allowing the medic to titrate oxygen delivery. Patients with significant traumatic brain injuries (Glasgow Coma Scale [GCS] < 12) are particularly susceptible to hypoxia. The occurrence of hypoxia in the head-injured patient (secondary insult) is associated with increased mortality. Supplemental oxygen should be utilized to maintain an oxygen saturation greater than 90% in these patients.

Dehydration

A problem unique to pressurized aircraft is the low relative humidity of the cabin environment. Cold, low-pressure air from outside the aircraft is compressed, heated, and vented into the cabin to provide pressurization. This process results in cabin air with negligible water-vapor content. Relative humidity in an aircraft cabin at cruising altitude can be as low as 10% to 20%.[6] The extremely low ambient humidity of the aircraft results in increased insensible water loss from both the casualty and the medical crew. The casualty must be kept adequately hydrated, as must the medic. Burn casualties are especially susceptible to insensible water loss because of the compromised dermal barrier. Specific care should be exercised to prevent thermal and fluid losses as well as to monitor intravascular volume and hydration status in the burn casualty during evacuation.

Thermal Stressors

As an aircraft ascends, the ambient temperature decreases. Most helicopters and fixed-wing aircraft have heating systems, but it frequently becomes cold in the aircraft, particularly on long-duration flights. In Operation Iraqi Freedom, medical evacuation crews were often challenged by severe extremes of both cold (flight operations) and heat (onload/offload ground operations). Medics should carefully package and prepare casualties so that appropriate thermal control and casualty comfort may be maintained through a wide range of temperatures. A coherent hypothermia prevention and reversal strategy is required during pre-mission planning. A layered approach should be used, taking into account weight, volume, power requirements, clinical effectiveness, and practicality (**Box 28-3**). All devices should be either disposable or a component of patient movement items, applicable at all levels of care, and capable of employment on any evacuation platform.

Electronic Equipment Considerations

Electronic monitoring equipment offers significant opportunity to increase situational awareness pertaining to the patient during en route care movement. However, it is critical for the safety of both the casualty and the flight crew that all such electronic equipment be tested and approved for use in the aeromedical environment. Aircraft electronic systems may interfere with monitors, giving rise to false readings or inoperative equipment. Of equal if not greater concern, electronic monitoring equipment may interfere with aircraft systems.[1,4] This is particularly true in rotary-wing platforms, in which medical monitors may be only inches from critical flight avionics equipment. For this reason, all electronic aeromedical equipment must be tested before use in flight. This type of testing for fixed-wing aircraft is performed by the U.S. Air Force at the 311th Human Systems Wing, Brooks

---

Box 28-3 Plan for Hypothermia Prevention as Casualty Is Moved to the Rear

At Role 1 Utilize:
1. Ready-Heat Blanket
2. Heat Reflective Shell

At Role 2 Utilize:
1. Ready-Heat Blanket
2. Heat Reflective Shell
3. Thermal Angel
4. Bair Hugger

At Role 3 Utilize:
1. Ready-Heat Blanket
2. Heat Reflective Shell
3. Thermal Angel
4. Bair Hugger
5. Belmont FMS 2000

On any Evacuation Platform Utilize:
1. Ready-Heat Blanket
2. Heat Reflective Shell
3. Thermal Angel

City-Base, Texas. Similar testing on rotary-wing aircraft is performed by the U.S. Army at Fort Rucker, Alabama.

Patient Movement Regulation

AE is a more formal, measured process than TACEVAC. In most cases, AE is arranged after the patient has been admitted and treated at a field medical facility. The sending medical unit initiates the process through the generation of a patient movement request (PMR). The PMR is subsequently routed through the patient movement requirement center (PMRC). The PMRC validates the PMR (basically finds the best-fit transportation option to meet the casualty's clinical needs) and hands the PMR to the theater Air Mobility Operations Control Center (AMOCC), which tasks the aircraft and crews to perform the mission.[10]

AE and CCATT patients are classified into one of three movement priority categories based upon the assessed medical conditions and requirements for further care: *routine* (the USAF AE standard is 72 hours); *priority* (the USAF AE standard is 24 hours); or *urgent* (the USAF AE standard is 1 hour but may be exceeded due to evacuation time required to reach the appropriate role of care).[5] All casualties moved by AE must be cleared for flight by a flight surgeon. The flight surgeon is responsible for assisting the medical team with considering and clearing the patient in preparation for flight. This clearance requires recognition of the stressors of the hypobaric environment and includes consideration of conditions like the evolution of trapped gas (pneumothorax, retrobulbar orbital air, pneumocephalus, etc.) and preparation for the stressors of AE discussed previously. This may be done by discussing the case with the theater validating flight surgeon by radio or phone if a flight surgeon is not available locally.[10]

Under usual circumstances casualties moved via routine AE must be stable. If critical or stabilized casualties need to be flown, a special transport team such as a CCATT may be requested to assist in the movement process.

SUMMARY

- The term *en route care* is employed to encompass and characterize a seamless continuum of medical care from the point of injury, through theater facilities, and onward to CONUS facilities.
- Although doctrinal differences exist among the service branches regarding terminology and definitions of phases of care, casualty movement in TCCC may be described as follows:
  - CASEVAC: Evacuation of a casualty from the battlefield to an MTF using tactical platforms.
  - MEDEVAC: Evacuation of a casualty from the battlefield to an MTF, or from one MTF to another within the tactical theater, using dedicated medical assets usually marked with a red cross.
  - TACEVAC: En route care from the battlefield to a theater Role 2 or Role 3 MTF, including both CASEVAC and MEDEVAC.
  - AE: A term most commonly utilized by the U.S. Air Force to designate the movement of a patient from a point of care within the theater to a more rearward location, such as a regional hospital or CONUS.
- In the process of AE, a wounded soldier is considered a casualty until he or she reaches the first point of definitive medical care. Once entered into the medical care system, the casualty is considered a patient.

SCENARIO RECAP

You are the senior flight nurse on an aeromedical evacuation team aboard a MEDEVAC C-130 transferring a patient from the Role 3 hospital in Kandahar, Afghanistan, to Craig Joint Theater Hospital in Bagram. As the aircraft makes its final approach, it comes under small arms fire. Two of your team members are wounded. Casualty 1 has sustained a gunshot wound to his right inguinal area with heavy bleeding. Casualty 2 has an injury to her left thigh with pulsatile bleeding. The aircraft banks away from the approach, and there is no further incoming fire.

SCENARIO SOLUTION

- **What phase of Tactical Combat Casualty Care (TCCC) are you in?**
  You are now in the TACEVAC phase of care. The incoming fire has ceased, and your aircraft will proceed to an alternate MTF.
- **You now need to do two things simultaneously. What are they?**
  Both casualties have external hemorrhage that may be lethal if not quickly controlled. You apply a limb tourniquet to the left thigh of Casualty 2 while directing another team member to apply Combat Gauze with direct pressure to the bleeding inguinal wound of Casualty 1.
- **What do you do next?**
  After ensuring that the limb tourniquet has stopped the bleeding from the thigh of Casualty 2, you move to apply a junctional tourniquet to provide more definitive control of Casualty 1's inguinal bleeding.

Two important points in this scenario are that anyone can become a casualty in a combat zone, and anyone may be called upon to provide lifesaving battlefield trauma care to a casualty.

References

1. Bagian JP, Allen RC. Aeromedical transport. In: Auerbach PS, ed. *Wilderness Medicine*. 4th ed. St. Louis, MO: Mosby; 2004.

2. Golbey SB. Dust off. *AOPA Pilot*. 1987;30:46.

3. Neel S. Army aeromedical evacuation procedures in Vietnam: implications for rural America. *JAMA*. 1968;204(4): 309-313.

4. Hurd WW, Jernigan JG. *Aeromedical Evacuation: Management of Acute and Stabilized Patients*. New York, NY: Springer-Verlag; 2003.

5. U.S. Joint Chiefs of Staff, *Joint Health Services,* Joint Publication 4-02 (Washington, DC: U.S. Joint Chiefs of Staff, 11 December 2017).

6. U.S. Joint Chiefs of Staff. *DoD Dictionary of Military and Associated Terms*. [Joint Publication 5-0]. Washington, DC: U.S. Joint Chiefs of Staff; August 2017.

7. DeLorenzo RA, Porter RS. *Tactical Emergency Care: Military and Operational Out-of-Hospital Medicine*. Upper Saddle River, NJ: Prentice-Hall; 1999.

8. U.S. Air Force. Air Force Instruction 41–307: Aeromedical Evacuation Patient Considerations and Standards of Care. 20 August 2003. http://govdocs.rutgers.edu/mil/af /AFI41-307.pdf. Accessed April 8, 2018.

9. U.S. Air Force. Technical Order 1C-130H-1. C-130H Flight Manual. 2002.

10. U.S. Air Force. Access to the aeromedical evacuation system. Air Mobility Command Pamphlet 11–303. November 2000.

CHAPTER **29**

Joint Trauma System and Military Roles of Care

Authors:
Col. Stacy Shackleford, MD
Col. (Ret) Brian Eastridge, MD

CHAPTER OBJECTIVES

At the completion of this chapter, you will be able to do the following:

- State the vision of the Joint Trauma System (JTS).
- List the components of the JTS mission.

- Describe the four roles of injury care in the military trauma system.

SCENARIO

Your platoon is on a mounted patrol in the Helmand Province of Afghanistan, about 100 miles (160 kilometers [km]) west of Kandahar, when the second vehicle in the convoy is attacked by a roadside improvised explosive device (IED). Upon securing the scene, you identify and treat the only critically injured casualty who received multiple fragment wounds to his right extremities and torso. The casualty is evacuated by an HH-60M medical evacuation (MEDEVAC) helicopter to the Role 3 hospital in Kandahar, and your platoon returns to base. Twenty-four hours later, your Commanding Officer requests an update on the casualty's whereabouts and condition.

- Which medical treatment facility (MTF) would you contact first?
- This facility informs you that your casualty was evacuated out of the theater of operations 12 hours ago after damage control surgery. He was in stable condition when he left. To which MTF would you direct your next call?
- You find out that your casualty is no longer in the intensive care unit (ICU) but is on a ward in stable condition. He is scheduled for evacuation to the San Antonio Military Medical Center (SAMMC) in 48 hours. There, he will receive convalescent and rehabilitative care. What role of care is SAMMC?

INTRODUCTION

Trauma care has evolved from a synergistic relationship between the military and civilian medical environments for the past 2 centuries.[1-4] Modern battlefield concepts of triage, evacuation, and tiered implementation of battlefield medical care were developed by Larrey during the Napoleonic era. During the Civil War, U.S. military physicians realized the need for prompt attention to the wounded, early debridement and amputation to mitigate the effects of tissue injury and infection, and evacuation of the casualty from the battlefield. World War I saw further advances in the concept of evacuation and the development of echelons of medical care.

During World War II, blood transfusion and resuscitative fluids were widely introduced into the combat environment, and surgical practice was improved to care for wounded soldiers. From his World War II experiences, Dr. Michael Debakey noted that wars have always promoted advances in trauma care due to the concentrated exposure of military hospitals to large numbers of injured people during a relatively short span of time. Furthermore, this wartime medical experience has fostered a fundamental desire to improve outcomes by improving practice.[5] During the Vietnam conflict, more highly trained medics treating casualties at the point of wounding and prompt prehospital transport contributed to a further decrease in battlefield mortality.[6] In 1966, the National Academy of Sciences (NAS) published "Accidental Death and Disability: The Neglected Disease of Modern Society," noting trauma to be one of the most significant public health problems faced by the nation.[7] Concomitant with advances on the battlefield and the conclusions of the NAS was the formal development of civilian trauma centers. In 1976, the American College of Surgeons produced the first iteration of injury care guidelines, the "Hospital Resources for the Optimal Care of the Injured Patient."[8] The concepts promoted therein rapidly evolved into the development of formal, integrated trauma systems. Trauma centers and trauma systems in the United States have had a remarkable impact on improving outcomes of injured patients, reducing mortality by up to 15% in mature systems.[3,6,9-11] In 2016, the National Academies of Sciences, Engineering, and Medicine recommended further integration of military and civilian trauma care into a national trauma system to achieve the aim of zero preventable deaths after injury.[12]

After civilian trauma systems demonstrated success in improving survival from traumatic illness, military conflicts brought attention to a similar need to apply a systematic approach to combat casualty care. Reports from Operation Desert Shield and Desert Storm in 1992 highlighted a number of opportunities to improve in the area of military trauma systems. Inadequacies were formally noted in both

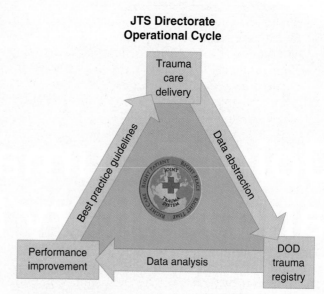

JTS Directorate Operational Cycle

Figure 29-1 Joint Trauma System operational cycle.
Courtesy of Dr. Brian Eastridge, Col., MC, USA (Ret).

preparation and delivery of trauma care in the combat environment.[4,13-15] Immediately after the terrorist attacks of September 11, 2001, the United States once again had large numbers of service men and women committed to armed conflict. Modeled after civilian trauma systems, the U.S. Central Command Joint Theater Trauma System (JTTS) was conceptualized as a deployable Combatant Command (COCOM) medical asset, incorporating a systematic and integrated approach to better organize and coordinate battlefield trauma care. It was designed to minimize morbidity and mortality and optimize the ability to provide essential care required by combat injuries. The JTTS evolved into a Department of Defense (DoD)-wide Joint Trauma System (JTS) with a mission to define best-practice trauma care for all deployed U.S. military forces. The mantra of the JTS is to improve battlefield trauma care by enabling the *right* patient, at the *right* place, and the *right* time to receive the *right* care (R4) (**Figure 29-1**).

This chapter will assist prehospital providers in understanding how prehospital trauma management is incorporated into the broader context of the military trauma care system.

The Joint Trauma System and the Department of Defense Trauma Registry

The JTS is the Department of Defense Center of Excellence for trauma. It provides the overarching organized and coordinated capability for injury prevention, care, and rehabilitation. It works in conjunction with the individual geographic command trauma systems to ensure optimal care across the continuum.

The vision of the JTS is that every service member injured on a full range of military operations has the optimal chance for survival and maximal potential for functional recovery. To attain this vision, the mission of the JTS includes the following:

- Improve organization and delivery of trauma care.
- Improve communication among providers in the evacuation chain to ensure continuity of care and access to patient care data.
- Develop and populate the Department of Defense Trauma Registry (DoDTR) to capture and report DoD injury demographics, evaluate care provided, and document outcomes.
- Provide a standardized repository to collect, store, and analyze battlefield casualty data for performance improvement on behalf of the entire DoD, and incorporate all trauma-relevant data throughout the entire continuum of care.
- Enable a joint strategic and tactical medical research program in support of the warfighter and injured service member by providing a structured and comprehensive trauma database.
- Facilitate movement, collection, and sharing of theater combat casualty data across all roles of care and all the Military Services.
- Evaluate and recommend new equipment or medical supplies for the Military Departments to improve efficiency, support clinical innovation, reduce cost, and improve outcomes.
- Facilitate medical performance improvement by promoting real-time, data-driven clinical process improvements and improved outcomes.
- Develop and maintain evidence-supported clinical practice guidelines.
- Recommend combat casualty care training requirements.
- Maintain trauma care and systems currency.
- Support the Military Services with trauma subject-matter expertise to optimize all aspects of trauma care across the DoD.

The components of a military trauma system, modeled after successful civilian counterparts,[15] include prevention (primary, secondary, and tertiary), prehospital care, acute injury care, evacuation, and rehabilitation (**Figure 29-2**). The JTS was developed to foster trauma education, leadership, communication, performance improvement, research, and information systems (**Figure 29-3**). The performance improvement mission of the JTS is facilitated by the DoDTR using data collection and analysis to support decision-making, clinical practice guidelines, and research to reduce morbidity and mortality.

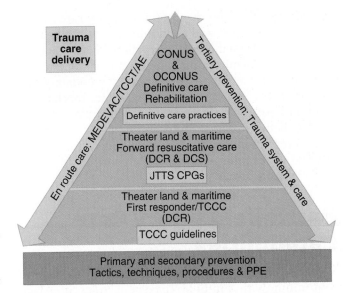

Figure 29-2 Joint Trauma System trauma care delivery.

Courtesy of Dr. Brian Eastridge, Col., MC, USA (Ret).

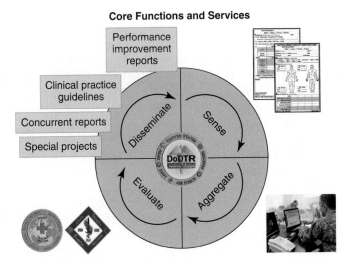

Figure 29-3 Joint Trauma System core functions.

Courtesy of Dr. Brian Eastridge, COL, MC, USA (Ret).

Prevention

Combat morbidity and mortality can be prevented by operational and medical leaders at multiple levels through (1) primary prevention: prevention of injury incident through physical and mental conditioning, TTPs (tactics, techniques, and procedures), and evidence-based findings from tactical and medical after-action reviews; (2) secondary prevention: mitigation of injury extent through contingency planning and personal protective equipment; and (3) tertiary prevention: establishment and maintenance of a system to optimize injury care starting at the point of injury and continuing through rehabilitation.[16-17] Data from the DoDTR are shared with numerous government organizations to help optimize operational injury prevention measures by constantly updating TTPs and protective equipment. Demographic, mechanistic, wounding pattern, and evacuation data are analyzed to develop better personal protection equipment, improve injury prevention strategies, and optimally allocate medical and evacuation resources in support of the operational Commander.

Battlefield Injury Care Capabilities

Military doctrine supports a battlefield trauma care continuum with multiple coexistent roles of triage, treatment, and evacuation. The current military combat casualty care paradigm consists of four discrete roles of injury care linked together by transport capabilities[19] (**Figure 29-4**). The system is designed to improve injury outcomes while responding to the realities of the resource-constrained environment of operations. Although constantly changing operational environments ensure that real-time roles of care rarely align perfectly with established doctrine, the tenets of early and definitive control of external hemorrhage, aggressive stabilization, resuscitation, staged treatment, and evacuation to progressively higher roles of care with robust en route care remain the core capabilities of a military trauma system.

Prehospital providers, using the concepts of tactical combat casualty care (TCCC), have had a substantial impact on the survival of combat casualties.[20-24] Advances in prehospital damage control resuscitation have delivered treatments previously reserved for in-hospital care to the point of injury on the battlefield.[25-26]

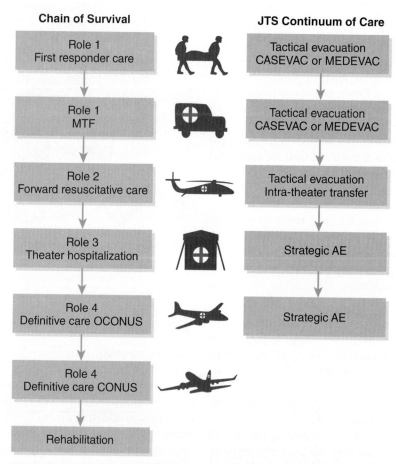

Figure 29-4 Military Trauma System roles of care: A well-developed military trauma system has multiple levels of care, however not all levels of care are available or utilized in every location or for every casualty.

Role 1 (First Responder Care)

Role 1 care includes care provided either by the casualty him- or herself or the medical or nonmedical first responder. Everyone on the battlefield should have received, as a minimum, the TCCC for All Combatants certification and be an expert with the contents supplied in their Joint First Aid Kit (JFAK) or service equivalent. Role 1 MTF care may vary somewhat by Military Service. It normally consists of a group of medics or corpsmen, one physician assistant (PA), and one nonspecific specialty military physician (e.g., battalion surgeon). Having one PA and one physician provides great flexibility for the operational commander and allows split operations to be conducted simultaneously. The U.S. Special Operations Command trains all of their medics, corpsmen, and pararescuemen above the paramedic level and these individuals will be able to perform various advanced procedures based their unit, training, and experience. All Role 1 providers are managed by their medical authorities and guided by unit-level standard operating procedures. All Role 1 first responders (medical and nonmedical) should receive TCCC tiered training in accordance with the TCCC skill sets outlined by the JTS (all service members, Combat Lifesavers, combat medic/corpsmen, and advanced providers) (**Figure 29-5**). Role 1 medical care is also provided at casualty collection points (CCPs) and in aid stations that have the capability to maneuver with the operational line units they support. The Role 1 organic medical staff have the capability to deploy forward in a mobile capacity and work out of a tent or a fixed facility of opportunity. Care at this resource-constrained role is mainly limited to TCCC and/or Advanced Trauma Life Support (ATLS) techniques, including external hemorrhage

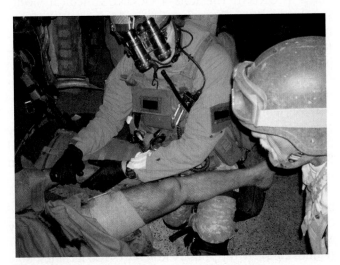

Figure 29-5 Role 1 trauma care by a combat medic.

Courtesy of Stephen Giebner, MD.

control, endotracheal intubation, surgical airway management, damage control resuscitation, administration of pain control and antibiotics, and splint stabilization of wounds and fractures. The goal of medical management at this role is to appropriately return less severely injured casualties to duty and to expeditiously address the immediate life-, limb-, and eyesight-threatening issues of severe and critically injured casualties, as well as to stabilize and evacuate those who are more severely injured. Some operational environments may lack expeditious evacuation capabilities, or weather or operational challenges may lead to situations requiring prolonged Role 1 care (prolonged field care) and Role 1 providers must be trained and equipped for this eventuality.

Role 2 (Forward Resuscitative Care)

Role 2 care includes damage control resuscitation and damage control surgical capabilities. The traditional size and configuration of an Army Forward Surgical Team, for example, is approximately 20 personnel and includes anesthesia, surgical, and nursing staff to run two operating room (OR) beds simultaneously. In response to operational needs, the Military Services have developed a variety of alternate Role 2 configurations. These include smaller surgical teams with more flexible capabilities, including highly mobile single-surgeon teams, mobile two-surgeon teams, and mobile four-surgeon teams, all with the capability to flex forward in support of operations. The two basic elements of Role 2 care are a damage control resuscitation capability that may include postoperative critical care and limited patient holding capacity and a small surgical element that has the capability to perform lifesaving resuscitative surgery for a limited number of casualties (**Figure 29-6**). Surgical team capabilities are directly related to the size of the team, with the smallest teams capable of temporizing damage control interventions to facilitate transport to a more robust surgical capability. Because of the resource-constrained forward-deployed environment, surgical procedures undertaken at Role 2 facilities are generally limited to damage control and temporizing procedures for life-, limb-, and eyesight-threatening injuries.

Role 3 (Theater Hospitalization)

Role 3 facilities are the most robust MTFs in a combat zone (**Figure 29-7**) and may be deployed in support of contingency operations if the operational tempo requires. Role 3 MTFs include a robust complement of hospital and provider resources extending beyond resuscitative surgery. Additional capabilities may include surgical specialists in neurosurgery, ophthalmology, oral and maxillofacial, cardiothoracic, vascular, plastic surgery, and

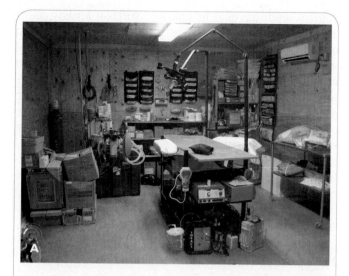

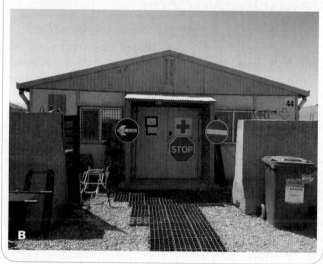

Figure 29-6 Deployed Role 2 facilities. **A.** Interior. **B.** Exterior.
Courtesy of Stephen Giebner, MD.

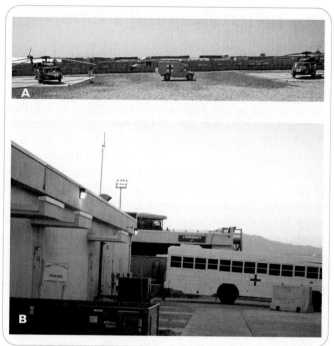

Figure 29-7 Deployed Role 3 facilities. **A.** Temporary. **B.** Fixed.
Courtesy of Stephen Giebner, MD.

2 facilities, but can also receive patients directly from Role 1 or point of injury. One or more of the Role 3 facilities in a theater of operations will typically function as the central evacuation point for fixed-wing aeromedical evacuation to Role 4.

Role 4 (Definitive Care)

Role 4 care is found in U.S.-based hospitals and robust overseas MTFs. Definitive surgery is typically initiated at a Role 4 MTF outside of the theater of operations, either outside (OCONUS) or within the continental United States (CONUS). The Role 4 OCONUS medical facility supporting U.S. Central Command and Africa Command is Landstuhl Regional Medical Center in Germany (**Figure 29-8**). The Role 4 OCONUS medical facility supporting U.S. Pacific Command is Tripler Army Medical Center in Hawaii. Role 4 facilities may care for casualties relatively soon after injury who require stabilization or temporizing surgical procedures and intensive care management. In other situations, the Role 4 facility may facilitate rapid transport to the continental United States or may initiate definitive care or rehabilitation interventions.

Definitive surgery, convalescent, restorative, and rehabilitative care are provided at Role 4 facilities within the continental United States. Walter Reed National Military Medical Center and San Antonio Military Medical Center (**Figure 29-9**) are the primary Role 4 CONUS facilities. Role 4 CONUS also includes other military medical centers, Department of Veterans Affairs (VA), and civilian hospitals.

others depending on the operational needs of the supported theater of combat operations. In addition, Role 3 facilities have anesthesiologists, critical care specialists, emergency medicine providers, critical care nursing, and technical support for continuous 24-hr activity. These facilities may represent the first location in the chain of evacuation that is located near a flight line capable of supporting large-frame fixed-wing aircraft necessary for longer inter- or intra-theater flights. During traditional land warfare, the roles of care are set up in linear fashion, with Role 1 being closest to the front lines of battle, and Roles 2 and 3 at successively farther distances rearward. In more modern and asymmetric combat operations, the echelons of care may adopt more of a "hub and spoke" arrangement, with the Role 3 facilities representing the central hub that receives patients from multiple Role

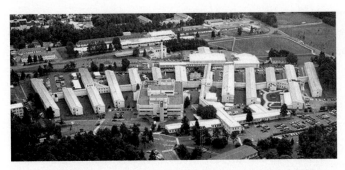

Figure 29-8 Landstuhl Regional Medical Center is a Role 4 facility located in Germany.
Courtesy of U.S. Department of Defense.

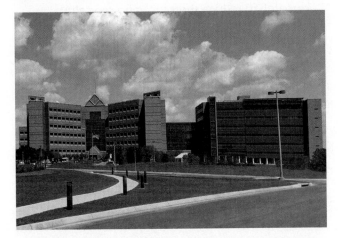

Figure 29-9 San Antonio Military Medical Center is a Role 4 CONUS facility located in San Antonio, Texas.
Courtesy of U.S. Department of Defense.

En Route Care

Evacuation of combat casualties progresses through a continuum within the trauma system. En route care provides the vital linkage between the roles of care necessary to sustain the patient during transport. Evacuation from the point of injury may occur by ground, air, or water. Casualty evacuation (CASEVAC) refers to the unregulated movement of a casualty by medical or nonmedical personnel aboard a land vehicle, aircraft, or boat. CASEVAC missions may be conducted using platforms of opportunity and medical personnel from the operational or supported unit. MEDEVAC traditionally refers to the transportation of casualties with predesignated vehicles temporarily staffed with intrinsic en route medical capability, moving patients from the point of injury to the first MTF or between MTFs within theater. Strategic aeromedical evacuation from a combat theater to a Role 4 facility is accomplished by fixed-wing aircraft. High-risk trauma patients are transported by Critical Care Air Transport Teams (CCATTs) with augmented medical resources to assure the best possible outcomes.

Continuum of Care

As the global trauma system in support of all of the DoD's missions, the JTS supports a continuum of care for the battlefield casualty that can spread over thousands of miles and bridge multiple roles of medical care, overseeing the trauma care delivered. Data-driven, real-time performance improvement initiatives within the JTS have led to improvements in combat injury outcomes.[27,28]

In 2017, the U.S. Congress directed that the JTS be moved to the Defense Health Agency and serve as the lead agency for trauma in the DoD.[29] In 2018, the improvements made by the U.S. military in caring for victims of trauma on the battlefield were recognized by the Defense Health Board,[30] the American College of Surgeons,[31-32] and the National Academies of Sciences, Engineering, and Medicine,[33] and transitioned to the civilian sector to benefit those injured in active-shooter incidents and terrorist bombings, as well as those injured in everyday trauma resulting from motor vehicle crashes and criminal violence. Implementation of military advances in trauma care into civilian trauma systems creates the potential for many additional lives to be saved through the use of combat casualty care concepts pioneered and refined by the JTS.[32,33]

SUMMARY

- The core capabilities of a military trauma system are early and definitive control of external hemorrhage, aggressive stabilization, resuscitation, staged treatment, and evacuation to progressively higher roles of care with robust en route care.
- The Joint Trauma System advises and supports the continuum of care to optimize injury outcomes while operating within resource constraints.

- Role 1 field care begins with TCCC at the point of injury and is divided into four individual TCCC skill sets (all service members, Combat Lifesaver, combat medic/corpsmen, and combat paramedics/providers).
- Role 1 medical care is provided at point of injury, casualty collection points (CCPs), or in aid stations.

(continued)

SUMMARY (CONTINUED)

Care at this level is mainly limited to stabilizing TCCC and/or ATLS techniques.

- Some operational environments may lack expeditious evacuation capabilities, or weather or operational challenges may lead to situations requiring prolonged Role 1 care (prolonged field care). Role 1 providers must be trained and equipped to support the DoD mission requirements.
- Role 2 care includes damage control resuscitation and damage control surgical capabilities and may include postoperative critical care and limited patient holding capacity. Surgical procedures undertaken at Role 2 are usually limited to damage control and temporizing procedures for life- and limb-threatening injuries.
- Role 3 facilities offer capabilities beyond resuscitative surgery, including surgical specialists, critical care specialists, nursing, and technical support for continuous 24-hour activity.
- Role 4 care is located outside of the active combat theater and may conduct resuscitative care, facilitate rapid transport to the continental

United States, or initiate definitive care or early rehabilitation interventions. Definitive surgery, convalescent, restorative, and rehabilitative care are provided at Role 4 facilities within the continental United States.

- The performance improvement mission of the JTS is facilitated by the DoD Trauma Registry, using data collection and analysis to support decision making, clinical practice guidelines, and research to reduce morbidity and mortality.
- Data from the DoD Trauma Registry are analyzed to develop better warrior protection, improve injury prevention strategies, and optimally allocate medical and evacuation resources to the battlefield.
- The continuum of care for combat casualties is spread over thousands of miles and multiple levels of medical care. The JTS provides coordination of patient care and movement across this continuum, with the goal of producing the optimal chance for survival and maximal potential for functional recovery.

SCENARIO RECAP

Your platoon is on a mounted patrol in Helmand Province, about 100 miles (160 km) west of Kandahar, when the second vehicle in the convoy is attacked by a roadside IED. Upon securing the scene, you identify and treat the only serious casualty, who received multiple fragment wounds to his right extremities and torso. The casualty is evacuated by helicopter to the Combat Support Hospital in Kandahar, and your platoon returns to base. Twenty-four hours later, your Commanding Officer requests an update on the casualty's whereabouts and condition.

SCENARIO SOLUTION

- **Which MTF would you contact first?**
  The Combat Support Hospital at Kandahar.

- **This facility informs you that your casualty was evacuated out of the theater of operations 12 hours ago after damage control surgery. He was in stable condition when he left. To which MTF would you direct your next call?**
  The Role 4 (OCONUS) facility that receives casualties from the U.S. Central Command theater, in this case, Landstuhl Regional Medical Center in Germany.

- **You find out that your casualty is no longer in the intensive care unit but is on a ward in stable condition. He is scheduled for evacuation to SAMMC in 48 hours. There, he will receive convalescent and rehabilitative care. What level medical facility is SAMMC?**
  Role 4 (CONUS).

References

1. Tracy EJ. Topics in emergency medicine. Combining military and civilian trauma systems: the best of both worlds. *Adv Emerg Nursing J.* 2005;27(3):170-175.

2. Trunkey DD. History and development of trauma care in the United States. *Clin Orthop Relat Res.* 2000;May(374):36-46.

3. Trunkey DD. In search of solutions. *J Trauma.* 2002;53(6):1189-1191.

4. DeBakey ME. History, the torch that illuminates: lessons from military medicine. *Mil Med.* 1996;161(12):711-716.

5. Hoff WS, Schwab CW. Trauma system development in North America. *Clin Orthop Relat Res.* 2004;May(422):17-22.

6. National Academy of Sciences. *Accidental Death and Disability: The Neglected Disease of Modern Society.* Washington, DC: National Academies Press; 1966.

7. Committee on Trauma of the American College of Surgeons Task Force. Hospital resources for optimal care of the injured patient. *Bull Am Coll Surg.* 1979;64(8):43-48.

8. Mullins RJ. A historical perspective of trauma system development in the United States. *J Trauma.* 1999;47(Suppl 3):S8-S14.

9. Mann NC, Mullins RJ, MacKenzie EJ, Jurkovich GJ, Mock CN. Systematic review of published evidence regarding trauma system effectiveness. *J Trauma.* 1999;47(Suppl 3):S25-S33.

10. Nathens AB, Jurkovich GJ, Rivara FP, Maier RV. Effectiveness of state trauma systems in reducing injury-related mortality: a national evaluation. *J Trauma.* 2000;48(1):25-30.

11. National Academies of Sciences, Engineering and Medicine. *A National Trauma Care System: Integrating Military and Civilian Trauma Systems to Achieve Zero Preventable Deaths after Injury.* Washington, DC: The National Academies Press; 2016.

12. Hinton HL Jr. *Operation Desert Storm: Full Army Medical Capability Not Achieved. GAO/NSIAD-92-175.* Washington, DC: U.S. General Accounting Office; 1992.

13. *War Time Medical Care: DOD Is Addressing Capability Shortfalls, but Challenges Remain. GAO/NSIAD-96-224.* Washington, DC: U.S. General Accounting Office; 1996.

14. *War Time Medical Care: Personnel Requirements Still Not Resolved. GAO/NSIAD-96-173.* Washington, DC: U.S. General Accounting Office; 1996.

15. American College of Surgeons. *Resources for Optimal Care of the Injured Patient.* Chicago, IL: American College of Surgeons; 2014.

16. Kotwal RS, Butler FK, Edgar EP, Shackelford SA, Bennett DR, Bailey JA. Saving lives on the battlefield: a Joint Trauma System review of prehospital trauma care in Combined Joint Operating Area Afghanistan (CJOA-A) executive summary. *J Spec Oper Med.* 2013;13(1):77-85.

17. Kotwal RS, Montgomery HR, Miles EA, Conklin CC, Hall MT, McChrystal SA. Leadership and a casualty response system for eliminating preventable death. *J Trauma Acute Care Surg.* 2017; 82(6 Suppl 1):S9-S15.

18. Joint Publication 4-02. Health Service Support. http://dtic.mil/doctrine/new_pubs/jp4_02.pdf. Accessed Sep 1, 2017.

19. Eastridge BJ, Mabry RL, Seguin P, et al. Death on the battlefield (2001-2011): implications for the future of combat casualty care. *J Trauma Acute Care Surg.* 2012;73(6 Suppl 5):S431-S437.

20. Kotwal RS, Montgomery HR, Kotwal BM, et al. Eliminating preventable death on the battlefield. *Arch Surgery.* 2011;146(12):1350-1358. doi:10.1001/archsurg.2011.213.

21. Kragh JF Jr, Walters TJ, Baer DG, Fox CJ, Wade CE, Salinas J, Holcomb JB. Survival with emergency tourniquet use to stop bleeding in major limb trauma. *Ann Surg.* 2009; 249:1-7.

22. Kotwal RS, Howard JT, Orman JA, et al. The effect of a golden hour policy on the morbidity and mortality of combat casualties. *JAMA Surg.* 2016;151(1):15-24.

23. Shackelford SA, del Junco DJ, Powell-Dunford NC, et al. Association of pre-hospital blood product transfusion during medical evacuation of combat casualties in Afghanistan with acute and 30-day survival. *JAMA.* 2017 Oct 24;318(16):1581-1591. doi:10.1001/jama.2017.15097.

24. Butler FK, Holcomb JB, Schrieber MA, et al. Fluid resuscitation for hemorrhagic shock in tactical combat casualty care. *J Spec Oper Med.* 2014;14(3):13-38.

25. Fisher AD, Miles EA, Cap AP, et al. Tactical damage control resuscitation. *Mil Med.* 2015;180(8):869-875.

26. Blackbourne LH, Baer DG, Eastridge BJ, et al. Military medical revolution: military trauma system. *J Trauma Acute Care Surg.* 2012;73(6)(Suppl 5):S388-S394.

27. Bailey JA, Morrison JJ, Rasmussen TE. Military trauma system in Afghanistan: lessons for civil systems? *Curr Opin Crit Care.* 2013;19(6):569-577.

28. National Defense Authorization Act for Fiscal Year 2017.

29. Dickey N. Combat Trauma Lessons Learned from Military Operations of 2001-2013. *Defense Health Board Report;* 9 March 15. https://health.mil/About-MHS/Defense-Health-Agency/Special-Staff/Defense-Health-Board/Reports. Accessed March 28, 2018.

30. Levy MJ, Jacobs LM. A call to action to develop programs for bystanders to control severe bleeding. *JAMA Surg.* 2016;151(12):1103-1104.

31. Jacobs L, Wade D, McSwain N, et al. Hartford Consensus: a call to action for THREAT, a medical disaster preparedness concept. *J Am Coll Surg.* 2014;218:467-475.

32. The National Academies of Sciences, Engineering, and Medicine. *A National Trauma Care System: Integrating Military and Civilian Trauma Systems to Achieve Zero Preventable Deaths After Injury.* Washington, DC: NASEM; June 2016.

33. Butler FK. Two decades of saving lives on the battlefield: Tactical Combat Casualty Care turns 20. *Mil Med.* 2017;182(3):e1563-e1568.

CHAPTER 30

© Ralf Hiemisch/Getty Images.

Triage in Tactical Combat Casualty Care

Authors:
Col. (Ret) John Holcomb, MD
Maj. Andy Fisher
Dr. Keith Gates

CHAPTER OBJECTIVES   At the completion of this chapter, you will be able to do the following:

- List the casualty categories used in battlefield triage, and describe each category.
- Identify the physiologic parameters of most importance in battlefield triage, and state how they
- are used to gauge a casualty's need for lifesaving intervention and the probability of survival.
- Given the physiologic data of primary interest on a casualty, place the casualty in the proper triage category.

SCENARIO

You are the only medic doing triage at a mass-casualty incident and are at least an hour from the closest surgical facility:

- Casualty 1 has a gunshot wound through his right thigh just above his knee, an obvious deformity, and massive bleeding. He can communicate with you appropriately and his radial pulse, though rapid, is strong. What is his initial triage category?
  - **A.** Minimal
  - **B.** Delayed
  - **C.** Immediate
  - **D.** Expectant
- Casualty 2 has a gunshot wound to the left chest. He is alert and has a weak and rapid radial pulse and increased respiratory rate. What is his initial triage category?
  - **A.** Minimal
  - **B.** Delayed
  - **C.** Immediate
  - **D.** Expectant
- Which casualty would you treat first?
  - **A.** Casualty 1
  - **B.** Casualty 2

(continued)

SCENARIO (CONTINUED)

- After Casualty 1 has undergone tourniquet application, his radial pulse is strong and no longer rapid, and he can converse normally though with pain from the tourniquet. What is his new triage category?
  - **A.** Minimal
  - **B.** Delayed
  - **C.** Immediate
  - **D.** Expectant

INTRODUCTION

Triage, a system of sorting, categorizing, and prioritizing casualties, was formalized by Baron Dominique Jean Larrey, surgeon-in-chief of the Napoleonic armies between 1797 and 1815. During this time, the baron initiated a system of battlefield stabilization, tourniquet use, and subsequent rapid evacuation to definitive care. He established this rule for the triage of war casualties: The wounded shall be treated according to the seriousness of their injuries and urgency of need for medical care, regardless of rank or nationality.[1]

Similarly, modern battlefield triage is a process for sorting casualties into groups based on their need for, or likely benefit from, immediate medical treatment (**Box 30-1**). Triage is most often used in mass-casualty

---

Box 30-1 Triage Categories

To be effective, triage requires appropriate categorization of casualties. These categories determine priority for treatment and evacuation. The four categories of tactical triage are:

- *Immediate.* This category includes those casualties who require an immediate lifesaving intervention (LSI) and/or surgery. Put simply, if medical attention is not provided they will die. The key to successful triage is to locate these individuals as quickly as possible. *Casualties do not remain in this category for an extended period. They are either found, triaged, and treated, or they die!* Hemodynamically unstable casualties with airway obstruction, chest or abdominal injuries, massive external bleeding, or shock deserve this classification. Some of these patients can be triaged into the delayed category once the LSI has been performed (e.g., extremity tourniquet application to an amputation, with no signs of shock).

- *Delayed.* This category includes those wounded who are likely to need surgery, but whose general condition permits delay in surgical treatment without unduly endangering the life, limb, or eyesight of the casualty. Sustaining treatment will be required (e.g., oral or IV fluids, splinting, administration of antibiotics and pain control), but can possibly wait. These casualties can often be overtriaged based on the anatomic injuries. However, their physiologic response should produce values for monitored parameters within acceptable limits. Examples of casualties in this category include those with no evidence of shock who have large soft-tissue wounds, fractures of major bones, intra-abdominal and/or thoracic wounds, and burns to less than 20% of total body surface area (TBSA). As noted previously, these comments are based on the assumption that the casualty has no life-threatening external hemorrhage, no airway compromise, and no respiratory distress.

- *Minimal.* Casualties in this category are often referred as the "walking wounded." Although these patients may appear to be in bad shape at first, it is their physiologic state that tells the true story. Casualties who fit into the minimal category may not present themselves until late in the triage process. These casualties have minor injuries (e.g., small burns, lacerations, abrasions, or small fractures) that can usually be treated with self-aid or buddy aid. These casualties should be utilized for mission requirements (e.g., scene security), to help treat and/or transport the more seriously wounded, or put back into the fight.

- *Expectant.* Casualties in this category have wounds that are so extensive, that even if they were the sole casualty and had the benefit of optimal medical resources, their survival would be highly unlikely. Even so, expectant casualties should not be neglected. They should receive comfort measures and pain medication if possible, and they deserve retriage as appropriate. An example of an expectant casualty is an unresponsive soldier with penetrating head trauma with obvious massive damage to the brain.

(MASCAL) situations because it is designed to provide the most good for the greatest number of casualties. It is a repetitious process whereby casualties are prioritized for treatment and evacuation, performed at every level of care. By reassessing the casualty frequently, the medic can identify changes in the casualty's status, determine the need for new interventions, or adjust previous interventions.

Triage in Tactical Combat Casualty Care

The realities of combat dictate that battlefield triage typically takes place in an environment of limited resources for treatment and transport. The treatment and evacuation priorities of combat casualties across the phases of Tactical Combat Casualty Care (TCCC) are outlined in previous chapters in this text. Triage of casualties during TCCC establishes order of treatment and movement, not which or whether treatment is provided (**Box 30-2**). The tactical situation and the need to continue with the mission may delay or proscribe treatment. Furthermore, effective triage may dictate that some do not receive immediate treatment and are returned to the fight.

Proper triage aids the field provider in deciding which casualties have the greatest probability of survival and in weighing the casualties' relative needs for LSIs, thus determining priority and urgency for treatment and evacuation.[2,3] Using a standardized approach to the triage of combat casualties will help combat medics correctly

---

Box 30-2 Triage in Tactical Combat Casualty Care (TCCC)

Triage in the Care Under Fire phase:

1. Direct those casualties who can to move to cover or provide self-aid.
2. Move casualties who are unresponsive or cannot provide their own care to cover, if possible.
3. Control life-threatening extremity hemorrhage with limb tourniquets.
4. Continue with the mission/fight.

Triage in the Tactical Field Care phase:

1. Perform an initial rapid assessment of the casualty for triage purposes. This should take no more than 1 minute per casualty. A casualty with altered mental status should immediately be disarmed and any communications gear and/or ordnance (e.g., hand grenades) that he or she might be carrying should be secured.
2. If a casualty can walk and has no significant internal or external hemorrhage or difficulty with airway/breathing, he or she will probably do well.
3. Remember the MARCH algorithm (massive bleeding, airway, respiration, circulation, head/hypothermia). Most preventable deaths on the battlefield are the result of failure to control external hemorrhage. It does no good to assure a good airway when the casualty has lost too much blood to survive.
4. Perform immediate LSIs as indicated, such as applying a tourniquet for life-threatening extremity hemorrhage, using Combat Gauze or junctional hemorrhage control devices for life-threatening external hemorrhage at a site

where a tourniquet cannot be applied, airway positioning, or needle decompression of a tension pneumothorax. Move rapidly.

5. Talk to the casualty while checking the radial pulse. If the casualty can talk easily, obeys commands, and has a strong radial pulse, he or she has an excellent chance of survival if there is no ongoing internal or external hemorrhage. This casualty is usually in the minimal or delayed category unless there is suspicion for noncompressible torso hemorrhage, as with penetrating torso trauma or a suspected pelvic fracture.
6. If the casualty obeys commands, but has a weak or absent radial pulse, he or she is at increased risk of dying and may benefit from an immediate LSI. This casualty is in the immediate category.
7. If the casualty cannot obey commands *and* has a weak or absent radial pulse, the casualty has a markedly increased chance of dying (>92%)[2,4,5] and may benefit from an immediate LSI. This casualty is in the immediate or possibly expectant category, depending on resource constraints and evacuation time.
8. Prepare casualties to move out of the area. Prevent hypothermia.

Nine Rules of Thumb for Determining Urgency for Evacuation During the Tactical Field Care phase:

1. Soft-tissue injuries are common and may look bad, but they typically do not result in death unless associated with shock.

(continued)

Box 30-2 Triage in Tactical Combat Casualty Care (TCCC) (*continued*)

2. Bleeding from most extremity wounds should be controllable with a tourniquet or hemostatic dressing. Tactical evacuation (TACEVAC) delays should not increase mortality if bleeding is fully controlled.

3. Casualties who are in shock should be evacuated as soon as possible.

4. Casualties with penetrating wounds of the chest who have respiratory distress unrelieved by needle decompression of the chest should be evacuated as soon as possible. If possible, place a chest tube.

5. Casualties with penetrating wounds of the chest or abdomen who are in shock have a high risk of dying and should be evacuated as soon as possible.

6. Casualties with blunt or penetrating trauma of the face associated with difficulty breathing should immediately receive definitive airway control and should be evacuated as soon as possible.

7. Casualties with blunt or penetrating wounds of the head in which there is obvious massive brain

damage and unconsciousness are unlikely to survive with or without emergent evacuation.

8. Casualties who have blunt or penetrating wounds to the head in which the skull has been penetrated but are still conscious should be evacuated as soon as possible.

9. Casualties with penetrating wounds of the chest or abdomen who are not in shock at their 15-minute evaluation have a moderate risk of developing late shock from slowly bleeding internal injuries. They should be carefully monitored and evacuated as soon as feasible.

Triage in the TACEVAC phase:

1. Triage casualties again. Categories and treatment requirements can and will change.

2. Electronic monitoring equipment should be available during TACEVAC care. Use it to help assess your casualties and assist in triage.

segregate, treat, and prioritize evacuation in the shortest possible time. Triage ensures the best care for the greatest number and the optimal utilization of medical personnel, equipment, and facilities, especially in a MASCAL event. Improved triage leads to improved survival. To be maximally effective, the most experienced medical provider available should perform initial triage and direct treatment. He or she is generally the one most familiar with the natural course of injuries, knows best when treatment is futile or emergently indicated, and is best able to identify those casualties who can be returned to battle. The senior provider should direct other resources (Combat Lifesavers, first aid providers) to assist with immediate treatment and movement to a casualty collection point (CCP) or evacuation platform.

Combat Triage Decision Algorithm

Civilian triage algorithms utilize physiologic, anatomic, and mechanism of injury (MOI) criteria because these are readily assessable at the point of injury and provide insight as to a casualty's current status and likely outcome.[2,6,8] Accuracy in triage depends on using only those criteria shown to predict outcomes and the need for immediate intervention. These criteria include (1) cursory evaluation, (2) physiologic status, and (3) anatomic criteria.

Cursory Evaluation

The purpose of the cursory evaluation is to rapidly detect those casualties with minor injuries and those who are mortally wounded. Those casualties with massive external hemorrhage should be identified in this step. By simply calling on casualties who can move to cover and/or treat themselves, you can identify those with minor wounds. However, as previously mentioned, they should receive follow-up triage to evaluate for any changes. Those with obvious mortal wounds should be placed in the expectant category. The remaining casualties require immediate evaluation.

Physiologic Status

The next step, an assessment of physiologic criteria, is intended to allow for rapid identification of critically injured patients by assessing level of consciousness (Glasgow Coma Scale [GCS]) and measuring vital signs (systolic blood pressure, respiratory status, and hemoglobin oxygen saturation).[2,4,6,7,10,11,]

Because the austere and often hazardous tactical environment precludes the use of sophisticated monitoring equipment, battlefield evaluation relies upon simple assessment tools. For triage in tactical situations, two criteria are highly predictive of outcomes: (1) whether the casualty can follow simple commands (from the motor component of the GCS) and (2) the radial pulse rate and character used as a surrogate for systolic blood pressure. Based on these criteria and other published data, a triage decision algorithm (**Figure 30-1**) has been developed for TCCC.[5-13] Unless there is significant external hemorrhage, airway or breathing difficulty, or a gunshot wound to the torso, the ability to ambulate usually places a casualty initially into the minimal category, whereas obvious signs of death will place a casualty in the expectant category. For those casualties who do not fall into either of these

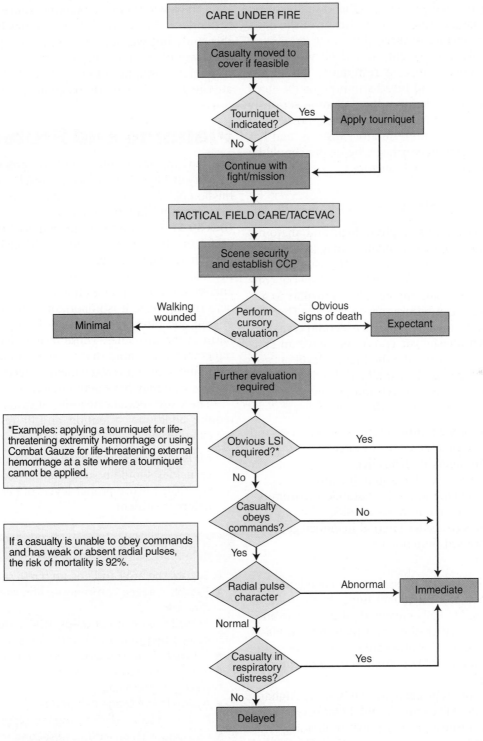

Figure 30-1 Triage algorithm for tactical combat casualty care (TCCC).

categories, further evaluation is required. All casualties requiring an LSI are placed initially in the immediate category. However, once the LSI is performed, a casualty must be retriaged. Again, triage is a continuous process and frequent reassessment is required—a casualty may move from one category to another at each assessment.

The provider doing triage should talk to the casualty while checking the radial pulse. If the casualty obeys commands and has a normal radial pulse, he or she has a greater than 95% chance of survival.[2,4,7]

Following this, the patient should be visually assessed for respiratory distress. A respiratory rate of less than 10 or greater than 30 breaths/minute or the need for ventilatory support identifies the patient as seriously injured.[10] If a casualty can obey commands, possesses a strong radial pulse, is in no respiratory distress, and has no significant external hemorrhage, he or she should be placed initially in the delayed category.

Anatomic Criteria

In civilian trauma care, using physiologic and anatomic criteria alone for triage of casualties may result in a high degree of undertriage, or assigning casualties to a lower-than-actual risk category. Inclusion of special considerations when assessing the need for transport to advanced trauma care can reduce that problem.[14] This also applies to combat trauma. For instance, certain casualties may have normal physiologic criteria but have an anatomic injury that might require the highest level of care. Providers doing triage on the battlefield should maintain a low threshold for early intervention and evacuation if any of the following injuries are identified:[10]

- Serious penetrating injuries to head, neck, torso, and extremities proximal to elbow or knee
- Chest wall instability or deformity
- Two or more proximal long-bone fractures
- Crushed, degloved, mangled, or pulseless extremity
- Amputation proximal to wrist or ankle
- Pelvic fractures (consider internal hemorrhage)
- Open or depressed skull fractures
- Paralysis

Mechanism of injury is also an independent predictor of mortality and functional impairment in blunt trauma casualties.[14,15] Falls greater than 20 feet (6 meters), high-risk vehicle crashes, and proximity to blasts are attended by a great risk of severe trauma. Serious injury and the need for rapid evacuation to definitive care should be anticipated.

A 2017 study of prehospital interventions in Afghanistan during MASCAL events found hemorrhage control, either with a tourniquet or pressure dressing, was the most commonly performed intervention. The second most common procedure was the administration of a pain medication (ketamine, morphine, or fentanyl) for pain management. The triage status for 10 MASCAL events with a total of 50 patients showed 24% (*n* = 12) were urgent, 8% (*n* = 4) were delayed, and 54% (*n* = 27) were minimal.[16] While there is often discussion of overwhelming urgent casualties, this study demonstrated that the majority of casualties will probably not require urgent care. However, there is a preponderance of undertriaging casualties in MASCALs,[17,18] which may be represented in this study but was not discussed. Field providers should be aware of the potential for undertriaging and should reevaluate casualties often and move them to appropriate categories if their criteria change.

Planning and Protection

In preparing for combat, with its propensity for mass-casualty incidents, many factors must be considered during mission planning and rehearsed in training to ensure mission accomplishment and proper care of the wounded (**Box 30-3**). Environment, mission, and timeline are critical factors that will affect the way triage is executed. How and where will the triage area and CCP be set up and security maintained? What are the evacuation assets available, and what is the response time frame? Furthermore, while performing triage it is important to remember to protect oneself and other rescuers as well as preventing further harm to the casualties. Those responsible for triage must remember at all times that triage is not a definitive treatment and constant reassessment is needed to identify casualties who may have deteriorated or improved.

There are special categories of casualties who should require additional attention and/or resources.[19] Below are examples with considerations:

- *Chemical or biologic contamination.* If at all possible, these casualties should be decontaminated before entering the CCP. Ensure proper levels of personal protection before treatment.

Box 30-3 Pearls for Mass-Casualty Triage

- Secure the area and ensure scene safety.
- Establish scene commander and medical director.
- Establish a Command Post (CP), casualty collection point (CCP), and routes of access.
- Estimate initial number and severity of casualties.
- Identify additional hazards (e.g., smoke, nuclear, biologic, chemical).
- Assign initial triage categories.
- Perform required lifesaving interventions.
- Retriage with an extended secondary survey as time permits.

- *Retained, unexploded ordnance.* While the casualty may be appropriately triaged, if there are multiple casualties, those with retained ordnance should be kept separate and at a safe distance to prevent harm to others if the ordnance detonates. This is recommended even though detonation has never been reported.[20]
- *Noncombatants.* Unfortunately, in combat, there are times when innocent persons are wounded. In these events, if mission and the tactical situation allow,

the noncombatant should be treated for any life-threatening wounds. Be aware of the evacuation plan (or lack thereof) and limitations of the local healthcare system when triaging.
- *Enemy prisoners.* Ensure any enemy casualties you treat are disarmed and guarded. They should also be searched for explosives or other ordnance, restrained as appropriate, and prevented from communicating with each other.

SUMMARY

- Triage is a process for sorting casualties into groups based on their need for, or potential benefit from, medical treatment.
- There are four triage categories: expectant, immediate, delayed, and minimal.
- The expectant category includes those with wounds that are so extensive that, even with optimal treatment, their survival would be highly unlikely.
- The immediate category includes those who require an immediate LSI and/or surgery.
- The delayed category includes those wounded who may need surgery, but whose general condition permits delay in surgical treatment without unduly endangering the life or limb of the casualty, although some sustaining treatment will probably be required.
- The minimal category includes those with minor injuries that can usually be cared for with self- or buddy aid.
- Obvious signs of death will place a casualty in the expectant category.
- Further evaluation is required for those casualties who do not fall into the minimal or expectant category upon initial triage. Casualties in all

categories require repeated triage—even those placed in the minimal and expectant categories may change.
- All casualties requiring an LSI are placed initially in the immediate category, and once the LSI is performed, the casualty must be retriaged.
- The ability to ambulate places a casualty immediately into the minimal category, unless there is significant external hemorrhage, airway or breathing difficulty, or a penetrating wound to the torso.
- If a casualty can obey commands, possesses a strong radial pulse, and is in no respiratory distress, he or she should be placed in the minimal or delayed category if no special circumstances such as those noted in the preceding bullet apply.
- The most experienced medical provider should perform initial triage because he or she is most familiar with the natural course of injuries and knows best when treatment will likely be futile.
- Triage is a continuous process. Frequent reassessment is needed to identify casualties who may have deteriorated or improved.
- Triage is not definitive treatment.

SCENARIO RECAP

You are the only medic doing triage at a mass-casualty incident, and you are at least an hour from the closest surgical facility.

SCENARIO SOLUTION

- **Casualty 1 has a gunshot wound through his right thigh just above his knee, an obvious deformity, and massive bleeding. He can communicate with you appropriately, and his radial pulse, though rapid, is strong. What is his initial triage category?**
  C. Immediate
- **Casualty 2 has a gunshot wound to the left chest. He is alert, and has a weak and rapid radial pulse and increased respiratory rate. What is his initial triage category?**
  C. Immediate
- **Which casualty would you treat first?**
  A. Casualty 1
- **After Casualty 1 has undergone tourniquet application, his radial pulse is strong and no longer rapid, and he can converse normally though with pain from the tourniquet. What is his new triage category?**
  B. Delayed

References

1. Bodemer CW. Baron Dominique Jean Larrey, Napoleon's surgeon. *Bull Am Coll Surg.* 1982;67(7):18-21.

2. Baxt WG, Jones G, Fortlage D. The trauma triage rule: a new, resource-based approach to the prehospital identification of major trauma victims. *Ann Emerg Med.* 1990;19(12):1401-1406.

3. McCoy CE, Chakravarthy B, Lotfipour S. Guidelines for field triage of injured patients: in conjunction with the *Morbidity and Mortality Weekly Report* published by the Centers for Disease Control and Prevention. *West J Emerg Med.* 2013;14(1):69-76.

4. McManus J, Yershov A, Ludwig D, et al. Radial pulse character relationships to systolic blood pressure and trauma outcomes. *Prehosp Emerg Care.* 2005;9(4):423-428.

5. Holcomb J, Niles S, Miller C, Hinds D, Duke J, Moore F. Prehospital physiologic data and lifesaving interventions in trauma patients. *Mil Med.* 2005;170(1):7-13.

6. Martinez B, Owings JT, Hector C, et al. Association between compliance with triage directions from an organized state trauma system and trauma outcomes. *J Am Coll Surg.* 2017 Oct;225(4):508-515. doi:10.1016/j.jamcollsurg.2017.06.016.

7. Butler FK, Hagmann J, Butler EJ. Tactical combat casualty care in special operations. *Mil Med.* 1996;161(Suppl):3-16.

8. Ekblad GS. Training medics for the combat environment of tomorrow. *Mil Med.* 1990;155(5):232-234.

9. Centers for Disease Control and Prevention. Guidelines for field triage of injured patients: recommendations of the National Expert Panel on Field Triage. *MMWR.* 2009;58(RR-1):1-35.

10. Centers for Disease Control and Prevention. Guidelines for field triage of injured patients: recommendations of the National Expert Panel on Field Triage. *MMWR.* 2012;61(RR-1):1-20.

11. Meredith W, Rutledge R, Hansen A, et al. Field triage of trauma patients based upon the ability to follow commands: a study in 29,573 injured patients. *J Trauma.* 1995;38(1):129-135.

12. Garner A, Lee A, Harrison K, Shultz C. Disaster medicine/domestic preparedness. *Ann Emerg Med.* 2001;38(5):541-548.

13. Eastridge BJ, Butler F, Wade CE, et al. Field triage score (FTS) in battlefield casualties: validation of a novel triage technique in a combat environment. *Am J Surg.* 2010;200(6):724-727.

14. Brown JB, Stassen NA, Bankey PE, Sangosanya AT, Cheng JD, Gestring ML. Mechanism of injury and special consideration criteria still matter: an evaluation of the National Trauma Triage Protocol. *J Trauma.* 2011;70(1):38-44; discussion 44-45. doi:10.1097/TA.0b013e3182077ea8.

15. Haider AH, Chang DC, Haut ER, Cornwell EE, Efron DT. Mechanism of injury predicts patient mortality and impairment after blunt trauma. *J Surg Res.* 2009;153(1):138-142. doi:10.1016/j.jss.2008.04.011.

16. Schauer SG, April MD, Simon E, Maddry JK, Carter R, Delorenzo RA. Prehospital interventions during mass-casualty events in Afghanistan: a case analysis. *Prehosp Disaster Med.* 2017;32(4):465-468.

17. Vassallo J, Smith J. Investigating the effects of under-triage by existing major incident triage tools. *Emerg Med J.* 2017;34(12):A871. doi:10.1136/emermed-2017-207308.16.

18. Cross KP, Petry MJ, Cicero MX. A better START for low-acuity victims: data-driven refinement of mass casualty triage. *Prehosp Emerg Care.* 2015 Apr-Jun;19(2):272-278. doi:10.3109/10903127.2014.942481.

19. Mass Casualty and Triage. In: Cubano MA, ed. *Emergency War Surgery.* Fifth United States revision. Fort Sam Houston, TX: Borden Institute; 2018: 23-40.

20. Lein B, Holcomb J, Brill S, Hetz S, McCrorey T. Removal of unexploded ordnance from patients: a 50-year military experience and current recommendations. *Mil Med.* 1999;164(3):163-165.

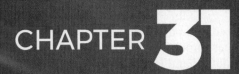

CHAPTER **31**

Injuries from Explosives

Author:
Dr. Howard Champion

CHAPTER OBJECTIVES

At the completion of this chapter, you will be able to do the following:

- List the five categories of mechanisms of explosion-related injury and give examples of each.
- Describe how explosion-related injuries differ from other types of injuries.

- Discuss the precautions that responders to explosive blast incidents need to take.
- Describe the major wounding effects of explosives and types of treatments typically required.

SCENARIO

While on foot patrol on a rural road, one member of a five-member team triggers an improvised explosive device (IED). One casualty is dead, two have minor injuries, and one has sustained significant injuries to his lower torso and right lower extremity. You are the person providing medical care.

- What are the tactical considerations in this situation?

INTRODUCTION

A contemporary understanding of injury from explosives is essential for all providers of emergency care in both military and civilian settings. Medical personnel need to understand the pathophysiology of injury caused by the improvised explosive devices (IEDs) that are widely used by insurgents and terrorists.

> Because of the increasing risk of terrorist IED attacks on civilians, non-military health care providers must become familiar with the characteristics of explosives and of explosions and of the nature of the injuries they may inflict.[1]

Explosions occur in homes (primarily due to gas leaks or fires) and are an occupational hazard of many industries, such as mining, and those involved in demolition, chemical manufacture, or handling fuel or dust-producing substances such as grain. Industrial explosions result from chemical spills, fires, faulty equipment maintenance, or electrical/machinery malfunctions, and they may produce toxic fumes, building collapse, secondary explosions, falling debris, and large numbers of casualties. As a whole, however, unintentional explosions are responsible for relatively few injuries and deaths[2] compared with the large numbers of injuries and deaths produced by explosives used by terrorists and military adversaries.

Explosives are the predominant cause of combat injury and death. In the postmaneuver insurgency phase in Iraq, they accounted for about 60% of injuries to American combatants.[3] The majority of U.S. troop deaths (72%) were caused by explosions.[4] In Afghanistan, the number of IED events (IEDs detected, disarmed, or detonated) increased more than 80% between 2009 and 2011 (from 9,300 to 16,800) and totaled 14,500 by mid-December 2012.[5] IEDs caused an average of 46% of all U.S. troop deaths in Afghanistan,[6] and, according to the Joint Improvised Explosive Device Defeat Organization (JIEDDO), were responsible for 63% of all U.S. casualties in Iraq and Afghanistan.[7]

Insurgents and terrorists worldwide are increasingly using bombs, especially IEDs, against civilian targets as well. In 2011, 10,283 terrorist attacks took place throughout the world, injuring almost 45,000 people and causing 12,533 deaths, of which 51% were civilians.[8] Almost half (43%) of the attacks and most (75%) of the deaths were caused by bombings, including suicide bombings, with IEDs implicated in most cases.[8] The reason for such widespread and increasing use of IEDs is because these devices are inexpensive, made from easily obtained materials (such as ammonium nitrate, which is derived from a common agricultural fertilizer and used in 70% of IEDs in Afghanistan[5]), and result in the devastating havoc that focuses international media exposure on their cause.

Explosive attacks typically result in mass-casualty incidents (MCIs), such as the 1995 attack on the Alfred P. Murrah Federal Building in Oklahoma City, which killed 168 and injured 518 people. Suicide bomb attacks in Israel, which occur both in open areas and confined spaces (buildings, buses), have produced limited mass-casualty events on a regular basis. Globally, however, countries such as Afghanistan, Iraq, Pakistan, Somalia, Nigeria, England, France, Spain, and the United States have been the sites of most terrorist attacks resulting in mass casualties.[8]

The U.S. Bomb Data Center serves as the national repository for explosives and arson-related incident data, having been established by the federal explosives laws and Attorney General designation.[9] These data can be accessed via the ATF Bomb Arson Tracking System (BATS). The BATS has 11,300 active users and contains information on more than 400,000 explosive- and arson-related incidents investigated by ATF, FBI, and other federal, state, and local law enforcement and public safety agencies.[9]

At present, the United States is not typically exposed to as many bomb attacks as other countries (**Figure 31-1**). However, because both civilian and military responders may be called upon during a bomb attack on civilian populations, all healthcare providers need to be familiar with their roles during these increasingly frequent occurrences and to be aware of and able to prevent or mitigate the attacks against first responders that often accompany terrorist bombings.[8]

From January 1, 2016, through December 31, 2016, the BATS captured a total of 15,943 explosives-related

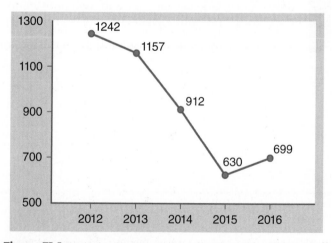

Figure 31-1 Explosion incidents chart, United States, 2012–2016.[10]

Data from: United States Bomb Data Center Explosives Incident Report. 2016. https://www.atf.gov/file/116371/download.

incidents. Of the reported incidents, there were 699 explosions, of which 439 were bombings, with California and Florida having the highest numbers.[11]

In 2014, there were 1,693 bomb threats reported; there were 1,670 in 2015 and 1,537 in 2016. Education and office/business properties remain the most commonly reported targets of bomb threats; however, the overall number of bomb threats to both have decreased since 2015.[11]

Overview

Injuries from explosions differ significantly from injuries from other mechanisms. They are also more complex than those typically seen in civilian practice. The most important differences are that explosions result in the following:

- *Cause injury by multiple mechanisms.* Unlike vehicular injury (blunt trauma) and injuries from bullets (gunshot), which apply relatively simple mechanisms to transfer energy to the human body, an explosion causes energy to be transferred in complex and multiple fashions. Energy from explosions is primarily designed to propel fragments (primary and secondary) at high velocity. Thus, the most significant cause of injury is multiple fragment wounds. However, primary blast overpressure, whole or partial body translocation, injury from building collapse (including crush injury), and injury from fireball and dust inhalation can all play a part in the complex anatomic and physiologic dysfunction.
- *Cause multiple injuries.* Unlike other mechanisms, survivors of explosive blasts tend to have multiple injuries involving numerous anatomic areas and organs.
- *Have multiple etiologies.* When a vehicle is hit by an IED, for example, the initial set of forces is a result of the explosion. However, the vehicle may be translocated and forcibly inverted or vectored into a tree or culvert, causing multiple blunt injuries that accompany the penetrating wounds and may be further modified by personal protective devices worn by vehicle occupants.

Furthermore, the rate of coupling of energy to the body from blast overpressure is much higher than, for instance, energy coupling in a car crash. This can cause unique tissue distortions and malfunctions.

When it comes to blast injury management, training of medical care professionals—from first responders to definitive care providers—is severely lacking. Also lacking is knowledge of the effects of combinations of multiple fragment injuries and blast overpressure on tissue reaction and implications for treatment. This chapter will acquaint the reader with contemporary practice and knowledge of this current health care imperative.

Explosive Agents
Categories

Explosives fall into one of two categories based on the velocity of detonation: low explosives and high explosives. IEDs may be made of high or low explosives or a combination.[12]

Low Explosives

When activated, low explosives (e.g., dynamite, gunpowder) change relatively slowly from a solid to a gaseous state, in an action more characteristic of deflagration (burning) than of detonation. Low explosives, which include pipe bombs and pure petroleum-based bombs such as Molotov cocktails, lack the highly compressed blast wave and shattering effect (brisance) that define high explosives.[11] Injuries caused by low explosives typically include fragment and thermal injuries, not the primary blast injuries (discussed later) that are often associated with high explosives.[13]

High Explosives

High explosives react almost instantaneously, in that they detonate rather than deflagrate, and their detonation velocity greatly exceeds the speed of sound.[12] The initial explosion creates an immediate rise in pressure, creating a shock wave that travels outward at supersonic speed (3,000–8,000 meters per second [mps; 9,843–26,247 feet per second). The shock wave is the leading front and an integral component of the blast wave, which is created upon the rapid release of enormous amounts of energy, with subsequent propulsion of fragments, generation of environmental debris, and often intense thermal radiation.

High explosives are frequently used in military ordnance and IEDs. Their sharp, shattering effect (brisance) can pulverize bone and soft tissue, create blast overpressure injuries (barotrauma), and propel primary and secondary fragments and debris at ballistic speeds. With conventional high explosives, the blast wave decays rapidly and is significantly affected by the environment. The rapid change in pressure and the duration of depressurization affect the severity of resultant primary blast injury (discussed later). The power of an explosive for military demolitions is expressed as its relative effectiveness (RE) factor, which is calculated based on its detonating velocity relative to that of TNT (which has an RE factor of 1.00).[14] Rate of detonation, given in feet per second (fps) and RE factors for typical high explosives used in IEDs are shown in **Figure 31-2**. A sampling of high explosives currently in use is given in **Table 31-1**.

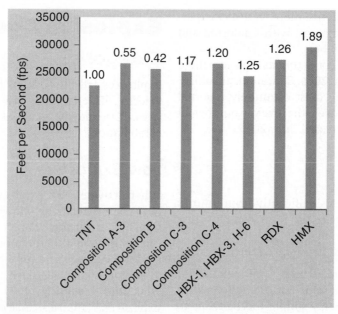

Figure 31-2 Velocity of detonation and relative effectiveness (RE) factors of typical high explosives used in IEDs.[14] In this figure, RE factors are shown above the bars and the reference point is TNT = 1.00.

Data from: U.S. Navy Salvage Engineer's Handbook, Volume 1 (Salvage Engineering). U.S. Navy Salvor's Handbook. S0300-A8-HBK-010. 1997.

Table 31-1 Sample of High Explosives Currently in Use[15-18]

Name Abbreviated	Expanded	Description
TNT	Trinitrotoluene	Conventional explosive; "TNT equivalent" is used as a measure of energy released from other explosives
AN	Ammonium nitrate	Often mixed with fuel oil; used in the 1995 Oklahoma City bombing
Tetryl	2,4,6 tetranitro-N-methylaniline	Used as a booster; placed next to detonator
Nitroglycerin		A liquid, unstable high explosive used as a component of dynamite
RDX	Cyclotrimethylene-trinitramine, $C_3H_6N_6O_6$	Second in strength to nitroglycerin among common explosive substances
PETN	Pentaerythritol tetranitrate	One of the strongest known high explosives
Semtex	PETN plus RDX	General-purpose, odorless plastic explosive
HMX	Cyclotetramethylene tetranitramine	Highest energy, mass-produced solid explosive made in the United States; a component of plastic-bonded explosives and rocket propellants; used as a high-explosive burster charge
TATP	Triacetone triperoxide	One of the most sensitive explosives (i.e., to impact, temperature change, friction); suspected agent in 2005 London bombings and suicide bomb attacks in Israel
EGDN	Ethylene glycol dinitrate	A liquid explosive typically found in dynamite explosives such as those used in the 2004 Madrid bombings

Types

Because this text is focused toward military healthcare providers, the primary emphasis will be on antipersonnel, rather than industrial explosives (examples of the former are given in **Table 31-2**). Both manufactured and improvised explosive devices (IEDs) will be considered here, with an emphasis on the latter because they have become the principal wounding agent of current conflicts[19,20] and of terrorists and insurgents.

Manufactured explosives refer to mass-produced, military-issued/tested weapons (land mines, mortars, grenades) whereas IEDs refer to devices made in small batches or adapted from existing weapons.[11] Of the three classes of conventional antipersonnel land mines (static, bounding, and horizontal spray), the static mine is most common throughout the world, and its mechanism of injury is unique.

The line between manufactured and improvised explosive devices blurs when manufactured explosives are adapted for use as IEDs, as described in the following:

Terrorists ... find it stunningly easy to obtain artillery shells, missile warheads, mortar rounds, and other high explosives for quick conversion to IEDs. ... The terrorists simply rig them with cheap RF [radiofrequency] detonators and bury them where military convoys or other targets of opportunity are likely to pass by. When the targets are in range, they trigger the explosives with radio signals from cell phones, garage-door openers, or other easily obtained devices.[22]

Table 31-2 Classifications of Major Explosive Weapons Currently in Use[21]	
Class	**Description**
Air-dropped bombs	Explosive weapons dropped from aircraft, including: ■ General purpose/high explosive (GP/HE) bombs ■ Penetration bombs ■ Carrier bombs (for delivery of other payloads, including submunitions)
Booby traps	Explosive weapons designed to be detonated by unsuspecting victims (also known as "victim-activated" explosive weapons
Demolition charges	Blocks of explosive for engineering or sabotage use
Grenades	Small explosive antipersonnel or antivehicle weapons that can be thrown or fired, e.g.: ■ Hand grenades (blast, fragmentation) ■ Antiarmor ■ Rifle ■ Spin-stabilized
Explosive projectiles	Explosive projectiles fired through a barrel after ignition of a propellant, e.g.: ■ Armor-piercing high explosive (APHE) ■ High explosive antitank (HEAT) ■ High explosive fragmentation (HE frag) ■ High explosive "squash head" (HESH) ■ Carrier (for delivery of other payloads such as submunitions)
IEDs	Explosive weapons of any class (e.g., grenade, bomb) that are not mass produced (although they may use mass-produced components), e.g.: ■ Person-borne (suicide) bombs ■ Vehicle-borne (VBIEDs) ■ Roadside IEDs
Land mines	Victim-activated explosive devices that include: ■ Antipersonnel mines ■ Antivehicle mines

(continued)

Table 31-2 Classifications of Major Explosive Weapons Currently in Use[21] (*continued*)

Class	Description
Missiles	Explosive devices with propulsion and guidance systems, including: ■ Air-to-air missiles ■ Air-to-surface missiles ■ Antitank guided missiles ■ Surface-to-air missiles (static, mobile, portable) ■ Surface-to-surface missiles
Mortars	Indirect fire weapons that are often muzzle loaded; these typically include: ■ High explosives ■ Carriers for delivery of other payloads such as submunitions
Rockets	Unguided munitions with propulsion systems, e.g.: ■ Air-launched rockets ■ Artillery rockets ■ Rocket-propelled grenades (RPGs)
Submunitions	Smaller explosive weapons delivered by carrier bombs, projectiles, or mortar bombs (often called "cluster munitions"), e.g.: ■ Antiarmor ■ High explosive fragmentation ■ Dual-purpose improved conventional munitions (DPICM)
Underwater	These include: ■ Depth charges ■ Limpet mines ■ Naval mines ■ Torpedoes

Moyers R. Explosive violence: The problem of explosive weapons. International Network on Explosive Weapons Web site. http://www.inew.org/site/wp-content/uploads/2011/06/Explosive-violence.pdf. August 11, 2009. Accessed May 7, 2018.

Manufactured Explosives

Manufactured explosives include grenades (including RPGs, the most widely used antitank weapon in the world), rocket launchers fitted with thermobaric or explosive fragmentation antipersonnel warheads,[23] and antipersonnel mines.[24]

Enhanced blast weapons (EBWs) are a type of manufactured explosive that originated with the military. They are incorporated into munitions that range from small grenades to large rockets and are a likely threat to military personnel in stabilization and peacekeeping operations.[25] The primary mechanism of injury of EBWs is blast overpressure, with secondary and tertiary effects similar to those of conventional bombs. EBWs may also create a vacuum effect, which can cause suffocation.[26] EBWs are increasingly deployed with thermobaric (TBX) and/or fuel-air explosives (FAEs), which generate significant thermal output and may contain toxic materials. An example is the Russian RPO-A, which may contain the carcinogen isopropyl nitrate.[26] Advanced thermobaric weapons

(also known as vacuum bombs) come in all sizes, from small, slide-action grenade launchers to long-range, multiple-barrel rocket launchers (MBRLs). An RPG-7 may be equipped with the thermobaric TBG-7V round, which "shreds and incinerates everyone within a 30-foot (ft; 9-meter [m]) radius of where it detonates."[27] These weapons are especially effective in urban environments because they can propagate around, into, under, and over objects, and their effects are magnified in enclosed spaces.[28]

Improvised Explosive Devices

The most common weapons in insurgency and terrorist warfare, however, are IEDs (**Figure 31-3**). These weapons are designed to increase the range of damage by propelling high-velocity, preformed fragments a greater distance and introducing a variety of wounding agents. An IED consists of an armoring/firing switch, a power source, a detonator, and a main charge (explosive or incendiary), and it can be triggered by a timer that can be set well in advance of the detonation, by remote control, or—in the case of suicide bomb attacks—by the assailant at the scene.[23] Primitive IEDs can be made from everyday items such as fertilizer and batteries, but most use a small amount of military- or industrial-grade explosive to trigger a larger amount of

lower-grade material, such as that contained in gas cylinders. An early example of the latter was used in the 1983 bombing of the U.S. Marine barracks in Lebanon. In that event, a truck carrying cylinders of compressed gas and 198 pounds (lb; 90 kilograms [kg]) of explosives collapsed a seven-story building, killing 241 U.S. military personnel.[29]

IEDs range in sophistication from simple pipe bombs to truck bombs containing thousands of kilograms of TNT equivalent.[30] They are categorized by the U.S. Technical Support Working Group (TSWG) based on size and destructive potential (**Figure 31-4**).[23]

IEDs are the preferred weapon of insurgents. In Iraq, with its modern system of paved roads, and where soldiers typically travel by vehicle, military-grade ordnance has been modified into IEDs for use in roadside attacks.[31] During the worst period of the Iraq war, approximately 50 IED attacks, mainly roadside attacks, occurred each day.[32] In more rural Afghanistan, which has few highways and paved roads, soldiers are more often on foot and are typically targeted with homemade IEDs using fertilizer components sourced from Pakistan.[33]

IEDs may be victim operated (e.g., mines and booby traps); operated on a time delay (including pipe and vehicle bombs); command operated (triggered by user); projected (launched like a rocket or mortar); or operated with a combination of firing methods (time-delay plus backup is common).[23] The panic and disruption associated with IEDs may also be caused by hoax IEDs and false (misreported) IEDs.[23] IED technology used in Iraq includes electronic triggering sensors and explosively formed projectile (EFPs), which are explosive-filled pipes sealed with a cone-shaped metal cap that, upon detonation, is propelled at a speed high enough to penetrate and shatter armor and vehicle compartment alike.[33] Another

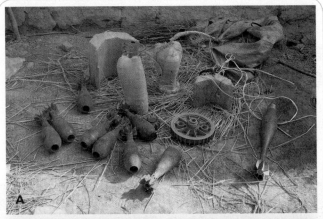
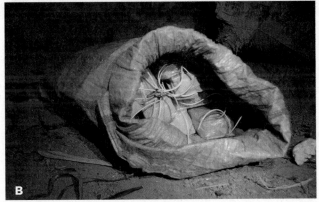

Figure 31-3 IEDs found in Afghanistan.

A: Courtesy of Stephen Giebner, MD; B: Image courtesy of Corporal Barry Lloyd, RLC.

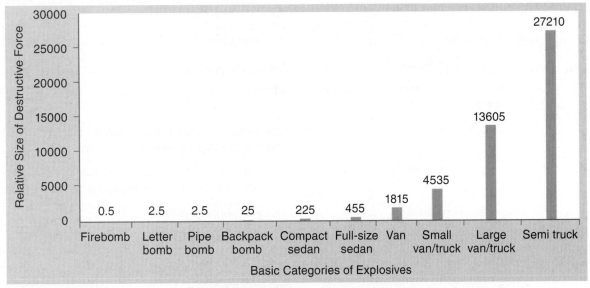

Figure 31-4 Relative size and destructive force (TNT-equivalent) of basic categories of explosives.[23]

Sullivan JP, Bunker RJ, Lorelli EJ, et al. *Jane's Unconventional Weapons Response Handbook*. Alexandria, VA: Jane's Information Group; 2002.

type of IED frequently used in Iraq is the "sticky IED," or IEDs that are attached by magnets to the bottom of vehicles.[34] In Afghanistan, however, IEDs currently are simpler devices that use fertilizer and crude triggers, contain less metal (making them harder to detect), and are less lethal compared to those used in Iraq.[34]

Positioning techniques used to maximize IED damage include coupling or daisy chaining and boosting (stacking underground to minimize detection and increase the force of the blast).[35,36] Other common practices are packing IEDs with fragments such as nuts, bolts, ball bearings, nails, and pieces of concrete—a frequent phenomenon in suicide bomb attacks in Israel.[37] IEDs are often camouflaged (e.g.,

to look like garbage along the side of the road) or hidden under rocks, in animal carcasses, etc., and may be detonated using direct wiring, remote devices such as doorbells, radio control, or by being thrown (e.g., from an overpass onto a vehicle) or launched.[38] Often, decoy devices are placed in plain sight so vehicles will stop near live, hidden IEDs.

Factors That Worsen Outcomes

The potency of an explosive device against a target can be increased in a variety of ways, as summarized in **Table 31-3**.[39]

Table 31-3 Prognostic Factors for Terrorist Bombings[44-46]		
Category	**Factor**	**Description**
Agent	Type of explosive used	C4, TNT, RDX, Semtex, etc.
	Amount of explosive used	The greater the TNT equivalent of an explosive, the greater its wounding potential
	Magnitude of explosion	A primary wounding factor
	Secondary effects of debris or shrapnel	Constitute most explosion-related injuries
	Presence of flame or hot gases	Burn injuries
	Presence of dust or smoke	Inhalation injuries or asphyxiation
Location	Presence of a barrier between victim and explosion	Does not mitigate primary blast but may reduce exposure to fragments
	Urban or remote setting	Influences emergency response factors
	Indoors or in contained space	Significantly more injuries and deaths than in open-space explosions, increased rates of tympanic membrane rupture and blast lung
	Building collapse	Crush injuries
	Entrapment under debris	Crush injuries
	Propulsion of victim and subsequent blunt trauma	Blunt injuries
	Distance from explosion	The closer to the point of detonation, the more severe the injury magnitude and type of injury
Victim	Body position during explosion	Those positioned perpendicular to blast wave are impacted more severely than those positioned horizontally
	Anatomic site of injury	Depends on above factors
Emergency response	Triage efficiency	Improves survival
	Reduced time to treatment	Improves survival
	Immediate presence of surgeons	Improves survival

The primary factors that influence outcomes include magnitude of and distance from the explosion, explosion within a confined space, and building collapse.[40,41] Fragments, which may be primary (i.e., part of the explosive device itself) or secondary (generated from the environment—e.g., glass, vehicle, or building debris) are the main cause of injury and death. Although proximity to the point of detonation clearly increases the risk of fragment injury, fragments are propelled great distances and can cause injury at distances far beyond the reach of blast overpressure.[43]

When an explosion occurs in an enclosed space, blast waves bouncing off structures collide with the primary blast wave, significantly increasing the damaging potential of the pressure waves. Furthermore, in buildings or vehicles with fire-suppression systems, toxic gases may be released.[30] In the 1995 Oklahoma City bombing, 82% of injuries and 87% of deaths occurred inside the building, compared to 18% of injuries and 5% of deaths occurring outside the building.[45,46] In the 1996 Khobar Towers bombing, almost all of the injuries and deaths occurred among individuals who had been in the building or on a balcony.[47] Detonation of a bomb on a bus or inside a vehicle is a prime example of how terrorists use a confined space to cause maximum injury to tight clusters of people through penetration by metal fragments from disintegrating vehicle parts. The vast increase in injury severity and mortality associated with this technique is illustrated in **Figure 31-5**, which shows severe injuries (expressed as an Injury Severity Score [ISS] greater than 15 or 16) and deaths associated with open-air and bus bombings in two Israeli studies.

Bombs detonated near or inside buildings often cause them to collapse (80% of the deaths in Oklahoma City were caused by collapse of the building structure rather than by the explosion itself), creating a high probability of secondary and tertiary injury effects. **Figure 31-6** shows the mechanism of blast-induced structural weakening and collapse. Structural collapse produces large numbers of casualties both inside and outside the structure, with increased frequency of inhalation and crush injury.[49]

ISS > 15* or 16** Mortality

Secondary explosions may be created by FAEs that disperse and ignite a spray of aerosol fuel, or cluster bombs that distribute "bomblets" that explode over a wider area. The term *secondary explosion* also refers to (1) a second round of explosions targeted at rescuers and first responders to the scene or (2) an initial blast setting off additional explosions. Secondary effects may also be initiated by snipers. Thus, it is important to exercise caution when approaching the scene of a blast to rule out the possibility of secondary attacks to providers and bystanders. Bystanders should be instructed to vacate the area.[50]

> Although most terrorist IED attacks outside war zones target civilians or symbols of authority and usually involve a single device, some are designed specifically to target emergency response personnel. The most common tactics involve using secondary or tertiary devices in tiered or sequential attacks intended to kill or maim response personnel after they arrive on the scene of an initial IED incident.[51]

Patterns of Injury

Explosions produce patterns of injury that are different from other types of trauma with respect to demographics of patients, distribution and severity of injuries, and frequent occurrence of injuries in several body regions or multiple injuries in the same body region.

When compared with patients injured via other types of trauma (e.g., gunshot wounds), victims of terrorist bombs are primarily in the 15 to 44 year age range,[53] have more severe injuries, require more surgical intervention, and have three times the rate of mortality.[54,55]

After exposure to an explosive device, most casualties with lethal injuries die immediately. Although the large majority of survivors do not have life-threatening injuries, 10% to 15% of casualties will have critical injuries and may be saved with appropriate management.[47,56,57] An analysis of 3,357 casualties of terrorist bombings worldwide yielded specific patterns of injury, as outlined in **Box 31-1**.[58] Comparison of patterns of injury in terrorist bombing victims versus trauma patients whose injuries were attributed to other causes revealed that terrorist bombing victims had increased incidence

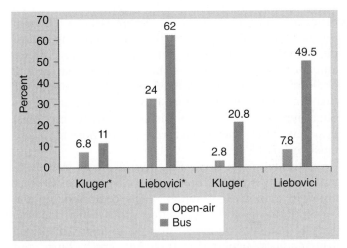

Figure 31-5 Injuries and deaths associated with open-air and enclosed-space (bus) explosions.[42,48]

Data from: Kluger Y. Bomb explosions in acts of terrorism—Detonation, wound ballistics, triage, and medical concerns. *Isr Med Assoc J.* 2003;5(4):235-240; and Liebovici D, Gofrit ON, Stein M, et al. Blast injuries: bus versus open-air bombings—a comparative study of injuries in survivors of open-air versus confined-space explosions. *J Trauma.* 1996;41(6):1030-1035.

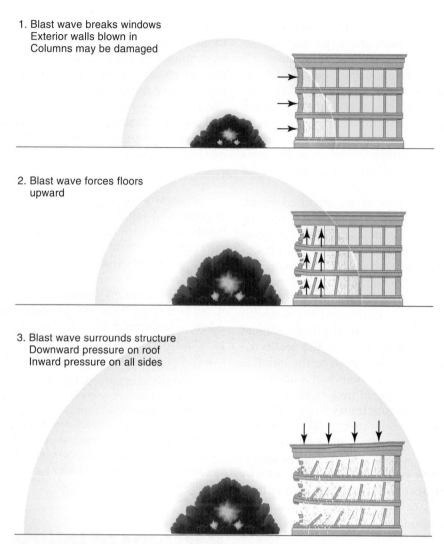

1. Blast wave breaks windows
Exterior walls blown in
Columns may be damaged

2. Blast wave forces floors
upward

3. Blast wave surrounds structure
Downward pressure on roof
Inward pressure on all sides

Figure 31-6 Chronology of blast-induced structural collapse.[52]

Primer to Design Safe School Projects in Case of Terrorist Attacks and School Shootings. FEMA 428/BIPS-07/January 2012. U.S. Department of Homeland Security, Federal Emergency Management Agency: Buildings and Infrastructure Protection Series, p. 4-9, Department of Homeland Security Web site. http://www.dhs.gov/xlibrary/assets/st/bips07_428_schools. pdf. Accessed May 7, 2018.

Box 31-1 Typical Injuries in Terrorist Bombings[58]

- Wounds tend to be either noncritical soft-tissue or skeletal injuries, or critical, with little middle ground
- Head injuries predominate among fatalities (50%–70%).
- Most head-injury survivors (98.5%) have noncritical injuries.
- Head injuries are disproportionate to exposed total body surface area.
- Most casualties with blast lung die immediately.
- Survivors have a low incidence of abdominal and chest wounds, burns, traumatic amputations, and blast lung, although specific mortalities are high (10%–40%).

Quenemoen LE, Davis YM, Malilay J, et al. The World Trade Center bombing: injury prevention strategies for high-rise building fires. *Disasters*. 1996;20(2):125-132.

---

of severe injury (29% vs. 10%; **Figure 31-7**), subsequent increased intensive care unit (ICU) use, prolonged hospital length of stay (LOS), more surgical interventions, and increased hospital mortality.[58] Approximately half of all initial casualties will need medical care within the first hour after the explosion. Those with minor injuries often bypass EMS providers and go directly to the closest hospitals, where they often arrive before those more seriously injured.[53]

Although most survivable injuries occur from fragments, many injuries from explosive devices result from multiple etiologies of injury, each compounding the condition to make the total effect more difficult for the body to handle. Combined/multiple injuries—including primary blast, penetrating fragment, crush, burn, and inhalation injuries—often occur, especially in urban warfare environments or in urban terrorist bombings. A comparison of casualties in the first and second phases of Operation Iraqi Freedom revealed more deaths, higher injury severity, more major injuries per patient, and more casualties with fragment wounds in the latter phase.[59,60]

Compared with nonterror-related trauma, civilian victims of terrorist bombings are generally more seriously injured, with more body regions injured (see **Figure 31-7**). For example, victims of suicide bomb attacks exhibit a characteristic combination of blunt injury, burns, and numerous

penetrating injuries with extensive soft-tissue damage,[63-65] with typical injuries including penetrating injuries to the head, extremities, and torso, as well as burns, open fractures, and blast lung.[64,65]

Whereas bomb injuries in military personnel previously followed a pattern characteristic of fragment injury, and civilian bomb injuries were distinguished by the addition of materials such as nails or bolts, the widespread use of IEDs against both military and civilian targets is now common. Differences between military and civilian casualties of bomb blasts include the following:[66]

- Military casualties are more likely to be a healthy male, 18 to 35 years old, whereas civilian casualties are more often young, old, or female and may be in poor health.
- Unlike their civilian counterparts, military casualties are often wearing protective gear, reducing the risk of head and upper torso injury. This can result in devastating limb injuries in casualties who would have died from injuries to protected areas.
- Bombs used against military targets are typically high-explosive military ordnance, whereas bombs used against civilians are both low- and high-explosive IEDs.

Certain patterns of injury have emerged from Iraq and Afghanistan as a result of explosive devices used in a particular manner in certain tactical situations. For example, an explosive device detonated under a Humvee can produce massive injury to seat occupants, including severe pelvic injury as a result of secondary fragmentation from the vehicle itself. Likewise, explosive devices detonated at the roadside will often injure the front-seat passenger who is riding with an arm and leg outside the vehicle, weapon at the ready. This results in injuries to the right arm, right leg, and face, with little injury to the other occupants. In Afghanistan, a new injury trend was identified in 2010, which is on the rise in dismounted patrols. This pattern, known as dismounted complex blast injury (DCBI), is characterized by a combination of high lower-extremity amputation, pelvic and genital injuries, and injuries to the spine.[67]

Triage

Accurate triage is essential in effective, timely matching of casualty need with available resources. In a tactical setting, this requires an accurate assessment of the urgency of the needs of each casualty. In general, uncontrolled hemorrhage and emergence of shock, as evidenced by vanishing radial pulse, require urgent treatment. However, if the bleeding can be stopped and resuscitation is seen to be effective in maintaining a radial pulse and a conversational level of consciousness, evacuation can be delayed for a limited period.

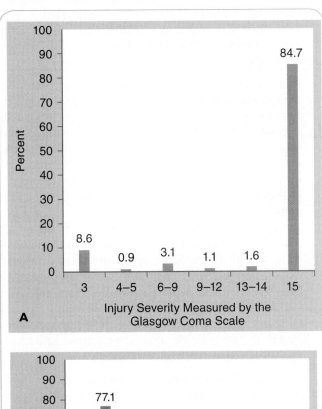

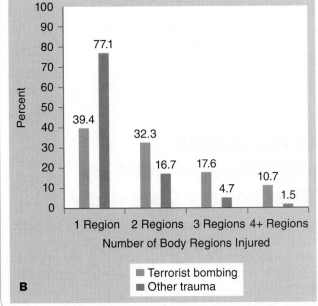

Figure 31-7 Patterns of injury in terrorist bombings: injury severity (**A**) and number of body regions injured (**B**).[68]

(A) and (B) Data from Frykberg ER. Medical management of disasters and mass casualties from terrorist bombings: How can we cope? *J Trauma.* 2002;53(2):201-212.

Mass-casualty triage presents different problems, especially when related to explosions. As discussed earlier, the distribution of injuries from a bomb explosion is normally a significant number of lightly wounded casualties and a significant number of deaths, with a smaller number of high-risk casualties requiring urgent medical treatment. The natural flow of individuals accessing a medical care system is often such that the "walking wounded" and lesser-injured casualties arrive at the emergency facility first, thus impeding access to care for the more critically injured casualties who follow. Therefore, it is essential that triage decisions be repeated and confirmed at every level of care so that overtriage and undertriage can be minimized.[68]

Overtriage is the assignment of unnecessarily high priority to lesser-injured individuals. Although this ensures prompt access to care, overtriage may deluge the health care system and allocate resources away from those who might be in desperate need. Overtriage can result in increased preventable mortality for casualties with an ISS greater than 15 (moderate injury).[64] Overtriage following explosions is often self-directed. Thus, it is vital to establish an outer perimeter around hospital facilities so that floods of patients with minor injuries cannot gain access to resources that might need to be reserved for the most severely injured who follow. Undertriage clearly needs to be avoided to ensure that more severely injured casualties receive prompt access to care.

Triage for MCIs (bomb attacks and other types) is performed with a focus on providing an acceptable quality of care to minimize morbidity and mortality with limited resources.[69,70] This means identifying from among the minimally wounded, dead, and expectant casualties the small subset of casualties with critical injuries who have a chance of survival and focusing scarce personnel and resources on them. This challenge, and that of identifying casualties at risk for occult injuries, can more effectively be met with a thorough understanding of the mechanics and patterns specific to explosion-related injury.[59] For example, understanding that explosions in confined spaces (e.g., vehicles) cause more primary blast effects, lung damage, and penetrating injuries than explosions in open areas will raise the index of suspicion for these types of injuries when encountering victims of confined-space explosions. It is important to keep in mind that survivors of blast explosions not initially considered to be critically injured should nonetheless be monitored to identify subtle signs of deterioration that may indicate the need for immediate care.[59]

Furthermore, with the complex injuries often sustained by blast victims—for example, devastating multimechanistic injuries to more than one body region or multiple injuries in the same body area—it is more important than ever to triage these patients for transport to the highest available level of care. This fundamental tenet of civilian trauma

systems[71] is becoming increasingly prioritized in the military arena,[72] but it faces challenges in operational settings that result in prolonged field, littoral, or shipboard care.

Taxonomy

"Blast injury" is a generalized term that is often used to refer to various injuries caused by an explosive device. However, it is important to differentiate among these injuries because they vary according to injury category. Injuries from explosions are generally classified as primary, secondary, tertiary, quaternary, and quinary after the injury taxonomy described in Department of Defense Directive 6025.21E[73] (**Table 31-4**)[74] as follows:

- Primary injuries, resulting from the blast wave or overpressure, which cause direct tissue damage or primary blast injury (PBI); unique to high explosives
- Secondary injuries, in which ballistic wounds are produced by missiles or primary fragments from the exploding weapon (shrapnel, preformed and unformed fragments) and secondary fragments, or projectiles from the environment (e.g., debris, vehicular metal)
- Tertiary injuries caused by propulsion of casualties onto the ground or into solid objects and structural collapse with concomitant crush and blunt trauma
- Quaternary injuries, including burns and toxicities from fuel, metals, septic syndromes from soil, and environmental contamination
- Quinary injuries, such as those caused by radiation, chemicals, or biologic agents; i.e., from radiation-enhanced explosives ("dirty bombs")

Although these categories are useful ways to think about explosion-related injuries, it is important to note that these injuries often occur in combination.[46] The greatest diagnostic challenges for clinicians at all levels of care in the aftermath of explosions are the large numbers of casualties and multiple penetrating injuries.[67,75]

Assessment and Management by Blast Injury Category

Plans for scene assessment and security must be worked out in advance, with the first priority being to ensure scene safety and lack of persistence of a threat. This is particularly important in the tactical or terrorist environment in which a small explosion can draw combatants into the field of a large explosion or to sniper fire. A well-known tactic of terrorists is to attract security and health care personnel into the environment and then explode a second device (see secondary explosions, discussed previously).

Table 31-4 Blast-Injury Categories[76]

Effect	Impact	Mechanism of Injury	Typical Injuries
Primary	Direct blast effects (over- and under-pressurization)	■ Produced by contact of blast shock wave with body ■ Stress and shear waves occur in tissues ■ Waves reinforced/reflected at tissue density interfaces ■ Gas-filled organs (lungs, ears, etc.) at particular risk	■ Tympanic membrane rupture ■ Blast lung ■ Eye injuries ■ Concussion ■ Traumatic amputation in foot-activated IEDs
Secondary	Projectiles propelled by explosion	Ballistic wounds produced by: ■ Primary fragments (pieces of exploding weapon) or ■ Secondary fragments (environmental fragments, e.g., glass)	■ Penetrating injuries ■ Traumatic amputations ■ Concussion ■ Lacerations
Tertiary	Propulsion of body onto hard surface or object or propulsion of objects onto individuals	■ Whole body translocation ■ Crush injuries caused by structural damage and building collapse	■ Blunt injuries ■ Crush syndrome ■ Compartment syndrome ■ Concussion
Quaternary	Heat and/or combustion fumes	■ Burns and toxidromes from fuel, metals ■ Septic syndromes from soil and environmental contamination	■ Burns ■ Inhalation injury ■ Asphyxiation
Quinary	Additives such as radiation or chemicals (e.g., dirty bombs)	Contamination of tissue from: ■ Bacteria, radiation, or chemical agents, or ■ Allogeneic bone fragments	■ Variety of health effects, depending on agent

DePalma RG, Burris DG, Champion HR, Hodgson MJ. Blast injuries. *N Engl J Med.* 2005;352(13):1335-1342.

As in any medical emergency, prehospital trauma life support (PHTLS) providers responding to the scene of an explosive blast should employ standard operating procedures of assessment and initial management, consisting of aggressive and definitive control of external hemorrhage, clearing the airway, promoting breathing, splinting fractures, etc. Because bomb explosions typically constitute an MCI, mass-casualty principles of triage and treatment should be used, with rapid evacuation to a medical facility as the primary objective.[76]

In this section, each injury category is described, and guidelines for assessment and management are given as needed. A summary of typical explosion-related injuries by organ system is given in **Table 31-5**.

General principles to aid in management of blast victims include the following:[1]

- Early mortality is caused primarily by multiple trauma, then by trauma to the head, thorax, and abdomen[77,78]

- Effective triage and prompt medical attention to those whose survival depends on it are essential; this entails delaying care for those with minor injuries and minimizing care for those with likely lethal injuries such as burns approaching 100% body surface area and those in cardiac arrest.[1,47,77]

- Initial history and physical exam should include the elements listed in **Table 31-6**.

It is predominantly with PBI that assessment and care will differ, because it is only at the scene of an explosion that providers will encounter such injuries. Fortunately, dominant PBI in survivors is not common. The secondary through quinary injuries described here, although characteristic of explosive blast, are also exhibited in other trauma, and, therefore, care will not differ for these injuries. As stated previously, the predominant issue with explosions is fragment injury and multisystem, multietiology injury.

Table 31-5 Summary of Typical Blast Injuries by Organ System[12]

System	Injury/Condition
Auditory	Tympanic membrane rupture, ossicular disruption, cochlear damage, foreign body implantation
Face and eye	Facial fracture, perforated globe, foreign body, retinal artery air emboli
Respiratory	Blast lung, hemothorax, pneumothorax, pulmonary contusion/hemorrhage, arteriovenous fistulas (source of air embolism), airway epithelial damage, aspiration pneumonitis, sepsis
Digestive	Bowel perforation, hemorrhage, ruptured liver or spleen, sepsis, mesenteric ischemia from air embolism
Circulatory	Cardiac contusion, myocardial infarction from air embolism, shock, vasovagal hypotension, peripheral vascular injury, other air embolism-induced injury
Central nervous system	Concussion, closed and open brain injury, stroke, spinal cord injury, air embolism-induced injury
Renal	Renal contusion, laceration, acute renal failure due to rhabdomyolysis, hypotension, and hypovolemia
Extremity	Traumatic amputation, fractures, crush injuries, compartment syndrome, burns, cuts, lacerations, acute arterial occlusion, air embolism-induced injury

Modified from Centers for Disease Control and Prevention. CDC Emergency Preparedness and Response: Explosions and blast injuries: A primer for clinicians. https://www.cdc.gov/masstrauma/preparedness/primer.pdf. Accessed May 7, 2018.

Table 31-6 Components of Rapid Assessment of Blast Victims[1,47,79,80]

History		Physical
Symptoms	**Circumstances**	Blood in external ear or nose
Deafness	Close proximity to blast	Cyanosis
Tinnitus	Enclosed-space explosion	Hemoptysis
Earache	Entrapment	Cough
Nausea	Crush	Rales
Retrograde amnesia	Compartment syndrome	Rhonchi
	Comorbid conditions	Abdominal tenderness, rigidity, guarding
	Underwater or underground	

Primary Blast Injury

PBI results from interaction of the blast wave with the body or tissue to produce stress and shear waves (**Table 31-7**). The strongest blast wave that can allow for a high probability of survival lasts a few milliseconds and has a peak pressure of approximately 300 pounds per square inch (psi).[30] Overpressure injury most often occurs in areas in which tissue densities change (e.g., tympanic membrane, lung air/tissue interfaces, or heart fluid/muscle interface).

The degree of primary blast-induced damage to the body is dependent on the intensity of the blast overpressure, which, in turn, depends on the size of the explosive,[79] proximity of the victim to the point of detonation, and whether or not the victim was in an enclosed space.[51,80] Backpack bombs, for example, have a range of serious injury of 33 to 98 ft (10–30 m), passenger vehicle bombs have a range of 1,476 to 2,756 ft (450–840 m), and large-scale truck bombs have a range of 3,773 to 6,496 ft (1,150–1,980 m).[54] After an attack in which conventional high explosives are used, few survivors close to the epicenter of the explosion have life-threatening PBI (rates of 0.1%–2% have been reported[81,82]) because they have typically been killed by fragments and fire.[83]

Peak overpressures inside enclosed, blast-loaded vehicles typically exceed the threshold for unprotected ear damage but stay below the threshold for blast lung injuries.

Table 31-7 Characteristics of Stress and Shear Waves

Stress Waves	Shear Waves
■ High frequency ■ Supersonic, longitudinal pressure waves ■ Create high local forces with small, rapid distortions ■ Produce microvascular injury ■ Are reinforced/reflected at tissue interfaces, thereby enhancing injury potential, especially in gas-filled organs such as the lungs, ears, and intestines ■ Cause injury via pressure differentials across delicate structures (e.g., alveoli), rapid compression/reexpansion of gas-filled structures, and reflection of the tension wave (a component of the compressive stress wave) at the tissue-gas interface ■ Cause mucosal/submucosal damage and serosal injury that may represent full-thickness damage	■ Low frequency ■ Transverse waves with a lower velocity and longer duration that cause asynchronous movement of tissues ■ Degree of damage depends on extent to which the asynchronous motions overcome inherent tissue elasticity, resulting in tearing of tissue and possible disruption of attachments.

Table 31-8 Short-Duration Pressure Effects From Blasts on Unprotected Persons[84]

Pressure (psi)	Effect		
	Eardrum Rupture	Lung Injury	Death
5	Possible		
15	50% chance		
30–40	Almost certain	Possible	
80		50% chance	
100–200			Possible
130–180			50% chance
200–250			Almost certain

psi = pounds per square inch.

Owen-Smith M. Bomb blast injuries: In an explosive situation. *Nurs Mirror*. 1979;149(13):35-39.

Because unprotected ear damage pressure levels are very low (5 psi; **Table 31-8**), hearing-based crew safety requirements are not appropriate. At present, it is not clear whether hearing threshold values are below that for neurologic injury.

Underwater Explosions

In water, the body reacts very differently to pressure waves and is more susceptible to injury. Close to the explosion, there is a rapid, high-pressure wave front. At greater distances, the waveform more closely approximates the low-frequency, continuous waveform. Water is approximately 800 times denser than air and approximately 10,000 times less compressible. A diver in shallow water or at the surface will receive not only the direct blast wave from the explosion, but also the reflected waves from the surface or seabed and any surrounding structures (**Figure 31-8**). Explosions underwater are estimated to be three times stronger than their counterparts on land,[87] and the deeper the subject is immersed, the greater the effect of the blast. Pulmonary hemorrhage is the most frequent injury related to underwater blast, followed by injury to the susceptible gas-filled intestines.

Assessment and Management

Knowledge of the characteristics of blast physics and PBI is helpful for effective initial evaluation, triage, and treatment of casualties with suspected PBI.

In severe blast injury, immediate death typically occurs, which may be attributed to a characteristic triad of physiologic responses to the primary blast overpressure:

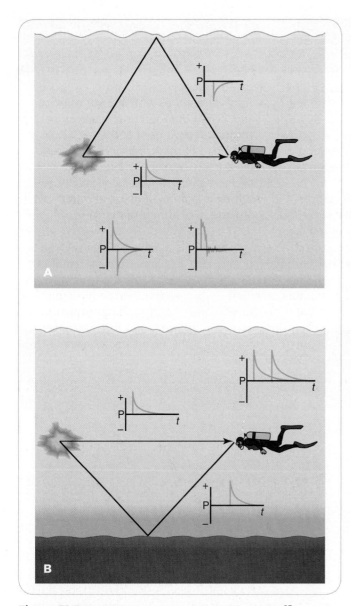

Figure 31-8 Blast effects on a diver in shallow water.[85]
A. Superimposition of direct- and surface-reflected blast waves.
B. Superimposition of direct- and bottom-reflected blast waves.

A. and **B.** Reproduced from: Cudahy E, Parvin S. The Effects of Underwater Blast on Divers. Naval Submarine Medical Research Laboratory. NSMRL Report 1218.

(1) bradycardia, (2) apnea, and (3) hypotension.[86] Immediate death has also been attributed to massive air embolism, which results from disruption of the alveolar wall and adjacent pulmonary capillaries with air emboli, primarily affecting cerebral and coronary vessels. In immediate survivors, dysrhythmias, signs of neurologic injury, and retinal artery air emboli have been noted.

In survivors, PBI can present with no outward signs of trauma or may present as perforated eardrums, ocular trauma, flash burns, traumatic amputation, or acute dyspnea.[68,87] Patients with these signs and symptoms may at first appear stable but may deteriorate quickly.

Blast testing has revealed thresholds of injury for organs classified as (1) air containing (lung, eardrum, gastrointestinal tract, larynx, trachea); (2) liver and spleen; and (3) kidney, pancreas, and gallbladder.[30] The first group is the most vulnerable, exhibiting the first signs of injury at the lowest threshold, followed by the second, and then the third group.[30] Of the air-containing organs, the tympanic membrane is the most frequent site of injury, followed by the lungs.

Use of the Trendelenburg position is not recommended for casualties of blast explosions because it may increase the risk of coronary air embolus. Immediate therapy is supplemental oxygen at the highest feasible fraction of inspired oxygen. Hyperbaric oxygen treatment—if available and initiated shortly after the onset of symptoms—typically results in rapid improvement of signs and symptoms. Alveolar-venous fistulas are thought to resolve in 24 hours but must be considered a continuing risk in casualties who require positive-pressure ventilation, especially with application of positive end-expiratory pressure (PEEP) typically used for hypoxic pathophysiology.[88]

Tympanic Membrane Rupture

The auditory system is very susceptible to blast and is the site of the most frequently detected blast injury.[89] Immediate, but often temporary, blast-induced deafness often occurs, which heightens anxiety and impedes communication; deafness may be permanent or may resolve within hours. Sensorineural hearing loss associated with high-pitched tinnitus frequently occurs immediately after a blast.

The tympanic membrane is the functional structure injured at the lowest pressure by blasts and, thus, may assist in detecting other primary blast effects. Higher overpressures may result in permanent hearing loss.[93] The presence of tympanic membrane rupture has traditionally been used as a marker of PBI, although its absence does not absolutely rule out lung injuries.[90,91] The incidence of tympanic membrane rupture increases with proximity to the epicenter and when the explosion occurs in an enclosed space.[91]

Perforation of the eardrum (in the anteroinferior part of the pars tensa) is the most common physical finding and may occur at pressures as low as 5 to 15 psi.[92,93] Deafness, tinnitus, and vertigo may indicate rupture and should heighten suspicion of rupture if the tympanic membrane cannot be visualized.

Examination of casualties with blast injury should include otoscopic identification of tympanic membrane rupture. Absence of rupture may lower (but not eliminate) the index of suspicion for PBI, except if the casualty exhibits abdominal pain, dyspnea, or respiratory distress.

Treatment of ruptured tympanic membrane is not a priority. Signs and symptoms include hearing loss and bleeding from the ears. The diagnosis may be confirmed by visualizing the eardrum with an otoscope. A large proportion (50%–80%) of ruptured tympanic membranes heal spontaneously.[94]

Although not a priority for treatment, auditory injury should be addressed within 24 hours and the auditory canal cleaned of all debris. Probing or irrigating the auditory canal, however, should be avoided. When the ear is full of contaminated debris, antibiotic eardrops should be administered.

With respect to the outer ear, traumatic blast amputation of an ear or earlobe has been shown to be almost uniformly associated with fatal injury.[95]

Pulmonary Injury

The lung is the second most susceptible organ to PBI.[96] Increased overpressure increases pulmonary damage, with overpressures of 200 psi uniformly fatal in open-air blasts.[88] Blast injury to the lungs is the most common cause of injury and death from the primary blast effect alone, although it occurs with variable frequency, ranging from 7% to 39% in several studies.[72,94,97] The effect of body armor in preventing the pulmonary effects of primary blast continues to be discussed.[100]

The pulmonary sequelae of blast wave exposure are collectively referred to as "blast lung." Although it occurs rarely among survivors,[98] blast lung is an often fatal combination of acute respiratory distress (dyspnea/apnea), bradycardia, and hypotension subsequent to a blast exposure.[11] Patients with blast lung may exhibit hypoxemia and hemoptysis and may require endotracheal intubation.

Reflection of stress waves at rigid interfaces of the lungs causes paramediastinal, peribronchial, and subpleural tissue disruption and hemorrhage. Primary blast effect on the chest wall also produces a classic pattern of contusion and hemorrhage on the surface of the lungs **(Figure 31-9)**. The index of suspicion for blast lung (if providers have access to this information) at charge sizes of 0.5, 4.5, and

45 lb (1, 10, and 100 kg) of TNT equivalent would occur at distances from the charge of approximately 11, 25, and 123 ft (3.5, 7.5, and 37.5 m), respectively, for blasts close to ground level. This is a general guideline that may be especially useful when patients have multiple injuries.[91]

Among survivors of PBI, clinical manifestations may be present immediately[99,100] or may have a delayed onset of 24 to 48 hours.[101] Bleeding from the ears is a sign of possible blast lung or hollow organ injury.[102] Intrapulmonary hemorrhage and focal alveolar edema result in frothy, bloody secretions and lead to ventilation/perfusion mismatch, increased intrapulmonary shunting, and decreased compliance. Hypoxia results from increased work of breathing and is pathophysiologically similar to pulmonary contusions induced by other mechanisms of nonpenetrating thoracic trauma.[103] Other injuries may include pneumothorax, hemothorax, subcutaneous and mediastinal emphysema, pneumoperitoneum, and tension pneumoperitoneum.[104,105]

PBI to the lung may not be immediately apparent yet may require complex ventilatory and fluid management and support. Recommended guidelines for care include the following:

1. Monitor for frothy secretions and respiratory distress.
2. Monitor early for hemodynamic parameters.
3. Provide oxygen, if available.
   - Use high-frequency ventilation, with liberal hypercapnia.
   - Limit peak inspiratory pressures, because elevated pressures increase the risk of air embolism or pneumothorax.
4. Carefully manage fluid administration, avoiding fluid overload; although the ideal fluid for resuscitation in blast injury is not known, the following guidelines are recommended:
   - Use whole blood as the resuscitation fluid of choice for blast casualties in hemorrhagic shock.
   - Use TXA for blast casualties with suspected noncompressible torso hemorrhage.
   - Resuscitate to a systolic blood pressure of 80-90 mm Hg unless TBI is present, in which case the target SBP should be 90 mm Hg or higher.
5. Continually monitor patient because edema is a common sequela in casualties with lung damage; if pneumothorax begins to develop, employ tube thoracostomy immediately.
6. Consider prophylactic tube thoracostomy if casualties must be evacuated by air or when close observation is impractical.
7. Do not remove impaled objects; shorten them to facilitate transport, and then wrap them carefully to prevent movement before surgical exploration.
8. If TBI is present, prevent/minimize hypercapnia to avoid intracranial hypertension.

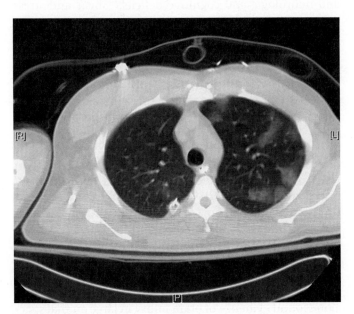

Figure 31-9 Classic pattern of blast on lungs.
Courtesy of H.R. Champion.

The role of antibiotics and corticosteroids is not currently defined.

Abdominal and Gastrointestinal Tract Injuries

Although much less common than massive lethal injuries, ear and lung injuries, and penetrating fragment injury, PBI to the intestines does occur, and casualties should be examined and monitored for delayed perforation or presentation of this condition. A review of U.S. Army collective animal data indicates that PBI to the gastrointestinal (GI) tract is as prevalent as pulmonary injuries in free-field blasts,[106] and when multiple detonations occur in a complex environment (i.e., inside a structure), the GI tract appears more susceptible to injury.[107] A review of the literature on terrorist bombings between 1996 and 2002 revealed that intestinal perforation was the most common type of PBI to the abdomen,[44] primarily occurring in suicide bombings (both in open air and in enclosed spaces).[108] Victims of underwater blasts are at greater risk of GI injury than lung injury, especially with partial submersion.[109]

The lower GI tract is often filled with gas. The ileocecal area is most susceptible to PBI, and the small intestine is generally spared. Blast-induced rapid compression and decompression damage the stomach wall, often creating a rupture that leads to peritonitis, hemorrhage, bleeding and devascularizing injury, and submucosal to transmural injury. Multifocal intramural hematoma is the characteristic injury, which begins in the submucosa and extends with increasing severity to become a large, transmural confluent hematoma that may involve the mesentery and vascular supply. Serosal injury should always be considered indicative of transmural injury.[110]

Symptoms include nausea and vomiting; pain in the abdomen, rectum, and testes; straining/inability to urinate or defecate; and, rarely, hematemesis. In primary blast with pulmonary injury, free-air and even tension pneumoperitoneum without intestinal injury have been reported.

Intestinal perforation, which is considered a closed injury, is common, but open injuries may occur as well. Signs and symptoms, which may be hard to discern in the immediate postblast period, may include pain in the abdomen, rectum, and testes. Treatment does not differ from treatment of GI injuries resulting from other mechanisms.[111]

A 2011 review of the literature on abdominal injury from primary blast revealed that, although the incidence was highly variable (1%–33%, and as high as 69% in underwater blasts), and less frequent than abdominal injury from fragments, it has a high risk of morbidity and death.[112] Reasons for this include the fact that issues may present days or weeks after injury—for example, perforation of a GI mural hematoma. Most affected are the terminal ileum and cecum. British combat casualty data (2003–2008) showed that vascular injuries to the abdomen and thorax were extremely rare (occurring in 2% of casualties who did not return to duty) but 100% fatal.[113]

Injuries to the liver, spleen, adrenal glands, kidneys, and testicles have all been reported in underwater blasts,[114] although solid-organ injury is less common in air blasts. These injuries are probably caused by shear forces, and they present similarly to solid-organ injury resulting from blunt trauma. Gallbladder, renal pelvis, and bladder injury secondary to primary blast have rarely been recorded, most likely because of their fluid contents.[115] These injuries present like hemorrhagic shock and should be treated accordingly.

Traumatic Brain Injury

TBI is a major cause of death in bomb attacks, historically accounting for 71% of early deaths and 52% of later deaths.[55] Between 2001 and 2009, TBI was the primary cause of death (83%) among U.S. combat casualties with injuries deemed nonsurvivable.[4] Lethal TBI is often caused by secondary and tertiary effects, but significant histologic damage and central nervous system dysfunction can occur with the primary blast overpressure.[116] Casualties may present with periods of loss of consciousness, agitation, excitability, and irrational behavior. Moderate and severe TBIs are incapacitating. Long-term sequelae and coexistent posttraumatic stress disorder (PTSD) have also been associated with TBI from primary blast mechanisms,[117] especially with repeated exposures.[118,119]

Visible wounds or obvious penetration of the skull may indicate "conventional" or penetrating TBIs, which are easily diagnosed. In the blast etiology of blunt head trauma, the initial high-pressure shock wave is followed closely by a gust of displaced air filling the vacuum. These extreme fluctuations in pressures, which may be 1,000 times greater than atmospheric pressure,[30] may cause concussion, loss of consciousness, loss of vision, deafness, and neurologic and cognitive deficits.[3] Shear and stress waves of the primary blast may cause concussion, hemorrhage, edema, diffuse axonal injury, and formation of gas emboli leading to infarction.[120] Signs and symptoms of TBI may include loss of consciousness, acute headache, amnesia, confusion, and disorientation.[121]

Mild TBI due to blast injury may initially be asymptomatic (loss of consciousness need not be present for mild TBI to occur[122]) but may cause cognitive and performance decrements with the passage of time, especially in the event of repeated exposures. Short- or long-term transient cognitive decrement associated with mild TBI is of significant concern in combat. Mild TBI can result from blunt head trauma or exposure to blast overpressure. In the past, researchers had difficulty differentiating mild TBI from psychological trauma,[125-128] but more recent studies have been able to document physical damage to the brain in animal studies.[129-131] A test series evaluating the effects of high-rate mechanical insults alone found evidence of brain injury in large animal specimens for short-duration blasts that do not result in fatal pulmonary injuries.[98] However, the etiology, mechanistic basis, and detailed progression of such brain injuries remain obscure and easily confused with other diagnoses.

The Defense Advanced Research Projects Agency (DARPA) and the Office of Naval Research sponsored a study to research TBI in Marines who use explosives to gain access to buildings. Results indicate that these individuals, known as "breachers," have neurologic deficits that are associated with long-term, repeated exposure to explosive blast events.[130]

> On 21 June 2010, guided in part by the breacher study, the Pentagon announced its first policies for identifying and treating people who may have TBI. Included were the first military-wide mandatory triggers for screening troops, including a rule that anyone within 50 meters of a blast had to be evaluated for signs of brain injury.[132]

To assess the impact of exposure to blast, the Department of Defense fielded the Military Acute Concussion Evaluation (MACE).[131] Updated in 2012, the MACE is a tool for small-unit commanders and medics to assess cognitive function following incidents to help evaluate immediate fitness for continued combatant function in a tactical setting.

After several years of surveillance in Iraq and Afghanistan, it became clear that large numbers of TBIs resulting from IED blasts in military personnel were going unrecognized.[78,132] In October 2015, the International Classification of Diseases was updated with improved surveillance definitions for TBI. The assistant secretary of defense also clarified TBI case definitions for the military. These changes meant that some cases previously categorized as "unclassifiable" severity would contribute to higher counts of moderate TBI. The Department of Defense Standard Surveillance Case Definition for TBI[133] lists the following classifications for severity:

> **Concussion/mild TBI is characterized by the following**: Confused or disoriented state which lasts less than 24 hours; or loss of consciousness for up to 30 minutes; or memory loss lasting less than 24 hours. Excludes penetrating TBI. A computed tomography (CT) scan is not indicated for most patients with a mild TBI. If obtained, it is normal.

> **Moderate TBI is characterized by the following**: Confused or disoriented state which lasts more than 24 hours; or loss of consciousness for more than 30 minutes, but less than 24 hours; or memory loss lasting greater than 24 hours but less than 7 days; or meets criteria for mild TBI except an abnormal CT scan is present. Excludes penetrating TBI. A structural brain imaging study may be normal or abnormal.

> **Severe TBI is characterized by the following**: Confused or disoriented state which lasts more than 24 hours; or loss of consciousness for more than 24 hours; or memory loss for more than 7 days. Excludes penetrating TBI. A structural brain imaging study may be normal but usually is abnormal.

> **Penetrating TBI, or open head injury, is characterized by the following**: A head injury in which the scalp, skull and dura mater (the outer layer of the meninges) are penetrated. Penetrating injuries can be caused by high-velocity projectiles or objects of lower velocity such as knives, or bone fragments from a skull fracture that are driven into the brain.

> Immediate treatment of TBI does not differ for blast-related injuries and includes immediate attention to hemorrhage control, securing of the airway, judicious fluid resuscitation, and attention to other immediately life-threatening injuries to prevent hypoxia and hypotension (and thus secondary injury).

Between 2000 and 2017, more than 379,000 U.S. service members suffered a TBI, with the incidence of mild TBI comprising 82.3% (**Figure 31-10**).[134] (These numbers represent medical diagnoses of TBI among U.S. forces located anywhere, including within the continental United States.)

Traumatic Amputation

Traumatic amputation resulting from a primary blast has traditionally been a marker of injury severity with few survivors.[99,135] In recent years, however, data show both improved survivability and increased severity in the form of more casualties losing multiple limbs. In the 2005 London train bombings, 24.5% of those with traumatic amputations survived.[136] Analysis revealed that survival in several cases was associated with being seated instead of standing because (1) seated victims were far enough away from the explosion to avoid receiving an incident pressure high

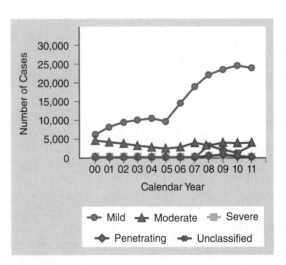

Figure 31-10 Traumatic brain injury incidence by severity, 2000–2017.

Data from: Armed Forces Surveillance Center, 2013.

enough to be fatal, but the pressure was magnified by the solid surface of the bench to create enough force to sever a limb; and (2) the legs of the seated victims were as much as a 1.6 ft (0.5 m) closer to the explosion than the chest. Combat casualty data show that in 2009, casualties evacuated to higher levels of care included 86 amputees (largely attributed to IED attacks), 63 with one limb amputated and 23 with multiple amputations. The following year, these numbers had risen to 187 amputees, with 115 having single and 72 having multiple limbs amputated. In an evaluation of 111 blast-related fatalities in 2010, 68 (61%) had multiple limbs amputated, up from 28% in 2007.[69]

> The ATO's [Afghanistan's] most dramatic changes in 2010 were the increased numbers of bilateral thigh amputations, triple and quadruple amputations, and associated genital injuries.[69]

Land mine explosions often cause traumatic amputations via the primary blast shock wave,[137] which fractures the bone before the limb is amputated by the blast wind.[40] The levels of amputation following explosions are counterintuitive, and, instead of occurring through joints as one might imagine, they tend to occur approximately 4 to 6 inches (10–15 cm) proximal or distal to the joint surfaces. In cases of traumatic amputation in a surviving casualty, the injury should be treated symptomatically.

Secondary Injury

Most injuries in explosions are from fragments. Fragment munitions are frequently designed to generate multiple small preformed fragments that weigh 0.35 to 0.70 ounce (oz; 1–2 g) and are 0.08 to 0.12 inches (2–3 millimeters [mm]) in diameter, whereas others may have larger fragments that weigh as much as 0.7 oz (20 g). Both lighter- and heavier-weight varieties have initial velocities of 1,500 mps (4,921 fps) that decelerate rapidly (especially in the presence of large, irregularly shaped fragments).

Secondary fragment injuries are caused by energy transfer and the velocity of the projectile and are the most common injuries sustained in bomb explosions. Fragments take the form of both the exploding pieces of the bomb itself along with shattered pieces of glass, wood, etc., from the environment,[43] and they frequently include metal from disintegrating vehicle interiors. Environmental debris such as glass, splinters, soil, and various structural particles are major causes of multiple fragment wounds (**Figure 31-11**). Glass is the most ubiquitous wounding agent among environmental fragments. For example, in the 1996 Khobar Towers bombing, 88% of injuries were caused by glass, especially from windows and patio doors.[49]

Magnitude of injury is thought to depend more on the inherent tissue characteristics of the affected organ than on the projectile itself, with clinical impact and priority of treatment determined by the tissue or organ involved. For example, the presence of numerous

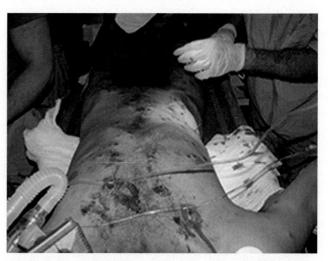

Figure 31-11 Fragmentation injury from environmental debris.
Courtesy of Maj. Scott Gering, Operation Iraqi Freedom.

extremity wounds does not usually have high associated morbidity or mortality, whereas wounds of the eyes or thorax are much more likely to be immediately disabling or life threatening, respectively.

The threat of injury from fragments exceeds that of the blast wave by a factor of 100. Therefore, in a free-field environment, one is unlikely to be affected by blast overpressure within ranges that usually result in potentially survivable fragment injury. For example, in an open-space detonation of a 155-mm (200-lb [91-kg]) shell, death from primary blast and fragments, as well as eardrum rupture, is likely to occur within 50 ft (15 m) of the detonation. At 80 ft (24 m), death from fragments is likely. At 130 ft (40 m), fragment injury and temporary hearing-threshold shift are likely, and at distances as far as 1,800 ft (549 m), fragment injury is still possible.

A diagram of projected injuries from terrorist bombs ranging from small bombs packed in luggage to large truck bombs shows that most injuries will be caused by glass fragments as well as structural collapse (**Figure 31-12**).[54] Fragment throw distance and blast overpressure are both functions of casing material thickness and net explosive weight. However, in a free-field environment, in which there are no structures to block the propagation of casing fragments, the dominant injury mechanism from a cased weapon is always fragment penetration.

Assessment and Management

Multiple Injuries

Fragment injuries from explosive blasts differ from other penetrating injuries in the type and quantity of penetrating agents, which often occur across multiple body regions. Ideally, each fragment injury would be treated as a specific injury based on its size, severity, and location. The unique aspect of explosive injuries is the massive number of individual injuries that can occur, making

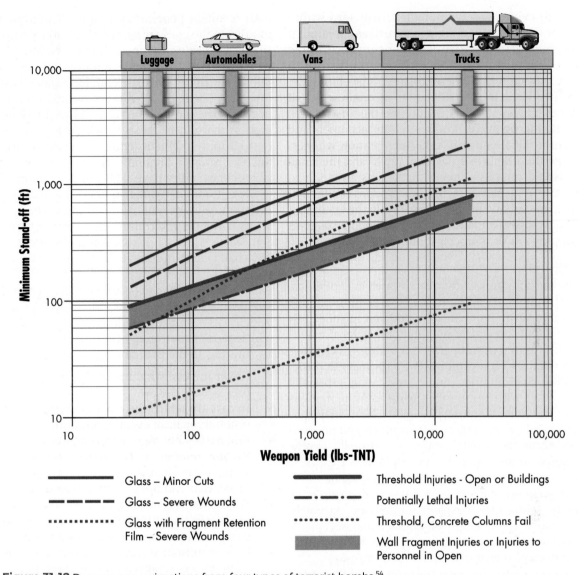

Figure 31-12 Damage approximations from four types of terrorist bombs.[54]

Reproduced from *Reference Manual to Mitigate Potential Terrorist Attacks Against Buildings.* FEMA 426. Figure 4-2, p.239. December 2003. http://www.fema.gov/pdf/plan/prevent/rms/428/fema428_ch4.pdf.

individualized treatment for each wound difficult, if not impossible, in certain settings (**Figure 31-13**). General treatment guidelines can be found in other chapters. General principles must apply, with attention to airway, control of bleeding, resuscitation, immobilization, and splinting.

For military personnel, the abdomen and chest have a greatly reduced incidence of secondary penetrating injury because they are protected by body armor. However, fragments can enter laterally and below the body armor and in junctions between the torso, arms, neck, and legs. Penetrating wounds entering the torso from explosions must be managed in the same way as any other penetrating injury, treating respiratory distress and shock as needed. The chest must be evaluated for penetration and pneumohemothorax. Abdominal wounds should be

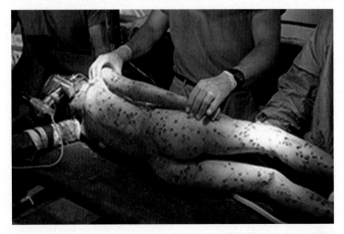

Figure 31-13 Multiple fragment wounds from cluster bomblet.

Photo courtesy of Maj. Scott Gering, Operation Iraqi Freedom, 2003.

dressed with a view to providing definitive therapy within 8 hours, or if shock occurs from hemorrhage, treatment must be provided as a matter of extreme urgency. In the absence of body armor, significant fragment injury can occur, with as many as 30 or 40 fragments lacerating the body. In the field, it is often difficult to ascertain which, if any, of these fragments have penetrated the torso.

Penetrating fragment wounds of the abdomen and thorax are no different from other penetrating wounds, except that the number of pieces of metal and the small size of visceral injuries demand meticulous attention to detail. Almost all penetrating thoracic wounds can be successfully managed by tube thoracostomy. In the event that wounds are grossly contaminated, as is common, standard infection prophylaxis protocols should be followed.

Limb Injuries

Limbs are the body areas most often injured in explosions. In combat, limb injury accounts for 70% of injuries. Such injuries vary from minor to massive and may include multiple amputations and near-amputations. A focal explosive force is exerted by antipersonnel mines, which often injure the limbs with a combination of primary and secondary blast. Such injuries can be devastating, especially if contaminated with dirt or other debris, causing tremendous pain and often requiring emergency hemostatic maneuvers, including application of tourniquets and pressure dressings. Scene and initial therapy should usually involve tourniquet(s) to stop hemorrhage. Definitive treatment for such injuries must include thorough debridement, often to the point of completing amputation of seriously injured limbs. Injuries from exploding mines are extremely serious, with a combination of primary and secondary blast wounds in localized body areas. Mine injuries often require extensive staged treatment and transfusions.

Casualties with long-bone fractures should be managed with temporary splinting to prevent further soft-tissue damage, minimize further neurovascular compromise and bleeding,[138,139] and reduce pain. No attempt should be made to reduce or manipulate fractures. Current practice is to apply a transport external fixator at Level II and transport to Level III. All open or compound fractures should be immobilized and covered with bulky sterile dressings, followed by administration of systemic, broad-spectrum antibiotics. Tetanus prophylaxis or booster injections should be given during initial treatment.

All war wounds are contaminated by soil, clothing, and skin, whereas low-velocity fragmentation wounds are minimally contaminated with debris. Bacterial contamination is common in fragmentation wounds,[140] although infection is uncommon in small, low-velocity extremity wounds. Standard protocol should be followed.

Injuries to the Eye

Although the eyes are extremely resistant to PBI, they are vulnerable to secondary and tertiary mechanisms, with resultant penetrating trauma. The most significant injuries to the eyes are caused by explosions that produce shattered glass or tiny metal fragments. Most injuries can be prevented by wearing eye protection. Secondary blast injuries include corneoscleral lacerations, orbital fractures, hyphema, lid lacerations, traumatic cataracts, optic nerve injury, serous retinitis, and rupture of the globe. A high proportion of these injuries are caused by minute (1- to 2-mm) fragments entering the eye, causing damage that can result in blindness. As many as 10% of all survivors of blast injury have significant eye injuries from projectile perforation, with symptoms that may include pain, irritation, sensation of a foreign body, changes in visual acuity, swelling, and contusions.[11] Among survivors of the September 11, 2001, attacks on the World Trade Center, 26% had ocular injuries attributed to smoke, dust, fumes, and debris.[141]

Ocular injuries can occur with all categories of mines. The primary mechanism of injury involves the products of detonation and environmental fragments and debris, which cause penetrating ocular wounds.[142]

Injuries to the eye should be treated as follows:

- Cover the eye with a rigid shield that does not place pressure on the eye.
- In cases in which the globe is exposed, consider provisional repair of eyelid laceration.
- Emergency enucleation is not advised.
- Do not remove objects penetrating the eye at the scene; cover the eye with a paper cup or other clean object that will not exert pressure on the globe.
- Treat chemical burns (such as those sustained from car battery acid) by at least 60 minutes of irrigation using sterile saline or the cleanest water available.
- If toxic substance release is suspected, wear eye protection such as polycarbonate goggles.

Tertiary Injury

Tertiary injuries, which result when a person is propelled into a hard surface or a hard surface is propelled onto a person, are the second most common type of injury among survivors of bomb attacks.[86] These injuries include closed head injuries, blunt trauma to the abdomen and thorax, spinal injury, fractures of the extremities, and less severe injuries such as dislocations, sprains, and strains.[49] The presence of rib fractures should increase suspicion of tertiary or quaternary injury to the thorax. Muscle, bone, and solid-organ injury are much more likely to result from the tertiary and quaternary effects of the blast than from the blast wave alone.[92]

Crush injuries and compartment syndrome are tertiary injuries that frequently accompany structural collapse. Compartment syndrome, initiated by the buildup of pressure in myofascial compartments, is an acute condition that can cause loss of limb, paralysis, or death.

Damage to muscle groups causes swelling, ultimate constriction by the unyielding fascia, compression on and reduced supply of oxygen and nutrients to nerves and blood vessels, and ultimately cell death.[143] Irreversible tissue death can occur in as few as 4 hours, depending on the location of the injury and the compartmental pressure. Compartment syndrome is distinguished from crush syndrome by its localized effects; crush syndrome has systemic effects.

Spinal injury may result when a patient is propelled onto a hard surface, shattering vertebrae. In Afghanistan, spinal injuries have increased due to roadside bombs that propel the military's mine-resistant ambush protected (MRAP) vehicles into the air, throwing the occupants against the interior, damaging (including causing crush injuries) spinal columns, and causing concussions and broken bones of feet and ankles.[144] This phenomenon was the catalyst for redesigning the vehicle seats to absorb the blast (blast mitigation seats) or to float above the floor and hull to isolate it from blast effects (suspended seats) and increase the headroom.[145]

Assessment and Management

Tertiary injuries may result in blunt injuries such as head and spinal cord trauma, and if structural collapse occurs, compartment syndrome or crush syndrome may result.

Compartment Syndrome

In compartment syndrome, the damaged muscle swells (creating pressure within its inelastic sheath) and becomes ischemic; then it continues swelling, increases compartment pressures, decreases tissue perfusion, and further increases ischemia. Left untreated, compartment syndrome causes local tissue necrosis, which may lead to paralysis, amputation, and death, and presages development of crush syndrome. Compartment syndrome usually involves the extremities but occasionally involves the buttocks[146,147] and abdominal muscles (e.g., rectus).[148] The most characteristic sign of compartment syndrome is pain out of proportion to visible injury. Other signs include pain when the affected muscles are stretched, tension and swelling involving the gluteal or rectus abdominis muscles, and absence of pulses in the affected area (**Box 31-2**).

Box 31-2 The Five Ps of Compartment Syndrome

Pain out of proportion to the injury
Pain with passive stretch
Pressure, tension, or swelling
Paresthesia, or loss of feeling below affected area
Pulselessness, usually in late stages

Field management of compartment syndrome should include the following:

- Administration of high-flow oxygen
- Splinting when long transport times are anticipated
- Expeditious transport to definitive care
- Fluid resuscitation
- Analgesia

No ice or elevation should be used. U.S. Army Reserve protocol for management of compartment syndrome includes performance of field fasciotomy.[145] Fasciotomy is the only definitive treatment for a patient with compartment syndrome.

Crush Syndrome

Crush syndrome occurs when the muscle is damaged, causing cell disruption, ischemia and leakage, and vascular compression of and reduced blood supply to tissues. Cell death occurs in muscle tissue after approximately 4 hours without blood. The lethality of crush syndrome is related to reperfusion, whereby toxins are released into the body. Oliguric renal failure, the most severe endpoint of crush syndrome, also causes potassium accumulation in addition to that released from damaged muscle. An illustrative case of crush syndrome involved a woman pinned for 12 hours in the wreckage after a train derailment in 1987. Although she remained conscious and oriented and her vital signs were stable, shortly after she was extricated, she went into cardiac arrest and died.[145]

Indicators of crush syndrome include compression for 1 hour or longer; involvement of large muscle mass; no pain in area of compression; shock; clammy, cool, pale skin; rapid, weak pulse; and no pulses or capillary refill.[145]

Treatment of crush syndrome includes the following:

- Maintenance of hydration and alkalization[149]
- Fluid therapy that maintains renal perfusion without fluid overload
- Airway management, including protection from dust
- Oxygenation
- Maintenance of body temperature
- Rapid transport to definitive care
- Maintenance of circulation
- Treatment of shock
- Fluid resuscitation
- Cardiac monitoring
- Analgesia
- Expeditious extrication

In most circumstances, immediately before extrication, the casualty should be given a 1- to 2-liter bolus of normal saline or lactated Ringer solution and two ampules of sodium bicarbonate.[145]

Spinal Injury

If signs and symptoms of spinal cord injury (e.g., numbness, inability to move or breathe independently, neck or back pain) are present, the cervical spine should be stabilized if the tactical situation allows, because injuries from explosives entail the potential of spinal fractures from tertiary blast effects. Spinal injury should also be assumed in a casualty who is unconscious from blast-related trauma. Often, however, stabilization may have to be delayed until a secure environment is obtained and preparations can be made for immediate evacuation to definitive neurosurgical support.

Quaternary Injury

Quaternary injuries include burns, inhalation injury, and asphyxiation resulting from fire or fumes. The flash (fireball) produced by the detonation of an explosion can reach temperatures >3,000°C (>5,432°F).[59] IEDs are the primary cause of burn injuries in recent conflicts, and they most often affect the head and hands (i.e., areas not covered by body armor).[150] Almost one-fifth (17%) of surviving casualties of terrorist bomb attacks have sustained burns in addition to their other injuries.[151]

Common substances causing inhalation injury after an explosion are smoke, nitrogen oxides, cyanide, phosgene, carbon monoxide, and heavy metal fumes. Inhalation injury occurs primarily in conjunction with fires or structural collapse. In the 1993 World Trade Center bombing, for example, almost all survivors had smoke inhalation, a result of both the ensuing fires and prolonged evacuation.[58] In the subsequent World Trade Center attack in 2001, half of immediate survivors had inhalation injury caused by fires and dust from the building collapse.[59]

Assessment and Management

Burns after an explosion should be treated as any other burn wounds. For field treatment guidelines, see the treatment of burn casualties chapter.

Quinary Injury

Quinary injuries include those caused by release of toxic (chemical, biologic, or radioactive) agents or by introduction of foreign bodies that have the potential to transmit disease. In suicide bomb attacks, fragments of body parts from the assailant or other bombing casualties may become projectiles, embedding in the bodies of victims and increasing the risk for transmission of bloodborne disease agents such as hepatitis B virus and human immunodeficiency virus (HIV).[97] Of six such cases in the medical literature, two resulted from suicide bombings; in one, embedded bone fragments tested positive for hepatitis B.[154-156]

Chemical agents may come in contact with skin or be inhaled and cause early effects such as coughing, itching, and eye inflammation. It may be difficult to tell if a chemical agent has been released because it may be odorless and cause no initial symptoms. Classifications of chemical agents include the following:

- *Nerve agents.* These are quickly absorbed through the skin and mucous membranes and cause an almost immediate, often lethal, reaction.[155] Signs and symptoms of nerve agent poisoning include pinpoint pupils, muscular twitching, unexplained nasal secretion, salivation, tightness of the chest, shortness of breath, or nausea and abdominal cramps. Treatment calls for immediate intramuscular injection of 2 mg atropine, combined if possible with oxime.[156] Indications of the presence of nerve agents such as sarin gas or Soman are advanced respiratory failure or victims who are dead but have no apparent major injuries.[157]
- *Blister/vesicant agents.* These agents burn and blister on contact and cause damage to the mucous membranes of the respiratory tract when inhaled. Of particular importance to note is that some blister agents (e.g., mustard gas or phosgene oxime) have a latent symptom-free period that may last 2 to 6 hours.[158,157]
- *Choking agents.* Signs and symptoms of exposure to choking agents (e.g., phosgene and chlorine) may include coughing, choking, tightness in the chest, vomiting, headache, and lacrimation. However, as with some blister agents, no symptoms may be evident immediately following exposure.[158]

Thus, in addition to dealing with the usual traumatic injuries expected from an explosive event, you may also be faced with victims who, after treatment for minor injuries at the site, may develop subsequent toxic, potentially lethal effects.[157]

Theoretically, drug-resistant bacteria, such as methicillin-resistant *Staphylococcus aureus* (MRSA), could also be disseminated through an explosive device. If a biologic agent (e.g., anthrax or ricin) is released, no immediate signs of illness will be apparent. As with some chemical agents, biologic agents have an initial symptom-free incubation period, which may last days instead of hours, depending on the agent.[157] Thus, it may not be possible to tell if such an agent has been released in an explosion, especially in the midst of the ensuing debris, dust, and fire.[158]

Contamination of an explosive with radioactive material results in radiation exposure that varies with the size and sophistication of the explosive, the type of material, weather conditions, and speed of evacuation from the scene.[158]

A noted quinary effect of explosions is the phenomenon of "human remains shrapnel," in which a bone fragment from the assailant (usually a suicide bomber) pierces the skin of a victim.[159] Management of injuries from bone projectiles depends on whether the bone belongs to the patient (autogeneic fragment) or from someone else (allogeneic fragment). Autogeneic bone penetration typically presents as an open fracture that is managed as any open fracture.

Penetration by allogeneic fragments, however, carries the risk of transmitting bloodborne diseases such as HIV or hepatitis B (discussed previously).[156] The latter are treated in a standard fashion, but personal protective equipment (PPE) must be worn, and the receiving facility must be notified.

Assessment and Management

Nerve Agents and Radioactive Material

Removal of shoes and clothing will reduce contamination by 90%, and particulate contaminants on the skin and hair can be washed off. Internal contaminants are not transmissible.[160] Antidotes are available for certain nerve agents (e.g., sarin gas).

Blister Agents

Treatment of casualties with blister agent exposure includes the following:

- Decontaminating affected areas
- Rinsing eyes
- Applying topical steroid creams and sprays
- Preventing secondary infection and pneumonia
- Administering analgesia

Choking Agents

Treatment may include the following:

- Decontaminating affected areas
- Rinsing eyes with normal saline or water for at least 3 minutes
- Monitoring hemoglobin oxygen saturation
- Administering oxygen as rapidly as possible
- If pulmonary edema is present, administering PEEP oxygen, diuretics, or bronchodilators[160]

Lessons for first responders from the 1995 release of sarin gas in the Tokyo subway system included the following:

- Wear PPE.
- Stand upwind and uphill of the toxic cloud.
- Communicate with victims remotely (e.g., via bullhorn) until the toxic agent is identified.
- Wait for the hazardous materials team.[161]

Until the agent has been identified, responders should treat exposed persons as their conditions (e.g., chemical burns, pulmonary edema, cardiorespiratory failure, neurologic damage, shock) dictate.[162]

Combination Injuries

> ... [T]he term multidimensional injury has been coined to describe the multiple sites and unusual complexity of injury from blasts (i.e., blunt and penetrating wounds from displaced objects or the body being displaced, primary blast lung or bowel disruption, burns from the thermal effects of the initial explosion fireball, combined effects of simultaneous chemical or radiologic contamination from dirty bombs) and the unusual level of severity of these injuries as a result of insult to multiple sites and to multiple organ systems.[42]

> These injury characteristics, which are not normally seen in routine trauma care, create difficult surgical challenges in triage decision making and treatment. ...[85]

Explosion-related injuries frequently occur in combinations of mechanisms and injury types/categories. Commonly seen penetrating combat injuries include soft-tissue fragment wounds, high-velocity penetration, blast injuries (mutilating or nonmutilating), and/or bilateral and multiple injuries that result from explosive devices, including IEDs. The cumulative effect of multiple injuries on mortality has been estimated at approximately 15% as each additional viscus is injured.[163] Devastating injuries to multiple areas of the body are characteristic of IED attacks. In two studies of military IED casualties, 13% to 51% had a combination of primary and secondary injuries.[168-168]

In several studies of terrorist bomb attacks, a majority of the victims had injuries that fell into more than one of these categories.[166-172]

> The hallmark of injuries after an SBA [suicide bombing attack] is the combination of blunt injury, multiple penetrating injuries with extensive soft tissue damage, and burns....[171,172,quoted in 174]

> The majority of victims of penetrating trauma sustain injuries to isolated parts of the body such as the head, chest, abdomen, or limbs. Blunt trauma is more commonly a multisite injury, the severity of which depends on the mechanism of injury. The injuries sustained by victims of suicide bombing attacks share the worst of both worlds. The multitude of heavy particles causes damage to a large surface area of the victim, much like blunt trauma. Each particle causes extensive tissue damage at the site of entry, much like penetrating trauma.... Survivors typically suffer a combination of wounds of varying severity and location, and the diagnostic work up is focused on determining the extent of damage caused by each missile.[173]

Another type of explosive that typically causes both primary and secondary injury is the land mine. The stress waves produced by the blast can propagate as far as the midthigh, with demyelination of nerves occurring 12 inches (30 centimeters [cm]) above the most proximal area of tissue injury. This effect, combined with fragments from the device, soil, and footwear, produces the classic land mine injury of complete tissue destruction distally, associated with traumatic amputation at the midfoot or distal tibia (**Figure 31-14**). Proximal to the variable level of amputation, there is complete stripping of tissue from the bony structures and separation of fascial

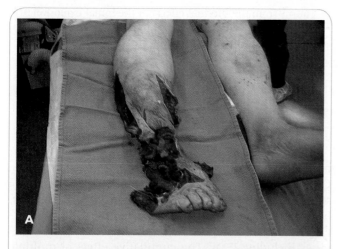

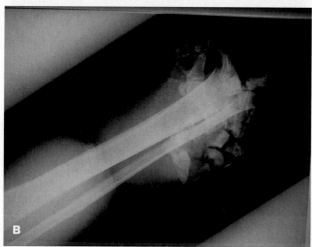

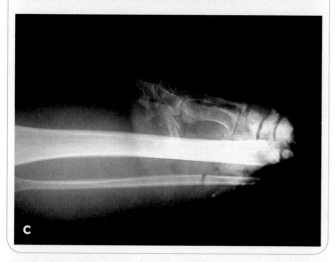

Figure 31-14 Classic pattern of land mine injury to lower leg, with radiographs.
Courtesy of H. R. Champion.

planes contaminated with soil, debris, microorganisms, and pieces of the device, footwear, and clothing.

Associated penetrating injury to the contralateral limb and perineum are common.[173] Land mine injuries

occur in three distinct patterns: (1) severe lower extremity, perineal, and genital injuries caused by contact with a buried mine; (2) less severe lower extremity injury, less traumatic amputation, and often head, thoracic, and abdominal injuries caused by a proximity-device explosion; and (3) severe head, face, and upper extremity injuries resulting from mine handling or clearing.[174]

Combined blast and penetrating injuries are almost always the most life threatening, and the basic principles of the ABCs should always be followed when dealing with multiple injuries.

Special Considerations

Personal Protection

Because of the initial symptom-free period after exposure to some toxic agents, it may not be possible to ascertain that chemical or biologic contamination has occurred. Thus, responders may inadvertently be exposed directly (e.g., in the case of choking agents such as phosgene) or via contact with patients.[158] Thus, in a bombing incident with suspected chemical or biologic agents, PPE should be worn that is commensurate with the suspected agent, degree of hazard, and individual role at the scene.[175]

Another protective measure that should be taken when responding to the scene of a bomb attack is to avoid, insofar as is possible, secondary bomb attacks that are often set to go off when first responders arrive at the scene.[176] Avoidance tactics include (1) not moving or handling any suspected item; (2) not operating radios, cell phones, or other electronic devices that may trigger a detonator; (3) being aware of the fact that explosives are often placed near flammable materials; and (4) staying alert for suspicious individuals.[23]

Casualties with retained, unexploded ordnance should be transported in the position found so as not to change the missile orientation; they always should be grounded to the airframe if evacuated by air. Such casualties should be isolated, and, in an MCI, they should be treated last because the removal of ordnance is time-consuming, and surgeons must attend to other casualties before placing themselves at risk. Closed-chest massage or defibrillation should never be attempted in these casualties, and during removal, any equipment emanating electrical energy, heat, vibrations, or sonic waves (e.g., electrocautery, ultrasound, blood warmers, power instruments) should not be used. These casualties should be placed in a protected area away from the main hospital, and all personnel in the immediate area should use body armor or explosive ordnance disposal (EOD) equipment. EOD personnel should be involved before removal to help identify the round and fuse. Furthermore, a plain radiograph helps in planning the

Box 31-3 Guidelines for Removal of Ordnance from Casualties

- Notify explosive ordnance disposal (EOD) team.
- Do not use cardiopulmonary resuscitation (CPR) or electric shock.
- Isolate casualty to protected area (sandbagged bunker).
- Ensure protective equipment is available for medical personnel.
- Do not use cautery, power equipment, or blood warmers.
- Avoid vibration, change in temperature, and change in missile orientation.
- Use plain radiography, not computed tomography (CT) or ultrasound.
- Perform only minimal anesthesia; anesthesia provider leaves after induction.
- Ensure surgeon and assistant (EOD) are only personnel present during removal.
- Remove ordnance without changing its orientation, and hand over to EOD.
- Move casualty to operating theater for definitive procedure.

operative removal and will not cause the round to explode. Anesthesia should be restricted to the minimum required and should be used in such a manner that the anesthesia provider need not be present during removal of the ordnance. The only personnel required during removal are the surgeon and an assistant, ideally EOD personnel. The round should be removed "en bloc" without touching the missile with metal instruments. Every effort should be employed to maintain the orientation of the missile until removed from the area by EOD. **Box 31-3** outlines the basic guidelines for removal of ordnance.[177]

Psychological Considerations

The vast majority of casualties, as well as health care personnel, typically sustain psychological damage as the result of their ordeal. Reactions range from acute stress reaction, to acute stress disorder, to PTSD. All casualties exhibiting decreased awareness, acute anxiety, dissociative symptoms (including a sense of time distortion), or other stress-related symptoms must be provided with screening for mild TBI and survivor counseling utilizing social work, chaplain, and psychiatric resources, as needed.

Evidence

Personnel who secure the scene of an explosion and manage casualties often need to realize that they are working within a crime scene from which evidence must be collected. Multidisciplinary rehearsals with security and medical care personnel should optimize the functions of both types of responders.

SUMMARY

- Explosive devices are the most common source of injury in both military and terrorist settings and can produce devastating casualties in small and large numbers.
- Mass-casualty explosion-related events, once the sole province of the battlefield hospital, now threaten the urban hospital, the civilian trauma surgeon, and health systems throughout the world.
- All medical providers need to bear the burden of preparing for influxes of overwhelming numbers of casualties with primary blast and penetrating wounds, as well as burns and crush injuries.
- It is important that prehospital care providers and medics (1) understand the nature of the explosive weapons that are being used to cause death and serious injuries with increasing frequency, (2) recognize the physiologic consequences of these weapons of war and terror, and (3) are prepared to provide care that will save lives and reduce morbidity.

SCENARIO RECAP

While on foot patrol on a rural road, one member of a five-member team triggers an IED. One casualty is dead, two have minor injuries, and one has sustained significant injuries to his lower torso and right lower extremity. You are the person providing medical care.

SCENARIO SOLUTION

- **What are the tactical considerations in this situation?**
  - Will an ambush or sniper fire follow?
  - Is there a second device?
  - Should the element set security and treat the casualty in place?
  - Where is the nearest effective cover? Is that cover safe?

  There is no immediate follow-on hostile fire. You and the other uninjured man use a two-man drag to move the seriously injured casualty to cover, stabilizing his neck as best you can. You pass by a derelict truck and elect to gather in a shallow depression behind a small mound of rocks and dirt. The uninjured man and the casualties with minor injuries set a perimeter, and you begin to treat the seriously wounded man.

- **Why did you bypass the derelict truck?**

  It was the most obvious cover, so it was also a likely place for a second IED.

- **What will you do initially for this casualty?**

  Identify and stop life-threatening bleeding. You quickly cut off the casualty's trousers. His right foot is missing, and his right lower leg is badly mangled. There are multiple large, bleeding wounds high on his right thigh, and there are several wounds in his perineum and right buttocks. You apply a Combat Ready Clamp to his right inguinal region, and that seems to control the severe bleeding from his thigh. He is breathing spontaneously, has a palpable radial pulse, and is unresponsive. The uninjured man is calling in for reinforcement and medical evacuation (MEDEVAC). Estimated time of arrival (ETA) is 20 minutes. You have taken no sniper fire so far.

- **Does the casualty need fluids?**

  You stopped the life-threatening bleeding, and his radial pulse is present, so his mental status decrement is probably due to TBI from blast injury. Intravenous (IV) fluid therapy is not indicated at this time, and it may make blast lung (if present) worse.

- **Do you need IV access?**

  Yes. Medications are warranted, and he may well need fluid resuscitation before you get him to the emergency department (ED). You cannot rule out internal bleeding from penetrating torso injury at this point, and you must be prepared to prevent hypotension in this casualty with a TBI. You place a sternal intraosseous (IO) device and attach an IV setup. The casualty's status is unchanged.

- **What next?**

  You administer tranexamic acid (TXA) 1 g in 100-ml normal saline (NS) IO followed by ertapenem 1 g IO.

- **With respect to blast as the source of the casualty's injuries, is his TBI a secondary or tertiary blast injury?**

  You carefully remove his helmet and examine his head. You find no indication of either penetrating or blunt trauma. His TBI is probably a PBI.

- **Should you be concerned about other PBIs?**

  Yes. The casualty is breathing normally at this time, his breath sounds are clear, and he is oxygenating well at 98%. Nevertheless, his respiratory status must be closely monitored throughout evacuation. You also find that both his tympanic membranes are ruptured.

- **Is C-spine immobilization indicated?**

  Yes. The casualty is breathing spontaneously, but you cannot test for sensation or mobility. Spinal cord injury cannot be ruled out, even though you believe his TBI to be primary (vs. secondary or tertiary) blast injury.

- **What else?**
  - Check for uncontrolled bleeding and other injuries.
  - Insert a nasopharyngeal airway (NPA).
  - Check his eyes, lids, and visible parts of his globes.
  - Check pulse oximetry.

SCENARIO SOLUTION (CONTINUED)

- Dress all known wounds.
- Check for burns.
- Keep the casualty warm.
- Continue to monitor closely.
- **What else would you do while waiting for MEDEVAC?**
  Document injuries, care rendered, and response to treatment on a Tactical Combat Casualty Care (TCCC) Casualty Card.

References

1. Lemonick DM. Bombings and blast injuries: a primer for physicians. *Am J Clin Med.* 2011;8(3):134-140.

2. Hall HR Jr. *Deaths due to unintentional injury from explosions.* National Fire Protection Association, Fire Analysis and Research Division. Quincy, MA: March 2008. Available from the NFPA Research Library: https://library.nfpa.org /GeniePLUS/GeniePLUS/Portal/Public.aspx?lang=en-US.

3. Eshel D. IED blast related brain injuries: the silent killer. *Defense Update.* http://www.defense-update.com/analysis /analysis_270507_blast.htm. Updated June 6, 2010. Accessed January 8, 2018.

4. Eastridge BJ, Hardin M, Cantrell J, et al. Died of wounds on the battlefield: causation and implications for improving combat casualty care. *J Trauma.* 2011;71(Suppl):S4-S8.

5. Statement by Lieutenant General Michael D. Barbero, Director, Joint Improvised Explosive Device Defeat Organization, United States Department of Defense before the United States Senate Committee on Foreign Relations Subcommittee on Near Eastern and South and Central Asian Affairs. December 13, 2012. https://www.jieddo.mil /content/docs/20121213_JIEDDO_SFR_S%20_Foreign _Relations_FINAL.pdf. Accessed January 9, 2018.

6. Livingston IS, O'Hanlon M, Brookings Institution. Afghanistan Index September 18, 2012. https://www.brookings .edu/wp-content/uploads/2016/07/index20120918.pdf. Accessed January 12, 2018.

7. Porter G. How the U.S. quietly lost the IED war in Afghanistan. *Inter Press Service.* October 9, 2012. http:// www.ipsnews.net/2012/10/how-the-u-s-quietly-lost -the-ied-war-in-afghanistan/. Accessed January 11, 2013.

8. National Counterterrorism Center. 2011 Report on Terrorism. http://www.nctc.gov/docs/2011_NCTC_Annual _Report_Final.pdf. Information available as of March 12, 2012. Accessed January 11, 2013.

9. Bureau of Alcohol, Tobacco, Firearms and Explosives: Fact sheet. U.S. Bomb Data Center. https://www.atf.gov /resource-center/fact-sheet/fact-sheet-us-bomb-data-center. Accessed September 22, 2017.

10. *Data from:* United States Bomb Data Center Explosives Incident Report. 2016. https://www.atf.gov/file/116371 /download.

11. United States Bomb Data Center (USBDC) Explosives Incident Report (EIR). https://www.atf.gov/explosives /docs/report/2016-explosives-incident-report/download. Accessed May 7, 2018.

12. Centers for Disease Control and Prevention. CDC Emergency preparedness and response: explosions and blast injuries: a primer for clinicians. https://www.cdc.gov/masstrauma /preparedness/primer.pdf. Accessed May 7, 2018.

13. Brevard SB, Champion H, Katz D. Weapons effects. In: Savitsky E, Eastridge B, eds *Combat Casualty Care: Lessons Learned From OEF and OIF.* Fort Detrick, MD: Borden Institute; 2012.

14. Explosives. Global Security.org. http://www.globalsecurity .org/military/systems/munitions/explosives.htm. Accessed May 7, 2018.

15. Explosives—Compositions. GlobalSecurity.org. http://www .globalsecurity.org/military/systems/munitions/explosives -compositions.htm. Accessed May 7, 2018.

16. Booster explosives. GlobalSecurity.org. http://www.global security.org/military/systems/munitions/explosives -booster.htm. Accessed May 7, 2018.

17. Explosives—Nitramines. GlobalSecurity.org. http://www .globalsecurity.org/military/systems/munitions/explosives -nitramines.htm. Accessed May 7, 2018.

18. Ostmark H, Wallin S, Pettersson A, Oser H. Real-time detection of IED explosives with laser ionization mass spectrometry. In: Schubert H, Rimski-Korsakov A. eds. *Stand-off Detection of Suicide Bombers and Mobile Subjects. NATO Security Through Science Series.* Dordrecht, Netherlands: Springer; 2006.

19. Wade AL, Dye JL, Mohrle CR, Galarneau MR. Head, face, and neck injuries during Operation Iraqi Freedom II: results from the U.S. Navy-Marine Corps Combat Trauma Registry. *J Trauma.* 2007;63:836-840.

20. Gondusky JS, Reiter MP. Protecting military convoys in Iraq: an examination of battle injuries sustained by a mechanized battalion during Operation Iraqi Freedom II. *Mil Med.* 2005;170:546-549.

21. Moyers R. Explosive violence: the problem of explosive weapons. International Network on Explosive Weapons website. http://www.inew.org/site/wp-content/uploads /2011/06/Explosive-violence.pdf. August 11, 2009. Accessed May 7, 2018.

22. Keller J. A COTS response to the IED threat. Military Aerospace and Electronics website. http://www.military aerospace.com/articles/print/volume-17/issue-11/depart ments/trends/a-cots-response-to-the-ied-threat.html. November 1, 2006. Accessed May 7, 2018.

23. Sullivan JP, Bunker RJ, Lorelli EJ, et al. *Jane's Unconventional Weapons Response Handbook*. Alexandria, VA: Jane's Information Group; 2002.

24. Horrocks CL. Blast injuries: biophysics, pathophysiology and management principles. *J R Army Med Corps*. 2001;147(1):28-40.

25. Murray SB, Anderson CJ, Zhang F, et al. Force protection against enhanced blast. Report No. DRDC-Suffield-SL-2006-174. Defense Research and Development Canada website. http://cradpdf.drdc-rddc.gc.ca/PDFS/unc53/p526381.pdf. January 1, 2006. Accessed May 7, 2018.

26. Bean JR. Enhanced blast weapons and forward medical treatment. *Army Med Dept J*. 2004;April–June:48-51. U.S. Army Academy of Health Sciences, Stimson Library website. http://cdm15290.contentdm.oclc.org/cdm/singleitem/collection/p15290coll3/id/179/rec/17. Accessed May 7, 2018.

27. Wilson J. Weapons of the insurgents. *Popular Mechanics*. 2004;(March):64-70. http://books.google.com/books?id=5NIDAAAAMBAJ&pg=PA64&lpg=PA64&dq=%22 weapons+of+the+insurgents%22+popular+mechanics +wilson&source=bl&ots=_C_nqK5nrx&sig=G2tOlvF8 ChJxByoJ0wYSfcWTktA&hl=en&sa=X&ei=XBT4UN 2FAaPy0wHA5IDgBA&sqi=2&ved=0CDAQ6AEwAA#v =onepage&q&f=false. Accessed May 7, 2018.

28. Phillips YY, Richmond DR. Primary blast injury and basic research: a brief history. In: Bellamy RF, Zajtchuk R, eds. *Conventional Warfare: Ballistic, Blast, and Burn Injuries*. Washington, DC: Office of the Surgeon General, Department of the Army; 1989:221-240.

29. Dugdale-Pointon T. Terrorist weapons: Bombs (IEDs). *Military History Encyclopedia on the Web* website. http://www.historyofwar.org/articles/weapons_terrorbomb.html. August 27, 2003. Accessed May 7, 2018.

30. Stuhmiller JH. Blast injury: translating research into operational medicine. In: Santee WR, Friedl KE, eds. *Military Quantitative Physiology: Problems and Concepts in Military Operational Medicine*. Washington, DC: Office of the Surgeon General, Department of the Army; 2008:267-302.

31. Murray W. IED detection/defeat. *Spec Ops Technol*. 2012;10(5):10-13. https://issuu.com/kmi_media_group/docs/sotech_10-5_final/20. Accessed May 7, 2018.

32. McEvers K. "Sticky IED" attacks increase in Iraq. *NPR News* website. http://www.npr.org/2010/12/03/131774133/Iraqi -Insurgents-Use-IEDs-To-Target-Iraqis. December 3, 2010. Accessed May 7, 2018.

33. Anderson J, Fainaru S, Finer J. Bigger, stronger homemade bombs now to blame for half of U.S. deaths. *Washington Post* website. http://www.washingtonpost.com/wp-dyn /content/article/2005/10/25/AR2005102501987.html. October 26, 2005. Accessed May7, 2018.

34. Neptune M, Quexada D. Analysis: Afghan IEDs have been somewhat different than those perfected in Iraq. United for Peace of Pierce County website. http://www.ufppc.org /us-a-world-news-mainmenu-35/9500-analysis-afghan -ieds-have-been-somewhat-different-than-those-perfected -in-iraq.html. March 31, 2010. Accessed May 7, 2018.

35. Improvised explosive devices (IEDs)/booby traps. Global Security website. http://www.globalsecurity.org/military /intro/ied.htm. Accessed May 7, 2018.

36. Wilson C. Improvised explosive devices in Iraq: effects and countermeasures. *CRS Report for Congress*. Congressional Research Service. Federation of American Scientists website. https://fas.org/sgp/crs/weapons/RS22330.pdf. November 23, 2005. Accessed May 7, 2018.

37. Bala M, Shussman N, Rivkind AI, et al. The pattern of thoracic trauma after suicide terrorist bombing attacks. *J Trauma*. 2010;69(5):1022-1029.

38. Improvised explosive devices (IEDs)—Iraq. Global Security website. http://www.globalsecurity.org/military/intro/ied -iraq.htm. Accessed May 7, 2018.

39. Harrisson SE, Kirkman E, Mahoney P. Lessons Learnt from Explosive Attacks. *J R Army Med Corps*. 2007;153(4):278-282.

40. Kluger Y. Bomb explosions in acts of terrorism—detonation, wound ballistics, triage, and medical concerns. *Isr Med Assoc J*. 2003;5(4):235-240.

41. Champion HR, Holcomb JB, Young LA, Wade CE. Injuries from explosions: physics, biophysics, pathology, and research focus needs. *J Trauma*. 2009;66(5):1468-1477.

42. Arnold JL, Tsai M-C, Halpern P, et al. Mass-casualty, terrorist bombings: epidemiological outcomes, resource utilization, and time course of emergency needs, Part I. *Prehosp Disaster Med*. 2003;18(3):220-234.

43. Stuhmiller JH, Phillips YY, Richmond DR. The physics and mechanism of primary blast injury. In: Bellamy RF, Jenkins DP, Zajtcjuk JT, et al., eds. *Conventional Warfare: Ballistic, Blast, and Burn Injuries*. Washington, DC: Office of the Surgeon General; 1991:241-250.

44. Briggs SM, Brinsfield KH. *Advanced Disaster Medical Response*. Boston, MA: Harvard Medical International Trauma & Disaster Institute; 2003.

45. Mallonee S, Shariat S, Stennies G, et al. Physical injuries and fatalities resulting from the Oklahoma City bombing. *JAMA*. 1996;276(5):382-387.

46. Prendergast J. Oklahoma City aftermath. *Civil Eng*. 1995; 65:40-45.

47. Thompson T, Brown S, Mallonee S, Sunshine D. Fatal and non-fatal injuries among U.S. Air Force personnel resulting from the terrorist bombing of the Khobar Towers. *J Trauma*. 2004;57(2):208-215.

48. Leibovici D, Gofrit ON, Stein M, et al. Blast injuries: bus versus open-air bombings: a comparative study of injuries in survivors of open-air versus confined-space explosions. *J Trauma*. 1996;41(6):1030-1035.

49. Halpern P, Tsai M-C, Arnold JL. Mass-casualty, terrorist bombings: implications for emergency department and hospital emergency response. Part II. *Prehosp Disaster Med*. 2003;18(3):235-241.

50. Occupational Safety and Health Administration. *Secondary Explosive Devices Guide*. OSHA website. https://www.osha .gov/SLTC/emergencypreparedness/guides/secondary.html. February 3, 2005. Accessed May 7, 2018.

51. National Counterterrorism Center. IED targeting of first response personnel: tactics and indicators. NCTC 2012-34a. Public Intelligence website. http://info.publicintelli

gence.net/NCTC-FirstResponderIEDs.pdf. August 7, 2012. Accessed May 7, 2018.

52. Primer to design safe school projects in case of terrorist attacks and school shootings. FEMA 428/BIPS-07/January 2012. U.S. Department of Homeland Security, Federal Emergency Management Agency: Buildings and Infrastructure Protection Series, p. 4-9, Department of Homeland Security website. http://www.dhs.gov/xlibrary/assets/st/bips07_428_schools.pdf. Accessed May 7, 2018.

53. Peleg K, Aharonson-Daniel L, Michael M, et al. Patterns of injury in hospitalized terrorist victims. *Am J Emerg Med.* 2003;21(4):258-262.

54. Bala M, Rivkind AI, Zamir G, et al. Abdominal trauma after terrorist bombing attacks exhibits a unique pattern of injury. *Ann Surg.* 2008;248(2):303-309.

55. Frykberg ER, Tepas III JJ. Terrorist bombings: lessons learned from Belfast to Beirut. *Ann Surg.* 1988;208(5):569-576.

56. Quenemoen LE, Davis YM, Malilay J, et al. The World Trade Center bombing: injury prevention strategies for high-rise building fires. *Disasters.* 1996;20(2):125-132.

57. Marshall TK. Injury by firearms, bombs, and explosives: explosion injuries. In: Tedeschi CG, Eckert WG, eds. *Forensic Medicine: A Study in Trauma and Environmental Hazards. Vol 1. Mechanical Trauma.* Philadelphia, PA: Saunders; 1977.

58. Kluger Y, Peleg K, Daniel-Aharonson L, et al. The special injury pattern in terrorist bombings. *J Am Coll Surg.* 2004;199(6):875-879.

59. Brethauer SA, Chao A, Chambers LW, et al. Invasion versus insurgency: U.S. Navy/Marine Corps forward surgical care during Operation Iraqi Freedom. *Arch Surg.* 2008;143(6):564-569.

60. Kelly JF, Ritenour AE, McLaughlin DF. Injury severity and causes of death from Operation Iraqi Freedom and Operation Enduring Freedom: 2003–2004 versus 2006. *J Trauma.* 2008;64(2)(Suppl):S21-S27.

61. Almogy G, Belzberg H, Mintz Y, et al. Suicide bombing attacks: update and modifications to the protocol. *Ann Surg.* 2004;239(3):295-303.

62. Aschkenasy-Steuer G, Shamir M, Rivkind A, et al. Clinical review: the Israeli experience: conventional terrorist and critical care. *Crit Care.* 2005;9(5):490-499.

63. Almogy G, Rivkind AI. Surgical lessons learned from suicide bombing attacks. *J Am Coll Surg.* 2006;202(2):313-319.

64. Wade CE, Ritenour AE, Eastridge BJ, et al. Explosion injuries treated at combat support hospitals in the Global War on Terrorism. In: Elsayed NM, Atkins JL, eds. *Explosion and Blast-Related Injuries: Effects of Explosion and Blast from Military Operations and Acts of Terrorism.* Burlington, MA: Elsevier Academic Press; 2008:41-72.

65. Almogy G, Mintz Y, Zamir G, et al. Suicide bombing attacks: can external signs predict internal injuries? *Ann Surg.* 2006;243(4):541-546.

66. Davis TE, Lee CY. Asymmetric war (terrorism) and the epidemiology of blast trauma. U.S. Department of Health & Human Services. Greater New York Hospital Association website. http://www.gnyha.org/65/File.aspx. November 3, 2005. Accessed January 29, 2013.

67. Dismounted Complex Blast Injury Task Force. Dismounted complex blast injury. https://armymedicine.health.mil/Reports. Accessed May 7, 2018.

68. Frykberg ER. Medical management of disasters and mass casualties from terrorist bombings: how can we cope? *J Trauma.* 2002;53(2):201-212.

69. Levi L, Michaelson M, Admi H, et al. National strategy for mass-casualty situations and its effects on the hospital. *Prehosp Disaster Med.* 2002;17(1):12-16.

70. Hamblin DL. Learning to treat terrorist attack victims. *Ortho Today Int.* 2008;11(3):16. Healio website. http://www.healio.com/orthopedics/trauma/news/print/orthopaedics-today-europe/%7B38fad9cb-3671-4fcf-8ec1-9d9c8a855ad7%7D/learning-to-treat-terrorist-attack-victims. Accessed May 7, 2018.

71. Hodgetts T, Smith J. Essential role of prehospital care in the optimal outcome from major trauma. *Emerg Med.* 2000;12(2):103-111.

72. Clarke JE, Davis PR. Medical evacuation and triage of combat casualties in Helmand Province, Afghanistan: October 2010–April 2011. *Mil Med.* 2012;177(11):1261-1266.

73. Department of Defense Directive 6025.21E: Medical research for prevention, mitigation, and treatment of blast injuries. Defense Executive Services Directorate website. http://www.esd.whs.mil/Portals/54/Documents/DD/issuances/dodd/602521p.pdf. July 5, 2006. Accessed May 7, 2018.

74. DePalma RG, Burris DG, Champion HR, Hodgson MJ. Blast injuries. *N Engl J Med.* 2005;352(13):1335-1342.

75. Beekley AC, Starnes BW, Sebesta JA. Lessons learned from modern military surgery. *Surg Clin N Am.* 2007;87(1):157-184.

76. Warden DL, French L. Traumatic brain injury in the war zone. *N Engl J Med.* 2005;353(6):633-634.

77. Stewart C. Blast injuries: preparing for the inevitable. *Emerg Med Prac.* EB Medicine website. April 2006. Accessed May 7, 2018.

78. Mines M, Thach A, Mallonee S, et al. Ocular injuries sustained by survivors of the Oklahoma City bombing. *Ophthalmology.* 2000;107(5):837-843.

79. Persaud R, Hajioff D, Wareing M, Chevretton E. Otological trauma resulting from the Soho nail bomb in London, April 1999. *Clin Otolaryngol Allied Sci.* 2003;28(3):203-206.

80. Gondusky JS, Reiter MP. Protecting military convoys in Iraq: an examination of battle injuries sustained by a mechanized battalion during Operation Iraqi Freedom II. *Mil Med.* 2005;170(6):546-549.

81. Katz E, Ofek B, Adler J, et al. Primary blast injury after a bomb explosion in a civilian bus. *Ann Surg.* 1989;209(4):484-488.

82. Avidan V, Hersch M, Armon Y, et al. Blast lung injury: clinical manifestations, treatment, and outcome. *Am J Surg.* 2005;190(6):926-931.

83. Ciraulo DL, Frykberg ER. The surgeon and acts of civilian terrorism. *J Am Coll Surg.* 2006;203(6):942-950.

84. Owen-Smith M. Bomb blast injuries: in an explosive situation. *Nurs Mirror.* 1979;149(13):35-39.

85. Cudahy E, Parvin S. The effects of underwater blast on divers. Naval Submarine Medical Research Laboratory. NSMRL Report 1218. Rubicon Foundation website. http://archive.rubicon-foundation.org/xmlui/bitstream/handle/123456789/7518/ADA404719.pdf?sequence=108 August 2, 2001. Accessed May 7, 2018.

86. Guy RJ, Glover MA, Cripps NP. The pathophysiology of primary blast injury and its implications for treatment. Part I. The thorax. *J R Nav Med Serv.* 1998;84(2):79-86.

87. Almogy G, Luria T, Richter E, et al. Can external signs of trauma guide management? Lessons learned from suicide bombing attacks in Israel. *Arch Surg.* 2005;240(4):390-393.

88. Guy RJ, Kirkman E, Watkins PE, Cooper GJ. Physiologic responses to primary blast. *J Trauma.* 45(6):983-987.

89. Ritenour AE, Wickley A, Ritenour JS, et al. Tympanic membrane perforation and hearing loss from blast overpressure in Operation Enduring Freedom and Operation Iraqi Freedom wounded. *J Trauma.* 2008;65(2 Suppl):S174-S178.

90. Mellor SG. The relationship of blast loading to death and injury from explosion. *World J Surg.* 1992;16(5):893-898.

91. Peters P. Primary blast injury: an intact tympanic membrane does not indicate the lack of a pulmonary blast injury. *Mil Med.* 2011;176(1):110-114.

92. Jensen JH, Bonding P. Experimental pressure induced rupture of the tympanic membrane in man. *Acta Otolaryngol.* 1993:113(1):62-67.

93. Kerr AG. Blast injury to the ear: a review. *Rev Environ Health.* 1987;7(1-2):65-79.

94. Kerr AG, Byrne JE. Concussive effects of bomb blast on the ear. *J Laryngol Otol.* 1975;89(2):131-143.

95. Stein M, Hirshberg A. Medical consequences of terrorism: the conventional weapon threat. *Surg Clin North Am.* 1999;79(6):1537-1552.

96. Bass C, Rafaels KA, Salzar RS. Pulmonary injury risk assessment for short-duration blasts. *J Trauma.* 2008; 65(3):604-615.

97. Mellor SG, Cooper GJ. Analysis of 828 servicemen killed or injured by explosion in Northern Ireland 1970-84: the Hostile Action Casualty System. *Br J Surg.* 1989;76(10):1006-1010.

98. Cooper GJ. Protection of the lung from blast overpressure by thoracic stress wave decouplers. *J Trauma.* 1996;40(3)(Suppl):105S-110S.

99. Caseby NG, Porter MF. Blast injury to the lungs: clinical presentation, management and course. *Injury.* 1976;8(1):1-12.

100. Leibovici D, Gofrit ON, Shapira SC. Eardrum perforation in explosion survivors: is it a marker of pulmonary blast injury? *Ann Emerg Med.* 1999;34(2):168-172.

101. Coppel DL. Blast injuries of the lungs. *Br J Surg.* 1976;63(10):735-737.

102. Pennardt A. Blast injuries clinical presentation. Medscape website. https://emedicine.medscape.com/article/822587-clinical#b4. February 14, 2016. Accessed May 7, 2018.

103. Cohn SM. Pulmonary contusion: review of the clinical entity. *J Trauma.* 1997;42(5):973-979.

104. Arnold L, Halperin P, Tsai MC, Smithline H. Mass-casualty terrorist bombings: a comparison of outcomes by bombing type. *Ann Emerg Med.* 2004;43(2):263-273.

105. Oppenheim A, Pizov R, Pikarsky A, et al. Tension pneumoperitoneum after blast injury: dramatic improvement in ventilatory and hemodynamic parameters after surgical decompression. *J Trauma.* 1998;44(5):915-917.

106. Johnson DL, Yelverton JT, Hicks W, Doyal R. Blast overpressure studies with animal and man: non-auditory damage risk assessment for simulated weapons fired from an enclosure. http://www.dtic.mil/dtic/tr/fulltext/u2/a280435.pdf. Accessed May 14, 2013.

107. Stuhmiller LM, Ho KH, Stuhmiller JH. Health hazards assessment for blast overpressure exposures. Defense Technical Information Center website. http://www.dtic.mil/cgi-bin/GetTRDoc?AD=ADA303649. Accessed May 14, 2013.

108. Paran H, Neufeld D, Shwartz I, et al. Perforation of the terminal ileum induced by blast injury: delayed diagnosis or delayed perforation? *J Trauma.* 1996;40(3):472-475.

109. Harmon JW, Haluszka M. Care of blast-injured casualties with gastrointestinal injuries. *Mil Med.* 1983; 148(7):586-588.

110. Cripps NP, Cooper GJ. Risk of late perforation in intestinal contusions caused by explosive blast. *Br J Surg.* 1997;84(9):1298-1303.

111. Blast related injuries. *FMST Student Manual—2008 Web Edition.* United States Marine Corps Field Medical Training Battalion, Camp Lejeune. Operational Medicine website. http://www.operationalmedicine.org/TextbookFiles/FMST_20008/FMST_1424.htm. Accessed May 7, 2018.

112. Owers C, Morgan JL, Garner JP. Abdominal trauma in primary blast injury. *Br J Surg.* 2011;98(2):168-179.

113. Stannard A, Brown K, Benson C, et al. Outcome after vascular trauma in a deployed military trauma system. *Br J Surg.* 2011;98(2):228-234.

114. Huller T, Bazini Y. Blast injuries of the chest and abdomen. *Arch Surg.* 1970;100(1):24-30.

115. Rossle R. Pathology of blast effects. In: *German Aviation Medicine in World War II.* Vol. 2. Washington, DC: U.S. Government Printing Office; 1950:1260-1273.

116. Kocsis JD, Tessler A. Pathology of blast-related brain injury. *J Rehab Res Dev.* 2009;46(6):667-672.

117. Trudeau DL, Anderson J, Hansen LM, et al. Findings of mild traumatic brain injury in combat veterans with PTSD and a history of blast concussion. *J Neuropsychiatry Clin Neurosci.* 1998;10(3):308-313.

118. Moore B. Blast injuries: a prehospital perspective. *J Emerg Prim Health Care.* 2006;4(1):1-13. https://ajp.paramedics.org/index.php/ajp/article/view/359/359. Accessed May 29, 2018.

119. Ruff RL, Riechers 2nd RG, Wang XF, et al. A case-control study examining whether neurological deficits and PTSD in combat veterans are related to episodes of mild TBI. *BMJ Open.* 2012;2(2):e000312.

120. Taber KH, Warden DL, Hurley RA. Blast-related traumatic brain injury: what is known? *J Neuropsychiatry Clin Neurosci.* 2006;18(2):141-145.

121. Rutland-Brown W, Langlois JA, Nicaj L, et al. Traumatic brain injuries after mass-casualty incidents: lessons from the 11 September 2001 World Trade Center attacks. *Prehosp Disast Med.* 2007;22(3):157-164.

122. Xydakis MS, Ling GS, Mulligan LP, et al. Epidemiologic aspects of traumatic brain injury in acute combat casualties at a major military medical center: a cohort study. *Ann Neurol.* 2012;72(5):673-681.

123. Mott FW. The effects of high explosives upon the central nervous system. *Lancet.* 1916;1:441-449.

124. Fabing HD. Cerebral blast syndrome in combat soldiers. *Arch Neurol Psychiatry.* 1947;57(1):14-57.

125. Cramer F, Paster S, Stephenson C. Cerebral injuries due to explosion waves, cerebral blast concussion; a pathological,

clinical and electroencephalographic study. *Arch Neurol Psychiatry.* 1949;61(1):1-20.

126. Macleod AD. Shell shock, Gordon Holmes and the Great War. *J R Soc Med.* 2004;97(2):86-89.

127. Cernak I, Savic J, Malicevic Z, et al. Involvement of the central nervous system in the general response to pulmonary blast injury. *J Trauma.* 1996;40(3 Suppl):S100-S104.

128. Cernak I, Wang Z, Jiang J, et al. Ultrastructural and functional characteristics of blast injury-induced neurotrauma. *J Trauma* 2001;50(4):695-706.

129. Cernak I, Wang Z, Jiang J, et al. Cognitive deficits following blast injury-induced neurotrauma: possible involvement of nitric oxide. *Brain Inj.* 2001;15(7):593-612.

130. Weinberger S. Bombs' hidden impact: the brain war. *Nature.* 2011;477:390-393. http://www.nature.com/news/2011/110920/full/477390a.html. September 21, 2011. Accessed May 7, 2018.

131. Military Acute Concussion Evaluation (MACE) Pocket Cards. Defense and Veterans Brain Injury Center website. http://www.dvbic.org/material/military-acute-concussion-evaluation-mace-pocket-cards. Accessed May 7, 2018.

132. Armonda RA, Bell RS, Vo AH, et al. Wartime traumatic cerebral vasospasm: recent review of combat casualties. *Neurosurgery.* 2006;59(6):1215-1225.

133. DoD standard surveillance case definition for TBI adapted for AFHSB use. Military Health System website. https://health.mil/Military-Health-Topics/Health-Readiness/Armed-Forces-Health-Surveillance-Branch/Epidemiology-and-Analysis/Surveillance-Case-Definitions. Accessed May 31, 2018.

134. DoD worldwide TBI numbers. Defense and Veterans Brain Injury Center website. https://dvbic.dcoe.mil/files/tbi-numbers/worldwide-totals-2000-2017_feb-14-2018_v1.0_2018-03-08.pdf. Updated February 14, 2018. Accessed May 7, 2018.

135. Hadden WA, Rutherford WH, Merrett JD. The injuries of terrorist bombing: a study of 1532 consecutive patients. *Br J Surg.* 1978;65(8):525-531.

136. Patel H, Dryden S, Gupta A, Ang SC. Pattern and mechanism of traumatic limb amputations after explosive blast: experience from the 07/07/05 London terrorist bombings. *J Trauma.* 2012;73(1):276-281.

137. Hull JB, Cooper GJ. Pattern and mechanism of traumatic amputation by explosive blast. *J Trauma.* 1996;40(3 Suppl):S198-S205.

138. Abarbanell NR. Prehospital midthigh trauma and traction splint use: recommendations for treatment protocols. *Am J Emerg Med.* 2001;19(2):137-140.

139. Wood SP, Vrahas M, Wedel SK. Femur fracture immobilization with traction splints in multisystem trauma patients. *Prehosp Emerg Care.* 2003;7(2):241-243.

140. Hill PF, Edwards DP, Bowyer GW. Small fragment wounds: biophysics, pathophysiology and principles of management. *J R Army Med Corps.* 2001;147(1):41-51.

141. Rapid assessment of injuries among survivors of the terrorist attack on the World Trade Center—New York City, September 11, 2001. *MMWR.* 2002;51(1):1-5. http://www.cdc.gov/mmwr/preview/mmwrhtml/mm5101a1.htm. Accessed June 1, 2018.

142. Dalinchuk MM, Lalzoi MN. [Eye injuries in explosive mine wounds.] [Article in Russian]. *Voen Med Zh.* 1989;8:28-30.

143. Bittenbender C. Compartment syndrome versus crush syndrome: the difference between each and their respective prehospital treatments. Presented at: National Collegiate EMS Foundation 10th Annual Conference, February 21–23, 2003; Arlington, VA. http://www.ncemsf.org/about/conf2003/lectures/bittenbender_crush.pdf. Accessed June 1, 2018.

144. Zoroya G. Spinal injuries up among troops. *USA Today.* November 4, 2009. http://usatoday30.usatoday.com/news/world/2009-11-03-afghanistan-ieds_N.htm. Accessed June 1, 2018.

145. Kauchak M. Land mines and IEDs are dangerous for the damage they cause with fragmentation but the more critical element is the ability to mitigate the energy transfer of the blast to the seat occupant. *Spec Ops Technol.* 2008;6(8).

146. Brumback RJ. Traumatic rupture of the superior gluteal artery, without fracture of the pelvis, causing compartment syndrome of the buttock: a case report. *J Bone Joint Surg Am.* 1990;72(1):134-137.

147. Su WT, Stone DH, Lamparello PJ, Rockman CB. Gluteal compartment syndrome following elective unilateral iliac artery embolization. *J Vasc Surg.* 2004;39(3):672-675.

148. O'Mara MS, Semins H, Hathaway D, Caushaj PF. Abdominal compartment syndrome as a consequence of rectus sheath hematoma. *Am Surg.* 2003;69(11):975-977.

149. Abassi ZA, Hoffman A, Better OS. Acute renal failure complicating muscle crush injury. *Semin Nephrol.* 1998;18(5):558-565.

150. Kauvar DS, Wolf SE, Wade CE, et al. Burns sustained in combat explosions in Operations Iraqi and Enduring Freedom (OIF/OEF explosion burns). *Burns.* 2006;32(7):853-857.

151. Aharonson-Daniel L, Klein Y, Peleg K. Suicide bombers form a new injury profile. *Ann Surg.* 2006;244(6):1018-1023.

152. Liebner ED, Weil Y, Gross E, et al. A broken bone without a fracture: traumatic foreign bone implantation resulting from a mass-casualty bombing. *J Trauma.* 2005;58(2):388-390.

153. Braverman I, Wexler D, Oren M. A novel mode of infection with hepatitis B: penetrating bone fragments due to the explosion of a suicide bomber. *Isr Med J.* 2002;4(7):528-529.

154. Wong JM, Marsh D, Abu-Sitta G, et al. Biological foreign body implantation in victims of the London July 7th suicide bombings. *J Trauma.* 2006;60(2):402-404.

155. Hanson D. Car bomb response. Cover report: disaster preparedness/terrorism response. EMS World website. http://www.emsworld.com/article/10324195/car-bomb-response. February 1, 2005. Accessed June 1, 2018.

156. Types of chemical weapons. Federation of American Scientists website. https://fas.org/programs/bio/chemweapons/cwagents.html. September 9, 2013. Accessed June 1, 2018.

157. Chemical and biological attacks, detection, and response FAQ. KI4U.Inc.website.http://www.ki4u.com/chemical_biological_attack_detection_response.htm. Updated January 1, 2011. Accessed June 1, 2018.

158. Philips GW, Nagel DJ, Coffey T. A primer on the detection of nuclear and radiological weapons. Defense Technical Information Center website. http://www.dtic.mil/dtic/tr/fulltext/u2/a436197.pdf. May 2005. Accessed June 1, 2018.

159. Singer P, Cohen J, Stein M. Conventional terrorism and critical care. *Crit Care Med.* 2005;33(1 Suppl):S61-S65.

160. Love JS, Dickinson ET. A review of chemical warfare agents and treatment options. http://www.jems.com /articles/print/volume-42/issue-9/features/a-review-of -chemical-warfare-agents-and-treatment-options.html ?c=1. September 1, 2017. Accessed June 1, 2018.

161. Committee on Confronting Terrorism in Russia. *High-Impact Terrorism: Proceedings of a Russian-American Workshop,* Washington, DC: National Academies Press; 2002.

162. Centers for Disease Control and Prevention, Strategic Planning Workgroup. Chemical and biological terrorism: strategic plan for preparedness and response. *MMWR.* 2000;49:1-14.

163. Wolff LH, Giddings WP, Childs SB, et al. Time lag and the multiplicity factor in abdominal injuries. In: DeBakey ME, ed. *Surgery in World War II, Vol. 2, General Surgery.* Washington, DC: Office of the Surgeon General, Department of the Army; 1955:103-117.

164. Cernak I, Savic J, Ignjatovic D, Miodrag J, Jevtic M. Blast injury from explosive munitions. *J Trauma.* 1999;47(1):96-103.

165. Chambers LW, Green DJ, Gillingham BL, et al. The experience of the U.S. Marine Corps' surgical shock trauma platoon with 417 operative combat casualties during a 12 month period of Operation Iraqi Freedom. *J Trauma.* 2006;60(6):1155-1164.

166. Chambers LW, Rhee P, Baker BC, et al. Initial experience of U.S. Marine Corps forward resuscitative surgical system during Operation Iraqi Freedom. *Arch Surg.* 2005;140(1):26-32.

167. Ad-El DD, Eldad A, Mintz Y, et al. Suicide bombing injuries: the Jerusalem experience of exceptional tissue damage posing a new challenge for the reconstructive surgeon. *Plast Reconstr Surg.* 2006;118(2):383-387.

168. Aharonson-Daniel L, Waisman Y, Dannon YL, Peleg K. Epidemiology of terror-related versus non-terror-related traumatic injury in children. *Pediatrics.* 2003;112(4): e280-e284.

169. Almogy G, Rivkind AI. Surgical lessons learned from suicide bombing attacks. *J Am Coll Surg.* 2006;202(2):313-319.

170. Bala M, Wilner D, Keidar A, et al. Indicators of the need for ICU admission following suicide bombing attacks. *Scand J Trauma Resusc Emerg Med.* 2012;20:19-24.

171. Almogy G, Belzberg H, Mintz Y, et al. Suicide bombing attacks: update and modifications to the protocol. *Ann Surg.* 2004;239(3):295-303.

172. Aschkenasy-Steuer G, Shamir M, Rivkind A, et al. Clinical review: The the Israeli experience: conventional terrorism and critical care. *Crit Care.* 2005;9(5):490-499.

173. Trimble K, Clasper J. Antipersonnel mine injury: mechanism and medical management. *J R Army Med Corps.* 2001;147(1):73-79.

174. Coupland RM, Korver A. Injuries from antipersonnel mines: the experience of the International Committee of the Red Cross. *BMJ.* 1991;303(6816):1509-1512.

175. Cox RD. Hazmat: personal protective equipment. Medscape website. https://emedicine.medscape.com/article/764812 -overview#a4. Updated August 14, 2015. Accessed June 1, 2018.

176. Erich J. Extreme EMS: training for terrorism response. *Emerg Med Serv.* 2003;32(3):60-62.

177. Lein B, Holcomb J, Brill S, et al. Removal of unexploded ordnance from patients: a 50-year military experience and current recommendations. *Mil Med.* 1999;164(3):163-165.

Treatment of Burn Casualties in Tactical Combat Casualty Care

Authors:

Col. Jennifer Gurney
Col. Booker King
Dr. John Graybill

Dr. Wylan Peterson
Col. Kevin Chung
Dr. Jonathan Lundy

Col. (Ret) Evan Renz, MD
Col. (Ret) Lee Cancio

CHAPTER OBJECTIVES

At the completion of this chapter, you will be able to do the following:

- Describe the Rule of Nines for estimation of burn size.
- Describe the modern classification system for burn depth.
- Understand the difference in clinical significance of partial- and full-thickness burns.
- Use the U.S. Army Institute of Surgical Research Rule of Tens to calculate the initial fluid resuscitation rate for an adult burn victim.
- Discuss the prehospital management of severe burn injuries.

SCENARIO

You are a medic assigned to an infantry platoon. Your unit is on a patrol in eastern Afghanistan when an improvised explosive device (IED) detonates underneath your vehicle, causing it to catch on fire. Three soldiers are injured in this incident. After the area is secured you begin to assess the casualties.

Soldier 1 is a 21-year-old male who is alert, following commands, and walking around. He has sustained burns to his whole face, the lower half of both arms, the lower part of both legs except for his feet. He has no other visible injuries. His radial pulse is 110 beats/min and strong, and his respiratory rate is 18 breaths/min. He weighs 154 pounds (lb; 70 kilograms [kg]).

Soldier 2 is a 27-year-old platoon sergeant who is confused and disoriented. His left foot is severely mangled and bleeding badly. He has burns to his lower right arm, left hand, and left lower leg. His radial pulse is strong at 135 beats/min, and he is breathing fast. He weighs 165 lb (75 kg).

Soldier 3 is 20 years old. He has partial traumatic amputations of both legs below the knees and is losing a lot of blood. He is completely unresponsive. There are burns to his face, both arms, both legs, and the lower third of his anterior and posterior torso. His radial pulses are not palpable, but he is breathing spontaneously, although slowly. He weighs 198 lb (90 kg).

- What is the triage category for each of these casualties?
- What is the initial management of each casualty?
- What is the extent of burn for each casualty (percentage of total body surface area [%TBSA])?
- Calculate the initial fluid resuscitation and describe how you will monitor the effectiveness of the resuscitation.

INTRODUCTION

Burn wounds are present in 5% to 15% of combat casualties. Burn patients are clinically challenging to manage even in the best of circumstances; management of burn patients during combat and deployment missions involves many additional challenges and considerations. Prehospital medical personnel not only must adapt to the combat environment but also must ensure casualties receive the best care from point of injury until they arrive at their final destination. During recent conflicts, U.S. armed forces have devised a global evacuation system that is unparalleled in the history of combat medicine. It has the capability to transport patients from the battlefield to the continental U.S. (CONUS) in as little as 48 hours, delivering high-quality medical care throughout the evacuation chain. The U.S. Army Institute of Surgical Research (USAISR) Burn Flight Team is a critical care air transport capability that evacuates burn casualties to the burn center in San Antonio. The burn flight team conducted over 90 burn casualty transports during Operation Iraqi Freedom and Operation Enduring Freedom. Significant advances have been made in the care of burn casualties since the start of these conflicts. Lessons learned during these conflicts have been analyzed, and improvements have been implemented in real time. The predeployment training that is provided to combat medics, nurses, physicians, and other medical personnel is essential to ensuring that they are equipped to deliver the best care to wounded warriors. A comprehensive guideline for burn care is available in the Joint Trauma System Clinical Practice Guideline for Burn Care at: www.usaisr.amedd.army.mil/cpgs.html.

Initial Assessment

Care Under Fire

The Tactical Combat Casualty Care (TCCC) guidelines state that, even when the unit is under hostile fire, it is imperative that casualties be extricated from burning vehicles or buildings and moved to places of relative safety. Whatever is necessary to stop the burning process should be accomplished immediately.

Tactical Field Care

A prehospital provider evaluating a thermally injured casualty should make sure he or she does not also become a casualty as a result of entering an environment that is unsafe. For example, the provider should don proper protective equipment before entering a chemically contaminated environment, ensure that the power is shut off before touching the casualty if the injury is electrical, and should approach any fire with extreme caution.

Prehospital assessment of the thermally injured casualty is similar to that of any injured patient. The acronym MARCH, which stands for Massive hemorrhage, Airway, Respiration, Circulation, and Hypothermia prevention, is appropriate for burn patients. A combination of burn and nonburn injuries must be considered in combat casualties. Examples include blast and burn injury in explosions, blunt injury and burns in motor vehicle collisions with fires or falls/jumping from burning structures, and patients injured by falling debris in a burning structure. The combination of burn and nonburn injuries results in a synergistic increase in mortality.[1] Even though burn injuries increase the mortality of other injuries, burn wounds are rarely immediately life threatening.

Massive Hemorrhage

During the initial assessment, it is important to remember that even though burn wounds can be dramatic and distracting, they are unlikely to result in immediate death, so initial focus must be on controlling life-threatening external hemorrhage.

Airway

The casualty should be quickly assessed for the need for intubation. This is especially important in patients with findings suggestive of inhalation injury. Risks for inhalation injury include thermal injury in an enclosed space such as a vehicle, a building, or a burning compartment in a ship at sea. Clinical findings suggestive of inhalation injury include facial burns, carbonaceous sputum, stridor, hoarseness, or cough. Direct thermal injury to the face or to a large total body surface area (TBSA) burn resulting in generalized edema, can make intubation extremely challenging. Burn casualties may also require intubation due to decreased mental status, which may be caused by low oxygen levels in the fire environment, inhalation of toxic gases (see later), head injury, or hypovolemic shock. Securing the endotracheal tube in casualties with facial burns is critical to prevent catastrophic airway loss, because adhesive tape does not stick to the skin in a burned casualty... *not even to normal skin.* Therefore, cotton ties (umbilical tape), or other devices for securing the tube all the way around the head and neck, are required. Some burn casualties are at increased risk of cervical spine injury. These include casualties who have sustained motor vehicle collisions, falls, high-voltage electric injuries, or blast injury. In these casualties, cervical spine stabilization is important.

Respiration

Assessment of bilateral breath sounds and pulse oximetry (hemoglobin oxygen saturation, or SpO_2) follows airway evaluation. Processes in combat casualties that may compromise breathing include: hemothorax, pneumothorax, rib fractures, open pneumothorax, tracheal injury, and pulmonary contusion. The presence of an inhalation injury may cause delayed respiratory failure that can occur 15 to 60 minutes after the injury. Burning compounds can release a variety of chemicals. Fires involving wood, charcoal, natural gas, petroleum, or similar compounds release carbon monoxide (CO). CO impairs the ability of hemoglobin to carry oxygen and can cause symptoms of decreased oxygenation ranging from nausea and headache to myocardial infarction, mental status changes, and death. It binds powerfully with hemoglobin, turning the blood bright red and producing misleading (i.e., not low) Spo_2 readings. Therefore, all burn patients should receive 100% oxygen until a measurement of the carboxyhemoglobin level and arterial oxygen partial pressure can be obtained in the emergency department.

Fires involving materials like plastics and foam may release cyanide (CN). CN gas is also a chemical warfare agent. CN compromises the cells' ability to use oxygen. No rapid test exists for diagnosis of CN poisoning. Signs include loss of consciousness, hypotension, lactic acidosis, and cardiopulmonary arrest. CN poisoning is treated with intravenous (IV) hydroxocobalamin (e.g., Cyanokit®), a form of high-dose vitamin B_{12}; any burn casualty that is unconscious from a burn injury in an enclosed space should receive a Cyanokit.

Full-thickness burns across the chest can impair breathing by inhibition of chest wall motion, creating a straightjacket-like effect. These patients will be difficult to ventilate using a bag-mask device due to chest wall restriction and may suffer cardiopulmonary arrest. In this situation, immediate chest escharotomy (by a qualified provider) is required to create room for the chest to expand.

Circulation

In combat trauma, bleeding from nonburn injuries may occur in combination with burns. In a burn casualty with hemorrhage, bleeding control takes priority. The source of the hemorrhage should be identified and controlled with direct pressure, tourniquets, hemostatic adjuncts (such as Combat Gauze or X-Stat), and/or junctional hemorrhage control devices (as described in previous chapters). Peripheral IV catheters should be placed to initiate blood and/or fluid resuscitation. Placing an IV line through unburned skin is preferable; placing it through burned skin is acceptable, if necessary. An intraosseous (IO) device may be placed if IV access cannot be obtained. All lines should be secured with tape, gauze, Coban™, or preferably suture to prevent inadvertent removal during transport and because tape does not stick to burn patients. Patients with deep, circumferential burns of an extremity can lose blood flow as swelling develops secondary to the burn wound and resuscitation. Monitor pulses in these extremities and elevate them as much as possible on pillows or blankets to slow the swelling process. Loss of pulses may indicate severe shock (requiring immediate blood and/or fluid resuscitation) or may be the result of a tourniquet-like effect of the circumferential burns (requiring rapid transport to a medical treatment facility [MTF] for escharotomy).

Hypothermia Prevention

During transport, hypothermia should be prevented by wrapping burn wounds in dry gauze and placing the casualty in a Heat Reflective Shell™ after the primary survey is complete. Vehicles or aircraft used for evacuation should be warmed during transport, if possible.

Additional Burn Assessments and Interventions

Any burning material, such as clothing, should be immediately removed. Dry chemicals should be brushed off; all chemically injured areas should undergo copious decontamination with water. This is particularly critical for casualties with acid or alkali exposure to the eyes which can require up to10 liters of irrigation to normalize ocular pH and prevent permanent damage. All burned areas should be exposed. Jewelry should be removed from all fingers because of the risk of swelling. There may be a role for immediate cooling of thermal burns with cold water in order to cease the burning process; however, this must be limited in duration (3–5 minutes) and extent, because burn victims are at high risk of hypothermia secondary to loss of thermoregulation.

A brief assessment of the casualty for any gross neurologic deficits should be carried out. A decreased level of consciousness (LOC) is abnormal even after a large burn, unless there is something else wrong with the casualty. Decreased LOC in burn victims is commonly associated with asphyxiation, CN exposure, CO exposure, or traumatic brain injury (TBI). Asphyxiation can occur in the fire environment as oxygen levels drop and carbon dioxide levels rise. Alternatively, casualties may inhale toxic gases; i.e., CO or CN (see previous). Burn victims should also be evaluated for motor deficits consistent with spinal cord injury. Casualties suffering high-voltage electrical injuries can be thrown from the power source and may sustain concomitant spinal trauma or direct electrical injury to the spinal cord resulting in paralysis; paralysis in electrical injury patients can be asymmetric and not necessarily be associated with a "spinal level."

After the primary survey is performed, reassessment of each portion of the MARCH algorithm should be repeated as deemed necessary. Caring for casualties suffering thermal and other traumas is a dynamic process, and they can deteriorate rapidly, especially from airway compromise.

The secondary survey is performed by examining the casualty from head to toe. A history of the events surrounding the injury should be obtained from the casualty and any witnesses whenever possible. The casualty's medical history, medications, allergies, last meal, and any other pertinent information should also be sought. Fluid resuscitation will be discussed later and should be begun as soon as IV/IO access is established. When available, analgesia following TCCC guidelines should be administered to treat the significant pain that can accompany burn wounds.

Physical Characteristics of the Burn Wound

The skin is the largest organ system in the human body. It is composed of two layers: the epidermis and the dermis. The thickness of the skin varies from region to region of the body, with the skin being thinnest at the eyelids and thickest on the soles of the feet. Skin thickness also varies based on age and gender.[2] The skin protects the body against fluid and electrolyte loss, infection, and radiant energy. It allows humans to maintain a constant interior temperature in response to changes in the environment and activity. These vital functions are impaired by burns.

Types of Burns

Thermal Burns

Mechanisms of burn injury that can be seen on the battlefield include thermal, chemical, and electrical. Thermal injury is the by far the most common and involves direct damage to skin and underlying structures by heat or flame.[3] Injury can result from contact with open flames, scalds from hot liquids, blast from explosive or incendiary devices, or direct contact with a heated object causing coagulation necrosis of the skin. Factors that affect the depth of a burn include the temperature of the heat source, duration of exposure, the age of the patient, and the location of the burn (variations in skin thickness throughout the body can alter the depth of the injury).

Chemical Burns

Chemical burns are caused by exposure to alkalis (bases), acids, petroleum products, or chemical munitions.[4] Chemical burns can be lethal when systemic absorption occurs, or a large area of skin is exposed. The severity of the injury is dependent upon the concentration of the chemical, the type of chemical, and the duration of the exposure.[5] The final extent of tissue damage from a chemical burn is extremely difficult to assess immediately after exposure because absorption of a chemical deposited on the skin may continue to cause tissue damage for hours. The key to chemical injury treatment is rapid and thorough decontamination with copious irrigation.

Most chemical compounds are removed by wiping off any dry material and irrigating the exposed areas with water. Hydrofluoric acid, commonly used in oil refining, glass manufacturing, and industrial cleaning agents, binds serum calcium and can lead to life-threatening hypocalcemia and tetany. In addition to irrigation with water, areas burned by hydrofluoric acid should be covered with 2.5% calcium gluconate gel (mix calcium gluconate with a lubricant like Surgilube). White phosphorus is an incendiary agent used in some munitions. It is also found in fertilizers, pesticides, and fireworks. Above 86°F (30°C), white phosphorus ignites spontaneously when in contact with air, producing a yellow flame and white smoke in the wound bed. To prevent spontaneous ignition, the wound should be immediately immersed in water or saline, and then placed in water- or saline-soaked dressings. Furthermore, phosphate may be absorbed into the body. Phosphate binds with calcium, causing potentially life-threatening reduction in the level of calcium in the blood (hypocalcemia) and/or hyperphosphatemia as early as 1 hour after a burn injury. The electrocardiogram and calcium levels should be monitored to prevent life-threatening arrythmias.[4]

Electrical Injury

Electrical injury is classified as low voltage or high voltage. Low-voltage injuries result from exposure to power sources less than 1,000 volts (V). Most wall sockets and residential electrical wiring are low voltage; they are 220 V or less, depending on the country. Low-voltage electrical injuries may cause arrhythmias in addition to burns. High-voltage power sources are greater than 1,000 V. High-tension wires are common high-voltage sources. High-voltage electrical injuries may result in occult injuries in addition to burns. For example, muscle can be severely damaged or even dead with minimal to no changes on the skin. Muscle breakdown can lead to rhabdomyolysis, kidney failure, and arrhythmias. It should be suspected in the presence of low urine output or tea-colored urine, even if red blood cells are absent on microscopic exam. Aggressive fluid resuscitation is the treatment for rhabdomyolysis. High-voltage sources also tend to project a casualty away from the power source, causing blunt trauma that may include fractures of any portion of the spine. Any victim of high-voltage injury should be evaluated for blunt trauma and should be transported with spinal precautions.

Burn Depth

Superficial Burn

Burn depth is classified by depth of injury (**Figure 32-1**). A superficial burn injures only the epidermis. Skin integrity

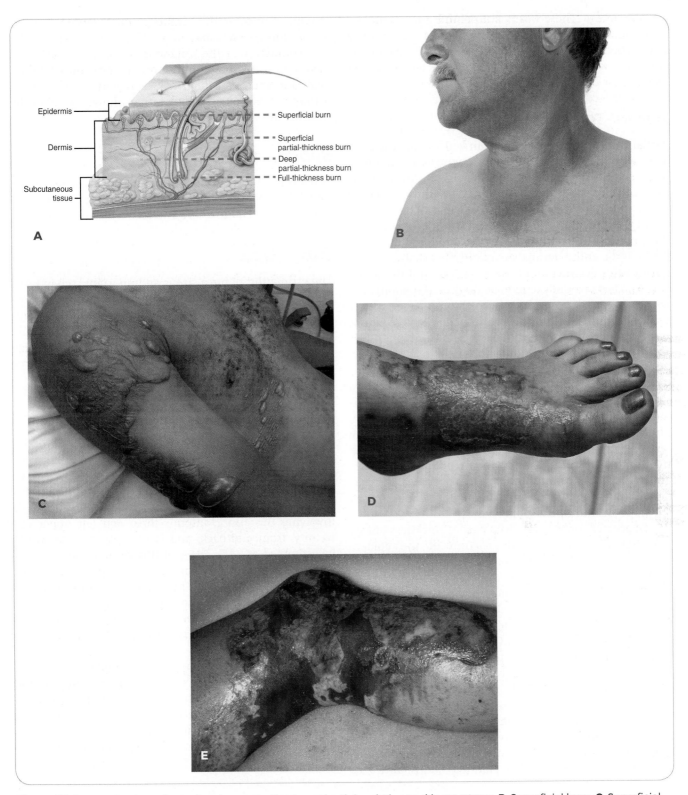

Figure 32-1 Burn depth. **A.** Illustration demonstrating burn depth in relation to skin structures. **B.** Superficial burn. **C.** Superficial partial-thickness burn. **D.** Deep partial-thickness burn. **E.** Full-thickness burn.

remains intact. These burns are painful and erythematous without blistering or open wounds. An example of a superficial burn is sunburn. Rapid wound healing occurs (< 1 week) without scarring. These burns are not included in the calculation of TBSA burned.

Partial-Thickness Burn

Partial-thickness burns are categorized as superficial or deep, and it can sometimes be challenging to discriminate between the two. Additionally, partial-thickness burns can evolve or convert to deeper burn wounds secondary to the thermal injury or because of inadequate (over or under) resuscitation. A partial-thickness burn destroys the epidermis and part of the dermis but does not extend through the entire dermis. A superficial partial-thickness burn causes destruction of the epidermis and the upper dermis. These wounds tend to be bright red to mottled in appearance, and wet to the touch. Blisters are commonly seen in superficial partial-thickness burns. Severe pain is caused by exposure of dermal nerve endings to air. It is important to leave blisters intact initially in the field because they act as a temporary "field dressing" for the injury. In the case of delayed evacuation or prolonged field care, the blisters should be debrided, the burn size reestimated, and sterile dressings placed over the burned tissue. These burns tend to weep fluid, contributing to volume loss. Additionally, patients may become hypothermic due to saturated dressings that may require frequent changes. Superficial partial-thickness burn wounds heal spontaneously with minimal scarring in 1 to 3 weeks, as long as adequate wound care is employed.

Of greater concern are deep partial-thickness burns. These involve complete destruction of the epidermis and a variable amount of the dermis. Wounds are characteristically dark red to yellowish-white in color, minimally blanching, less moist than superficial partial-thickness burns, and exhibit decreased sensation to skin prick. Blisters can occur but are less common at this depth. Pain can vary, but in general they hurt less secondary to destruction of pain fibers in the dermis. Blood flow to areas with deep partial-thickness burns is compromised allowing for increased risk of infection and wound conversion to full-thickness injury. Wound healing may take weeks to months with increased risk of hypertrophic scarring if treated nonoperatively. Excision and grafting is commonly warranted to expedite wound healing, and decrease pain and contracture risk in these casualties.

Full-Thickness Burn

Full-thickness burns are characterized by injury of the epidermis, dermis, and underlying skin structures (hair follicles and glands). The burned tissue appears charred or whitish in color, dry, leathery, and insensate. Thrombosed blood vessels may be visible. This eschar is a potent stimulator of the inflammatory response and is a medium for microorganism growth. These burns do not heal, and there is a high risk of hypertrophic scarring if they are not excised, but rather allowed to close by contraction.

Subdermal Burn

Subdermal burns extend through subcutaneous tissue into fascia, muscle, and even bone. These patients require specialized burn care and reconstructive surgery.[5]

Burn Size

The estimation of burn size is an important step in burn care. Mortality is directly related to burn size and most importantly, for the prehospital phase of management, burn size dictates the volume of fluid required to resuscitate the patient. Burn size is expressed as a percentage of total body surface area (%TBSA). Superficial burns are not included in the determination of %TBSA.

Burn injuries in the prehospital and early Role 1 phase of management should initially be mapped using the Rule of Nines. The Rule of Nines assigns percentages in intervals of 9% to different areas of the body[6] (**Figure 32-2**). Use the diagram in Figure 32-2 to calculate the %TBSA involved by second- and third-degree burn wounds. Do *not* include first-degree wounds in this assessment. Example: Second- and third-degree wounds involving the entire anterior torso and left upper extremity, front and back, and front of right thigh would be estimated as 32% TBSA. If this wound had scattered areas of unburned skin and/or first-degree burns, adjust the %TBSA downward. The %TBSA is an estimate using this rule; final burn mapping is done after wounds have been cleaned and debrided. Both over- and underestimates have potential negative impacts on a patient's resuscitation.

This mapping technique must be modified for use in children, whose heads occupy a larger percentage of the body surface area and whose lower extremities occupy a smaller percentage. The Lund and Browder chart is a more detailed burn diagram suitable for use in hospitals when the burn wounds have been debrided and can be more accurately mapped (**Figure 32-3**).[7]

Fluid Resuscitation for Burn Injury

Burn injury involving approximately 20% TBSA or more can result in massive fluid shifts, and patients can

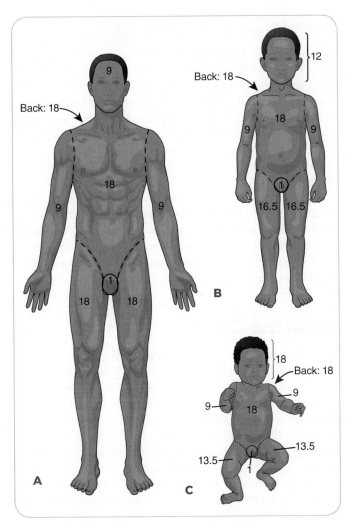

Figure 32-2 The Rule of Nines for burn area estimation.
A. Adult. **B.** Child. **C.** Infant.

develop hypovolemic shock. The inflammatory response that causes the dramatic hemodynamic changes varies among casualties, which can be confusing in the prehospital, and even in the hospital environment. During the immediate postinjury period, a hypotensive burn casualty should always be considered to be in hemorrhagic shock, although other forms of shock in a burn casualty must be ruled out.

Fluid shifts in burn patients can cause hypovolemic shock during the first 48 hours. Delayed or inadequate replacement of volume results in poor tissue perfusion, burn wound conversion, renal failure, and possibly death. Over-resuscitation may cause complications just as morbid that are associated with tissue edema (which can result in conversion of burn wounds to full thickness), pulmonary complications, extremity compartment syndrome, abdominal compartment syndrome, and even death. *The goal of fluid resuscitation after severe burn is to replace the losses with just enough fluid to maintain adequate tissue perfusion throughout the 48-hour period following injury.* There are several formulas for estimating how much fluid to give in this situation. For example, IV fluid can be given at a rate based on the modified Brooke formula: total volume to be infused over the first 24 hours = 2 milliliters (ml) × weight in kg × TBSA, with one-half administered over the first 8 hours post burn, and one-half over the second 16 hours. To simplify this calculation, the USAISR Burn Center advocates the Rule of Tens formula for adult patients **Box 32-1**.

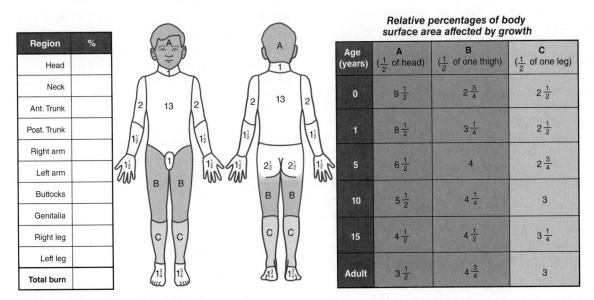

Figure 32-3 Lund and Browder burn area map.

Data from Lund CC, Browder NC. The estimation of areas of burns. *Surg Gynecol Obstet.* 1944;79:352-358.

Region	%
Head	
Neck	
Ant. Trunk	
Post. Trunk	
Right arm	
Left arm	
Buttocks	
Genitalia	
Right leg	
Left leg	
Total burn	

Relative percentages of body surface area affected by growth

Age (years)	A ($\frac{1}{2}$ of head)	B ($\frac{1}{2}$ of one thigh)	C ($\frac{1}{2}$ of one leg)
0	$9\frac{1}{2}$	$2\frac{3}{4}$	$2\frac{1}{2}$
1	$8\frac{1}{2}$	$3\frac{1}{4}$	$2\frac{1}{2}$
5	$6\frac{1}{2}$	4	$2\frac{3}{4}$
10	$5\frac{1}{2}$	$4\frac{1}{4}$	3
15	$4\frac{1}{2}$	$4\frac{1}{2}$	$3\frac{1}{4}$
Adult	$3\frac{1}{2}$	$4\frac{3}{4}$	3

To illustrate, if one is faced with resuscitating three patients with varying burn sizes of 30%, 50%, and 70%, initial fluid rates of 300, 500, and 700 ml/hr of fluid would be initiated.[8] Lactated Ringer (LR) solution is the preferred fluid for resuscitation of burn victims. Normal saline is less desirable because of the increased risk for hyperchloremia and kidney injury. If LR is not available, resuscitation can be initiated with normal saline and transitioned to LR as soon as possible. Though LR is currently the fluid of choice, IV fluid resuscitation in burn patients is an active area of research. Enteral resuscitation and fresh frozen plasma are being investigated as potential therapies that may decrease the resuscitation morbidities seen with crystalloids. Optimal care requires adjusting the LR rate *every* hour, with the goal of maintaining a urine output of 30 to 50 ml/hr in adults—no more and no less. Insertion of a Foley catheter and hourly measurement of urine output, fluid input, and vital signs are required. In an effort to help standardize care, burn resuscitation guidelines were devised along with a burn resuscitation flow sheet to help better document the resuscitation during evacuation and minimize resuscitation morbidity (**Figure 32-4**). Both are available at https://jts.amedd.army.mil/assets/docs/cpgs/JTS_Clinical_Practice_Guidelines_(CPGs)/Burn_Care_11_May_2016_ID12.pdf.

Pediatric Casualties

Children require proportionally larger volumes of IV fluid than adults with similar sized burns. The Rule of Ten is designed for *adults only* and thus should not be utilized for children. For children, the following formula should be used. Total volume of LR to infuse over the first 24 hours post burn = 3 ml × weight in kg × %TBSA. Give half of this amount over the first 8 hours, and half over the second 16 hours.[10] Additionally, very young children and infants may not be able to maintain their glucose levels during periods of stress. They should receive D_5 ½NS at a standard maintenance rate in *addition* to the burn resuscitation fluids using the following formula:

- 0 to 10 kg: 4 ml/kg/hr
- 10 to 20 kg: 40 ml/hr + 2 ml/kg/hr
- > 20 kg: 60 ml/hr + 1 ml/kg/hr

Special Circumstances

In the presence of polytrauma, inhalation injury, or electrical injury, fluid needs will be greater. It is imperative to keep the potential complications of these circumstances in mind during resuscitation. Blood loss resulting in massive transfusion may dominate the fluid resuscitation requirements in patients with both burn and nonburn trauma. In cases where patients can tolerate oral intake, encourage oral hydration with a glucose-containing liquid. If sufficient IV fluids are not available, oro- or nasogastric tube resuscitation can be used to resuscitate patients with burns of up to about 30% TBSA.[9] Oral (or enteral, with the use of a nasogastric tube) resuscitation fluids can be prepared by adding 8 teaspoons (tsp) of sugar and 1 tsp of salt to each liter of clean, potable water.[11]

Wound Care

Many factors affect the treatment of burn casualties on the battlefield, including availability of medical evacuation, capabilities of the medical treatment facility, training of the provider, and external tactical threats. Regardless, clinical outcomes will be determined to a large extent by the quality of medical treatment provided in the theater of operations. Therefore, predeployment training in courses such as the American Burn Association (ABA) Advanced Burn Life Support (ABLS) course, Department of Defense (DoD) Joint Forces Combat Trauma Management Course (JFCTMC), and the Emergency War Surgery (EWS) course are critical for relaying the basic knowledge needed to treat this special population of casualties. The physical appearance of burn injuries can be distracting and may cause an inexperienced provider to overlook other less obvious but more immediately life-threatening injuries. Therefore, early emphasis must be placed on identifying and treating all life-threatening injuries. This becomes particularly important for polytrauma patients injured by IEDs.

As noted previously, during the Care Under Fire phase, the most important aspect of care is to remove the casualty from the burning vehicle or building and immediately halt the burning process. This may be done with nonflammable liquid, dropping and rolling, smothering the flames with a blanket, or any other expedient means that may be at hand.

In the Tactical Field Care phase, burns should be covered with dry, sterile dressings. After appropriate lifesaving interventions are accomplished, casualties with extensive burns may be placed in a Heat Reflective Shell, which will both cover the burned areas with a clean material and help to prevent hypothermia. The medic, corpsman, or pararescueman (PJ) should then

JTS Burn Resuscitation Flow Sheet – page 1 of 3

Date		Initial Treatment Facility				
Name		SSN	Pre-burn estimated weight (kg)	%TBSA (Do not include superficial 1st degree burn)	Calculate Rule of Tens (if >40<80kg, %TBSA x 10 = starting rate for LR	Calculate max 24hr volume (250ml x kg) Avoid over-resuscitation, use adjuncts if necessary

Date &Time of Injury					BAMC/ISR Burn Team DSN 312-429-2876: Yes No		
Tx Site/ Team	HR from burn	Local Time	Crystalloid* (LR) /Colloid	Total	UOP (Target 30-50ml/hr)	Base Deficit/ Lactate	Heart Rate	MAP (>55) / CVP (6-8mmHg)	Pressors (Vasopressin 0.04 u/min) Bladder Pressure (Q4)

Tx Site/Team	HR from burn	Local Time	Crystalloid*(LR)/Colloid	Total	UOP (Target 30-50ml/hr)	Base Deficit/Lactate	Heart Rate	MAP(>55)/CVP(6-8mmHg)	Pressors (Vasopressin 0.04 u/min) Bladder Pressure (Q4)
	1st								
	2nd								
	3rd								
	4th								
	5th								
	6th								
	7th								
	8th								
	9th								
	10th								
	11th								
	12th								
	13th								
	14th								
	15th								
	16th								
	17th								
	18th								
	19th								
	20th								
Total Fluids:					*Titrate LR hourly to maintain adequate UOP (30-50ml/hr) and perfusion				

Figure 32-4 Joint Trauma System burn resuscitation flow Chart.

estimate the %TBSA burned using the Rule of Nines described earlier, remembering that first-degree burns are not included in this calculation. Fluid resuscitation, if needed to prevent burn shock (> 20% TBSA), should be initiated as soon as IV/IO access is established. Resuscitation for hemorrhagic shock, if present, takes precedence over burn resuscitation and should be administered per TCCC guidelines for shock. Analgesia in accordance with TCCC guidelines should be administered as needed for burn pain. Antibiotic therapy in the field for burn wounds alone is not recommended, but antibiotics may be given per TCCC guidelines if indicated to prevent infection in penetrating wounds. The key to successful treatment of burn casualties is urgent transport to definitive care. Care of the burn casualty is similar in the Tactical Evacuation Care (TACEVAC) phase except that additional emphasis should be placed on hypothermia prevention and close airway monitoring if casualties have facial burns.

At Role 2 and Role 3 military treatment facilities, fluid resuscitation is continued, and initial wound care is performed in addition to addressing other life-threatening injuries. The surgical management of burn wounds in deployed settings focuses on cleansing the wounds and preventing complications from resuscitation such as compartment syndrome. Burn wounds should be cleansed with chlorhexidine gluconate (Hibiclens™) solution, removing all surface debris and contamination. Patients with circumferential deep burns of the extremities are at risk of edema causing constriction of blood flow. To prevent this, a surgeon makes an incision into the burned skin (escharotomy) along the medial and lateral lines of the limb (**Figure 32-5**). After debridement, burn wounds should be dressed with topical antimicrobial agents to prevent infection. A variety of topical agents can be used, including silver sulfadiazine cream, 11% mafenide acetate

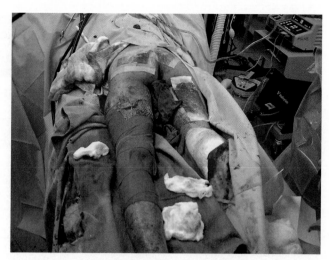

Figure 32-6 Silver-impregnated nylon dressings.
Courtesy of U.S. Army Burn Center.

cream, honey dressings, and 5% mafenide acetate solution.[13] Silver-impregnated nylon (Silverlon) dressings are an excellent alternative, that do not require twice-daily dressing change (**Figure 32-6**). These dressings are easy to apply and may not have to be changed for 3 to 5 days if the wounds are clean when the Silverlon is applied. Burned extremities (especially upper extremities) should be elevated to reduce edema. The outer gauze dressings (e.g., Kerlix [Covidien]) should be moistened (not soaked) at least daily with sterile or clean water.

Fire can also cause eye injuries, so irrigation with sterile water or saline is performed to remove any debris from the eye, and the corneas are examined with a Wood's lamp. Once these patients reach a higher level of care, ophthalmology consultation should be obtained.

Evacuation of Burn Patients

In comparison with previous conflicts, U.S. military medical care during the conflicts in Iraq and Afghanistan has been characterized by rapid aeromedical evacuation out of the theater of operations. The average time elapsed from point of injury in these theaters to arrival in CONUS was 96 hours. All attempts are made to evacuate burn victims as expeditiously as possible, but severe respiratory and hemodynamic compromise can delay transport. Most of these patients have been stabilized and burn resuscitation has been completed by the time they arrive at the U.S. Army Burn Center located at the USAISR in San Antonio, Texas. Patients with severe burn injury or respiratory status that precludes conventional mechanical ventilation

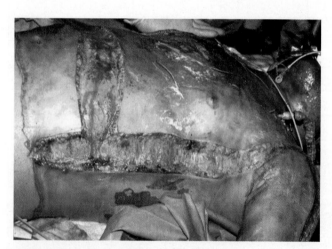

Figure 32-5 Escharotomies.
Courtesy of U.S. Army Burn Center.

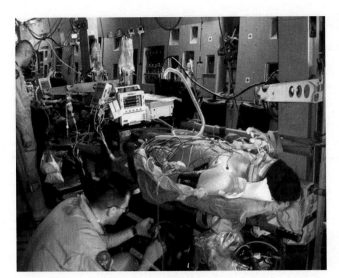

Figure 32-7 U.S. Army Burn Flight Team transport setup.
Courtesy of U.S. Army Burn Center.

may require transatlantic aeromedical evacuation by the USAISR Burn Flight Team (BFT) (**Figure 32-7**).

Casualties are rarely triaged to the expectant category based on burn size. Patients with a TBSA exceeding 95% have survived with a good quality of life.[12]

U.S. Army Institute of Surgical Research Burn Flight Team

The BFT was created in the 1950s and was instrumental in evacuating burn casualties from Vietnam. Since that time, the BFT has been activated for both humanitarian and wartime missions. The BFT consists of five personnel: burn surgeon, registered nurse, licensed practical nurse, respiratory therapist and operations noncommissioned officer. The BFT typically transports patients with greater than 40% TBSA burns, with inhalation injury, and/or with both burns and multiple nonburn injuries from combat trauma. Recently, the BFT has acquired in-flight capabilities such as continuous renal replacement therapy and extracorporeal membrane oxygenation. The BFT has expertise in transporting patients with severe pulmonary compromise secondary to burn injury and uses specialized ventilators for lung rescue strategies. The BFT usually transports patients on C-17 or C-121 aircraft and relies on U.S. Air Force Aeromedical Evacuation Squadrons for logistical support. Since 2003, the BFT has conducted over 100 missions and has evacuated over 350 combat casualties to the U.S. Army Burn Center.[14]

SUMMARY

- The proper management of the thermally injured combat casualty requires a unique set of skills as well as recognition of the pitfalls of resuscitation.
- The initial assessment is key to identifying life-threatening injuries and beginning lifesaving therapies.
- Knowledge of basic burn wound care is imperative in a deployed environment.

- The care that burn casualties receive in the early stages of their injury will largely determine their outcomes.
- The ability to determine the percentage of body surface area burned and an understanding of burn resuscitation is crucial so that care of the casualty is not delayed.

SCENARIO RECAP

You are a medic assigned to an infantry platoon. Your unit is on a patrol in eastern Afghanistan when an IED detonates underneath your vehicle, causing it to catch on fire. Three soldiers are injured in this incident. After the area is secured you begin to assess the casualties.

Soldier 1 is a 21-year-old male who is alert, following commands, and walking around. He has sustained burns to his whole face, the lower half of both arms, the lower part of both legs except for his feet. He has no other visible injuries. His radial pulse is 110 beats/min and strong, and his respiratory rate is 18 breaths/min. He weighs 154 lb (70 kg).

SCENARIO RECAP (CONTINUED)

Soldier 2 is a 27-year-old platoon sergeant who is confused and disoriented. His left foot is severely mangled and bleeding badly. He has burns to his lower right arm, left hand, and left lower leg. His radial pulse is strong at 135 beats/min, and he is breathing fast. He weighs 165 lb (75 kg).

Soldier 3 is 20 years old. He has partial traumatic amputations of both legs below the knees and is losing a lot of blood. He is completely unresponsive. There are burns to his face, both arms, both legs, and the lower third of his anterior and posterior torso. His radial pulses are not palpable, but he is breathing spontaneously, although slowly. He weighs 198 lb (90 kg).

SCENARIO SOLUTION

- **What is the triage category for each of these casualties?**
  - Soldier 3 is in the Immediate category because he cannot walk or talk, and immediate hemorrhage control and intubation are indicated.
  - Soldier 2 has an altered mental status and is hemorrhaging from an extensive wound. His radial pulse is still palpable, but fast. His mental status decrement may be due to TBI or blood loss that may be compensated for the moment. He should be placed in the Immediate category.
  - Soldier 1 is walking, talking, and obeying commands, but has serious burn injury. He is in the delayed category.
    - A potential pitfall with this casualty is not being acutely aware that respiratory compromise secondary to facial burns may occur within the first hour of injury. He should be reassessed after the other soldiers are stabilized, and his head should be kept elevated to decrease facial edema.
- **What is the initial management of each casualty?**
  - Soldier 3 initially needs tourniquets on both legs, and blood via the IV or IO route. If blood is not available, he should receive a LR or Hextend bolus to maintain a palpable pulse. Airway should be immediately obtained with a supraglottic airway, endotracheal intubation, or cricothyrotomy. Ventilatory support should be provided with a bag-mask device. Tranexamic acid (TXA) should be administered as an adjunct to hemorrhage control that was performed initially. The cervical spine should be stabilized due to the mechanism of injury. Antibiotics can be administered if the casualty will not arrive at a higher level of care shortly after injury.
  - Soldier 2 should have a tourniquet placed above his injured left foot, IV or IO access established, and cervical spine stabilization. You should anticipate his near-term need for a definitive airway and fluid resuscitation for hemorrhagic shock. IV antibiotics are indicated, and if he should need fluid resuscitation, he will also need TXA. Avoid opioid medications in this casualty; use ketamine if analgesia is required.
  - Soldier 1 may soon need significant analgesia. Avoid opioid medications in this casualty; use ketamine if analgesia is required. Although initially stable, he could develop the need for an airway depending on the extent of his facial burns; it is always optimal and easier to obtain an airway in patients with a significant facial burn early and electively instead of emergently. Facial and airway edema can make obtaining an airway significantly challenging. This patient's face should be assessed and frequently reassessed for edema. His airway should also be assessed and frequently rechecked for patency. His head should remain elevated. It is imperative, and much safer, to obtain an airway in facial burn patients prior to it becoming emergent secondary to airway compromise.
- **What is the extent of burn for each casualty (%TBSA)?**
  With deductions for the back of the head and the amputations, the calculated burn surface area for Soldier 3 is about 70%. For Soldier 2 it is approximately 15%. It is 31% for Soldier 1.

(continued)

SCENARIO SOLUTION (CONTINUED)

- **Calculate the initial fluid resuscitation and describe how you will monitor the effectiveness of the resuscitation.**
  - For Soldier 3, calculated burn resuscitation is:
    - 70% TBSA × 10 = 700 ml/hr
    - Add 100 ml/hr for the extra 10 kg over 80 kg = 800 ml/hr
    - Monitor urine output and adjust fluids to achieve and maintain 30 to 50 ml/hr.
  - The TBSA for Soldier 2 is 15%, so resuscitation for burn fluid shift per se is not indicated.
  - For Soldier 1, TBSA = 31%, so rounded to the nearest ten, 30 × 10 = 300 ml/hr. He weighs 70 kg, so the initial rate is not increased. Urine output should be monitored hourly and fluid rate adjusted as needed to maintain 30 to 50 ml/hr.

Note: All three of these casualties should have their burn wounds dressed after secondary assessment, and Soldier 2 and Soldier 3 should be given supplemental oxygen as soon as it becomes available in the evacuation process. They should also be protected from hypothermia.

References

1. Santaniello JM, Luchette FA, Esposito TJ, et al. Ten-year experience of burn, trauma, and combined burn/trauma injuries comparing outcomes. *J Trauma.* 2004;57(4):696-700.

2. Bishop JF. Burn wound assessment and surgical management. *Crit Care Nurs Clin N Am.* 2004;16(1):145-177.

3. American Burn Association. National Burn Repository 2005 Report. http://www.ameriburn.org/NBR2005.pdf. Accessed May 17, 2013.

4. Barillo DJ, Cancio LC, Goodwin CW. Treatment of white phosphorus and other chemical burn injuries at one burn center over a 51-year period. *Burns.* 2004;30(5):448-452.

5. American Burn Association. *Advanced Burn Life Support Course Provider Manual.* Chicago, IL: American Burn Association; 2001.

6. Knaysi GA, Crikelair GF, Crosman B. The rule of nines: its history and accuracy. *Plast Reconstr Surg.* 1968;41(6):560-563.

7. Lund CC, Browder NC. The estimation of areas of burn. *Surg Gynecol Obstet.* 1944;79(4):352-358.

8. Chung KK, Salinas J, Renz EM, et al. Simple derivation of the initial fluid rate for the resuscitation of severely burned adult combat casualties: in silico validation of the Rule of Ten. *J Trauma.* 2010;69(Suppl 1):S49-S54.

9. Pham TN, Cancio LC, Gibran NS. American Burn Association practice guidelines: burn shock resuscitation. *J Burn Care Res.* 2008;29(1):257-266.

10. Chung KK, Blackbourne LH, Wolf SE, et al. Evolution of burn resuscitation in Operation Iraqi Freedom. *J Burn Care Res.* 2006;27(5):606-611

11. Cancio LC, Kramer GC, Hoskins SL. Gastrointestinal fluid resuscitation of thermally injured patients. *J Burn Care Res.* 2006;27:561-569.

12. White CE, Renz EM. Advances in surgical care: management of severe burn injury. *Crit Care Med.* 2008;36(7)(Suppl):S318-S324.

13. Borden Institute. *Emergency War Surgery, The Third United States Revision.* Fort Dietrich, MD: Borden Institute; 2004.

14. Renz EM, Cancio LC, Barillo DJ, et. al. Long range transport of war-related burn casualties. *J Trauma.* 2008;64(2)(Suppl):S136-S145.

CHAPTER 33

Casualty Response Planning in Tactical Combat Casualty Care

Authors:
Col. (Ret) Russ Kotwal, MD
Master Sgt. (Ret) Harold Montgomery

CHAPTER OBJECTIVES

At the completion of this chapter, you will be able to do the following:

- Identify the core components of a medical threat assessment.
- List six sources of medical intelligence suitable for pre-mission planning.
- Discuss the importance of alternate planning.
- List the five types of mission rehearsals, and define each.
- Discuss the site characteristics of a good casualty collection point.

INTRODUCTION

The tactical environment encompasses the actions of armed personnel who are actively engaged in or directly maneuvering to kill or capture one another, or seize one another's terrain or assets. It is that part of the battlefield where forces are limited on everything, and nothing is truly secure or safe. Environmental factors influence the battle and can make or break the day. The fight may range from a few hundred meters to hand-to-hand combat. Decisions and actions are measured in seconds. Outcomes are measured by success, disaster, and anything in between.

Combat operations and realistic training for them will inevitably result in casualties. Tactical casualty scenarios can range from one casualty to dozens, with degrees of trauma from minor to massive, and usually a mix of these. The tactical situation or prosecution of the mission may overrule medical decisions. Time is usually critical for the mission and for the casualties.

Trauma care is optimized by minimizing the time between wounding and the meeting of the wounded with a treatment capability sufficient to the injury sustained. This capability is dependent upon the availability of adequate equipment and supplies combined with the knowledge and skills necessary to perform the inherent tasks. Tactical leaders can significantly reduce the number of casualties who are killed in action or die of their wounds by simply positioning optimal medical capability in close proximity to the point of wounding. Survival of the combat casualty lies mostly in the hands of the person who initiates treatment. Managing casualty response, including contingency planning, casualty collection points, and tactical evacuation, is a tactical leader's task; supplying medical expertise throughout the casualty's care on and evacuation from the battlefield is a combat medic's task.

Casualty Response System

Both tactical leaders and tactical medical advisors must be intimately familiar with the tactics, techniques, and procedures involved in the implementation of a Casualty Response System. This is not a medical system; instead, it is a tactical system of tiered casualty management that integrates the expertise of nonmedical and medical personnel in order to achieve the best possible outcomes for both the mission and the casualties. In the tactical environment, anyone has the potential to be a first responder. Therefore, all who engage in combat operations must understand the basic tenets of Tactical Combat Casualty Care (TCCC). If all personnel are well versed in appropriate levels of TCCC, they will be able to provide casualty care collectively, as a team, while minimizing interference with the unit's tactical flow during combat operations. In warfare, the majority of all combat deaths have historically occurred prior to casualties receiving advanced trauma care.

Training

Actions conducted in training equate to actions conducted in combat. Implementing a Casualty Response System should be viewed as a battle drill. It should be integrated into all combat training exercises and rehearsed to the greatest extent possible. If rehearsals are performed to standard, the novelty of a real casualty will be mitigated. Realistic training will save lives on the battlefield. Safety is paramount, but risk reduction in training should not be purchased with preventable death in combat.

Training should be conducted to standard and not to time. The basics of casualty management can be mastered through repetition and conditioning, and as in any serious training regimen, discipline precludes shortcuts. The more conditioned a person and a team become through training, the more likely they will achieve optimal outcomes for their casualties on the battlefield. The true success of a Casualty Response System will be defined by a team's ability to successfully prosecute the mission while minimizing morbidity and mortality.

Focus on the Possible

In planning and training for combat casualty management, the focus should be on the possible, not the impossible. Essentially, there are three groups of casualties that will be encountered. In the first group, no matter what you do, the wounded will live. In the second group, no matter what you do, they will die. In the third group, if you do the right thing, at the right time, your treatment will make the difference between life and death or between greater and lesser disability. The Casualty Response System should focus its efforts on this third group because there is a much greater probability of positively affecting their outcomes.

Decisions in tactical casualty management should not be made by people who are far removed from the fighting. The Casualty Response System should be a flattened organization with decentralized decision making that empowers first responders, tactical leaders, and

medical providers at all levels. When those who must implement the system far forward also direct its operation far forward, they are likely to invest in realistic casualty management training in order to become more efficient and effective at and near the point of injury. Ultimately, this will equate to lives saved.

Medical Planning

Medical planning in line units relies heavily on the experience and knowledge of unit physician assistants and senior medics. *All* tactical medics, from the most junior to the most senior, should become skilled planners. Effective medical planning requires that the planner be well integrated into the unit's (company/battalion/brigade/regimental) mission planning staff. Many medical issues that arise during planning are regulated, decided, or solved by other members of the staff, including the S3 (Operations), S3 (Air), S4 (Logistics), Commanders, Executive Officers, First Sergeants, and Platoon Sergeants. Good working relationships and effective communications must be maintained for successful medical planning.

Medical planners must be fluent in the unit's planning sequences (compressed or deliberate) and have a good understanding of the role they play therein. Medical planners should be involved as early as possible in planning sequences for *all* training exercises and real-world contingencies. It is a good idea to make a planning checklist and timeline of planning events or milestones for every exercise and operation.

The medical plan should include an overall casualty response plan in which every unit member has a role. When a casualty occurs, it is not just the medic's problem; it is a tactical problem that must be planned for and solved by the entire unit. Units should integrate a casualty response phase into all of their tactical battle drills. Unit members and leadership must be well versed in the casualty response plan. Medical personnel have a tendency to focus on providing critical patient care once they begin treating casualties and, as such, may not be able to maintain sufficient situational awareness to execute the plan. The unit must be able to execute the casualty response plan around the medic while the medic treats the wounded.

Predeployment Requirements

The unit should conduct predeployment medical training and casualty response drills during training exercises. The time to ponder what can be done during the Care Under Fire phase is not when real bullets are flying. A comprehensive medical skills training program will enable units to prepare for casualties sustained in combat operations. Individual operators should be trained in first responder TCCC skills and equipped appropriately long before launching on the combat mission. A unit that conducts TCCC skills training for individual operators and integrates casualty response drills into unit exercises will reduce preventable combat deaths (**Box 33-1**).

Medical Threat Assessment

The medical planner must assess all medical threats the unit may face during the operation. This assessment includes environmental health hazards as well as specific threats from enemy weapons systems. Through the medical threat assessment, the medical planner will identify preventive measures the unit can employ to minimize these threats. Once the preventive measures appropriate to the mission have been selected, medical planners must be prepared to make recommendations to unit commanders, leaders, and members on how to employ them. The overall goal is to have healthy operators ready to perform a mission, to keep them healthy during the mission, and to bring healthy operators back home.

Identify the Area of Operations (AO)

The medical planner must develop a clear understanding of medical threats and assets in the countries, regions, and environments in which the operation will be conducted. The locations of targets, staging bases, etc., must be known in order to adequately plan for medical threats. The most important area to assess is the target area. This is the area or region in which the unit will be conducting tactical missions. The host country or staging area must also be evaluated. This is the secure region used as a base of operations. The threats here may or may not be the same as those of the target area.

Identify Medical Intelligence and Health Threats

Medical intelligence is a key component of all training and contingency operations. Information on hazardous plants and animals, prevalent diseases, required immunizations and chemoprophylaxis, climatology, as well as medical and hospital capabilities in the areas involved should be gathered. The National Center for Medical Intelligence (NCMI) is a primary source for medical intelligence. NCMI collects and disseminates information on disease occurrence, medical capabilities, health services, and environmental health hazards specific to regions around the world. The internet address for the NCMI is: www.ncmi.detrick.army.mil/. It is available to active duty and civilian government employees who hold a common access card. Other sources for medical intelligence online are as follows:

- Centers for Disease Control and Prevention (CDC)
  - www.cdc.gov/
- U.S. State Department Travel Warnings and Consular Information
  - https://travel.state.gov/content/travel/en/404.html
- World Health Organization (WHO) homepage
  - www.who.int/en/
- U.S. Army Public Health Center
  - https://phc.amedd.army.mil/Pages/default.aspx/

The medical planner must also maintain an awareness of the unit's medical readiness status. A review of immunization and health records should be conducted well before the operation begins.

The types of enemy weapons the unit may encounter, including chemical and biologic weapons, must also be determined. The planner should make recommendations to prevent and treat the injuries these weapons may inflict, such as the use of body armor, chemoprophylaxis, or protective masks.

Higher Headquarters Orders and Guidelines

Higher Headquarters Medical Guidelines and Requirements

The operational headquarters often publishes specific guidelines regarding casualty evacuation and hospitalization as well as preventive medicine requirements in its operations orders (OPORDs). The planner must determine if unit members will have to take medications before, during, and after the mission to prevent illnesses like malaria. A key question that must be asked is, "Does the unit need to change anything from their normal procedures to meet higher headquarters requirements?"

Requests for Information (RFI)

Medical planners should be familiar with the processes for requesting updates to dated information about disease or environmental threats. Sources for such periodic reports and publications may lie within the chain of command or may be external, such as international health organizations. Maps, imagery, and information on medical facilities in the staging or target areas may also be needed.

Determine Medical Assets

On a given operation, the unit will be supported by its internal medical assets. External medical personnel, equipment, or units may also be attached as needed. A thorough understanding of all medical assets assigned to the mission is crucial. This includes the proper unit designations or names; number of personnel by specialty, treatment, and evacuation capabilities; logistical requirements; task organization; and command and control. It is important to ensure that all external medical assets are well connected into the unit's structure operationally, logistically, and administratively.

Evacuation Assets

There are two basic types of evacuation conducted during combat operations: casualty evacuation (CASEVAC) and medical evacuation (MEDEVAC). CASEVAC implies the use of nonmedical platforms to evacuate casualties. These mission platforms are ground vehicles, watercraft, or aircraft typically used by the unit for infiltration, exfiltration, or resupply. These vehicles do not usually have medical personnel or equipment onboard unless previously assigned in the operational plan. These assets are more suited for routine evacuation of nonemergent casualties, but prestaged medical personnel and equipment can facilitate the treatment and transport of the more seriously wounded. Medical planners should plan for the use of CASEVAC assets as much as possible, as these assets are often the most readily available for rapid evacuation. Furthermore, these vehicles are usually armed and, thus, are better prepared to conduct evacuation while the fight with the enemy is ongoing.

MEDEVAC refers to the use of dedicated medical platforms whose primary mission is the evacuation of casualties. Most often conducted by aircraft, MEDEVAC can also be carried out using medically staffed and equipped frontline ambulances (FLAs). MEDEVAC platforms are usually assigned to a regulated region, are not under the direct control of the tactical unit, and must be requested through operational channels. Controllers in operations centers receive MEDEVAC requests and launch or divert MEDEVAC assets as required on a prioritized basis.

Unit medical planners should determine the casualty evacuation assets that will likely be needed to support the unit's mission whether by air, ground, or water. Assets should be matched to the expected needs in pre-mission planning.

Requesting Evacuation

MEDEVAC requests are normally transmitted using the standard NATO nine-line MEDEVAC request format (**Table 33-1**).

The MEDEVAC request provides controllers in operations centers with the critical information needed to launch and manage MEDEVAC platforms. CASEVAC requests can be tailored specifically to the unit mission and operating area, but typically consist of the first five lines of a MEDEVAC request. This works for CASEVAC platforms since they are normally already part of the tactical operation, and the drivers have a clear understanding of the battle space through previous coordination and ongoing communications.

Familiarization With Evacuation Assets

In pre-mission planning, key questions must be answered concerning CASEVAC and MEDEVAC. How many and what type of platforms are available? What are the capabilities, limitations, and restrictions of the platforms? Are air evacuation assets capable of hoist or high-angle extractions? What medical equipment is on board each platform? Who are the assigned medical personnel and to what levels are they trained?

Rehearsals With External Assets

The unit's leaders and tactical medics should coordinate face-to-face with external evacuation personnel prior to mission execution to assure a clear understanding of procedures by all personnel. If possible, live rehearsals with evacuation assets should be conducted to prepare for smooth handover of casualties. Unit operators should practice with the evacuation platforms as aid-and-litter teams. During the real evacuation of a wounded and bleeding operator is not the time to learn how to secure a litter inside an aircraft.

Surgical and Area Medical Support Assets

The medical treatment facilities to which combat casualties will be transported should be identified and their capabilities and capacities (especially surgical) documented.

Line	Item	Brevity Codes
1	Location/grid	Grid
2	Frequency and call sign of requesting unit	FM freq Call sign
3	Number of patients by precedence	A—Urgent B—Urgent surgical C—Priority D—Routine E—Convenience
4	Special equipment needed	A—None B—Hoist C—Extraction equipment D—Ventilator
5	Number of patients by type (litter and ambulatory)	L—Number of litter patients A—Number of ambulatory patients
6 (wartime)	Security at pick-up site (wartime)	N—No enemy troops in area P—Possibly enemy troops in area E—Enemy troops in area (use caution) X—Enemy troops in area (armed escort required)
6 (peacetime)	Number and type of wounded, injured, or ill	Description of each
7	Method of marking pick-up site	A—Panels B—Pyrotechnic signal C—Smoke signal D—None E—Other (specify)
8	Patient nationality and status	A—U.S. military B—U.S. civilian C—Non-U.S. military D—Non-U.S. civilian E—Enemy prisoner of war
9 (Wartime)	NBC contamination (wartime)	N—Nuclear B—Biologic C—Chemical
9 (Peacetime)	Terrain description (features in and around the landing site)	

Table 33-1 MEDEVAC Request Format*

*Use lines 1–5 for precoordinated CASEVAC cequests using organic assets.

Reproduced from the *Ranger Medic Handbook*, © William Donovan.

With this knowledge, planners can predict how many of what type of casualties could overwhelm a given facility, and casualty flow can be directed accordingly. Furthermore, casualties can be routed directly to facilities with greater capabilities if dictated by the severity of their injuries. For casualties with severe injuries, evacuation to a fully capable combat support hospital has been found to produce better outcomes than evacuation to a treatment facility with limited surgical and intensive care capabilities if the evacuation times are comparable.

It is highly desirable to visit the supporting medical facilities to gain an understanding of their physical layouts and unique equipment. Face-to-face coordination with appropriate staff personnel is most important. Also, unit medical personnel must know how to follow up with the unit casualties as commanders will require serial reports on their status.

Deployed troops will suffer routine illnesses and noncombat injuries that may require medical attention exceeding the tactical medic's scope of practice. Area medical support assets are those facilities that provide medical services other than combat trauma care to meet these needs. Established policies and procedures for operators' care at area medical support facilities should be conveyed to unit leaders and medical personnel.

Primary and Alternate Planning

As with all military operations, the unit and the medical planner should always have backup plans. A unit should never launch on a combat mission with only one planned means of casualty evacuation, for example. In this instance, alternatives for all possible routes of evacuation (e.g., air, ground, water) should be written into the medical plan. Alternate receiving facilities should be identified in case mass-casualty situations occur or conditions prohibit evacuation to primary facilities. Additionally, weather and environmental conditions can have detrimental effects on preplanned evacuation operations that can be mitigated by a good alternate plan.

Tactical Medical Support Plan Development

Understand the Tactical Commander's Plan

The tactical medical planner must understand the overall scheme of maneuver of the forces arrayed on the battlefield. This understanding is gained by attending all of the operations planning meetings and ensuring that medical operations are well synchronized into the tactical plan. Tactical plans may evolve rapidly, so the medical planner must keep abreast of changes, and should participate in

course of action development to determine if the various options can be supported medically.

Casualty Estimation

Medical and tactical planners should predict where casualties are likely to occur and develop casualty management and evacuation plans for all phases of the operation (infiltration, assault, clear/secure, consolidation, exploitation, defense, and exfiltration). Computer-based planning tools such as the Medical Course of Action Tool (MCOAT) can assist medical planners in forecasting attrition during military operations. Other key elements to consider are the layout of the target and template of enemy positions as projected by intelligence and operations staffs. Understanding the commander's tactical plan will indicate how best to develop the medical support plan.

Casualties should be expected and planned for in all phases of the tactical operation. The following questions will help develop casualty management plans: Where on the target is taking casualties foreseen? What types of injuries are expected based on the type of operation and enemy weapons? Where is the most critical location for unit medics to be positioned? Do you need to task organize the medical team to separate locations or to separate fighting elements? Where does the unit need to establish casualty collection points (CCPs) based on the expectations of casualties? What evacuation methods should be considered? Where are the nearest helicopter landing zones (HLZs) or ambulance exchange points (AXPs) to high casualty areas? Where should medical assets or augmentation be staged? How will casualties be moved from point to point on the target prior to evacuation from the target?

The casualty estimation also includes projecting disease and nonbattle injury (DNBI), the potential for nonbattle-related illness and injury calculated from known medical threats, unit activities, previous events, and individual health profiles. DNBIs include trauma, such as parachute landing injuries, that did not occur as a result of combat. The MCOAT can assist with casualty estimations for injuries of this type, too.

Issue Initial Medical Planning Guidance to Subordinates

Medical planners should constantly disseminate information to subordinate elements and junior medics. Information provided should be as comprehensive as possible consistent with operational security considerations. Planning guidance should include the medical threat analysis, medical assets, copies of higher OPORDs/OPLANs, and information that will assist subordinates with medical planning at their level. Guidance from above helps junior medics better prepare themselves and their equipment for tactical operations.

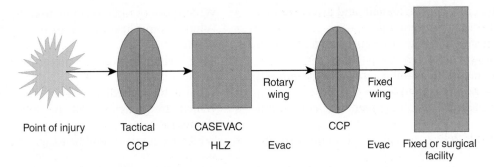

Figure 33-1 Casualty flow from target to hospitalization.

Reproduced from the *Ranger Medic Handbook*, © William Donovan.

Determine Casualty Flow From Target to Hospitalization

If possible, casualty flow should be planned from the point of injury all the way back to admission to a medical facility in the continental United States (CONUS). However, in an established combat theater, a casualty may be admitted, treated, and even released from an intermediate facility between the battlefield and CONUS (**Figure 33-1**). At a minimum, the tactical medic should always have a detailed understanding of the casualty flow up to two levels above themselves, including patient regulating, casualty accountability, and hospitalization requirements. For example, a platoon medic should have a good understanding of where a casualty goes after leaving the CCP or battalion aid station.

Several issues need to be addressed and questions answered in order to establish the tactical casualty flow:

- To what location will the unit's casualties be evacuated?
- Will evacuation be conducted by ground or air (or water) assets to a CCP?
- How will evacuation be conducted to casualty transload points?
- What are the distances and times of travel?
- Will expected casualties be able to make it that far? If not, which parts of the plan need to be corrected?
- Who will evacuate the casualties?
- Will medical assets be properly positioned to ensure continuity of care?

Determine Key Locations

Key locations for medical assets are determined based on the casualty estimation and the commander's tactical assault plan:

- Where should the CCP be located?
- Where should patient exchanges (HLZs, AXPs) be located?
- Where are the projected fighting positions, blocking positions, roadblocks, and checkpoints?

- Where will Command and Control be located?
- Who will be in charge of each key location?
- Are both primary and alternate locations for all medical functions within the plan established?
- What are the planned ground movement routes?

Establish the Tactical Medical Support Plan

The medical support plan can be developed alongside tactical plans, but often it is difficult to lock in the medical plan until tactical planners have settled on the preferred course of action. A basic tactical medical support plan should include the following elements:

1. The distribution, task organization, and tactical movement (infiltration/exfiltration) of medical elements, all synchronized with each other and the overall tactical plan.
2. The casualty flow plan from point of injury through evacuation to a medical treatment facility, including primary and secondary evacuation routes, methods, and modes (aid and litter, air, ground, water).
3. Primary and alternate sites for CCPs, casualty evacuation points (CEPs), HLZs, and possible casualty exchange points (CXPs).
4. A medical communications plan (Will medical nets be required? Will medics carry radios? How will casualty information and evacuation requests be relayed from element to element?).
5. A medical resupply plan if the operation will continue for a length of time.
6. Management plans for wounded hostile combatants and noncombatant casualties.

Air Tactical Evacuation Plan

The following information should be gathered in the formulation of a tactical air evacuation plan:

- What aircraft types will be used, and what is the maximum casualty load of each type?

- How will the casualties be loaded, and are there any patient packaging requirements?
- Are there specific loading procedures and approach procedures to the aircraft?
- What is the medical capability aboard each aircraft (equipment and personnel)?
- Is any special casualty management equipment required?
- Can the aircraft deliver prepackaged medical resupply bundles?
- What are the request procedures, and who is the launch authority?
- What are the landing requirements (landing zone dimensions, markings required, and special equipment required)?

Ground Tactical Evacuation Plan

A ground tactical evacuation plan has two major sections. The first section comprises those actions required to move casualties within the target area. This section applies even if moving casualties to an AXP. The other section describes the actions required to evacuate casualties from the target area to a medical facility by ground vehicles. The security of the ground element is a critical aspect of moving casualties within or out of the target area. The unit must ensure that a fighting element will protect the evacuation asset from enemy attack.

Ground tactical evacuation at the objective consists of moving casualties from their points of injury to CCPs or evacuation points. Aid-and-litter teams should be formed by personnel within the fighting elements. These personnel should be trained and equipped to conduct this secondary mission prior to launching the tactical mission. Vehicles of opportunity such as abandoned or captured enemy vehicles on the target can be used to move casualties. For instance, in an airport seizure, the unit could use baggage carts to move casualties.

Planning for evacuation by ground from the objective to a medical facility incorporates the same kind of information as planning for air evacuation, except for questions that are unique to the vehicles. One critical aspect of ground evacuation, however, is whether the unit will conduct the evacuation using its own assets or call on another unit.

Medical Communications

The tactical medical support plan includes a plan for medical communications. In formulating this plan, the following should be considered:

- Will all medics have radios? If not, how will the radios be assigned among the medics?
- Will a medic be able to contact a higher-level care provider for guidance?

- What types of radios will be used?
- What communications security requirements will be in effect?
- How will medical Command and Control be delineated?
- What will the medical call signs be?
- Which frequencies will be assigned to medical elements?
- Which frequencies will be assigned to the evacuation assets?
- Who will be responsible for reporting casualties, to whom, and in what format?

Medical Resupply Requirements and Methods

Medical planners must first develop a thorough understanding of the unit's normal medical equipage, supplies, load plans, and pre-mission shortages. For the medical support plan, determinations are made regarding the equipment and supplies that will be initially carried into the target, and a further plan established for a first and second echelon of resupply. For exercises, Class VIII (medical supply) accounts at medical treatment facilities near the training area can be established. Although not normally a unit function, tactical medical planners should also understand the acquisition and availability of blood products, special vaccines, antidotes, and antivenins as required.

Briefs, Rehearsals, and Pre-combat Inspections

Briefs

Typically, the OPORD at all levels should include the tactical medical support plan. The medical brief for this plan should include the following items, at a minimum:

- All identified health threats
- An overview of the Casualty Response System
- Casualty flow
- Key locations (CCPs, HLZs, AXPs, etc.)
- Requesting procedures (CASEVAC, MEDEVAC, assistance, resupply)
- Medic call signs and frequencies
- Tracking and reporting casualties

Rehearsals

Rehearsals allow unit members to familiarize themselves with the briefed plan and to visualize the expected action. Depending on the level and repetition of rehearsal, unit members can develop a thorough familiarity with the sequence of events that will be executed. A rehearsal should be conducted as a scripted event that lays out the operational plan in a sequence of overlapping events. Contingencies and complications can be injected to assess unit member reactions and to practice alternate plans.

Full dress rehearsals provide the most detailed understanding of the operation and involve all unit members executing their expected tasks, flowing through the expected timeline of the event. A full dress rehearsal is essentially a military field exercise—a training event preparing for the real event at a similar location layout. Obviously, full dress rehearsals are the most time- and resource-intensive and cannot be undertaken for short-notice or compressed operational timelines.

A reduced force rehearsal involves only key leadership of subordinates and operational units. Although such rehearsals are less time- and resource-consuming, they are dependent on leaders driving nearly all actions.

Terrain model rehearsals, also known as "rock drills" or "sandbox drills," use miniature depictions of the operational area. Historically, terrain model rehearsals are probably the most commonly used method for rehearsal of military operations. A terrain model can be as simple as sticks and rocks arranged on the ground or as elaborate as scale models of buildings and vehicles. Although miniaturized, a terrain model can provide unit members with a reasonable visualization of the objective and the operational area. Leaders at all levels should use the model to rehearse their missions with subordinates.

Map rehearsals can be used virtually anywhere, using actual maps or sketches of operational areas. Similar to a terrain model, a map rehearsal provides visualization of the objective, but with limits. A map rehearsal usually involves a small number of people who must squeeze together to see the map, and symbols are often used to depict objects and units. Map rehearsals are best left to the most time-sensitive or austere situations, when elaborate exercises or terrain models are simply not possible.

A radio or communications rehearsal, also known as a COMMEX, is a combination of testing communications systems and unit members running through the sequence of events through radio calls. For the communications equipment tests, using the same equipment, same frequencies, and same distances specified in the operational plan will provide the unit with the best insight into whether their equipment will function as needed. If possible, line-of-sight obstacles such as buildings or terrain should be interposed between radios to exactly replicate conditions at the target. For the sequence of event radio calls, the unit should utilize an execution checklist that prescribes a specific sequence of events and deviations with specific code words so that unit members know something has been completed or complicated.

If possible, the unit should exercise the Casualty Response System by rehearsing expected and possible actions on the objective such as the following:

- First responder drills
- Squad casualty response drills (Care Under Fire, TACEVAC request and loading)
- Aid-and-litter team drills
- CCP operations (assembly, security and movement, casualty movement, CCP markings, vehicle parking, link-up procedures, casualty tracking and recording, and triage, treatment, and management of casualties)
- Mass casualty plan
- COMMEX—communications exercise/radio test
- Casualty tracking/accountability

Pre-combat Inspections

Every combat unit should conduct pre-combat inspections (PCIs) prior to launching on a mission. PCI is conducted from the lowest leadership levels to the highest; no one should ever be exempted. Medically this includes the following:

- Individual unit members
  - First aid kits
  - Individual preventive medicine (water purification, chemoprophylaxis)
- Squad casualty response kit
  - Team first responder bags
  - Evacuation equipment (Skedco, litters, etc.)
  - Vehicle-mounted aidbags
- Medic aidbags (pack and/or reconfigure as required)
  - Select appropriate aidbag system for mission requirements
  - Ensure packing list agrees with recommended stockage
- Resupply packages (pack and/or reconfigure per mission requirements)
  - Reconfigure in accordance with mission specifics (ground, air, etc.)
  - Utilize bundles or pull-off configuration as required
  - Pre-position as required with aircraft and vehicles or at staging base with logistics teams
- Medic individual equipment (weapon, night vision device, radio, mission-specific gear)
- Evacuation assets (quads, vehicles, etc.)

Casualty Collection Point Operations

The following is a checklist for the establishment and operation of tactical CCPs.

CCP Site Selection

- Should be reasonably close to the fight.
- Located near areas where casualties are likely to occur.
- Must provide cover and concealment from the enemy.
- Inside a building or on hardstand (an exclusive CCP building limits confusion).
- Should have access to evacuation routes (foot, vehicle, aircraft).
- Proximal to "lines of drift" or paths across terrain that are the most likely to be used when going from one place to another; these are paths of least resistance that offer the greatest ease while taking into account obstacles and modes of transit on the objective.
- Adjacent to tactical choke points (breeches, HLZs, etc.).
- Avoid natural or enemy choke points.
- Choose an area providing passive security (inside the perimeter).
- Good drainage.
- Accessible to evacuation assets.
- Expandable if casualty load increases.

CCP Operational Guidelines

- First Sergeant (1SG) or Platoon Sergeant (PSG) is responsible for casualty flow and everything outside the CCP.
  - Provides for CCP structure and organization (color coded with chemlights).
  - Maintains command and control and battlefield situational awareness.
  - Controls aid-and-litter teams and provides security.
  - Strips, bags, tags, organizes, and maintains casualties' tactical gear outside the treatment area.
  - Accountable for tracking casualties and equipment into and out of CCP and reports to higher command.
  - Moves casualties through CCP entrance/exit choke point, which should be marked with an IR chemlight.
- Medical personnel are responsible for everything inside the CCP.
  - Triage officer sorts and organizes casualties at choke point into appropriate treatment categories.
  - Medical officers and medics organize medical equipment and supplies and treat casualties.
  - EMTs, first responders, and aid-and-litter teams assist with treatment and packaging of casualties.
- Minimal casualties should remain with original element or assist with CCP security if possible.
- KIAs (soldiers, sailors, airmen, or marines killed in action) should remain with original element.

Guidelines for Establishing CCP Inside a Building

- Ensure building is cleared and secured.
  - Enter and assess the building prior to receiving casualties.
  - Use largest rooms.
  - Consider litter/Skedco movement (Can you do it in the area?).
  - Are separate rooms for treatment categories available?
  - Determine location of choke point/triage.
  - Minimize congestion.
- Remove/relocate furniture or obstructions.
- Color code rooms to treatment categories (mark doors, etc.).

CCP Duties and Responsibilities

Tactical Medics

- Triage, treatment, monitoring, and packaging.
- Delegation of treatment.
- Request assistance from other medical or unit assets.
- Provide guidance and recommendations to leadership on casualty management and evacuation.

Unit Leadership and Medical Planners

- Establish and secure CCPs.
- Provide assistance to medics with augmentation and directing aid-and-litter teams.
- Gather and distribute casualty equipment and sensitive items.
- Provide accountability and reporting to higher authority.
- Request evacuation and establish CASEVAC or MEDEVAC link-up points.
- Manage KIA remains.

General Guidelines for CCP Personnel

- Maintain security.
- Maintain command and control.
- Maintain appropriate medical treatment.
- Maintain situational awareness.
- Maintain organization.
- Maintain control of equipment and supplies.
- Maintain accountability.

General CCP Layout Templates

Figure 33-2 through **Figure 33-7** depict common configurations for casualty collection points.

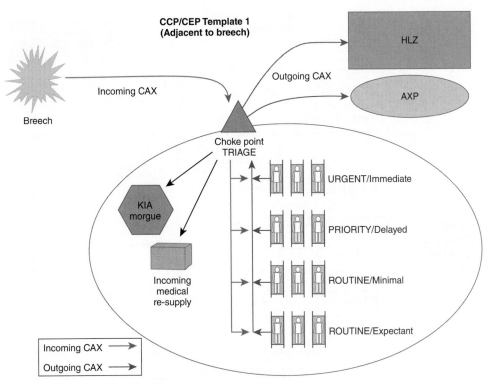

Figure 33-2 CCP/CEP Template 1: Adjacent to breech.

Reproduced from the *Ranger Medic Handbook,* © William Donovan.

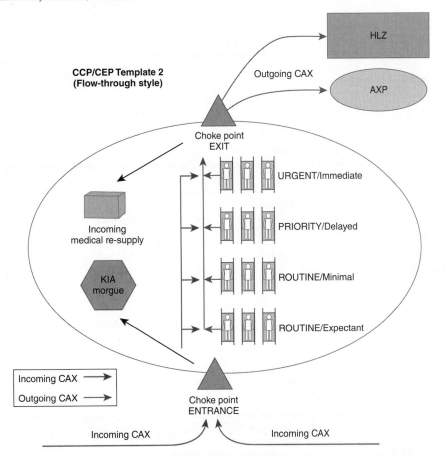

Figure 33-3 CCP/CEP Template 2: Flow-through style.

Reproduced from the *Ranger Medic Handbook,* © William Donovan.

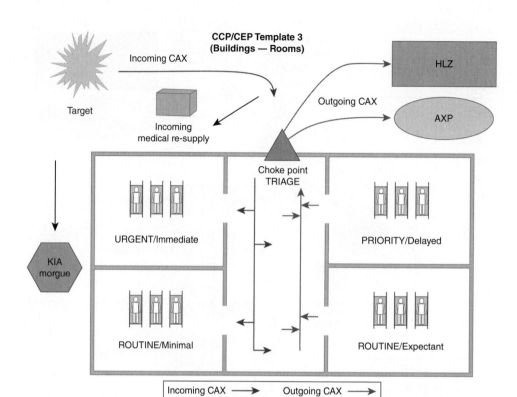

Figure 33-4 CCP/CEP Template 3: Building—rooms.
Reproduced from the *Ranger Medic Handbook*, © William Donovan.

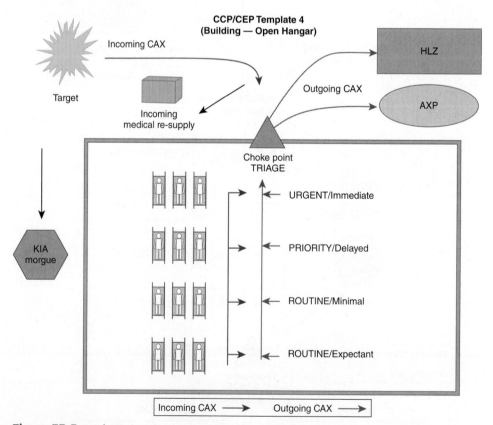

Figure 33-5 CCP/CEP Template 4: Building—open hanger.
Reproduced from the *Ranger Medic Handbook*, © William Donovan.

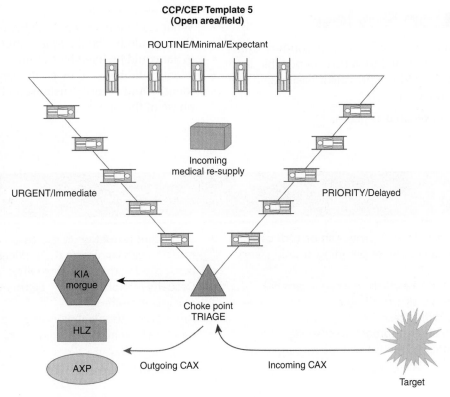

Figure 33-6 CCP/CEP Template 5: Open area/field.

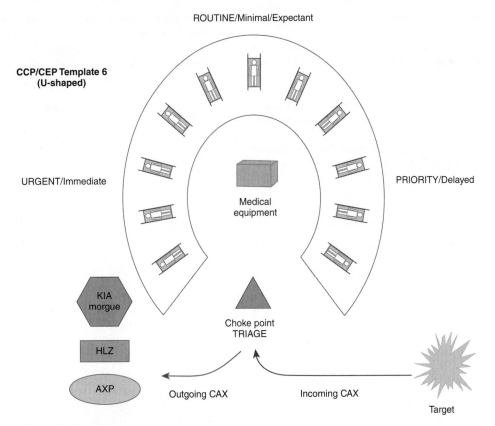

Figure 33-7 CCP/CEP Template 6: U-shaped.

After-Action Review

After each operation, an assessment of its conduct from beginning to end is conducted to gather all possible lessons. The questions listed here provide a basic topic list for the after-action review (AAR):

- Was the mission executed as planned?
- What went right?
- What went wrong?
- What could have been done better?
- What could be fixed by planning/preparation?
- What could be fixed by training?
- What could be fixed by equipment modification?
- Identify and record "sustains and improves" in each phase of the operation.

SUMMARY

- Suboptimal casualty outcomes can be reduced through casualty response planning, training, and rehearsals.
- Directing casualty response management is a tactical leader's task; providing medical expertise is a combat medic's task.
- An integrated team approach to casualty management can directly translate into a significant reduction in the casualty fatality rate and can minimize the tactical turbulence associated with taking casualties.
- Casualty response should be thoroughly exercised in mission training.
- Pre-mission medical planning should cover casualty flow from the point of injury to definitive care.

Suggested Reading

1. Center for Army Lessons Learned. *Medical Planning Newsletter* 04–18, December 2004.
2. Dupuy TN. *Attrition: Forecasting Battlefield Casualties and Equipment Losses in Modern War.* Falls Church, VA: Nova; 1995.
3. Kotwal RS, Meyer DE, O'Connor KC, et al. Army Ranger casualty, attrition, and surgery rates for airborne operations in Afghanistan and Iraq. *Aviat Space Environ Med.* 2004;75(10):833-840.
4. Kotwal RS, Montgomery HR, Hammesfahr JF. *Ranger Medic Handbook.* 3rd ed. Midlothian, TX: Cielo Azul Publications; 2007.
5. Kotwal RS, Montgomery HR, Mechler KK. A prehospital trauma registry for tactical combat casualty care. *J Spec Oper Med.* 2011;11(3):127-128.
6. Shahbaz BA. *Medical Course of Action Tool.* Ver 8b. Alexandria, VA: Altavum Institute; 2006.
7. U.S. Department of Defense. *U.S. Army Ranger Handbook.* New York, NY: Skyhorse Publishing; 2006.

CHAPTER 34

© Ralf Hiemisch/Getty Images.

Medical Support of Urban Operations

Author:
Col. Robert Mabry, MD

CHAPTER OBJECTIVES

At the completion of this chapter, you will be able to do the following:

- List and describe the four distinct levels of urban battle space.
- Describe the effects of urban terrain on communications, navigation, and logistics in combat operations.

- Discuss the injury patterns likely to be encountered during urban operations.
- Discuss adjustments in medical support that should be anticipated for urban combat operations.

SCENARIO

Your platoon is patrolling the streets of Mogadishu on foot when you are suddenly attacked at an intersection by multiple hostiles firing from the street ahead and from windows above. The platoon quickly takes cover in the lobby of an abandoned, shot-up apartment building. Two rocket-propelled grenades (RPGs) strike the outside of the wall that you and two others are kneeling behind, and the wall collapses. The legs of the soldier beside you are trapped by reinforced concrete and cinder blocks. The casualty is alert but in great pain.

The platoon's fire forces the hostiles back. The lobby is secured, and you have good cover from sniper fire. Your platoon leader calls for vehicular extraction; the estimated time of arrival (ETA) is 40 minutes. You are the medic, and you have three casualties to care for.

Casualty 1 has a massive wound to the right side of his head. Heavily disrupted brain tissue is visible. He is unresponsive, has no palpable carotid pulse, and is not breathing.

Casualty 2 is the soldier trapped by the fallen rubble. He is screaming in pain and asking for help to get his legs free. His radial pulse is strong and rapid. Two platoon members are digging him out.

Casualty 3 has a fragment wound to the left side of his neck and mandible, with heavy bleeding from his neck wound. He is leaning forward with blood draining out of his mouth, holding direct pressure on his neck wound with his hand. He is alert and responds to instructions but cannot talk.

- What do you do?

"The future of warfare lies in the streets, sewers, high-rise buildings, industrial parks and the sprawl of houses, shacks, and shelters that form the broken cities of our world."

—Ralph Peters[1]

INTRODUCTION

Warfare in cities is inevitable. Historically, military planners have sought to avoid combat in cities, preferring to isolate, bypass, or avoid them. Urban combat places tremendous demands on resources and manpower, often resulting in large numbers of casualties. Nevertheless, some of the most intense battles in our history have occurred in and around urban areas. Stalingrad, Achen, Manila, Hue, Sarajevo, Mogadishu, Grosny, Fallujah; the very names of these cities conjure images of brutal house-to-house combat.

Since the fall of the Berlin Wall and the end of the Cold War, many new and different threats have emerged. Global terrorism, international criminal activity, the illegal drug trade, and regional despotisms such as Iran and North Korea have replaced the monolithic Soviet military as challenges to our security. Rogue nations and shadowy international terrorist groups like Al-Qaeda, lacking the resources to fight a conventional war against the United States or other western powers, instead seek battles that exploit weaknesses in conventional military power while emphasizing their own strengths. During these "asymmetric" conflicts, terrorism, insurgency, and unconventional guerilla warfare are tactics commonly used by a weaker opponent against a stronger conventional force. The rapidly urbanizing developing world will likely be the setting for many of these future conflicts.

Cities have historically been "centers of gravity" during war. They serve as control points, centers of finance, population, and industry. If current demographic trends continue, by 2030 more than 600 cities will have populations greater than 1 million. By 2025, more than 85% of the world's population will live in and around cities. The modern spectrum of urban conflict is vast; from Stalingrad to the LA riots, there have been an estimated 1.6 million casualties. U.S. military forces must be prepared to fight a determined enemy in the urban environment. General Charles Krulak, former Commandant of the U.S. Marine Corps (USMC), described a "three-block war" wherein we would conduct humanitarian assistance, peacekeeping operations, and intense, highly lethal urban combat in separate parts of the same city.[2]

This chapter provides an overview of planning considerations for health care providers supporting urban operations. Characteristics of the urban battlefield, an overview of likely types of casualties, and training and planning considerations will be discussed. It is difficult to develop specific tactics, techniques, and procedures applicable to all combat medics and corpsmen who may fight in a city. No one-size-fits-all solution is presently available. In future urban battles, combatants and medical providers alike will be required to quickly adapt to the current mission, terrain, and situation.

Urban Terrain

The USMC manual on Military Operations in Urbanized Terrain (MOUT), MCWP 3-35.3, and the Joint Publication 3-06, Doctrine for Joint Urban Operations, are both excellent references for planning urban operations and for descriptions of tactical considerations encountered in urban terrain.

The urban battlefield is a three-dimensional, 360-degree battle space encompassing great variations in terrain. A single city may include deep, dense "urban canyons" with large blocks of tall, multistory buildings with hundreds of rooms and corridors typical of core areas of larger cities; large blocks of industrial areas with factories and warehouses; and sprawling suburban residential areas. Each of these has distinctive characteristics that present unique challenges.

MOUT divides the urban battle space into four distinct levels:

1. **Subterranean level**: consists of sewers, tunnels, networks, subway systems, and underground garages. Here, forces can move unobserved beneath an enemy to attack his rear or flank. Subterranean systems in large cities may be extensive—for example, the New York City subway system or the London Underground.

2. **Street level**: includes broad avenues and highways or narrow back streets and alleys. Generally this level will provide a rapid avenue of approach but will also channelize combatants, making them vulnerable to ambush (**Figure 34-1**). Confined on either side by buildings and structures, the street level can be easily blocked by obstacles such as rubble or disabled vehicles.

3. **Building level**: provides numerous locations for cover and concealment, serving as a vertical barrier to attacking forces while providing multiple fighting positions for defenders. The many rooms and windows of multistory structures offer a variety of positions for snipers while the upper floors provide excellent locations for

antiarmor weapons to be fired down onto vehicles, exploiting weaknesses in their armor.

4. Air level: serves as a high-speed avenue of approach for the insertion and extraction of forces. Aircraft will be vulnerable to manmade obstacles on buildings and rooftops such as power lines, antennae, and radio towers. They will also be subject to small arms and antiaircraft fire from buildings and rooftops (**Figure 34-2**). Aircraft ambushes in urban areas, conducted successfully in the past against U.S. forces in Mogadishu and Russian forces in Chechnya, will make urban air operations difficult and dangerous.

It is likely that on the modern urban battlefield, combat will take place on all of these levels simultaneously.

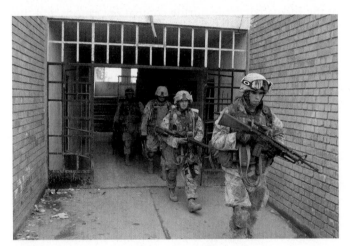

Figure 34-1 The concrete and masonry construction of walls, streets, and buildings form "bullet funnels."

Courtesy of L.Cpl. James J. Vooris/U.S. Marine Corps/Official DoD Photo.

Characteristics of Urban Combat

Urban operations are characterized by intense small-unit, infantry engagements. Fighting will take place at close range, often hand-to-hand (**Figure 34-3**). Because of the three-dimensional nature of the battlefield and the density of numerous man-made structures, troops are often dispersed into small teams.

This greater dispersion of forces will make it difficult for leaders to see and control their forces. Difficulties in communication will increase chaos and confusion. Troops fighting in built-up areas require strong small-unit leaders who possess a high level of situational awareness, flexibility, and initiative.

Operations in built-up areas are manpower, resource, and time intensive. Whereas military planners normally recommend a 3:1 friendly force versus hostile force manpower ratio to conduct offensive operations, urban operations may require a 5:1 ratio. In one war-game scenario conducted by the USMC entitled "Urban Canyon," it was estimated that a dense city "core" area 20 by 20 square blocks with 20- to 60-story buildings would require 49 infantry battalions 10 days to clear, assuming only 10 seconds per room. An operation of this scale would require every squad of infantry in the U.S. Army and Marine Corps.

Radio communications are often degraded by steel and concrete structures. Troops operating in the subterranean level may have no communication capability outside their immediate area. Poor electronic communications combined with the greater dispersion and isolation of forces increases the risk of friendly fire casualties.

Navigation in cities may be challenging. Many cities in developing countries lack organized urban planning.

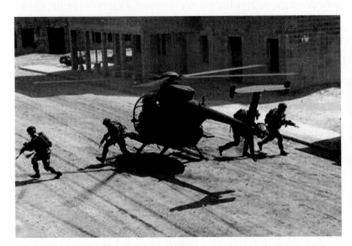

Figure 34-2 Helicopters provide rapid means of infiltration into the urban battlefield but are vulnerable to small arms fire, rocket-propelled grenades, and surface-to-air-missiles.

Courtesy of U.S. Department of Defense.

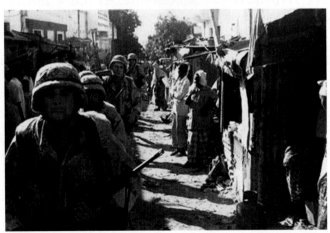

Figure 34-3 The close-quarters nature of urban combat places significant psychological stress on combatants.

Courtesy of U.S. Department of Defense.

As a result, many areas lack street signs and are poorly mapped. Physical factors that interfere with radio communications may also render global positioning systems (GPS) unreliable. Overhead imagery and human intelligence will be crucial for accurate navigation.

The highly intense nature of urban warfare places extraordinary demands on logistical support systems. Requirements for ammunition, fuel, water, food, and medical supplies are significantly higher than those required for a conventional rural battle. Support troops and supply trains will be targeted as they try to deliver food, water, and ammunition to forces in urban combat. Lightly armed logistical and support units may not be able to deliver supplies to areas near intense fighting. Delivery by heavy armored vehicle or by hand may be required, making resupply difficult. Logistical demands will be further increased by the requirement to provide humanitarian relief during the course of the fighting.[3]

Armored vehicles are vulnerable to ambush if not supported by infantry,[4,5] so traditional heavy weapons such as armor and artillery may be of limited use for fighting in cities. For example, during the early stages of the Russian conflict in Chechnya, the Russian 131st Brigade lost 20 of its 26 tanks and 102 of its 120 armored personnel carriers. Its commander and almost 1,000 officers and men died, and 74 were taken prisoner. The Chechens allowed the armored columns, unsupported by dismounted infantry, to enter the city, and lured them into narrow, confined streets. Small groups of Chechen fighters with antitank rockets then attacked the lead and rear vehicles. The columns, effectively isolated from friendly forces and immobilized, were then methodically destroyed.

The Chechens also used "three-tiered" ambushes, directing fire from positions in basements, street-level windows, upper stories, and rooftops simultaneously. Their positions in the subterranean and upper floors were out of the elevation and depression ranges of the Russian guns.[4] Rockets were fired down onto the tanks and armored personnel carriers, exploiting the relatively thin armor of the tops of these vehicles.

During the battle of Stalingrad, the Soviet forces maintained their lines in close opposition to those of the Germans, sometimes as near as 164 feet (50 meters). This tactic not only placed constant psychological stress on the German forces, who feared constant close-range attack, but also negated their substantial air superiority. Chechen forces fighting in Grozny adopted similar tactics.

Restrictive Rules of Engagement

Civilian populations encountered in urban warfare may be armed and hostile, like those encountered by U.S. Army Rangers in Somalia in October 1993. On the other hand, they may simply be innocents caught in the cross fire. Insurgents and terrorists will likely blend in with civilian populations, making target discrimination difficult and increasing the likelihood of unintentional civilian injuries.

U.S. forces and our allies operate with restrictive rules of engagement reflecting morals and values considered proper for a civilized society. Unfortunately, the tactical advantage will often go to the belligerent who disregards or actively endangers the safety of civilians. Civilians may be targeted or held hostage on an urban battlefield by an enemy wishing to create a humanitarian crisis or to manipulate the media. Shocking images of maimed and dead women and children, burned homes, and mourning families will be disproportionately featured by media outlets. This practice will be manipulated by hostile forces, who may stage and time attacks on military or civilian targets to maximize media exposure in order to degrade popular and political support for the conflict. The effects of the media coverage during combat operations and the need to respond to it will often be variables in the decision making of senior military and political leaders.

The unacceptability to the American people of high U.S. casualty rates is another important political consideration. The first Persian Gulf War created a (perhaps false) perception that military operations, relying on high-technology equipment, can be conducted cleanly without casualties or collateral damage.[6]

Casualties

Casualty rates in mid- to high-intensity urban operations are higher than in most conventional operations. The types of injuries encountered in urban fighting vary according the weapons and tactics used by the combatants, although several trends can be identified. In operations where armored vehicles were used extensively, such as the Battle for Grozny during the Russian campaign in Chechnya, injuries from fragments and blasts are common, reflecting the use of antitank munitions, explosive shells from tanks, mortars, artillery, and land mines. Where troops operate in dismounted formations, gunshot wounds from machine gun and assault rifles produce the most serious casualties. During Operation Iraqi Freedom (OIF) and Operation Enduring Freedom (OEF), enemy forces used IEDs to initiate ambushes, resulting in a mix of mutilating blast injuries and penetrating trauma.

Snipers are a common and significant threat when fighting in urban areas (**Figure 34-4**). Urban terrain provides the sniper with numerous hide sites and cover for moving from one position to the next. The sniper can engage at much closer ranges, increasing accuracy. The vulnerable anterior head, face, and neck are often hit.

In Chechnya, snipers prevented rapid medical evacuation, and the wounded frequently could not be moved until nightfall.[3]

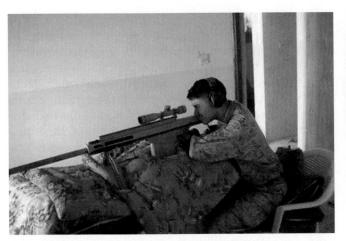

Figure 34-4 Snipers are able to engage targets at much closer ranges, increasing lethality on the urban battlefield.
Courtesy of U.S. Department of Defense.

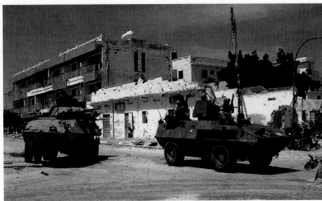

Figure 34-5 Troops mounted on vehicles while fighting in urban areas are not only vulnerable to penetrating and blast injuries but also to blunt trauma from vehicular accidents.
Courtesy of U.S. Department of Defense.

Penetrating Injury

Body armor is critical for survival on the urban battlefield. Contemporary body armor (with front and back plates) used in OEF and OIF has greatly reduced thoracic and upper abdominal injuries. However, improvements in armor for the head and torso have paradoxically resulted in an increased number of severe extremity injuries such as traumatic amputations. U.S. Army Rangers fighting in Somalia experienced nearly 60% fewer fatal chest injuries compared to Vietnam. The incidence of fatal abdominal wounds was not significantly different from the Vietnam conflict because missiles entered through the hips, groin, and abdomen below the area covered by armor. Lethal head injury rates were the same.[7] Future innovations in body armor should make it stronger, lighter, and cooler, while adding coverage to vulnerable areas such as the face, groin, and pelvis.

Other individual protective equipment such as eye protection, gloves, and knee and elbow pads will prevent injury as combatants fight through streets and buildings strewn with rubble. The current emphasis on eye protection during OEF/OIF has saved the sight of many U.S. service members.

Blunt Trauma

Although penetrating wounds from small arms and blasts will produce the greatest number and severity of injuries, severe *blunt* trauma injury must be anticipated in urban combat. Soldiers will fall while climbing up and down buildings. Explosive munitions will create numerous unstable structures that will crush and trap victims. Vehicle crashes, a result of hostile fire or operator fatigue, will produce injuries like those seen daily on American highways (**Figure 34-5**).

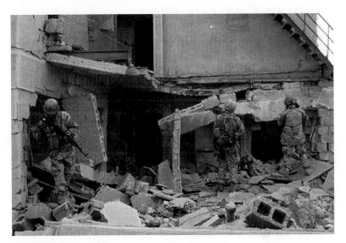

Figure 34-6 Buildings and other structures are subject to collapse when targeted by explosive munitions. Locating and extracting casualties trapped in these structures during a battle will be extremely difficult and dangerous.
Courtesy of U.S. Department of Defense.

Tools used during peacetime urban search and rescue operations such as pry bars, jacks, ropes, and cutting tools, will be needed to extricate wounded soldiers from wrecked vehicles and collapsed structures. Search and rescue is difficult and dangerous enough in a peacetime environment. Locating and rescuing soldiers trapped in collapsed structures during combat will be an incredible challenge (**Figure 34-6**).

Psychological Injury

The intense nature of urban combat may produce more psychological casualties than conventional operations. The Russians experienced more psychiatric casualties while fighting in Chechnya than in their war in Afghanistan. Troops were generally poorly trained conscripts who fought under horrendous conditions. Psychiatric screening of Russian troops who had served in Chechnya revealed that 72% suffered some type of psychological disorder such as insomnia, lack of motivation, anxiety, fatigue, or hypochondriacal fixation.[8] While these findings may not be applicable to professional, well-trained U.S. forces, they do reflect the conditions experienced during intense urban combat. Combat at close range, the constant threat of sniper fire and hidden improvised explosive devices (IEDs), shadowy enemies mixed into the civilian population, and prolonged exposure to the dead and dying will require a regular rotation of not only combat troops but also the medical personnel supporting them. Medical planners should anticipate an increase in combat stress casualties and augment units with mental health professionals trained to treat combat stress disorders.

Civilian Casualties

Large numbers of civilian casualties may be encountered. Medical planners must anticipate the need to care for them. In some instances, civilians can be directed to current and existing local health care facilities. In others, especially in extremely poor countries, large numbers of injured civilians may quickly overwhelm U.S. military medical capabilities and impede their ability to support warfighters. A clear plan for civilian casualty care must be in place before hostilities begin.

Health care providers anticipating battlefield trauma should also be prepared to manage pediatric and geriatric trauma, tropical diseases, nutritional diseases, and poorly managed chronic medical conditions like diabetes.

Medical Preparation for Urban Combat

Wide dispersal of personnel in small units will decrease direct access to casualties by combat medics. Medics will be spread thin and may not be able to reach a wounded soldier only a few meters away during intense fighting. They may also be quickly overwhelmed by multiple casualties. Units fighting in cities must be very well trained in self- and buddy-aid[9] using the principles of tactical combat casualty care (TCCC).

A robust individual first aid kit (IFAK) should include a functional and easily applied field tourniquet, a field dressing, a hemostatic agent, and the medications recommended by the Committee on Tactical Combat Casualty Care (CoTCCC). Units receiving more advanced medical training, such as Special Operations forces, could further augment IFAKs in accordance with their higher level of training.

Units fighting in cities should augment their organic medical capabilities at all levels. For instance, because moving patients over broken, irregular terrain is difficult and hazardous to the casualty, an aid-and-litter team should be designated for each infantry squad. Team members should receive additional medical training with emphasis on TCCC, and each team should be issued a robust squad medical kit including lightweight litters. Support personnel at company and battalion level can be trained in TCCC and serve as additional litter teams.[9] Mounted troops should have an advanced medical kit in every vehicle in case the primary medical vehicle is disabled or destroyed. Individual combat medics should be placed at strong points, at key positions, and with isolated units. During combat in and around Grozny, the Russians augmented each maneuver company with a physician assistant and each battalion with a physician and an ambulance company. Surgeons, anesthetists, and additional nurses manned the regimental medical post.[10] Aid stations and Forward Surgical Teams (FSTs) should be located as far forward as possible, in locations that provide adequate cover, security, and vehicle access such as an underground parking garage or basement.[3]

Medical support personnel present easy, "soft" targets for enemy forces fighting an asymmetric conflict. If medical personnel are to be located well forward, they must be able to provide appropriate security, and they must possess the same battlefield awareness and survival skills as the combatant forces.

Evacuation

Evacuating casualties from the urban battlefield will be difficult and time consuming. Casualties may have to be carried by hand to a secure consolidation point. As discussed earlier, it may take hours to move a litter patient a few hundred yards over broken, exposed terrain covered by enemy fire. Unarmored vehicles and ambulances will likely be targeted as they evacuate casualties. Even armored vehicles are vulnerable. The M113 armored personnel carrier was called a "death trap" for evacuation of casualties during the 1982 conflict in Beirut.[5] They were attacked from the upper floors of buildings with RPGs that penetrated the thinner armor on the top of the vehicle. Heavy armor such as the battle tank was used successfully to evacuate casualties during the Battle of Beirut[5] and by U.S. Marines fighting the Battle for Hue during the Tet Offensive in Vietnam. The fighting in Grozny[11] and Mogadishu[12] proved the need for an armored ambulance resistant to small arms and RPG fire that can maneuver over rubble-strewn streets. The Army's Stryker medical evacuation vehicle, for example, can transport four patients on standard NATO litters or six ambulatory patients, in addition to an ambulance team of three.

Helicopter evacuation is more dangerous in urban conflict than during conventional operations. The density of urban structures and the proximity of hostile combatants allow few landing zones. Even when a physically adequate landing zone is available, it is likely to be covered by enemy fire from rooftops and upper floors. Helicopters have been downed by small arms fire during numerous urban battles. RPGs, Stingers, and machine-gun fire proved effective in disabling moving aircraft in both Afghanistan and Iraq. During the Russian fighting in Grozny, the wounded were normally evacuated to the regimental medical post by armored ambulance. Evacuation by helicopter was used far less than in the Russo-Afghani conflict, especially after several MEDEVAC helicopters were lost to enemy fire.[10]

Infectious Disease

Infectious disease is a major threat during urban conflicts. Many areas of the developing world where future conflicts are likely have poor public health infrastructure, contaminated water supplies, poor sanitation, and high levels of endemic disease. Military conflict will overwhelm the meager health and sanitation infrastructures of large poverty-stricken cities that compose much of the third world (**Figure 34-7**).

Humanitarian crises generated by armed conflict in these settings can be massive and may endanger tactical and strategic aims.

Soldiers interacting with civilians and enemy prisoners will be exposed to endemic diseases such as tuberculosis, malaria, and leishmaniasis. Sexually transmitted diseases such as gonorrhea, syphilis, hepatitis, and HIV will also pose a serious risk to soldiers if they mix socially with locals. Barrier and personal protective measures should be provided as a force health protection measure.[8]

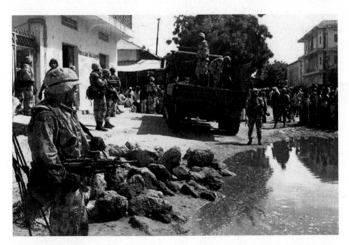

Figure 34-7 Sanitation may be nonexistent in areas affected by urban conflict.
Courtesy of U.S. Department of Defense.

Disease vectors such as rats, lice, ticks, and mosquitoes, as well as feral animals and unburied bodies, will present additional public health hazards.

Potable Water

Potable water will be scarce. Troops engaged in urban and mountainous operations can potentially consume up to 5 to 6 quarts (qt; 4.7–5.7 liters) per day (about 20–24 8-ounce glasses) depending on the soldier's level of physical activity and the weather conditions. As the weather warms, daily consumption can be expected to increase substantially. Less active troops will need to drink about 5 to 7 qt (4.7–6.6 liters) per day; more active troops, 7 to 9 qt (6.6–8.5 liters) per day. Supplying front-line troops with enough water during urban combat will be difficult. Logistical units may not be able to deliver enough water near intense fighting for reasons already mentioned. Water resupply may have to be carried by hand or by armored vehicle, severely limiting quantity and consuming valuable manpower. Thirsty troops may be tempted to drink from local sources that may be heavily contaminated by infectious diseases like hepatitis, intestinal parasites, or industrial waste. In one Russian brigade in Chechnya, 15% of the unit was sick with hepatitis at one time.[13]

The Future

The end of the Cold War left the United States as the sole remaining superpower, with no other nation currently able to match American might on a conventional battlefield. Future struggles will likely see our forces drawn into cities as terrorists, criminals, regional despots, and rogue nations seek to engage and bog us down in asymmetric battles intended to erode the national will. Military and medical planners will continue to struggle to appropriately train and equip our forces in the face of finite resources; to minimize friendly and innocent civilian casualties while isolating and destroying the enemy; to both prevent and mitigate complex humanitarian crises; and to manage intense and often one-sided media scrutiny, all while holding true to the mores and ethics of our military and our society. Tactical and even strategic success in future urban conflicts may well be determined by the thoughtful, deliberate, and proactive execution of medical support.

"They are . . . the post-modern equivalent of jungles and mountains—citadels of the dispossessed and irreconcilable. A military unprepared for urban operations across a broad spectrum is unprepared for tomorrow."

—Ralph Peters[1]

SUMMARY

- Urban combat can involve action on four levels: subterranean, street, building, and air.
- Urban operations are characterized by intense small-unit infantry engagements and are manpower, resource, and time intensive. Navigation, communication, and logistics are all more difficult.
- Engagements are often at close range due to the wide variety and ready availability of cover and concealment in urban environments. Closer engagement allows for more accurate fire.
- Insurgents and terrorists can blend in with the civilian populations. Civilians may be innocents caught up in the conflict or may be armed and hostile.
- Casualty rates are higher in urban as opposed to conventional operations. Penetrating, blunt, and blast trauma should be expected and planned for. Psychological casualty rates may also be higher.
- Medical planning for support of urban operations should include preparations for civilian casualties, complex ground evacuation, infectious diseases, poor sanitation, and advanced first responder care training and equipage.

SCENARIO RECAP

Your platoon is patrolling the streets of Mogadishu on foot when you are suddenly attacked at an intersection by multiple hostiles firing from the street ahead and from windows above. The platoon quickly takes cover in the lobby of an abandoned, shot-up apartment building. Two RPGs strike the outside of the wall that you and two others are kneeling behind, and the wall collapses. The legs of the soldier beside you are trapped by reinforced concrete and cinder blocks. The casualty is alert but in great pain.

The platoon's fire forces the hostiles back. The lobby is secured and you have good cover from sniper fire. Your platoon leader calls for vehicular extraction; the estimated time of arrival (ETA) is 40 minutes. You are the medic, and you have three casualties to care for:

Casualty 1 has a massive wound to the right side of his head. Heavily disrupted brain tissue is visible. He is unresponsive, has no palpable carotid pulse, and is not breathing.

Casualty 2 is the soldier trapped by the fallen rubble. He is screaming in pain and asking for help to get his legs free. His radial pulse is strong and rapid. Two platoon members are digging him out.

Casualty 3 has a fragment wound to the left side of his neck and mandible, with heavy bleeding from his neck wound. He is leaning forward with blood draining out of his mouth, holding direct pressure on his neck wound with his hand. He is alert and responds to instructions but cannot talk.

SCENARIO SOLUTION

- **What do you do?**
  You must first decide where to begin.

- **Who should you treat first and why?**
  First treat Casualty 3 because he may bleed to death in the next few minutes, and the best lifesaving intervention can be applied quickly. Casualty 1 is dead, and you can do nothing further for Casualty 2 until he is freed.

  While you are applying Combat Gauze to the neck wound of Casualty 3, you note an open fracture of the jaw, which is slowly oozing dark red blood. You stop the external bleeding, but the patient continues to lean forward with blood dripping from his mouth.

- **What do you do next?**
  Check for other wounds. There are none.

- **Does he need an IV?**
  Yes. You controlled the bleeding before he went into shock, so he does not need IV fluid resuscitation at this point, but he probably should not try to swallow antibiotic pills. Antibiotics can be given intramuscularly, but he may have already lost significant blood volume and may lose more during evacuation, so you elect to start an IV.

  You place a field-appropriate IV line and give ertapenem, 1 g IV.

- **What else do you want to do?**
  Provide analgesia, if needed. Ketamine can be given via the IV if pain is severe. Monitor the casualty's breathing after ketamine is given.

- **Should you lay the patient down?**
  No.

- **Why not?**
  He is maintaining a patent airway on his own. If he is forced to lie on his back, the blood now dripping from his mouth will drain into his airway.

- **If the patient becomes unconscious, what should you do?**
  Unconsciousness may be from either airway obstruction or blood loss. First place him in the rescue position and listen for continued spontaneous respiration while you look quickly to determine if heavy bleeding has resumed. Address any life-threatening hemorrhage, and then attend to his airway. A pulse oximeter may help to identify hypoxia, if present.

- **Even if the casualty breathes on his own in the rescue position, you would probably have to secure his airway to transport him while unconscious. How would you do it?**
  Cricothyrotomy.

  At this point, the enemy's fire remains ineffective. Casualty 2 has just been freed from the rubble. He is still complaining loudly of great pain in his legs, and his radial pulse is strong. You remove his boots and socks and cut his pant legs open. His left lower leg has been badly crushed, and there is diffuse oozing of blood over the calf. There is gross instability and crepitance at the mid-tibial level. His left foot looks normal when you take off his boot, and the dorsalis pedis pulse is normal. He cannot, however, feel your touch on his foot or wiggle his toes. His right calf is badly bruised diffusely, but skeletal, vascular, and neurologic exams of the right lower leg and foot are normal.

- **What do you do first?**
  You check him carefully for other injuries and find none.

- **What do you do next?**
  Dress and splint the left lower leg.

  You reassess vascular and neurologic status, which are unchanged.

- **What else does he need?**
  Administer moxifloxacin and oral transmucosal fentanyl citrate.

- **What about an IV?**
  He does not need one at this point, but a saline lock would not hurt since you have time and security.

  Your platoon leader has called for reinforcements and tactical evacuation for the casualties. The ETA has been delayed and is still 50 minutes away. Your platoon is keeping the hostiles at bay.

- **What do you do during this interval?**
  You should repeatedly reassess the casualties, and you might want to dress the head wound of the deceased. Ensure the casualties are protected from hypothermia.

References

1. Peters R. Our soldiers, their cities. *Parameters, US Army War College Quarterly*. 1996;26(1):43-50.

2. Krulak, CC. The three block war: fighting in urban areas. *Vital Speeches of the Day*. 1997;139.

3. Grau, LW, Thomas, TL. "Soft log" and the concrete canyons: Russian urban combat logistics in Grozny. *Marine Corps Gazette*. 1999;Oct:67-75.

4. Grau, LW. *Changing Russian Urban Tactics: The Aftermath of the Battle for Grozny*. Washington, DC: INSS Strategic Forum; 1995:38.

5. Yheskel B. *Military Operations in Urbanized Terrain (MOUT), Medical Aspects, Lebanon War 1982-A Case Study*. Bethesda, MD: Uniformed Services University of the Health Sciences; 1985.

6. Akers FH, Singleton GB. *Task Force Ranger: A Case Study Examining the Application of Advanced Technologies in Modern Urban Warfare*. Oak Ridge, TN: National Security Program Office, Oak Ridge Y-12 Plant; 2000.

7. Mabry RL, Holcomb JB, Baker AM, et al. US Army Rangers in Somalia. *J Trauma*. 2000;49:515-528.

8. Novikov VS. The psychophysiological support of the combat activities of servicemen. *Voen Med Zh*. 1996;317(4): 37-40.

9. Grau LW, Gbur CJ. Mars and Hippocrates in megapolis: urban combat and medical support. *Army Med Dept J*. 2003;(PB 8-03-1/2/3 Jan/Feb/Mar):19-26.

10. Grau LW, Jorgensen WA. Handling the wounded in a counter-guerrilla war: the Soviet/Russian experience in Afghanistan and Chechnya. *Army Med Dept J*. 1998;Jan/Feb:2-10.

11. Savvin Y. Za zhizni voinov [For the lives of warriors]. *Armeyskiy sbornik* [Army Digest]. 1995;45.

12. Butler FK, Hagmann JH, Richards DT. Tactical management of urban warfare casualties in special operations. *Mil Med*. 2000;165(Suppl 4):1-48.

13. Grau LW, Jorgensen WA. Viral hepatitis and the Russian war in Chechnya. *Army Med Dept J*. 1997;(May/Jun):2-5.

CHAPTER 35

© Ralf Hiemisch/Getty Images.

Ethical Considerations for the Combat Medic

Authors:
Col. (Ret) Frank Anders, MD
Capt. (Ret) Frank Butler, MD

It is the duty of any military force to wage war, and in the absence of war, to prepare for it.

—General Douglas MacArthur[1]

INTRODUCTION

First, a clarification: Some individuals believe that combat medical personnel are exclusively medics and not combatants; this is not true. Combat medics, corpsmen, and pararescuemen are an integral part of their unit's fighting force who have an additional mission to treat the combat wounded. In the U.S. military today, medics wear no red cross on their helmet or chest, and they typically carry the same weapons as other unit members.

Ethics in Conflict

War is prosecuted by killing people and destroying things. It ends when the enemy capitulates or is totally annihilated, whichever comes first. We are charged as combat medics to render care in order to relieve pain and suffering, to friend and foe alike. This seems like a paradox, especially in the Special Operations setting where the medic is also a belligerent. In fact, it is not. Although some argue that combat itself is so highly unethical as to defy attempts to apply ethical precepts, some cultures have specific ethical principles for engaging in combat.[2]

The focus of every soldier in combat, medic or not, should be support of his fellow warriors in completion of their primary mission. Once the tactical situation is secure, attention can be turned to those in need of care. The practical sense of this approach is borne of the

historical fact that those with medical expertise in hostile engagements are always a small minority. If the medic becomes a casualty, the quality of care in the local theater drops dramatically. Therefore, it is clear that for the sake of those who might benefit from his or her attention, the medic should predicate his or her actions on the tactical situation. Articles 12 and 13 of the First Geneva Convention of 1949 dictate that the wounded should be cared for in the order of severity of their wounds without regard to their status as friendly or hostile.[3] However, this is not to suggest that a medic should abandon his duty to his mission to tend enemy wounded before the immediate fight has ended.

In every war—save some specific battles—succor, however meager, has been afforded to surviving enemy combatants. The first war in which medical care and transport of wounded was organized and standardized was the American Civil War. Both sides had high morbidity and mortality rates, and tragically, both sides were American. Over 400,000 were wounded and over 204,000 killed.[4] Both sides had Surgeons General and Medical and Ambulance Corps. In 1863, at the height of that terrible war, Major General J.E.B. Stuart issued Cavalry Tactic, General Order number 26: "The Ambulance Corps alone will be allowed to remove the wounded, and all will bear in mind that our first duty to our wounded is to win the victory."[5] The goal of the combat medic should be to give aid to as many who need it as possible within the limits of time available and the tactical situation. It is not necessary to hate one's enemy in order to kill him or love him in order to treat his wounds. It is simply expeditious and proper to remember your duty to your country, comrades in arms, and your fellow man and to apply your talent, skills, and training as opportunity presents. Triage and treatment require judgment and decisiveness to be maximally effective.

The principles and ethics of triage for medical personnel are written about at length in Chapter 7 of Part I of the *Textbook of Military Medicine*.[2] This historical review gives much food for thought regarding those factors that are influential in the formation ethical precepts. In part, it reads:

> In ordinary emergency situations the most seriously ill might be allowed to die so that limited medical resources can be devoted to salvaging the lives and limbs of the seriously injured. In combat settings, this might be carried a step further in rendering care first to those most likely to carry out the combat mission, that is, the lightly wounded combat stress casualties. The military is mission driven and resource scarce, and this creates ethical dilemmas in terms of individual survival. Differing perspectives on impairment result in a conflict between putting the mission first versus the risk of increased morbidity. The principle of military triage holds that individual soldiers' interests can be sacrificed when necessary either for the medical welfare of other soldiers or to further military goals. Yet, triage and different degrees of risk taking by certain groups is less than fully analogous. When triage takes place, no group is singled out on the basis of some pre-existing characteristic that subjects some to a greater risk of morbidity or death.

Ethics, like judgment, can be taught but not guaranteed.

Ethics and Prisoners of War

Incarceration, isolation, and even physical restraints are methods sometimes necessary to deny the enemy the opportunity to continue hostile acts. These are not to be misconstrued as acts of torture or abuse. Admiral Raphael Semmes captured or sank 67 enemy vessels with the single unescorted ship he commanded during the American Civil War, a record that stands unbroken. He took many prisoners, including wounded. When the tactical situation dictated (i.e., more prisoners than crew to guard them), he put them in irons. Because his side lost and he had been extraordinarily effective as a Confederate naval commander, the victorious government of the North charged him after the war with being a "privateer" (pirate) during the war. Many of his former prisoners were called to testify during his several-month-long trial. Not a single one alleged mistreatment or torture despite the irons or meager rations for weeks when shipboard rations were short. He was completely exonerated.[6] When applied, the Golden Rule is truly golden.

Management of Wounded Hostile Combatants

As outlined in the preceding chapters in this text, combat medical personnel face the unique challenge of integrating the medical care they provide to combat wounded with the specifics of their unit's tactical situation. Thus, during Care Under Fire—an active battle with hostile forces—no care is rendered to hostile combatants. Even members of the medic's unit are treated only with limb tourniquets, preferably self-applied, for life-threatening extremity hemorrhage. Furthermore, if the casualty is able, he or she is expected to continue to assist in carrying out the unit's mission and engaging with hostile forces. During Tactical Field Care and Tactical Evacuation Care, the medic renders to care to all wounded combatants who require it, both hostile and friendly, *after* the hostile combatants have indicated surrender, have been searched for weapons and explosives, and have been appropriately restrained so that they no longer present a threat to the treating medic or to the other members of the medic's unit. After these essential steps have been taken, combat medical personnel treat all the wounded based on the immediacy of their need for lifesaving interventions. It is essential that medical personnel providing treatment throughout the continuum of care remember that a wounded enemy combatant may continue to have hostile intent and do whatever is possible to harm friendly forces.

SUMMARY

Merriam-Webster's Collegiate Dictionary defines *ethics* as: (a) "a set of moral principles or values" and (b) "the principles of conduct governing an individual or group of individuals."[7] The history of the application of principles of conduct, moral and otherwise, among humans fills many volumes. Those ethics range from "Kill 'em all and let God sort 'em out" to "Treat friend and foe with equal love and kindness." It is not the purpose of this text to dictate a particular ethic but to remind military caregivers that those who may someday sit in judgment of their actions will certainly use a set of values by which to measure the appropriateness of those actions.

As outlined in the preceding chapters in this text, combat medical personnel face the unique challenge of integrating the medical care they provide to combat wounded with the specifics of their unit's tactical situation. Thus, during Care Under Fire—an active battle with hostile forces—no care is rendered to hostile combatants. Even members of the medic's unit are treated only with limb tourniquets, preferably self-applied, for life-threatening extremity hemorrhage. Furthermore, if the casualty is able, he or she is expected to continue to assist in carrying out the unit's mission and engaging with hostile forces. During Tactical Field Care and Tactical Evacuation Care, the medic renders care to all wounded combatants who require it, both hostile and friendly, *after* the hostile combatants have indicated surrender, have been searched for weapons and explosives, and have been appropriately restrained so that they no longer present a threat to the treating medic or to the other members of the medic's unit. After these essential steps have been taken, combat medical personnel treat all the wounded based on the immediacy of their need for lifesaving interventions. It is essential that medical personnel providing treatment throughout the continuum of care remember that a wounded enemy combatant may continue to have hostile intent and do whatever is possible to harm friendly forces.

When treating wounded hostile combatants on the battlefield, care is rendered according to medical need to both friendly and hostile forces. Medical care for wounded hostile combatants, however, is rendered only after those individuals have dropped their weapons; indicated their wish to surrender; have been searched to ensure that they have no more weapons or explosive charges; and have been restrained and denied the ability to communicate with others as tactically appropriate.

References

1. McArthur D. Public Address 1949. In: Taylor RL, Rosenbach WE, eds. *Military Leadership: In Pursuit of Excellence.* 4th ed. Boulder, CO: Westview Press; 2000.

2. Department of the Army. *The Textbook of Military Medicine.* Washington, DC: Borden Institute, Office of the Surgeon General, U.S. Army; 1994.

3. International Committee of the Red Cross. Convention (1) for the Amelioration of the Condition of the Wounded and Sick in Armed Forces in the Field. http://www.icrc.org/ihl.nsf/full/365?opendocument. Accessed April 18, 2013.

4. Kuz JE, Bengston BP. *Orthopaedic Injuries of the Civil War: An Atlas of Orthopaedic Injuries and Treatments during the Civil War.* Kennesaw, GA: Kennesaw Mountain Press; 1996:10.

5. McClellan HB. General Orders, No. 26, Hdqrs. Cav. Div., Army Northern VA, July 30, 1863. In: Commander United States War Department. *The War of the Rebellion: A Compilation of the Official Records of the Union and Confederate Armie.* Washington, DC: Government Printing Office; 1880-1901: Series 1, Vol. XXVII, Part III:1055. http://ebooks.library.cornell.edu/cgi/t/text/pageviewer-idx?c=moawar;cc=moawar;idno=waro0045;node=waro0045%3A2;view=image;seq=1057;size=100;page=root. Accessed April 19, 2013.

6. Spencer WF. *Raphael Semmes: The Philosophical Mariner.* Tuscaloosa, AL: University of Alabama Press; 1997.

7. *Merriam-Webster's Collegiate Dictionary.* Ethics. Springfield, MA: Merriam-Webster.

Abbreviated Injury Scale (AIS) An injury categorization system that assigns injuries a value between 1 and 6, with (1) being minor, (2) being moderate, (3) being serious, (4) being severe, (5) being critical, and (6) being unsurvivable.

abuse The willful infliction of injury, unreasonable confinement, intimidation, or cruel punishment resulting in physical or psychological harm or pain, or the withholding of services that would prevent these events.

acetylcholine A chemical that functions as a neurotransmitter, released at the end of nerve cells to transmit a nervous system impulse.

acid A chemical substance that has a pH less than 7 and that will neutralize an alkali.

acidosis Accumulation of acids and decreased pH of the blood.

active strategy When referring to injury prevention, prevention steps that require the active participation of the individual; e.g., wearing a helmet.

acute mountain sickness (AMS) A constellation of symptoms that result from travel to high altitude (usually above 8,000 feet [2,400 meters]).

acute radiation syndrome The physiologic consequences of whole-body radiation; characterized initially by acute nausea and vomiting, followed by damage to the bone marrow (hematologic syndrome), the gastrointestinal tract, and the cardiovascular/central nervous system.

acute respiratory distress syndrome (ARDS) Respiratory insufficiency as a result of damage to the lining of the capillaries and alveoli in the lung, leading to the leakage of fluid into the interstitial spaces and alveoli.

acute tubular necrosis (ATN) Acute damage to the renal tubules, usually due to ischemia associated with shock.

advance directive A written declaration that describes end-of-life treatment wishes and appoints medical decision makers in the event that the patient is unable to make a medical decision for himself or herself. The two types of written advance directives most often encountered are a living will and a medical power of attorney.

aerosol Solid particles and liquid particles that are suspended in air.

afterload The pressure against which the left ventricle must pump out (eject) blood with each beat.

air density As used in this text, the property of organs having approximately the same weight and density as air; e.g., lung tissue.

air-purifying respirator (APR) A device that uses a filter, canister, or cartridge to remove contaminants from ambient air that passes through the air-purifying component and makes the air safe to breathe.

alpha particle A particle emitted during the decay of a radioactive material; consists of two protons and two neutrons, thus giving the particle a positive charge.

alveoli The terminal air sacs of the respiratory tract where the respiratory system meets the circulatory system and gas exchange occurs.

anastomosis A connection between two structures such as two blood vessels or adjacent bowel.

anhidrosis The absence of sweating.

anisocoria Inequality of pupil size.

antecedent Something that occurred earlier in time.

anterior cord syndrome Damage to the anterior portion of the spinal cord, usually as a result of bony fragments or pressure on spinal arteries.

aortography An x-ray study of the aorta in which a radio-opaque contrast material is injected into the circulatory system to show the aorta.

apneic The absence of breathing.

appendicular skeleton That portion of the skeleton that includes the shoulders and arms as well as the pelvis and legs.

arachnoid mater Spiderweb-like transparent membrane between the dura mater and the pia mater; the middle of the three meningeal membranes surrounding the brain.

aspiration pneumonitis Inflammation and pneumonia caused by inhaling gastric contents or vomitus.

assist control (A/C) ventilation A form of mechanical ventilation; breaths may be assisted by the ventilator if the patient triggers the device by adequately attempting to breathe in or will automatically occur if the patient does not breathe.

atelectasis Collapse of alveoli or part of the lung.

atherosclerosis A narrowing of the blood vessels; a condition in which the inner layer of the artery wall thickens while fatty deposits build up within the artery.

atlas The first cervical vertebra (C1); the skull perches upon it.

atropine A chemical that competitively inhibits the effect of acetylcholine at parasympathetic nerve endings; anticholinergic medication; used to treat victims of nerve agent poisoning.

austere environment A setting in which resources, supplies, equipment, personnel, transportation, and other aspects of the physical, political, social, and economic environments are extremely limited.

autonomic nervous system The part of the central nervous system that directs and controls the involuntary functions of the body.

autonomy A competent adult patient's right to direct his or her own health care free from interference or undue influence.

autoregulation The biologic process of detecting change within the system and adjusting for that change; in the circulatory system, the process of maintaining a constant blood flow as blood pressure changes.

awareness level In hazardous materials training, the basic level of knowledge a responder should have, involved recognition of an incident, isolation and protection from exposure, and notification that the incident is happening.

axial loading The force acting on or applied to the long axis of an object; typically refers to force applied to the spine from the head downward; may also result from the weight of the body being applied to the lower part of the spine, as would occur in a fall from a height landing on the feet.

axis The second cervical vertebra (C2); its shape allows for the wide possible range of rotation of the head. Also, an imaginary line that passes through the center of the body.

baroreceptor A sensory nerve ending that is stimulated by changes in blood pressure. Baroreceptors are found in the walls of the atria of the heart, vena cava, aortic arch, and carotid sinus.

barotrauma Injury to air-containing organs that results from a change in air pressure.

basal level Baseline or minimal level.

basal metabolic rate The number of calories the body burns while at rest, resulting in heat production as a by-product of metabolism.

base A chemical with a pH greater than 7; dissolves in water and releases hydroxide ions or accepts hydrogen ions; causes liquefaction necrosis of tissue.

basilar skull fracture A fracture of the floor of the cranium.

behavioral regulation An individual's conscious response to environmental thermal change and the physical actions taken to keep warm or cool.

beneficence An ethical term that means "to do good"; requires prehospital care providers to act in a manner that maximizes the benefits and minimizes the risks to the patient.

beta particle A high-speed or high-energy electron emitted from radioactive decay.

biologic agent A bacterium, virus, or toxin that can be used as a weapon of mass destruction.

blast lung injury (BLI) Results from exposure to high-order explosive blast overpressure wave; lung damage varies from scattered petechiae to contusions and pulmonary hemorrhage.

blast overpressure Pressure exceeding normal atmospheric pressure that results from a high-order explosive detonation.

blast wave A sharply defined wave front of increased pressure that propagates outward from the center of an explosion.

blast wind The result of the sudden displacement of air from an explosion.

blind nasotracheal intubation (BNTI) A technique of inserting an endotracheal tube through the nares into the trachea without visualizing the larynx and vocal cords.

blister agent A chemical that creates burnlike injuries; used as a weapon of mass destruction.

blunt trauma Nonpenetrating trauma caused by a rapidly moving object that impacts the body.

bradypnea Abnormally slow breathing rate; usually less than 12 breaths per minute.

brain stem The stemlike part of the brain that connects the cerebral hemispheres with the spinal cord.

bronchioles The small divisions of the bronchial tubes through which air passes to the alveoli.

Brown-Séquard syndrome A condition caused by penetrating injury that involves hemitransection of the spinal cord; only one side of the cord is involved.

capillary The smallest type of blood vessel. These minute blood vessels are only one cell wide, allowing for diffusion and osmosis of oxygen and nutrients through the capillary walls.

capnography The method of measuring and monitoring the partial pressure of carbon dioxide in a sample of gas. It can correlate to the arterial partial pressure of carbon dioxide ($Paco_2$).

cardiac output The volume of blood pumped by the heart (reported in liters per minute).

cardiac tamponade Compression of the heart from an accumulation of fluid in the pericardium surrounding the heart; in the case of trauma, the fluid is usually blood; the accumulation of fluid prevents normal blood return to the heart by compressing the heart, thus impairing circulation.

care under fire (CUF) A phase of care in tactical casualty care; refers to the limited medical care that can be provided to a trauma victim while in a hostile situation such as an active shooter incident; also referred to as direct threat care.

casualty collection point A location used for the collection, triage, treatment, and evacuation of casualties from a multiple-casualty incident.

cataract A condition of the eye in which the lens becomes progressively more opaque and blocks and distorts light entering the eye and blurs vision.

catecholamines A group of chemicals produced by the body that work as important nerve transmitters. The main catecholamines made by the body are dopamine, epinephrine (also called adrenalin), and norepinephrine. They are part of the body's sympathetic defense mechanism used in preparing the body to act.

caudad Toward the tail (coccyx).

cavitation The act of forcing tissues of the body out of their normal position; to cause a temporary or permanent cavity (e.g., when the body is struck by a bullet, the acceleration of particles of tissue away from the missile produces an area of injury in which a large temporary cavity occurs).

cellular respiration The use of oxygen by the cells to produce energy.

central cord syndrome Damage to the central portion of the spinal cord that usually occurs with hyperextension of the cervical area; characterized by weakness or paralysis of the upper extremities but not the lower extremities.

central neurogenic hyperventilation Pathologic rapid and shallow ventilatory pattern associated with head injury and increased intracranial pressure.

cerebellum A portion of the brain that lies beneath the cerebrum and behind the medulla oblongata and is concerned with coordination of movement.

cerebral perfusion pressure The amount of pressure needed to maintain cerebral blood flow; calculated as the difference between the mean arterial pressure (MAP) and the intracranial pressure (ICP).

cerebrospinal fluid (CSF) A fluid found in the subarachnoid space and dural sheath; acts as a shock absorber, protecting the brain and spinal cord from jarring impact.

cerebrum The largest part of the brain; responsible for the control of specific intellectual, sensory, and motor functions.

chemical energy The energy, usually in the form of heat, that results from the interaction of a chemical with other chemicals or human tissue.

chemoreceptor A sensory nerve ending that is stimulated by and reacts to certain chemical stimuli; located outside of the central nervous system. Chemoreceptors are found in the large arteries of the thorax and neck, the taste buds, and the olfactory cells of the nose.

chemosis A watery swelling of the covering (conjunctiva) of the eye.

chilblains Red or purple skin lesions on the skin that are itchy and painful and appear after cold exposure, particularly in patients with poor underlying circulation.

choke A constriction in the barrel of a shotgun to decrease the amount of pellet spread after firing.

chronic traumatic encephalopathy (CTE) A progressive degenerative brain disease thought to occur primarily in athletes with a history of repetitive brain trauma and primarily seen with contact sport athletes. Symptoms include deteriorating attention, concentration, and memory; disorientation and confusion; and occasional dizziness and headaches.

cilia Hairlike processes of cells that propel foreign particles and mucus from the bronchi.

circumferential burn A burn that encompasses an entire body part such as the arm, leg, or chest.

classic heatstroke A disorder that results from exposure to high humidity and high temperature, characterized by elevated body temperature above 104°F (40°C) and neurologic abnormalities (altered mental status).

closed fracture A fracture of a bone in which the overlying skin is not interrupted.

coagulative necrosis The type of tissue damage that results from acid exposure; the damaged tissue forms a barrier that prevents deeper penetration of the acid.

coagulopathy Impairment in the normal blood-clotting capabilities.

cold-induced diuresis Increased urine production as a result of peripheral vasoconstriction from exposure to cold.

cold-induced vasodilation (CIVD) Physiologic response that occurs once an extremity has been cooled to 50°F (10°C) in an effort to provide some protection from the cold.

command staff The public information officer, safety officer, and liaison officer; they report directly to the incident commander.

command The first component of the incident command system, responsible for all incident oversight and management. It is the only position in the incident command system that must always be staffed.

commission A purposeful act.

commotio cordis Sudden cardiac dysrhythmia, often fatal, that results from a blow to the anterior chest or sternum.

compartment syndrome The clinical findings noted from ischemia and compromised circulation that can occur from vascular injury, causing hypoxia of muscles in an extremity compartment. The cellular edema produces increased pressure in a closed fascial or bony compartment.

competence (1) A legal term referring to a person's general ability to make good decisions for himself or herself; (2) the ability, skill, knowledge, and qualification to do something successfully.

complete cord transection Complete damage and severing of the spinal cord; all spinal tracts are interrupted, and all normal neurologic functions distal to the site are lost.

comprehensive emergency management The steps needed to manage an incident, consisting of four components: mitigation, preparation, response, and recovery.

compressibility The ability to be deformed by the transfer of energy.

compression injury An injury caused by severe crushing and squeezing forces; may occur to the external structure of the body or to the internal organs.

compression The type of force involved in impacts resulting in a tissue, organ, or other body part being squeezed between two or more objects or body parts.

conduction The transfer of heat between two objects in direct contact with each other.

confidentiality The obligation of health care providers to not share patient information that is disclosed to them within the patient–provider relationship to anyone other than those the patient has authorized, other medical professionals involved in the patient's care, and agencies responsible for processing state and/or federally mandated reporting.

conjunctiva The clear (usually) mucous membrane that covers the sclera (white part of the eye) and lines the eyelids.

contact wound The type of wound that occurs when the muzzle of a gun touches the patient at the time of discharge, resulting in a circular entrance wound, often associated with visible burns, soot, or the imprint of the muzzle.

convection The transfer of heat from the movement or circulation of a gas or liquid, such as the heating of water or air in contact with a body, removing that air (such as by wind) or water, and then having to heat the new air or water that replaces what left.

cord compression Pressure on the spinal cord caused by swelling, bone fragments, or hematoma, which may result in tissue ischemia and, in some cases, may require decompression to prevent a permanent loss of function.

cord concussion The temporary disruption of the spinal cord functions distal to the site of a spinal cord injury.

cord contusion Bruising or bleeding into the tissue of the spinal cord, which may also result in a temporary loss of cord functions distal to the injury.

cord laceration An injury that occurs when spinal cord tissue is torn or cut.

core temperature (1) The temperature at which vital organs are maintained and function best; (2) the measured temperature of the deep structures and organs of the body.

cornea The dome-shaped transparent outer portion of the eye that covers the pupil and colored iris.

coup-contrecoup injury (brain injury) An injury to the brain that occurs when the head strikes a fixed object, causing an injury at the site of impact (coup) and an injury on the opposite side (contrecoup), where the brain collides with the opposite side of the skull.

cranial vault The space within the skull or cranium.

crepitus A crackling sound made by bone ends grating together.

critical incident stress management (CISM) A group of intervention strategies used to help prevent and manage stress after an incident.

Cushing phenomenon The combination of increased arterial blood pressure and the resultant bradycardia that can occur with increased intracranial pressure.

cyanosis Blue coloring of skin, mucous membranes, or nail beds indicating unoxygenated hemoglobin and a lack of adequate oxygen levels in the blood; usually secondary to inadequate ventilation or decreased perfusion.

debridement The removal, usually surgically, of dead or damaged tissue.

decerebrate posturing Characteristic posture that occurs when a painful stimulus is introduced; the extremities are stiff and extended and the head is retracted. One of the forms of pathologic posturing (response) commonly associated with increased intracranial pressure.

decomposition A state of decay or rotting.

decompression sickness (DCS) A group of disorders that result from the effects of increased pressure on gases in a diver's body.

decontamination Reduction or removal of hazardous chemical, biologic, or radiologic agents.

decorticate posturing A characteristic pathologic posture of a patient with increased intracranial pressure; when a painful stimulus is introduced, the patient is rigidly still with the back and lower extremities extended while the arms are flexed and fists clenched.

deep frostbite Freezing of tissue that affects skin, muscle, and bone.

delayed primary closure Delayed suturing of a wound for 48 to 72 hours to allow any swelling to go down and to ensure that there are no signs of infection.

delayed-sequence intubation (DSI) A technique of medication-assisted intubation that emphasizes preoxygenation with CPAP and apneic oxygenation during intubation.

delirium An abrupt change in mental status secondary to an acute medical condition; generally reversible once the underlying acute process is corrected.

dementia The general term for a decrease in cognitive capabilities that causes interference with daily life.

denuded Having the covering or surface layer removed.

dependent lividity The settling or pooling of blood in the lowest lying portions of a deceased body.

dermatome The sensory area on the body for which a nerve root is responsible. Collectively, they allow the body areas to be mapped out for each spinal level and to help locate a spinal cord injury.

dermis The layer of skin just under the epidermis made up of a framework of connective tissues containing blood vessels, nerve endings, sebaceous glands, and sweat glands.

designated incident facility An assigned location where specific incident command system functions are performed; for example, incident command is located at the incident command post.

devitalized Lifeless or dead.

diaphragm The dome-shaped muscle that divides the chest and abdomen and that functions as part of the breathing process.

diastole Ventricular relaxation (ventricular filling).

distraction The pulling apart of two structures; e.g., pulling apart the fractured components of a bone or part of the spine.

diverter A device on a shotgun to spread the pellets into a wider, horizontal path when fired.

do-not-resuscitate (DNR) order (out-of-hospital medical order) An order given by a physician to ensure that prehospital care providers do not perform CPR on a terminally ill patient at home or in some other community or nonclinical setting against the patient's wishes.

dorsal root The spinal nerve root responsible for sensory impulses.

DUMBELS A mnemonic that represents the constellation of symptoms associated with the muscarinic effects of nerve agent toxicity (diarrhea, urination, miosis, bradycardia, bronchorrhea, bronchospasm, emesis, lacrimation, salivation, sweating).

dura mater The outer tough membrane covering the spinal cord and brain; the outer of the three meningeal layers. Literally means "tough mother."

dynamic pressure The component of an explosion that is directional and felt as a blast wind.

dysarthria Difficulty speaking.

dysbarism The changes that result physiologically as a result of changes in ambient environmental pressure.

ecchymosis A bluish or purple irregularly formed spot or area resulting from a hemorrhagic area below the skin.

eclampsia A syndrome in pregnant women that includes hypertension, peripheral edema, and seizures; also called toxemia of pregnancy.

edema A local or generalized condition in which some of the body tissues contain an excessive amount of fluid; generally includes swelling of the tissue.

edentulism The absence of teeth.

effective ventilation Total minute ventilation minus dead space ventilation.

elasticity The ability to stretch.

electrical energy The result of movement of electrons between two points.

endotracheal (ET) tube A plastic tube that is inserted into the trachea to ensure an open airway and used to assist a patient to breathe.

environmental temperature The thermal temperature of the air surrounding an individual.

epidermis The outermost layer of the skin, which is made up entirely of dead epithelial cells with no blood vessels.

epidural hematoma Arterial bleeding that collects between the skull and dura mater.

epidural space Potential space between the dura mater surrounding the brain and the cranium. Contains the meningeal arteries.

epiglottis A leaf-shaped structure that acts as a gate or flapper valve and directs air into the trachea and solids and liquids into the esophagus.

epinephrine A chemical released from the adrenal glands that stimulates the heart to increase cardiac output by increasing the strength and rate of contractions.

epithelial Any tissue that covers a surface or lines a cavity.

eschar Thick scab of dead tissue, often resulting from a burn.

escharotomy An incision made into an eschar to allow the tissues underlying the tough, leathery damaged skin created by severe burns to expand as they swell.

esophagus The muscular tube that connects the mouth to the stomach.

eucapnic state A condition in which the blood carbon dioxide level is within a normal range.

eupnea Normal, unlabored, quiet breathing or respiration.

evaporation Change from liquid to vapor.

event phase The moment of the actual trauma.

evisceration A condition in which a portion of the intestine or other abdominal organ is displaced through an open wound and protrudes externally outside the abdominal cavity.

exercise-associated hyponatremia (EAH) A life-threatening condition associated with excessive consumption of water (1.5 quarts [1.4 liters] or greater per hour) during prolonged activities leading to marked lowering of the sodium concentration in blood.

exercise-associated hyponatremic encephalopathy (EAHE) A life-threatening condition of cerebral edema resulting from lowered sodium concentration in blood from excessive consumption of water (1.5 quarts [1.4 liters] or greater per hour) during prolonged activities.

exertional heatstroke (EHS) A condition of elevated body temperature, usually in males working or exercising in the heat and humidity, characterized by pale, sweaty skin, elevated body temperature, and altered mentation.

exsanguination Total loss of blood volume, producing death.

extracellular fluid All body fluid that is not contained within cells.

extramural (extraluminal) pressure Pressure in the tissue surrounding the vessel.

extreme altitude An elevation higher than 18,045 feet (5,500 meters).

face-to-face intubation A technique for endotracheal intubation in which the endotracheal tube is inserted orally while the intubator is facing the patient instead of being located at the usual location above the head of the patient.

fascia A flat band of tissue that separates different layers; a fibrous band of tissue that encloses muscle.

field exercise A training event that involves the actual execution and performance of the community disaster-response plan.

finance/administration section The section responsible for all costs and financial actions of the incident.

first phase of death Deaths from traumatic injury that occur within seconds to minutes after the injury.

first-degree frostbite Epidermal injury limited to skin that had brief contact with cold air or metal; involved skin appears white or as yellowish plaque; there is no blister or tissue loss; skin thaws quickly, feels numb, and appears red with surrounding edema; healing occurs in 7 to 10 days.

flail chest A chest with an unstable segment produced by multiple ribs fractured in two or more places or including a fractured sternum.

flail sternum A variation of flail chest that involves fracture of the ribs on both sides of the sternum, allowing the sternum to float freely.

fontanelle The soft, membranous space between the unfused bones of an infant's skull; often referred to as the "soft spot."

foramen magnum The opening at the base of the skull through which the medulla oblongata passes.

foramina A small opening; singular is *foramen*.

fourth-degree frostbite A freezing injury that involves the skin, underlying tissue, muscle, and bone.

fragmentation The breaking up of an object to produce multiple parts or shrapnel.

frostbite The freezing of body tissue as a result of exposure to freezing or below-freezing temperatures.

full thickness burn A burn to the epidermis, dermis, and subcutaneous tissue (possibly deeper). Skin may look charred or leathery.

galea aponeurotica A tough, thick layer of tissue underneath the scalp that covers the cranium.

gamma ray A ray of high-energy electromagnetic radiation released as a result of radioactive material decay.

grand mal seizures A generalized seizure that involves loss of consciousness and muscle contractions; also known as tonic-clonic seizure.

group training Disaster response training directed at specific response groups.

Haddon Matrix A table that shows the interaction of host, agent, and environmental factors in an incident.

heat stress index The combination of ambient temperature and relative humidity.

heat syncope Fainting or light-headedness after standing for prolonged periods in a hot

environment; results from vasodilation and venous blood pooling in the legs, causing low blood pressure.

hemiparesis Weakness limited to one side of the body.

hemiplegia Paralysis on one side of the body.

hemothorax Blood in the pleural space.

high altitude An elevation above 5,000 to 11,480 feet (1,500 to 3,500 meters).

high explosive A type of explosive designed to detonate and release its energy very quickly; capable of producing a shock wave, or overpressure phenomenon, that can result in primary blast injury.

high-altitude cerebral edema (HACE) A life-threatening complication of brain swelling that results from travel to high altitude (usually above 8,000 feet [2,400 meters]).

high-altitude pulmonary edema (HAPE) A life-threatening complication of fluid accumulating in the lungs that results from travel to high altitude (usually above 8,000 feet [2,400 meters]).

homeostasis A constant, stable internal environment; the balance necessary to maintain healthy life processes.

homeotherm A warm-blooded animal.

hydrofluoric acid A type of acid; exposure to even small amounts can lead to life-threatening lowering of the serum calcium levels and cardiac dysrhythmias.

hyper-rotation Excessive rotation.

hypercarbia An increased level of carbon dioxide in the body.

hyperchloremic acidosis A type of metabolic acidosis (decrease in blood pH) associated with an increase in the amount of chloride ion in the blood; may result from the administration of large amounts of normal saline.

hyperextension Extreme or abnormal extension of a joint; a position of maximum extension. Hyperextension of the neck is produced when the head is extended posterior to a neutral

position and can result in a fracture or dislocation of the vertebrae or in spinal cord damage in a patient with an unstable spine.

hyperflexion Extreme or abnormal flexion of a joint. A position of maximum flexion. Increased flexion of the neck can result in a fracture or dislocation of the vertebrae or in spinal cord damage in a patient with an unstable spine.

hypertension A blood pressure greater than the upper limits of the normal range; generally considered to exist if the patient's systolic pressure is greater than 140 mm Hg.

hypertonic saline Any solution of sodium chloride in water with a concentration of sodium chloride greater than physiologic saline, which is 0.9% sodium chloride, the same as body fluid.

hyphema A collection of blood in the anterior chamber of the eye, between the clear cornea and the colored iris.

hypobaric hypoxia Hypoxia caused by the decrease in atmospheric pressure and the partial pressure of oxygen at increasingly higher altitudes.

hypochlorite solution A solution used in the production of household bleaches and industrial cleaners.

hypopharynx The lower portion of the pharynx that opens into the larynx anteriorly and the esophagus posteriorly.

hypothalamus The area of the brain that functions as the thermoregulatory center and the body's thermostat to control neurologic and hormonal regulation of body temperature.

hypothermia A condition characterized by core body temperature below normal range, usually between 78°F and 90°F (26–32°C).

iatrogenic Caused by the treatment.

ICS general staff The chiefs of each of the four major sections of the incident command system (ICS): operations, planning, logistics, and finance/administration.

immersion foot A nonfreezing cold exposure injury caused by prolonged immersion of extremities in wet and moisture that is cool to cold; also referred to as trench foot.

impact phase The phase of the disaster cycle that involves the actual incident or disaster.

incident action plan (IAP) A continuously updated outline of the overall strategy, tactics, and risk management plans developed by the incident commander or the incident command system staff.

incident command post (ICP) The location at which incident command functions are performed.

incident command system (ICS) A system that defines the chain of command and organization of the various resources that respond during a disaster.

incident commander (IC) The individual responsible for all aspects of a response to an incident, including developing incident objectives, managing all incident operations, setting priorities, and defining the incident command system organization for the particular response; the IC position will always be filled.

incomplete cord transection Partial transection of the spinal cord in which some tracts and motor/sensory functions remain intact.

independent learning Studying on one's own.

inferior vena cava A major vein that carries deoxygenated blood from the lower half of the body back to the heart.

inhalation The process of drawing air into the lungs.

injury process Similar to disease, a process involving a host, an agent (in the case of injury the agent is energy), and an environment or situation that allows the host and agent to interact.

Injury Severity Score (ISS) An injury categorization system that categorizes injuries into six anatomically distinct body regions, with (1) being the head and neck, (2) being the face, (3) being the chest, (4) being the abdomen,

(5) being the extremities, (6) being external injuries.

injury A harmful event that arises from the release of specific forms of physical energy or barriers to normal flow of energy.

inner perimeter A geographic boundary at a hazardous incident surrounding the area of highest danger and potential lethality.

insensible loss The unmeasured loss of water and heat from exhaled air, skin, and mucous membranes.

integrated communications A communications system that allows all responders at an incident to communicate with supervisors and subordinates.

intentional injury Injury associated with an act of interpersonal or self-directed violence.

intercostal muscles The muscles located between the ribs that connect the ribs to one another and assist with breathing.

interdisaster period (quiescent period) The time in between disasters or mass-casualty incidents during which risk assessment and mitigation activities are undertaken and when plans for the response to likely events are developed, tested, and implemented.

intermediate-range wound A penetrating gunshot wound that occurs at a distance of approximately 6 to 18 feet (1.8 to 5.5 meters).

intermittent mandatory ventilation (IMV) A form of mechanical ventilation that delivers a set rate and tidal volume to patients.

interstitial fluid The extracellular fluid located between the cell wall and the capillary wall.

intervertebral foramen A notch through which nerves pass in the inferior lateral side of the vertebra.

intracellular fluid Fluid within the cells.

intracranial pressure The pressure exerted against the inside of the skull by brain tissue, blood, and cerebrospinal fluid; usually less than

15 mm Hg in adults and 3 to 7 mm Hg in children.

intramural (intraluminal) pressure The pressure exerted against the inside of the walls of blood vessels by the intravascular fluids and blood pressure cycle.

involuntary guarding Rigidity or spasm of the abdominal wall muscles in response to peritonitis.

ionization The process by which a molecule becomes charged by gaining or losing an electron.

iris The colored portion of the eye that contains the adjustable opening of the pupil.

justice That which is fair or just; in medicine, usually refers to how medical resources are distributed with regard to health care.

kill zone The area of greatest risk in a hazardous incident; the area within the inner perimeter.

kinetic energy (KE) Energy available from movement. Function of the weight of an item and its speed: KE = 1/2 of the mass × the velocity squared.

kyphosis A forward, humplike curvature of the spine commonly associated with the aging process. Kyphosis may be caused by aging, rickets, or tuberculosis of the spine.

lactated Ringer solution An intravenous crystalloid solution that is isotonic with blood and used to replenish circulating volume and electrolytes; contains water, sodium, chloride, calcium, potassium, and lactate.

laryngeal mask airway (LMA) An airway management device; the distal end that is inserted into the patient's mouth is shaped like an oval mask to cover the supraglottic structures and isolate the trachea to allow for air passage.

larynx The structure located just above the trachea that contains the vocal cords and the muscles that make them work.

law of conservation of energy A law of physics stating that energy cannot be created or destroyed but only changed in form.

lewisite An oily liquid used as a chemical weapon to produce burnlike blisters; it is a blister agent (vesicant).

liaison officer A command staff member who assists or coordinates with multiple agencies; serves as an intermediary between the incident commander and outside agencies.

Lichtenberg's figures A branching or fernlike reddish skin marking that is painless and results from being struck by lightning.

ligament A band of tough, fibrous tissue connecting bone to bone.

liquefaction necrosis The type of tissue injury that occurs when an alkali damages human tissue; the base liquefies the tissue, which allows for deeper penetration of the chemical.

living will A form of advance directive that expresses a patient's end-of-life treatment wishes, such as whether mechanical ventilation, CPR, dialysis, or other types of life-prolonging or life-sustaining treatments are desired; generally does not go into effect until the patient lacks decision-making capacity and has been certified by a health care professional, usually a doctor, to be either terminally ill or permanently unconscious.

logistics section chief The position responsible for directing the logistics function for the incident commander.

logistics section The section responsible for providing all services, equipment, and facilities for the incident.

long-range wound A penetrating gunshot wound that occurs at a distance greater than 18 feet (5.5 meters).

low explosive A type of explosive that changes relatively slowly from a solid or liquid to a gaseous state (in an action more characteristic of burning than of detonation); because they release their energy much more slowly, low explosives do not produce blast overpressure.

maceration Softening of the skin as a result of exposure to constant moisture; the skin turns white and breaks down and can easily become infected.

maculopapular rash A skin rash characterized by areas of reddish discoloration (macules) in association with small, raised bumps (papules).

magnesium A highly flammable chemical element used to make incendiary weapons; also an essential electrolyte in human physiology.

mammalian diving reflex A reflex that occurs with submersion in cold water (less than 70°F [21°C]) resulting in rapid slowing of the body's metabolism, spasm of the larynx, shunting of blood from the periphery to the heart and brain, and a marked decrease in heart and respiratory rate.

mass-casualty incident (MCI) response The postevent actions taken to minimize damage, morbidity, and mortality resulting from the incident.

mass-casualty incident (MCI) An incident (such as a plane crash, building collapse, or fire) that produces a large number of victims from one mechanism, at one place, and at the same time; also referred to as multiple-casualty incident.

mean arterial pressure (MAP) The average pressure in the vascular system, estimated by adding one-third of the pulse pressure to the diastolic pressure.

mechanical energy The energy that an object contains when it is in motion.

mediastinum The middle of the thoracic cavity containing the heart, great vessels, trachea, main bronchi, and esophagus.

medical power of attorney (MPOA) An advance directive document used by competent adults to appoint someone to make medical decisions for them in the event that they are unable to make such decisions for themselves. Unlike living wills, MPOAs go into effect immediately any time a patient is incapable of making his or her own decision, regardless of preexisting condition, and become inactive again when/if the patient regains decision-making capacity.

meninges Three membranes that cover the brain tissue and the spinal cord: the dura mater, arachnoid, and pia mater.

minute ventilation The amount of air exchanged each minute; calculated by multiplying the volume of each breath (tidal volume) by the number of breaths per minute (rate).

minute volume The amount of air exchanged each minute; calculated by multiplying the volume of each breath (tidal volume) by the number of breaths per minute (rate).

mitigation In emergency medicine, a reduction in the loss of life and property by lessening the impact of disasters.

Monro-Kellie doctrine The sum of the volume of brain tissue, blood, and cerebrospinal fluid must remain constant within an intact skull.

MTWHF A mnemonic that represents the constellation of symptoms associated with stimulation of nicotinic receptors, usually after nerve agent exposure; MTWHF stands for mydriasis (rarely seen), tachycardia, weakness, hypertension, hyperglycemia, fasciculations.

mucocutaneous Made up of or pertaining to both skin and mucous membranes.

multisystem trauma patient A patient with injury to more than one body system.

muscarinic site An acetylcholine receptor found primarily in smooth muscle and glands.

myocardial hypertrophy An increase in the heart's muscle mass and size.

myoglobin A protein found in muscle that is responsible for giving muscle its characteristic red color.

myoglobinuria The release of myoglobin into the bloodstream in considerable amounts, causing a reddish or tea-colored urine, toxicity to the kidneys, and kidney failure.

nasopharyngeal airway (NPA) An airway that is placed in the nostril and follows the floor of the nasal cavity directly posterior to the nasopharynx in order to lift the tongue off of the back of the pharynx and open the airway. This airway is commonly tolerated by patients with a gag reflex.

nasopharynx The upper portion of the airway, situated above the soft palate.

neural arches Two curved sides of the vertebrae.

neutral position The position of a joint that allows for maximal movement; neither flexed nor extended.

Newton's first law of motion A fundamental law of physics stating that a body at rest will remain at rest, and a body in motion will remain in motion unless acted on by an outside force.

Newton's second law of motion A fundamental law of physics stating that the acceleration of an object is directly proportional to the magnitude of the force applied, in the same direction as the force applied, and inversely proportional to the mass of the object.

Newton's third law of motion A fundamental law of physics stating that for every action, there is an equal and opposite reaction.

nicotinic site An acetylcholine receptor found primarily in skeletal muscle.

nitrogen mustard An oily chemical used as a chemical weapon to produce burnlike blisters; can also damage the respiratory tract, gastrointestinal tract, and bone marrow; blister agent; vesicant; also used as an anticancer medication.

nonfreezing cold injury (NFCI) A syndrome resulting from damage to peripheral tissues, caused by prolonged (hours to days) exposure to wet/cold; also called immersion foot or trench foot.

nonmaleficence An ethical principle that obligates the medical provider to not take actions that may harm the patient or place the patient in harm's way.

norepinephrine A chemical released by the sympathetic nervous system that triggers constriction of the blood vessels to reduce the size of the vascular container and bring it more closely into proportion with the volume of the remaining fluid.

normal saline An intravenous crystalloid solution comprising water and sodium chloride in a concentration of 0.9%.

obtunded A condition in which the patient's mental capacity is dulled or diminished; mild to moderate decreased level of consciousness with impaired sensory perception.

oculomotor nerve The third cranial nerve; controls pupillary constriction and certain eye movements.

omentum A fold of peritoneum that covers and connects the stomach to other intra-abdominal organs.

omission The failure to act.

oncotic pressure Pressure that determines the amount of fluid within the vascular space.

open fracture A fracture of a bone in which the skin is broken.

open globe A penetrating injury to the eye; injury that involves the full thickness of the cornea or the sclera of the eye.

open pneumothorax A penetrating wound to the chest that causes the chest wall to be opened, producing a preferential pathway for air moving from the outside environment into the thorax.

operations level In hazardous materials training, the level of knowledge and training that a responder should have when involved in the response to and control of an incident involving chemical spills or release.

operations section chief The position responsible for managing all operations activities in the incident command system.

operations section The section responsible for all tactical operations at the incident.

oropharyngeal airway (OPA) An airway that, when placed in the oropharynx superior to the tongue, holds the tongue forward to assist in maintaining an open airway; used only in patients with no gag reflex.

oropharynx The central portion of the pharynx lying between the soft palate and the upper portion of the epiglottis.

orotracheal intubation A method of securing an open and patent airway that involves insertion of a plastic tube through the mouth into the trachea.

osmosis The movement of water (or other solvent) across a membrane from an area that is hypotonic to an area that is hypertonic.

osteoarthritis (OA) A degenerative condition that affects joints, leading to damage of the cartilage in joints that normally provide smooth surfaces for joint movement.

osteophytosis The development of bony outgrowths, usually along joints, particularly of the spine; also referred to as bone spurs.

osteoporosis A loss of normal bone density with thinning of bone tissue and the growth of small holes in the bone. The disorder may cause pain (especially in the lower back), frequent broken bones, loss of body height, and various poorly formed parts of the body. Commonly a part of the normal aging process.

outer perimeter The geographic boundary that defines the "safe zone" where no threat should exist at a hazardous incident.

overpressure phenomenon The sudden increase in atmospheric pressure or shock wave that occurs in proximity to the detonation of a high explosive.

oxygenation The process of providing, treating, or enriching with oxygen.

paradoxical pulse A condition in which the patient's systolic blood pressure drops more than 10 to 15 mm Hg during each inspiration, usually due to the effect of increased intrathoracic pressure such as would occur with tension pneumothorax or from pericardial tamponade.

parasympathetic nervous system The division of the nervous system that maintains normal body functions.

paresthesias Abnormal skin sensations that include tingling, "pins and needles," burning, prickling, and crawling.

parietal pleura A thin membrane that lines the inner side of the thoracic cavity.

partial thickness burn A burn that involves both the epidermis and the dermis. Skin presents with reddened areas, blisters, or open, weeping wounds.

passive strategy In injury prevention, a prevention method that requires no action on the part of the individual; e.g., vehicle air bags.

patent airway An open, unobstructed airway of sufficient size to allow for normal volumes of air exchange.

patent Open and clear.

patient care report (PCR) The written report documenting the prehospital care provided to a patient; includes the history, assessment, prehospital interventions, reassessment, and patient response to treatment.

peak overpressure value The maximum value of pressure experienced at a given location at the moment a blast wave from a high explosive reaches the location.

pediatric assessment triangle (PAT) A rapid assessment tool of pediatric patients utilized at the first point of contact; prehospital care providers assess the patient's appearance, work of breathing, and circulation to the skin.

pelvic ring The round shape that comprises the pelvis; made up of the ilium, ischium, pubis, sacrum, and coccyx; also referred to as the pelvic girdle.

penetrating trauma Trauma that results when an object penetrates the skin and injures underlying structures. Generally produces both permanent and temporary cavities.

percutaneous transtracheal ventilation (PTV) A procedure in which a 16-gauge or larger needle through which the patient is ventilated is inserted directly into the lumen of the trachea through the cricothyroid membrane, or directly through the tracheal wall.

percutaneous Occurring through the skin; e.g., a needlestick.

pericardiocentesis A procedure that involves insertion of a needle into the pericardial space to remove accumulated blood or fluid.

peritoneal cavity The space in the anterior abdominal cavity that contains the bowel, spleen, liver, stomach, and gallbladder. The peritoneal space is covered by the peritoneum.

peritonitis Inflammation of the peritoneum.

pharynx The throat; a tubelike structure that is a passage for both the breathing and digestive tracts. Oropharynx—area of the pharynx posterior to the mouth; nasopharynx—area of the pharynx beyond the posterior nares of the nose.

physician's order for life-sustaining treatment (POLST) An advance directive that expresses a patient's end-of-life treatment wishes and allows for the acceptance or refusal of a wide variety of life-sustaining treatments, such as CPR, medical nutrition and hydration, and ventilator support. A POLST allows prehospital care providers to access an active physician order regarding the end-of-life wishes of the terminally ill and frail elderly. Also known as medical orders on scope of treatment (MOST) and physician's orders on scope of treatment (POST).

physiologic reserve The excess functional capacity of an organ or organ system.

physiologic thermoregulation The process by which the body's temperature is controlled; involves dilation and constriction of blood vessels to help remove or conserve body heat.

pia mater A thin vascular membrane closely adhering to the brain and spinal cord and proximal portions of the nerves; the innermost of the three meningeal membranes that cover the brain.

planning section chief The ICS position responsible for collecting and evaluating information and assisting in planning with the incident commander.

planning section The ICS section responsible for the collection and evaluation of information related to the incident.

pneumothorax An injury that results in air in the pleural space; commonly producing a collapsed lung. A pneumothorax can be open, with an opening through the chest wall to the outside, or closed, resulting from blunt trauma or a spontaneous collapse.

polypharmacy A term used to describe patients taking more than five medications.

positive end-expiratory pressure (PEEP) The pressure in the lungs above atmospheric pressure at the end of expiration; also refers to a ventilatory technique to assist breathing in which an increased amount of pressure is applied to the lungs at the end of expiration to increase the amount of air remaining in the lungs and enhance gas exchange.

postevent phase The phase beginning as soon as the energy from the crash is absorbed and the patient is traumatized; the phase of prehospital care that includes response time, Golden Period, and transport time.

posttraumatic endophthalmitis Infection of the intraocular contents, usually as a result of penetrating trauma to the eye.

posttraumatic stress disorder (PTSD) A mental health condition that results from exposure to a horrific or terrifying event and leads to flashbacks to the incident, nightmares, anxiety, and uncontrollable thoughts about the incident.

powered air-purifying respirator (PAPR) A protective respiratory device that draws ambient air through a filter canister and delivers it under positive pressure to a face mask or hood.

pre-event phase The phase that includes all of the events that precede an incident (e.g., ingestion of drugs and alcohol) and conditions that predate the incident (e.g., acute or preexisting medical conditions). This phase includes injury prevention and preparedness.

preference The manner in which the principle of care is achieved in the time given and by the prehospital care provider available.

preload The volume and pressure of the blood coming into the heart from the systemic circulatory system (venous return).

preparedness A step of comprehensive emergency management that involves identifying, in advance of an incident, the specific supplies, equipment, and personnel that would be needed to manage an incident, as well as the specific action plan that would be taken if an incident were to occur.

presbycusis A condition characterized by a gradual decline in hearing.

primary blast injury An injury that is caused by exposure to the blast overpressure wave from the detonation of a high explosive (e.g., pulmonary bleeding, pneumothorax, perforation of the gastrointestinal tract).

primary contamination Exposure to a hazardous substance at its point of release.

primary hypothermia A decrease in body temperature that occurs when healthy individuals are unprepared for overwhelming acute or chronic cold exposure.

principle An element that must be present, accomplished, or ensured by the health care provider in order to optimize patient survival and outcome; also refers to the four ethical concepts of autonomy, nonmaleficence, beneficence, and justice.

principlism The use of the four ethical principles of autonomy, nonmaleficence, beneficence, and justice, which provide a framework for one to weigh and balance the benefits and burdens of treating a specific patient in order to do what is in the patient's best interest.

privacy The right of patients to control who has access to their personal health information.

prodrome (predisaster) phase (warning phase) The phase in the disaster cycle in which a specific event has been identified as inevitably going to occur and in which specific steps can be taken to mitigate the effects of the ensuing events.

profile A penetrating object's initial size and the degree of change in size that occurs at the time of impact.

public health impact of injury The totality of the impact of injury on the health of the public; includes deaths, injury, disability, and financial considerations.

public information officer (PIO) The incident command structure (ICS) command staff officer responsible for interacting with the public and media and distributing information.

pulmonary contusion A bruising of the lungs; can be secondary to blunt or penetrating trauma.

pulse oximeter A device that measures arterial oxyhemoglobin saturation. The value is determined by measuring the absorption ratio of red and infrared light passed through the tissue.

pulse pressure (1) The increase in pressure (surge) that is created as each new bolus of blood leaves the left ventricle with each contraction; (2) the difference between the systolic and diastolic blood pressures (systolic pressure minus diastolic pressure equals pulse pressure).

pulseless electrical activity A condition characterized by organized electrical activity on cardiac monitoring without an associated palpable pulse.

quaternary blast injury An injury from a blast or explosion that includes burns and toxicities from fuel, metals, trauma from structural collapse, septic syndromes from soil, and environmental contamination.

quaternary effects See *quaternary blast injury*.

quinary blast injury A hyperinflammatory state in blast victims thought to result from bacteria, chemicals, or radioactive materials added to the explosive device and released upon detonation.

radiation energy Any electromagnetic wave that travels in rays and has no physical mass.

radiation The direct transfer of energy from a warm object to a cooler one by infrared radiation.

radiologic dispersion device (RDD) A conventional explosive with a radionuclide (radioactive material) attached that is detonated to disperse the radioactive material.

rapid and remote assessment methodology (RAM) An assessment algorithm utilized to maximize the opportunity to extract and treat a salvageable casualty while minimizing risk to tactical emergency medical service providers.

rapid-sequence intubation (RSI) A technique of medication-assisted intubation that utilizes sedative medications and a fast-acting paralytic agent to render the patient unconscious and unresponsive to minimize the period of risk of aspiration.

rebound tenderness A physical examination finding that occurs by pressing deeply on the abdomen and then quickly releasing the pressure, causing more severe pain when the abdominal pressure is suddenly released.

recovery or reconstruction phase The period during the disaster cycle that addresses the community's resources to endure, emerge, and rebuild from the effects of the disaster through the coordinated efforts of the medical, public health, and community infrastructure (physical and political); this period is usually the longest, lasting months, and perhaps years, before a community fully recovers.

remote assessment A process by which tactical operators and providers gather information without revealing their position or intent to the hostile force; includes remote observation with binoculars, remote acoustic surveillance, and thermal imaging.

rescue, emergency, or relief phase The period during the disaster cycle immediately following the impact, during which response occurs and appropriate management and intervention can save lives.

resource management Agreements and procedures that enable local, state, and federal agencies to work together under one command during a large-scale incident.

respiration The total ventilatory and circulatory processes involved in the exchange of oxygen and carbon dioxide between the outside atmosphere and the cells of the body. Sometimes in medicine limited to meaning breathing and the steps in ventilation.

reticular activating system The central nervous system control center responsible for maintaining the level of consciousness and alertness.

retroperitoneal space The space in the posterior abdominal cavity that contains the kidneys, ureters, bladder, reproductive organs, inferior vena cava, abdominal aorta, pancreas, a portion of the duodenum, colon, and rectum.

rhabdomyolysis The breakdown of muscle tissue with the release of intracellular muscle components into the circulation.

rheumatoid arthritis (RA) An inflammatory disorder caused by an autoimmune response; can lead to joint swelling and deformity.

rifling Grooves on the inside of the barrel that spin a single missile (bullet) in a stable flight pattern toward the target.

rigor mortis The temporary stiffening and rigidity of muscles and joints that occurs after death; typically begins within 2 to 4 hours of death and lasts approximately 36 to 48 hours.

riot control agent A chemical agent used to rapidly and briefly disable those exposed to it by causing irritation to the skin, mucous membranes, lungs, and eyes.

sacrum Part of the spinal column below the lumbar spine containing the five sacral vertebrae (S1–S5), which are connected by immovable joints to form the sacrum. The sacrum is the weight-bearing base of the spinal column and is also a part of the pelvic girdle.

safety officer The incident command structure (ICS) command staff officer who is responsible for monitoring, assessing, and ensuring the safety of emergency personnel.

SAMPLE history A mnemonic to remember the components of the history; stands for symptoms, allergies, medication, past medical and surgical history, last meal, and events leading up to the injury.

sclera The dense, fibrous, white outer layer of the eyeball.

second phase of death Deaths from traumatic injury that occur within minutes to a few hours after the injury.

second-degree frostbite A freezing injury due to cold exposure that involves the epidermis and superficial dermis; initially appears similar to first-degree injury, but frozen tissues are deeper; after thawing, results in superficial skin blisters surrounded by erythema and edema; there is no permanent loss of tissue; healing occurs in 3 to 4 weeks.

secondary blast injury Injury that results from shrapnel, flying debris, and bomb fragments; typically causes penetrating ballistic injury.

secondary contamination Exposure to a hazardous substance after it has been carried away from the point of origin by a victim, a responder, or a piece of equipment.

secondary hypothermia A decrease in body temperature as a consequence of a patient's systemic disorder, including hypothyroidism, hypoadrenalism, trauma, carcinoma, and sepsis.

secondary impact syndrome The sudden deterioration in neurologic status in patients who have sustained a concussion and then have a second concussion before the symptoms from the first one have fully resolved.

self-aid The provision of medical care to one's self after sustaining an injury.

self-contained breathing apparatus (SCBA) A personal protective device consisting of a mask and portable supply of air, used in environments that are oxygen-deficient or pose a risk of toxic inhalation.

self-contained underwater breathing apparatus (SCUBA) A portable breathing device for underwater use, consisting of a mask with tubes connecting to a tank of compressed air.

senescence The process of aging.

sepsis Infection that has spread to involve the entire body.

sequela An aftereffect or complication of a disease or injury; plural is *sequelae*.

shear force Energy applied to the body that tends to move an organ or part of the body in one direction while the adjacent part moves in a different direction or remains fixed in place.

shear wave Energy applied to the body that tends to move an organ or part of the body in one direction while the adjacent part moves in a different direction or remains fixed in place.

shear Change-of-speed force resulting in a cutting or tearing of body parts.

shock front The boundary between the blast overpressure wave created by a high explosive detonation and normal atmospheric pressure.

shock wave See *shock front*.

simple pneumothorax The presence of air within the pleural space.

simulations A form of training that involves the imitation, enactment, or representation, verbally or with models, of the management of an incident or patient.

single command A command structure in which a single individual is responsible for all of the strategic objectives of the incident. Typically used when an incident is within a single jurisdiction and is managed by a single discipline.

single-system trauma patient A patient who has experienced trauma that involves injury to only one body system.

sniffing position A slightly superior anterior position of the head and neck to optimize ventilation as well as the view during endotracheal intubation.

solar keratitis Burns to the cornea of the eye that result from exposure to ultraviolet light, commonly as a result of reflection off of snow; also referred to as snow blindness.

solid density Tissue density consistent with bone.

span of control In an incident command system, the number of subordinates who report to one supervisor at any level within the response organization; in most situations, one person can effectively supervise only three to seven people or resources.

specialist level In hazardous materials incidents, an individual who is trained to provide command and support skills.

spinal shock An injury to the spinal cord that results in a temporary loss of sensory and motor function.

spinal stenosis Narrowing of the spinal canal.

spinous process The tail-like structure on the posterior region of the vertebrae.

spray The dispersal pattern of pellets fired from a shotgun.

spread See *spray*.

staging area A predetermined area where resources, equipment, and personnel can be located safely and at the ready for assignment.

START triage algorithm A method of evaluating patients and assigning priority for treatment and transport during a mass-casualty incident; involves evaluating the respiratory status, perfusion status, and mental status of the patient.

status epilepticus A life-threatening condition in which a seizure persists for greater than 5 minutes or in which two or more seizures occur without a period of wakening in between.

stellate (starburst) wound A star-shaped wound.

stipple Multiple small dots resulting from gunpowder from point-blank gunshot wounds.

stopping distance The distance over which a moving object comes to a stop; a measure of how quickly energy is dissipated or transferred.

stress wave A supersonic, longitudinal pressure wave that (1) creates high local forces with small, rapid distortions; (2) produces microvascular injury; and (3) is reinforced and reflected at tissue interfaces, thereby enhancing injury potential, especially in gas-filled organs such as the lungs, ears, and intestines.

stroke volume The volume of blood pumped out by each contraction (stroke) of the left ventricle.

subarachnoid hematoma A collection of blood in the cerebrospinal fluid-filled space beneath the arachnoid membrane.

subarachnoid hemorrhage (SAH) Bleeding into the cerebrospinal fluid-filled space beneath the arachnoid membrane.

subconjunctival hemorrhage Bleeding found between the clear conjunctiva covering the eye and the white sclera.

subcutaneous emphysema Accumulation of air in the soft tissues of the body.

subdermal burn A burn injury that involves all layers of the skin, as well as the underlying fat, muscles, bone, or internal organs.

subdural hematoma A collection of blood between the dura mater and the arachnoid membrane.

sublimation A process in which solids emit vapors, bypassing the liquid state.

subluxation A partial or incomplete dislocation.

sulfur mustard An oily, clear to yellow-brown liquid that can be aerosolized by a bomb blast or a sprayer; a vesicant or blister agent used as a weapon of mass destruction.

superficial burn A burn to the epidermis only; red, inflamed, and painful skin.

superficial frostbite A freezing injury due to cold exposure that affects the skin and subcutaneous tissues, resulting in clear blisters when rewarmed.

superior vena cava A major vein that carries deoxygenated blood from the upper portion of the body back to the heart.

supplied air respirator (SAR) A personal protective device consisting of a mask and source of air that is not carried by the responder; used in environments that are oxygen-deficient or pose a risk of toxic inhalation.

supraglottic airway An airway device inserted blindly into the mouth and pharynx; designed to isolate the trachea from the esophagus; none of these devices provides a complete seal of the trachea, so the risk of aspiration is lowered but not completely prevented.

surgical cricothyrotomy A procedure to open a patient's airway that is accomplished by making an incision into the cricothyroid membrane in the neck to open the airway into the trachea.

surveillance The process of collecting data within a community, usually for infectious diseases.

suspension syndrome A cascade of events that ultimately culminates as a state of shock caused by blood pooling in dependent lower extremities while the body is held upright without any movement for a prolonged time.

sympathetic nervous system The division of the nervous system that produces the fight-or-flight response.

systemic vascular resistance The amount of resistance to the flow of blood through the vessels. It increases as the vessel constricts. Any change in lumen diameter or vessel elasticity can influence the amount of resistance.

systolic blood pressure Peak blood pressure produced by the force of the contraction (systole) of the ventricles of the heart.

tachypnea An increased breathing rate.

tactical casualty care (TCC) The emergency medical care provided in a hazardous or tactical situation.

tactical emergency medical support (TEMS) An out-of-hospital system of care dedicated to enhancing the probability of special operations law enforcement mission success, reducing mission medical liability and risk, and promoting public safety.

tactical evacuation care The phase of care in tactical casualty care in which medical care is provided once the threat or hazard has been completely addressed, similar to a conventional emergency medical services (EMS) situation; also referred to as evacuation care.

tactical field care The phase of care in tactical casualty care in which medical care is provided when the threat or hazard has been contained but could resume; also referred to as indirect threat care.

tamponade The closure or blockage of a wound or blood vessel; also, the compression of the heart by the accumulation of blood or fluid in the pericardium.

technician level In hazardous materials incidents, an individual trained to work within the hazardous area and stop the release of hazardous materials.

tendon A band of tough, inelastic, fibrous tissue that connects a muscle to bone.

tension pneumothorax A condition in which the air pressure in the pleural space exceeds the outside atmospheric pressure and cannot escape, the affected side becomes hyperinflated, compressing the lung on the involved side and shifting the mediastinum to the opposite side to partially collapse the other lung; usually progressive

and is an imminently life-threatening condition.

tentorium cerebelli An infolding of the dura that forms a covering over the cerebellum. The tentorium is a part of the floor of the upper skull just below the brain (cerebrum).

tertiary blast injury An injury that occurs from an explosion when the victim becomes a missile and is thrown against some object; injuries, usually blunt, are similar to those sustained in ejections from vehicles, in falls from significant heights, or when the victim is thrown against an object by the force wave resulting from an explosion.

thermal energy Energy associated with increased temperature and heat.

thermal equilibrium The transfer of heat from a warmer object to a colder object in an effort to create the same temperature between them.

thermal gradient The difference in temperature (high vs. low temperature) between two objects.

thermite An incendiary compound that consists of powdered aluminum and iron oxide that burns furiously at 3,600°F (1,982°C) and scatters molten iron.

thermoregulatory center The area of the brain (hypothalamus) that controls body temperature.

third phase of death Deaths from traumatic injury that occur several days or weeks after the initial injury; most often caused by sepsis and organ failure.

third-degree frostbite A freezing injury due to cold exposure that involves the epidermis and dermis layers; skin is frozen with restricted mobility; after tissue thaws, skin swells and develops blood-filled blisters (hemorrhagic bullae), indicating vascular trauma to deep tissues; skin loss occurs slowly, leading to mummification and sloughing; healing is slow.

tidal volume The normal volume of air exchanged with each ventilation. About 500 ml of air is exchanged between the

lungs and the atmosphere with each breath in a healthy adult at rest.

torcula The confluence of sinuses.

total lung capacity The total volume of air in the lungs after a forced inhalation.

toxidrome A collection of clinical signs and symptoms that suggest exposure to a certain class of chemical or toxin.

tracheal shift Movement or displacement of the trachea away from the midline of the neck.

transesophageal echocardiography A technique of performing ultrasound of the heart using an ultrasound probe inserted into the esophagus.

transmission-based PPE The personal protective equipment used, in addition to standard precautions, to prevent transmission of disease; includes aerosol, contact, and droplet precautions.

transmural pressure state Difference between the pressure inside a blood vessel and the pressure outside the vessel.

transverse process A protuberance at each side of a vertebra near the lateral margins.

trauma chin lift A maneuver used to relieve a variety of anatomic airway obstructions in patients who are breathing spontaneously; accomplished by grasping the chin and lower incisors and then lifting to pull the mandible forward.

trauma jaw thrust A maneuver that allows opening of the airway with little or no movement of the head and cervical spine; the mandible is thrust forward by placing the thumbs on each zygomatic arch and placing the index and long fingers under the mandible and at the same angle, thrusting the mandible forward.

traumatic asphyxia Blunt and crushing injuries to the chest and abdomen with marked increase of intravascular pressure, producing rupture of the capillaries; characterized by a purplish discoloration of the skin of the upper torso and face along with petechiae of the skin.

trench foot A nonfreezing cold exposure injury caused by prolonged immersion of extremities in wet and moisture that is cool to cold; also referred to as immersion foot.

triage officer An individual trained to oversee the process of assigning injury severity categories and prioritization of treatment and transport.

triage French word meaning "to sort"; a process in which a group of patients is sorted according to their priority of need for care. When only several patients are involved, triage involves assessing each patient, meeting all of the patients' highest priority needs first, and then moving to lower priority items. In a mass-casualty incident with a large number of patients involved, triage is done by determining both urgency and potential for survival.

tumble An end-over-end motion. Bullets commonly tumble when resistance is met by the leading edge of the missile.

unified command An ICS command structure in which the incident commanders of all of the various agencies responding to an event work together to manage the incident.

unintentional injury An injury that was unplanned and did not involve intent to harm.

unity of command An incident command system management concept in which each responder has only one direct supervisor.

vapor A solid or liquid in a gaseous state, usually visible as a fine cloud or mist.

vertebral foramen Hole or opening in the bony structure of the vertebrae through which blood vessels and nerves pass.

very high altitude Elevation levels between 11,480 and 18,045 feet (3,500 and 5,500 meters).

vesicant A chemical agent such as sulfur mustard and lewisite used as a weapon of mass destruction; also referred to as blister agent because these agents create an injury that is visually similar to a burn.

vestibular folds The false vocal cords that direct airflow through the vocal cords.

vestibular nuclei The areas of the brain from which the vestibular nerves responsible for balance arise.

viral hemorrhagic fever (VHF) A clinical syndrome caused by several different viruses; typified by the clinical presentation of fever, malaise, and hemorrhagic symptoms.

viscera The internal organs of the body.

visceral pleura A thin membrane that covers the outer surface of each lung.

volatility The likelihood that solids or liquids will vaporize into a gaseous form at room temperature.

voluntary guarding An assessment finding in which the patient tenses the abdominal muscles when the provider palpates a tender area of the abdomen.

water density Organs that have a tissue density similar to that of water; e.g., liver, spleen, muscle.

weapon of mass destruction (WMD) A chemical, biologic, radiologic, or explosive agent designed to create significant damage and large numbers of casualties.

white blood cells Nearly colorless blood cells in the circulation responsible for responding to invading microorganisms.

white phosphorus An incendiary agent used in the production of munitions.

work of breathing The physical work or effort performed in moving the chest wall and diaphragm to breathe.

years of potential life lost (YPLL) An estimate of the impact of an injury calculated by subtracting age at death from a fixed age of the group under examination, usually 65 or 70 years, or the life expectancy of the group.

zone of coagulation The region of greatest tissue destruction in a full-thickness burn; the tissue in this zone is necrotic (dead) and is not capable of tissue repair.

zone of hyperemia The outermost zone in a full-thickness burn; it has minimal cellular injury and is characterized by increased blood flow secondary to an inflammatory reaction initiated by the burn injury.

zone of stasis The region next to the zone of coagulation; blood flow to this region is stagnant, and the cells in this zone are injured, but not irreversibly. If they are subsequently deprived of the delivery of oxygen or blood flow, these viable cells will die and become necrotic. Timely and appropriate burn care will preserve blood flow and oxygen delivery to these injured cells.

airway (Continued)

anatomy
lower airway, 200
organs of respiratory system, 201f
sagittal section through nasal cavity and pharynx, 202f
upper airway, 200
vocal cords, 202f

assessment of ventilation and
chest rise, look for, 207
obstructions, examine airway for, 207
position of airway and patient, 206–207
upper airway sounds, 207

categories for airway adjuncts and procedures
complex, 209
endotracheal tubes and supraglottic airways, 210f
manual, 208
methods of airway management, 211
nasopharyngeal airways, 208f
oropharyngeal airways, 208f
simple, 208
trauma chin lift, 208, 208f
trauma jaw thrust, 208, 208f

continuous quality improvement in intubation, 230

CUF in, 757

evaluation
capnography, 229–230, 230f
pulse oximetry, 229, 229f

management, 73, 172, 172f, 715–716, 716f
airway control, 207
based on spontaneous ventilation rate, 173f
essential skills, 207–209
methods of, 211

management and ventilation skills
alternate trauma jaw thrust, 236f
bag-mask ventilation, 241–243f
face-to-face orotracheal intubation, 251f
I-gel laryngeal mask airway, 245–246f
ILMA, 247–248f
intubation with airtraq channeled video laryngoscope, 253–254f
nasopharyngeal airway, 240–241f
oropharyngeal airway, 237–239f
supraglottic airway, 243–245f
surgical cricothyroidotomy, 252–253f
trauma chin lift, 237f
trauma jaw thrust, 235f
visualized orotracheal intubation of the trauma patient, 248, 249–250f

manual clearing
manual maneuvers, 209
suctioning, 209, 211, 211f

manual maneuvers
trauma chin lift, 209
trauma jaw thrust, 209

oxygen tank size and duration, 231t

oxygenation and ventilation of trauma patient
external respiration, 204–205
internal (cellular) respiration, 205
oxygen delivery, 205

pathophysiology
airway obstruction in trauma patient, 205–206, 206f
cause of upper airway obstruction, 205
endotracheal (ET) tube, 206

physiology
aerobic metabolism, 203–204
diaphragm, 200, 202
effective ventilation, 204
intrapulmonary pressure during phases of ventilation, 203f
minute volume, 204
oxygen and carbon dioxide diffusion, 203f
oxygen moves into red blood cells from alveoli, 203f
oxygenation and ventilation of trauma patient, 204–205

prolonged transport, 230–231

suctioning, 209, 211, 211f

tactical field care
overview of, 776–778
procedures, 778–782, 779f

techniques synopsis, 212

ventilation. See ventilation

airway management, 859–860t

all-risk and all-hazard system, 526

alternobaric vertigo, 650–651

alveoli, 200, 347, 347f

AMA. See American Medical Association

ambulances, flying, 4

American Academy of Orthopaedic Surgeons (AAOS), 5

American Academy of Pediatrics (AAP), 466

American College of Emergency Physicians (ACEP), 25, 741

American College of Surgeons Committee on Trauma (ACS-COT), 731, 740

American Heart Association (AHA)
guidelines for cardiopulmonary resuscitation and emergency cardiovascular care science, 616–618

modified from AHA hypothermia algorithm, 617f

American Medical Association (AMA), 6

amputations, 409
field, 410–412
management, 410
phantom pain, 409
primary survey algorithm, 411f
right leg after entangled in machinery, 410f

AMS. See acute mountain sickness

anaerobic metabolism, 48
by-product of, 49–50

analgesia, 432, 863–864t, 870
considerations, 720
TCCC Triple-Option plan
background of, 820
benzodiazepines, 825
combat wound medication pack, 820–823
emerging evidence, 825–826
ketamine, 824–825
morphine, 825
nausea and vomiting management, 825
NSAIDs, 826
OTFC in, 823–824

anatomy, entrance and exit wounds, 132–133, 132–133f

anemia, 269

angular impact, 118, 119f

anisocoria, 271t

anterior cord syndrome, 302, 302f

anthrax, 563–564

antibiotics, 826–828, 864t

antidiuretic hormone (ADH), 55

aortography, 365

ARDS. See acute respiratory distress syndrome

Army Special Missions Unit, 735

arterial bleeding, 171

arterial gas embolism (AGE), 652, 653

aspiration pneumonitis, 476

assist control ventilation, 227

atherosclerosis, 477

ATLS. See Advanced Trauma Life Support

ATN. See acute tubular necrosis

ATP. See adenosine triphosphate

atropine, 559

auscultation, 384

austere environment, mass-casualty incident management, 524

autoinjectors, 699

automated blood pressure monitoring, 178

autonomic nervous system, 54